Andrews' Diseases of the Skin
Clinical Atlas

Andrews' Diseases of the Skin
CLINICAL ATLAS

Robert G. Micheletti, MD
Associate Professor of Dermatology and Medicine
Chief of Hospital Dermatology
Chief of Dermatology at Pennsylvania Hospital
Perelman School of Medicine at the University of Pennsylvania
Philadelphia, Pennsylvania
USA

William D. James, MD
Paul R. Gross Professor of Dermatology
Department of Dermatology
Perelman School of Medicine at the University of Pennsylvania
Philadelphia, Pennsylvania
USA

Dirk M. Elston, MD
Professor and Chairman
Department of Dermatology and Dermatologic Surgery
Medical University of South Carolina
Charleston, South Carolina
USA

Patrick J. McMahon, MD
Assistant Professor of Pediatrics and Dermatology
Children's Hospital of Philadelphia and University of Pennsylvania School of Medicine
Philadelphia, Pennsylvania
USA

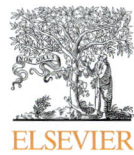

ELSEVIER

Elsevier
3251 Riverport Lane
St. Louis, Missouri 63043

ANDREWS' DISEASES OF THE SKIN
CLINICAL ATLAS, SECOND EDITION   ISBN: 978-0-323-79013-0

Copyright © 2023 by Elsevier, Inc. All rights reserved.

No part of this publication may be reproduced or transmitted in any form or by any means, electronic or mechanical, including photocopying, recording, or any information storage and retrieval system, without permission in writing from the publisher. Details on how to seek permission, further information about the Publisher's permissions policies and our arrangements with organizations such as the Copyright Clearance Center and the Copyright Licensing Agency, can be found at our website: www.elsevier.com/permissions.

This book and the individual contributions contained in it are protected under copyright by the Publisher (other than as may be noted herein).

Notice

Practitioners and researchers must always rely on their own experience and knowledge in evaluating and using any information, methods, compounds or experiments described herein. Because of rapid advances in the medical sciences, in particular, independent verification of diagnoses and drug dosages should be made. To the fullest extent of the law, no responsibility is assumed by Elsevier, authors, editors or contributors for any injury and/or damage to persons or property as a matter of products liability, negligence or otherwise, or from any use or operation of any methods, products, instructions, or ideas contained in the material herein.

Previous edition copyrighted 2018.

Cover images
Front cover
Top:
Fig. 15.100 Aspergillosis (Courtesy Yung-Tsu Cho, MD)
Bottom, left to right:
Fig. 22.25 Acrodermatitis enteropathica
Fig. 33.135 Acral lentiginous melanoma (Courtesy Dr Liao, National Cheng Kung University, Taiwan)
Fig. 12.26 Desquamative gingivitis caused by lichen planus
Fig. 27.36 Proteus syndrome (Courtesy Curt Samlaska, MD)
Fig. 9.2 Scleromyxedema (Courtesy National Cheng Kung University, Taiwan)

Back cover, left to right:
Fig. 10.21 Psoriasis
Fig. 11.43 Punctate palmoplantar keratoderma (Courtesy Curt Samlaska, MD)
Fig. 14.90 Scrub typhus (tsutsugamushi fever) (Courtesy Kaohsiung Chang Gang Memorial Hospital, Taiwan)
Fig. 29.68 Paget disease of the breast
Fig. 32.89 Rosai-Dorfman disease (Courtesy National Cheng Kung University, Taiwan)

Senior Content Strategist: Charlotta Kryhl
Senior Content Development Manager: Laura Schmidt
Publishing Services Manager: Deepthi Unni
Senior Project Manager: Manchu Mohan
Senior Book Designer: Bridget Hoette

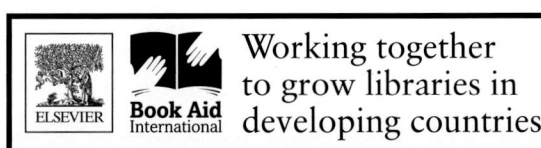

Printed in India
Last digit is the print number: 9 8 7 6 5 4 3 2 1

To my loving family:
My wife Ann, son Dan, daughter Becca, daughter-in-law Wynn, grandsons Declan and Driscoll, and sister Judy and her husband Cal.
You have given me a wonderful life!
–Bill James

Dorothy, Andrew, and Elisa: I am so proud of you all. You are a true source of love, joy, and inspiration. To my dad Gil, a dermatologist: thank you for setting me on this path.
–Robert Micheletti

To my family — you are my greatest joy — and to my teachers and students, past and present, who have made every day a pleasure.
–Dirk Elston

Thank you to my wonderful wife Kate and loving children Bridget, Brendan, Colin, and Molly for their support and for being up for any adventure.
–Pat McMahon

PREFACE

It is our pleasure to bring you this atlas of skin disorders. We are hopeful that by seeing this wide array of images, you may more easily recognize and diagnose skin conditions in your own patients. If our efforts result in a better outcome for one patient, then they were worthwhile. Our atlas is an accompanying volume to *Andrews' Diseases of the Skin*. The chapters and entities follow the organization of *Andrews'*, making explanatory text unnecessary and allowing you to enjoy the superior photographs in an uncluttered fashion.

Dermatologic diagnostic abilities are learned through repetitive exposures to patient presentations. The present volume of over 3000 pictures, combined with the main textbook, will be an outstanding resource to learn the depth and breadth of our specialty.

The four authors have benefitted by spending a combined 60 years in academic medicine, taking photographs along the journey. Additionally, the resources of our institutions and many friends have allowed a stunning array and variety of presentations to be represented. Bill James recognizes Richard Odom, MD, my teaching chief, who allowed myself and fellow resident Robert Horn to make copies of his best slides. Bill also thanks past residents and faculty of the Walter Reed Army Medical Center. Tim Berger has shared photographs from his experiences at the University of California at San Francisco. Bill and Rob both wish to thank the faculty and residents at the University of Pennsylvania, who generously shared their expertise. Dirk thanks the members of Brooke Army Medical Center who have contributed to the image collection in San Antonio. Pat wishes to recognize that the considerable resources of Paul Honig, MD's personal collection, as well as the combined image database of the current faculty at Children's Hospital of Philadelphia, were made fully available. These photos of pediatric patients enhance the atlas considerably. Finally, James Fitzpatrick, MD, also generously shared photographs taken by the faculty and staff of Fitzsimmons Army Medical Center. We call out all of these wonderful people, as they are not recognized individually in most of the photographs. In some cases when a photograph was obtained from a specific faculty member or resident, their names appear in a "Courtesy" line under the image.

You will find over 50 contributors individually recognized in the figure legends. These range from institutions in Taiwan, Brazil, and Japan, to individuals in Singapore, India, Thailand, Portugal, and the Philippines, to the National Institutes of Health and faculty from a variety of academic centers around the country. Several individuals deserve special mention: Steven Binnick, MD, is a superb dermatologist from Plymouth Meeting, Pennsylvania. When asked if he would make available some of his excellent photographs for this atlas, he simply donated his collection and was happy they would be used to educate others. Curt Samlaska, MD, trained at Walter Reed with Bill. He is an outstanding dermatologic photographer and contributed many photos of his patients from Hawaii and his practice in Henderson, Nevada. Doctors Shyam Verma and Archana Singal, close friends from India, shared many of their wonderful images. Dr. Leonard Swinyer took many outstanding photographs during his years in private practice. He gave his collection to the Dermatology Departments at the University of Utah and the Oregon Health Sciences Center. We thank all of them for their generosity.

This wide array of altruistic physicians and many others individually recognized in the atlas have allowed us to demonstrate entities rarely seen in the United States. More important, we had the full spectrum of patient ages, skin types, morphologies, classic examples, and disease subtypes available to us in choosing the best 3000+ images that make up this volume.

Charlotta Kryhl, Laura Schmidt, and Manchu Mohan from Elsevier assumed primary roles in the compilation of the book in a most expert and responsive manner.

No words of thanks could be complete without acknowledging the personal sacrifices of our families in allowing us the opportunity to pursue our professional dreams. Those include all of the individuals listed in the dedication.

Finally, to all of our past patients who generously allowed us to take their photographs, we hope this work helps fulfill your desire to aid future sufferers of skin disease recover more rapidly through earlier recognition and diagnosis of their conditions.

CONTENTS

1. Structure and Function — 1
2. Cutaneous Signs and Diagnosis — 15
3. Dermatoses Resulting from Physical Factors — 27
4. Pruritus and Neurocutaneous Diseases — 41
5. Atopic Dermatitis, Eczema, and Noninfectious Immunodeficiency Disorders — 53
6. Contact Dermatitis and Drug Eruptions — 65
7. Erythema and Urticaria — 87
8. Connective Tissue Diseases — 101
9. Mucinoses — 119
10. Seborrheic Dermatitis, Psoriasis, Recalcitrant Palmoplantar Eruptions, Pustular Dermatitis, and Erythroderma — 125
11. Pityriasis Rosea, Pityriasis Rubra Pilaris, and Other Papulosquamous and Hyperkeratotic Diseases — 139
12. Lichen Planus and Related Conditions — 153
13. Acne — 169
14. Bacterial Infections — 185
15. Diseases Resulting From Fungi and Yeasts — 203
16. Mycobacterial Diseases — 229
17. Hansen Disease — 239
18. Syphilis, Yaws, Bejel, and Pinta — 251
19. Viral Diseases — 263
20. Parasitic Infestations, Stings, and Bites — 291
21. Chronic Blistering Dermatoses — 309
22. Nutritional Diseases — 323
23. Diseases of Subcutaneous Fat — 331
24. Endocrine Diseases — 339
25. Abnormalities of Dermal Fibrous and Elastic Tissue — 351
26. Errors in Metabolism — 361
27. Genodermatoses and Congenital Anomalies — 379
28. Dermal and Subcutaneous Tumors — 405
29. Epidermal Nevi, Neoplasms, and Cysts — 437
30. Melanocytic Nevi and Neoplasms — 463
31. Macrophage/Monocyte Disorders — 479
32. Cutaneous Lymphoid Hyperplasia, Cutaneous T-Cell Lymphoma, Other Malignant Lymphomas, and Allied Diseases — 501
33. Diseases of Skin Appendages — 517
34. Diseases of Mucous Membranes — 543
35. Cutaneous Vascular Diseases — 561
36. Disturbances of Pigmentation — 583

Index — 595

Structure and Function

The diagnosis of skin disease is based on color, morphology, and distribution of cutaneous lesions. The structure of the skin and associated appendages relates directly to these characteristics.

Folliculitis presents with papules or pustules. Follicular accentuation is characteristic of any eruption in darker-skinned races. In patients with miliaria, involvement of the sweat gland ostia results in erythematous papules, pustules, or superficial vesicles in areas of heavy sweating. The vesicles of miliaria crystallina are irregular in shape because the stratum corneum fails to impede the spread of the blister in random directions. This is in stark contrast to spongiotic and subepidermal blisters, which are distinctly round—as in acute dyshidrotic eczema or bullous pemphigoid.

The color of a cutaneous eruption relates to various pigments. Brown pigments include melanin, lipofuscin, and hemosiderin. Brown pigments located deeper in the dermis impart a blue hue because of diffraction of light. This is evident in blue nevi as a result of deep melanin and as a result of lipofuscin present in the sweat within nodular hidradenomas. Red pigment relates to oxygenated hemoglobin and blue to deoxygenated hemoglobin. Dilatation or proliferation of blood vessels and the rapidity of blood flow produce various shades of red and blue. Yellow pigments relate to lipid deposition or carotenoids dissolved in the cytoplasm of epithelial cells and histiocytes. In granulomatous disease, diascopy removes the visible appearance of oxygenated hemoglobin, allowing the observer to see the apple jelly yellow appearance of carotenoids within the cytoplasm. This section of the atlas will focus on the structure of the skin and how that structure translates to clinical manifestations of disease.

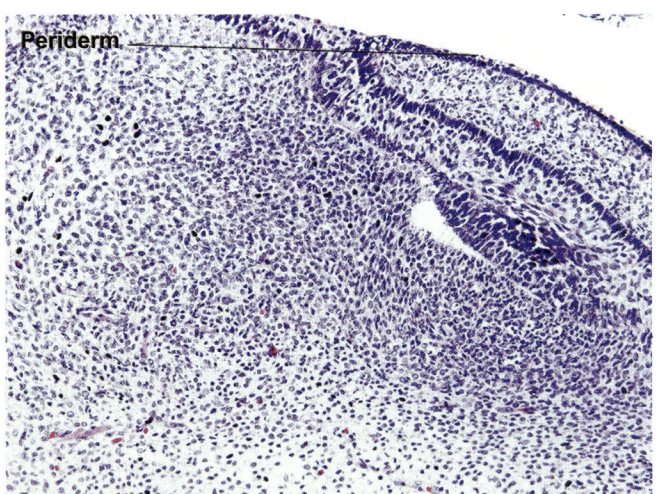

Fig. 1.1 In early fetal life, a cuboidal periderm is present rather than an epidermis. Fetal skin, H&E × 40.

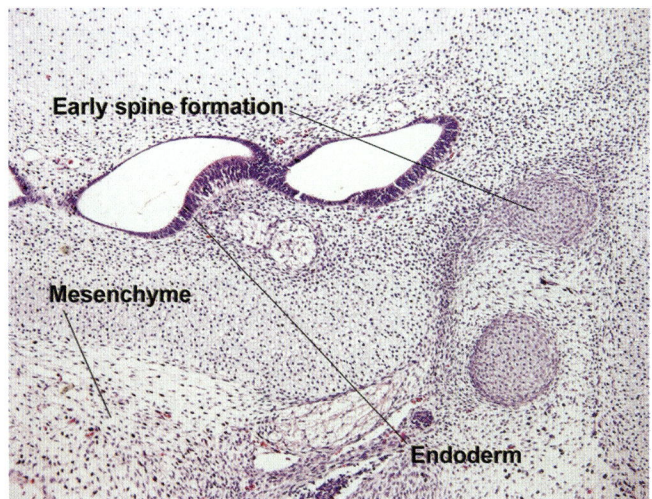

Fig. 1.2 In early fetal life, the spine is composed of cartilage, and mesenchyme is present rather than a dermis. Mesenchyme heals without scar formation. Once dermis forms, scars will occur after injury. Fetal skin, H&E × 40.

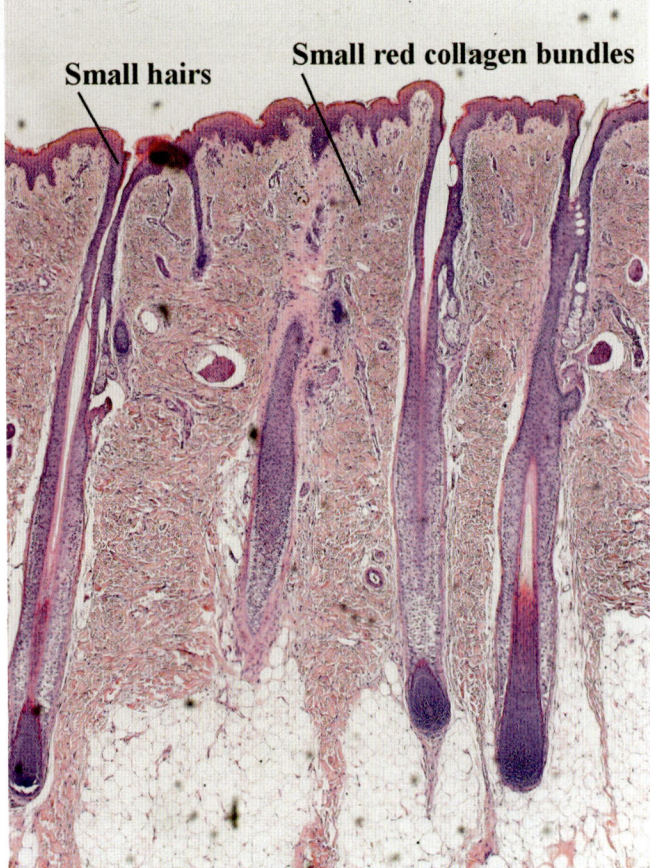

Fig. 1.3 Skin in young children is characterized by small adnexal structures and fine dermal collagen bundles that stain deep red in contrast to the thick, pink collagen bundles of an adult. Many plump fibroblasts are present in the dermis, actively synthesizing collagen. Childhood skin, H&E × 20.

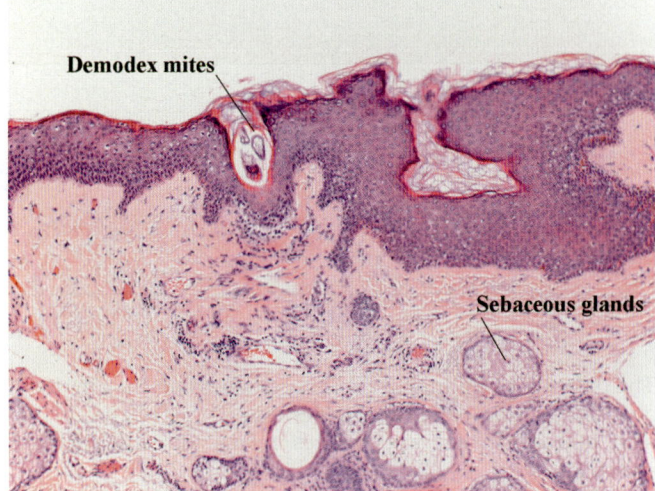

Fig. 1.4 Facial skin is characterized by prominent sebaceous follicles, often containing *Demodex* mites. Facial skin, H&E × 40.

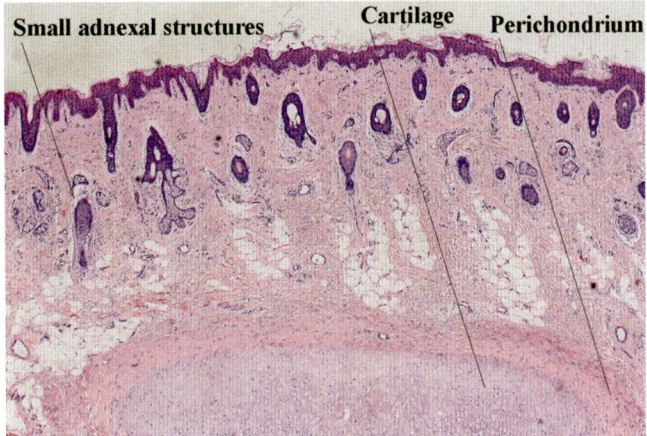

Fig. 1.5 Skin of the ear demonstrates small adnexal structures with an elastic cartilage surrounded by a red perichondrium. Ear skin, H&E × 20.

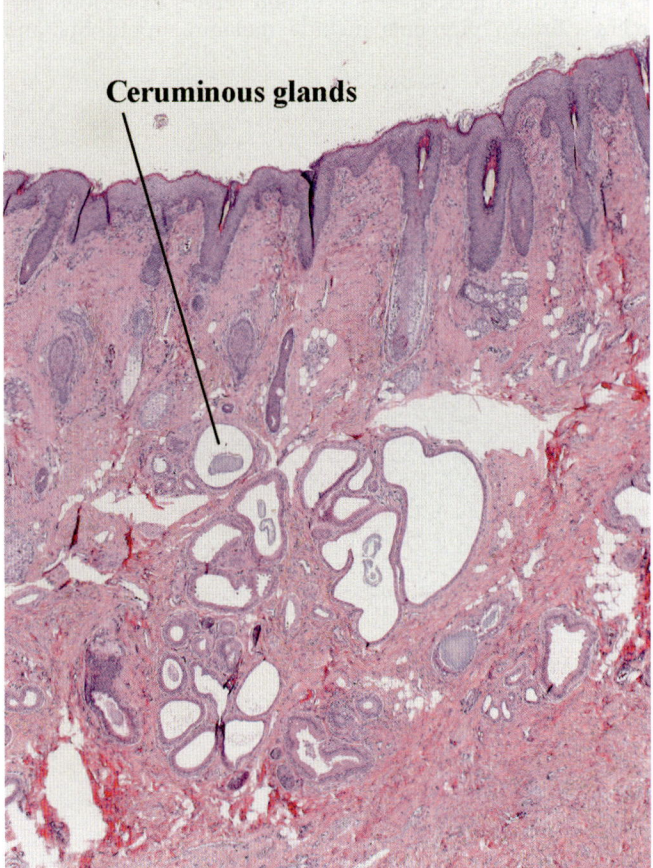

Fig. 1.6 The structure of the ear canal is similar to other parts of the ear, except for the presence of ceruminous glands, which represent modified apocrine glands. Ear canal skin, H&E × 20.

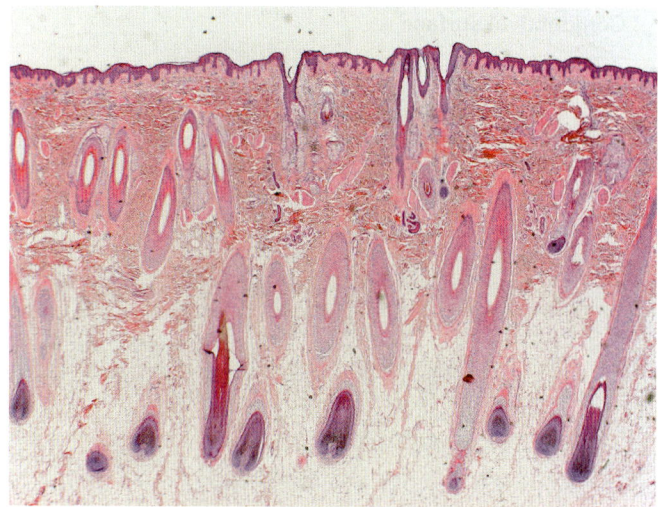

Fig. 1.7 Scalp skin demonstrates many terminal hair follicles. The inferior segment of each follicle sits within the subcutaneous fat. Scalp skin, H&E × 40.

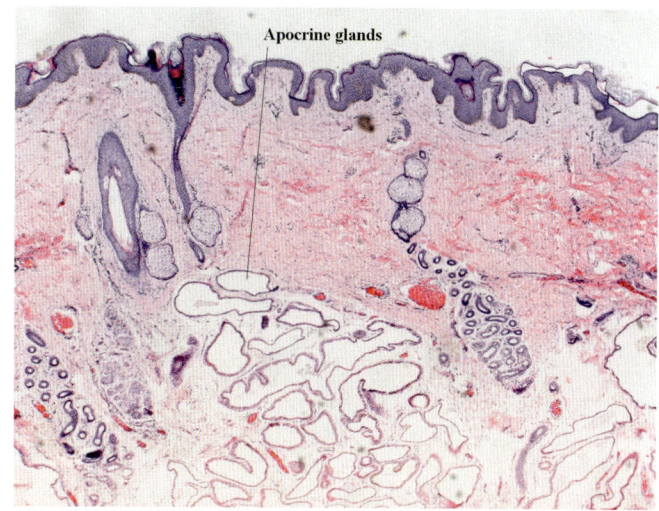

Fig. 1.8 Axillary skin is rugose and demonstrates large apocrine glands. Axillary skin, H&E × 40.

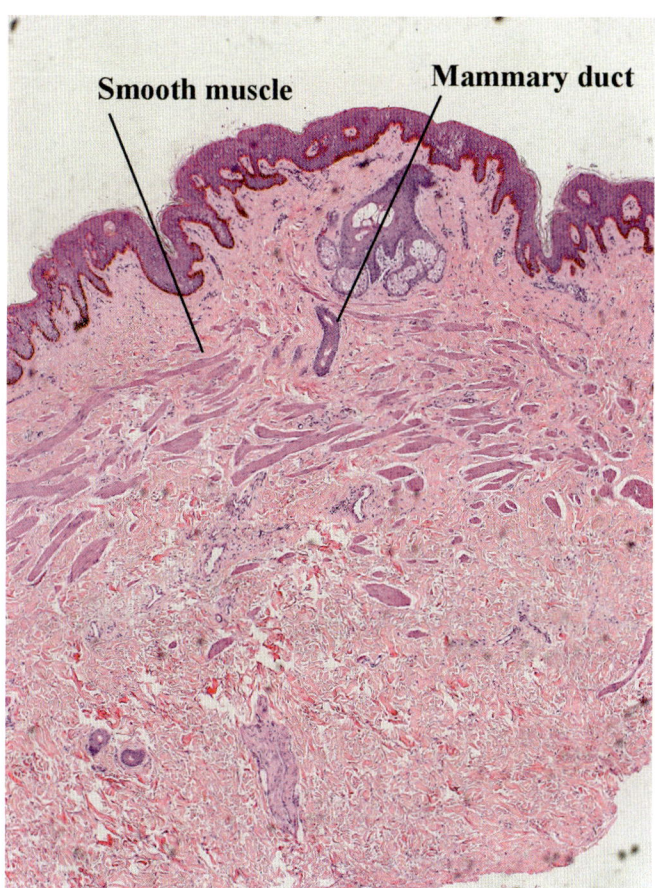

Fig. 1.9 Breast skin demonstrates numerous smooth muscle bundles. Breast skin, H&E × 20.

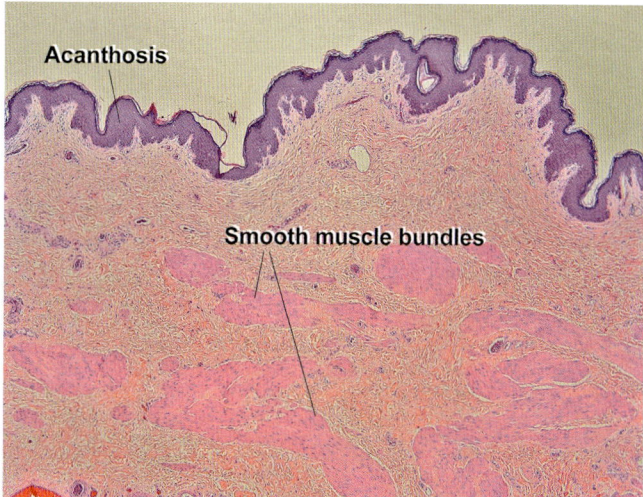

Fig. 1.10 Nipple skin demonstrates smaller smooth muscle bundles. The mammary duct resembles a large sweat duct. Breast skin, H&E × 20.

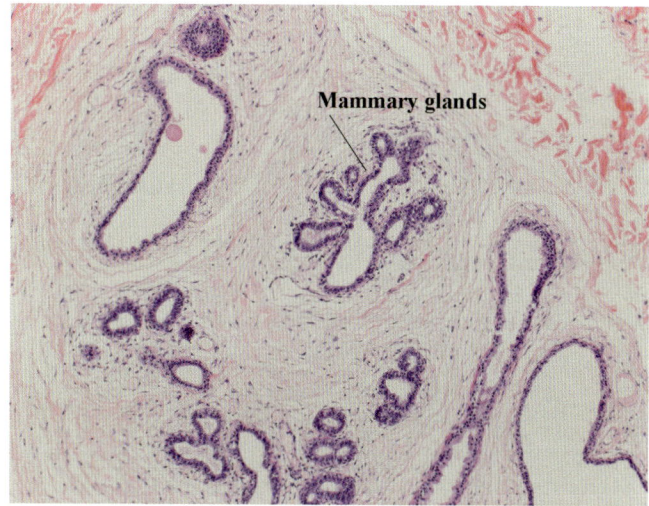

Fig. 1.11 The secretory portion of mammary glands demonstrates columnar epithelium forming complex lumens. Breast skin, H&E × 100.

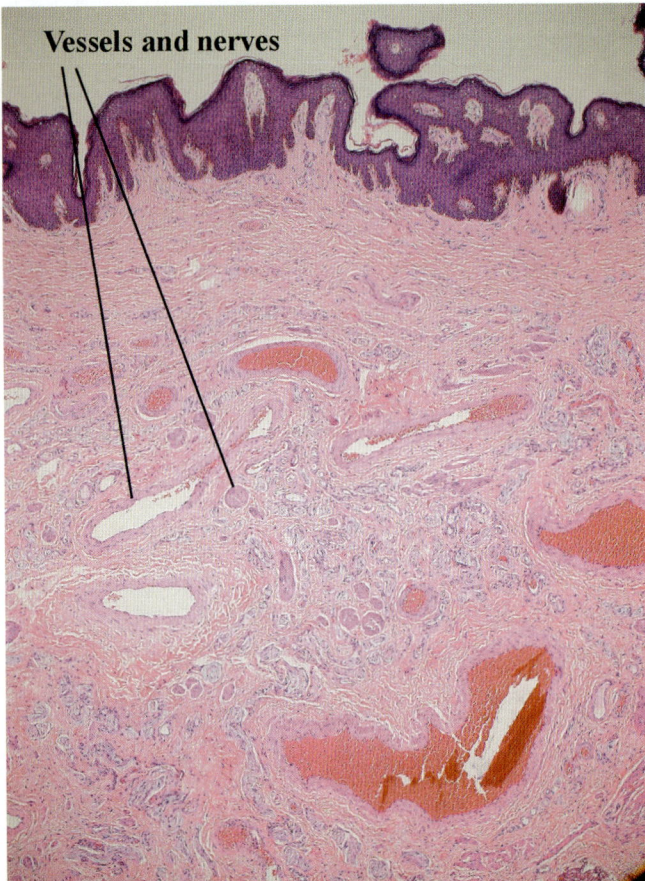

Fig. 1.12 Prepuce demonstrates a rugose appearance with many smooth muscle fascicles and high vascularity. Prepuce, H&E × 20.

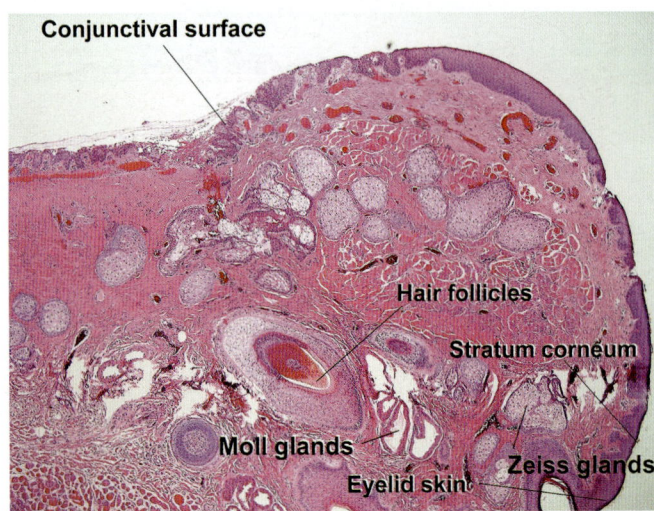

Fig. 1.13 Eyelid anatomy, below the conjunctiva; the densely fibrous tarsal plate contains sebaceous glands (meibomian glands), H&E × 100.

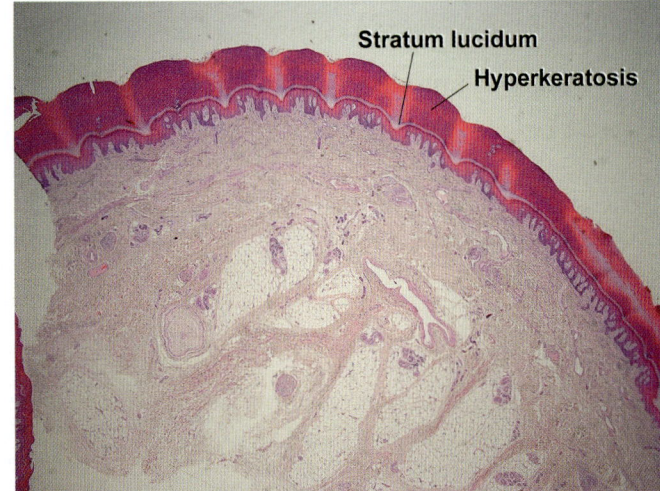

Fig. 1.15 Volar skin demonstrates a thick stratum corneum and lack of hair follicles, low power, H&E × 40.

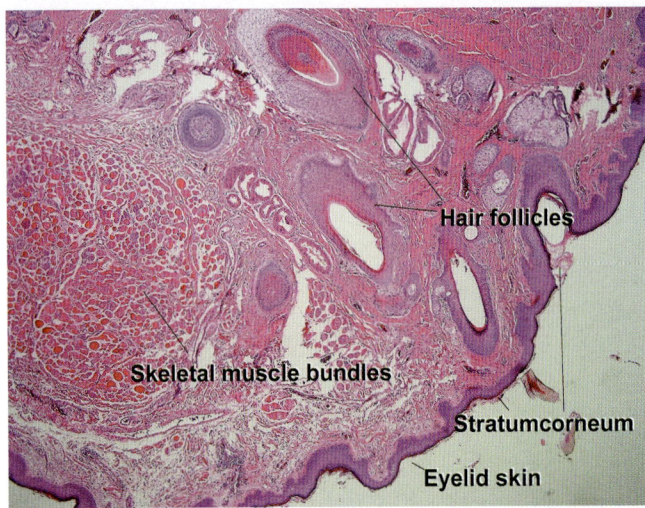

Fig. 1.14 The lid margin; on the cutaneous surface of the lid, a layer of striated muscle is present below the epidermis, H&E × 10.

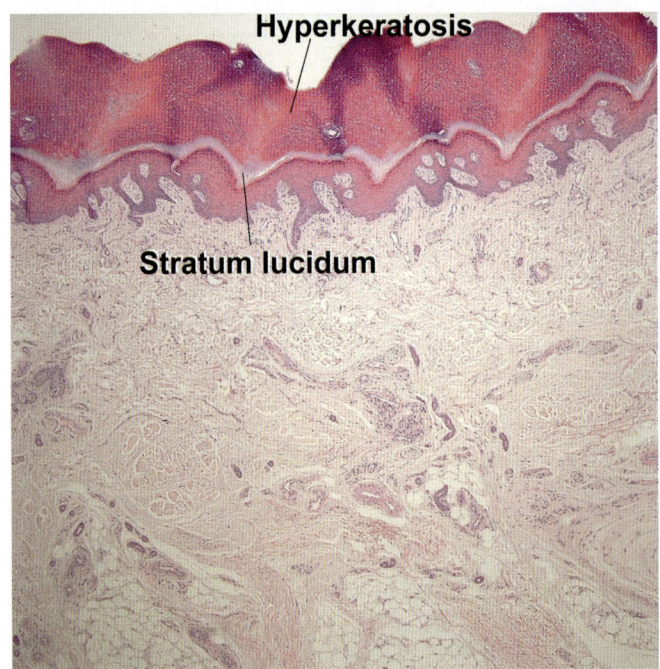

Fig. 1.16 Volar skin demonstrating a thick corneum and dermis, H&E × 100.

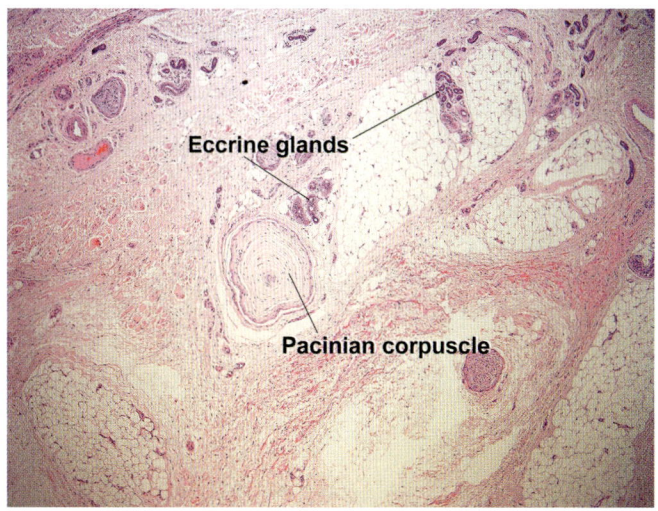

Fig. 1.17 Volar skin, with deep tissue demonstrating Pacinian corpuscles, H&E × 100.

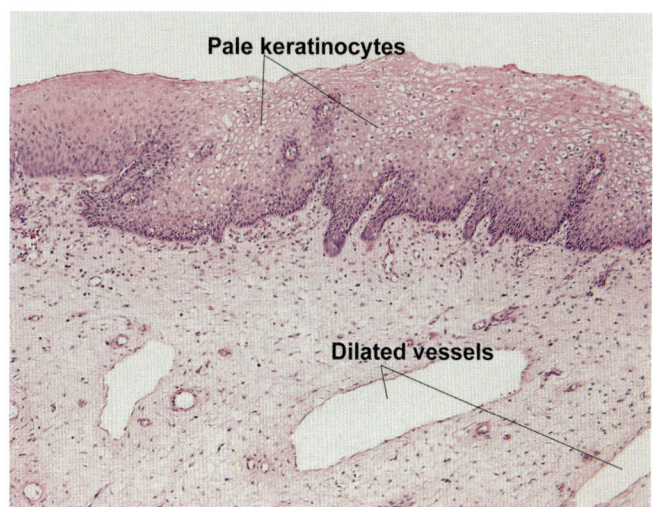

Fig. 1.18 Mucosal surface demonstrating nonkeratinizing epithelium and submucosa, H&E × 200.

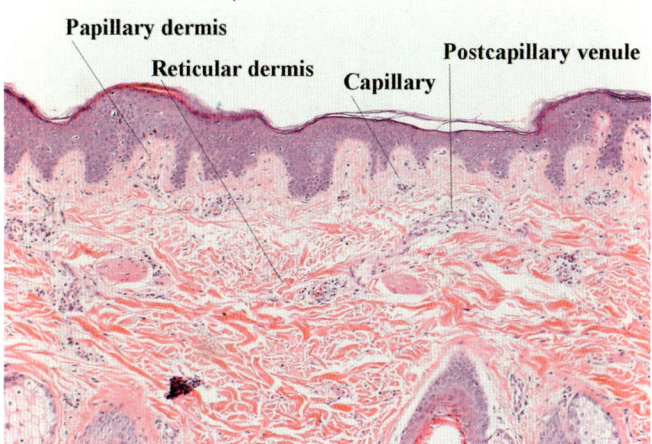

Fig. 1.19 Below the epidermis, the papillary dermis is composed of fine, nonbundled collagen. Capillaries are present within the papillary dermis, and the postcapillary venule sits at the junction of the papillary and reticular dermis. H&E × 40.

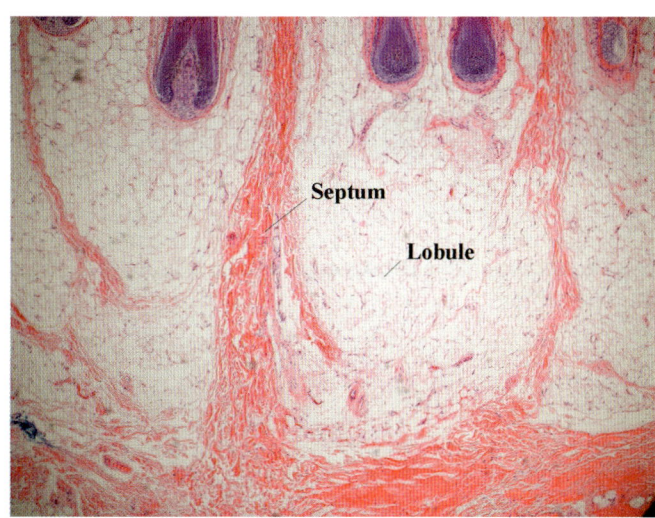

Fig. 1.20 The lobules of the subcutaneous fat are separated by fibrous septae. H&E × 40.

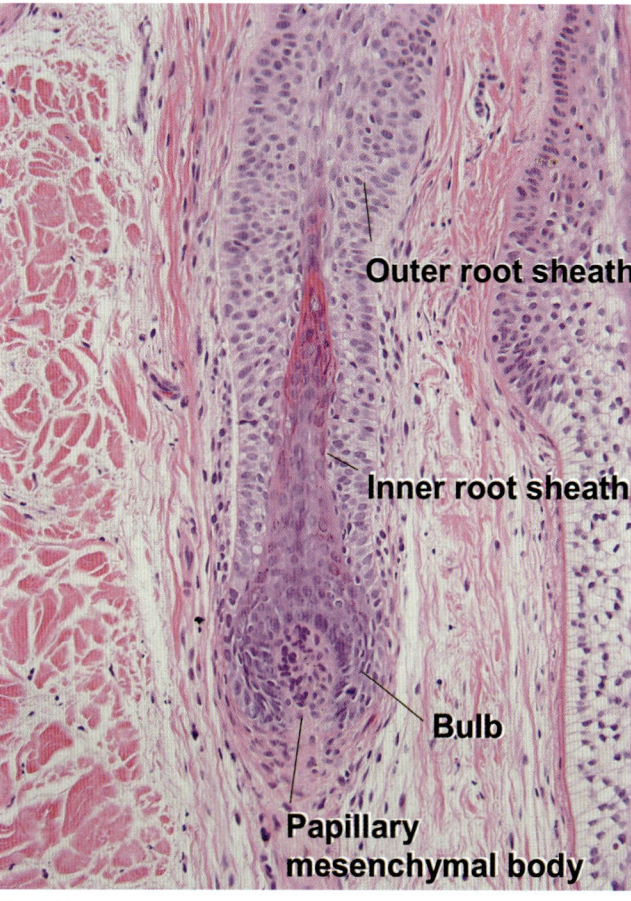

Fig. 1.21 Hair anatomy, vertical, H&E × 200.

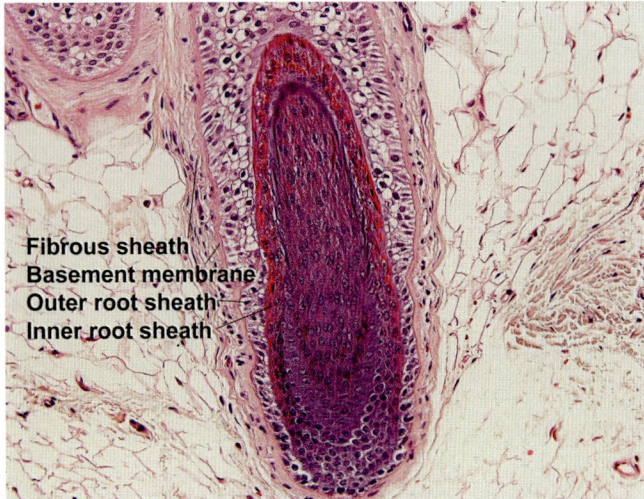

Fig. 1.22 In the inferior segment, the hair bulb gives rise to the inner and outer root sheath, H&E × 200.

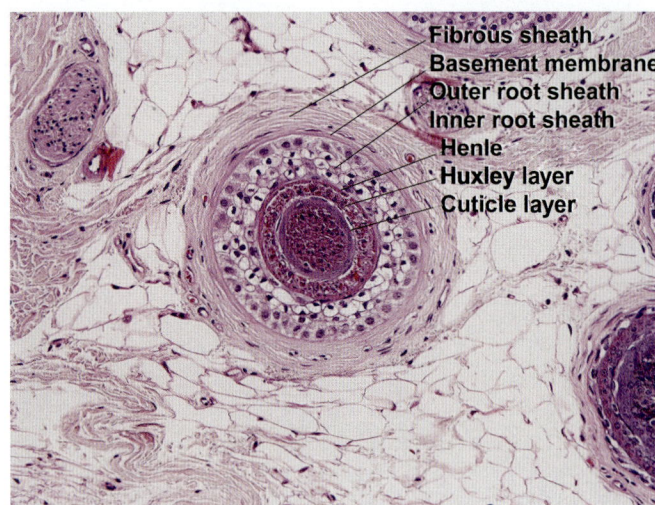

Fig. 1.23 Hair anatomy, transverse, H&E × 200.

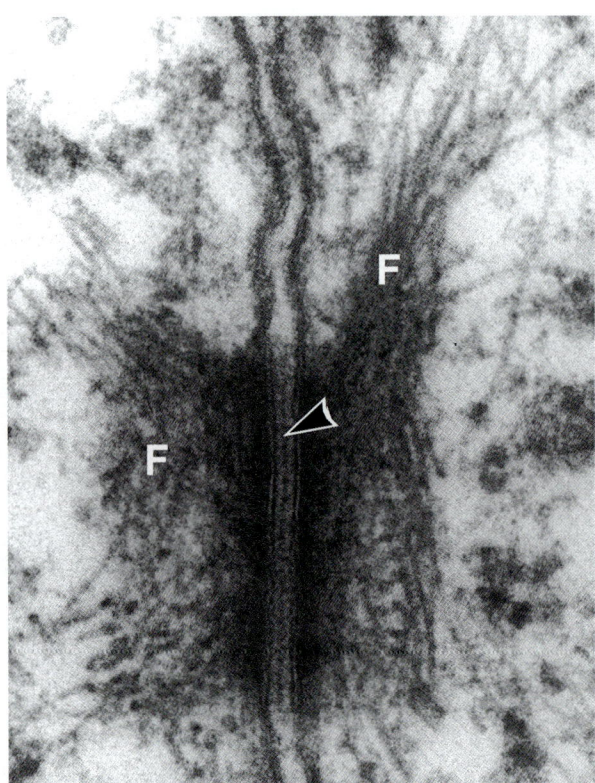

Fig. 1.24 Desmosome: A classic desmosome showing the following features: (1) Uniform gap of 20 to 30 nm between the apposed trilaminar plasma membranes with an intermediate line (*arrow*) in this gap. (2) Sharply delineated dense plaques into which tonofibrils (F) converge. *Courtesy Sunita Bhuta, MD.*

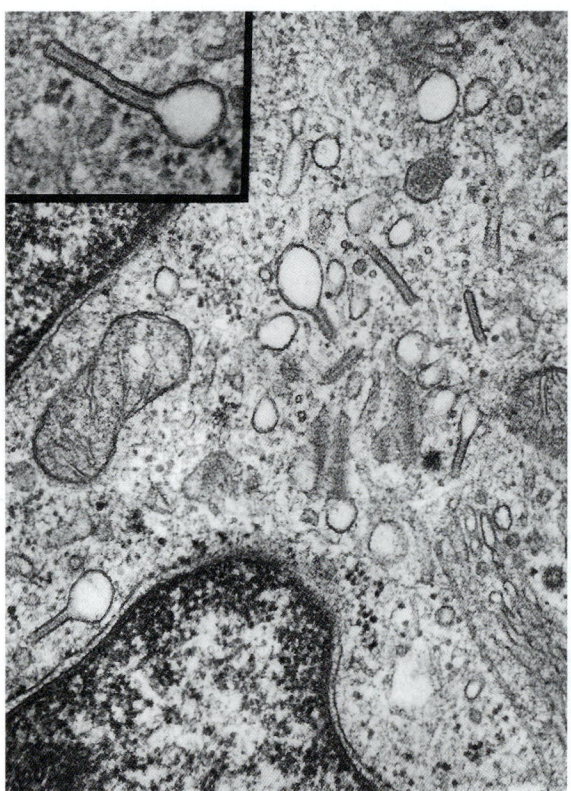

Fig. 1.25 Langerhans cell with Birbeck granules. This electromicrograph shows characteristic racket-shaped profiles of the granules in the cytoplasm (*inset* with higher magnification of the Birbeck granule). *Courtesy Sunita Bhuta, MD.*

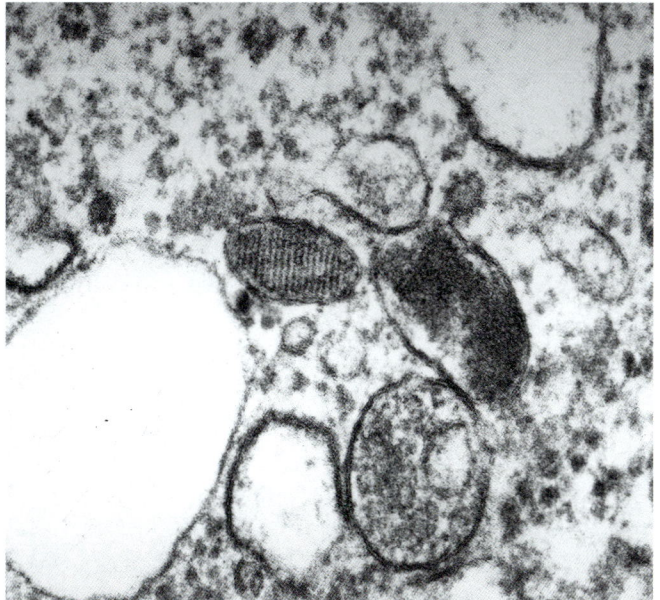

Fig. 1.26 Premelanosome: Solitary melanosome with characteristic internal striated structure. *Courtesy Sunita Bhuta, MD.*

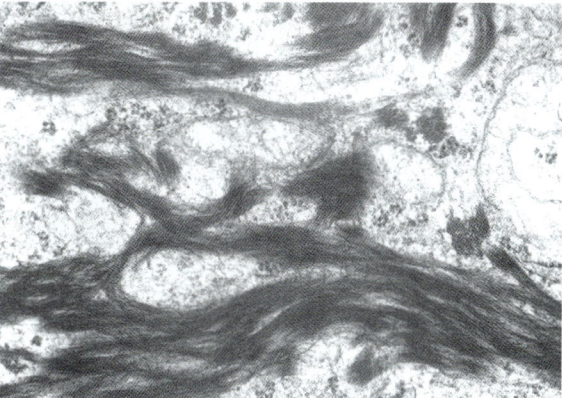

Fig. 1.27 Tonofibrils: Tonofibrils (intermediate filaments) lying free in the cytoplasm of a squamous cell. *Courtesy Sunita Bhuta, MD.*

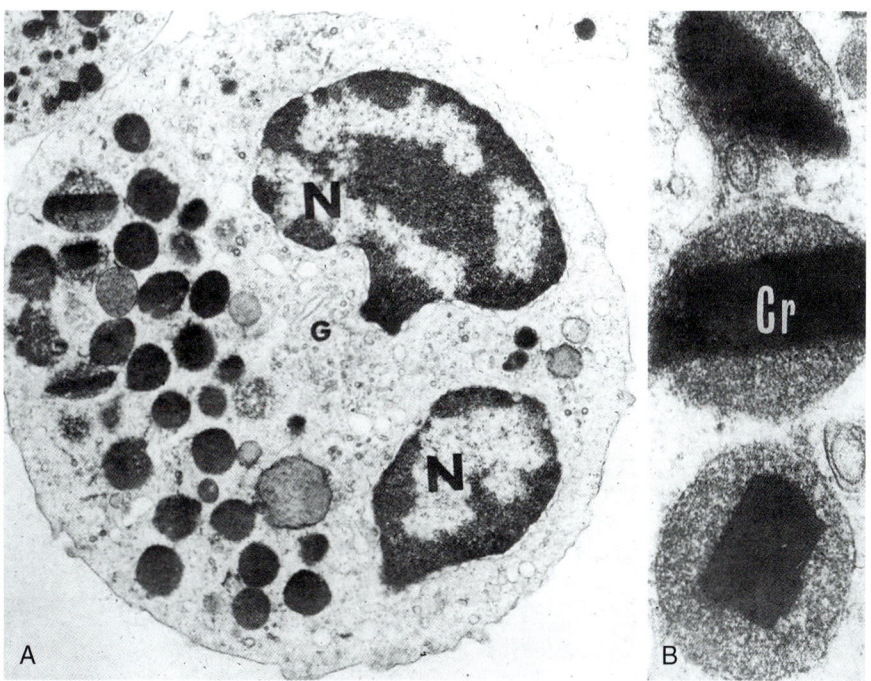

Fig. 1.28 Eosinophil: (A) Binucleate (N) with intracytoplasmic specific granules. (B) Specific granules have a finely granular matrix and a crystalline core. *Courtesy Sunita Bhuta, MD.*

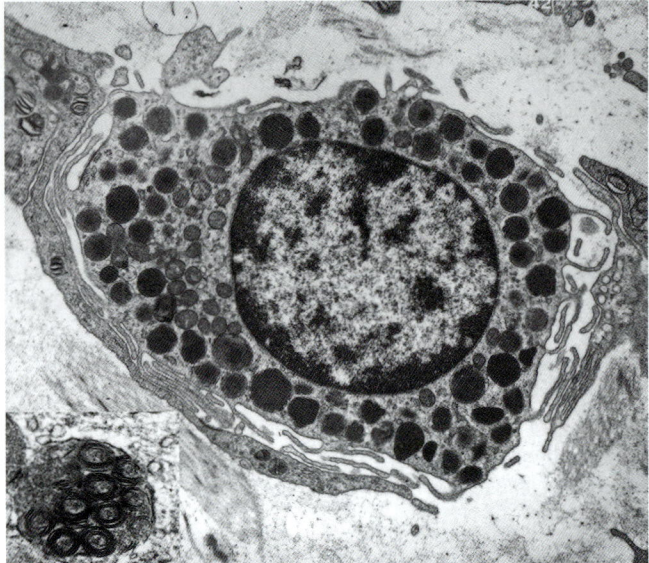

Fig. 1.29 Mast cell: Mast cell with numerous electron-dense granules. The inset shows internal structure of granules with membranous whorls (scrolls). *Courtesy Sunita Bhuta, MD.*

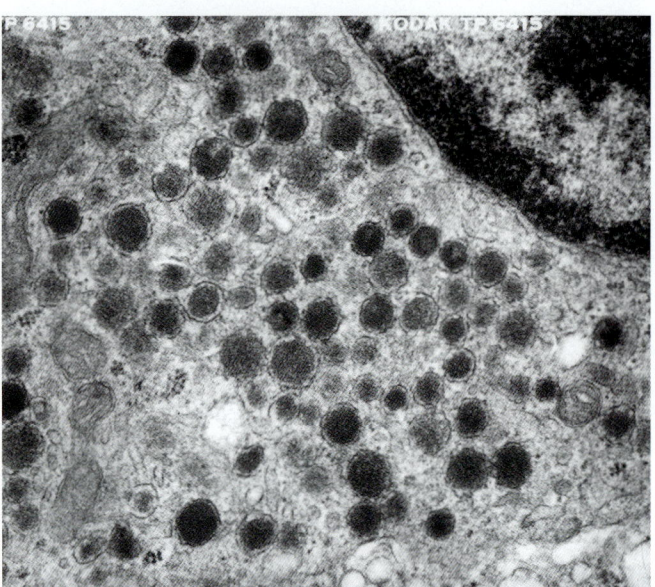

Fig. 1.30 Merkel cell: Merkel cell with intracytoplasmic membrane bound, electron-dense granules with a halo (neurosecretory granules). *Courtesy Sunita Bhuta, MD.*

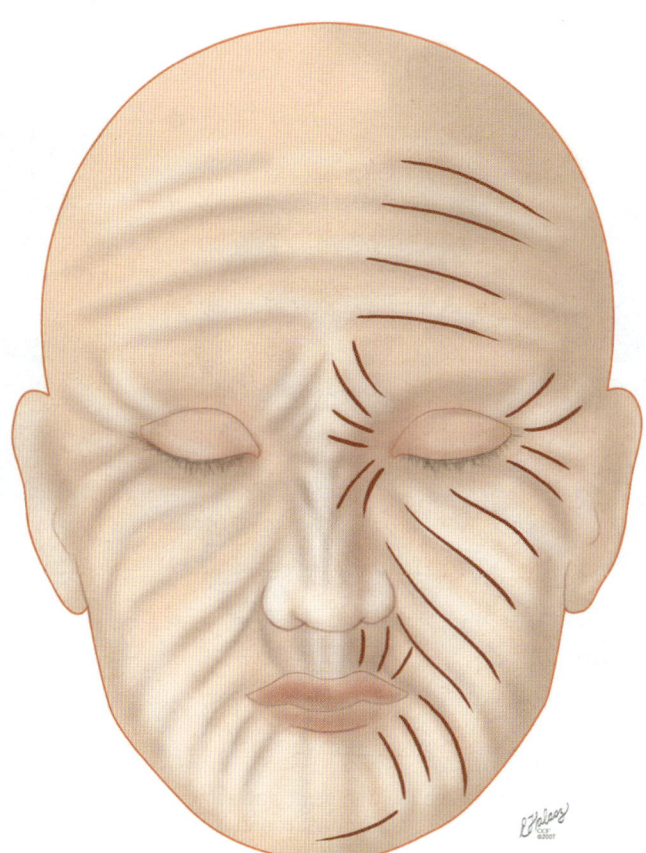

Fig. 1.31 Skin tension lines relate to creases visible in older skin. They relate to passive skin tension, as well as active contraction of superficial muscular aponeurotic system muscle. Optimal surgical results can be achieved by aligning incisions along these lines.

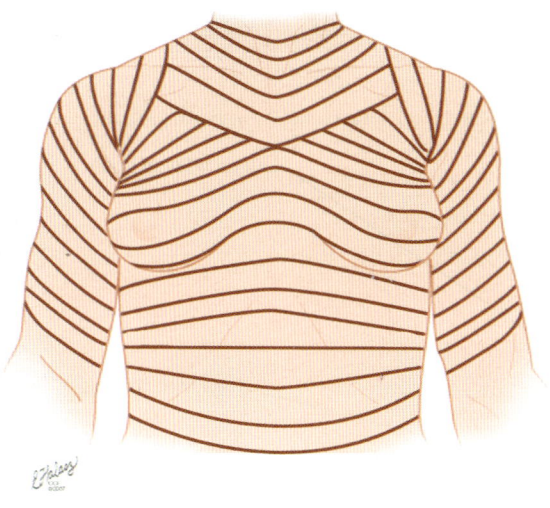

Fig. 1.32 Skin tension lines on the trunk.

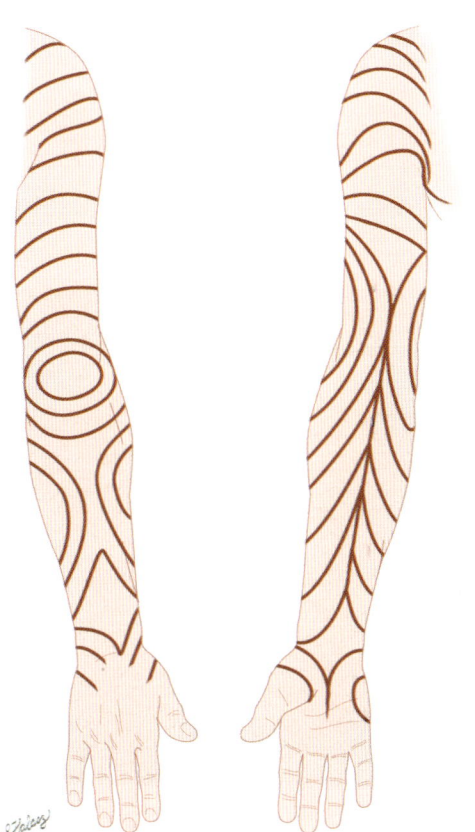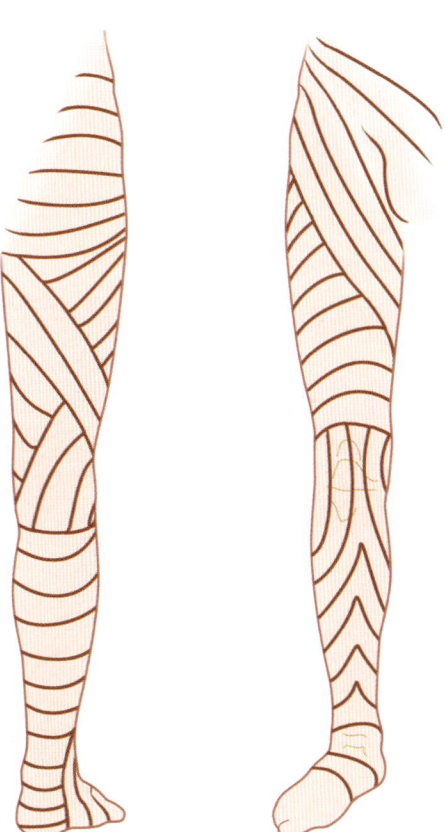

Fig. 1.33 Skin tension lines on the extremities.

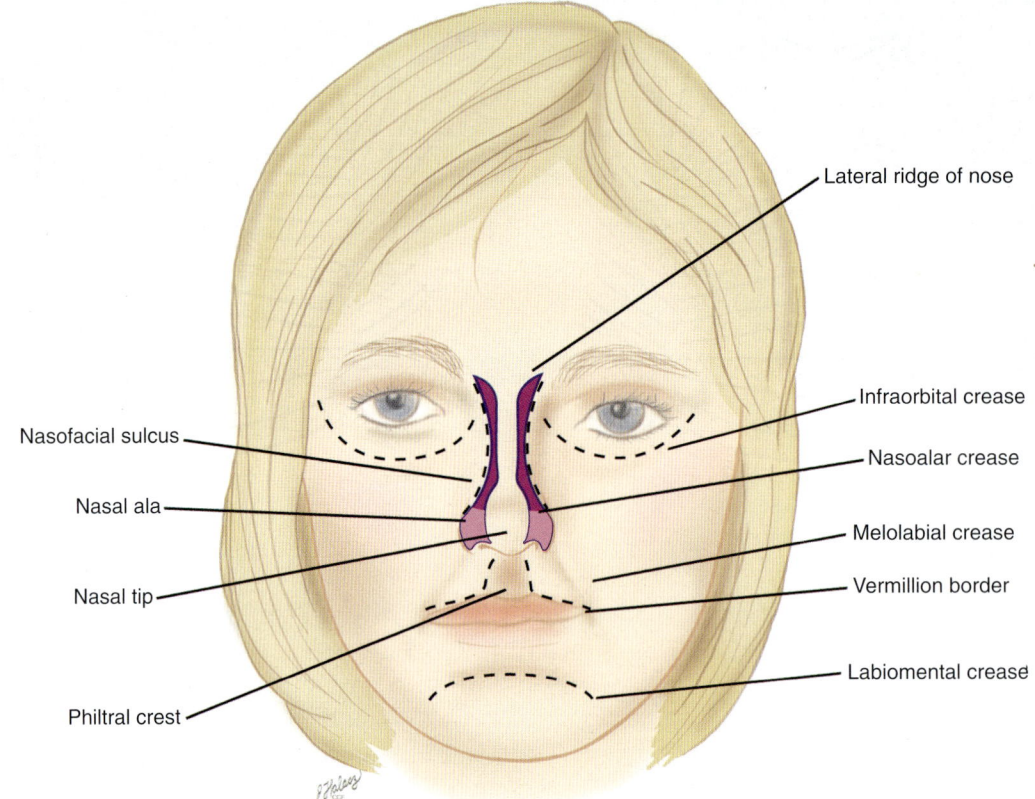

Fig. 1.34 Major anatomic landmarks.

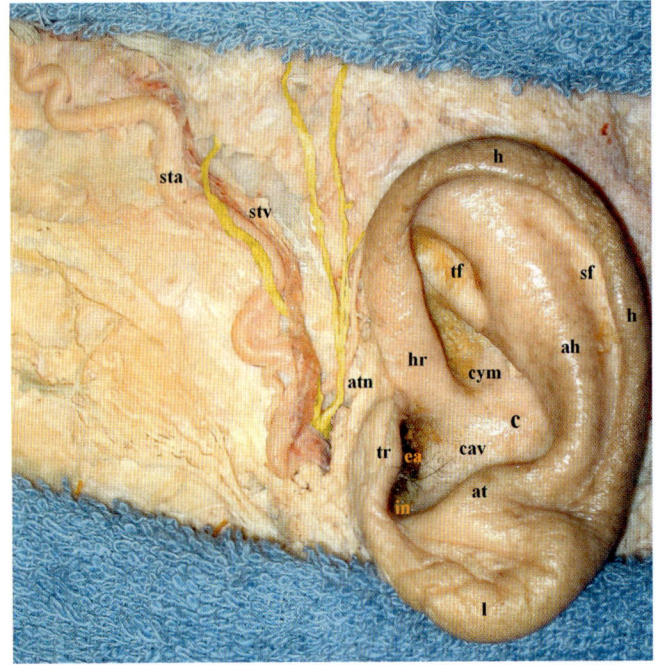

Fig. 1.35 Anatomy of the ear, superficial temporal artery, and auriculotemporal nerve. *Courtesy Joseph F. Greco, MD, and Christopher Skvarka, MD.*

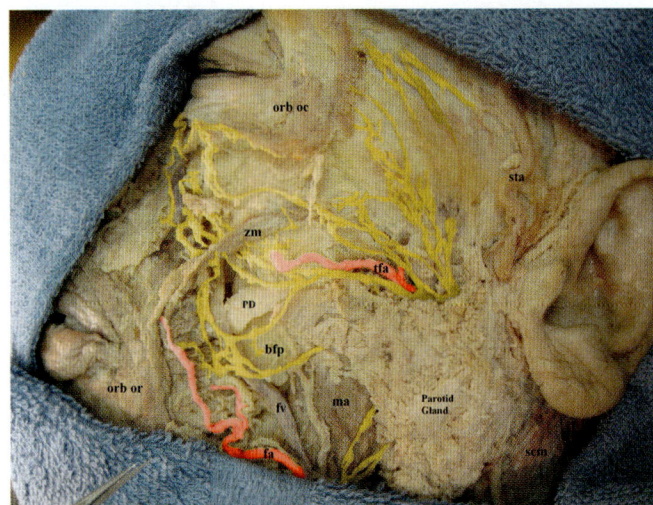

Fig. 1.36 Anatomy of the parotid gland and related structures. *Courtesy Joseph F. Greco, MD, and Christopher Skvarka, MD.*

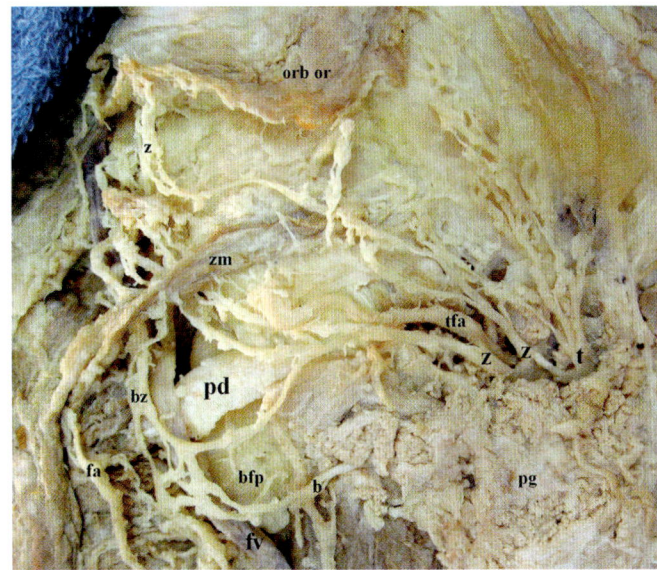

Fig. 1.37 Anatomy of the parotid duct and facial nerve. *Courtesy Joseph F. Greco, MD, and Christopher Skvarka, MD.*

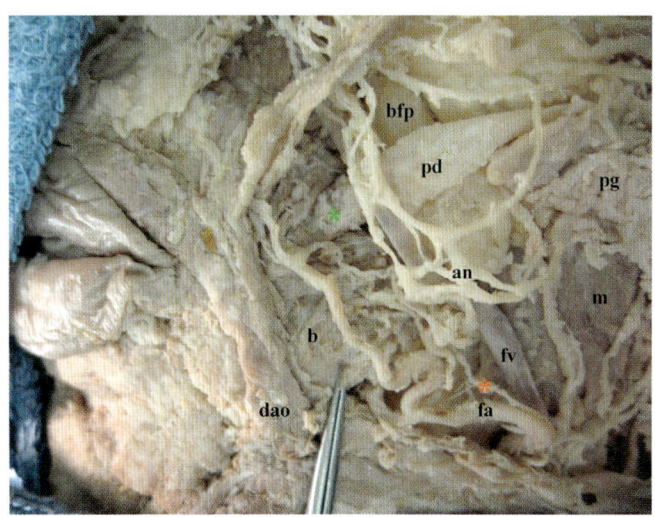

Fig. 1.38 Parotid duct as it pierces the buccinators muscle. *Courtesy Joseph F. Greco, MD, and Christopher Skvarka, MD.*

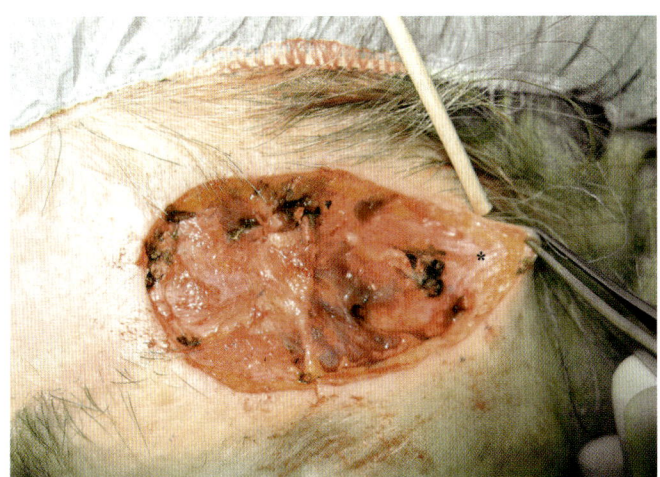

Fig. 1.39 Superficial muscular aponeurotic system. *Courtesy Joseph F. Greco, MD, and Christopher Skvarka, MD.*

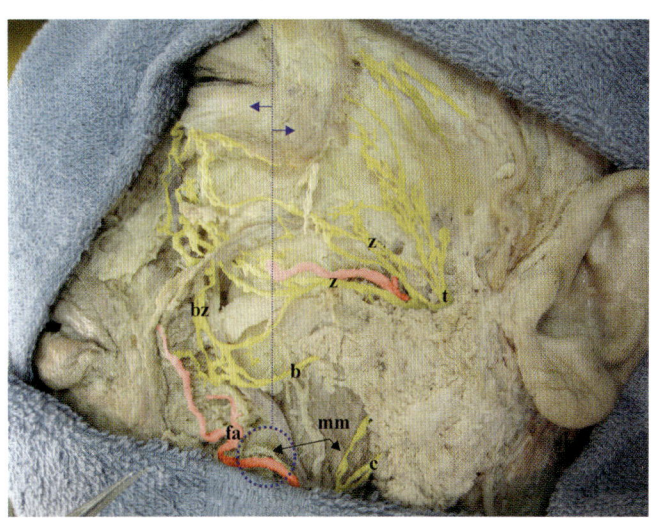

Fig. 1.40 Anatomy of the facial nerve. *Courtesy Joseph F. Greco, MD, and Christopher Skvarka, MD.*

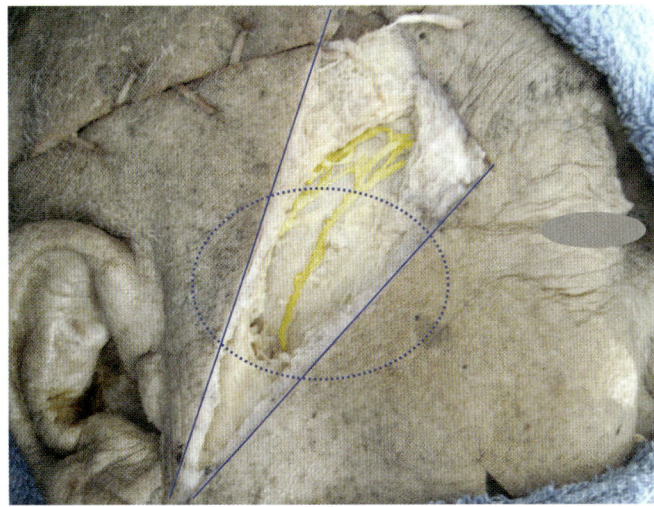

Fig. 1.41 The facial nerve: Danger zone for dermatologic surgery. *Courtesy Joseph F. Greco, MD, and Christopher Skvarka, MD.*

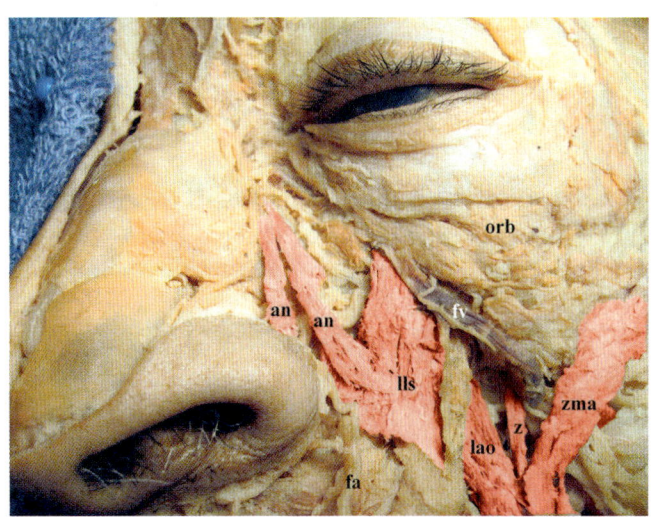

Fig. 1.42 Muscles of facial expression. *Courtesy Joseph F. Greco, MD, and Christopher Skvarka, MD.*

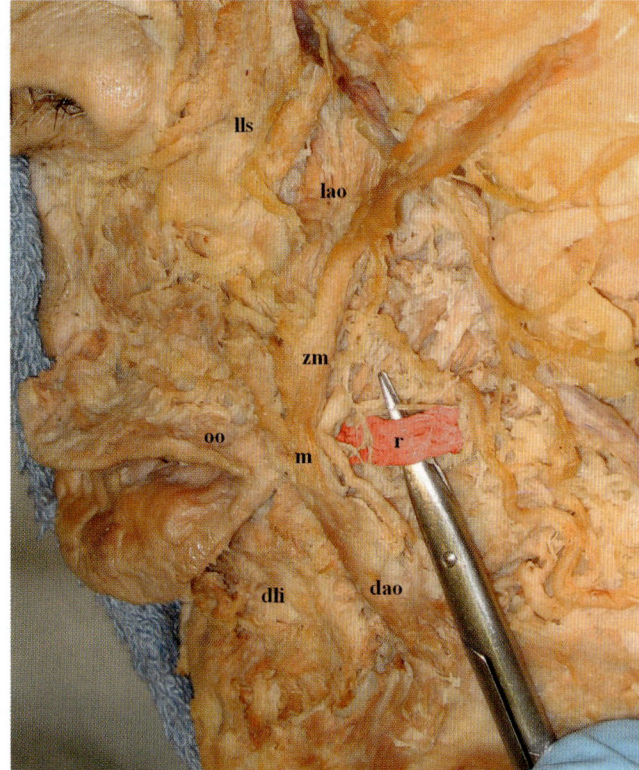

Fig. 1.43 Modiolus, elevators, and depressors. *Courtesy Joseph F. Greco, MD, and Christopher Skvarka, MD.*

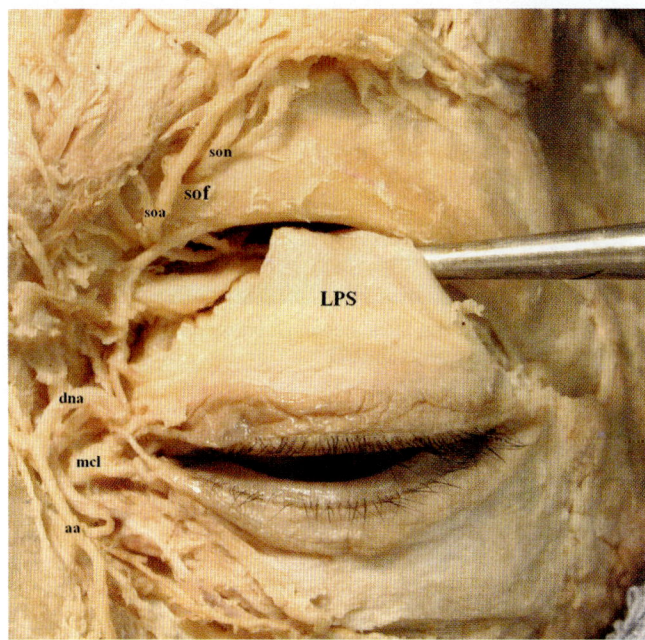

Fig. 1.45 Levator palpebrae superioris. *Courtesy Joseph F. Greco, MD, and Christopher Skvarka, MD.*

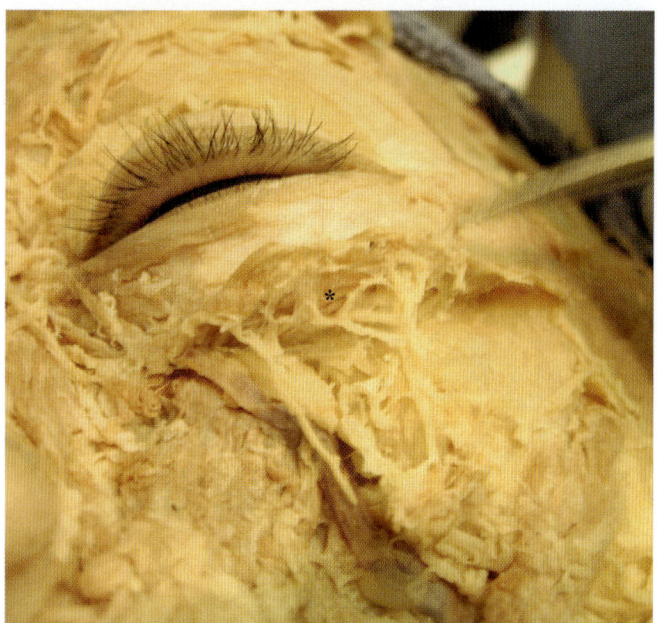

Fig. 1.44 Innervation of the facial skin. *Courtesy Joseph F. Greco, MD, and Christopher Skvarka, MD.*

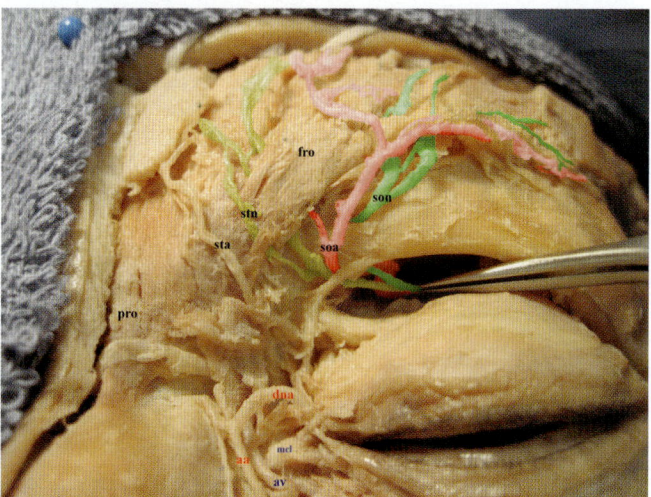

Fig. 1.46 Medial forehead: Supraorbital and supratrochlear neurovascular structures. *Courtesy Joseph F. Greco, MD, and Christopher Skvarka, MD.*

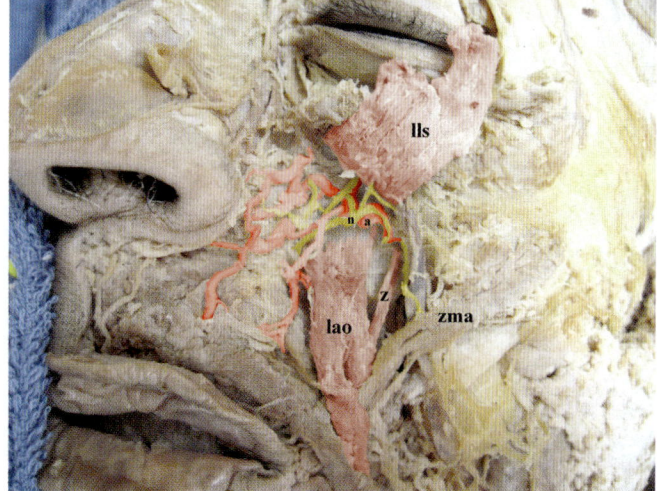

Fig. 1.47 Infraorbital foramen and related structures. *Courtesy Joseph F. Greco, MD, and Christopher Skvarka, MD.*

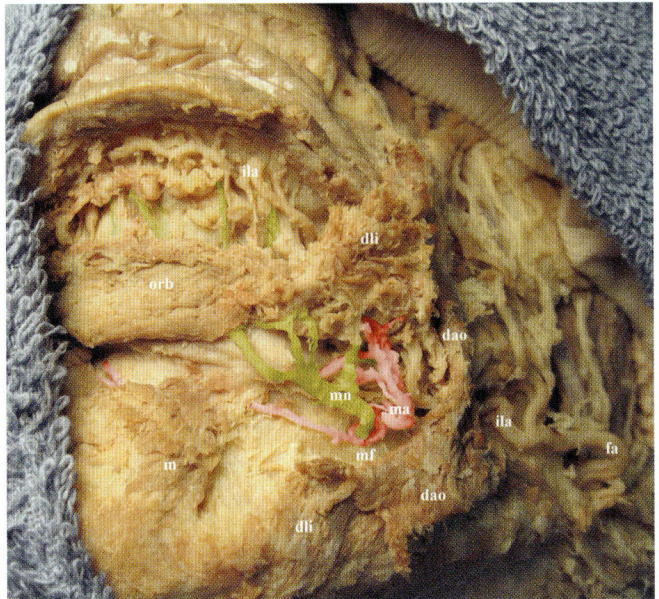

Fig. 1.48 Mental foramen and related structures. *Courtesy Joseph F. Greco, MD, and Christopher Skvarka, MD.*

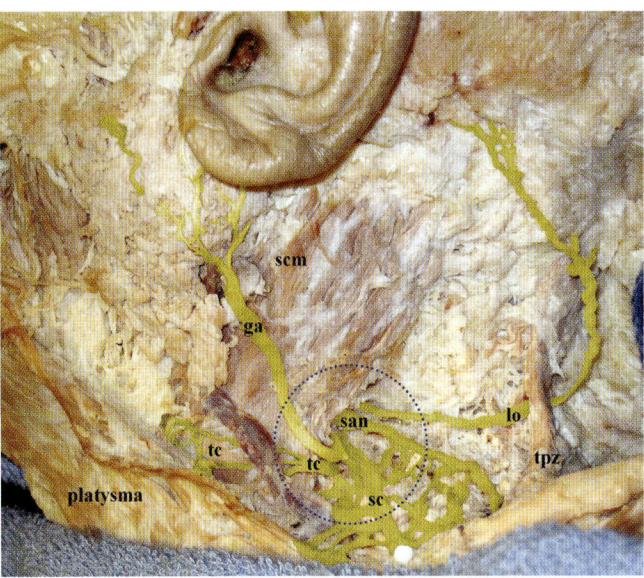

Fig. 1.49 Anatomy of the posterior triangle of the neck (Erb point). *Courtesy Joseph F. Greco, MD, and Christopher Skvarka, MD.*

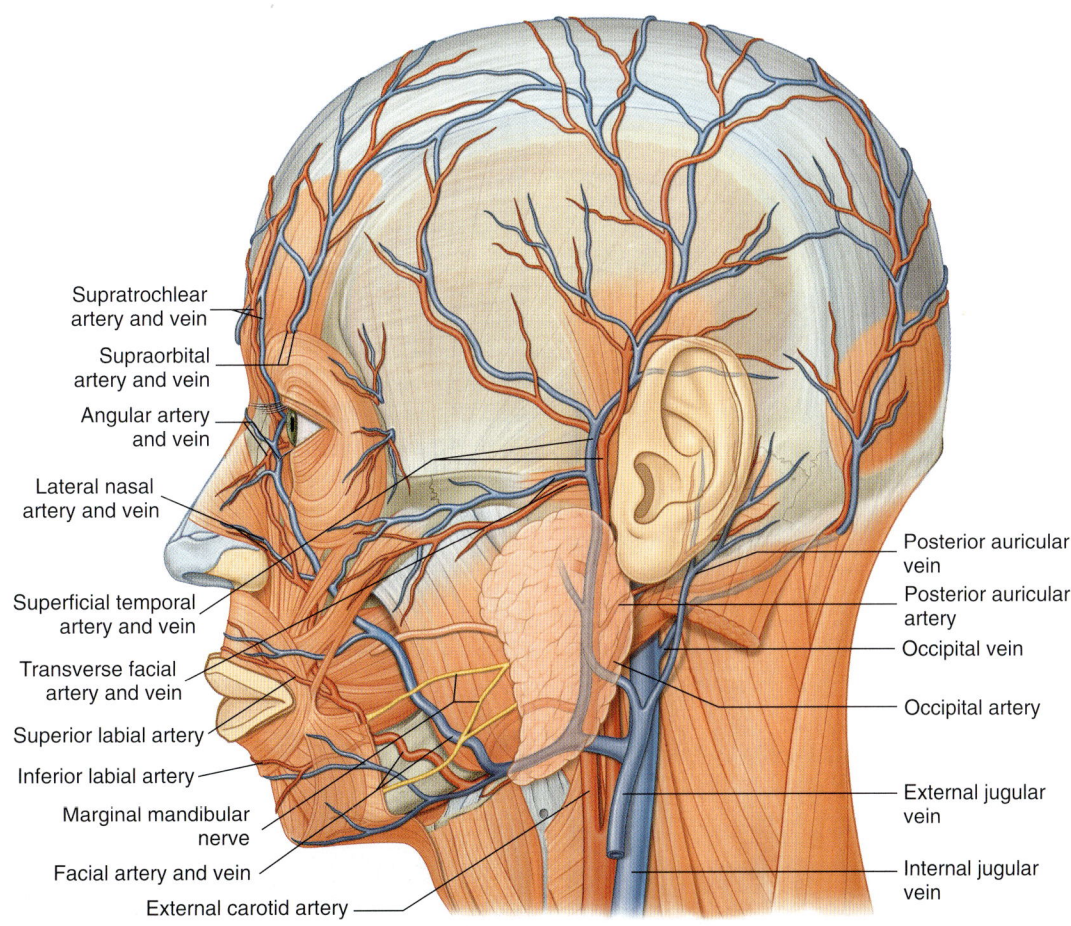

Fig. 1.50 Arterial and venous supply of the face.

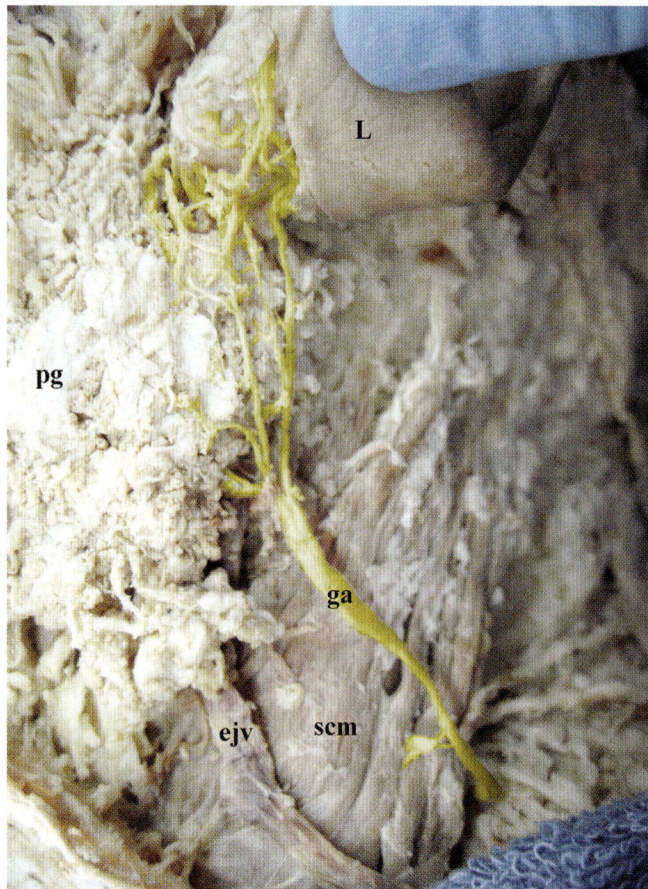

Fig. 1.51 Great auricular nerve and external jugular vein. *Courtesy Joseph F. Greco, MD, and Christopher Skvarka, MD.*

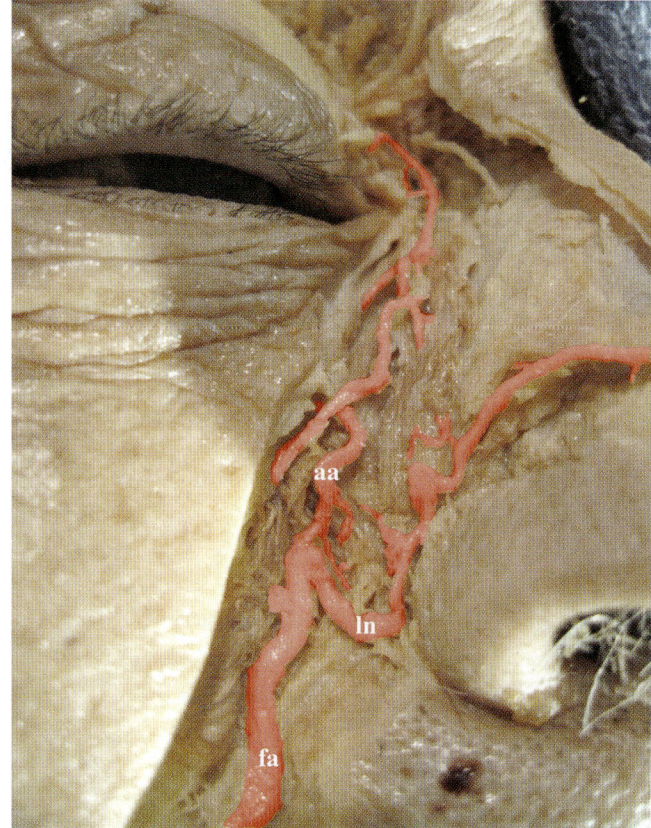

Fig. 1.52 Facial artery with angular artery. *Courtesy Joseph F. Greco, MD, and Christopher Skvarka, MD.*

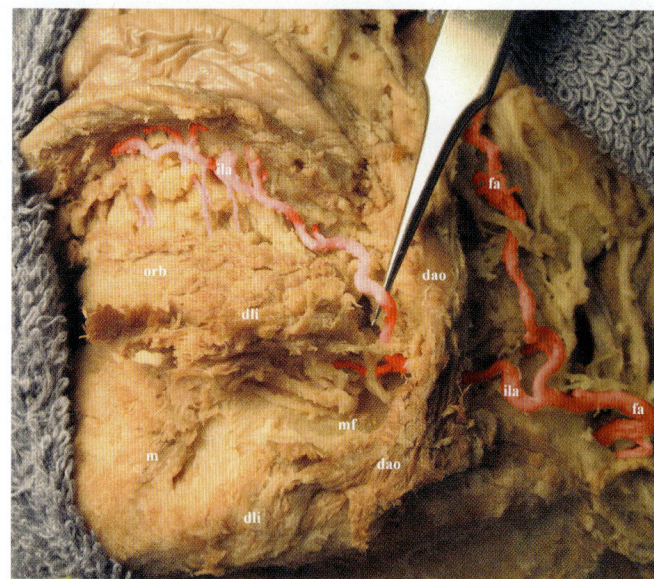

Fig. 1.53 Inferior labial artery and related structures of the lower lip and chin. *Courtesy Joseph F. Greco, MD, and Christopher Skvarka, MD.*

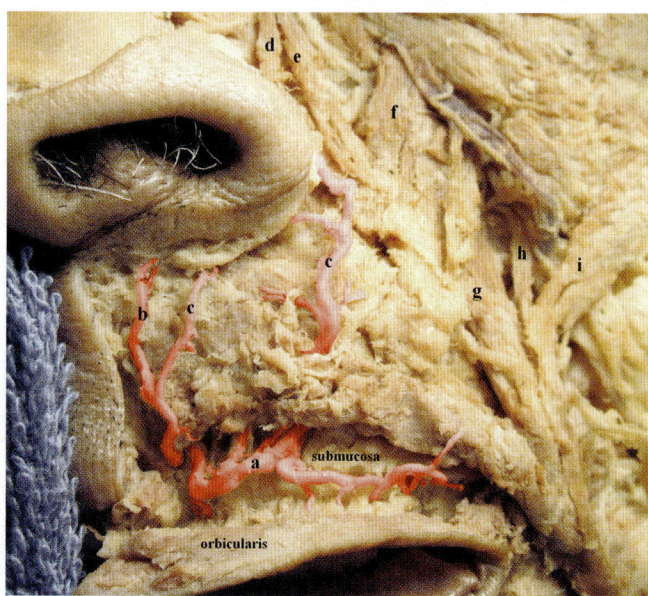

Fig. 1.54 Superior labial artery and related structures of the upper lip and cheek. *Courtesy Joseph F. Greco, MD, and Christopher Skvarka, MD.*

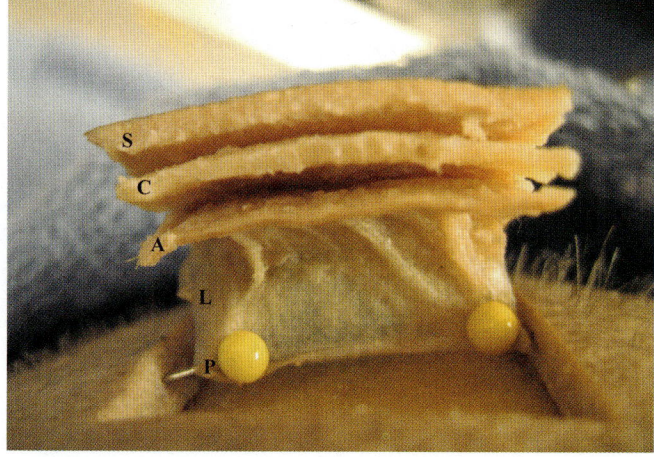

Fig. 1.55 Layers of the scalp. *Courtesy Joseph F. Greco, MD, and Christopher Skvarka, MD.*

Cutaneous Signs and Diagnosis   2

The astute clinician uses the appearance of the eruption and its accompanying symptoms to arrive at an accurate diagnosis. A symptom, such as itch or pain, is something that the patient reports. In contrast, a sign is elicited by the physician during examination. Pain is a symptom; tenderness to palpation is a sign.

This chapter will focus on the morphologic patterns skin lesions may have primarily or acquire over the course of time. The latter are called *secondary characteristics* and are not as helpful diagnostically as those present at the onset of the condition. Examples of each primary and secondary lesion are included, as well as other findings that are utilized to narrow the differential diagnosis such as the configuration, grouping, and color.

Finally, examples throughout will emphasize that the astute clinician should utilize all observable findings, inducing those of the hair, nails, and mucous membranes.

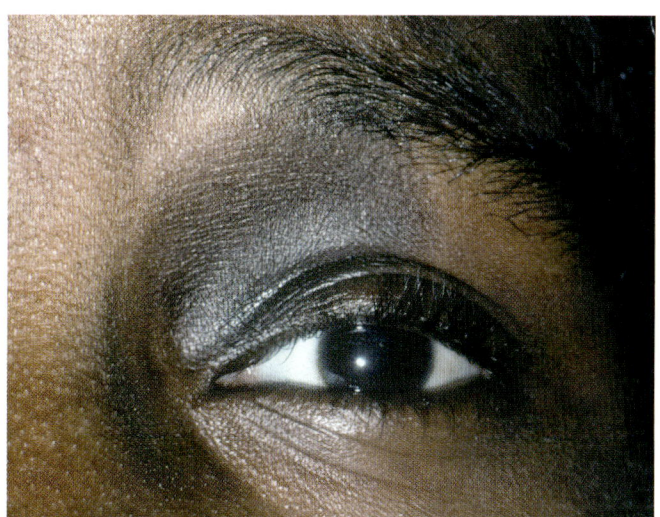

Fig. 2.1 Nevus of Ota (macule). *Courtesy Steven Binnick, MD.*

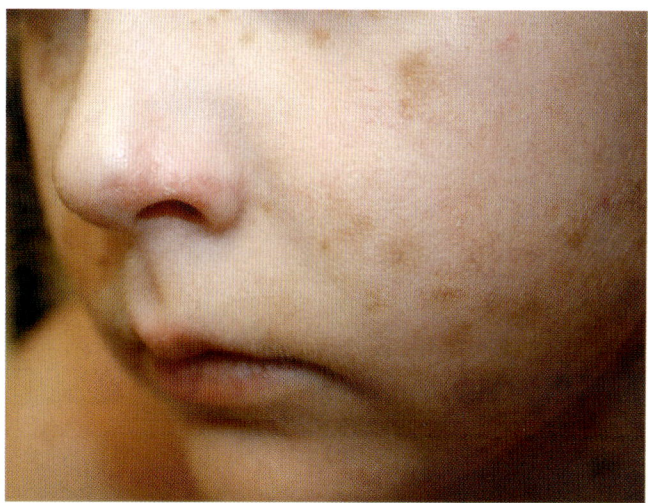

Fig. 2.3 Voriconazole-induced lentigines (macules). *Courtesy Jennifer Huang, MD.*

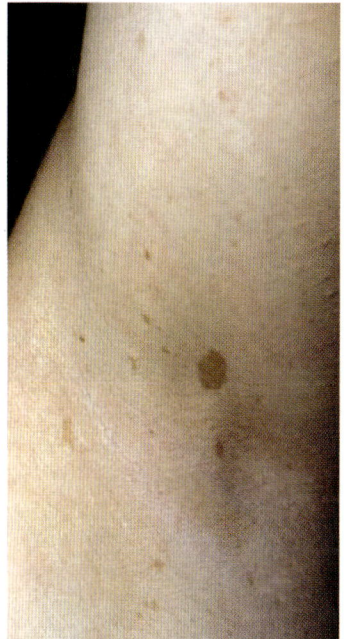

Fig. 2.2 Axillary freckling neurofibromatosis (macules).

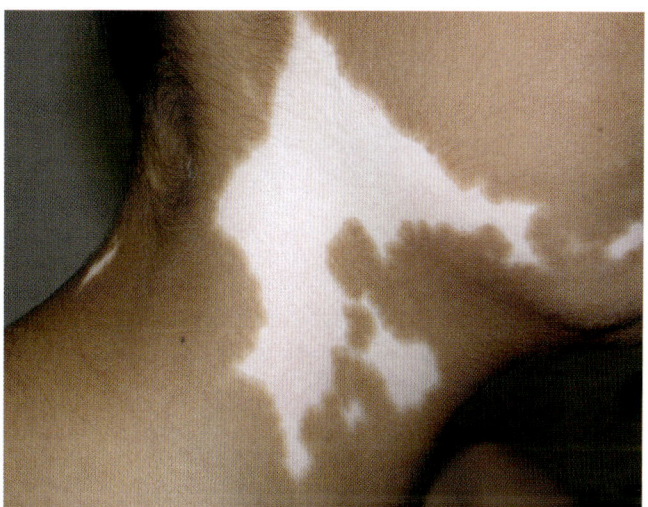

Fig. 2.4 Vitiligo (patch).

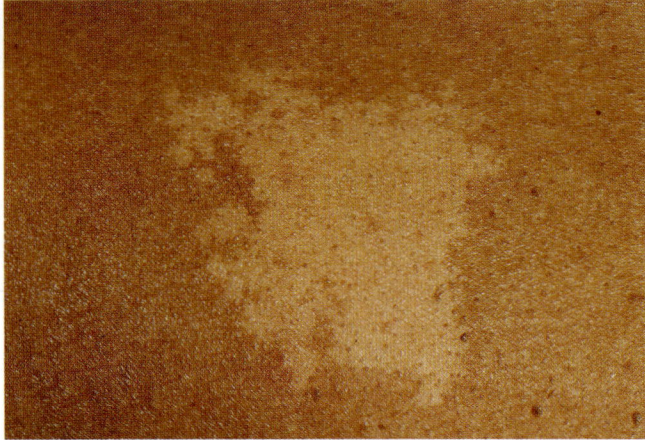

Fig. 2.5 Nevus depigmentosus (patch).

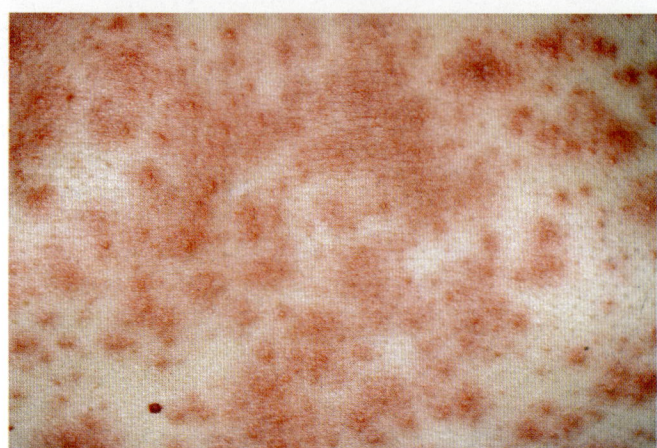

Fig. 2.6 Drug eruption (macules, some small papules present surmounting the erythema).

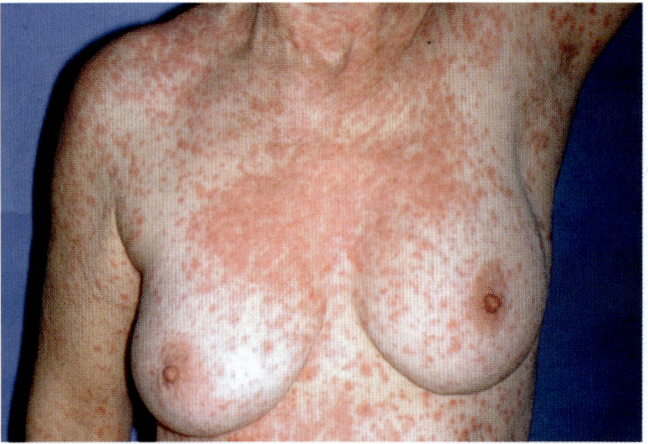

Fig. 2.7 Drug eruption (morbilliform appearance).

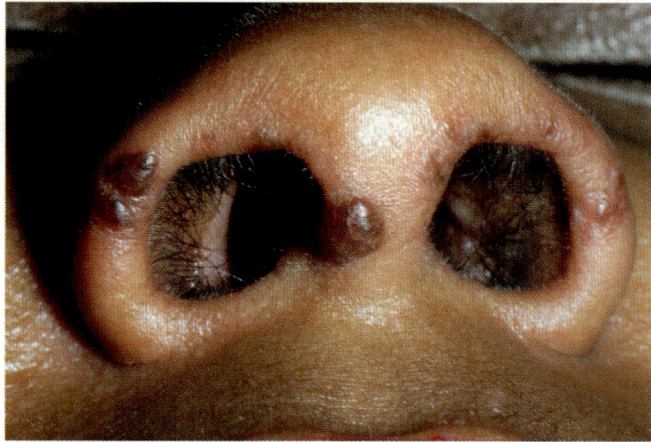

Fig. 2.8 Sarcoidosis (papules).

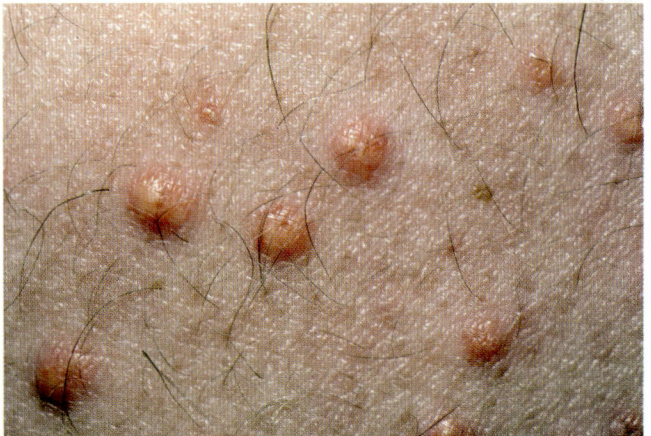

Fig. 2.9 Eruptive xanthomas (papules). Yellow color is uncommon in the skin and helps to narrow the differential diagnosis.

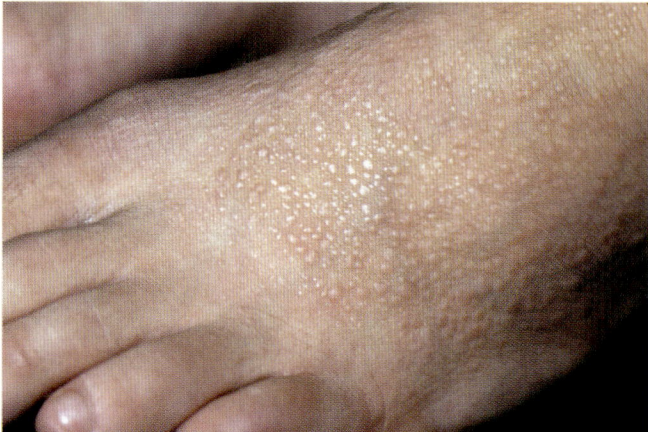

Fig. 2.10 Darier disease (papules).

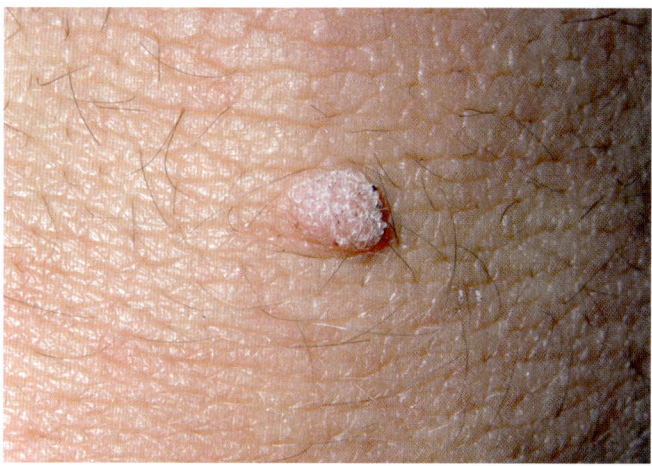

Fig. 2.11 Verruca vulgaris (scaly papule).

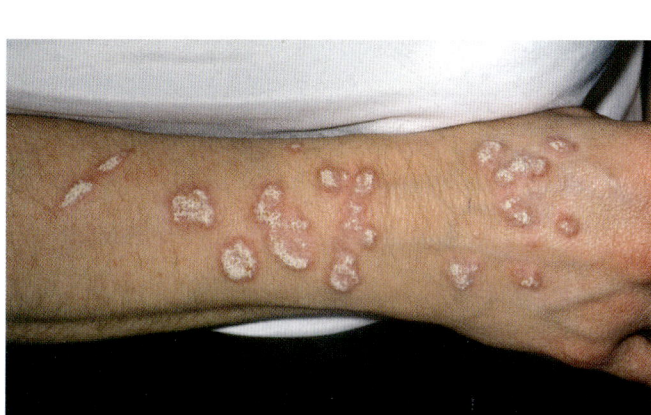

Fig. 2.12 Hypertrophic lupus erythematosus (scaly papules and plaques). *Courtesy Steven Binnick, MD.*

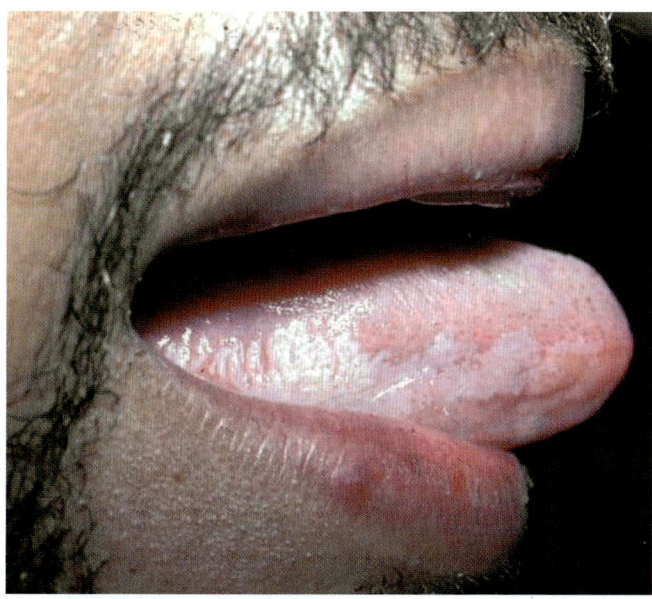

Fig. 2.13 Oral hairy leukoplakia (plaques).

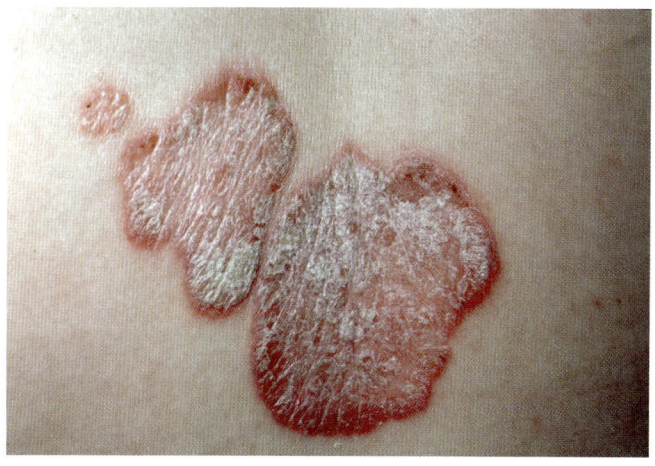

Fig. 2.14 Psoriasis (plaques). *Courtesy Steven Binnick, MD.*

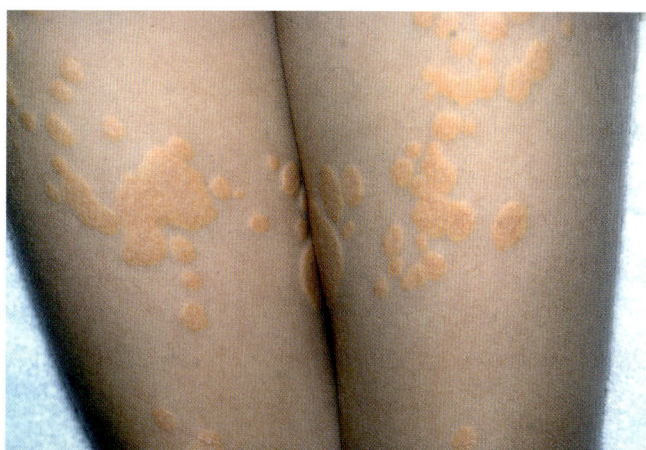

Fig. 2.15 Xanthomas in homozygous familial hypercholesterolemia (plaques of yellow color).

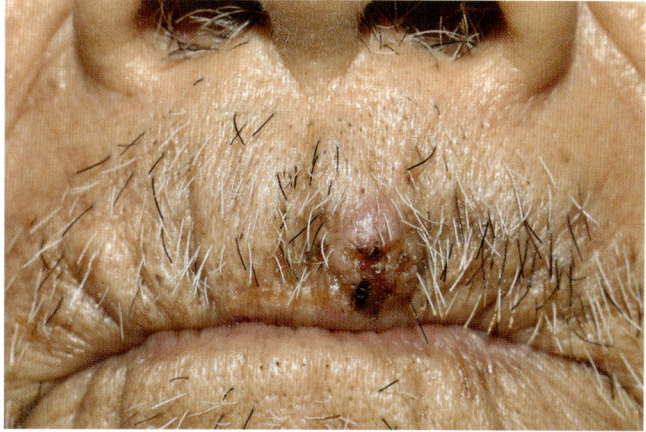

Fig. 2.16 Squamous cell carcinoma (eroded nodule). *Courtesy Dr. Yi-Shuan Sheen.*

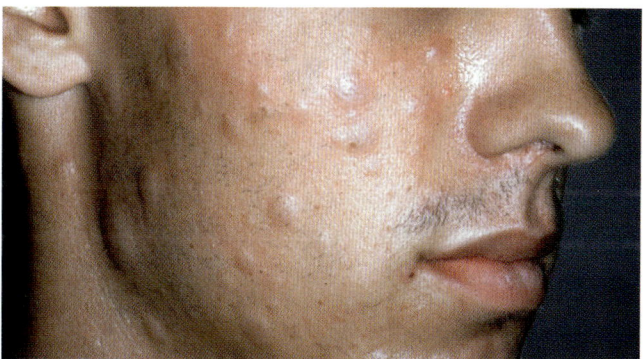

Fig. 2.17 Acute myelogenous leukemia (nodules).

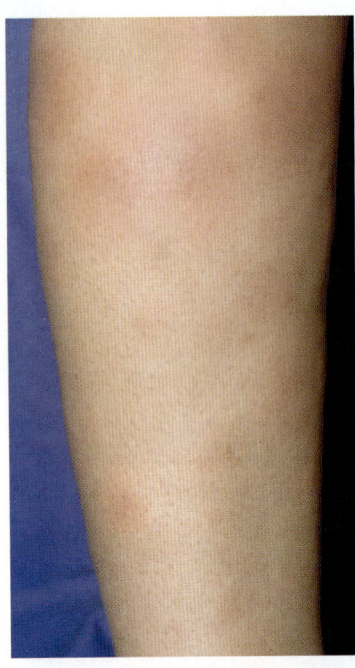

Fig. 2.18 Erythema nodosum (subcutaneous nodules).

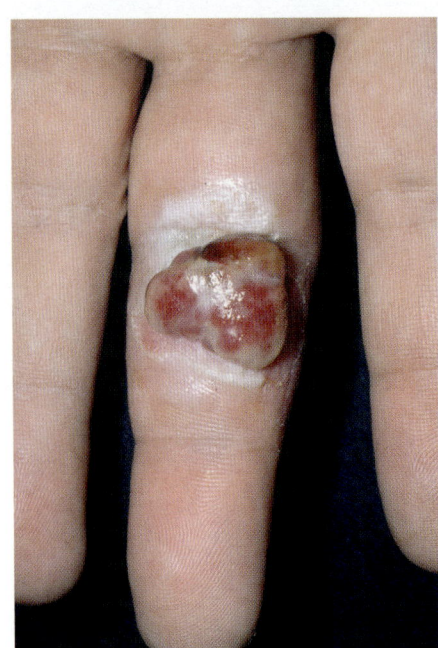

Fig. 2.19 Pyogenic granuloma (tumor). *Courtesy Curt Samlaska, MD.*

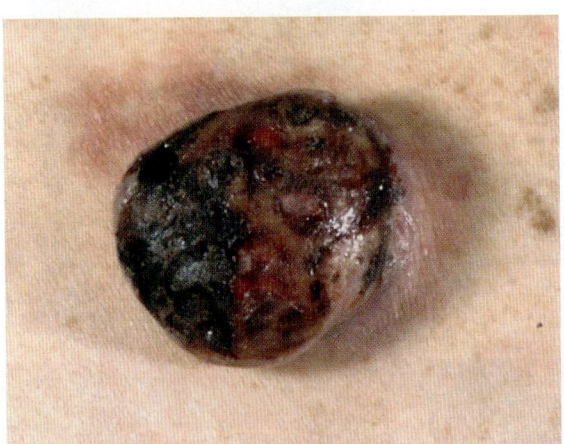

Fig. 2.20 Melanoma (tumor). *Courtesy Chris Miller, MD.*

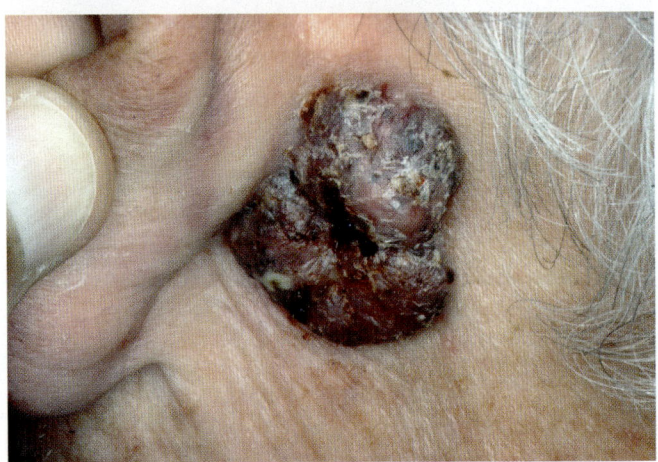

Fig. 2.21 Basal cell carcinoma (tumor).

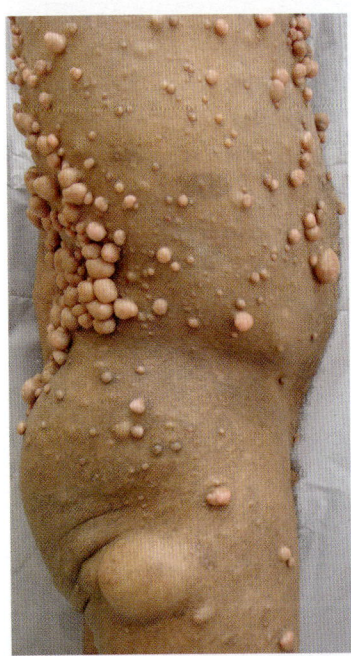

Fig. 2.22 Neurofibromatosis (macular hyperpigmentation, papules, tumors).

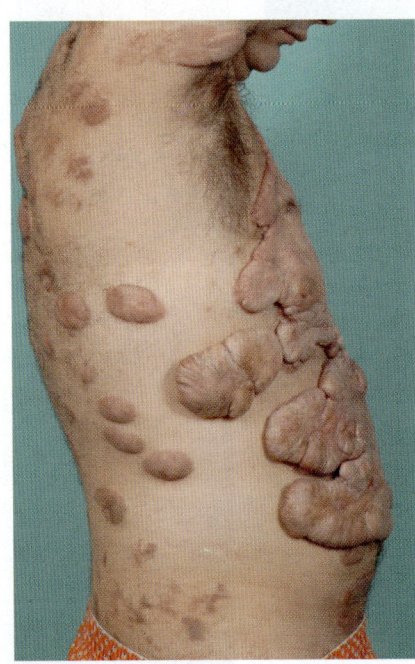

Fig. 2.23 Keloids (plaques and tumor).

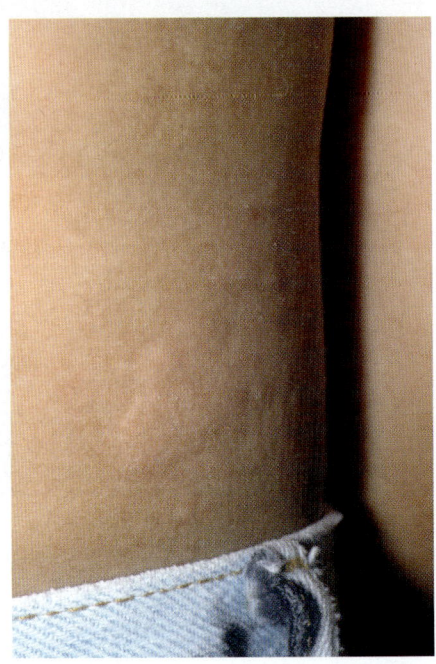

Fig. 2.24 Acute urticaria (wheal). *Courtesy Curt Samlaska, MD.*

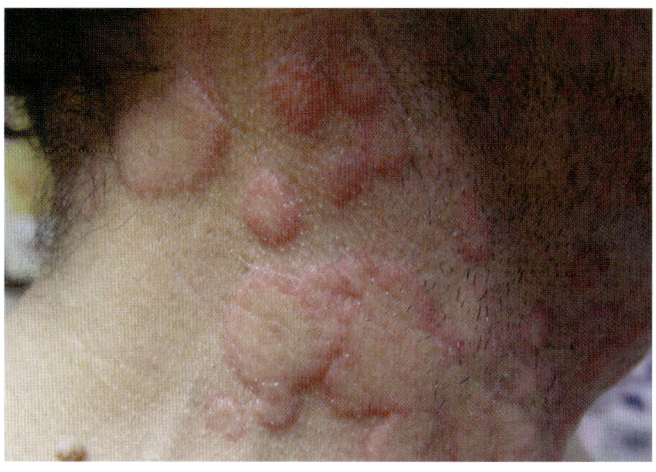

Fig. 2.25 Urticaria (wheal). *Courtesy Dr. Rui Carlos Taveres Bello.*

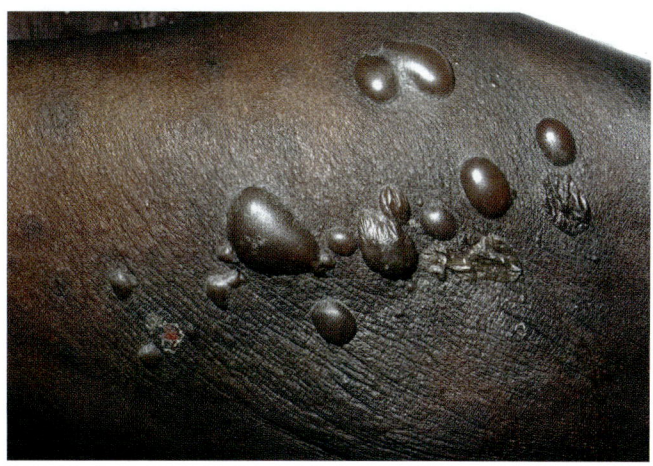

Fig. 2.28 Bullous pemphigoid (vesicles and bullae).

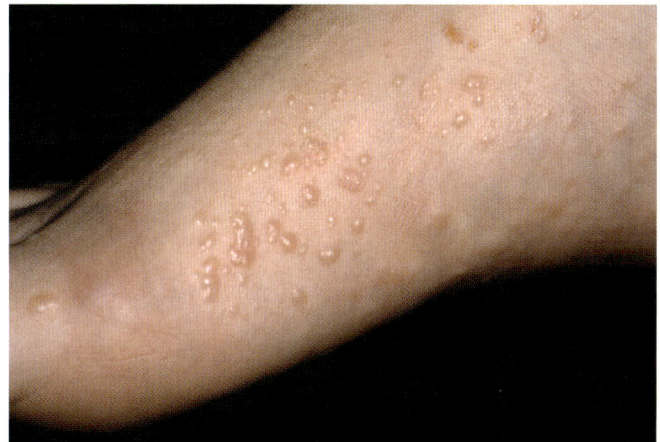

Fig. 2.26 Dyshidrosis (vesicles).

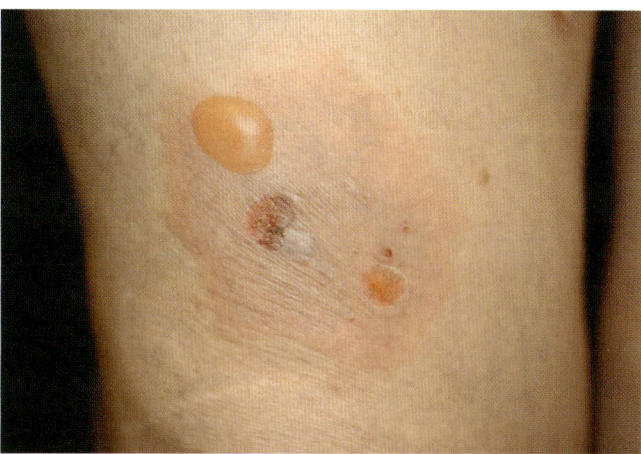

Fig. 2.29 Bullous pemphigoid (bulla and erosions on an erythematous base). *Courtesy Kaohsiung Chang Gang Memorial Hospital, Taiwan.*

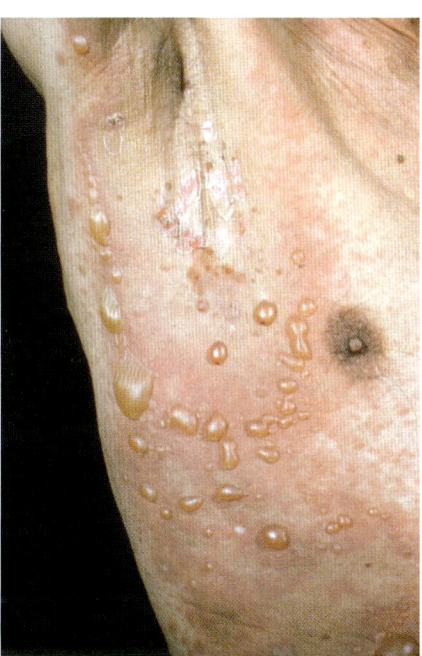

Fig. 2.27 Bullous pemphigoid (vesicles and bullae).

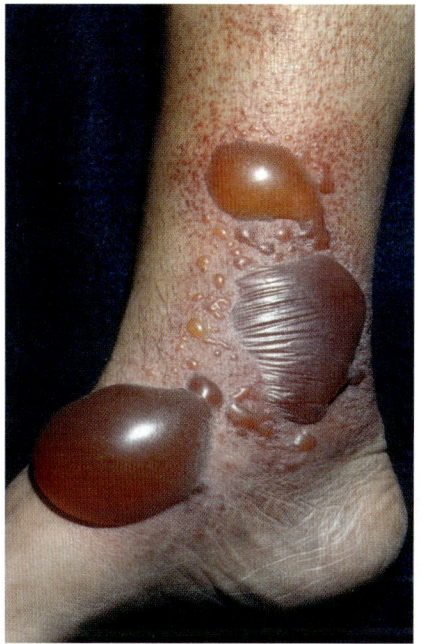

Fig. 2.30 Piroxicam hypersensitivity (vesicles and bullae, some with hemorrhage).

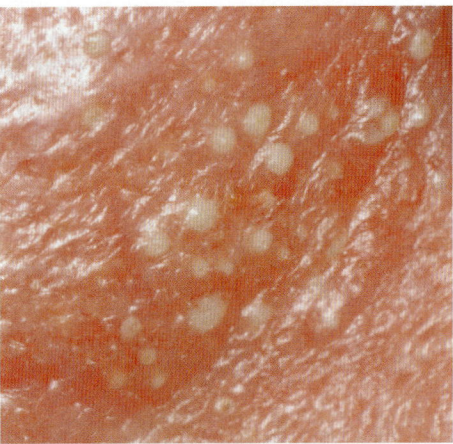

Fig. 2.31 Staphylococcal folliculitis (pustules).

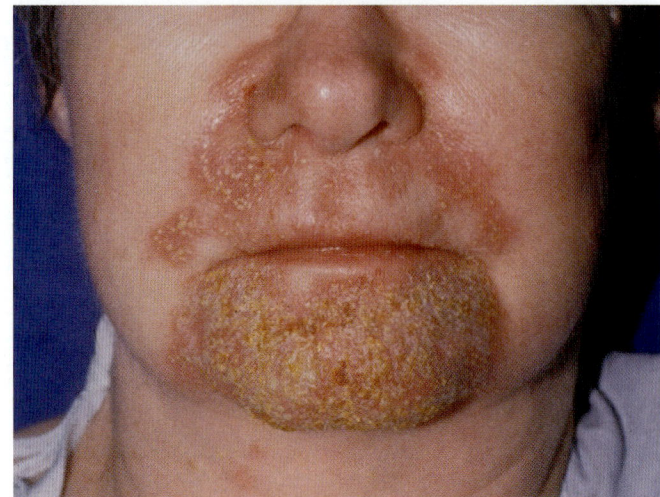

Fig. 2.34 Staphylococcal folliculitis and impetigo (pustules and crusts).

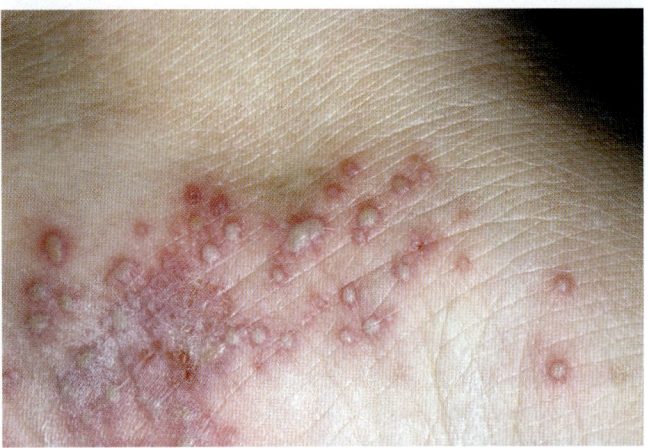

Fig. 2.32 Plantar pustulosis (pustules).

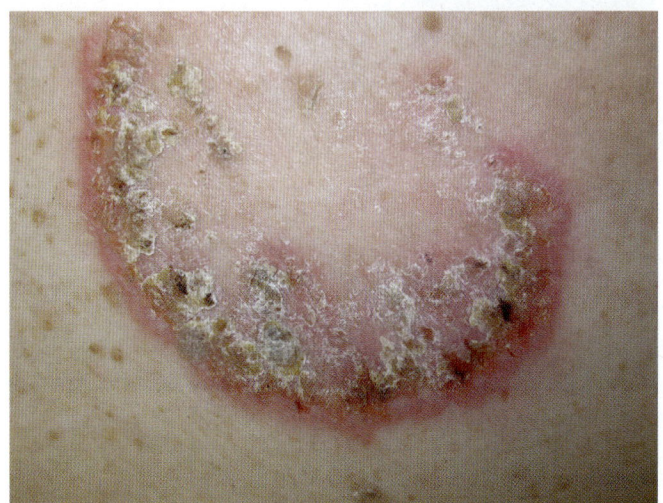

Fig. 2.35 Hailey-Hailey disease (crusts).

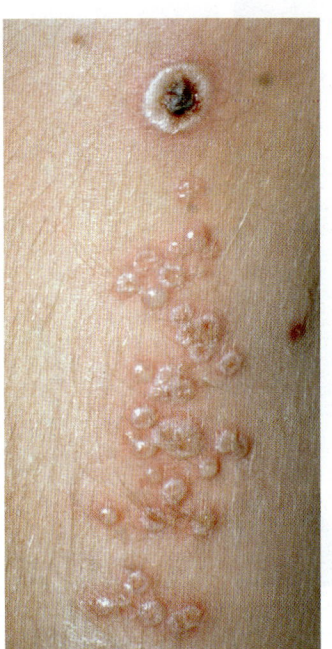

Fig. 2.33 Autoinoculation vaccinia (umbilicated pustules).

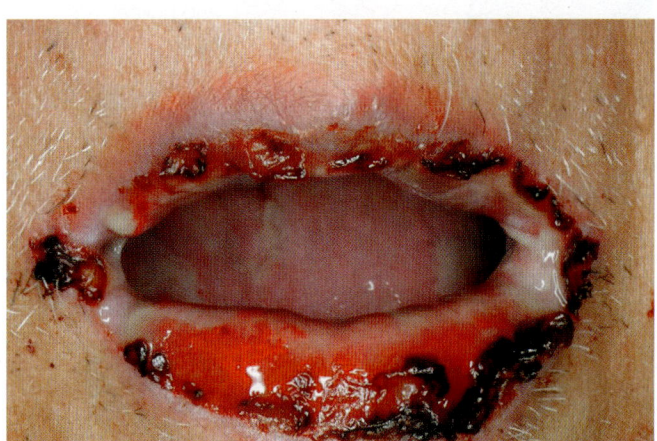

Fig. 2.36 Paraneoplastic pemphigus (hemorrhagic crusts). *Courtesy Department of Dermatology, Keio University School of Medicine, Tokyo, Japan.*

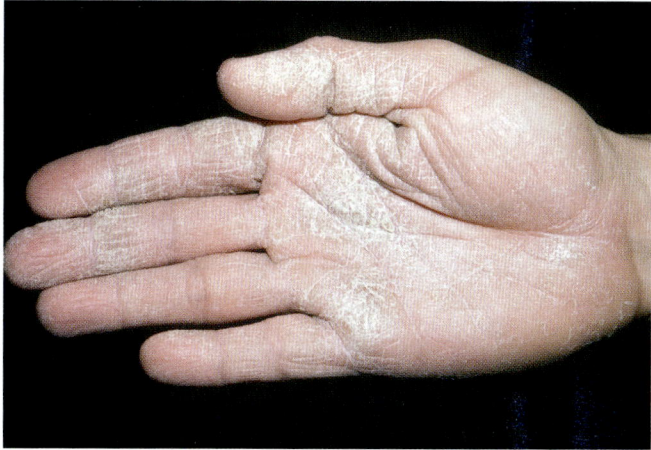

Fig. 2.37 Chronic hand dermatitis from cement (scale).

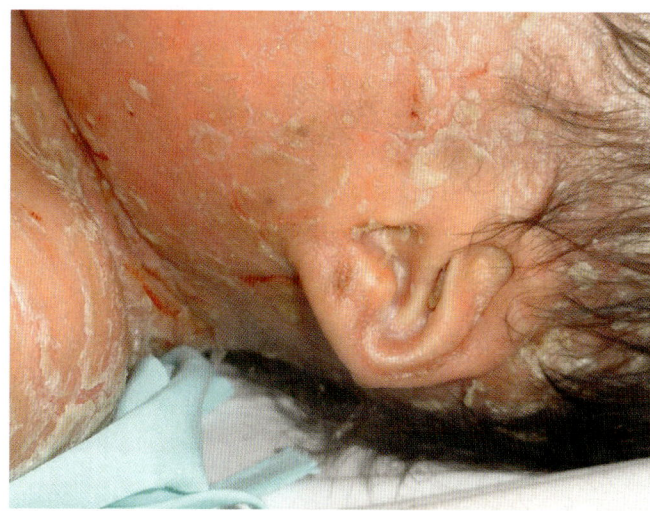

Fig. 2.40 Congenital ichthyosiform erythroderma (scale with desquamation). *Courtesy Scott Norton, MD.*

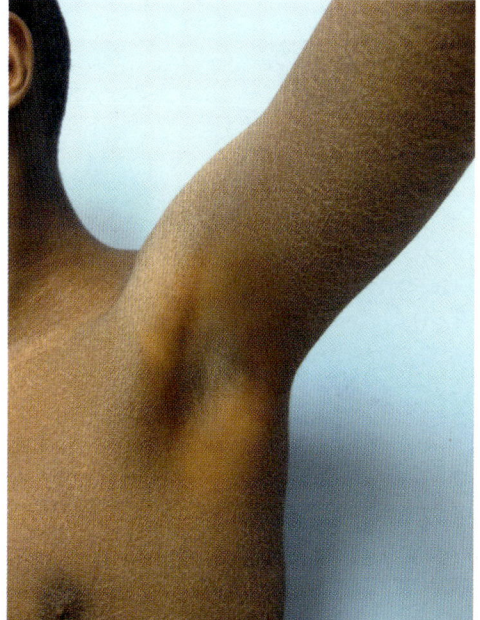

Fig. 2.38 X-linked ichthyosis (scale).

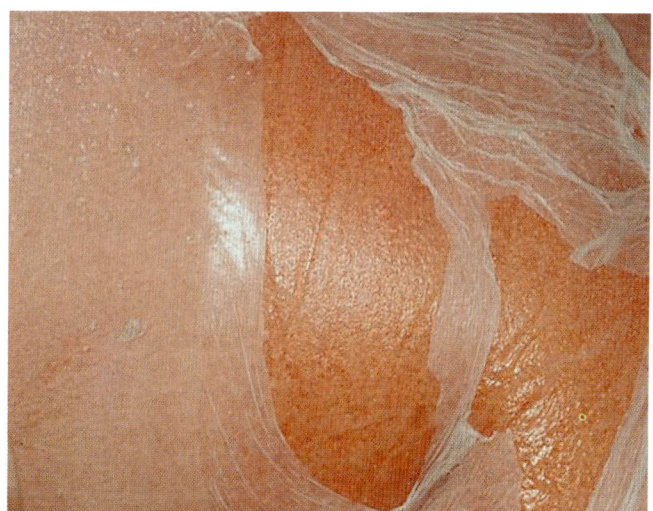

Fig. 2.41 Toxic epidermal necrolysis (sheets of desquamation).

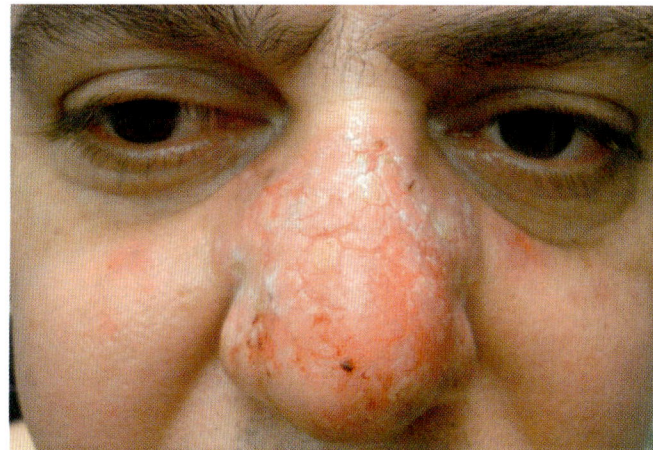

Fig. 2.39 Fogo selvagem (scale). *Courtesy Dermatology Division, University of Campinas, Brazil.*

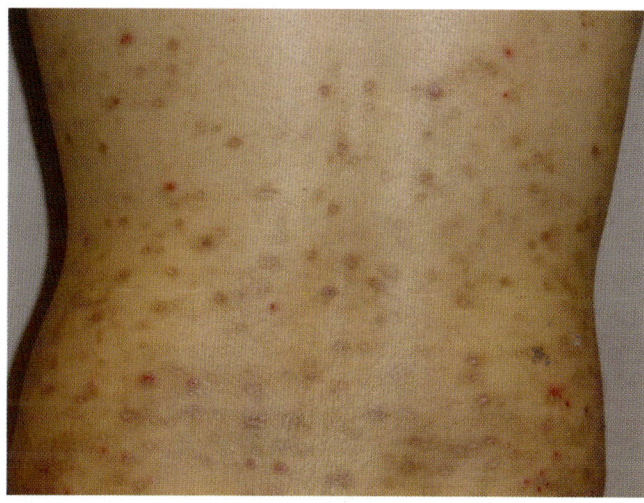

Fig. 2.42 Morgellons disease (excoriations). *Courtesy Scott Norton, MD.*

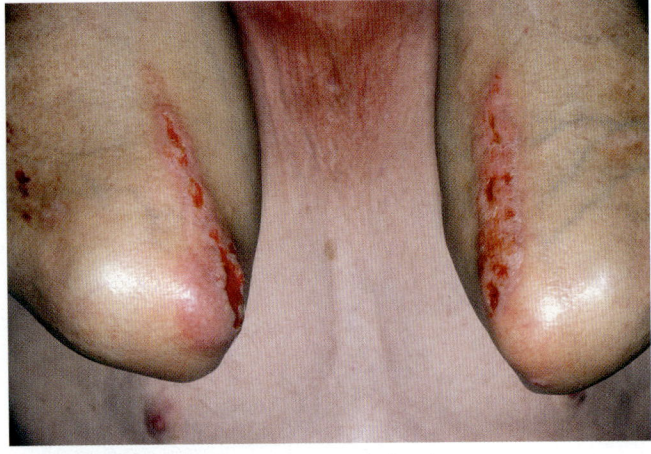

Fig. 2.43 Chronic pruritus (linear excoriations).

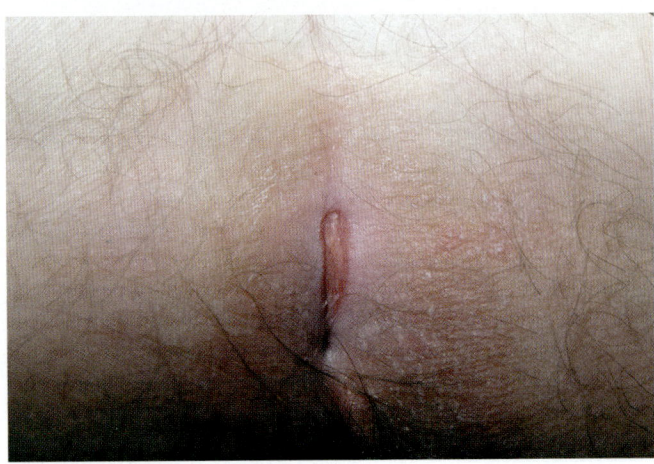

Fig. 2.44 Perianal fissure (fissure).

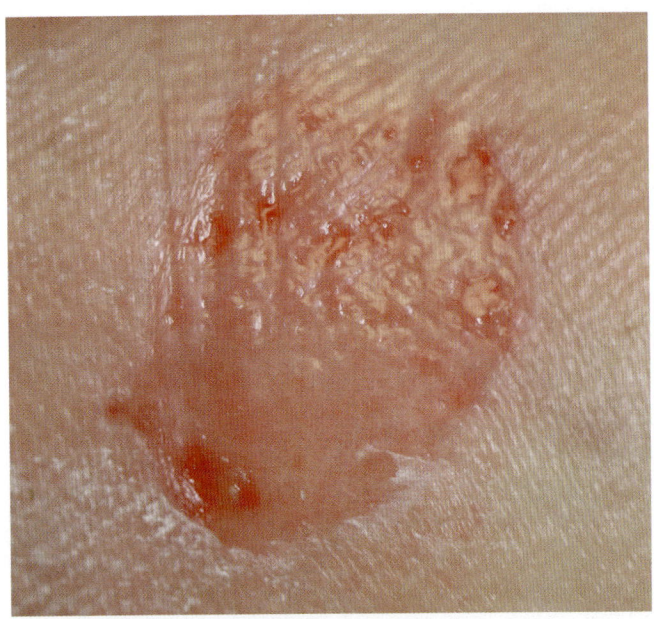

Fig. 2.45 Bullous pemphigoid (erosion).

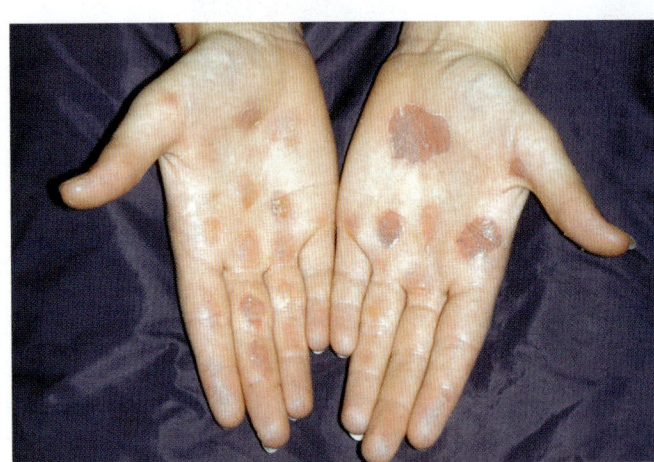

Fig. 2.46 Isotretinoin skin fragility in a college crew team member (erosions).

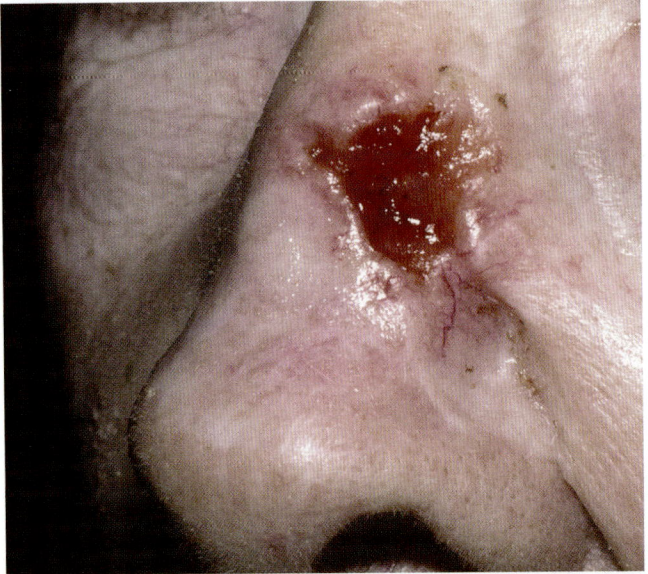

Fig. 2.47 Basal cell carcinoma (ulcer). *Courtesy Steven Binnick, MD.*

Fig. 2.48 Pyoderma gangrenosum (ulcer).

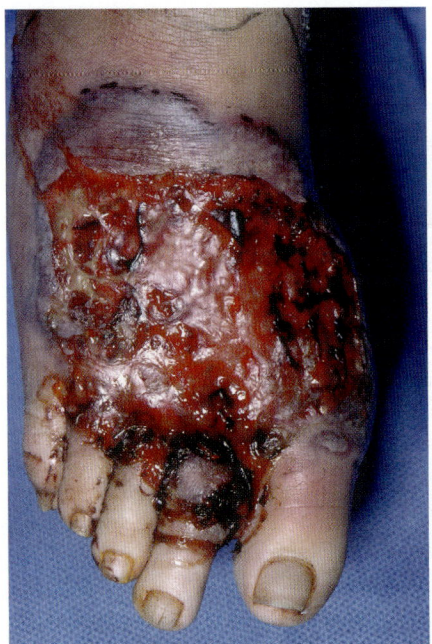

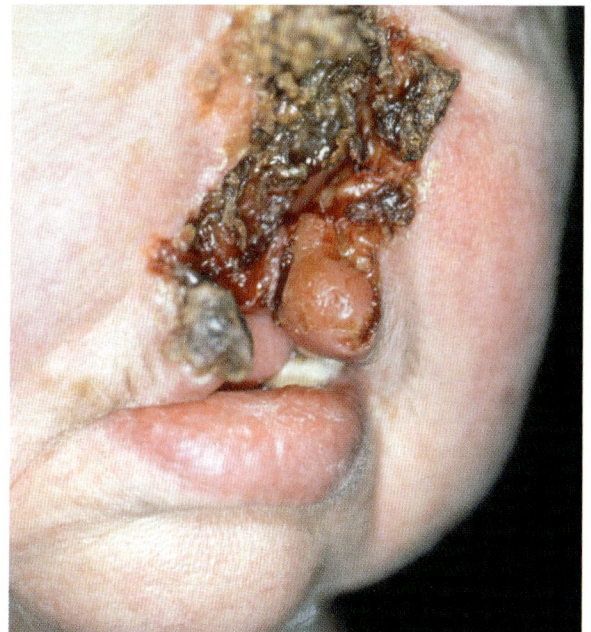

Fig. 2.49 Basal cell carcinoma (ulcer).

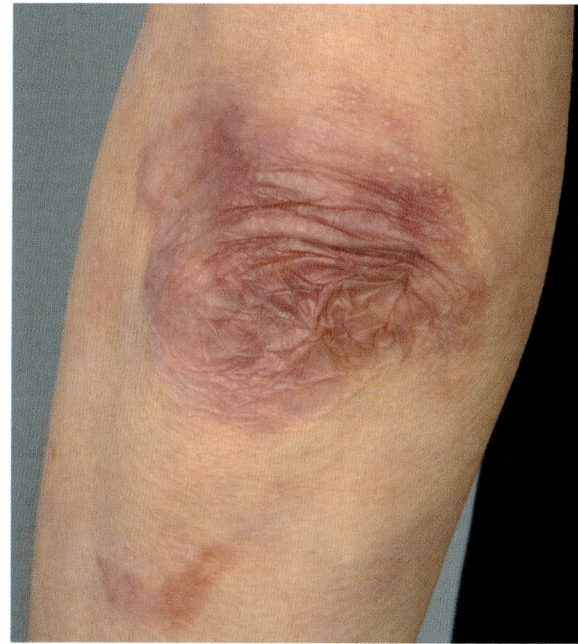

Fig. 2.50 Epidermolysis bullosa (atrophy). *Courtesy Scott Norton, MD.*

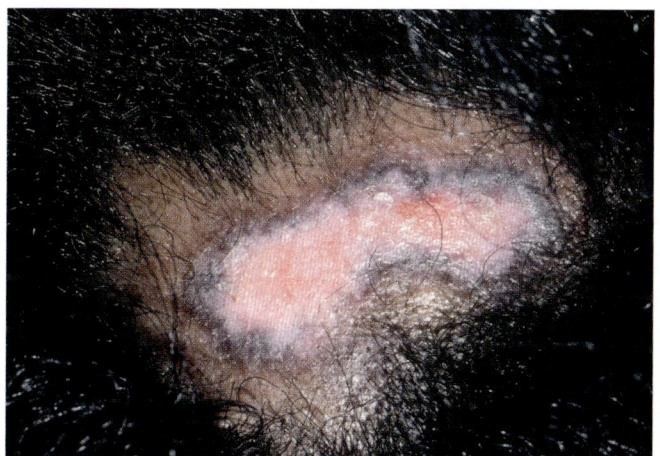

Fig. 2.51 Discoid lupus erythematosus (scarring alopecia). *Courtesy Steven Binnick, MD.*

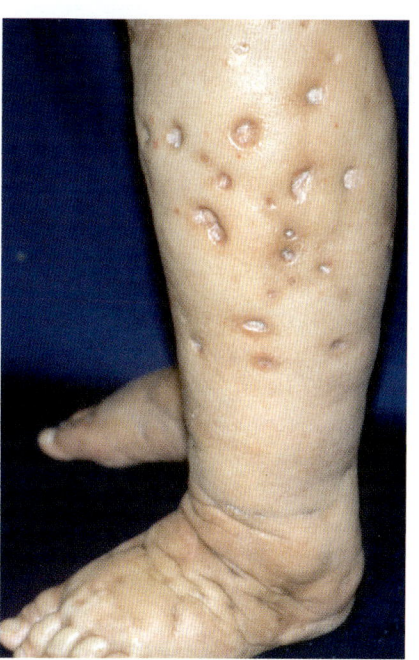

Fig. 2.52 Rounded scars and edema from skin popping.

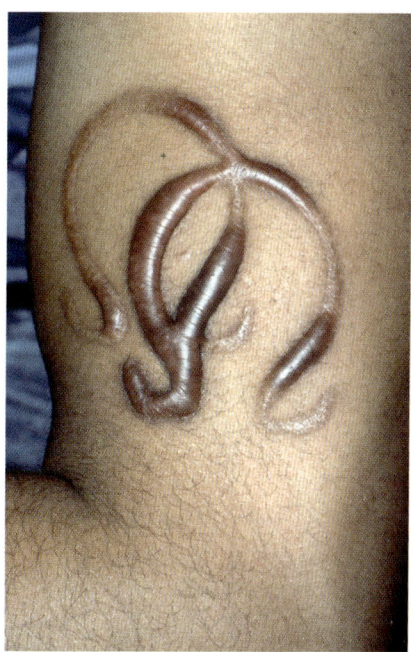

Fig. 2.53 Scarring after intentional trauma. *Courtesy Scott Norton, MD.*

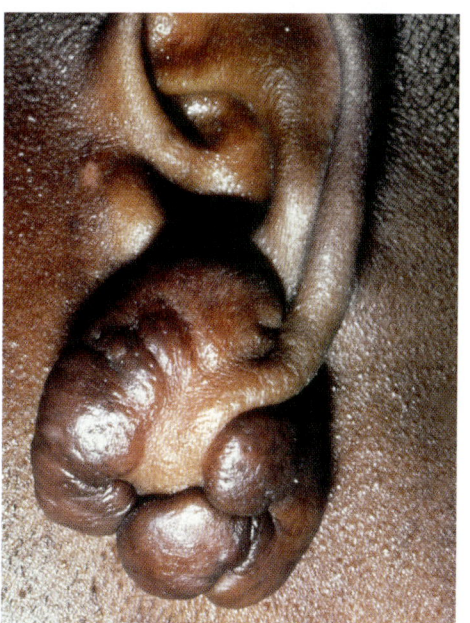

Fig. 2.54 Keloid.

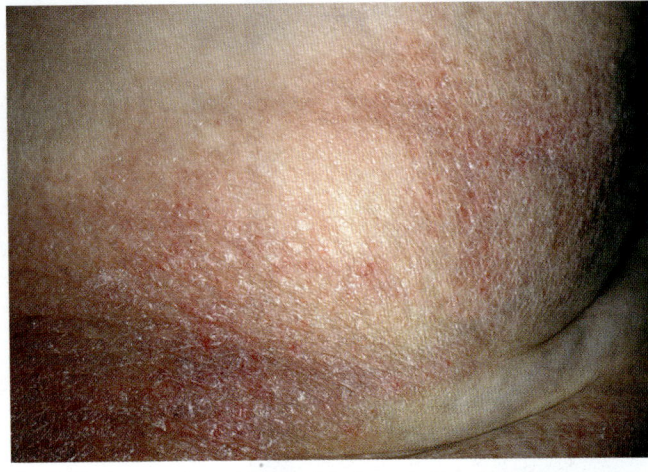

Fig. 2.55 Mycosis fungoides (poikiloderma). *Courtesy Steven Binnick, MD.*

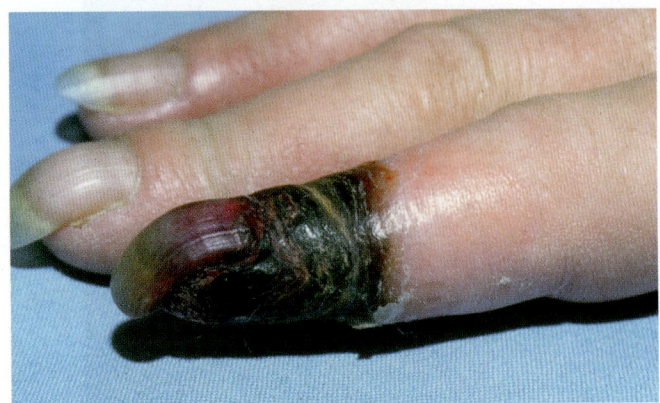

Fig. 2.56 Limited scleroderma, CREST (gangrene).

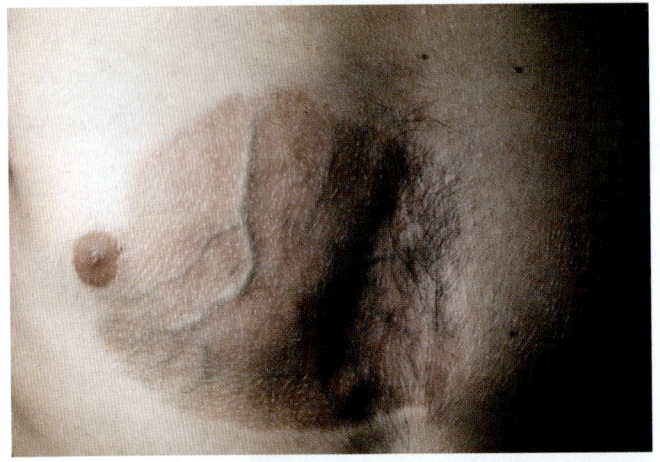

Fig. 2.57 Atrophoderma (atrophy). *Courtesy Steven Binnick, MD.*

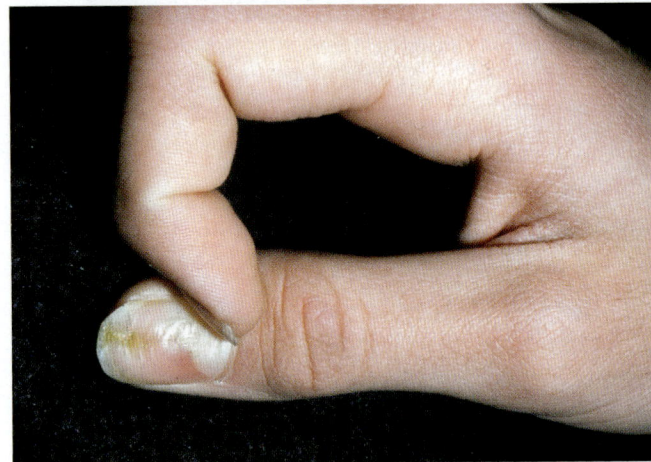

Fig. 2.58 Reeve sign (the reenactment of the cause of the condition during examination). Washboard nail dystrophy.

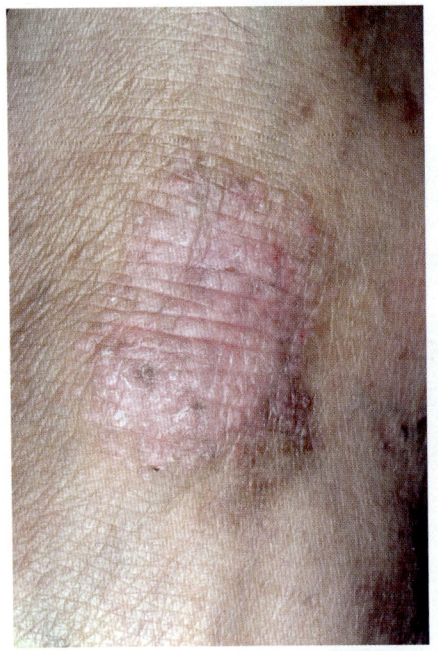

Fig. 2.59 Lichen simplex chronicus (lichenification).

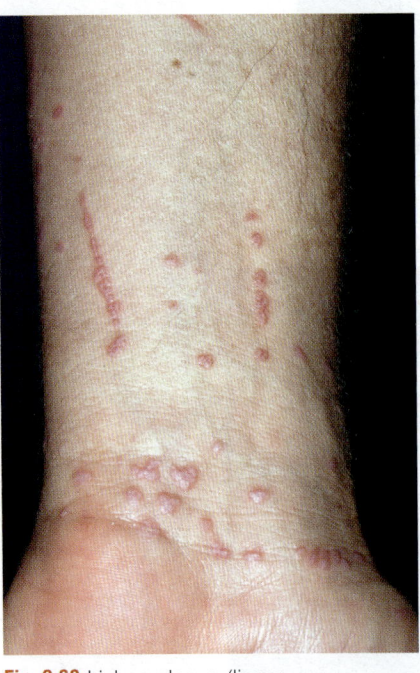

Fig. 2.60 Lichen planus (linear, koebnerization).

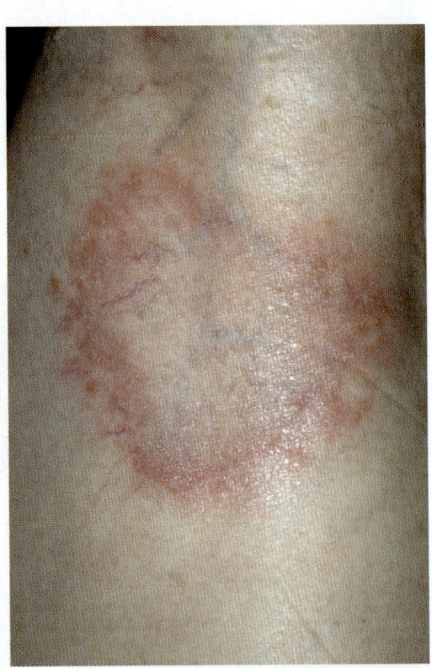

Fig. 2.61 Granuloma annulare (annular).

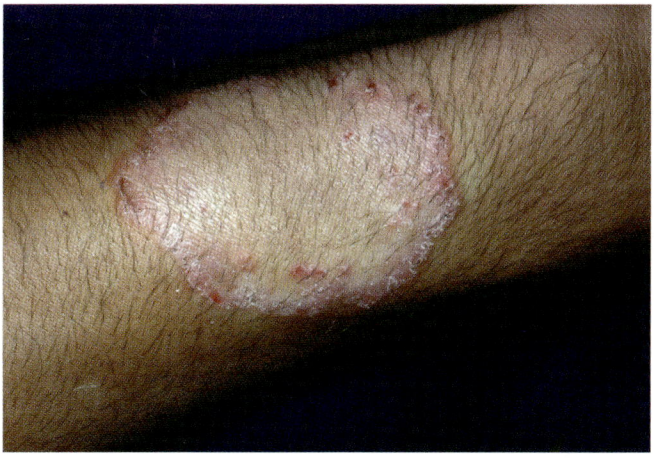

Fig. 2.62 Tinea corporis (annular).

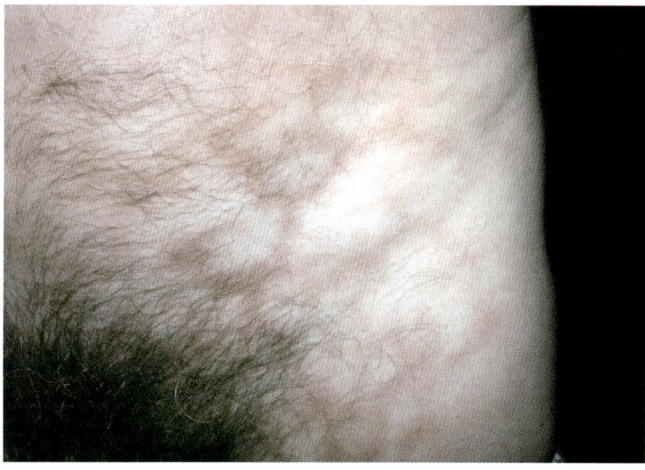

Fig. 2.63 Erythema ab igne (retiform).

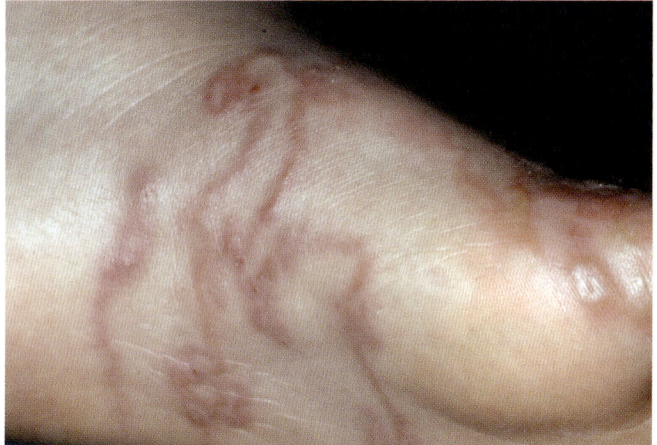

Fig. 2.64 Cutaneous larva migrans (serpiginous).

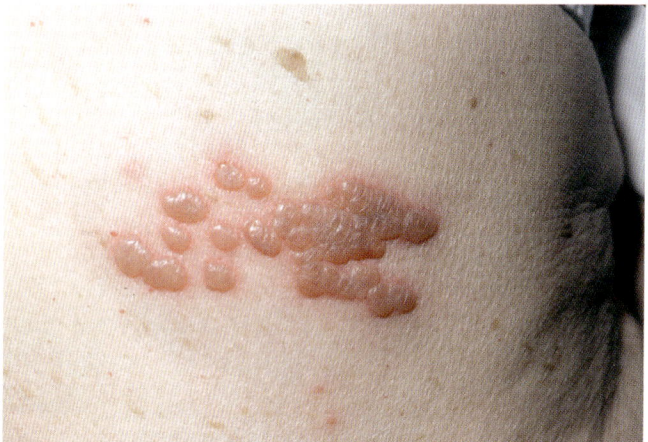

Fig. 2.65 Herpes simplex (grouped).

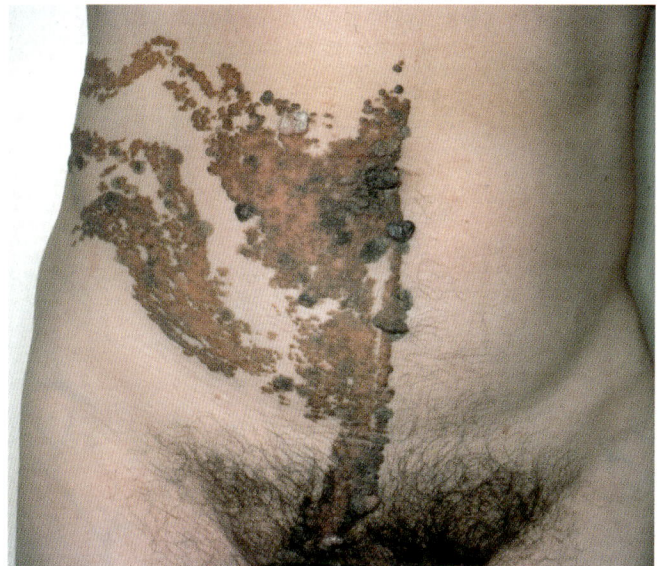

Fig. 2.66 Linear epidermal nevus (blaschkoid).

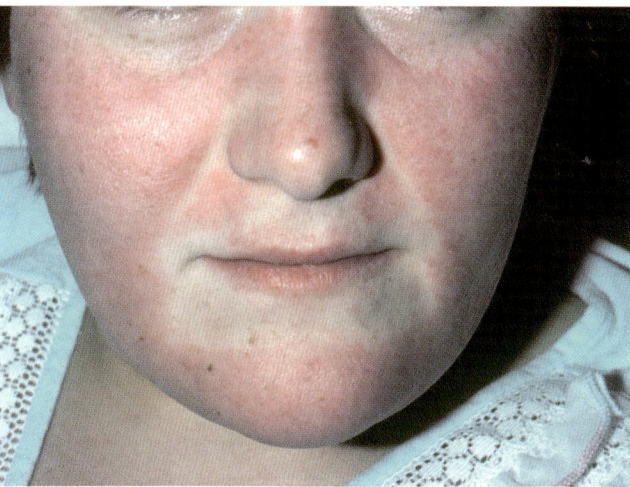

Fig. 2.67 Systemic lupus erythematosus (photosensitivity pattern sparing nasolabial folds, under nose, under mouth). *Courtesy Steven Binnick, MD.*

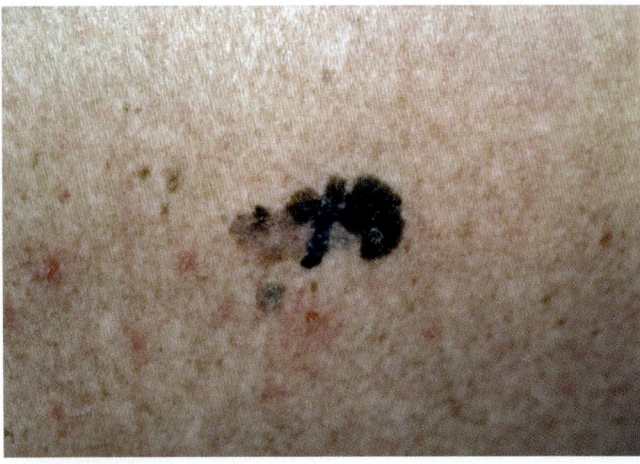

Fig. 2.68 Melanoma (color variegation).

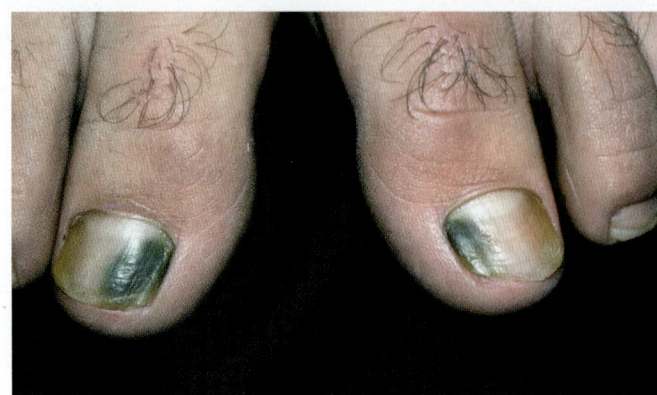

Fig. 2.69 Green nails from *Pseudomonas* infection (unusual color helps with the diagnosis).

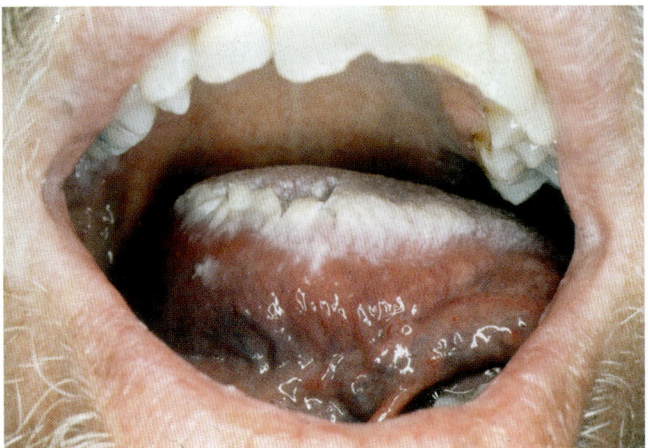

Fig. 2.70 Pachyonychia congenita (oral).

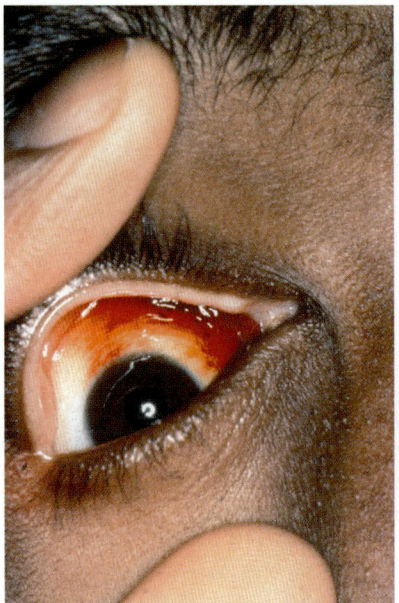

Fig. 2.71 Kaposi sarcoma (conjunctiva).

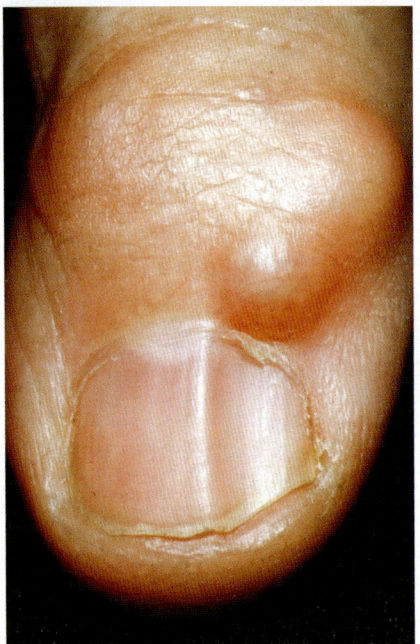

Fig. 2.72 Nail groove from mucous cyst (nail).

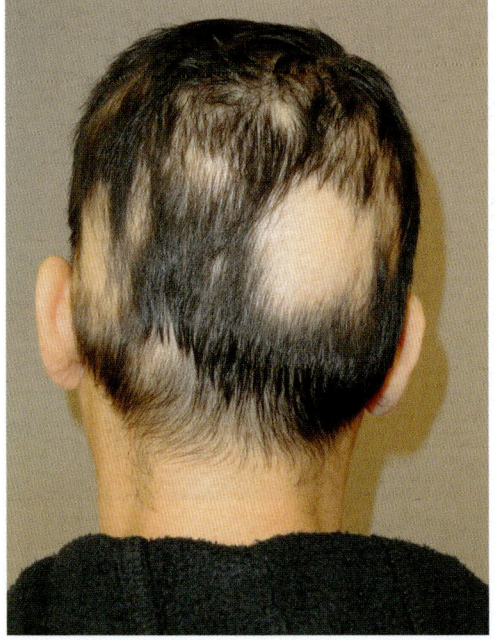

Fig. 2.73 Alopecia areata (hair). *Courtesy Scott Norton, MD.*

Dermatoses Resulting from Physical Factors

3

This chapter catalogues many examples of how the skin reacts to the external environment from which it protects the body. Exposure to physical factors such as heat, cold, moisture, ultraviolet light, radiation, mechanical trauma and imbedded foreign bodies can manifest as uniquely patterned skin findings.

Of particular note are the many examples of photo-distributed eruptions, symmetrically involving the face, chest, dorsal hands and forearms, as this pattern can be an important physical exam clue to one of many specific photosensitive conditions. Those who spend significant amounts of time outdoors are particularly susceptible to acute and chronic sun damage and may also sustain temperature-related (cold or hot) injuries at acral sites.

The distribution of mechanical injuries and foreign body reactions, however, is usually asymmetric. In this chapter, appreciate the geometric shapes and unnatural configurations that can be produced on the skin as a result of physical abuse, radiotherapy or phytophotodermatitis. The patient history, and at times tissue analysis, can help to confirm the diagnosis that was suspected after a thorough physical examination.

This portion of the atlas features examples of dermatoses and skin lesions resulting from physical factors.

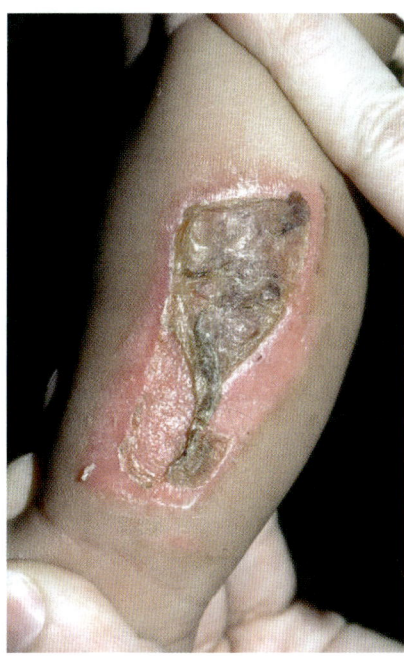

Fig. 3.1 Thermal burn from child abuse. *Courtesy Paul Honig, MD.*

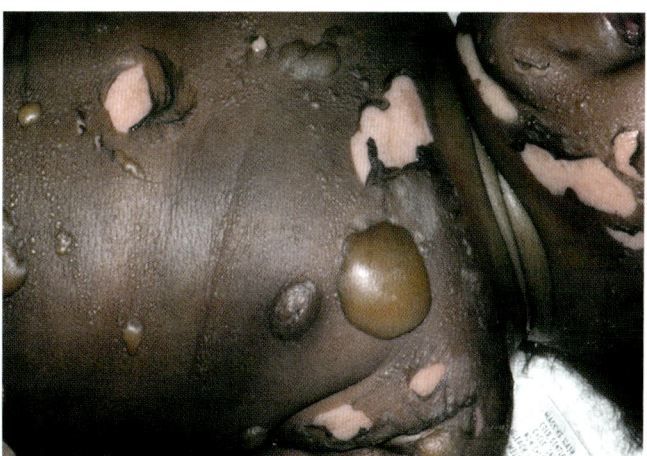

Fig. 3.2 Hot water burn. *Courtesy Steven Binnick, MD.*

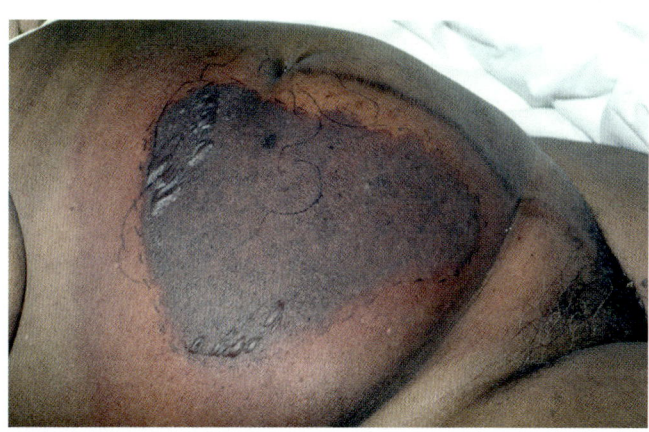

Fig. 3.3 Hot water bottle injury. *Courtesy Steven Binnick, MD.*

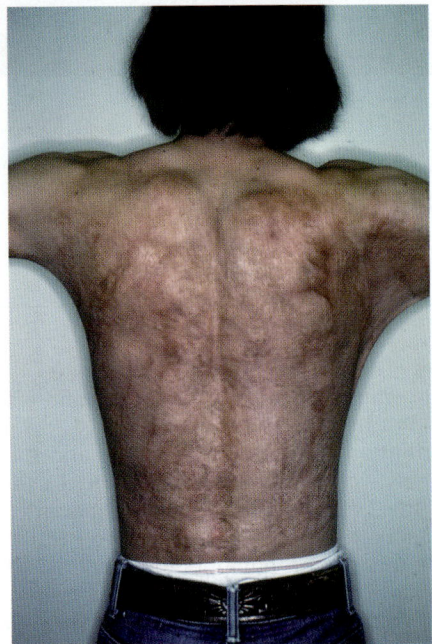

Fig. 3.4 Burn scar.

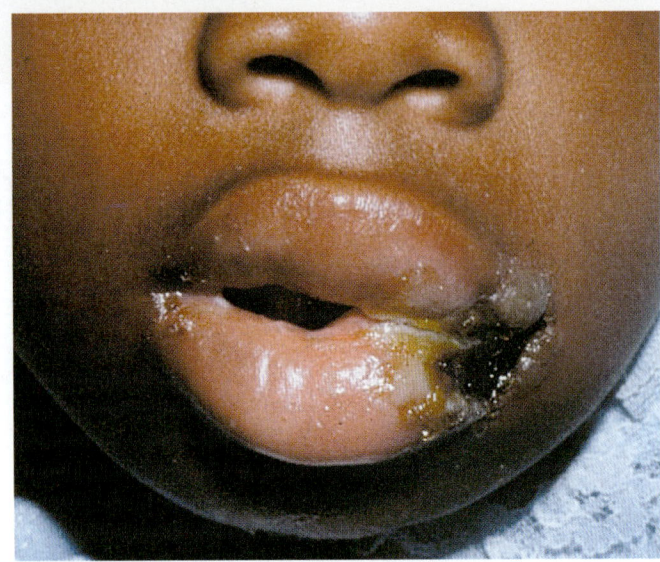

Fig. 3.5 Electrical burn from biting electrical cord. *Courtesy Paul Honig, MD.*

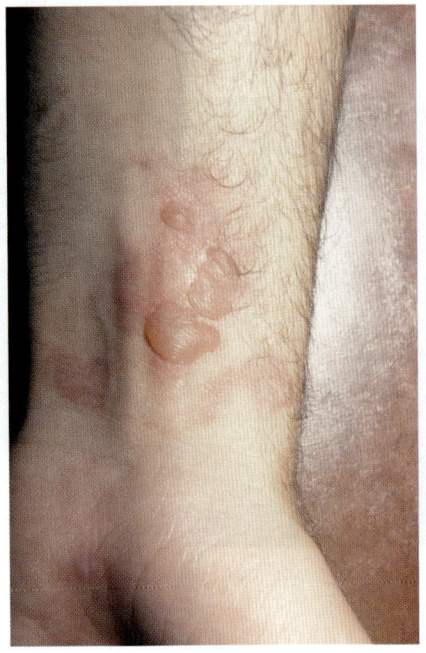

Fig. 3.6 Hot oil burn. *Courtesy Steven Binnick, MD.*

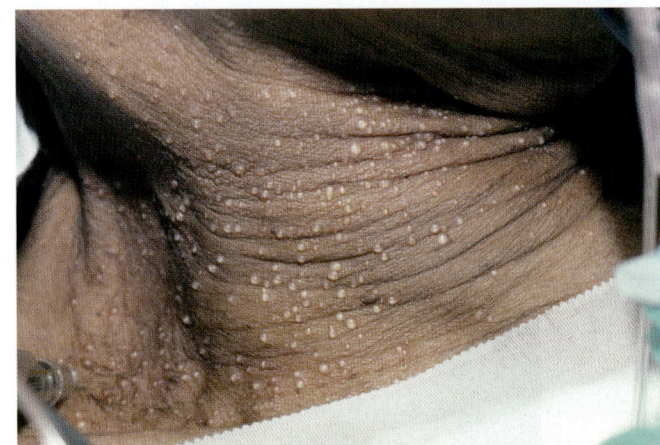

Fig. 3.7 Miliaria crystallina. *Courtesy Steven Binnick, MD.*

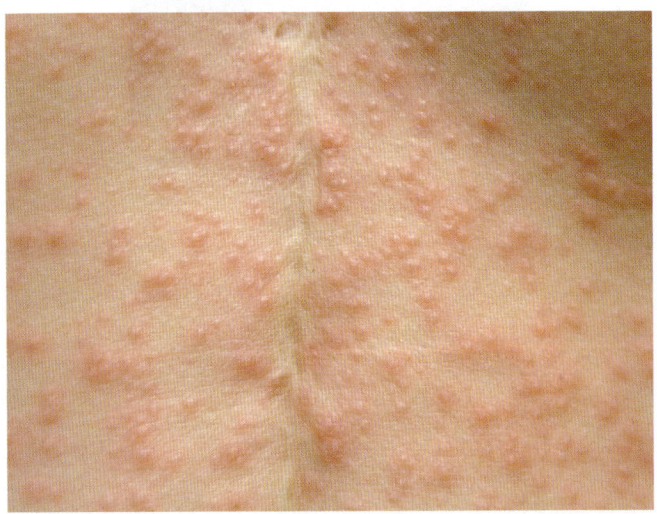

Fig. 3.8 Miliaria rubra.

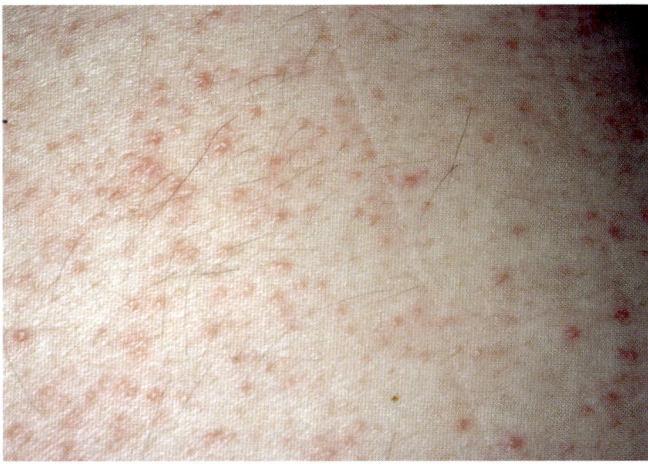

Fig. 3.9 Miliaria rubra.

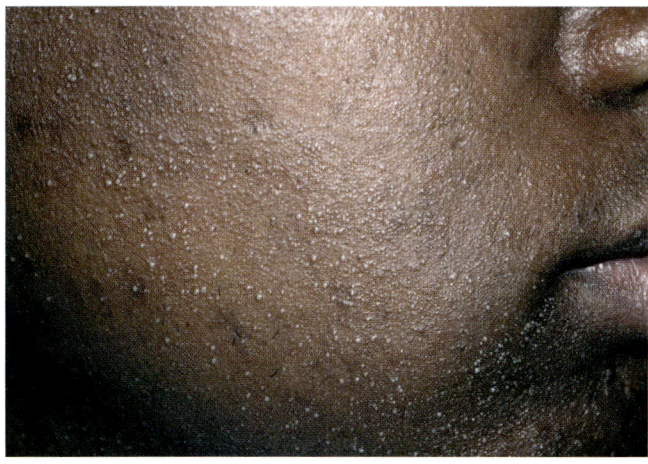

Fig. 3.10 Miliaria pustulosa secondary to childbirth. *Courtesy Curt Samlaska, MD.*

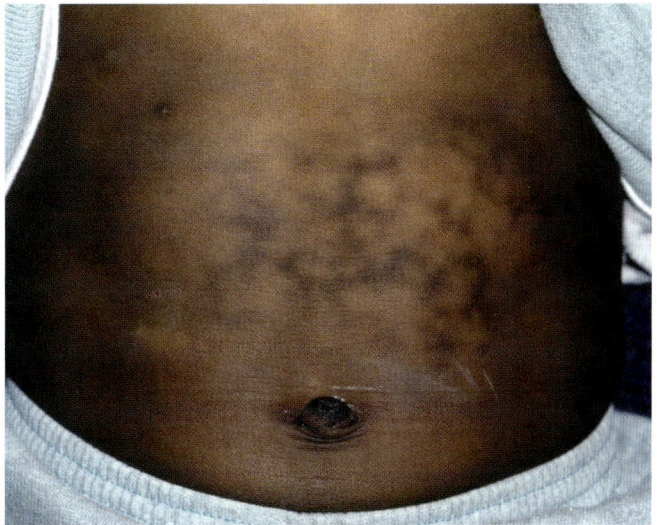

Fig. 3.11 Erythema ab igne. *Courtesy Paul Honig, MD.*

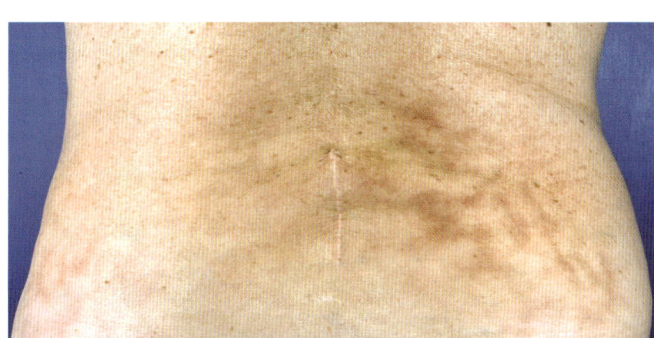

Fig. 3.12 Erythema ab igne. *Courtesy Curt Samlaska, MD.*

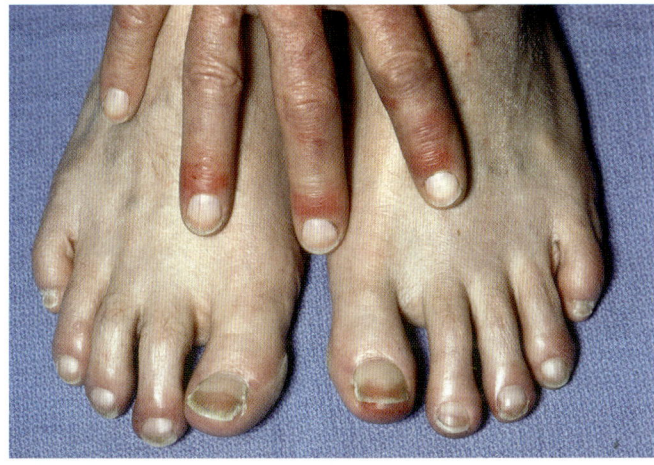

Fig. 3.13 Pernio. *Courtesy Steven Binnick, MD.*

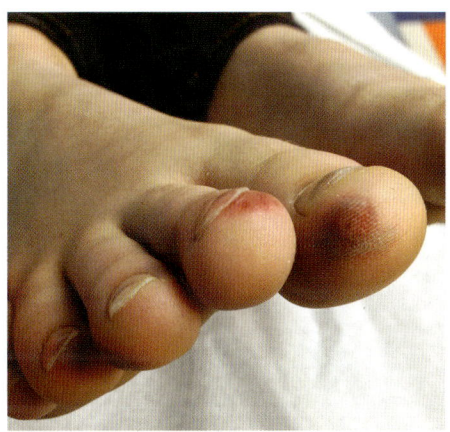

Fig. 3.14 Pernio.

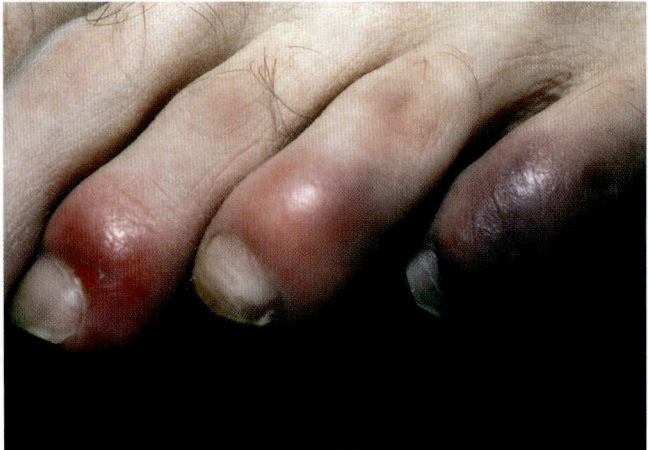

Fig. 3.15 Pernio. *Courtesy Steven Binnick, MD.*

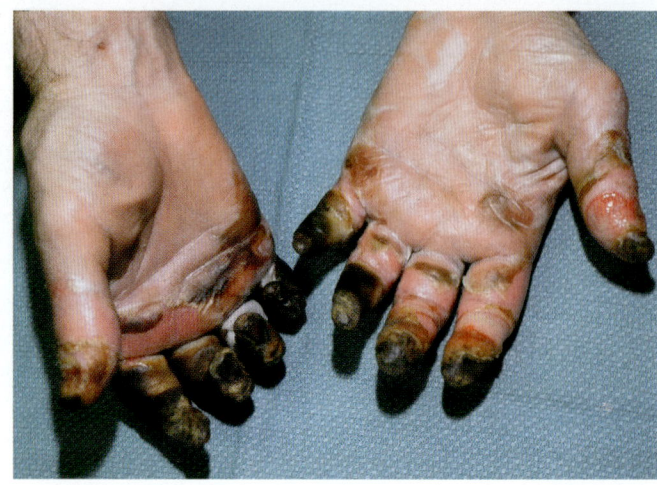

Fig. 3.16 Frostbite.

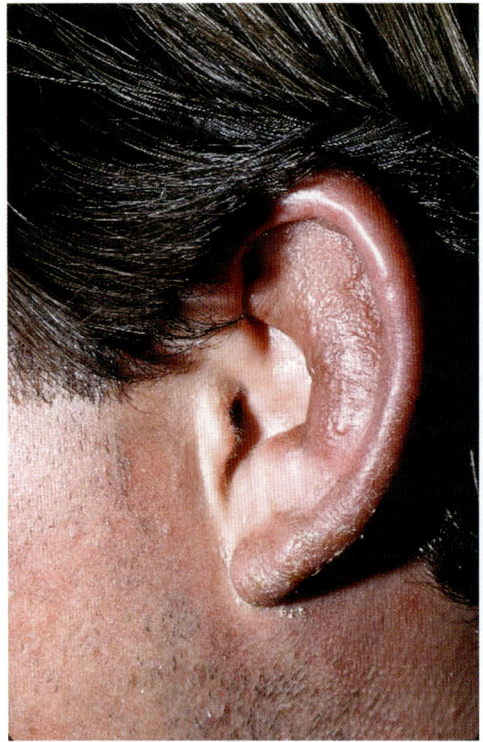

Fig. 3.17 Frostbite. *Courtesy The University of Utah and Oregon Health Sciences University Leonard Swinyer MD image collection.*

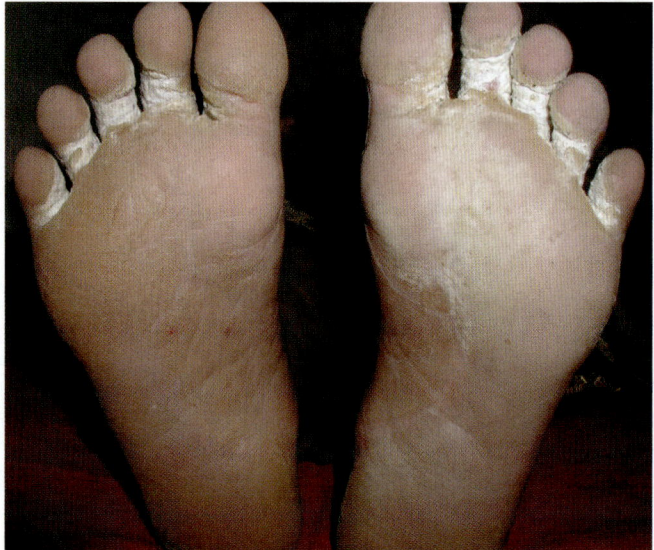

Fig. 3.18 Tropical immersion foot. *Courtesy Shyam Verma, MBBS, DVD.*

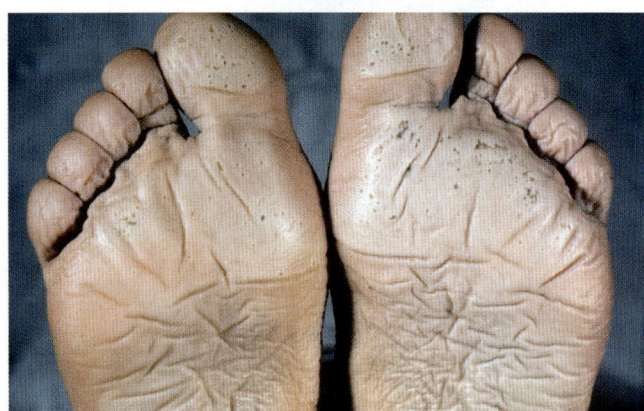

Fig. 3.19 Tropical immersion foot. *Courtesy Steven Binnick, MD.*

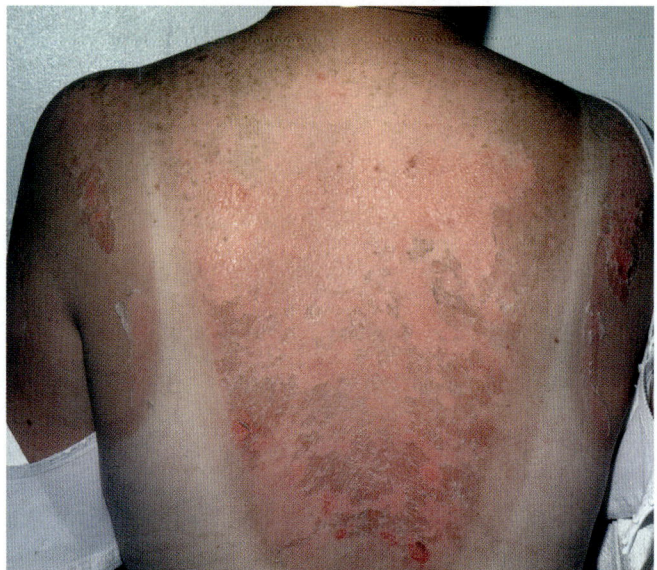

Fig. 3.20 Sunburn. *Courtesy Steven Binnick, MD.*

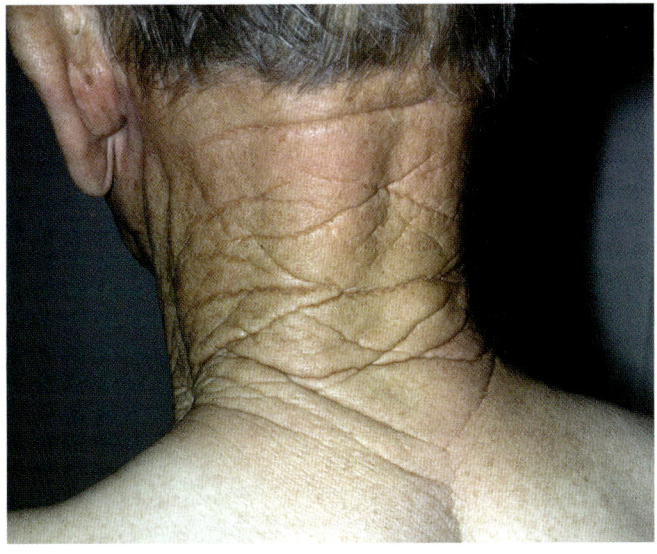

Fig. 3.21 Cutis rhomboidalis nuchae.

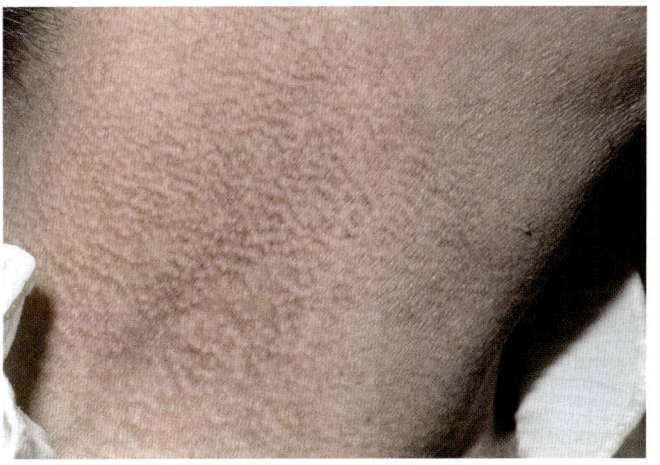

Fig. 3.22 Poikiloderma of Civatte.

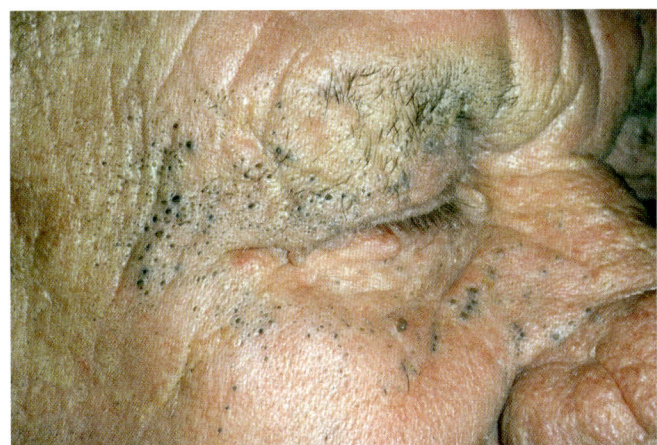

Fig. 3.23 Favre-Racouchot.

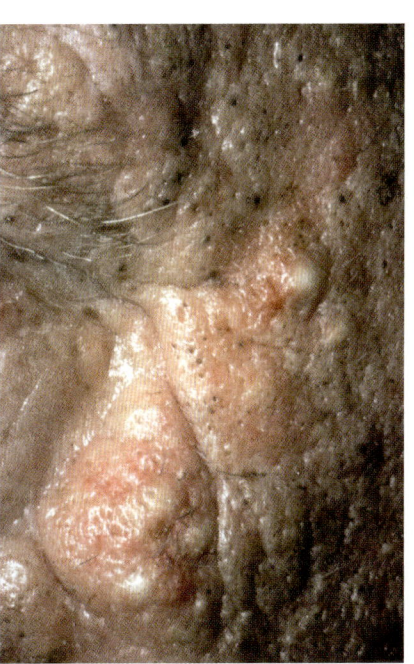

Fig. 3.24 Favre-Racouchot with solar elastotic nodules.

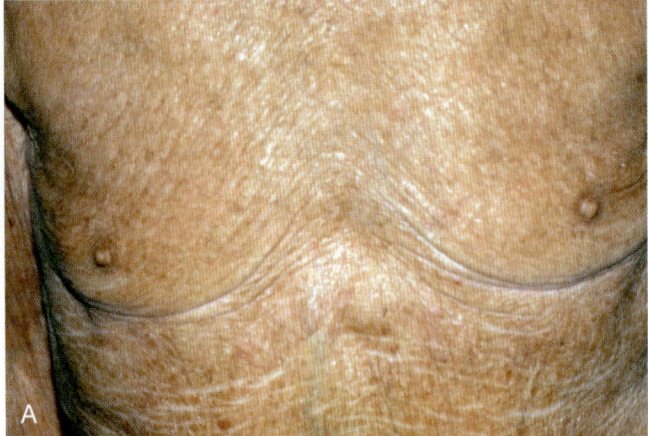
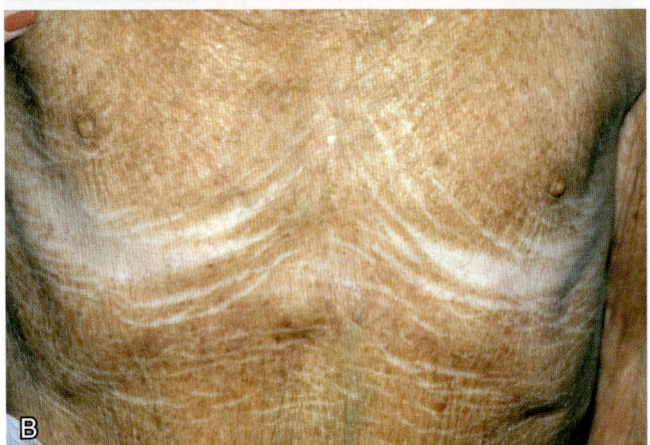

Fig. 3.25 (A) Chronic solar damage. (B) With upward traction, normal non–sun-exposed skin is revealed.

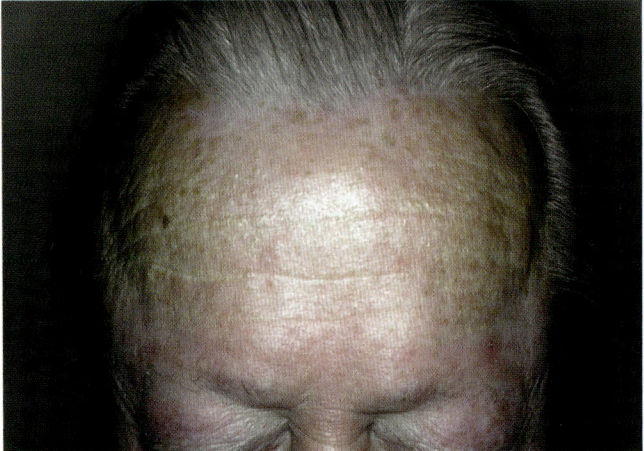

Fig. 3.27 Solar elastosis of the forehead.

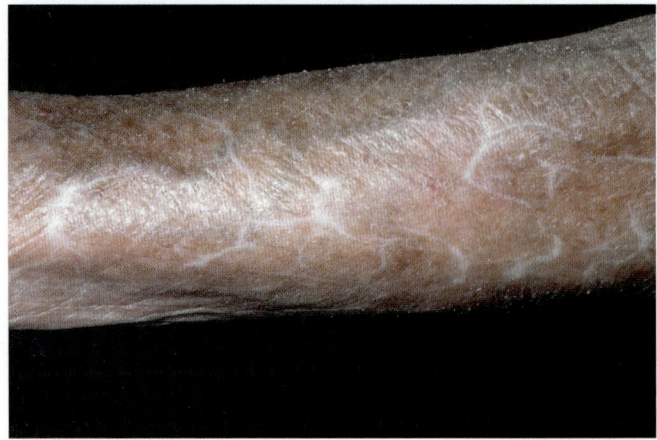

Fig. 3.26 Stellate pseudoscars.

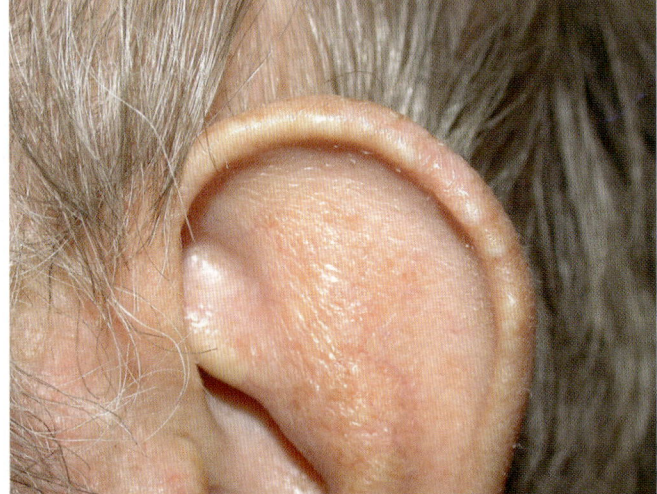

Fig. 3.28 Weathering nodules.

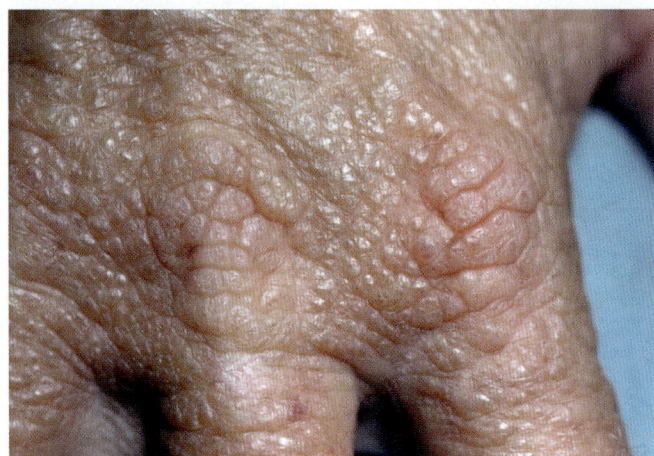

Fig. 3.29 Colloid milium. *Courtesy Ken Greer, MD.*

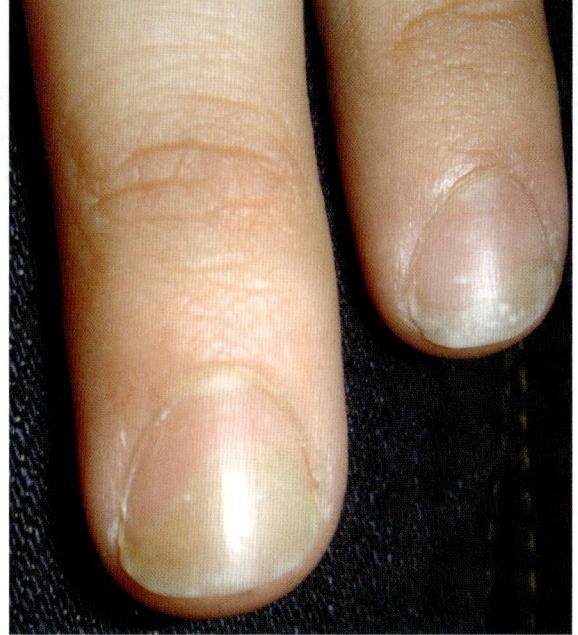

Fig. 3.30 Photo onycholysis secondary to doxycycline. *Courtesy Lindsay Ackerman, MD.*

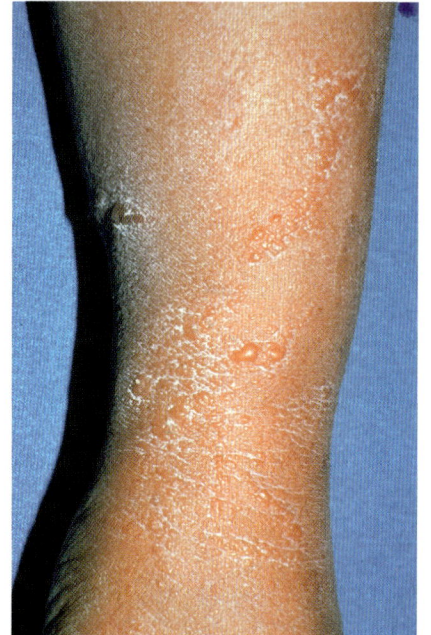

Fig. 3.31 Phytophotodermatitis.

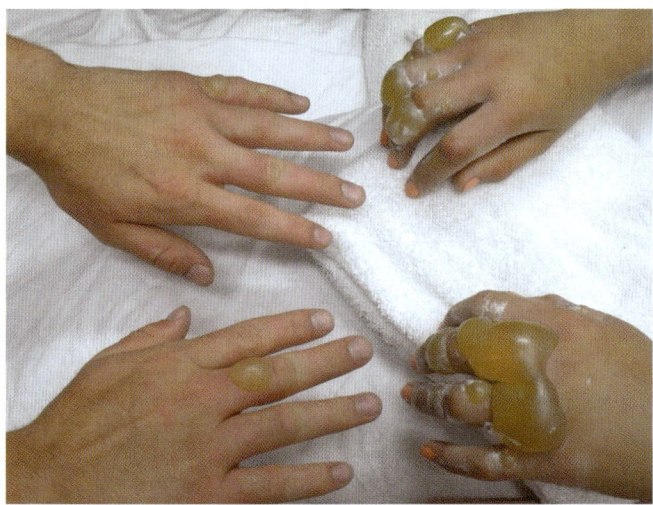

Fig. 3.32 Two friends who made limeade in the sun to sell in the summer.

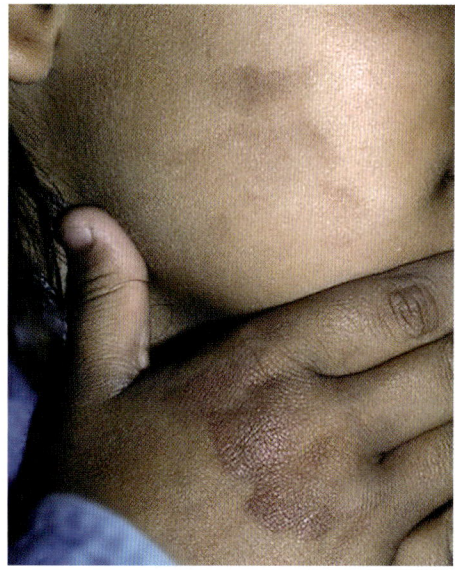

Fig. 3.33 Hyperpigmentation of the hand and cheek after phytophotodermatitis. *Courtesy Paul Honig, MD.*

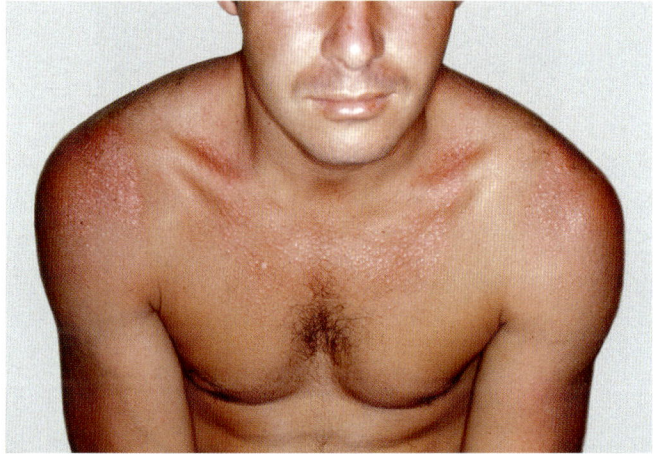

Fig. 3.34 Polymorphous light eruption, papular type.

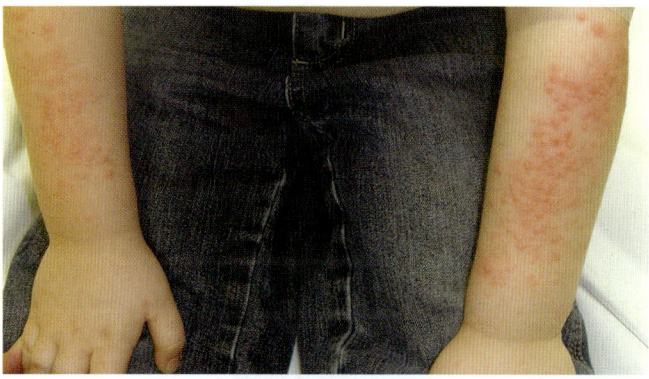

Fig. 3.35 Polymorphous light eruption, papular type.

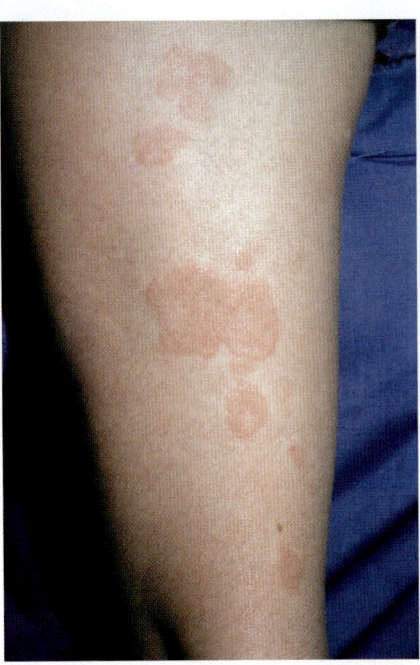

Fig. 3.36 Polymorphous light eruption, plaque type.

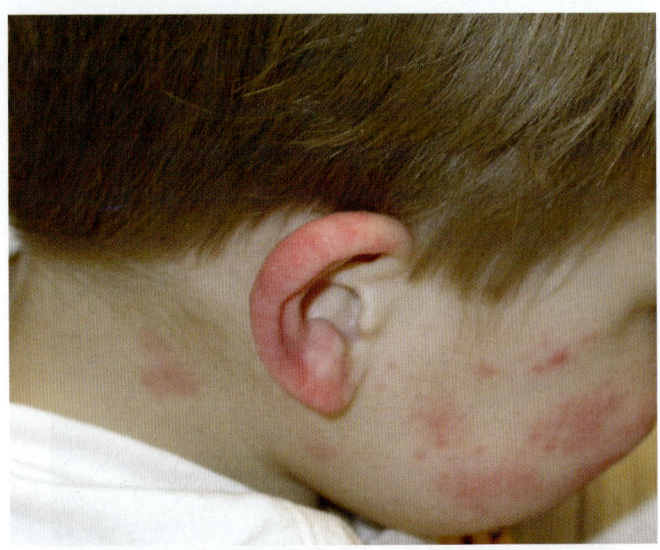

Fig. 3.37 Polymorphous light eruption, juvenile spring eruption type.

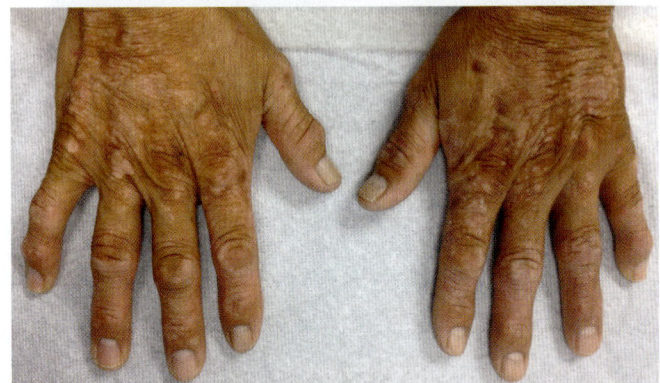

Fig. 3.39 Actinic prurigo. *Courtesy Campbell Stewart, MD.*

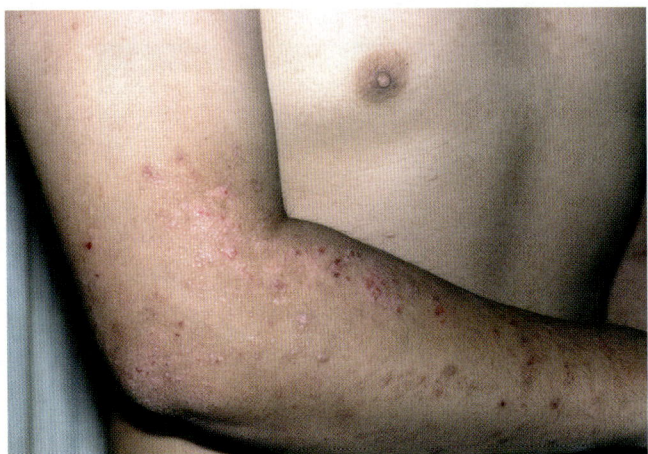

Fig. 3.38 Actinic prurigo. *Courtesy Steven Binnick, MD.*

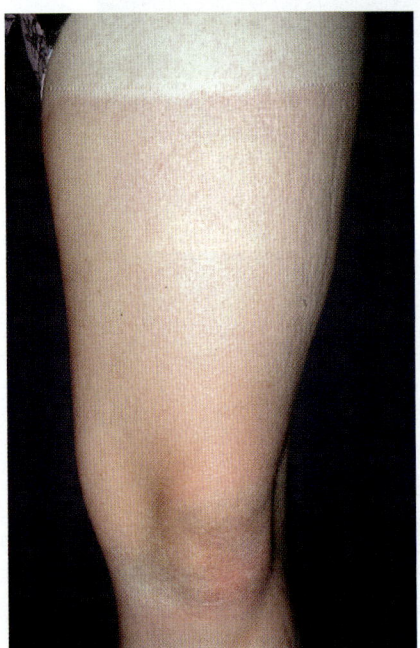

Fig. 3.40 Solar urticaria.

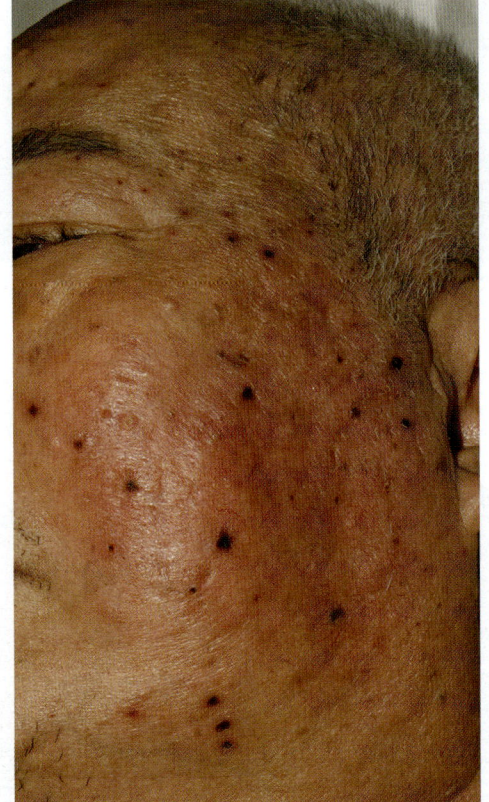

Fig. 3.41 Hydroa vacciniforme. *Courtesy National Taiwan University Hospital.*

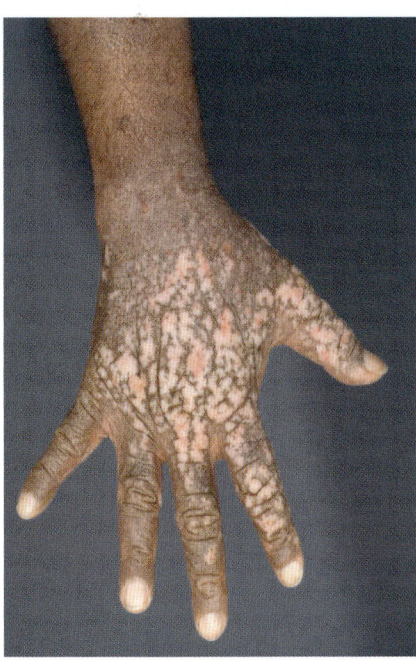

Fig. 3.42 Chronic actinic dermatitis.

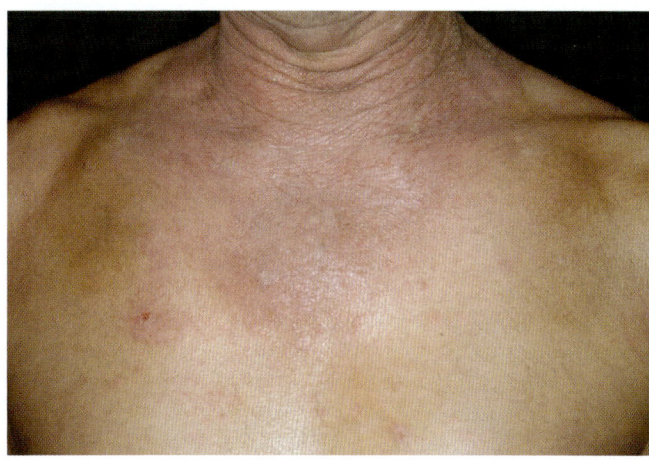

Fig. 3.43 Chronic actinic dermatitis. *Courtesy Kaohsiung Chang Gang Memorial Hospital, Taiwan.*

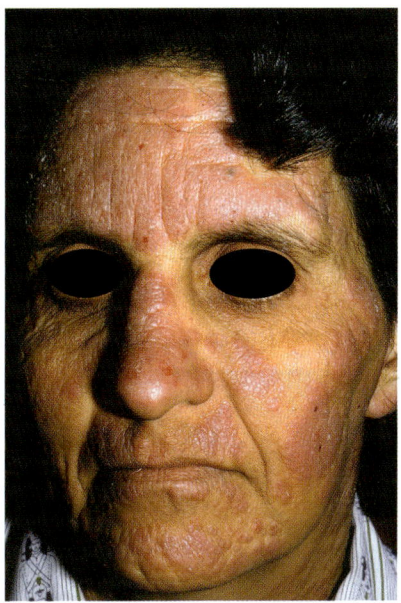

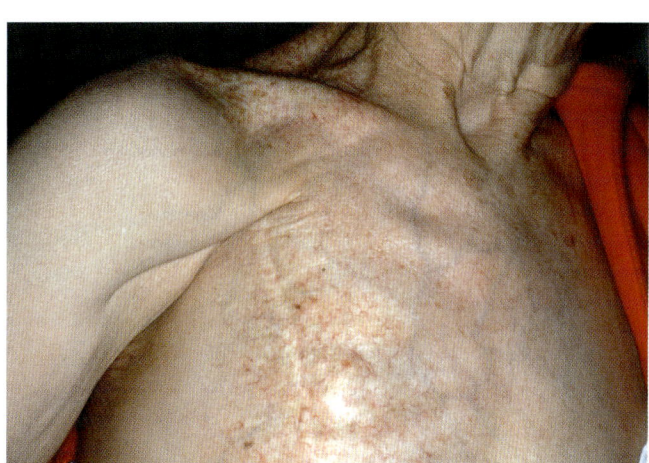

Fig. 3.45 Chronic radiation dermatitis.

Fig. 3.44 Chronic actinic dermatitis. *Courtesy The University of Utah and Oregon Health Sciences University Leonard Swinyer MD image collection.*

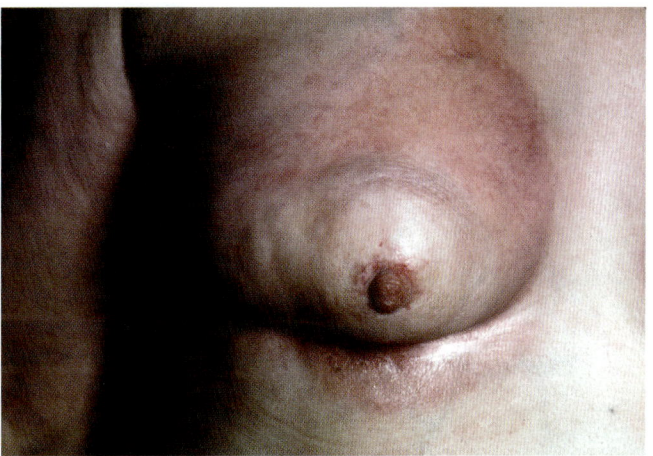

Fig. 3.46 Chronic radiation dermatitis. *Courtesy Steven Binnick, MD.*

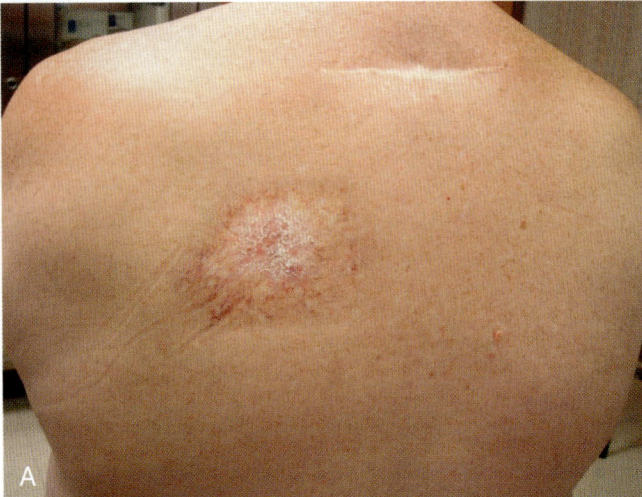

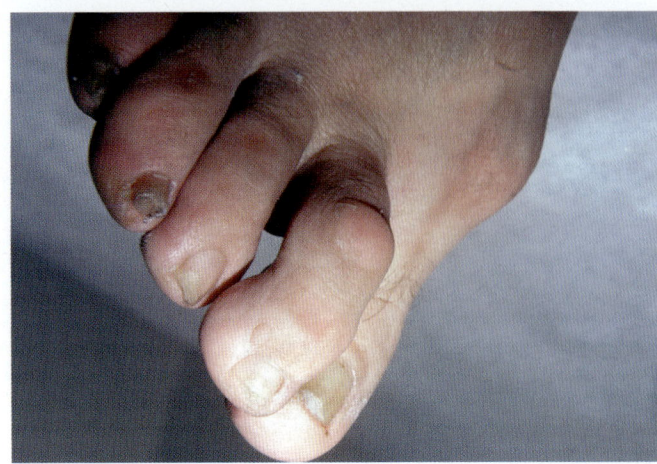

Fig. 3.48 Hard corn. *Courtesy Steven Binnick, MD.*

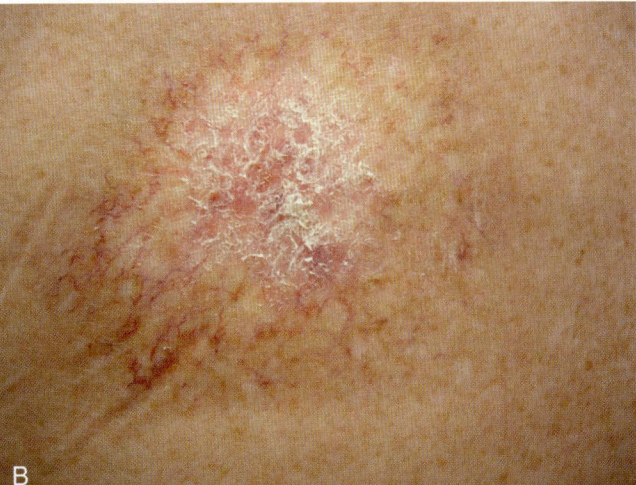

Fig. 3.47 (A) Fluoroscopy-induced radiodermatitis. (B) Close-up of A.

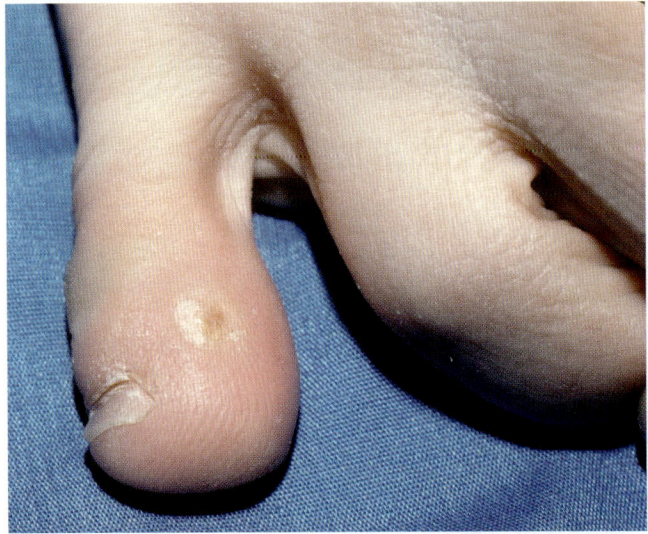

Fig. 3.49 Soft corn. *Courtesy Steven Binnick, MD.*

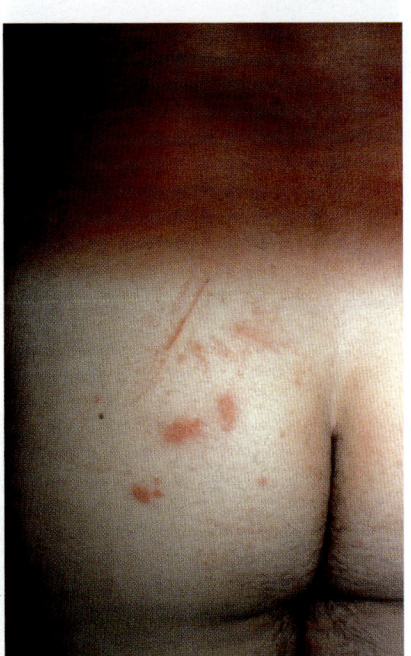

Fig. 3.50 Fire coral cuts. *Courtesy Steven Binnick, MD.*

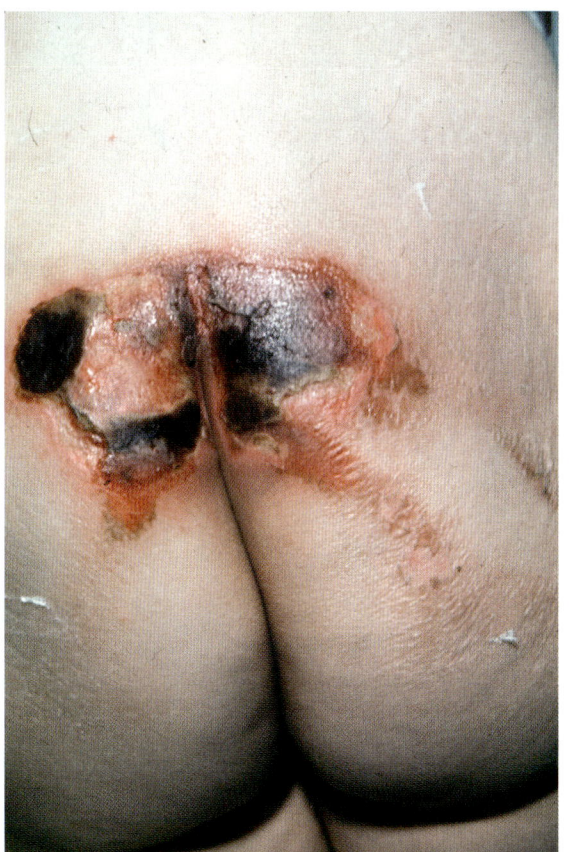

Fig. 3.51 Decubitus ulcer. *Courtesy Steven Binnick, MD.*

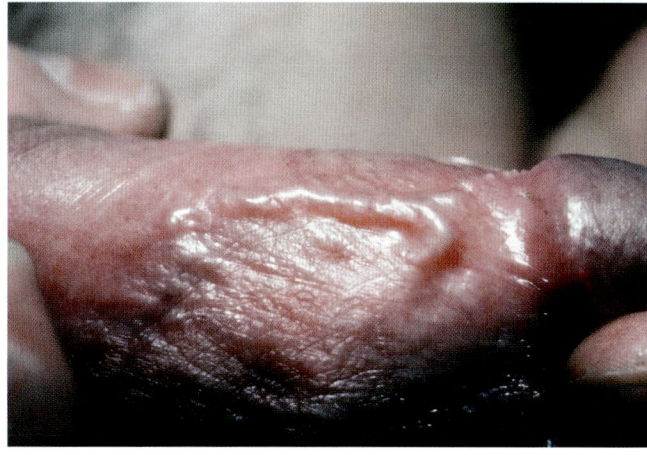

Fig. 3.52 Sclerosing lymphangitis.

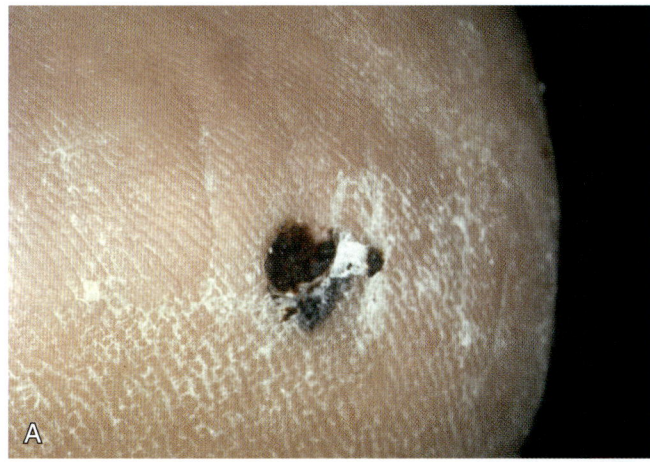

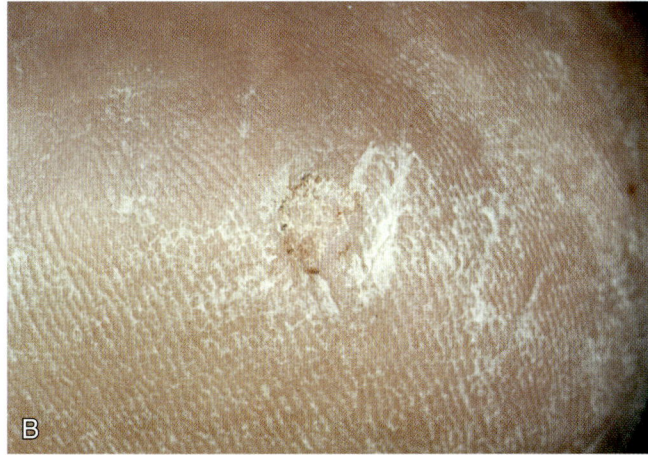

Fig. 3.53 (A) Black heel. (B) Immediately after scraping off blood from black heel.

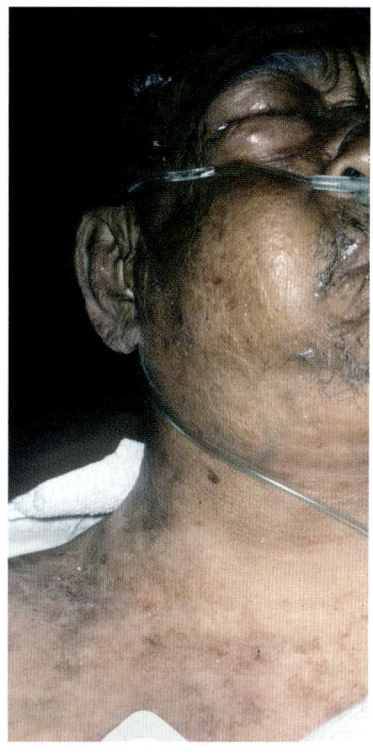

Fig. 3.54 Subcutaneous emphysema. *Courtesy Curt Samlaska, MD.*

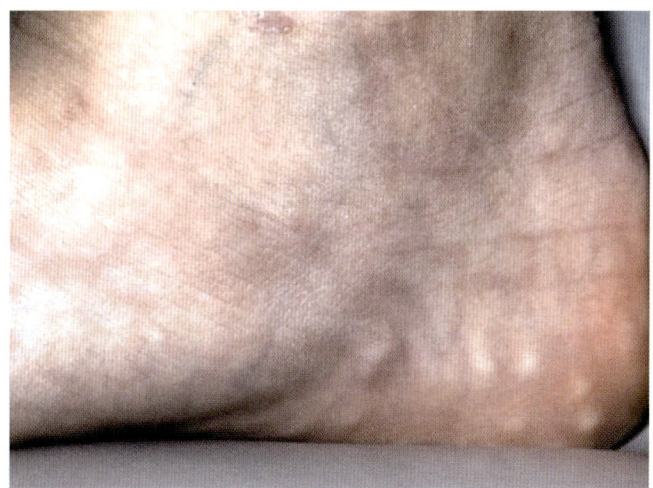

Fig. 3.55 Piezogenic papules. *Courtesy Paul Honig, MD.*

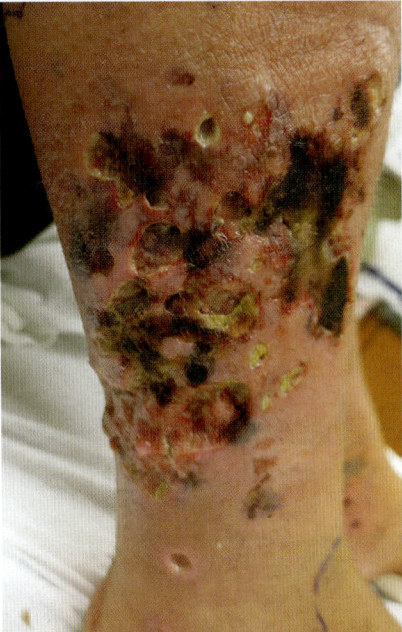

Fig. 3.56 Ulcerations and bacterial superinfection secondary to skin popping.

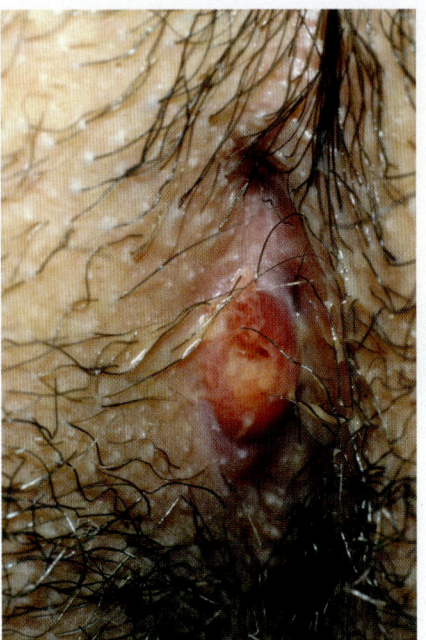

Fig. 3.57 Cotton granuloma.

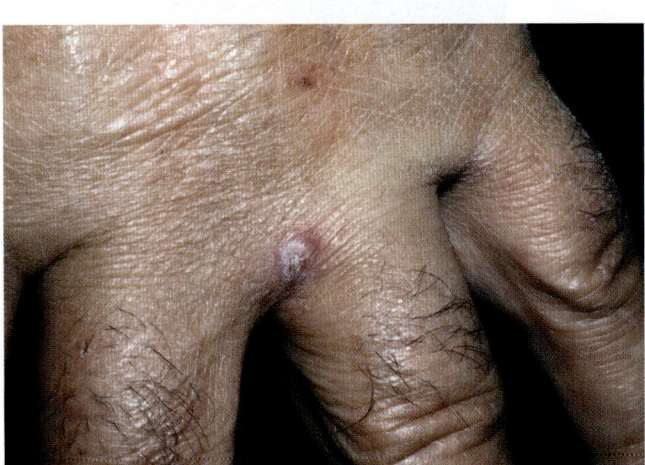

Fig. 3.58 Hair granuloma in a barber.

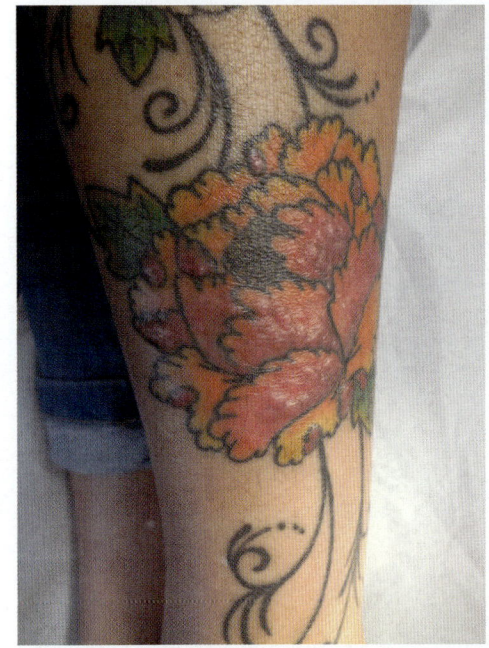

Fig. 3.59 Red tattoo reaction. *Courtesy Rui Tavares Bello, MD.*

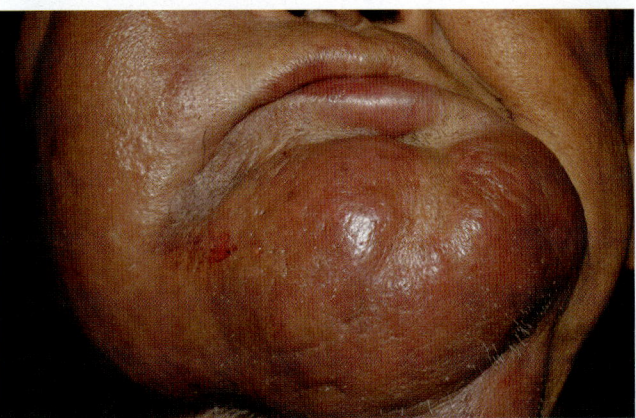

Fig. 3.60 Silicone granuloma. *Courtesy National Cheng Kung University, Taiwan.*

Fig. 3.61 Mercury granuloma from thermometer.

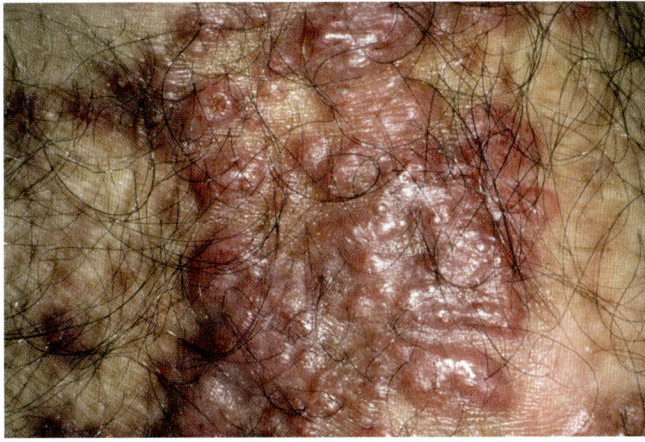

Fig. 3.62 Silica granuloma.

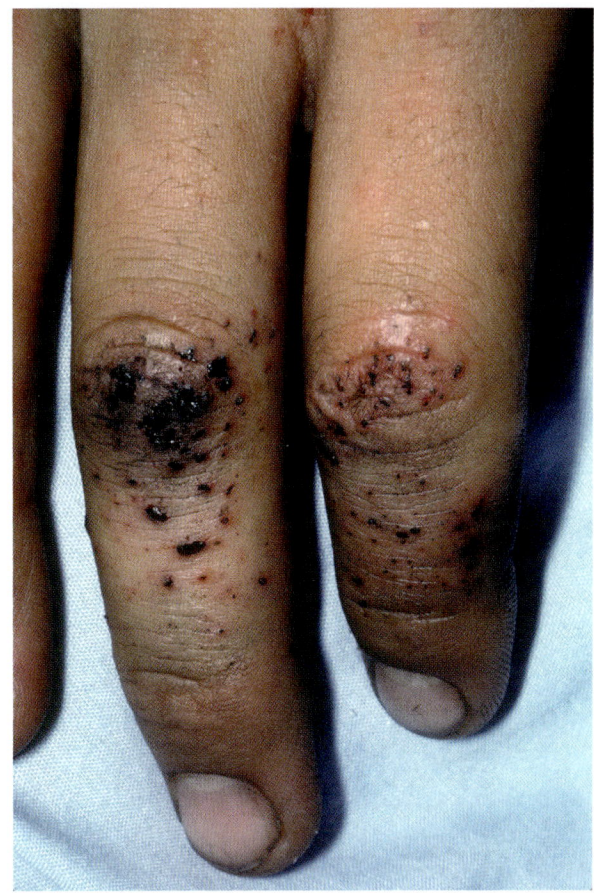

Fig. 3.63 Carbon stain, gunshot wound.

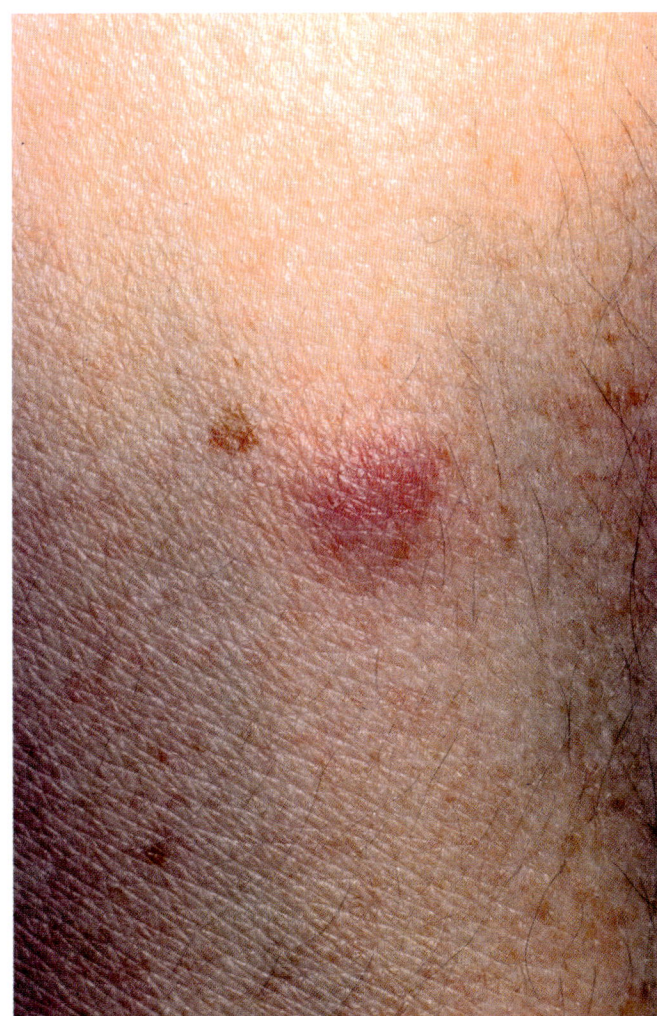

Fig. 3.64 Zyplast granuloma, test site.

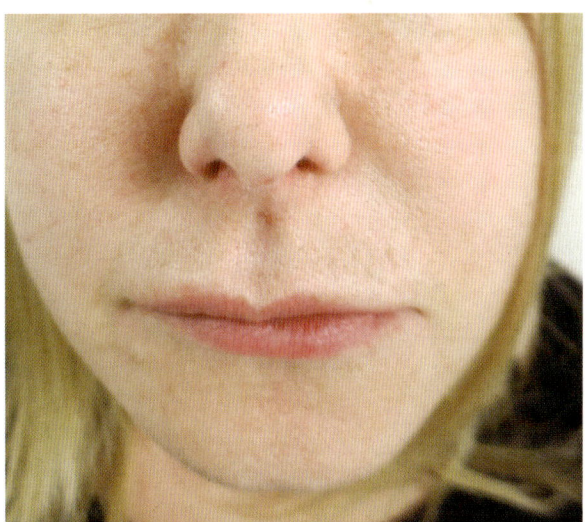

Fig. 3.65 Facial swelling reaction to hyaluronic acid filler.

Pruritus and Neurocutaneous Diseases

Pruritus often produces distinctive skin lesions, characterized by angulated borders. Endogenous diseases (in common parlance, an "inside job") tend to produce lesions that are rounded in character, whereas exogenous caustic agents, scratching, and other forms of external trauma tend to produce angulated, linear, or geometric shapes (signs of an "outside job").

Pruritus can also result in the isomorphic (Koebner) phenomenon, where lesions of an endogenous disease localize in areas of trauma. These lesions often demonstrate a hybrid morphology, suggesting both endogenous origin and external trauma.

Lichenification results from chronic scratching or rubbing and is characterized by hyperkeratosis and papillary dermal fibrosis. The resulting clinical morphology includes slight induration and accentuation of skin markings. Excoriation results in eosinophilic necrosis of the granular layer. The corneum can remain intact, but more severe excoriation results in loss of the corneum and viable epidermis. More pronounced trauma can result in ulceration, in which the injury extends to the level of the dermis.

Broad areas of lichenification are characteristic of lichen simplex chronicus. Discrete papules with focal evidence of excoriation are typical of prurigo nodularis and arthropod bites, including those caused by bedbugs. This portion of the atlas will guide you through the clinical manifestations related to pruritic disorders.

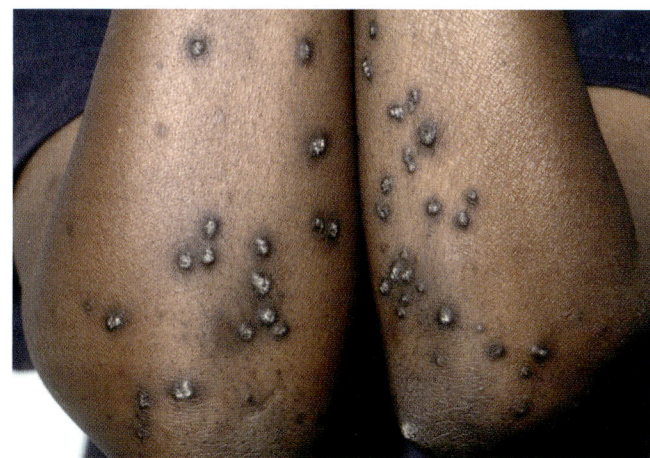

Fig. 4.2 Acquired perforating disease in renal failure.

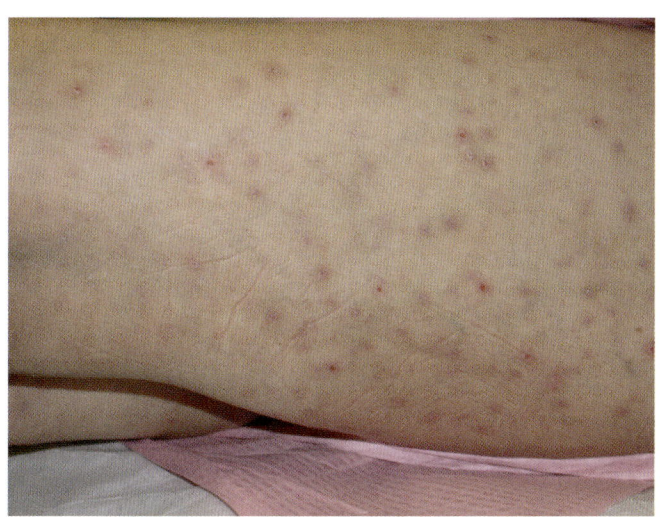

Fig. 4.1 Excoriations secondary to pruritus of Hodgkin disease.

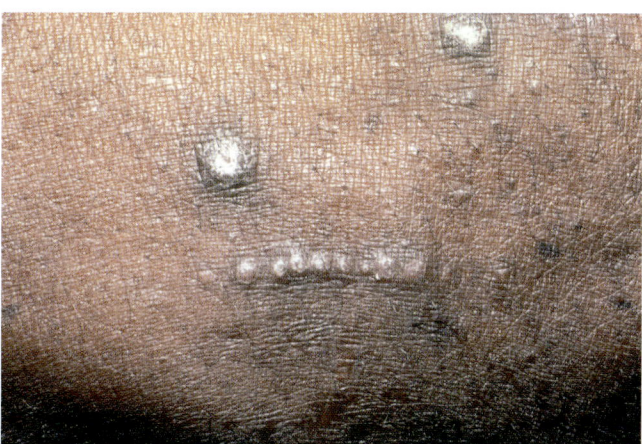

Fig. 4.3 Acquired perforating disease in renal failure.

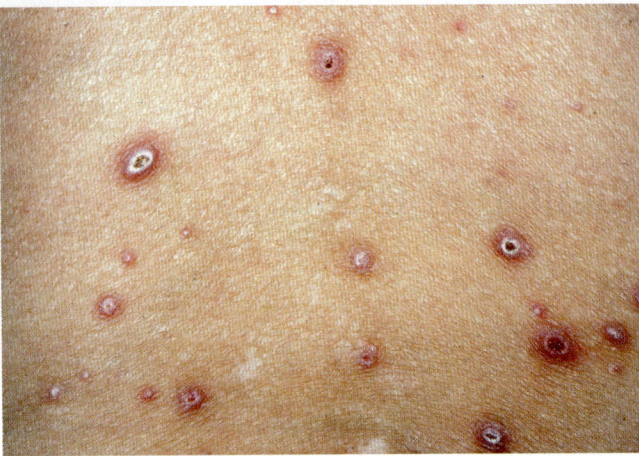

Fig. 4.4 Acquired perforating disease in renal failure. *Courtesy Steven Binnick, MD.*

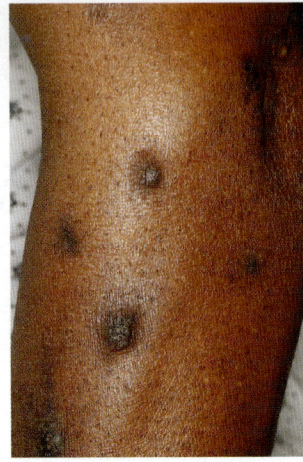

Fig. 4.5 Prurigo nodularis in a patient with chronic pruritus.

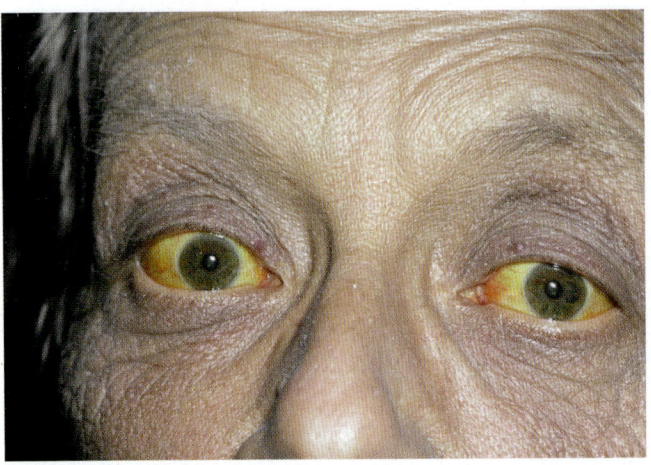

Fig. 4.6 Jaundice.

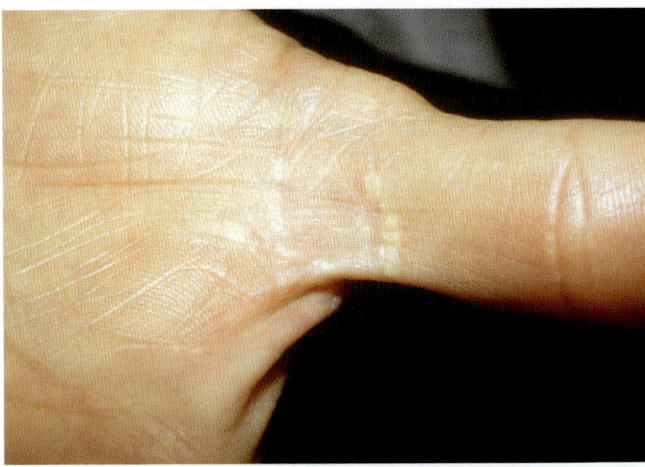

Fig. 4.7 Palmar xanthomas in hepatic cholestasis.

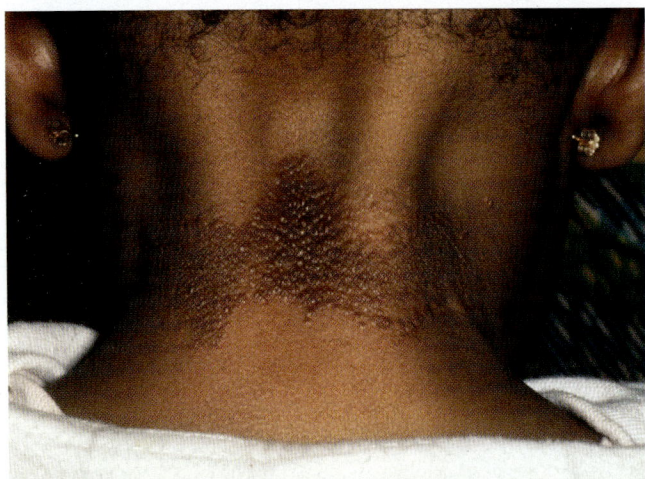

Fig. 4.8 Lichen simplex chronicus in Alagille disease.

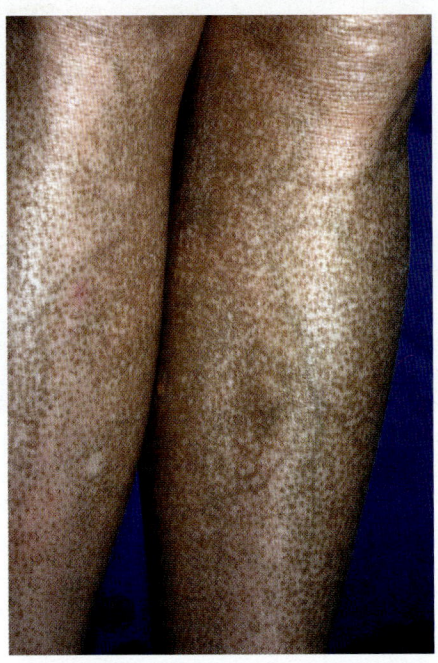

Fig. 4.9 Hyperpigmentation in primary biliary cirrhosis.

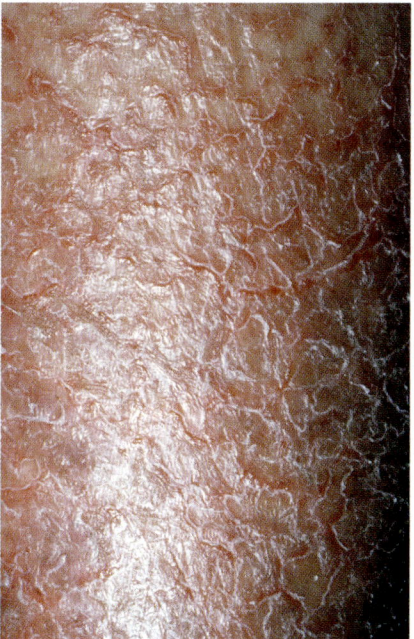

Fig. 4.10 Winter itch.

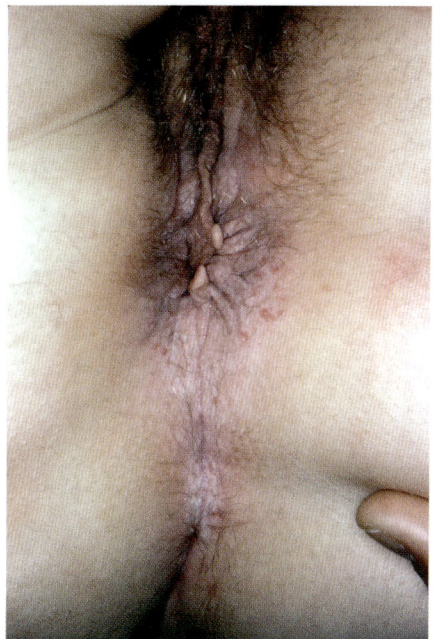

Fig. 4.11 Lichen simplex chronicus in pruritus ani.

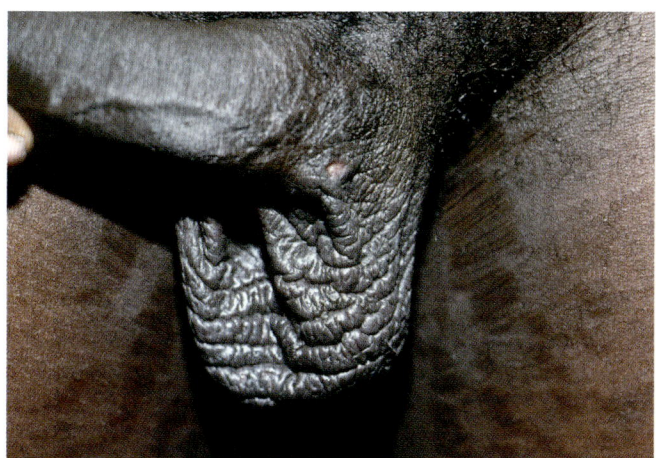

Fig. 4.12 Lichen simplex chronicus of the scrotum.

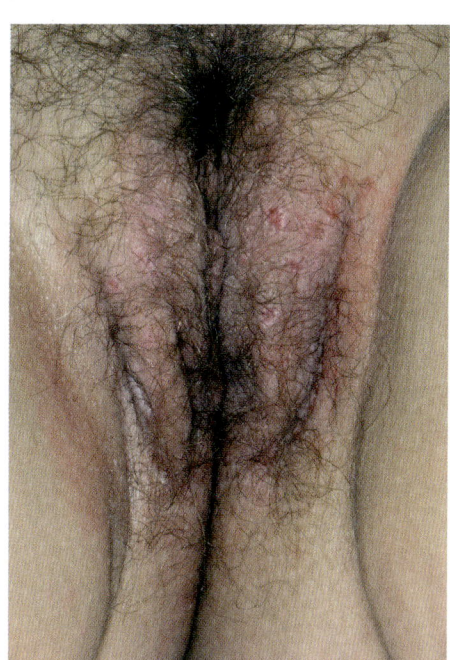

Fig. 4.13 Lichen simplex chronicus of the vulva.

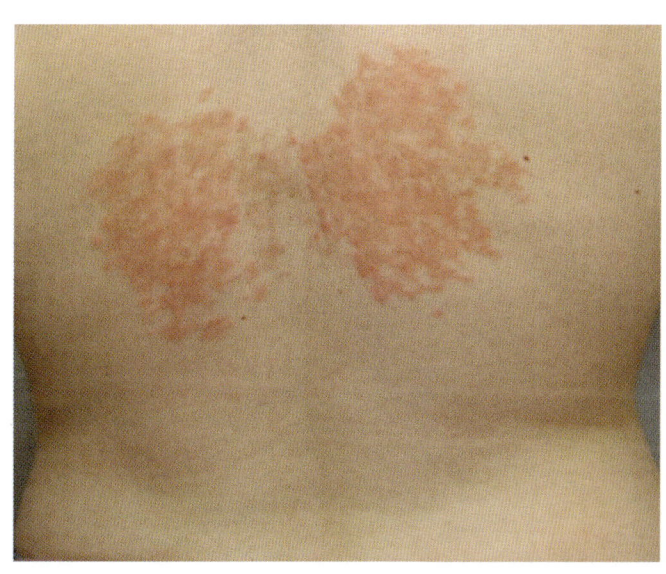

Fig. 4.14 Prurigo pigmentosa.

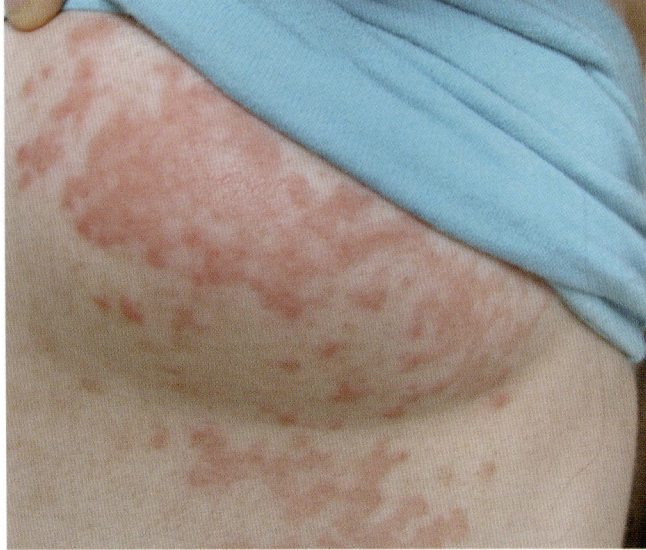

Fig. 4.15 Prurigo pigmentosa. *Courtesy Stephen D. Hess, MD, PhD.*

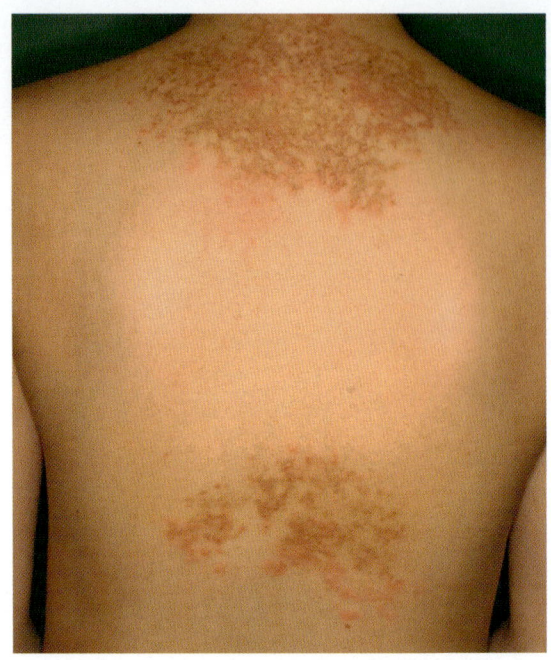

Fig. 4.16 Prurigo pigmentosa. *Courtesy Department of Dermatology, Keio University School of Medicine, Tokyo, Japan.*

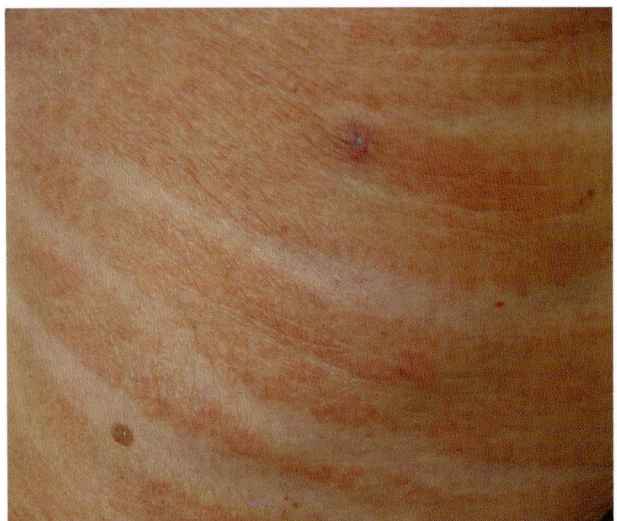

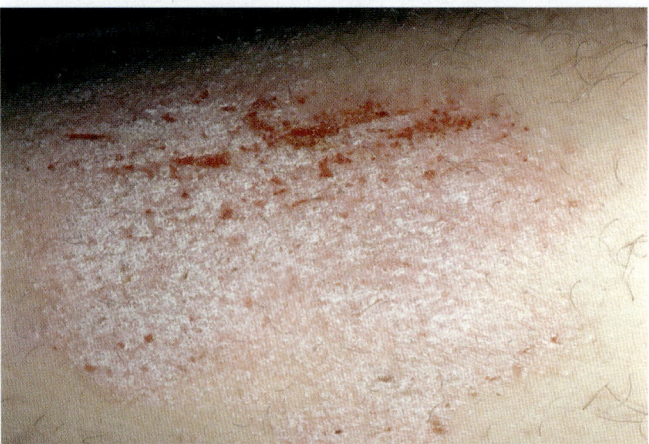

Fig. 4.18 Lichen simplex chronicus.

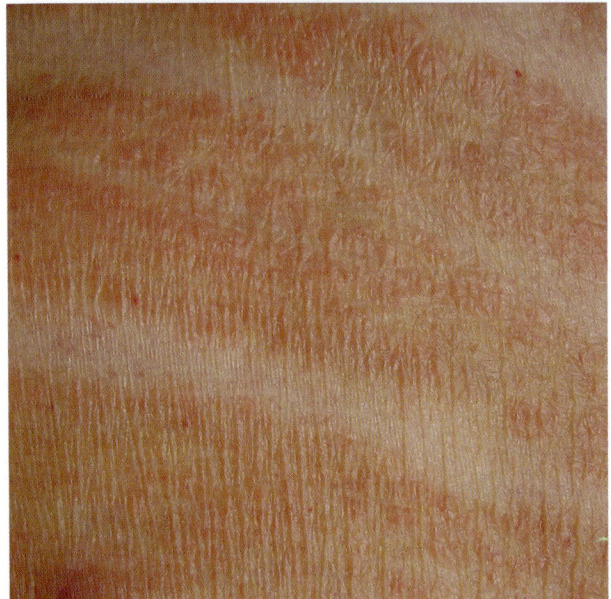

Fig. 4.17 A and B. Papuloerythroderma of Ofuji showing the deck chair sign. *Courtesy Dr. Rui Carlos Taveres Bello.*

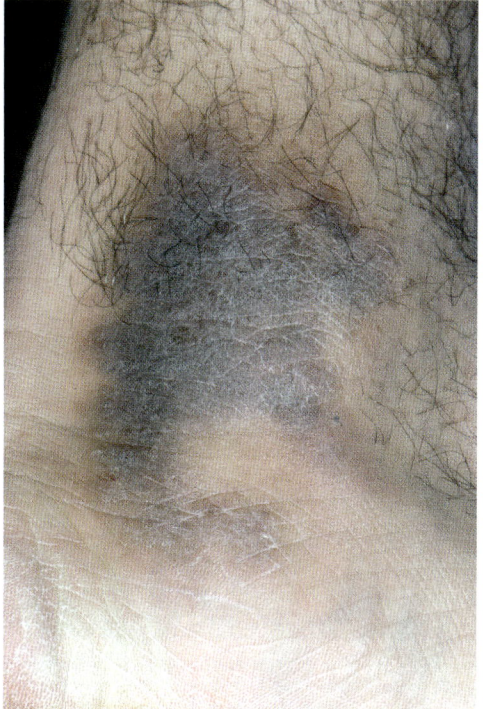

Fig. 4.19 Lichen simplex chronicus.

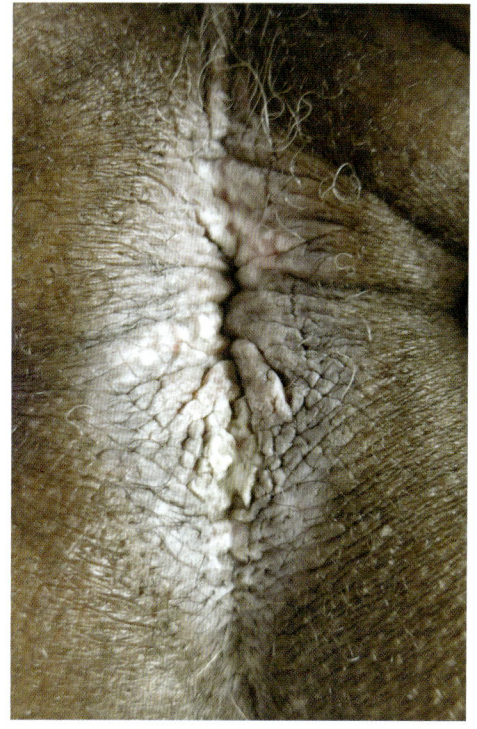

Fig. 4.20 Lichen simplex chronicus.

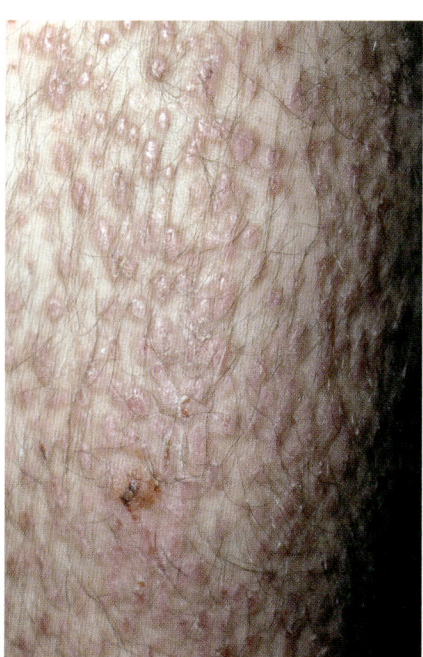

Fig. 4.21 Lichen simplex chronicus. *Courtesy Steven Binnick, MD.*

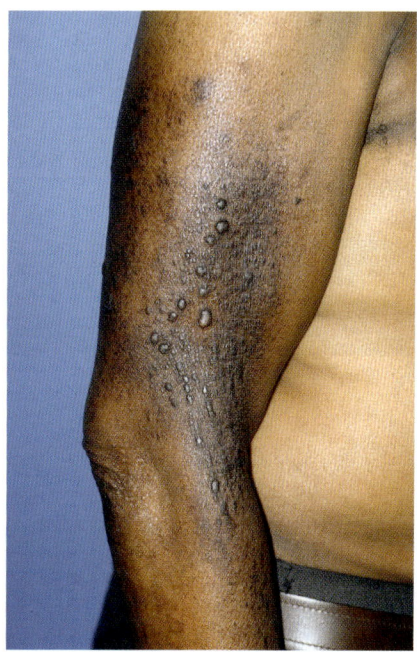

Fig. 4.22 Lichen simplex chronicus with dyspigmentation and early nodule formation.

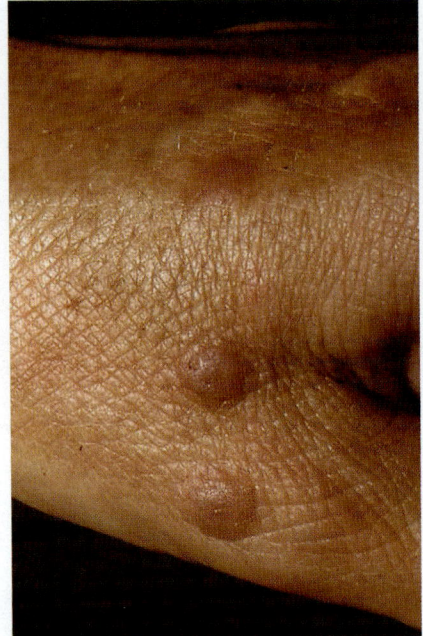

Fig. 4.23 Prurigo nodularis. *Courtesy The University of Utah and Oregon Health Sciences University Leonard Swinyer MD image collection.*

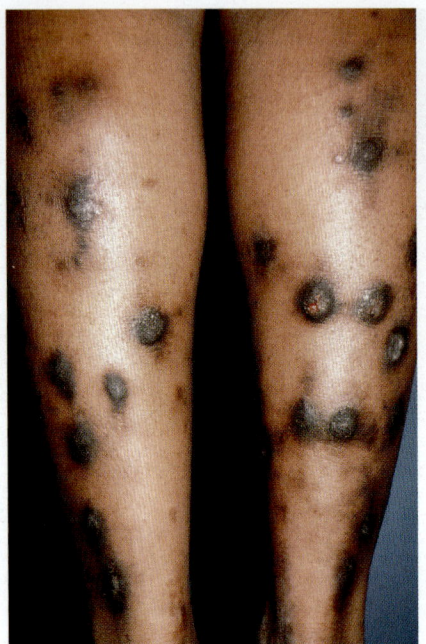

Fig. 4.24 Prurigo nodularis with excoriation.

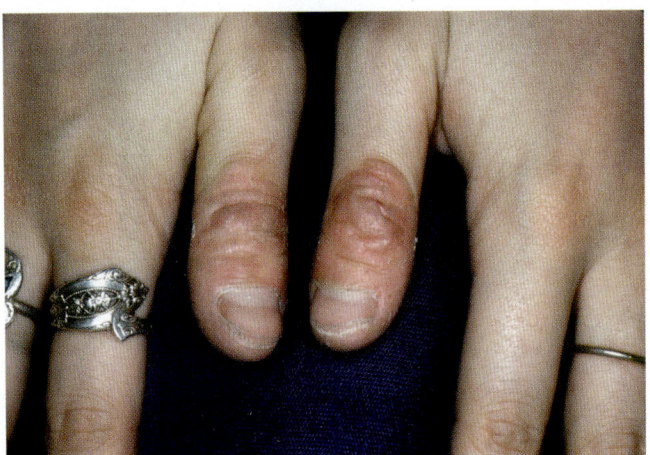

Fig. 4.25 Compulsive finger biting.

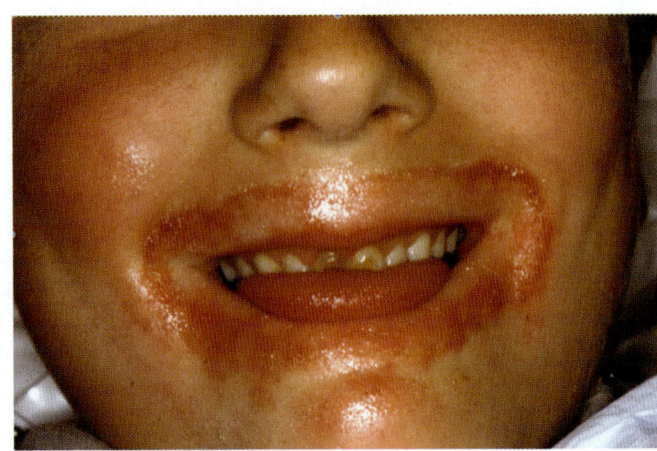

Fig. 4.26 Chronic lip licking habit. *Courtesy Ginat Mirowski, DMD, MD.*

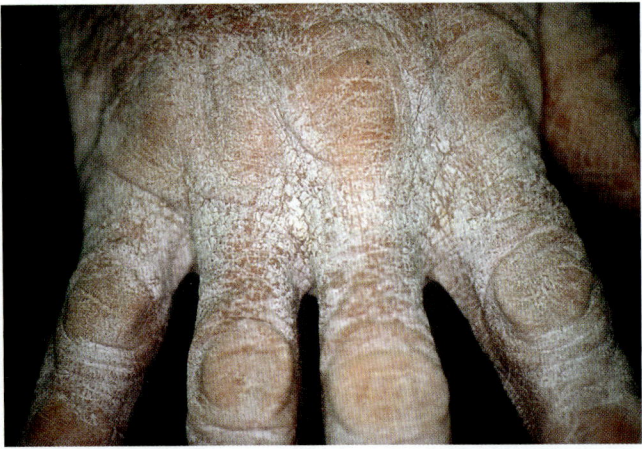

Fig. 4.27 Dryness secondary to compulsive hand washing.

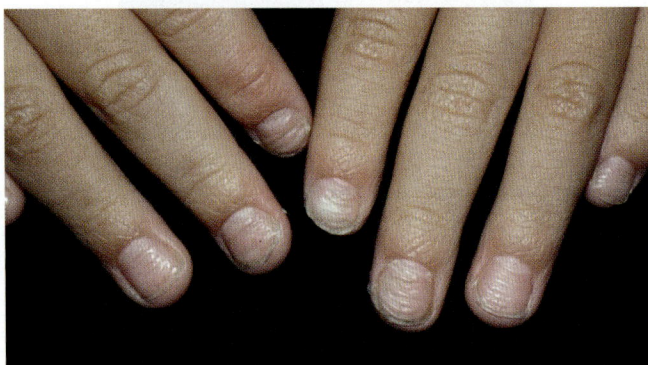

Fig. 4.28 Washboard nails secondary to habitual trauma to the matrix.

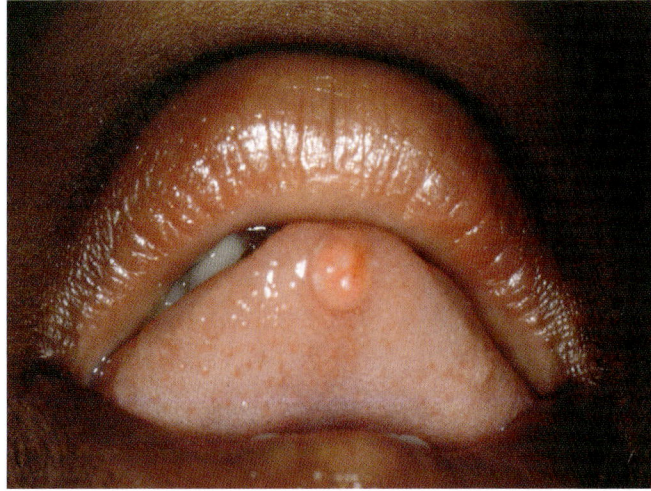

Fig. 4.29 Fibroma secondary to chronic tongue biting. *Courtesy the Department of Oral Medicine, the University of Pennsylvania School of Dental Medicine.*

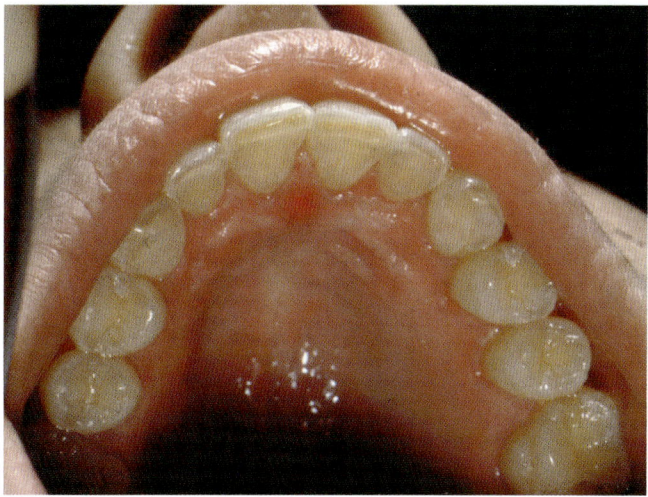

Fig. 4.30 Enamel erosion secondary to vomiting with bulimia. *Courtesy the Department of Oral Medicine, the University of Pennsylvania School of Dental Medicine.*

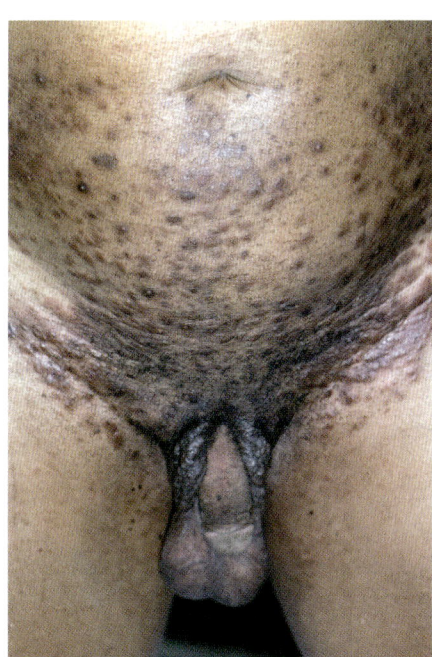

Fig. 4.31 Delusions of parasitosis.

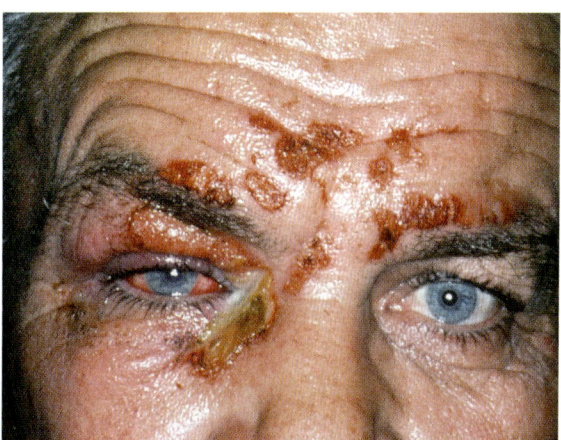

Fig. 4.32 Delusions of parasitosis.

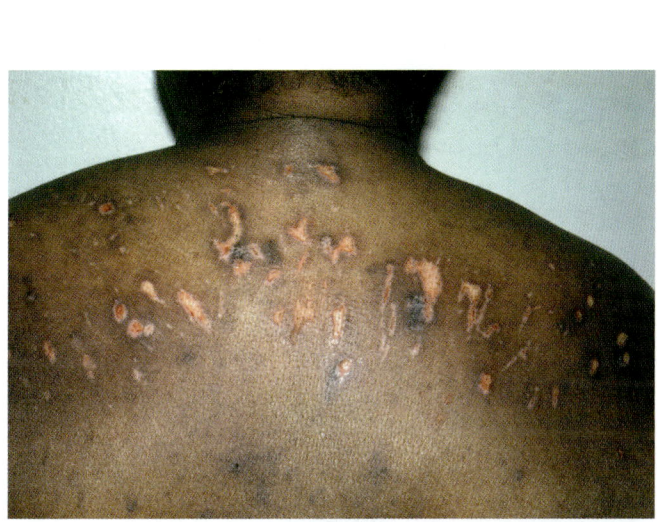

Fig. 4.33 Psychogenic excoriations. *Courtesy Steven Binnick, MD.*

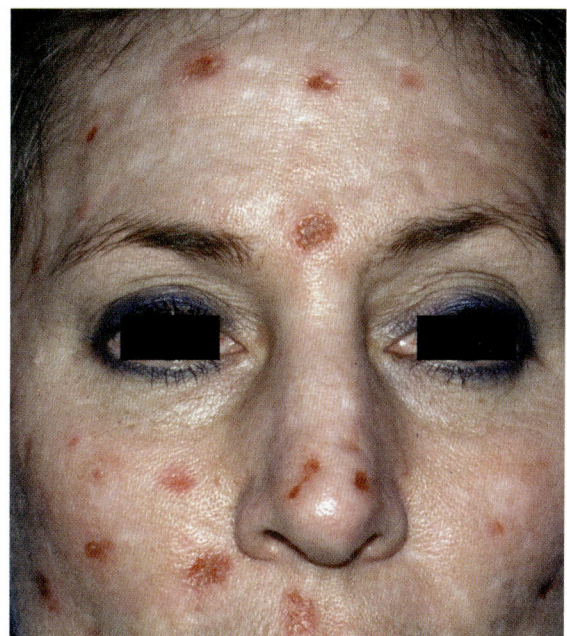

Fig. 4.34 Psychogenic excoriations. *Courtesy Curt Samlaska, MD.*

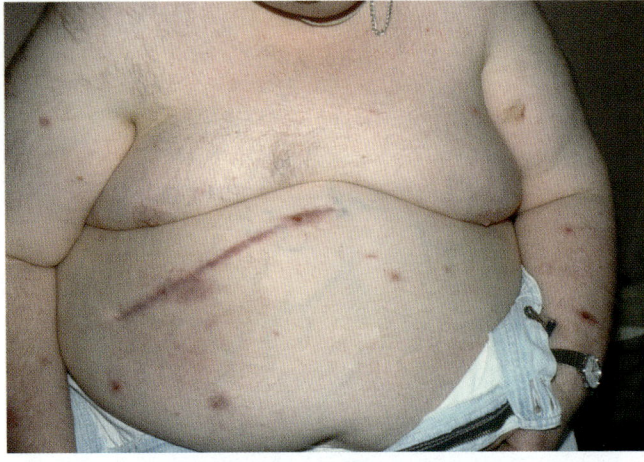

Fig. 4.35 Skin picking in Prader-Willi syndrome. *Courtesy Robert Horn, MD.*

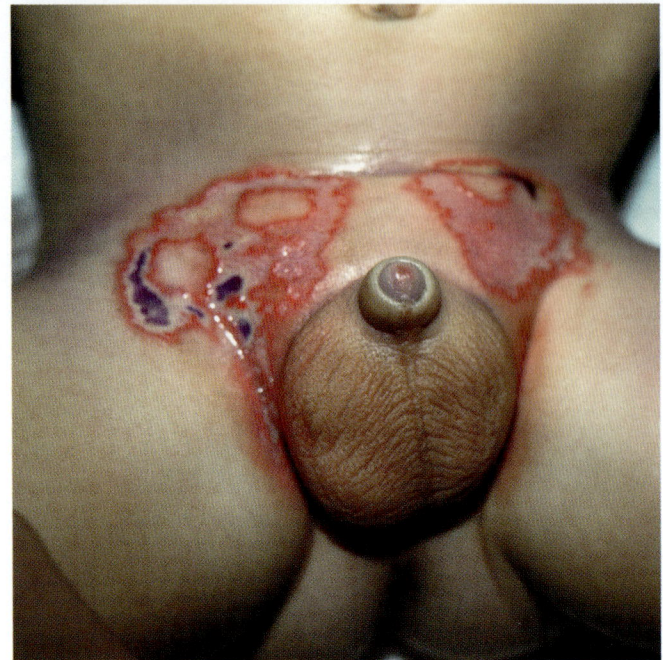

Fig. 4.36 Factitial ulcers induced by parents.

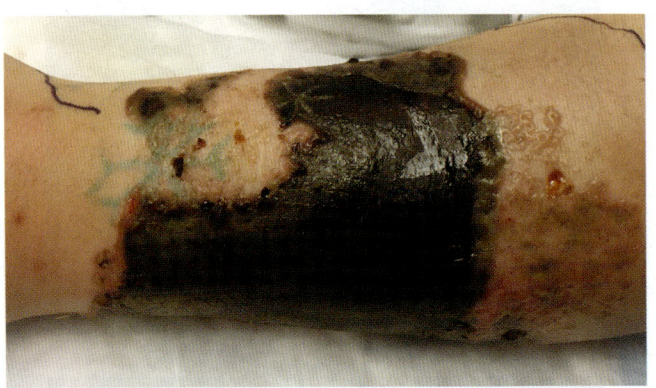

Fig. 4.37 Factitial dermatitis.

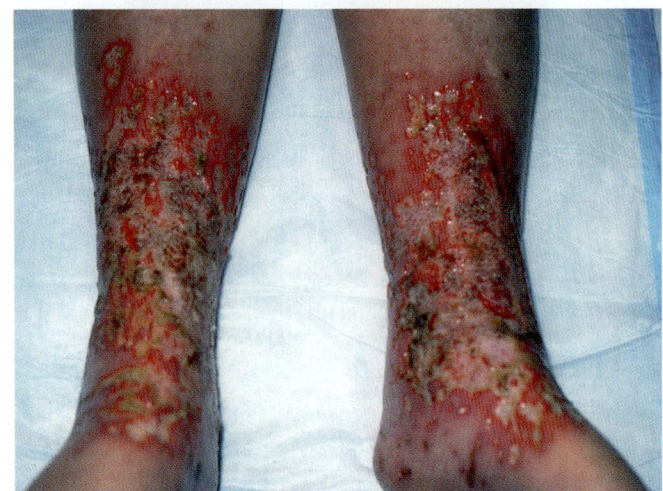

Fig. 4.38 Factitial ulcers.

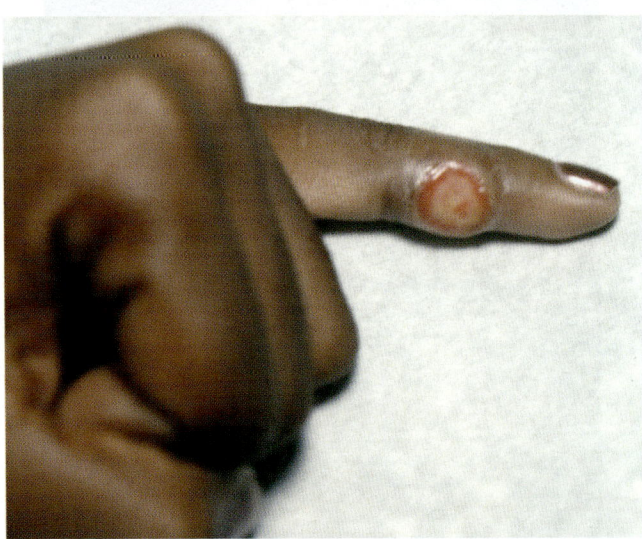

Fig. 4.39 Cigarette burn, factitial.

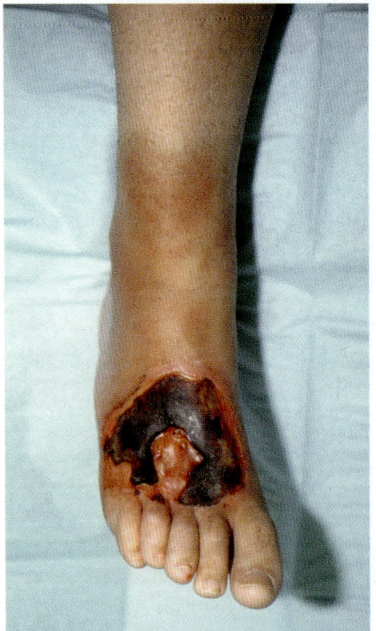

Fig. 4.40 Factitial ulcer.

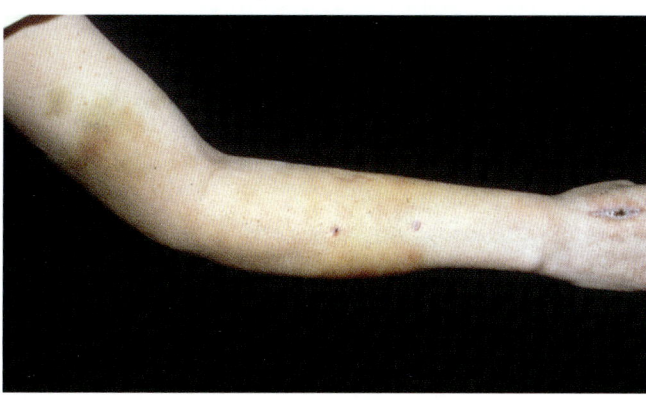

Fig. 4.41 Factitial bruising.

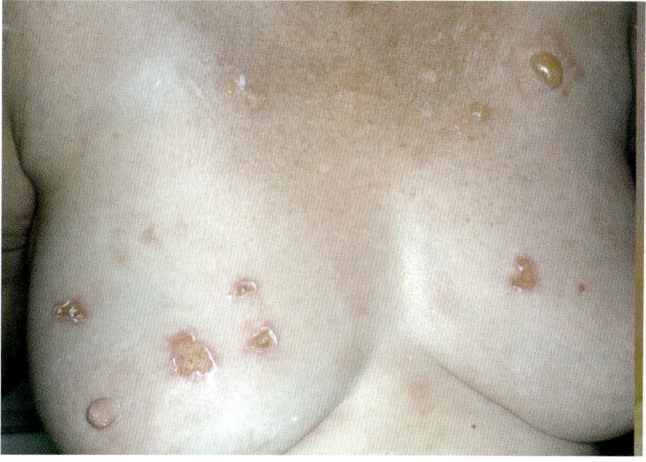

Fig. 4.42 Factitial blisters and erosions. *Courtesy Steven Binnick, MD.*

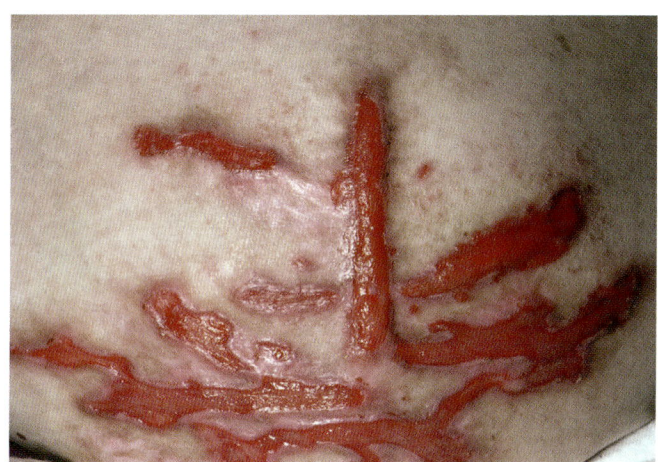

Fig. 4.43 Factitial scarring.

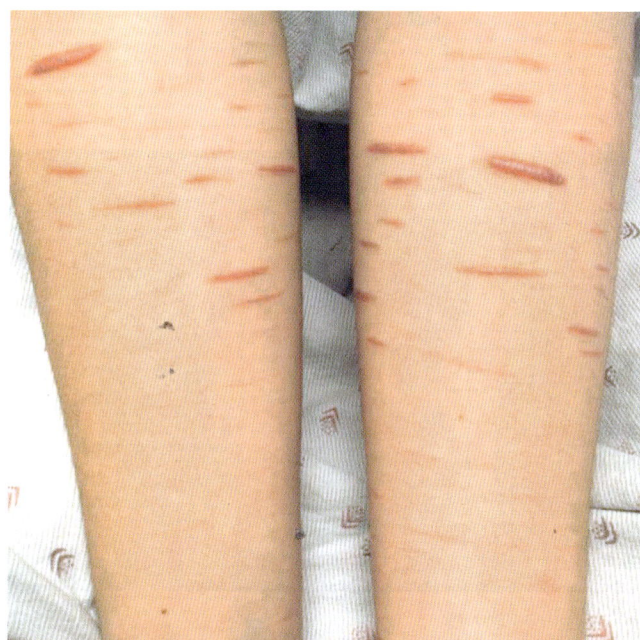

Fig. 4.44 Healed factitial lacerations. *Courtesy Sheilagh Maguiness, MD.*

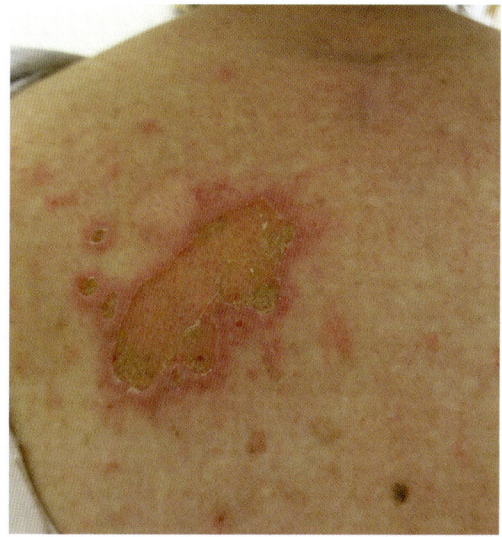

Fig. 4.45 Factitial ulcers and scarring on the back.

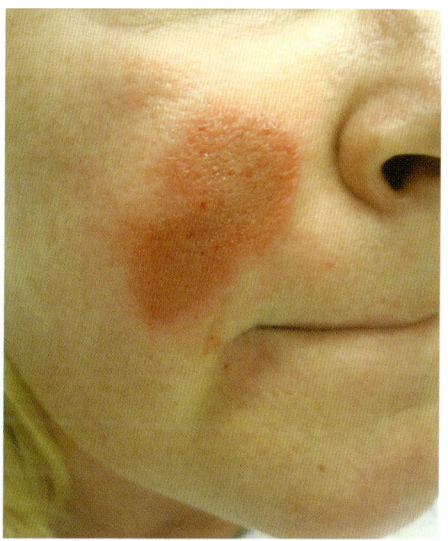

Fig. 4.46 Factitial erosion secondary to friction.

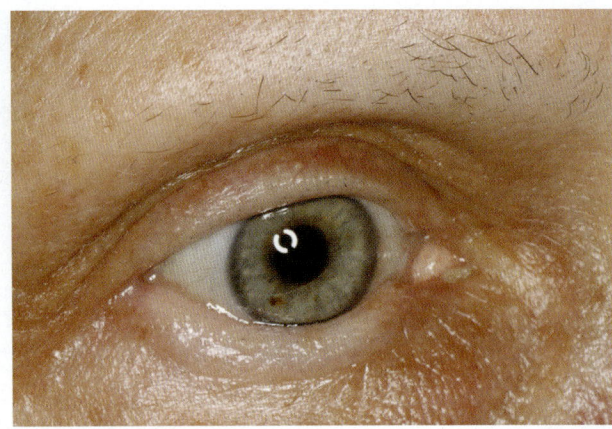

Fig. 4.47 Trichotillosis.

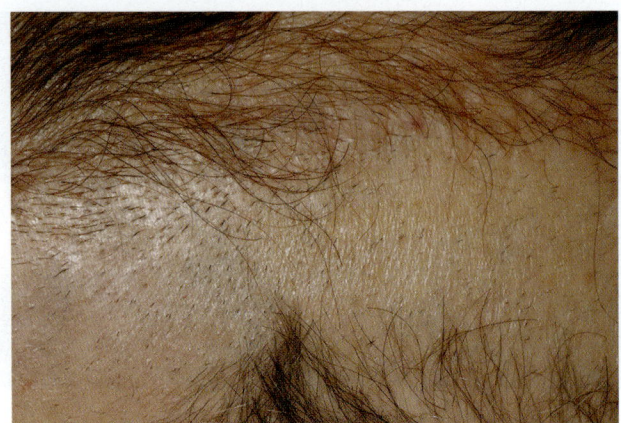

Fig. 4.48 Trichotillosis.

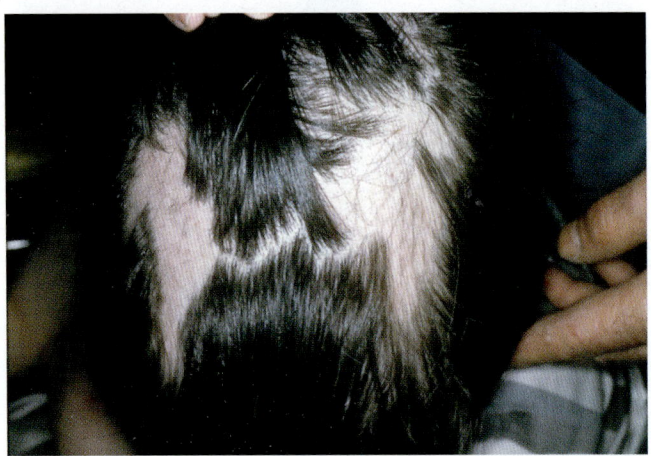

Fig. 4.49 Trichotillosis.

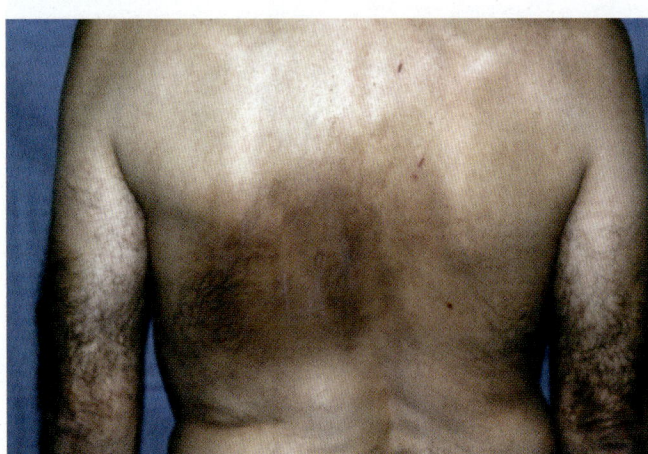

Fig. 4.50 Notalgia paresthetica. *Courtesy Curt Samlaska, MD.*

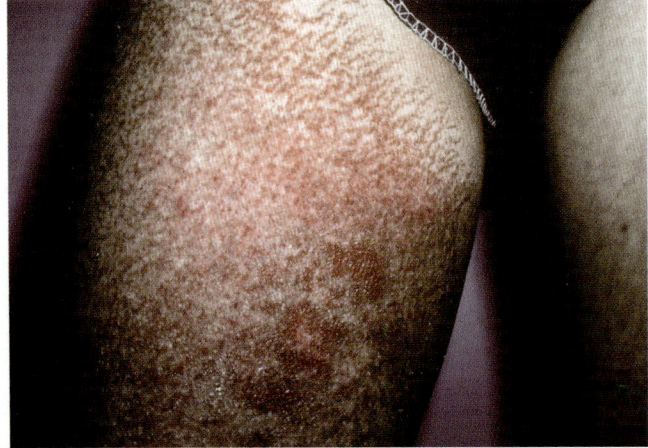

Fig. 4.51 Complex regional pain syndrome.

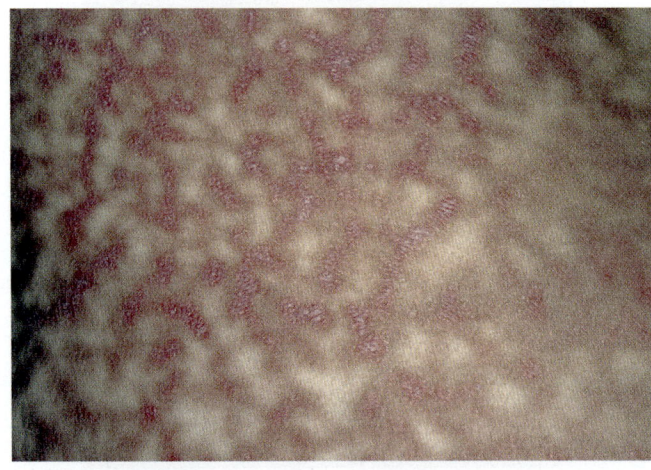

Fig. 4.52 Complex regional pain syndrome.

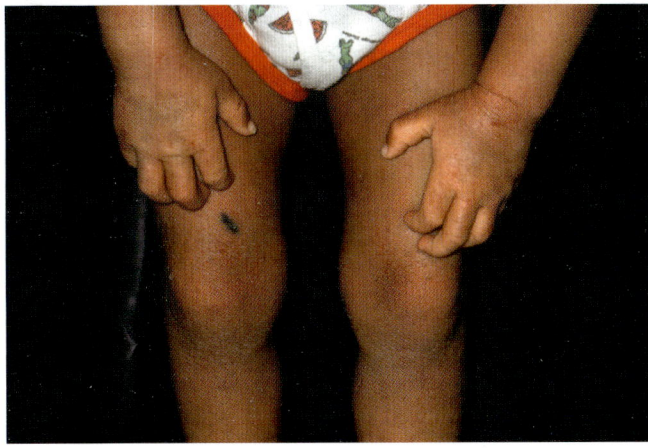

Fig. 5.3 Atopic dermatitis.

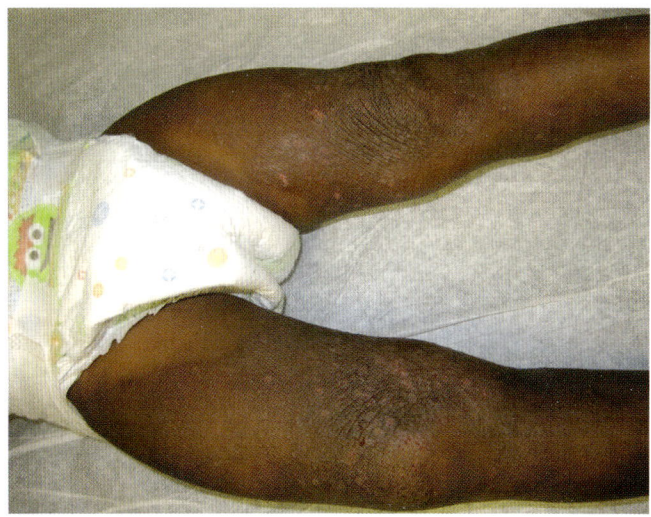

Fig. 5.4 Chronic atopic dermatitis.

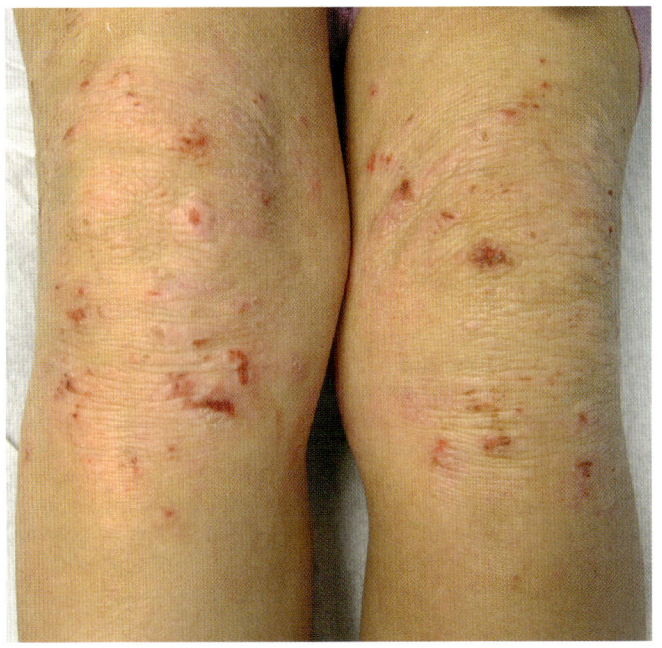

Fig. 5.5 Atopic dermatitis with excoriations.

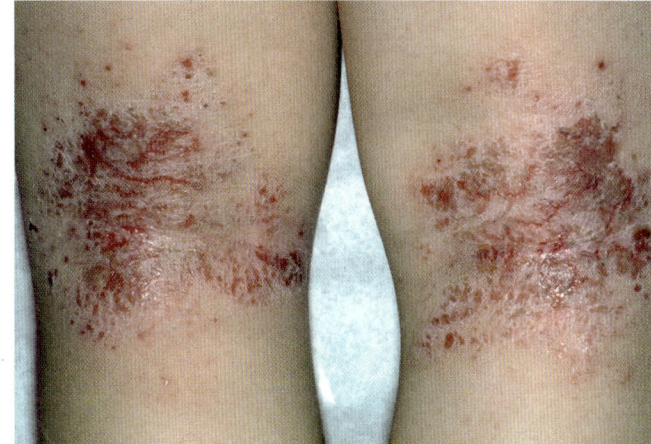

Fig. 5.6 Atopic dermatitis with secondary infection. *Courtesy Steven Binnick, MD.*

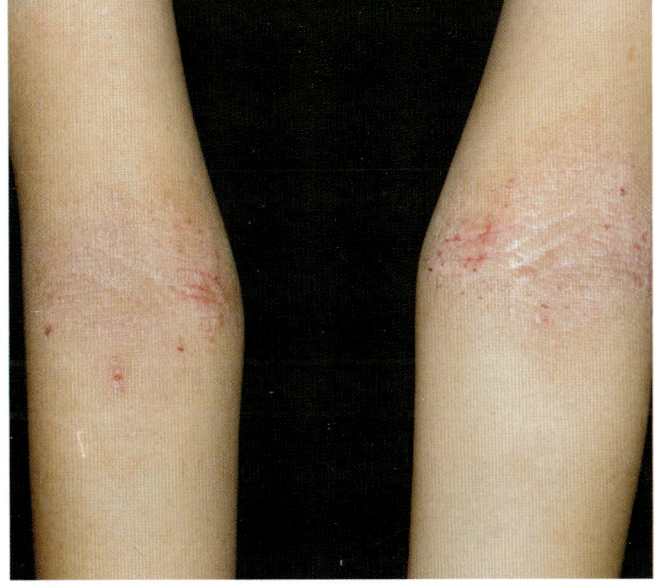

Fig. 5.7 Atopic dermatitis.

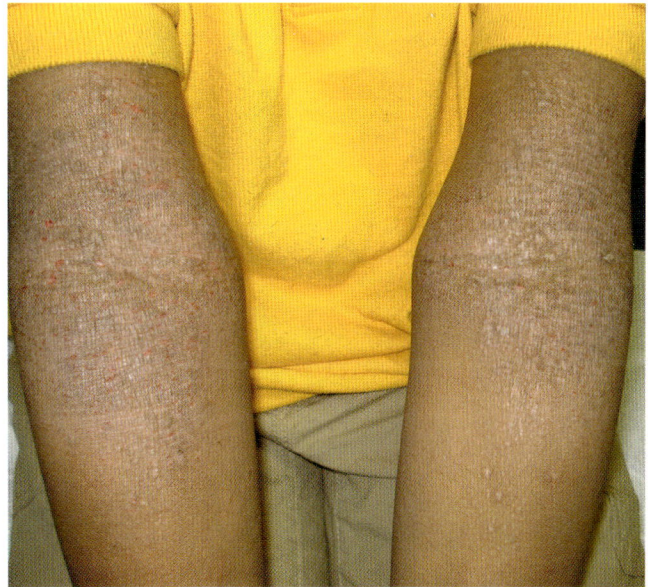

Fig. 5.8 Atopic dermatitis.

Atopic Dermatitis, Eczema, and Noninfectious Immunodeficiency Disorders

5

Dermatitis can present with a variety of physical examination findings ranging from exuberant oozing to dry scale. These findings represent the acute and chronic inflammation that defines a variety of dermatitides and eczematous conditions. Intense itching that accompanies these conditions can lead to overlying excoriations and eventually thickening of the skin known as *lichenification*. Ultimately, constant itching and a poor epidermal barrier predispose patients with these eczematous conditions to repeated skin infections from bacteria and viruses, which can present with pustules, vesicles, crusting, erosions, or painful nodules. Screening for signs of such infections is an important part of the physical examination for all patients with dermatitis, especially those with any underlying immunodeficiency.

Although most cases will not require a skin biopsy for a diagnosis, the spongiosis of acute dermatitis or the acanthosis of the epidermis seen in chronic dermatitis can be confirmatory in scenarios wherein other diagnoses that affect the epidermis are being considered, such as nutritional deficiencies, graft-versus-host disease, or psoriasis.

The anatomic location of atopic dermatitis (AD) can vary depending on age. Infantile AD tends to affect the cheeks and can have impressive overlying exudation and crusting even in the absence of infection. In infants, AD can also be quite widespread with predilections for extensor surfaces and notable sparing of the diaper region and nose, the so-called *headlight sign*. Childhood AD may be more localized to the flexors and can begin to take on a more lichenified appearance. Many people with AD will outgrow a more widespread dermatitis, but may have chronic hand dermatitis or other more localized flares of their AD. Associated features of AD found on physical examination include Dennie-Morgan lines (accentuated folds of the lower eyelids), keratosis pilaris, general xerosis, follicular accentuation, and signs of atopy such as hyperpigmentation around the eyes known as *allergic shiners*.

Other forms of eczema may take on different patterns on the body, including the coin-shaped, scaly, and exudative plaques of nummular eczema or the diffuse, dry, and cracked appearance of xerotic eczema (eczema craquelé). Even in patients without a history of AD, localized forms of eczema may arise on the eyelids or nipples, or on the hands as vesiculobullous hand eczema (pompholyx). Finally, some forms of immunodeficiency disorders can present with relatively nonspecific exfoliative erythroderma, as in severe combined immunodeficiency (SCID), or an atopic dermatitis-like eruption, as in hyper–immunoglobulinemia E (IgE) syndrome, Wiskott-Aldrich syndrome (WAS), or DiGeorge syndrome. In these cases, the astute clinician will observe distinctive clinical findings such as the pustular eruption of hyper-IgE syndrome, dysmorphisms of DiGeorge syndrome, or petechiae within the dermatitis of patients with WAS. This portion of the atlas will highlight the range of clinical findings seen in patients with atopic dermatitis and other forms of eczema, along with rarer findings seen in patients with immunodeficiency syndromes.

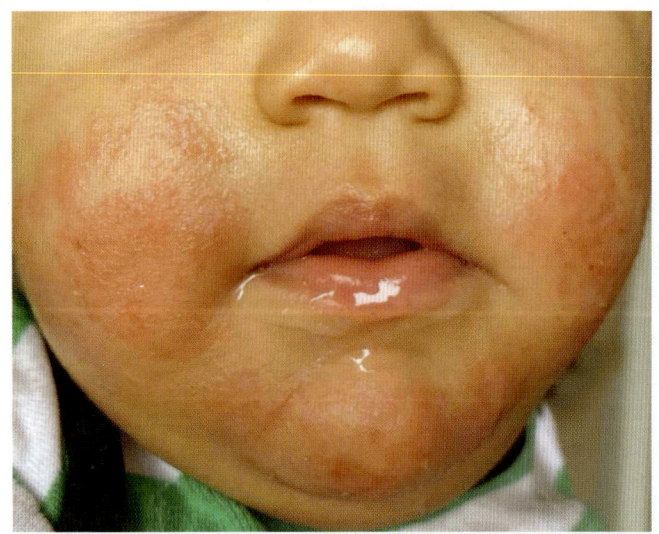

Fig. 5.1 Atopic dermatitis.

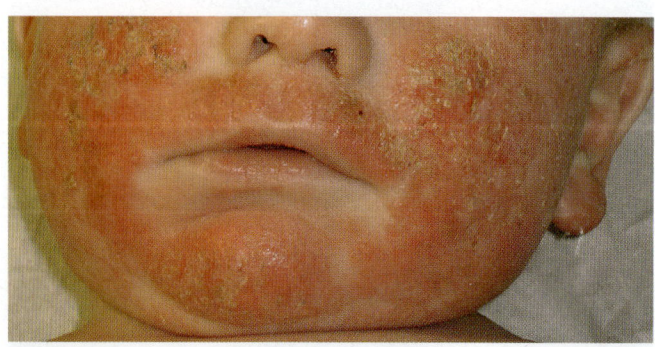

Fig. 5.2 Atopic dermatitis.

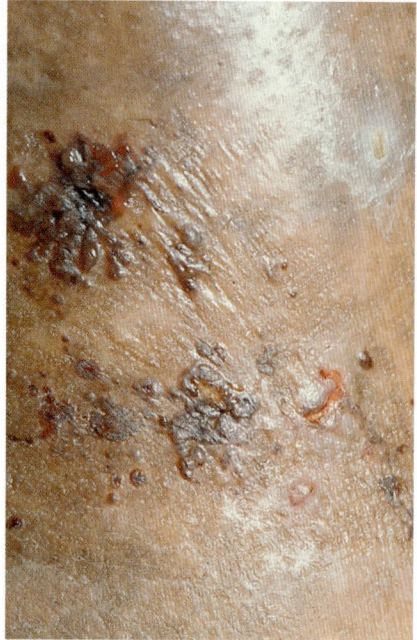

Fig. 4.53 Blistering and atrophy, complex regional pain syndrome.

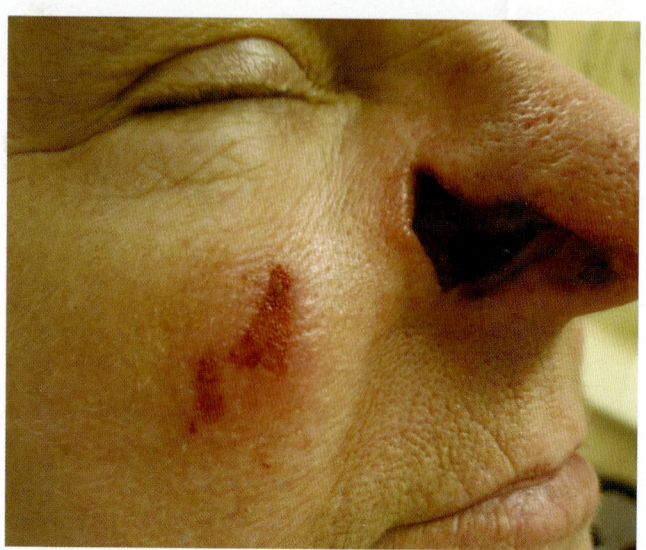

Fig. 4.54 Trigeminal trophic syndrome.

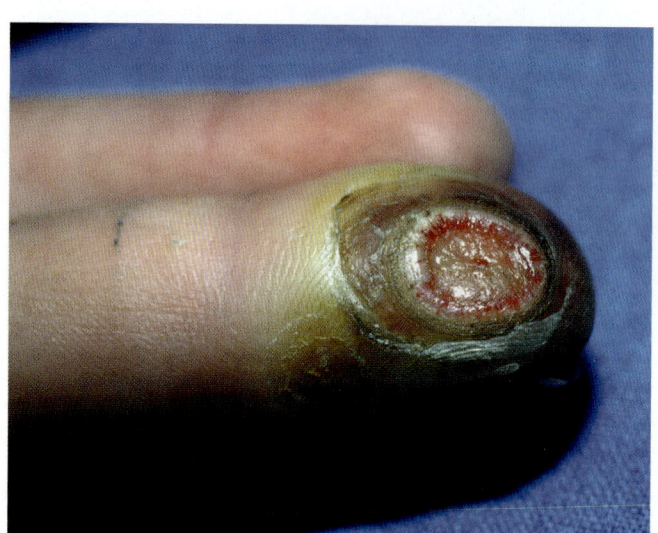

Fig. 4.55 Neuropathic ulcer of the hand in a patient with diabetes.

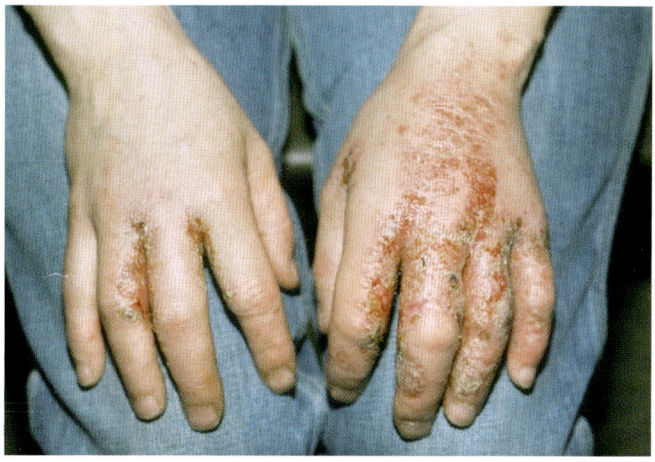

Fig. 5.9 Atopic dermatitis with secondary infection.

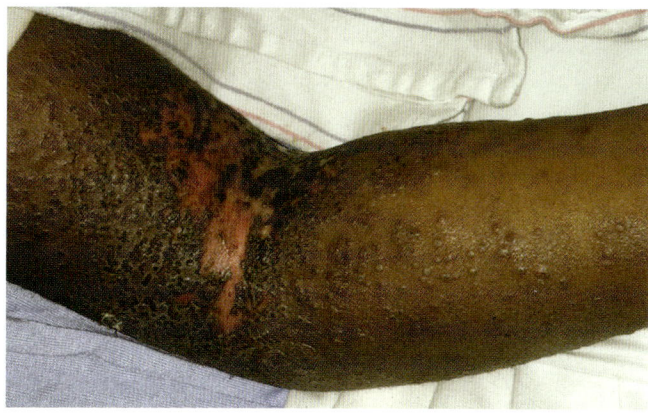

Fig. 5.10 Atopic dermatitis infected with *Staphylococci* and *Streptococci*.

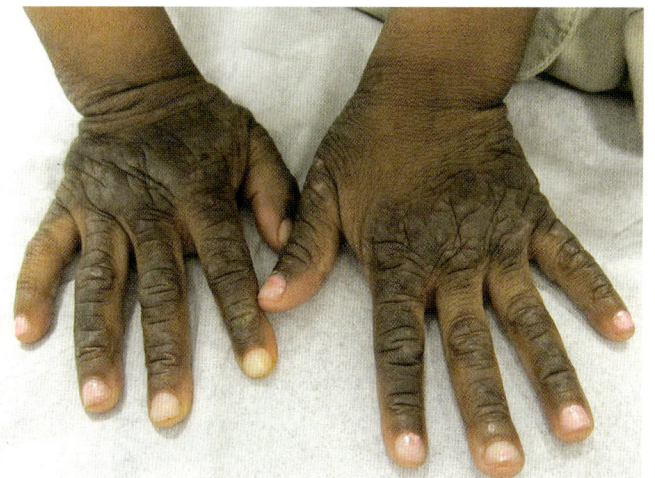

Fig. 5.11 Chronic atopic dermatitis.

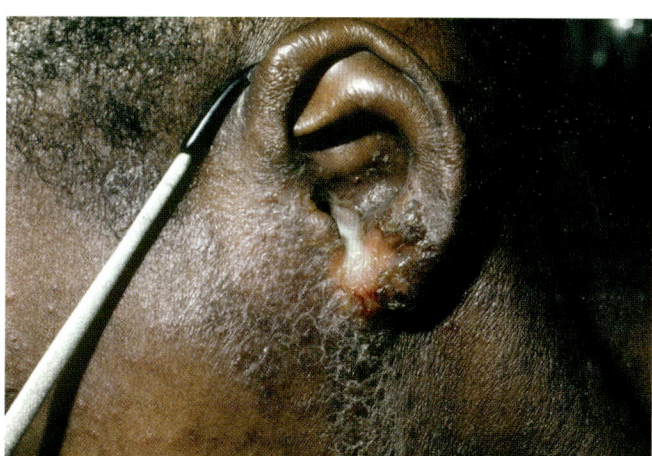

Fig. 5.12 Atopic dermatitis with secondary infection. *Courtesy Steven Binnick, MD*.

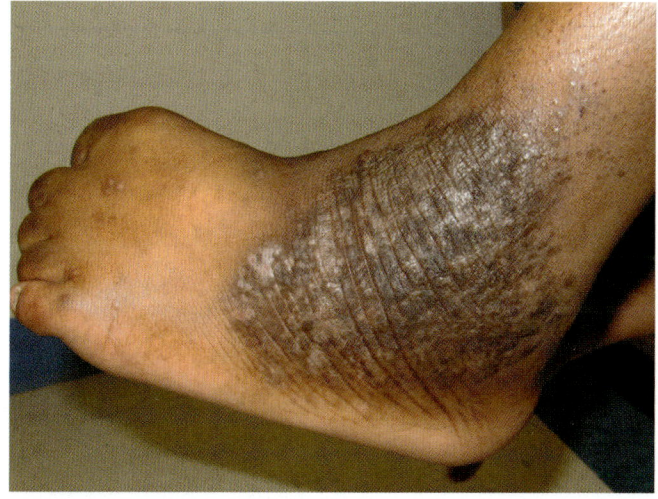

Fig. 5.13 Chronic atopic dermatitis with hyperpigmentation.

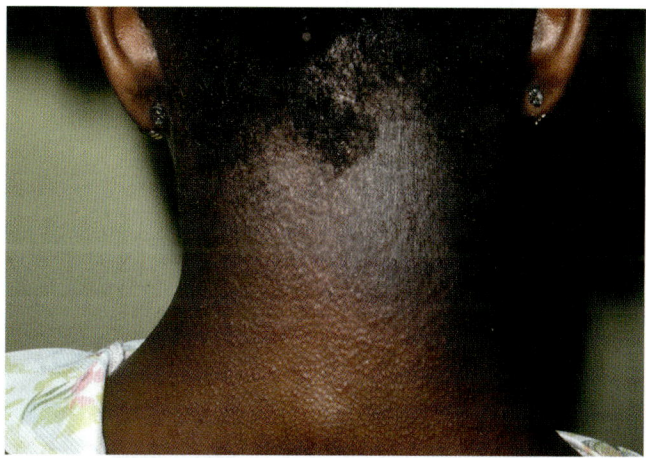

Fig. 5.14 Atopic dermatitis, lichenification. *Courtesy Steven Binnick, MD*.

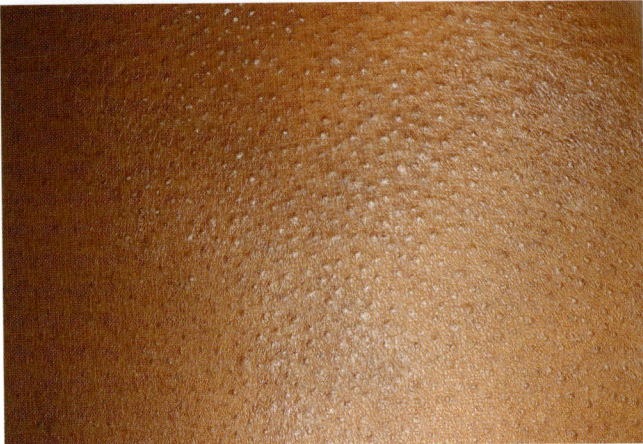

Fig. 5.15 Atopic dermatitis, follicular pattern.

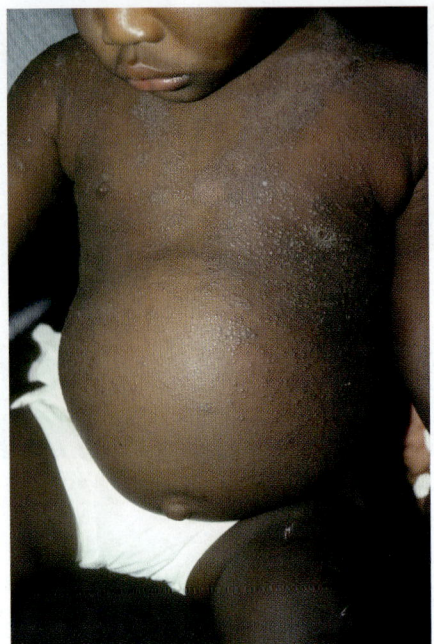

Fig. 5.16 Papular atopic dermatitis. *Courtesy Steven Binnick, MD.*

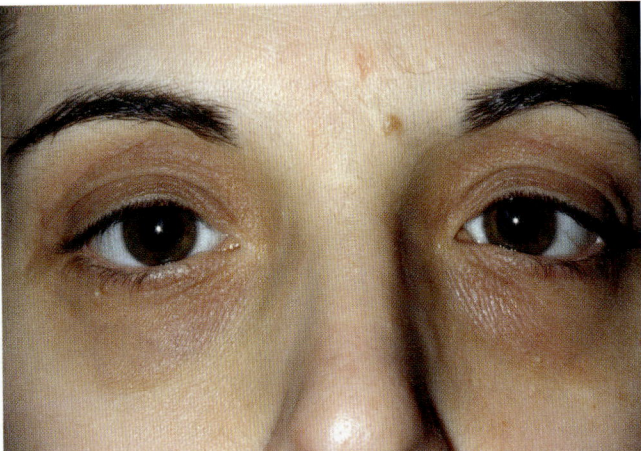

Fig. 5.17 Atopic dermatitis with Dennie-Morgan lines. *Courtesy Steven Binnick, MD.*

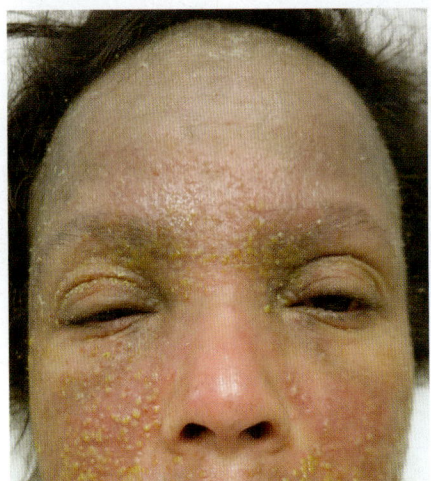

Fig. 5.18 Impetiginized atopic dermatitis.

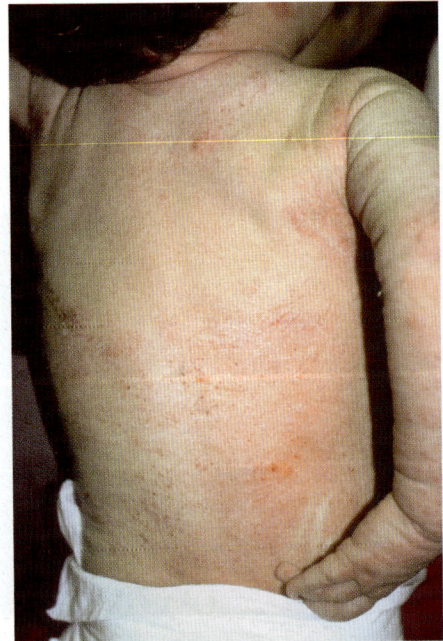

Fig. 5.19 White dermatographism.

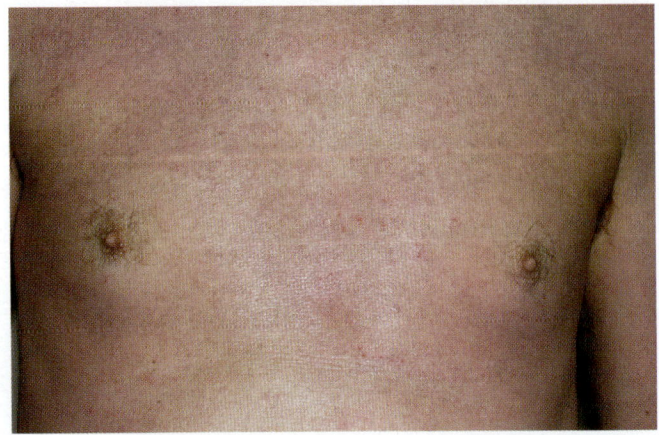

Fig. 5.20 Erythroderma from atopic dermatitis.

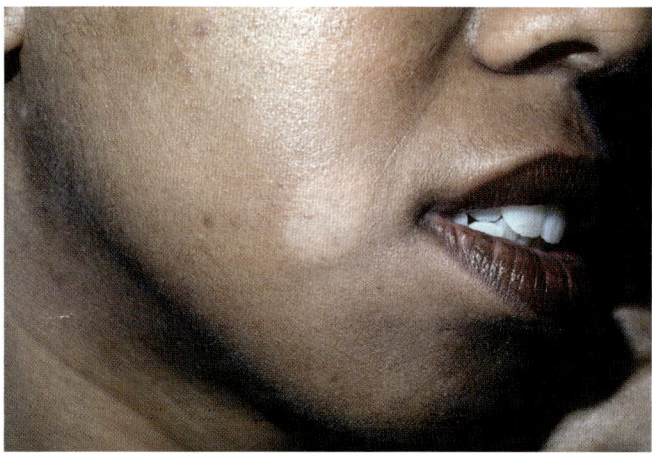

Fig. 5.21 Pityriasis alba. *Courtesy Steven Binnick, MD.*

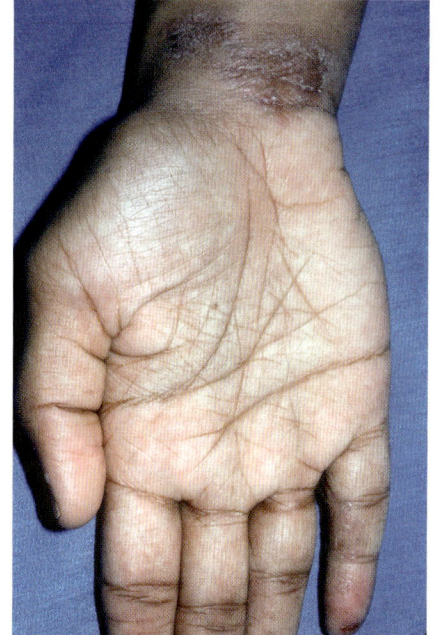

Fig. 5.22 Hyperlinear palms in a patient with active atopic dermatitis. *Courtesy Steven Binnick, MD.*

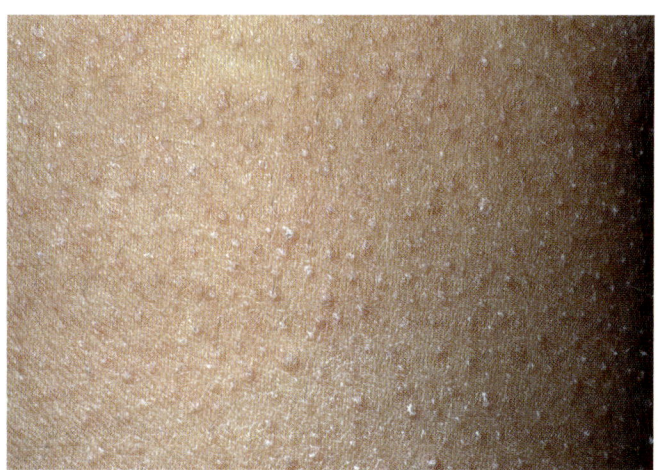

Fig. 5.23 Keratosis pilaris. *Courtesy Steven Binnick, MD.*

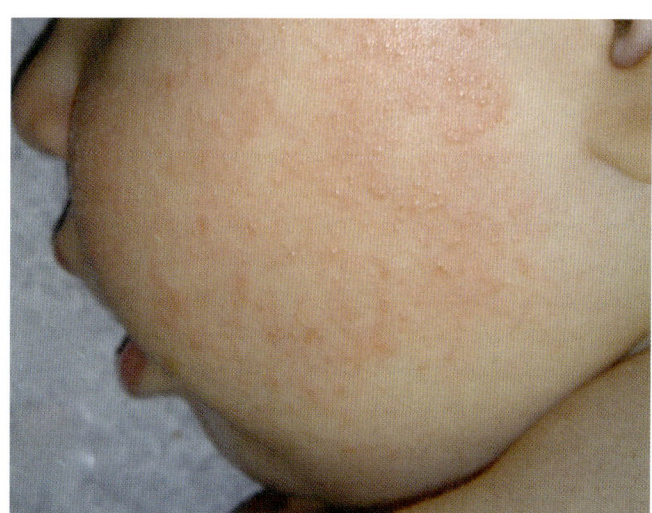

Fig. 5.24 Keratosis pilaris.

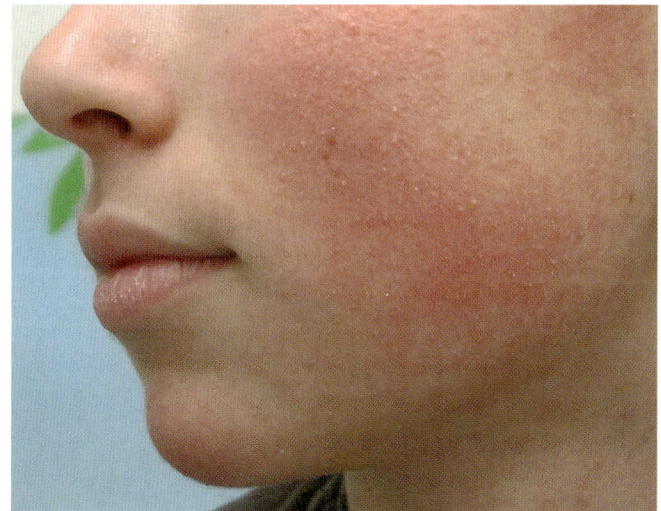

Fig. 5.25 Keratosis pilaris rubra faciei.

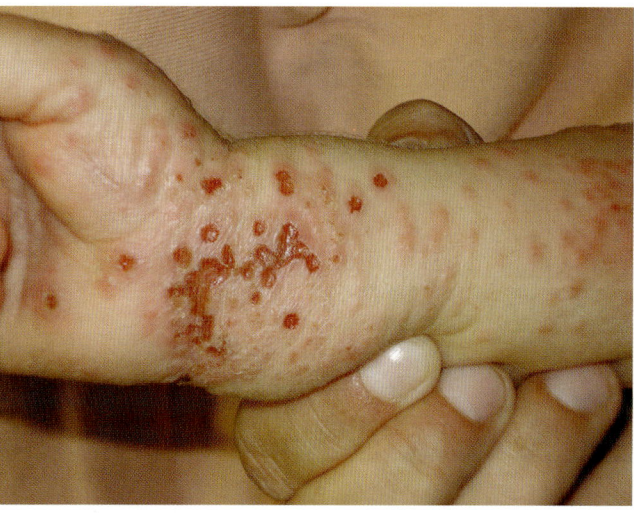

Fig. 5.26 Eczema herpeticum.

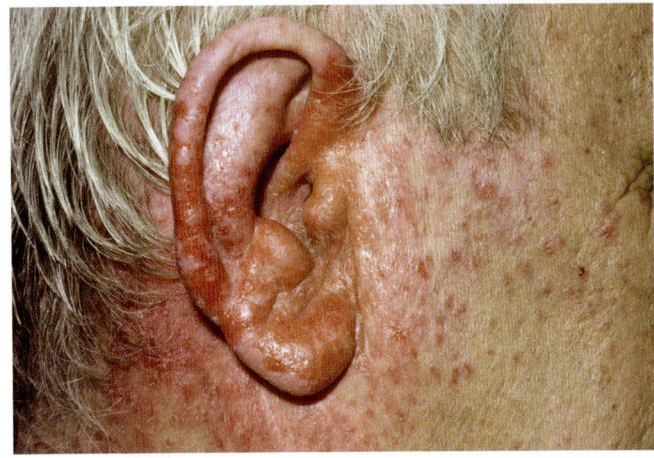

Fig. 5.27 Ear eczema.

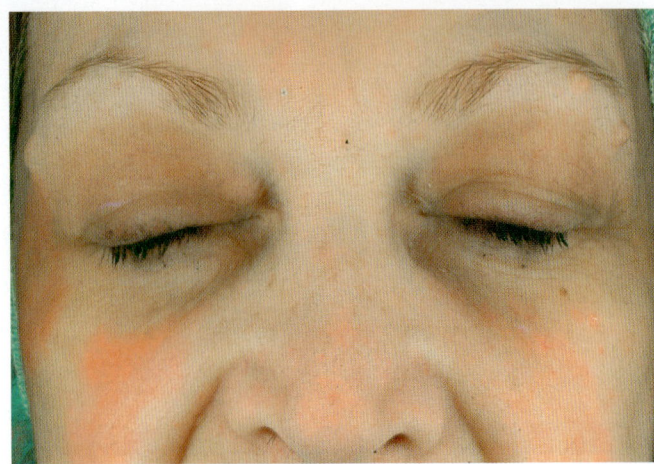

Fig. 5.28 Eyelid eczema.

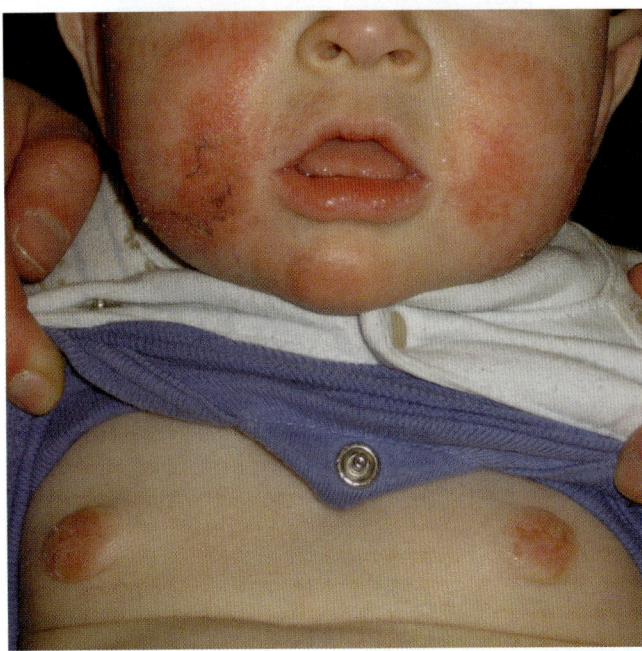

Fig. 5.29 Nipple eczema in an atopic child.

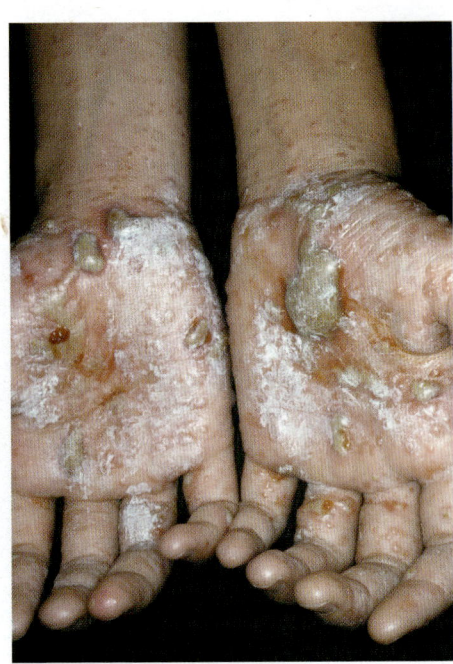

Fig. 5.30 Hand dermatitis with secondary infection.

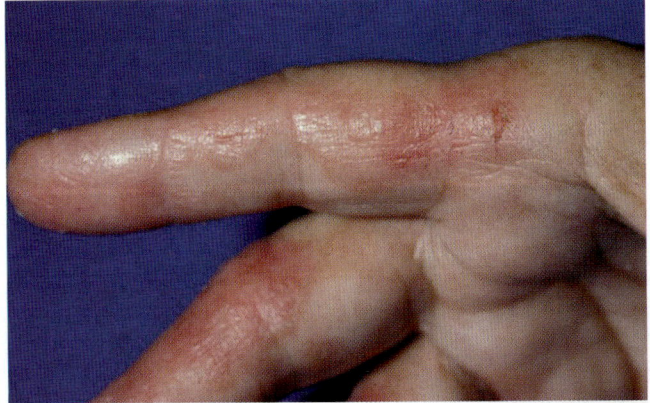

Fig. 5.31 Finger dermatitis from primrose allergy.

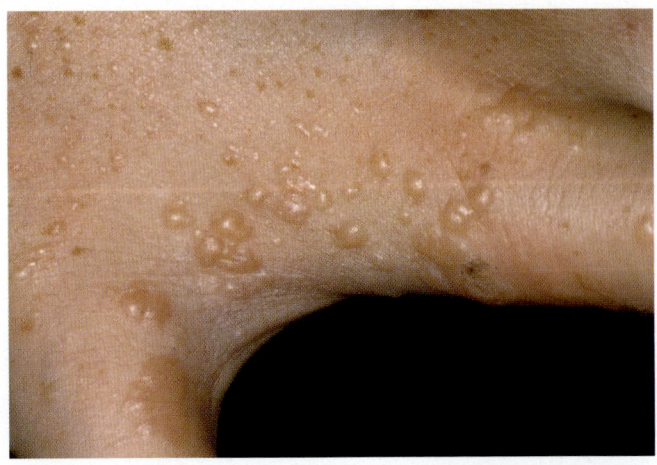

Fig. 5.32 Pompholyx.

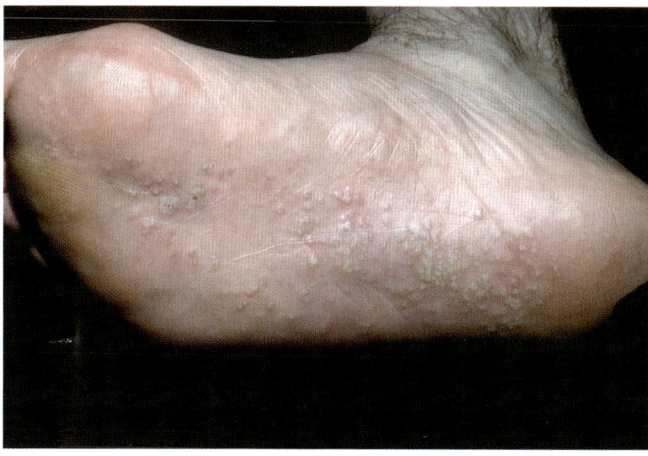

Fig. 5.33 Pompholyx. *Courtesy The University of Utah and Oregon Health Sciences University Leonard Swinyer MD image collection.*

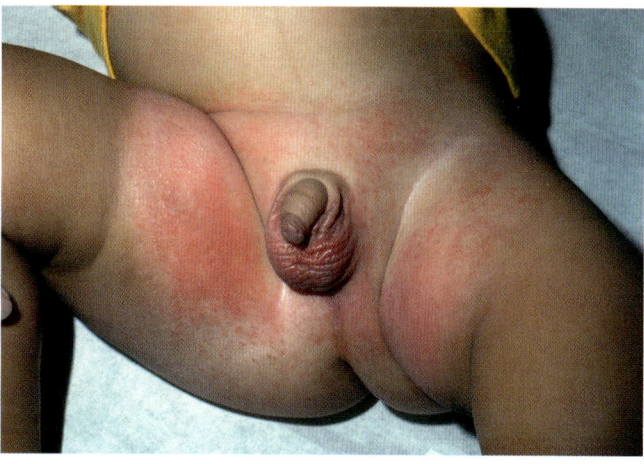

Fig. 5.34 Irritant diaper dermatitis. Note sparing of folds.

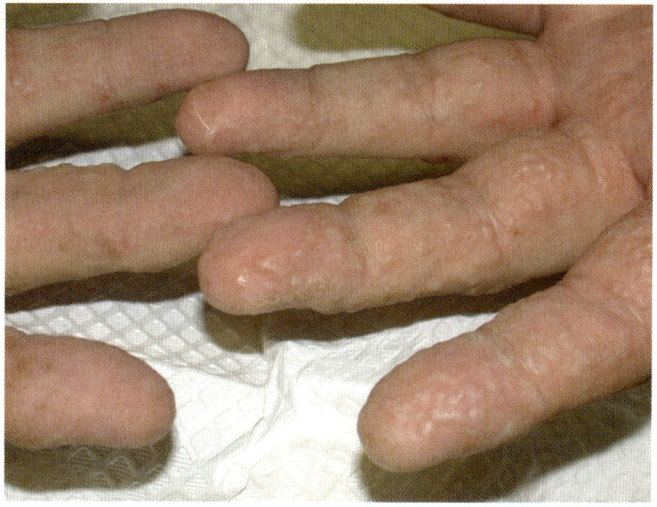

Fig. 5.35 Id reaction.

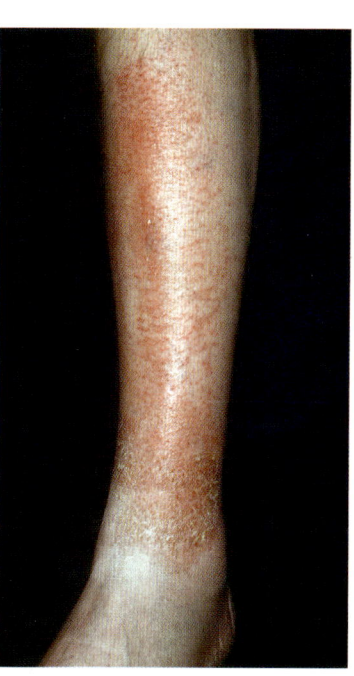

Fig. 5.36 Eczema craquelé.

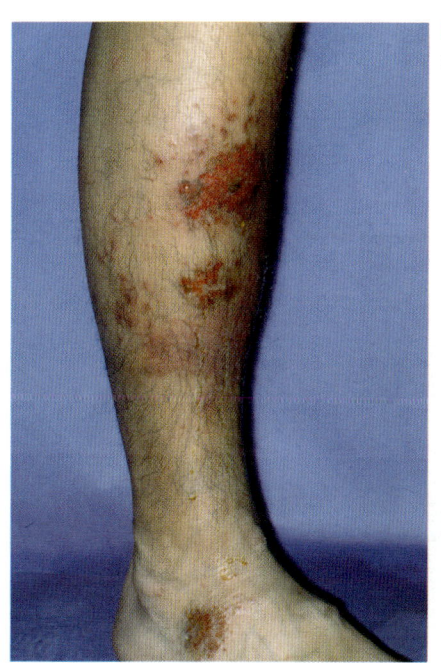

Fig. 5.37 Nummular eczema.

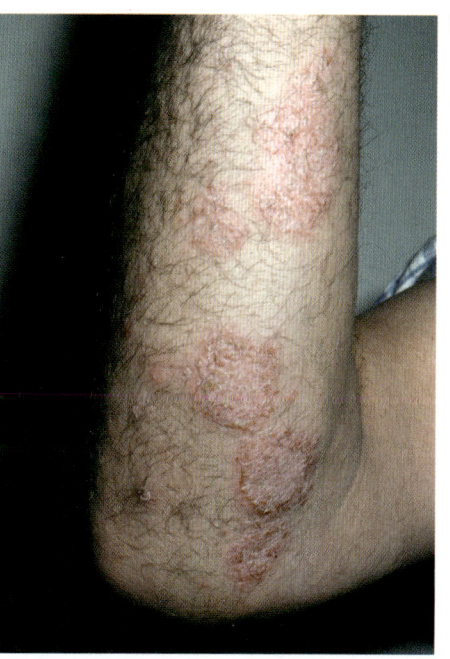

Fig. 5.38 Nummular eczema. *Courtesy Steven Binnick, MD.*

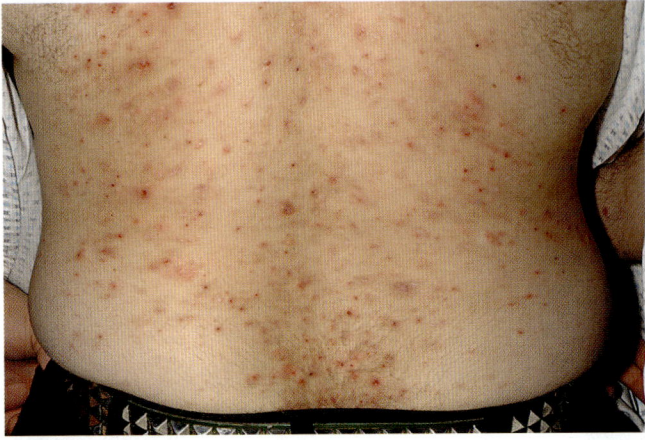

Fig. 5.39 Job's syndrome. *Courtesy Edward W. Cowen, MD.*

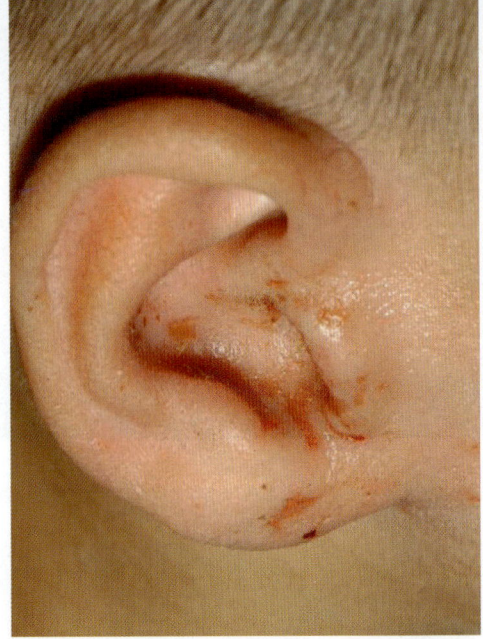

Fig. 5.40 Job's syndrome. *Courtesy Edward W. Cowen, MD.*

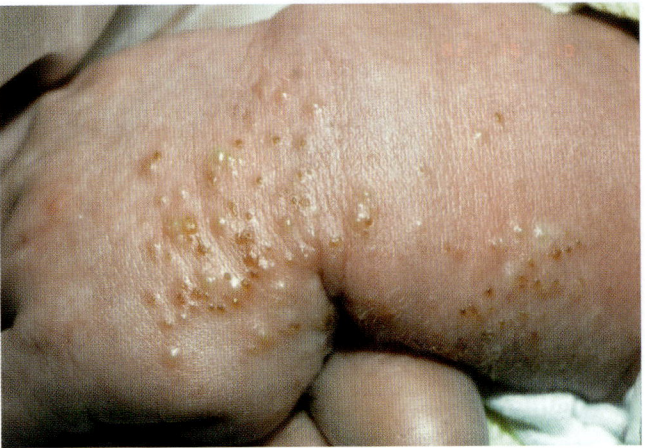

Fig. 5.41 Job's syndrome with secondary infection. *Courtesy Paul Honig, MD.*

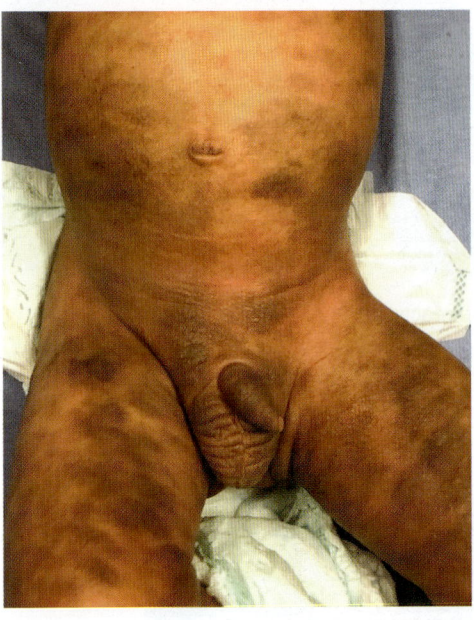

Fig. 5.42 Wiskott-Aldrich syndrome.

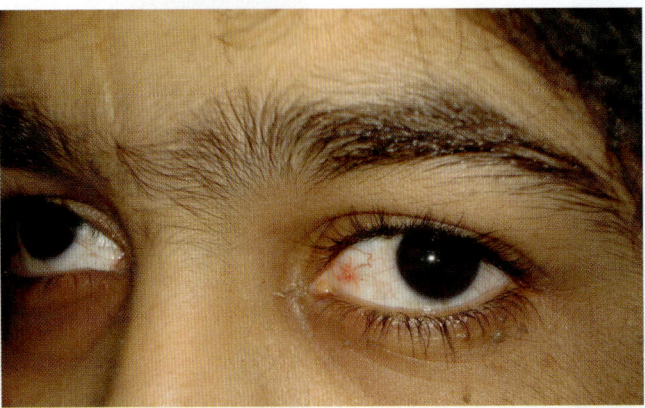

Fig. 5.43 Ataxia telangiectasia.

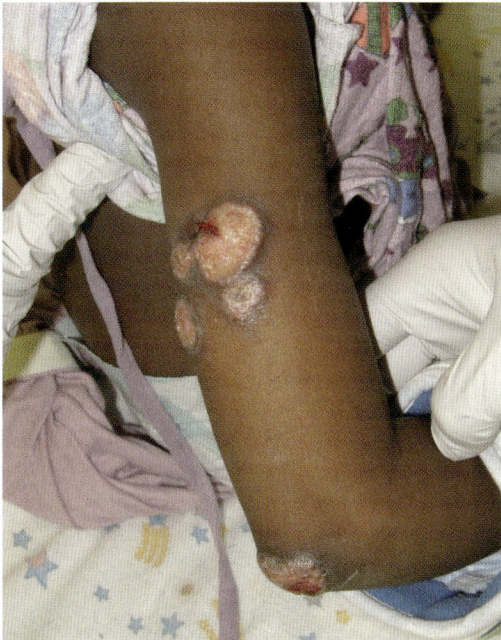

Fig. 5.44 Granulomatous lesions in ataxia telangiectasia.

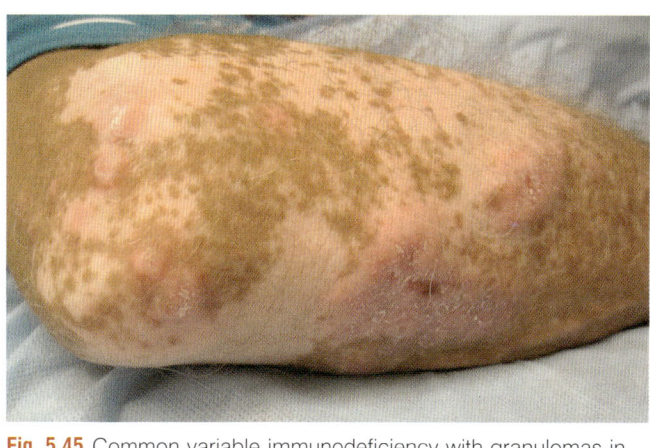

Fig. 5.45 Common variable immunodeficiency with granulomas in vitiligo.

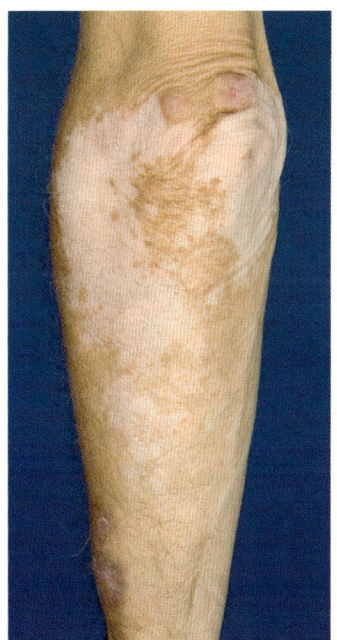

Fig. 5.46 Common variable immunodeficiency with granulomas in vitiligo.

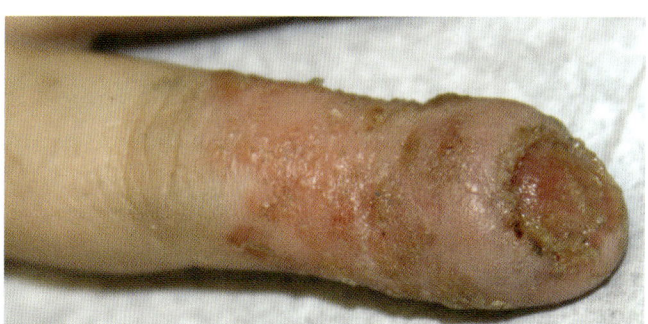

Fig. 5.47 Common variable immunodeficiency with chronic candidiasis.

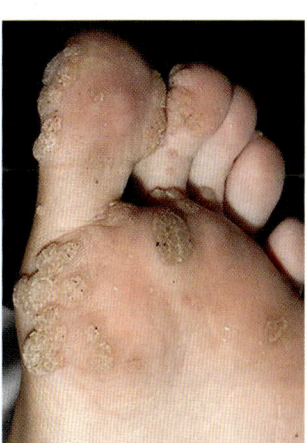

Fig. 5.48 Warts in DOCK8 immunodeficiency. *Courtesy Edward W. Cowen, MD.*

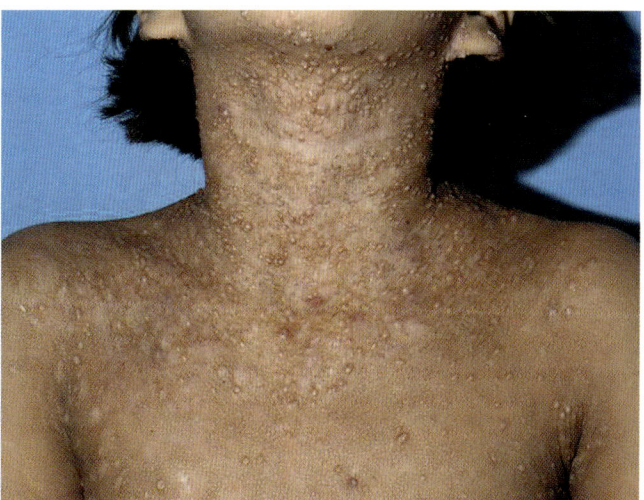

Fig. 5.49 Warts in DOCK8 immunodeficiency. *Courtesy Edward W. Cowen, MD.*

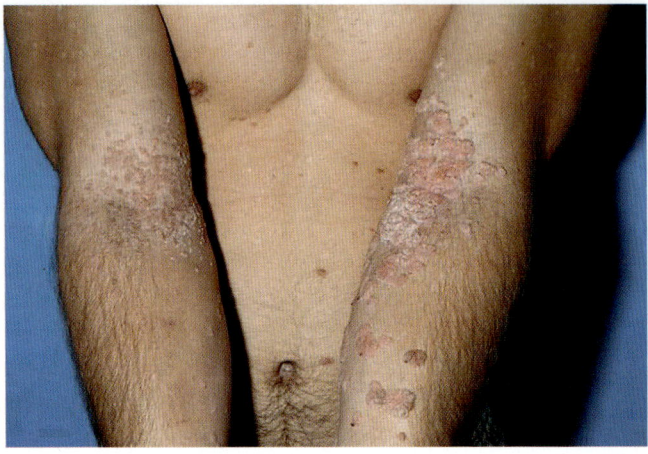

Fig. 5.50 Warts in DOCK8 immunodeficiency. *Courtesy Edward W. Cowen, MD.*

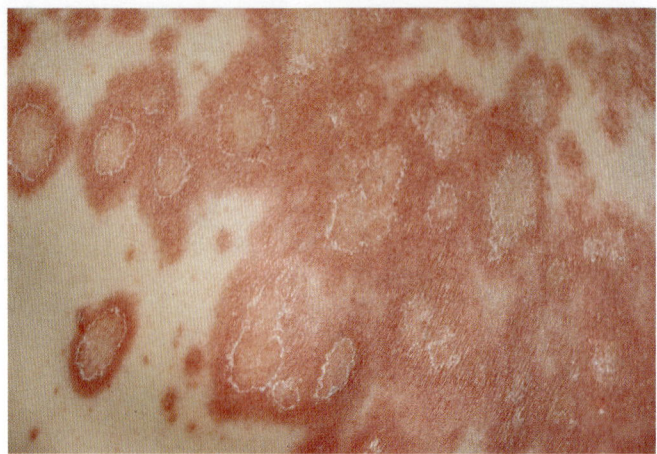

Fig. 5.51 Subacute lupus erythematosus as can be seen in complement deficiency disorders.

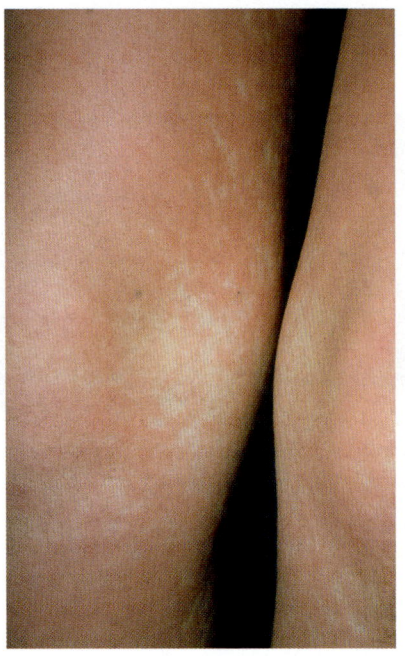

Fig. 5.52 Acute graft-versus-host disease.

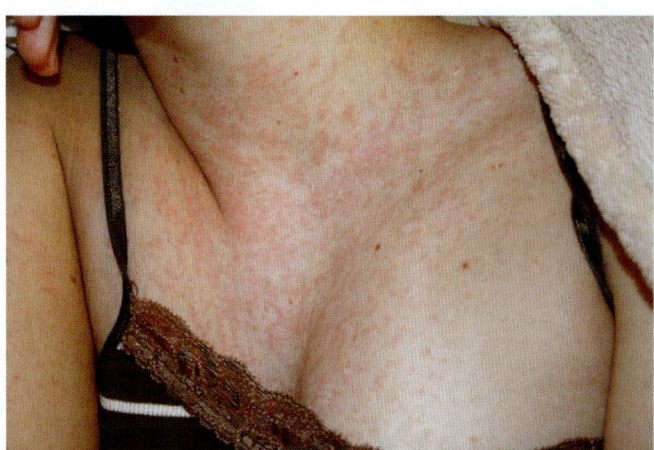

Fig. 5.53 Acute graft-versus-host disease, grade 2. *Courtesy Jennifer Huang, MD.*

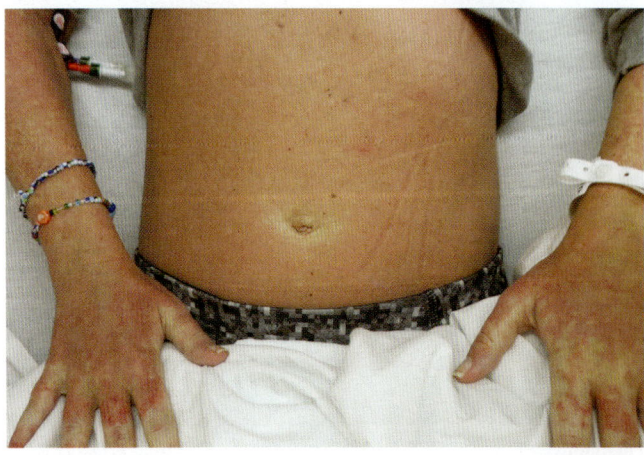

Fig. 5.54 Erythrodermic acute graft-versus-host disease, grade 3.

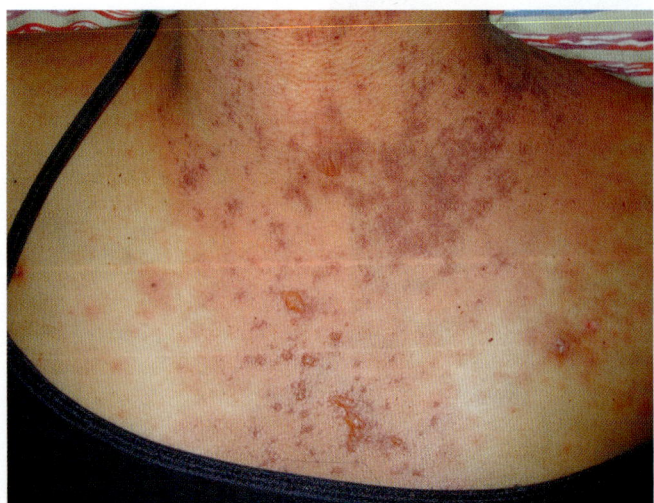

Fig. 5.55 Acute graft-versus-host disease, grade 4. *Courtesy Jennifer Huang, MD.*

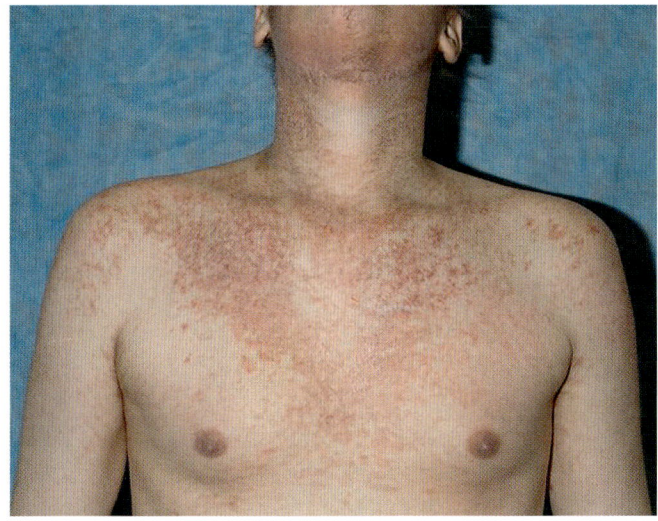

Fig. 5.56 Acute graft-versus-host disease. *Courtesy Edward W. Cowen, MD.*

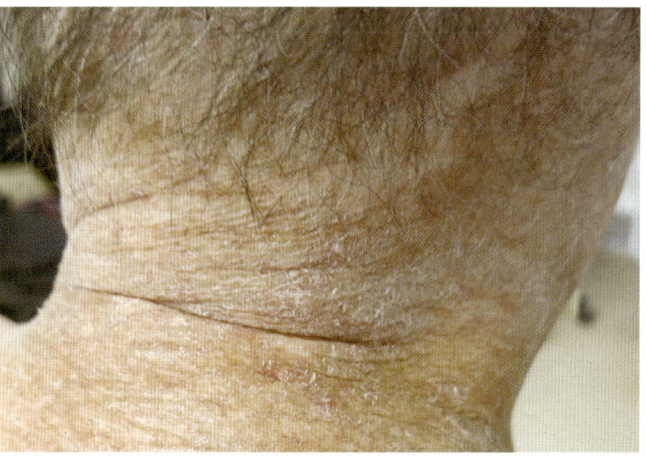

Fig. 5.57 Lichen planus–like chronic graft-versus-host disease.

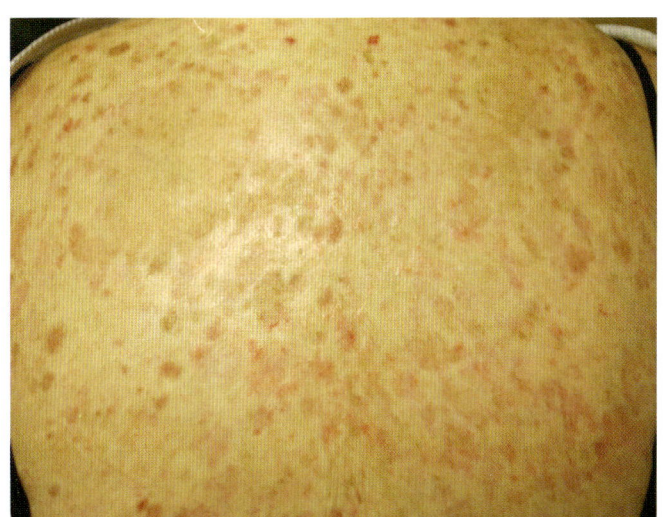

Fig. 5.58 Chronic graft-versus-host disease.

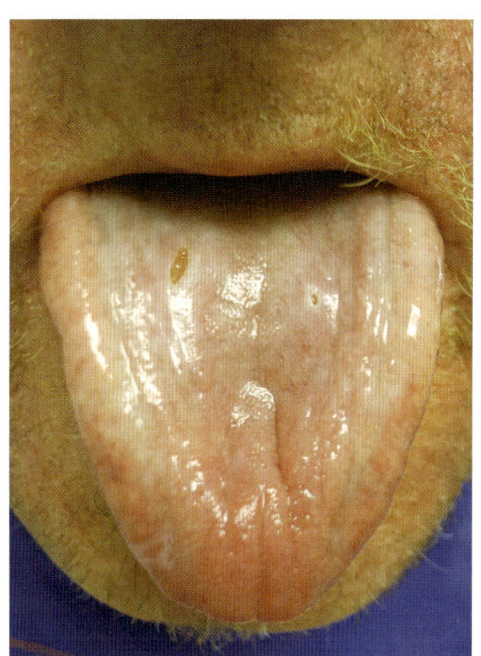

Fig. 5.59 Chronic graft-versus-host disease, oral.

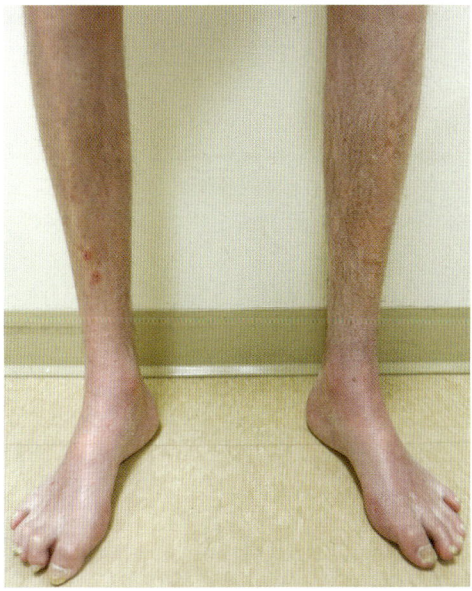

Fig. 5.60 Chronic graft-versus-host disease, scleroderma-like.

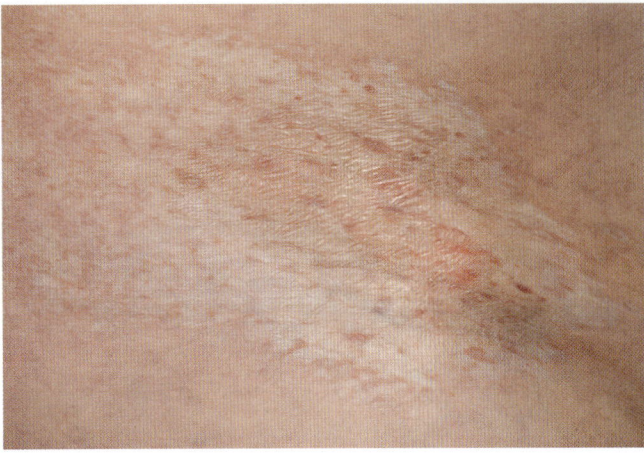

Fig. 5.61 Chronic graft-versus-host disease. *Courtesy Edward W. Cowen, MD.*

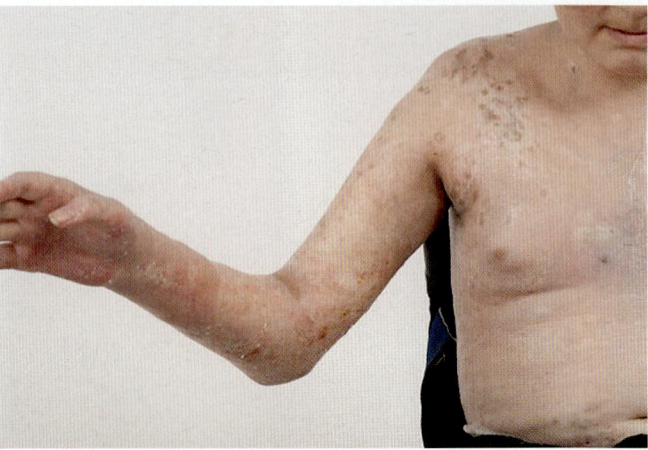

Fig. 5.62 Sclerodermoid graft-versus-host disease. *Courtesy Edward W. Cowen, MD.*

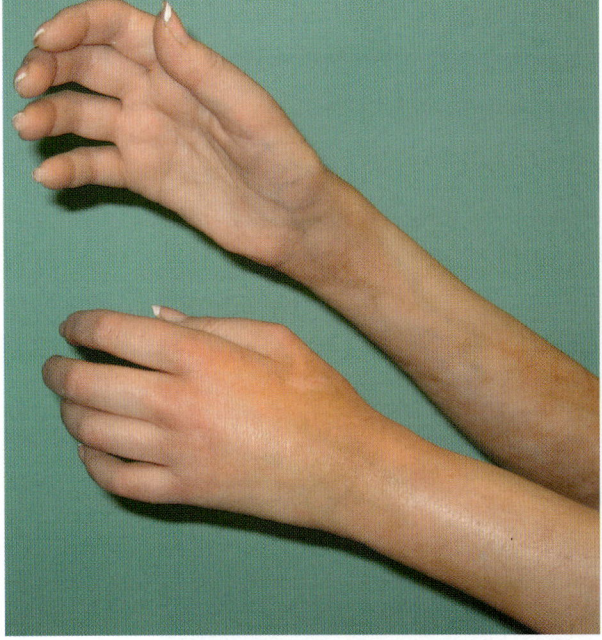

Fig. 5.63 Sclerodermoid graft-versus-host disease. *Courtesy Edward W. Cowen, MD.*

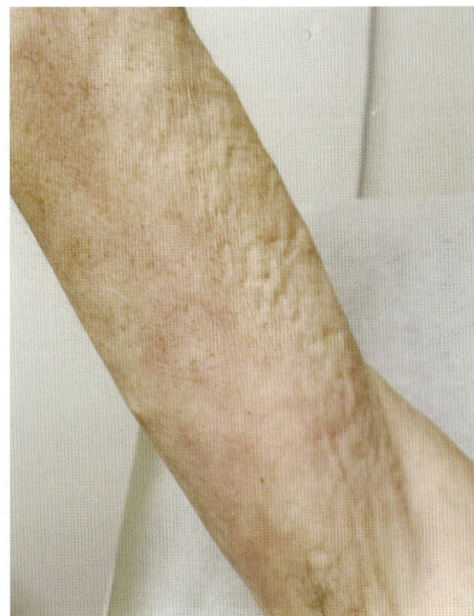

Fig. 5.64 Fasciitis in chronic graft-versus-host disease.

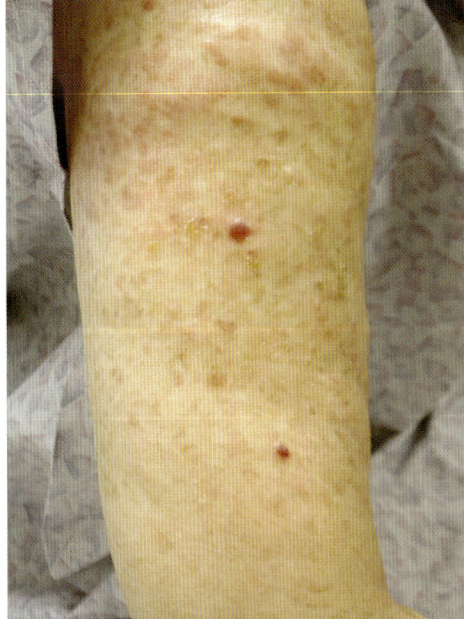

Fig. 5.65 Angiomatosis associated with chronic graft-versus-host disease.

Contact Dermatitis and Drug Eruptions

Contact dermatitis and cutaneous drug eruptions are both skin conditions triggered by external agents that are either in direct contact with the skin or ingested. Contact dermatitis shares many features with atopic dermatitis and eczema, including pruritus, erythema, scaling, oozing, and crusting. However, in the case of contact dermatitis, major clues to the diagnosis are the shapes found on the skin that demonstrate the particular locations of contact by the external irritant or allergic stimuli. These shapes can be classically *linear* like *Toxicodendron dermatitis* (poison ivy); *geometric* such as seen secondary to adhesives; in a *splattered pattern* secondary to liquid irritants (e.g., acids); or in the case of airborne triggers such as fragrances, concentrated on the face, neck, and other exposed regions of the body. Noting the location of the affected body part or parts is especially helpful in diagnosing contact dermatitis, such as the lower abdomen and ears in nickel dermatitis, dorsal feet in shoe dermatitis, and eyelids in dermatitis secondary to ingredients in nail polish. Other contact reactions can be more widespread, as is the case in some patients with atopic dermatitis and concomitant contact dermatitis due to preservatives or fragrances in lotions and detergents, respectively.

Cutaneous drug eruptions can be quite varied in their presentations, ranging from the sheets of micropustules overlying patches of broad erythema seen in acute generalized exanthematous pustulosis to the hemorrhagic mucosal erosions and vesicobullous lesions seen in Stevens-Johnson syndrome and toxic epidermal necrolysis. It is imperative to screen patients for associated features on physical examination such as fever, lymphadenopathy, and facial edema that can help distinguish a systemic drug hypersensitivity reaction such as drug reaction with eosinophilia and systemic symptoms (DRESS) from a simple morbilliform drug eruption. Blood work may also be needed in some patients with suspected DRESS to screen for eosinophilia, atypical lymphocytes, and evidence of end organ damage. Other drug eruptions may be more unique, such as the striking, deeply erythematous, circular patches and plaques of fixed drug eruptions or painful palmoplantar plaques of toxic erythema of chemotherapy. Because new medications are being produced every year, it is also important to remain knowledgeable about the diverse idiosyncratic drug eruptions such as the erosive psoriasiform scalp and posterior auricular plaques seen in individuals treated with tumor necrosis factor inhibitors.

This portion of the atlas will highlight the cutaneous patterns created by contact dermatitis, as well as the variety of skin findings seen in the setting of both mild and severe drug eruptions.

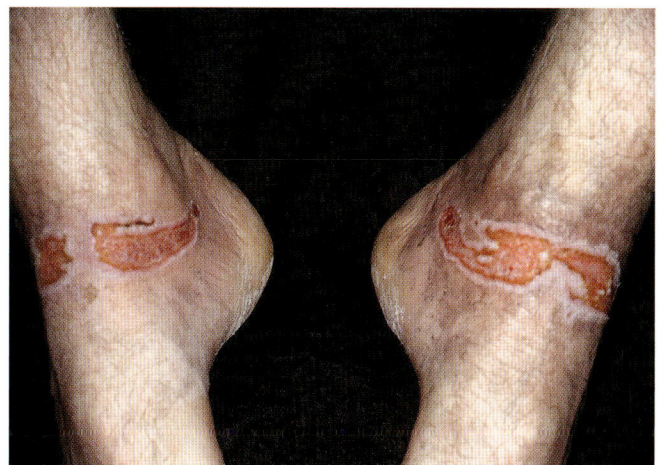

Fig. 6.1 Cement burns. *Courtesy Steven Binnick, MD.*

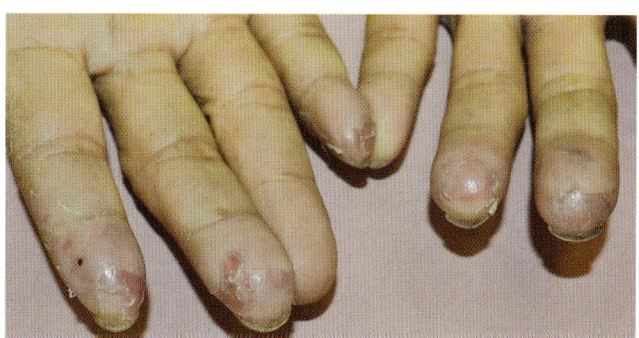

Fig. 6.2 Hydrofluoric acid burn. *Courtesy National Cheng Kung University, Taiwan.*

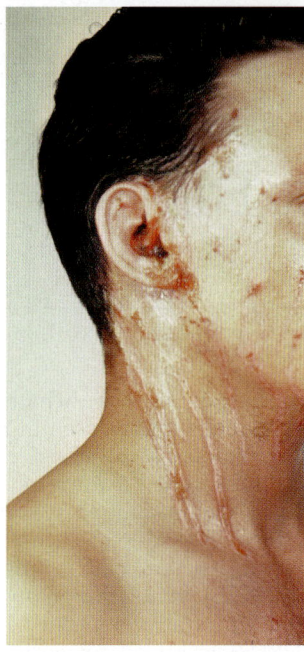

Fig. 6.3 Drip burn from acid solution.

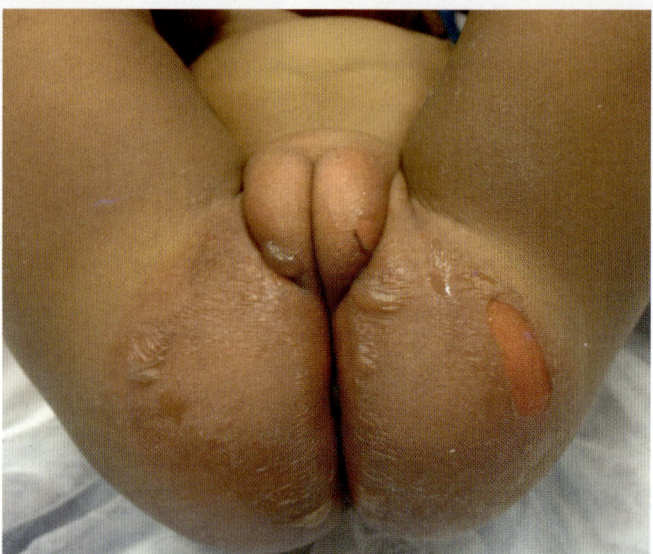

Fig. 6.4 Senna burn.

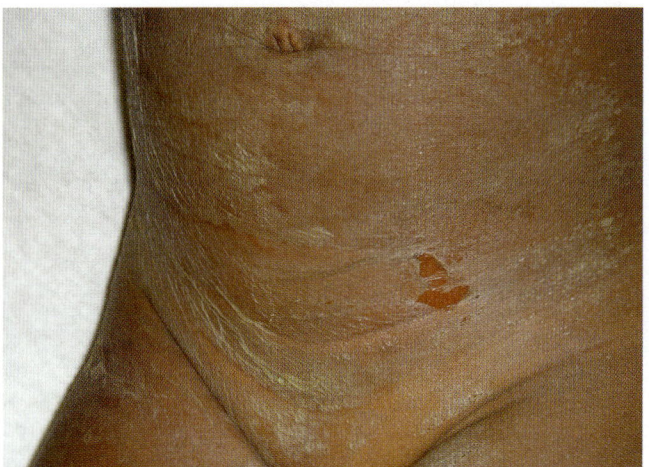

Fig. 6.5 Pesticide burn.

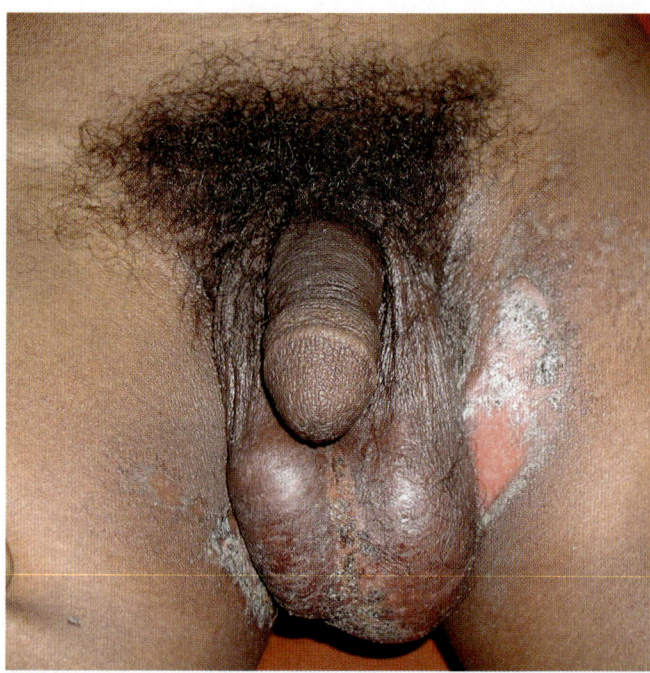

Fig. 6.6 Irritant dermatitis from kerosene. *Courtesy Shyam Verma, MBBS, DVD.*

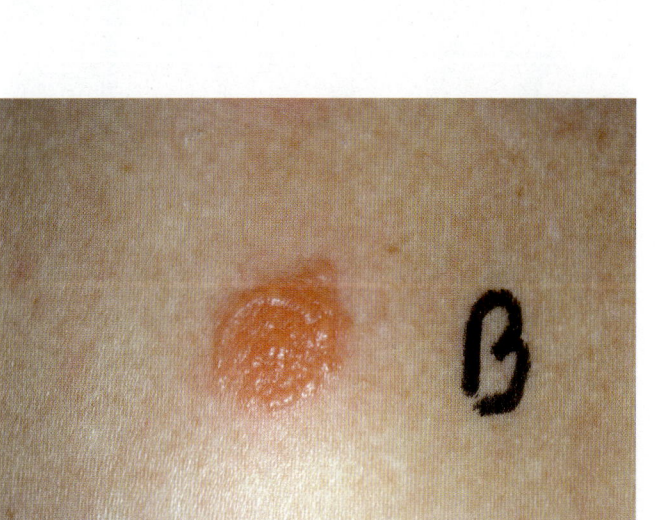

Fig. 6.7 Positive patch test result.

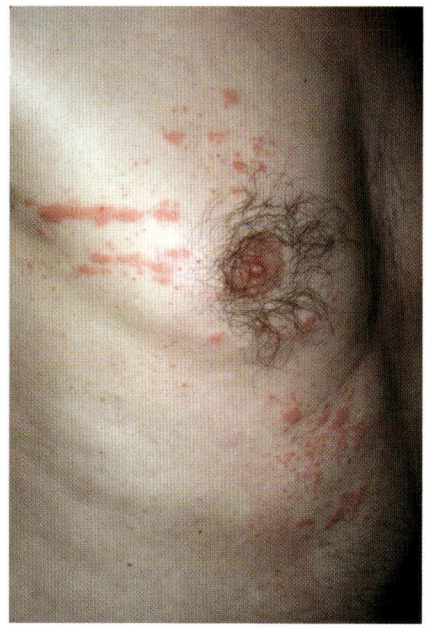

Fig. 6.8 Poison ivy dermatitis; note linear lesions.

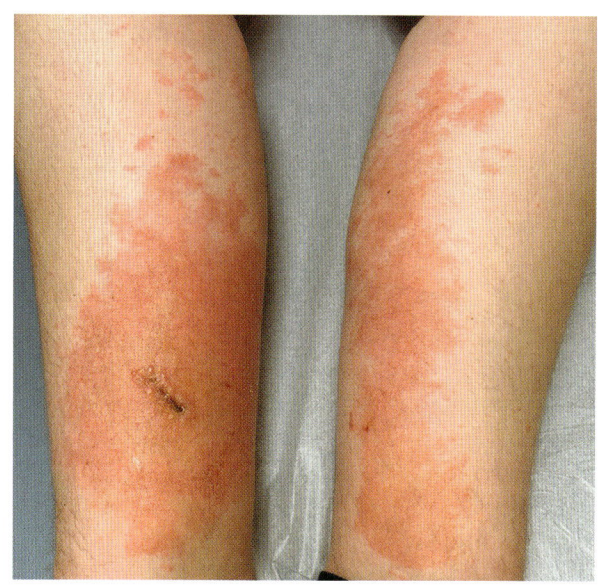

Fig. 6.9 Black dot poison ivy dermatitis.

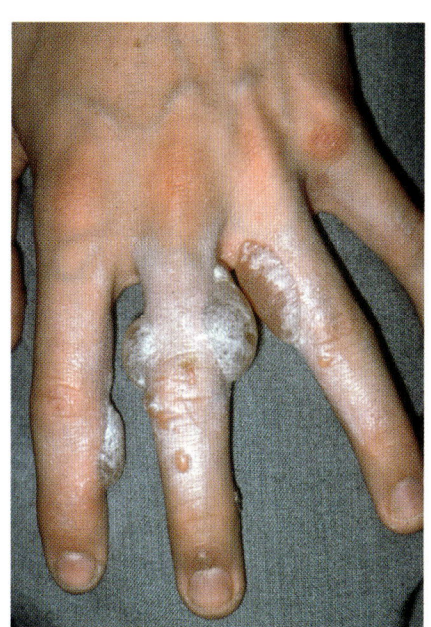

Fig. 6.10 Poison ivy dermatitis.

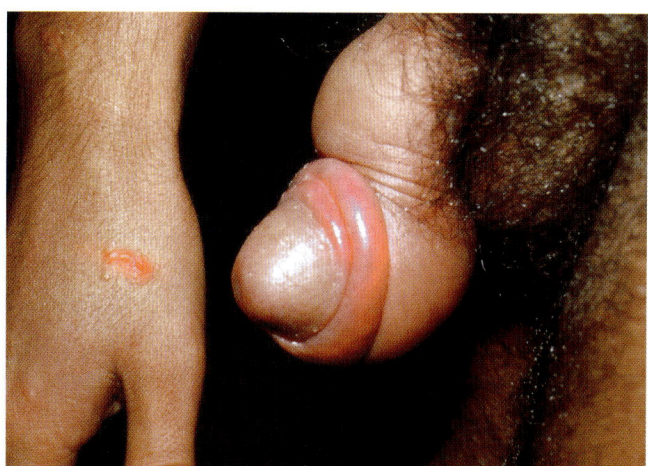

Fig. 6.11 Poison ivy dermatitis.

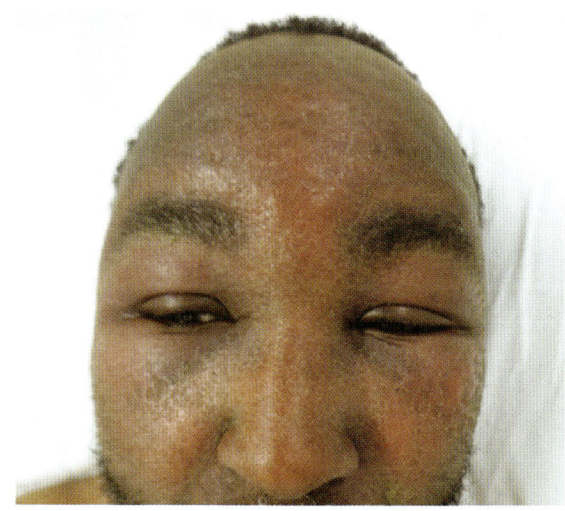

Fig. 6.12 Aerosolized contact dermatitis.

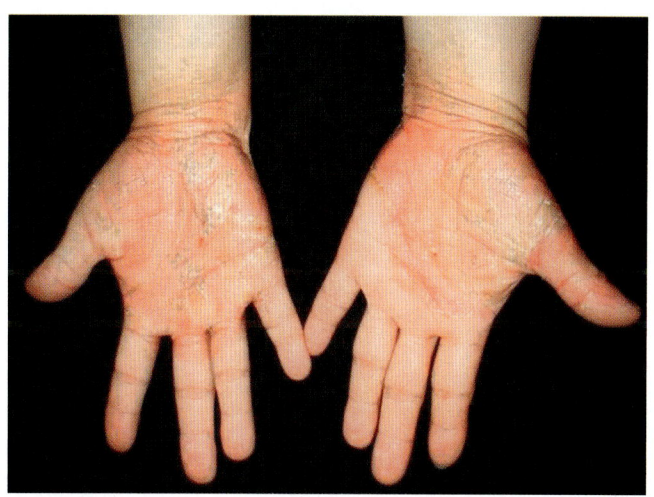

Fig. 6.13 Tea tree oil dermatitis. *Courtesy Glen Crawford, MD.*

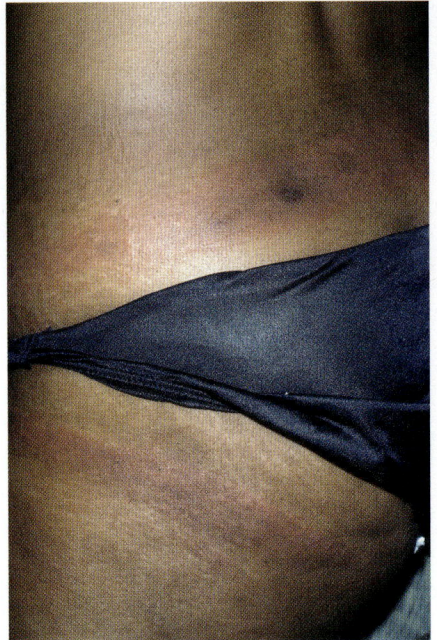

Fig. 6.14 Clothing contact dermatitis.

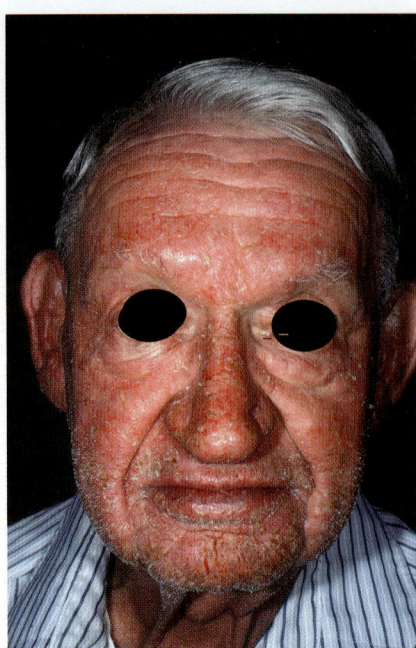

Fig. 6.15 Compositae dermatitis. *Courtesy The University of Utah and Oregon Health Sciences University Leonard Swinyer MD image collection*

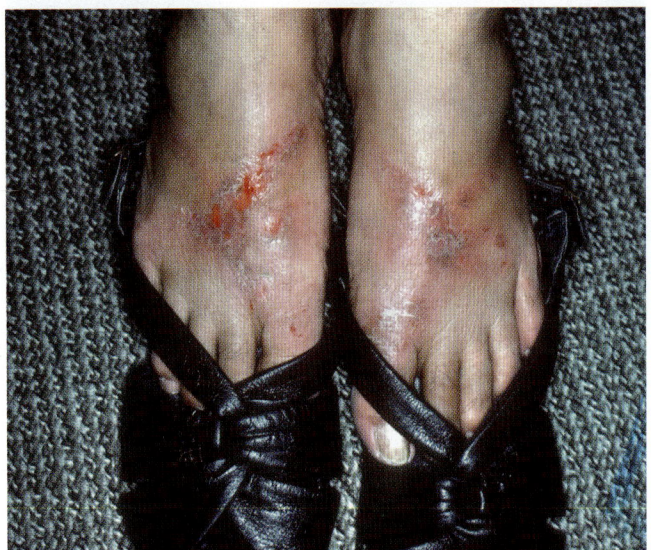

Fig. 6.16 Acute shoe dermatitis.

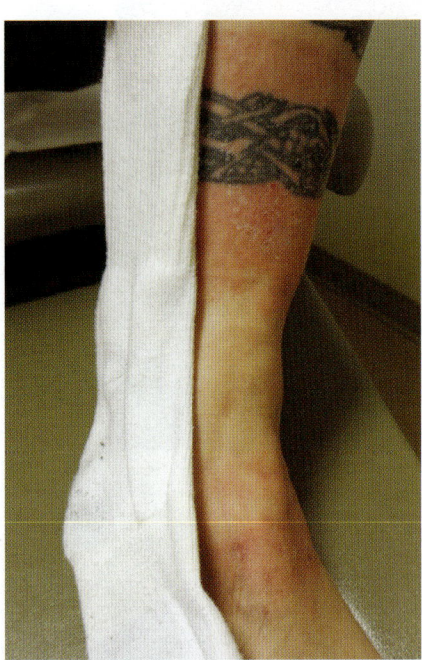

Fig. 6.17 Contact dermatitis caused by elastic in sock.

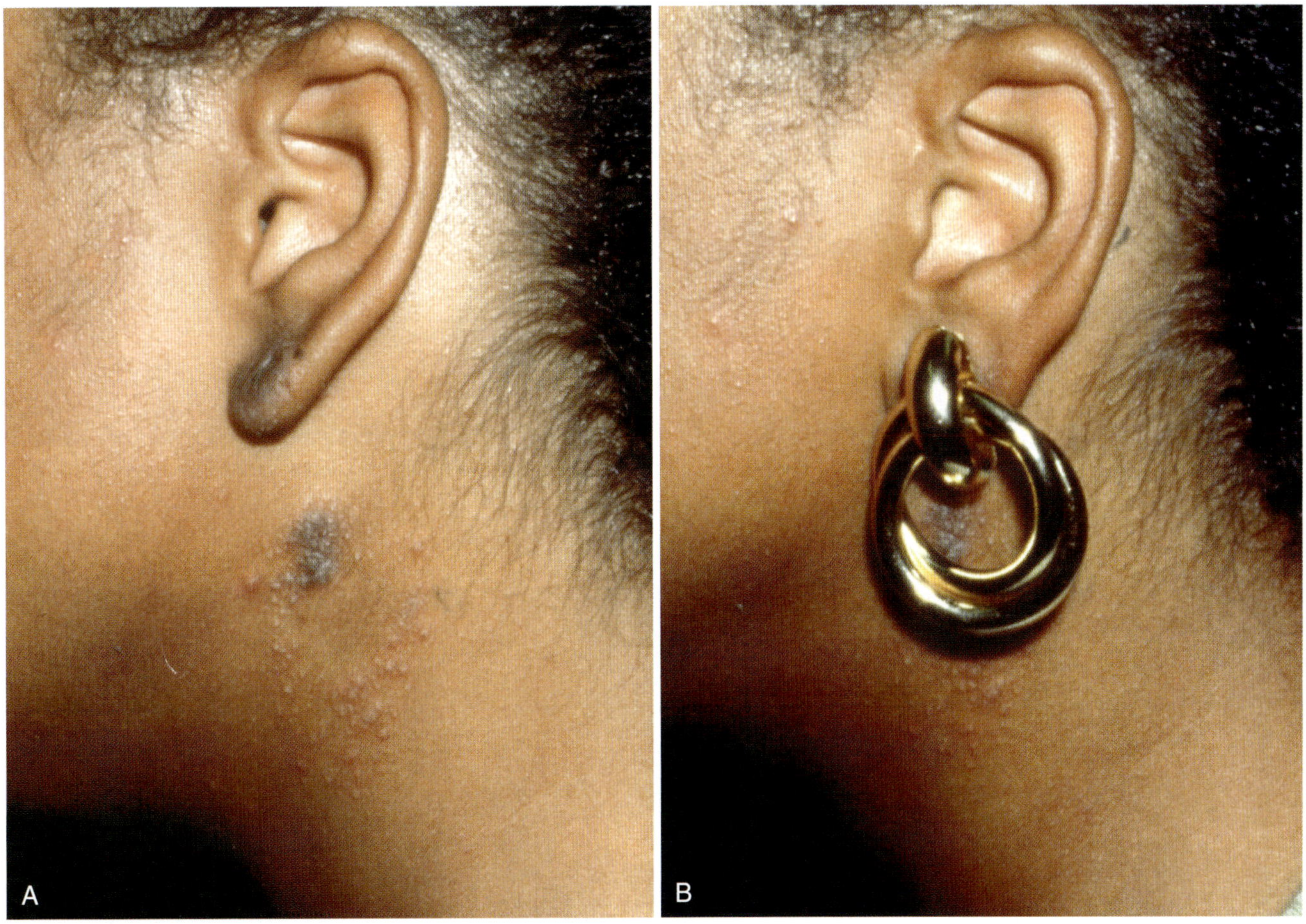

Fig. 6.18 (A) Nickel dermatitis. (B) With earrings on.

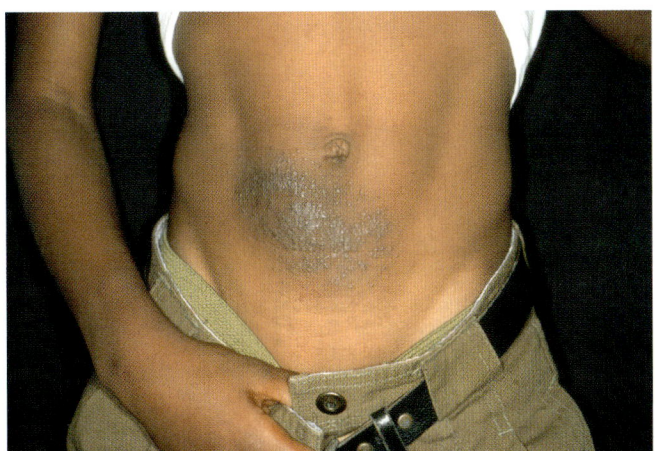

Fig. 6.19 Nickel dermatitis.

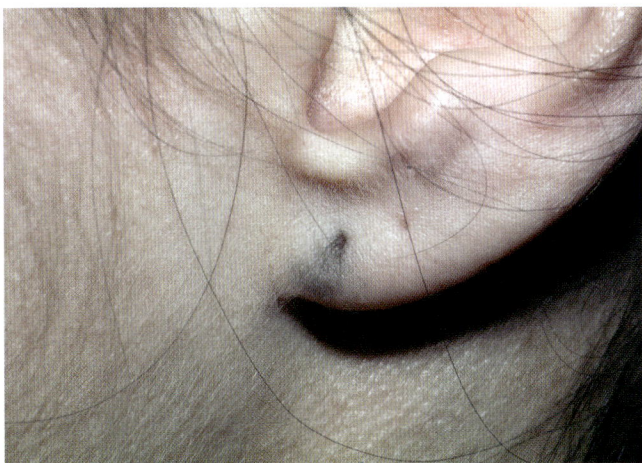

Fig. 6.20 Black dermatographism. *Courtesy Steven Binnick, MD.*

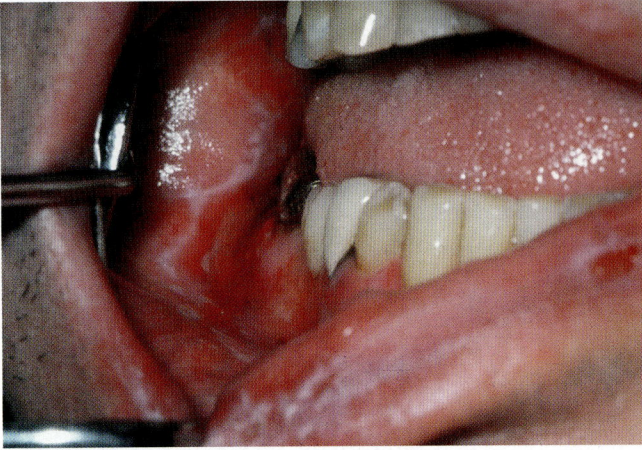
Fig. 6.21 Oral lichenoid dermatitis caused by gold.

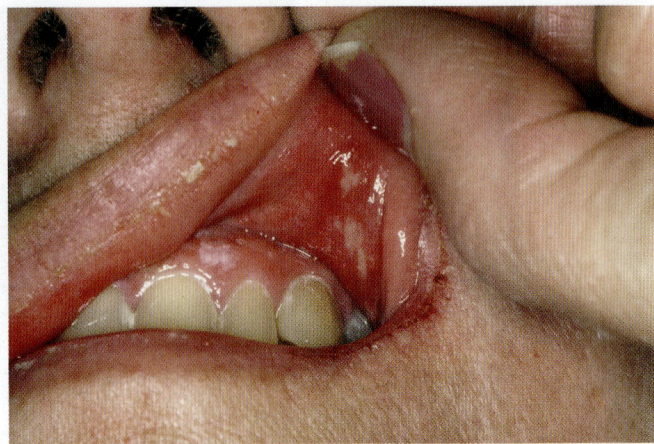
Fig. 6.22 Stomatitis caused by dental impression material allergy.

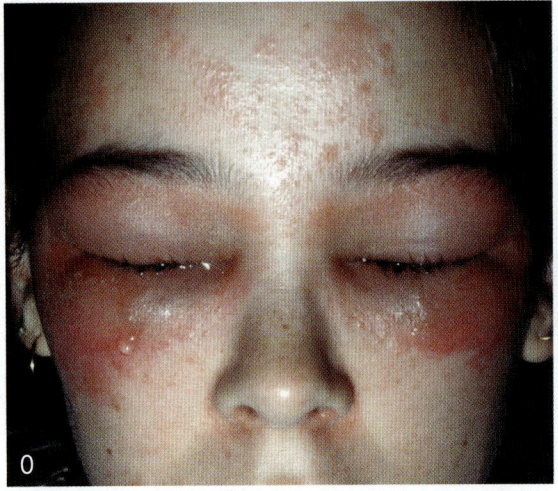
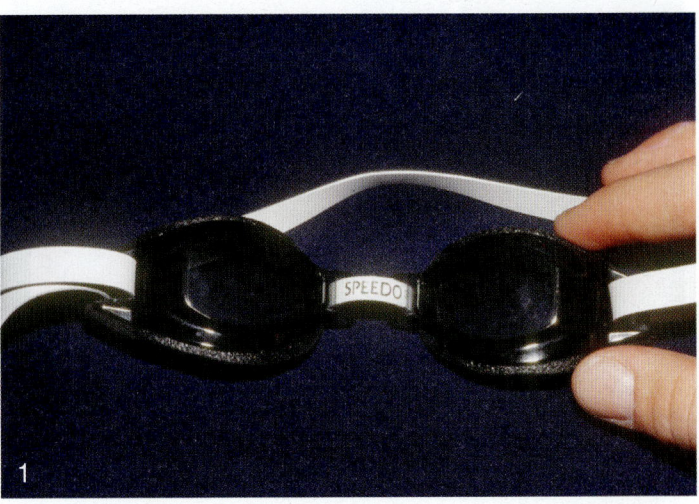
Fig. 6.23 (A) Rubber dermatitis. (B) Culprit swim goggles.

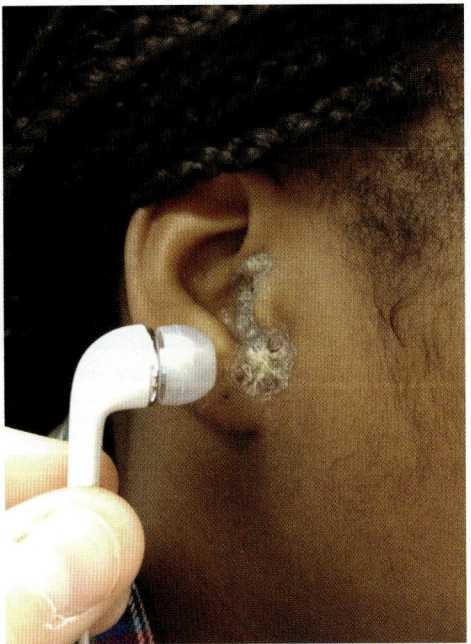
Fig. 6.24 Earbud dermatitis.

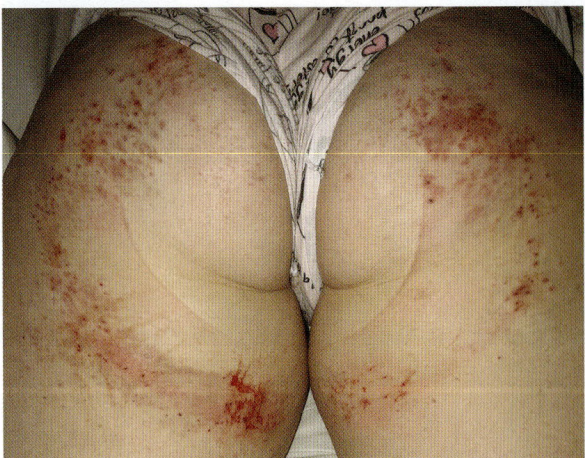
Fig. 6.25 Contact dermatitis caused by toilet seat cleaner.

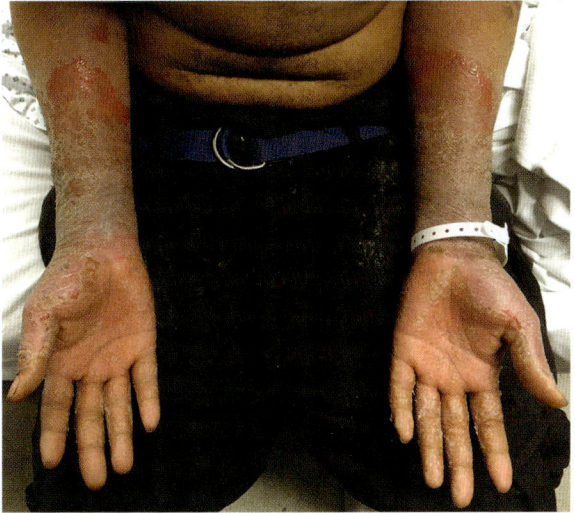

Fig. 6.26 Patient seen in the emergency department for occupational contact dermatitis (gloves).

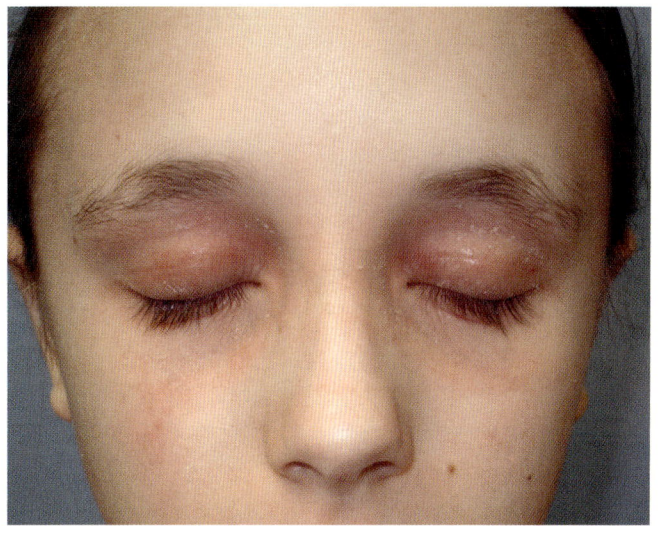

Fig. 6.27 Eyelid dermatitis secondary to nail polish.

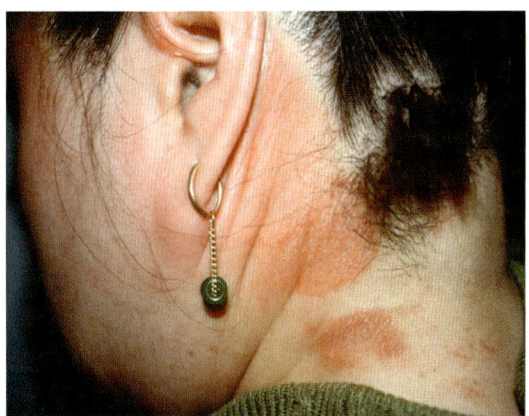

Fig. 6.28 Parapheylenediamine allergy from hair dye. *Courtesy Chia-Yu Chu, MD, PhD.*

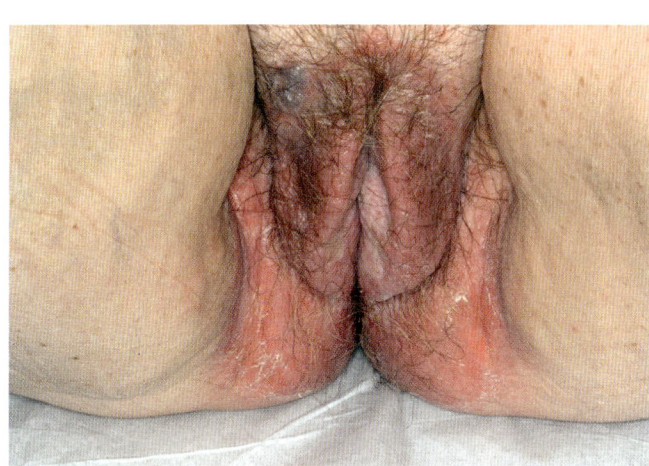

Fig. 6.29 Vulvar dermatitis secondary to preservatives.

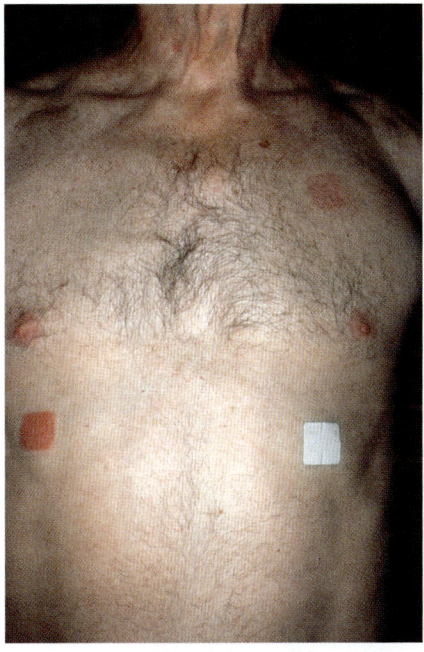

Fig. 6.30 Clonidine patch allergy.

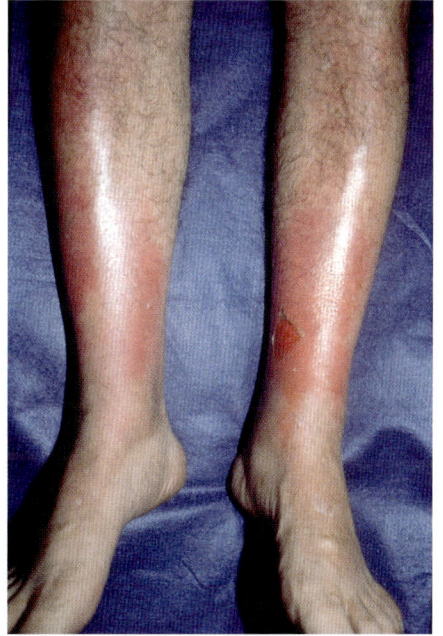

Fig. 6.31 Allergy to benzocaine.

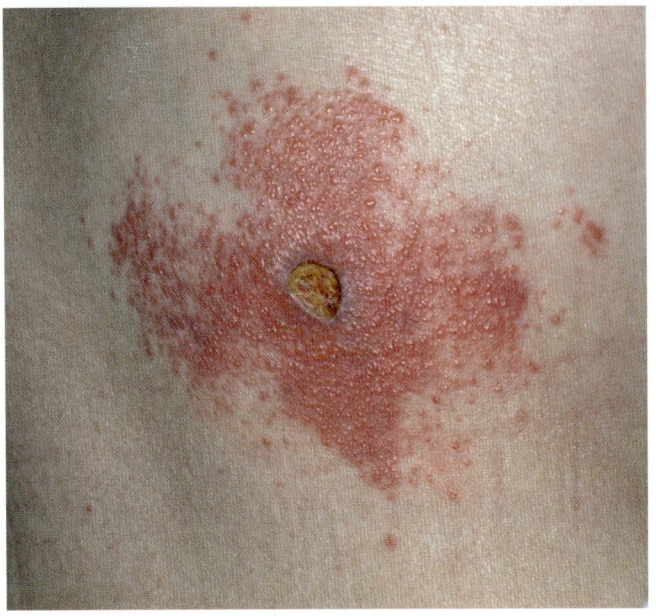

Fig. 6.32 Allergy to topical antibiotic.

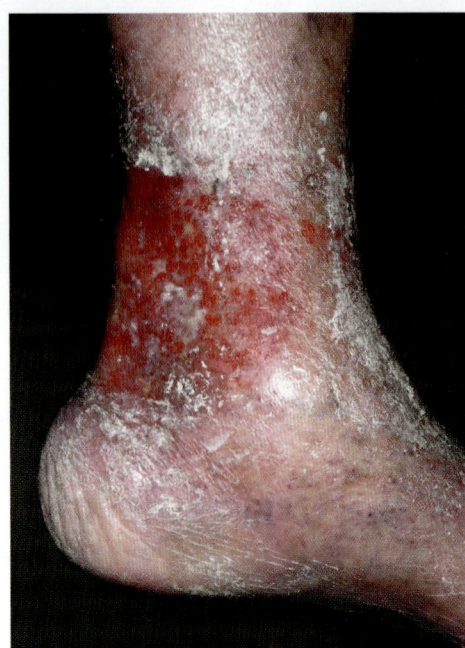

Fig. 6.33 Leg ulcer with contact dermatitis caused by topical antibiotic allergy.

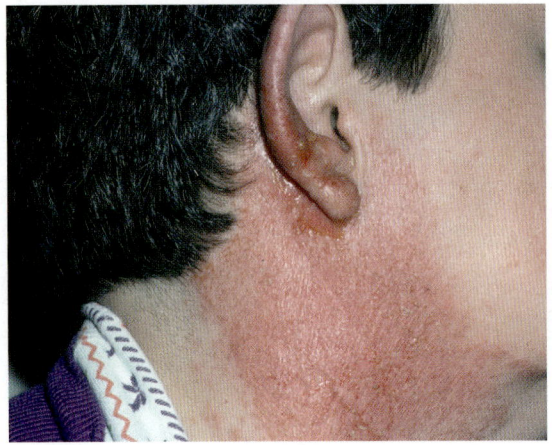

Fig. 6.34 Contact allergy to topical steroids.

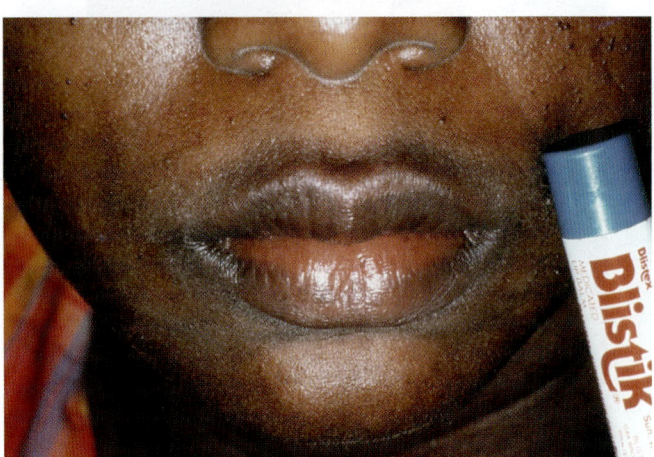

Fig. 6.35 Contact cheilitis to Blistik.

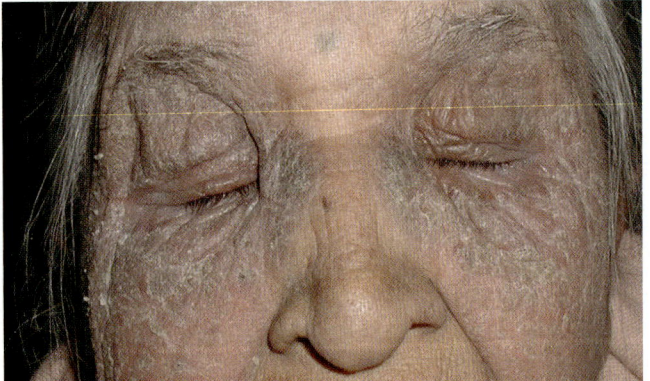

Fig. 6.36 Contact dermatitis to eye drops. *Courtesy Shyam Verma, MBBS, DVD.*

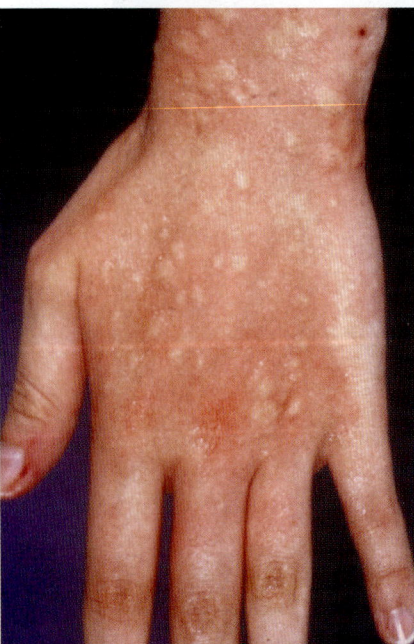

Fig. 6.37 Contact urticaria to surgical gloves. *Courtesy Arto Lahti, MD.*

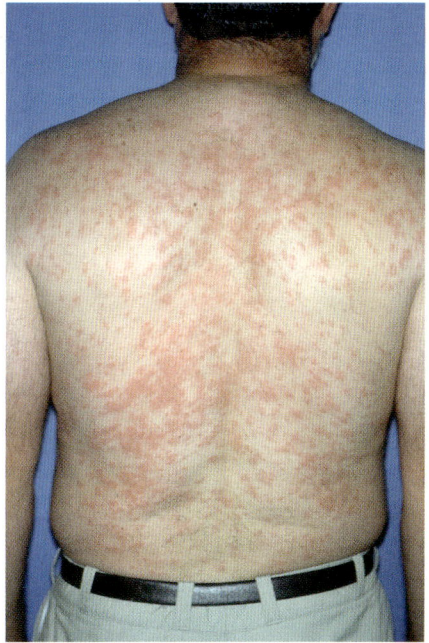

Fig. 6.38 Drug eruption.

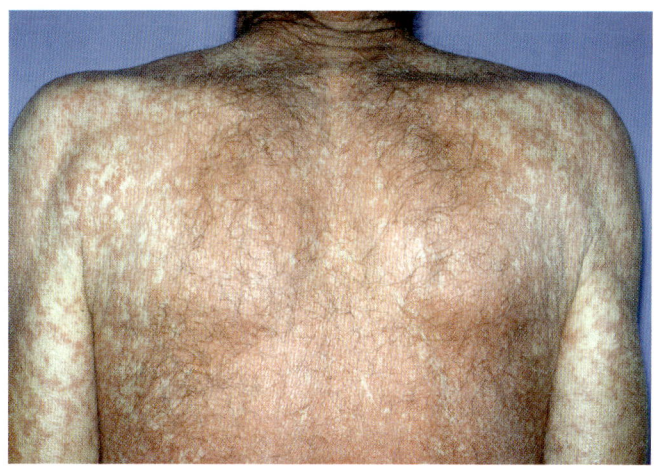

Fig. 6.39 Drug eruption.

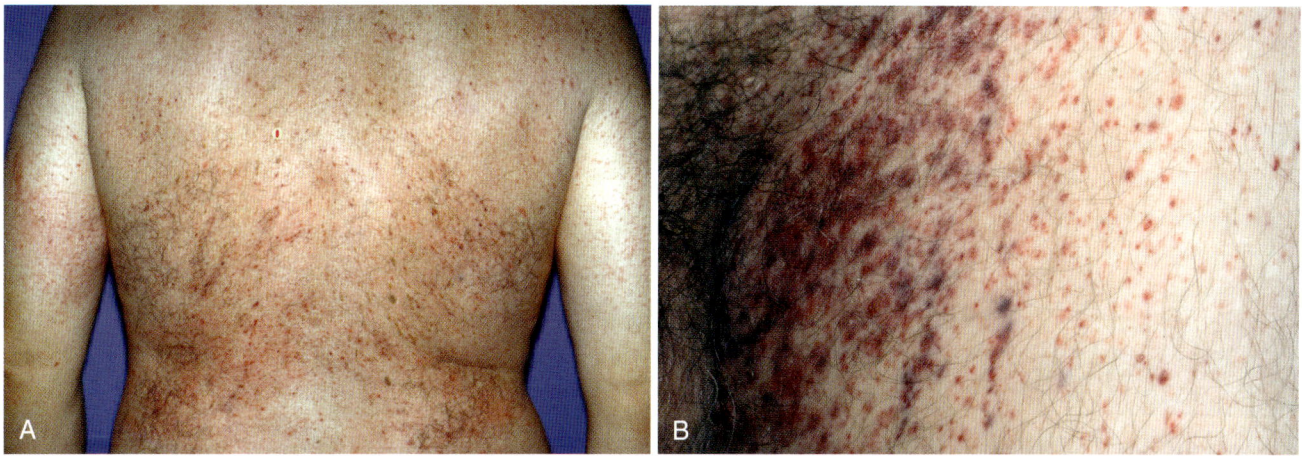

Fig. 6.40 (A) Drug eruption in leukemic patient. (B) Drug eruption in leukemic patient with low platelet count. The exanthem may be purpuric.

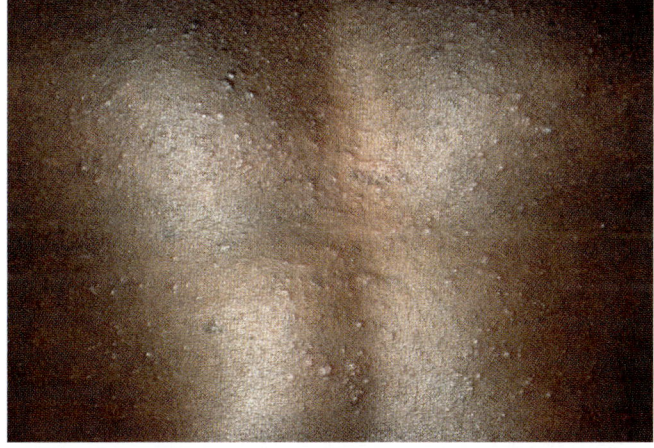

Fig. 6.41 Phenytoin-induced drug reaction with eosinophilia and systemic symptoms.

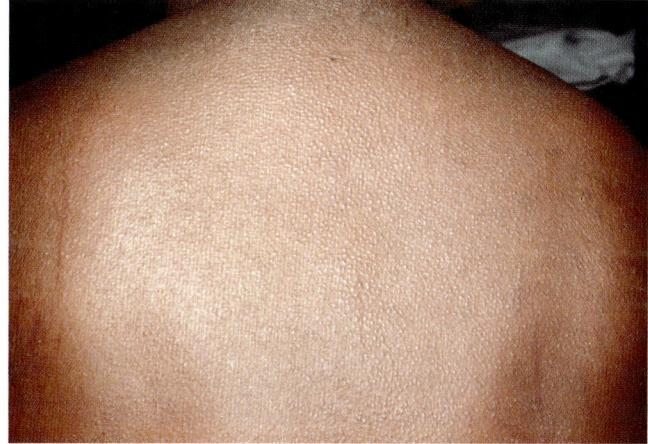

Fig. 6.42 Phenytoin-induced drug reaction with eosinophilia and systemic symptoms.

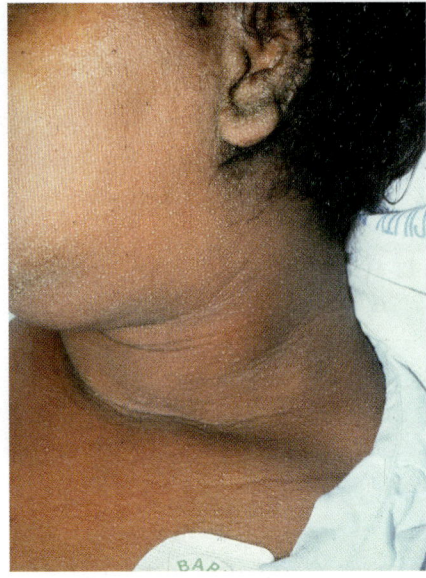

Fig. 6.43 Phenytoin-induced drug reaction with eosinophilia and systemic symptoms.

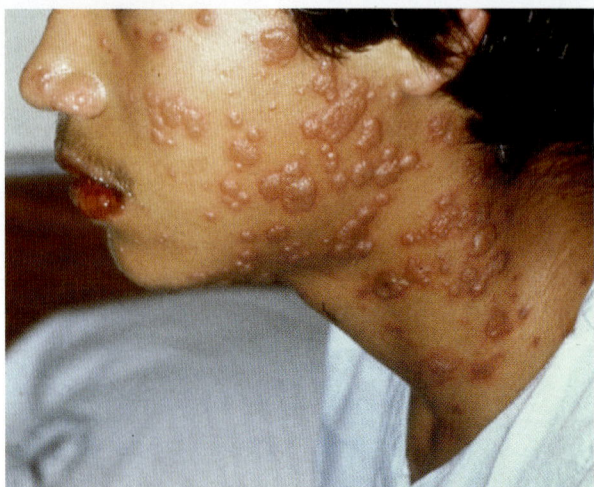

Fig. 6.44 *Mycoplasma*-induced rash and mucositis (formerly *Mycoplasma*-induced Stevens-Johnson syndrome).

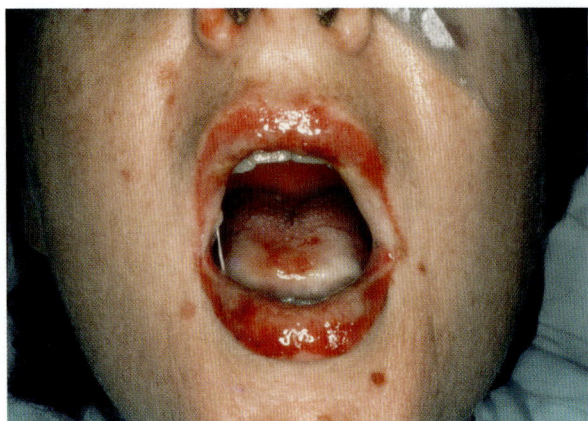

Fig. 6.45 Stevens-Johnson syndrome.

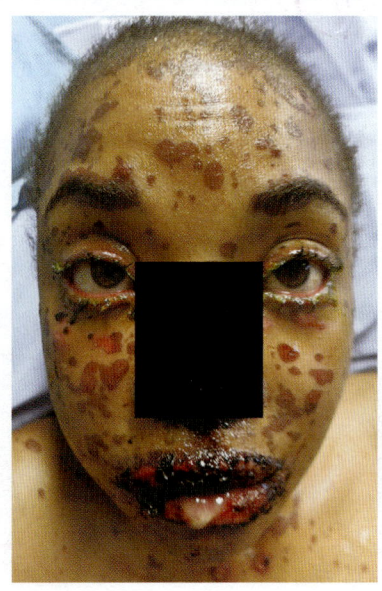

Fig. 6.46 Stevens-Johnson syndrome.

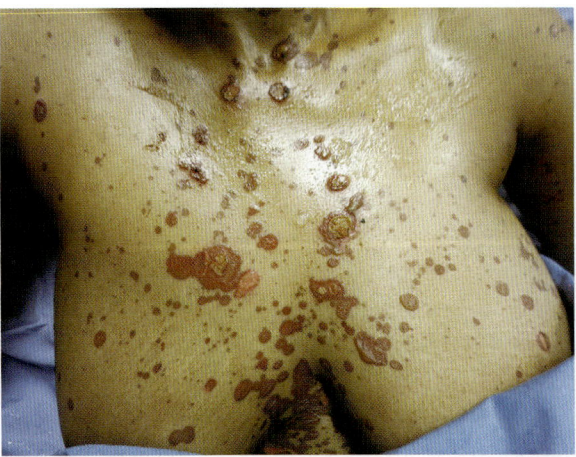

Fig. 6.47 Stevens-Johnson syndrome.

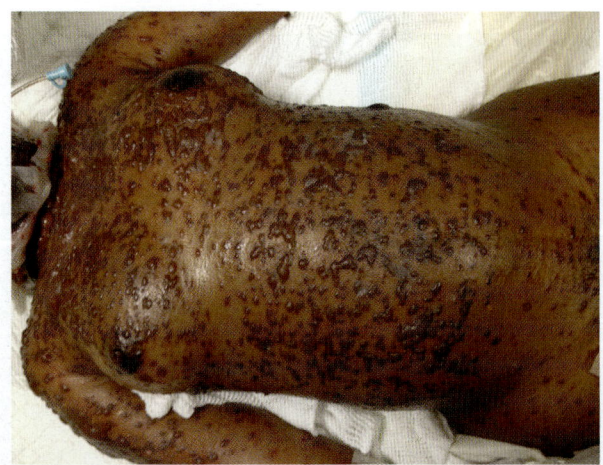

Fig. 6.48 Toxic epidermal necrolysis to lamotrigine.

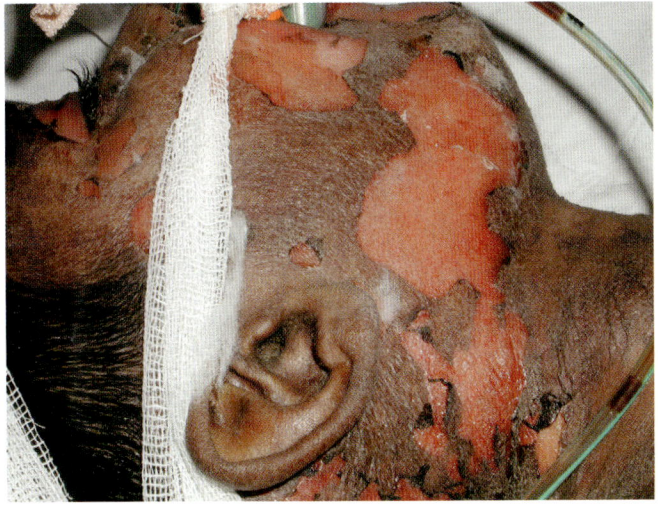

Fig. 6.49 Toxic epidermal necrolysis to lamotrigine.

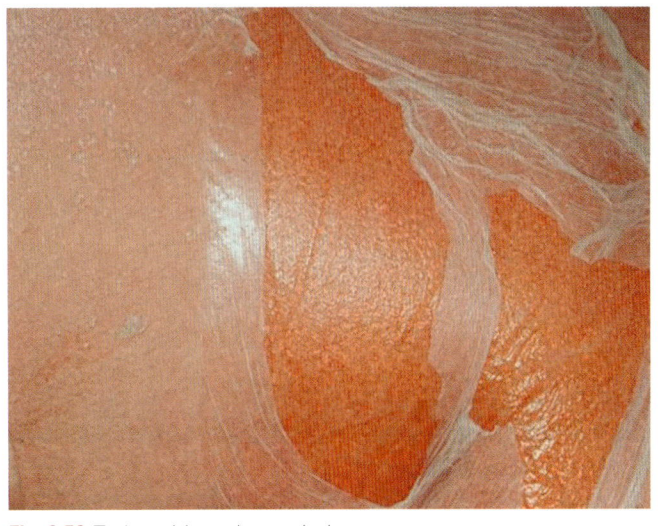

Fig. 6.50 Toxic epidermal necrolysis.

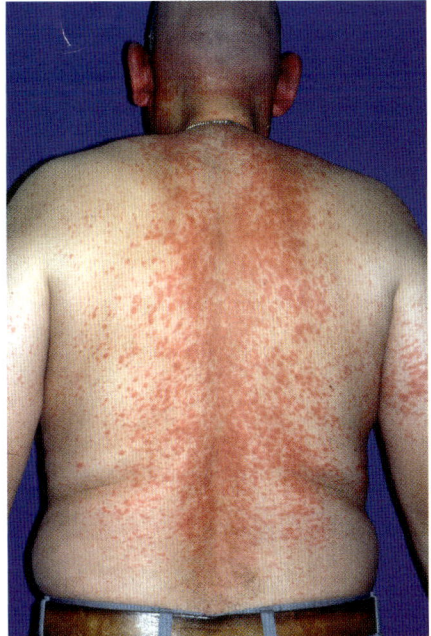

Fig. 6.51 Phenytoin plus radiation-induced reaction.

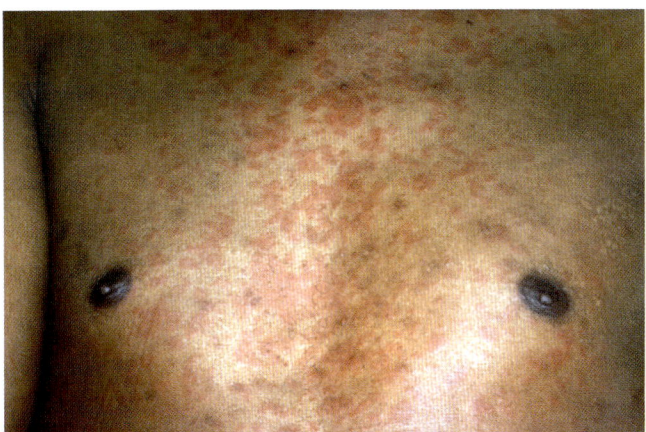

Fig. 6.52 Sulfa allergy in an HIV-infected patient.

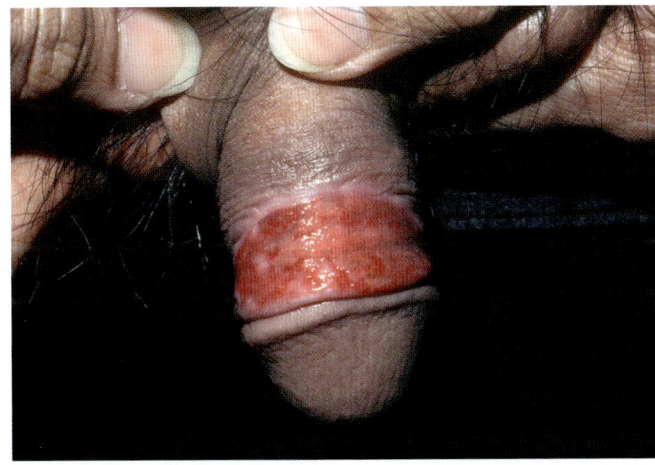

Fig. 6.53 Fixed drug reaction. *Courtesy Steven Binnick, MD.*

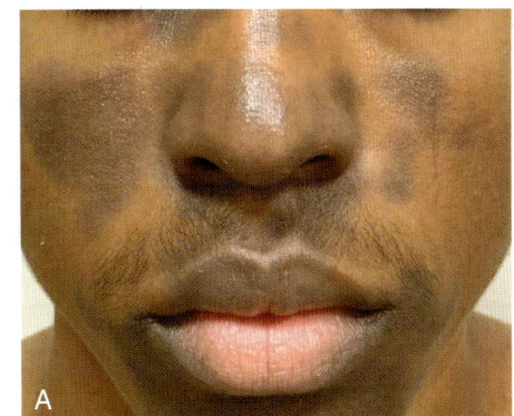
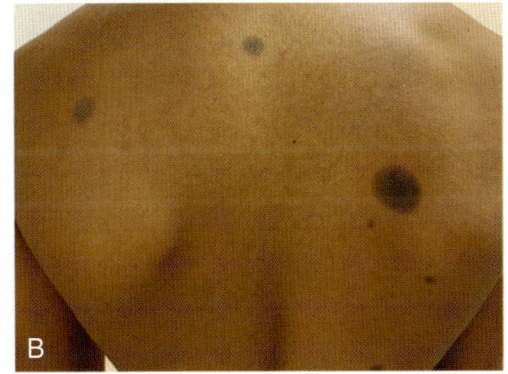

Fig. 6.54 (A) and (B) Fixed drug reaction.

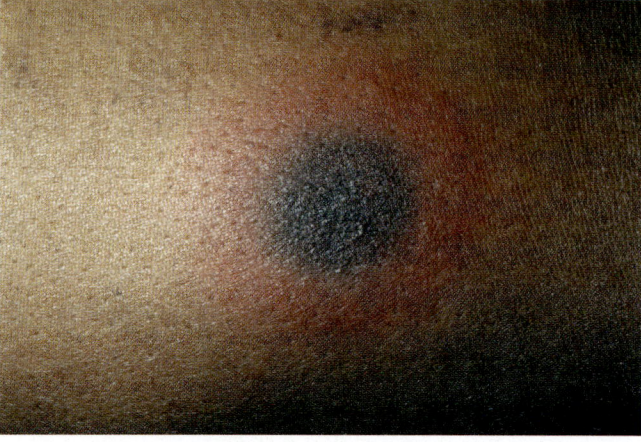

Fig. 6.55 Fixed drug reaction.

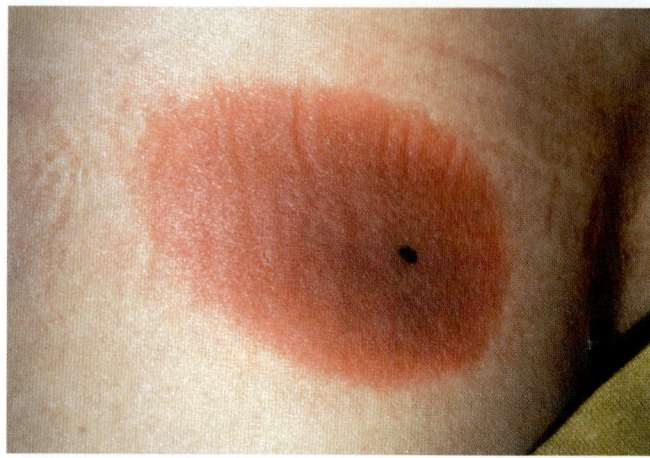

Fig. 6.56 Fixed drug reaction.

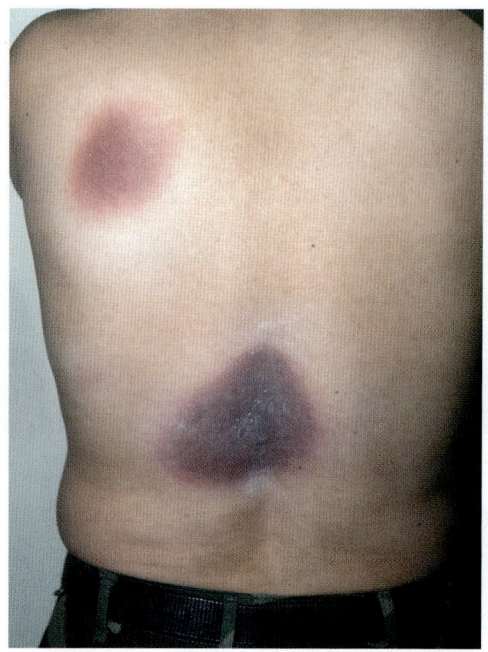

Fig. 6.57 Fixed drug reaction. *Courtesy Steven Binnick, MD.*

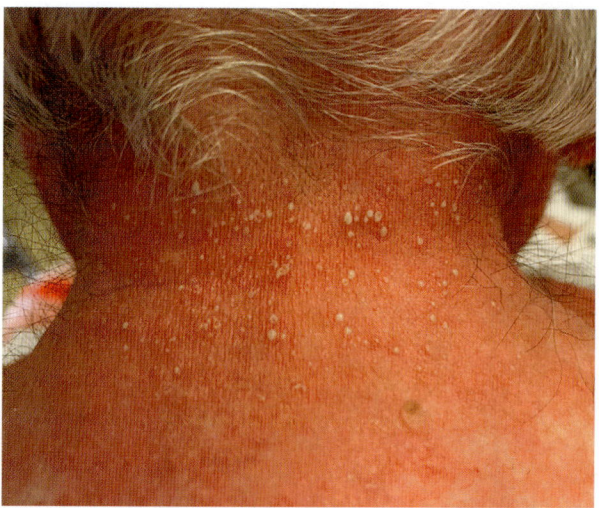

Fig. 6.58 Acute generalized exanthematous pustulosis.

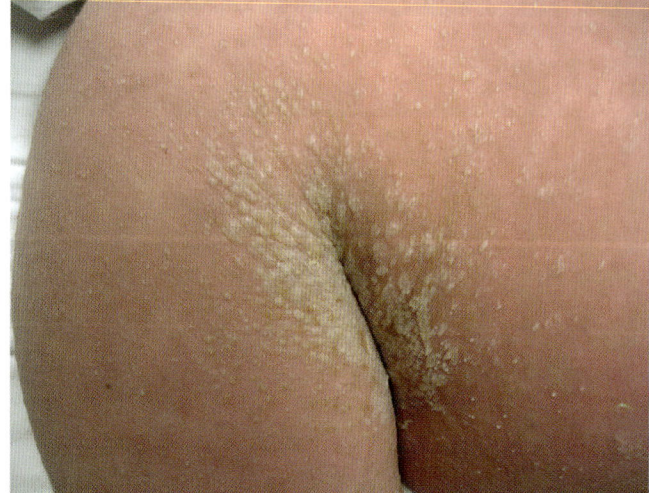

Fig. 6.59 Acute generalized exanthematous pustulosis.

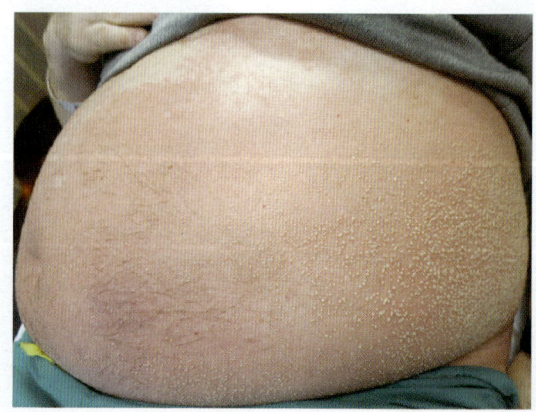

Fig. 6.60 Acute generalized exanthematous pustulosis.

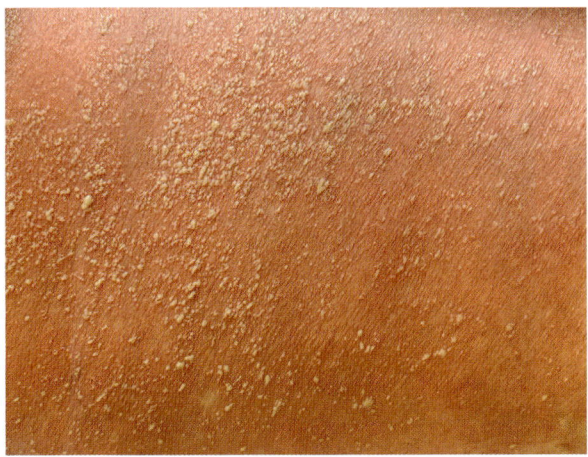

Fig. 6.61 Acute generalized exanthematous pustulosis.

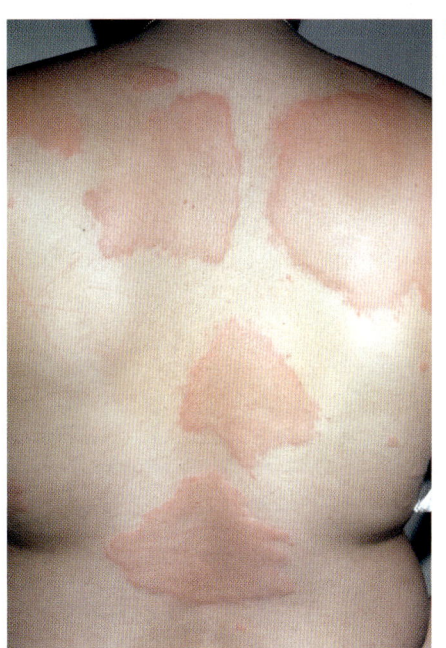

Fig. 6.62 Urticaria. *Courtesy Steven Binnick, MD.*

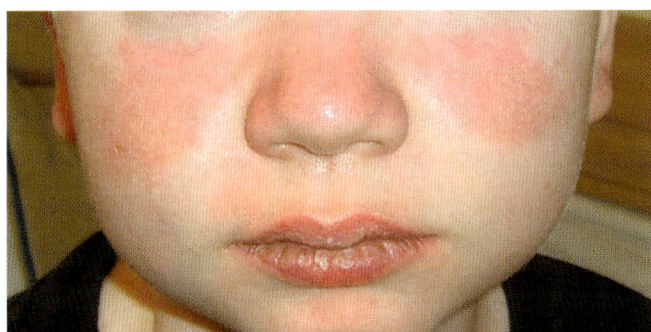

Fig. 6.63 Voriconazole phototoxicity. *Courtesy Jennifer Huang, MD.*

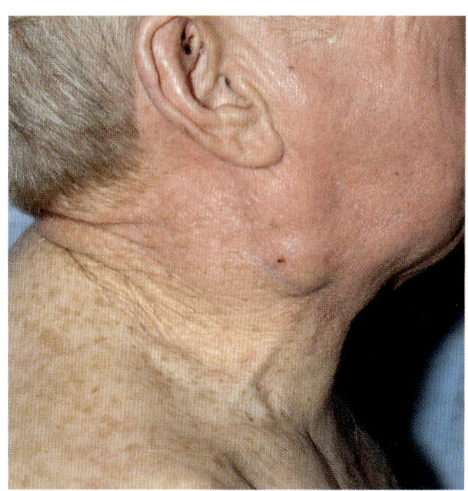

Fig. 6.64 Voriconazole phototoxicity. *Courtesy Edward W. Cowen, MD.*

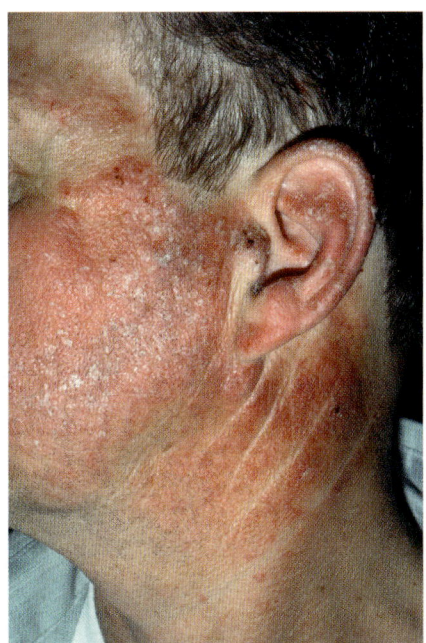

Fig. 6.65 Minocycline-induced photosensitivity.

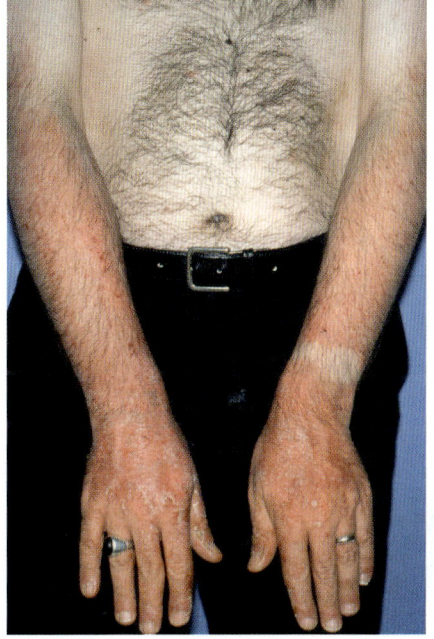

Fig. 6.66 Piroxicam photosensitivity.

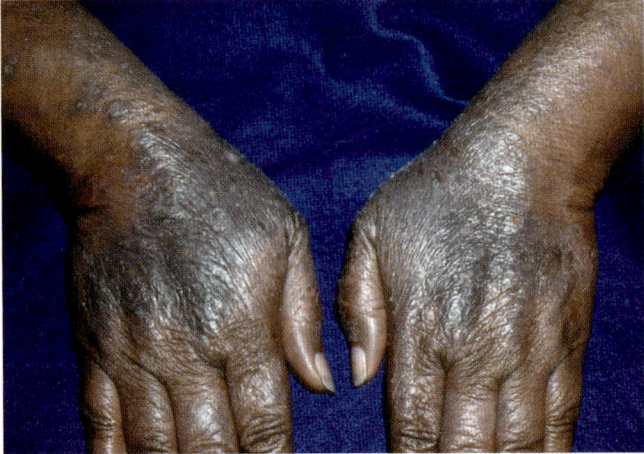

Fig. 6.67 Photosensitivity to quinine.

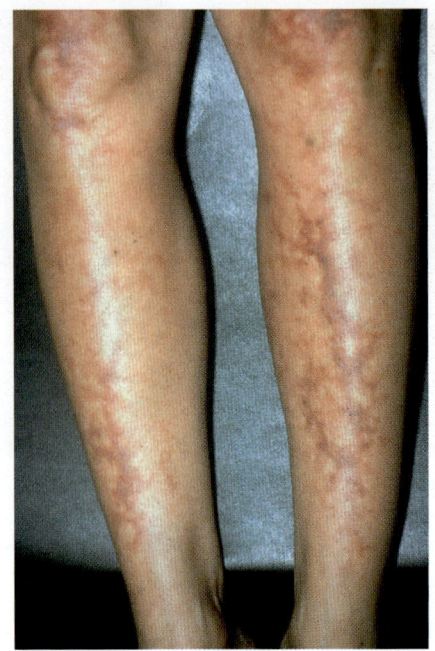

Fig. 6.68 Quinidine photo-induced livedo reticularis.

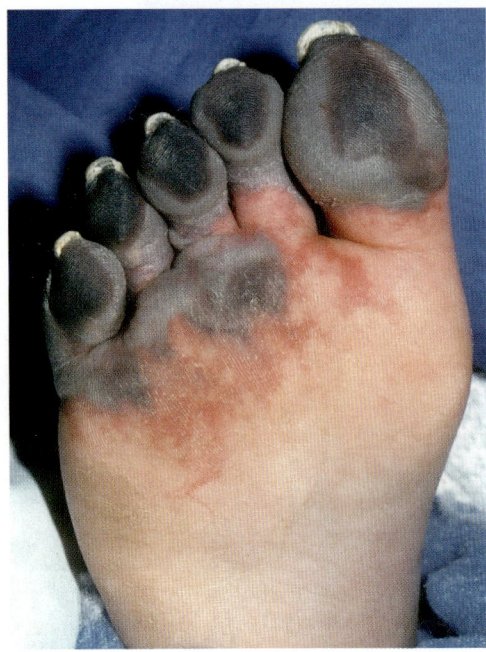

Fig. 6.69 Warfarin-induced necrosis. *Courtesy Steven Binnick, MD.*

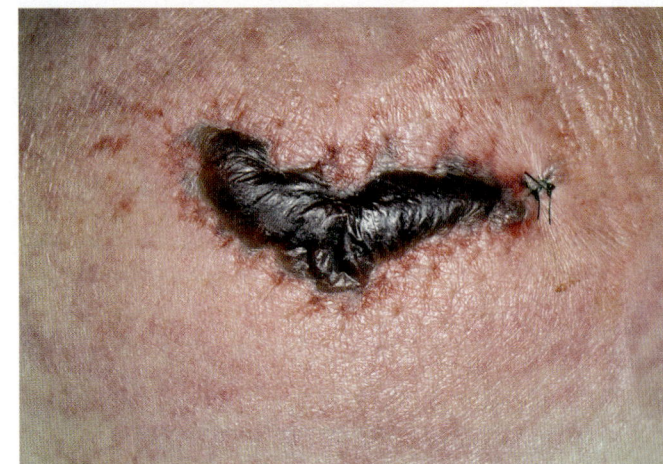

Fig. 6.70 Warfarin-induced necrosis. *Courtesy Steven Binnick, MD.*

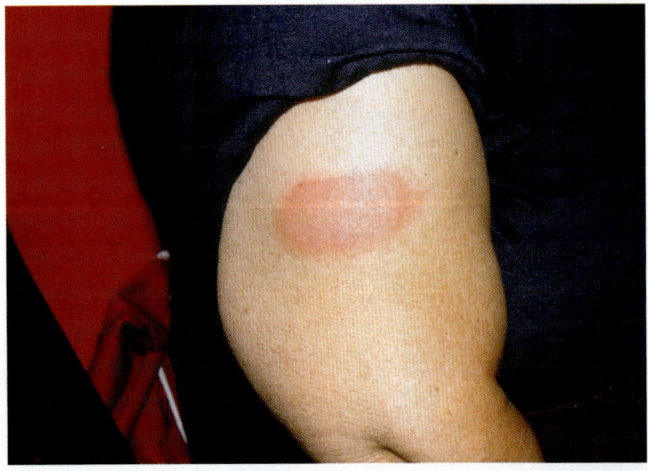

Fig. 6.71 Vitamin K injection site reaction.

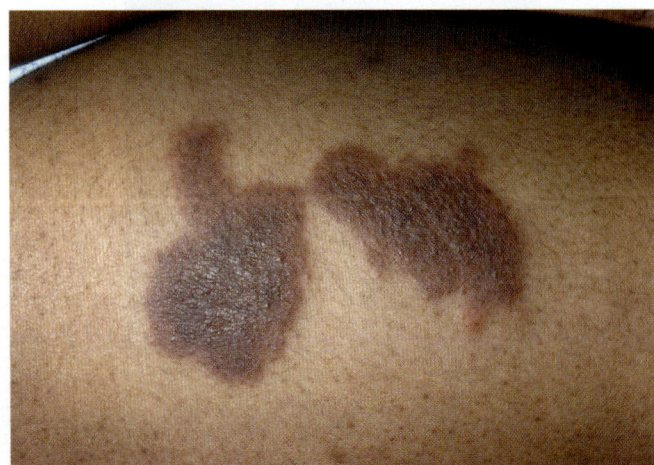

Fig. 6.72 Vitamin K injection site reaction.

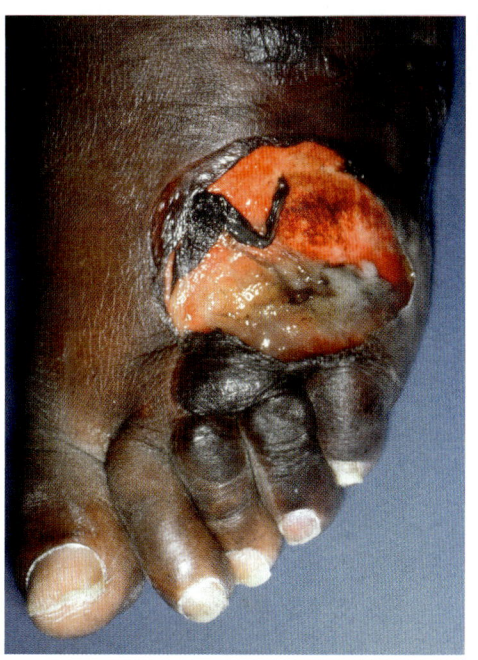

Fig. 6.73 Intravenous extravasation with necrosis.

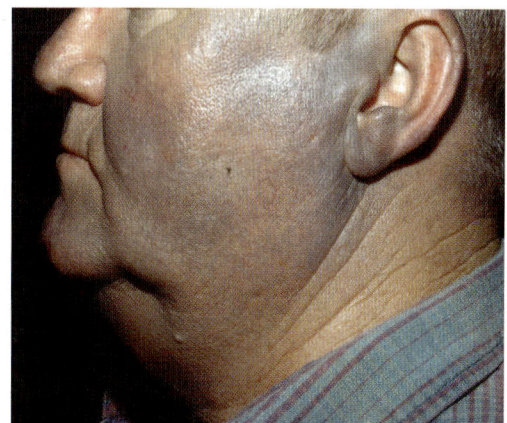

Fig. 6.74 Amiodarone hyperpigmentation.

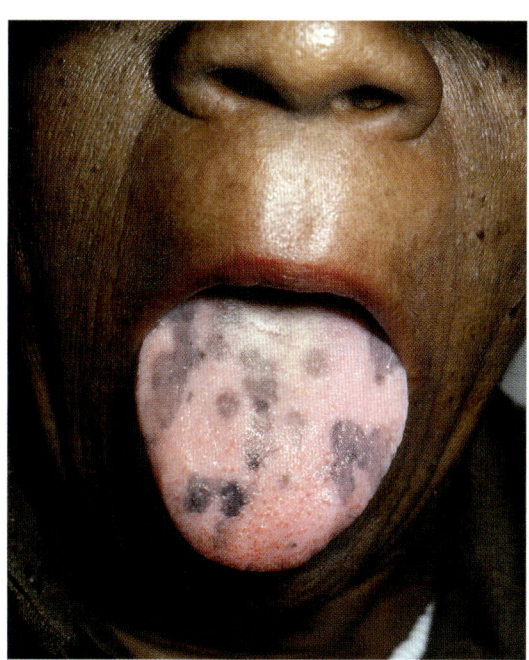

Fig. 6.75 Doxorubicin hyperpigmentation.

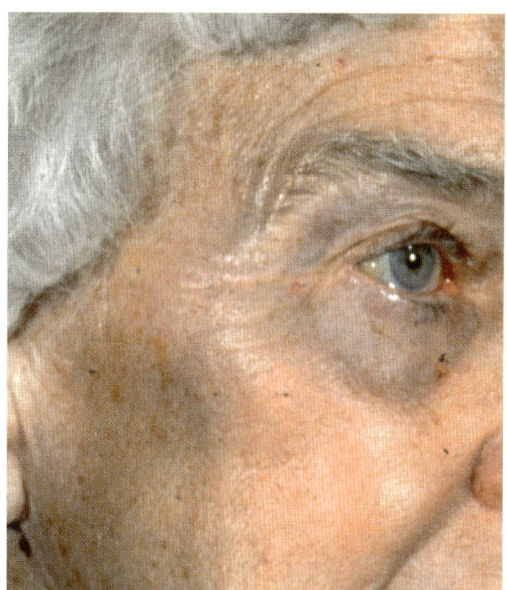

Fig. 6.76 Chrysiasis.

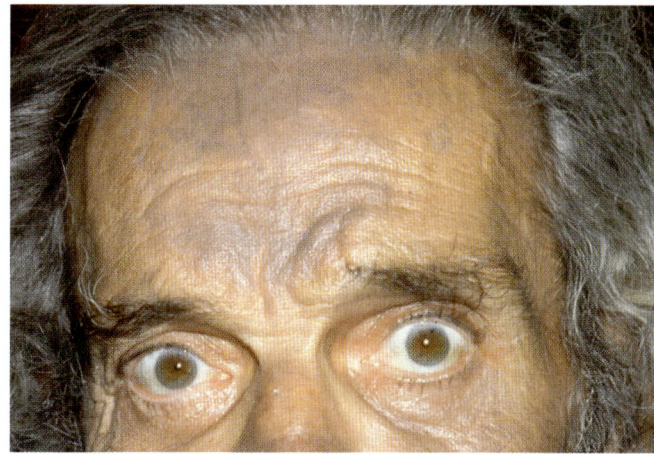

Fig. 6.77 Chlorpromazine hyperpigmentation.

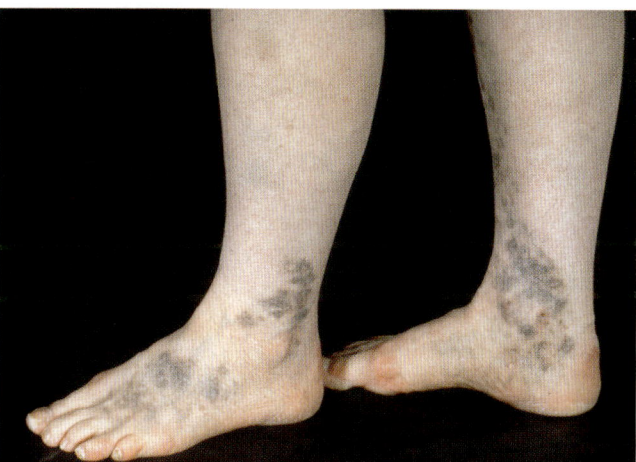

Fig. 6.78 Minocycline hyperpigmentation.

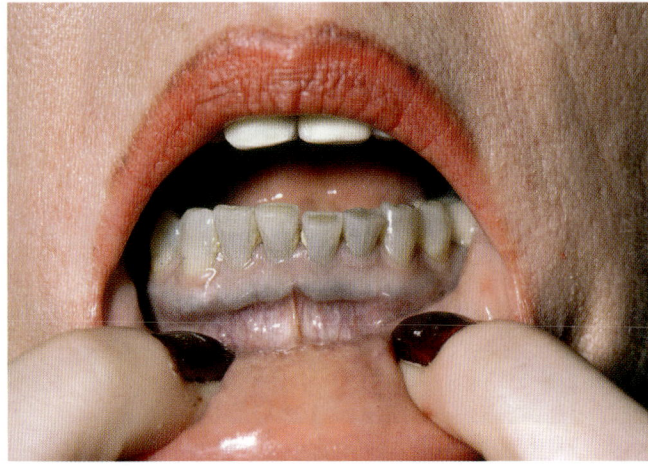

Fig. 6.79 Minocycline hyperpigmentation.

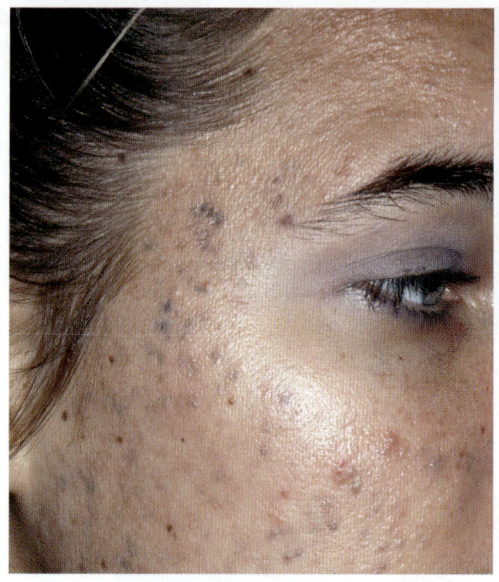

Fig. 6.80 Minocycline hyperpigmentation.

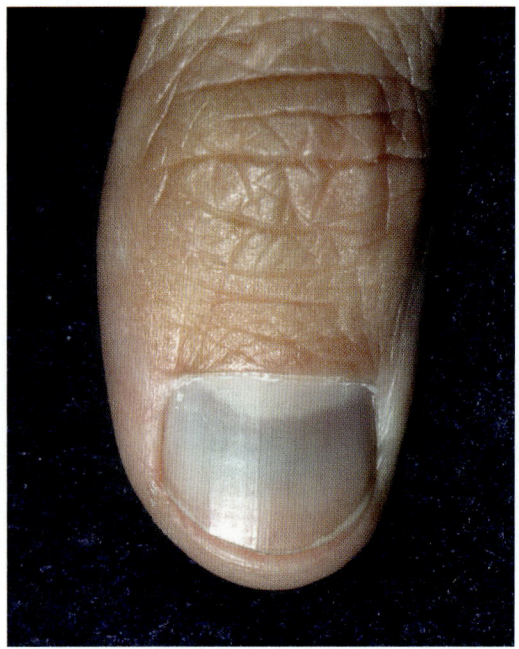

Fig. 6.81 Minocycline hyperpigmentation.

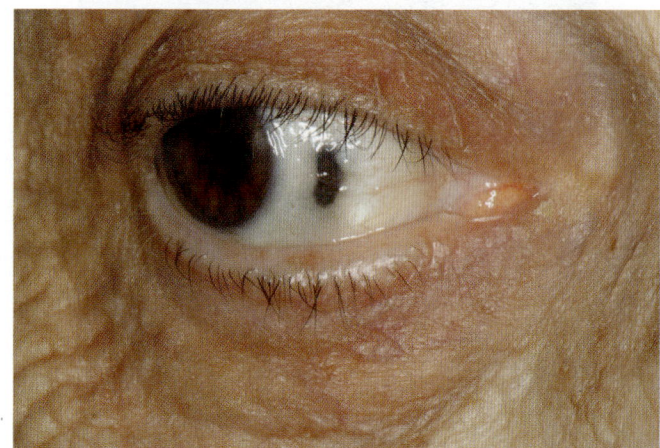

Fig. 6.82 Minocycline hyperpigmentation.

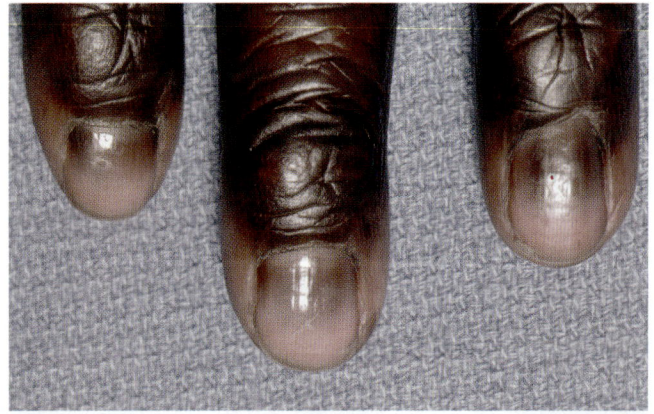

Fig. 6.83 Doxorubicin hyperpigmentation.

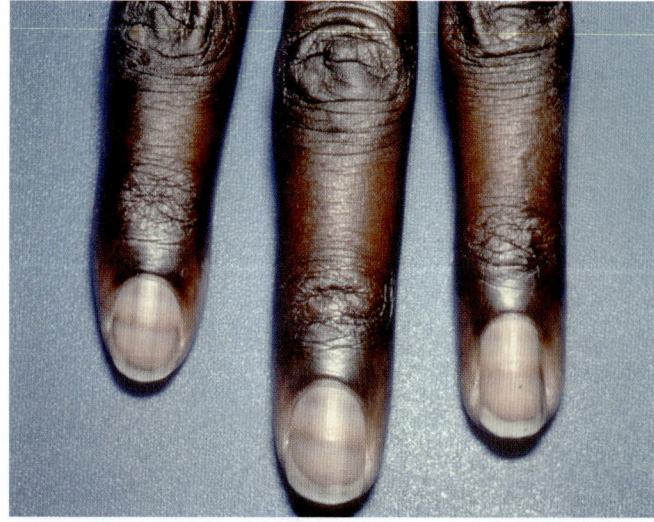

Fig. 6.84 Chemotherapy-induced transverse nail hyperpigmentation.

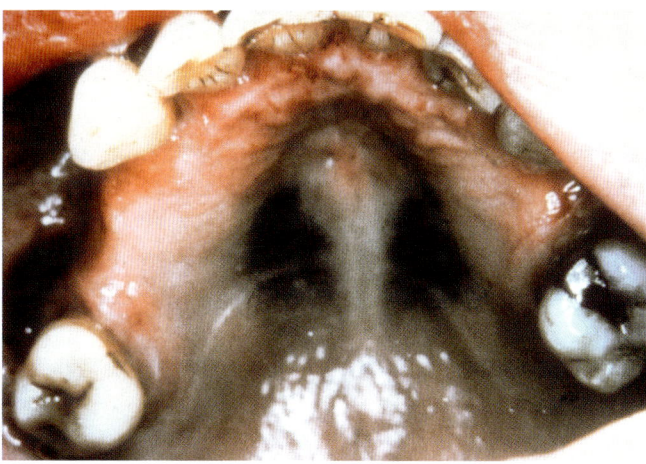

Fig. 6.85 Chloroquine hyperpigmentation.

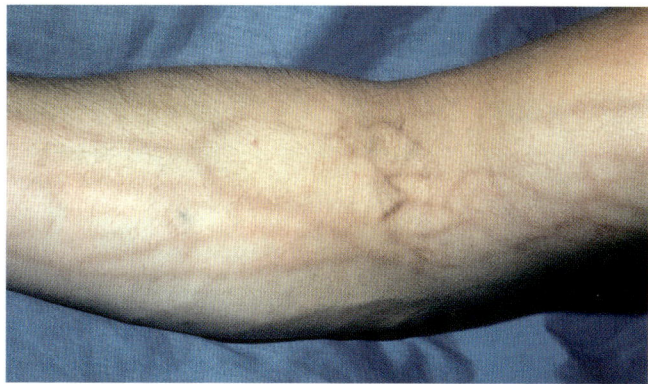

Fig. 6.86 Methotrexate-induced vascular hyperpigmentation. *Courtesy Steven Binnick, MD.*

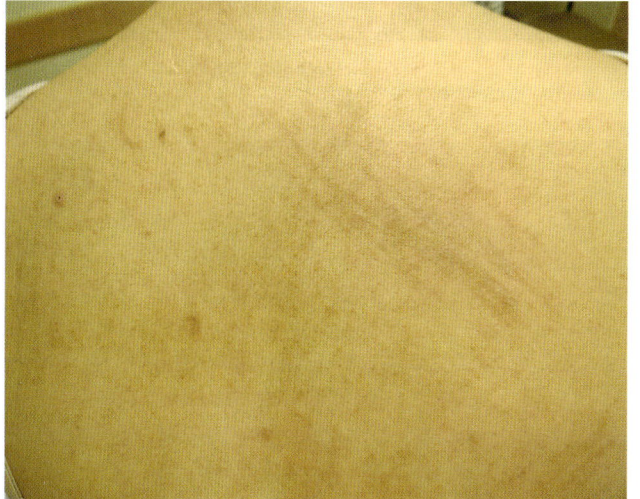

Fig. 6.87 Bleomycin-associated flagellate hyperpigmentation.

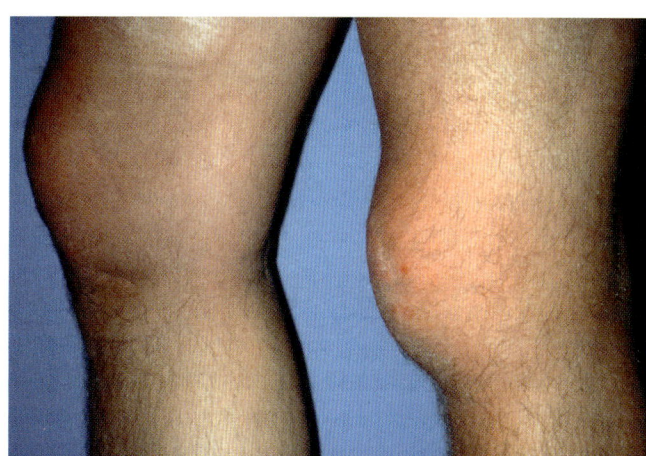

Fig. 6.88 Serum sickness–like reaction.

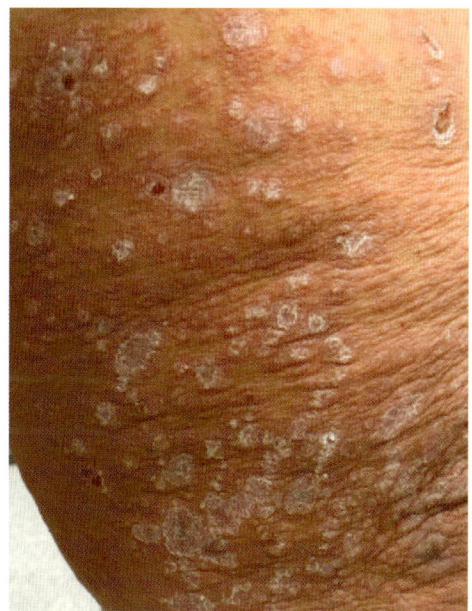

Fig. 6.89 Lichenoid drug reaction.

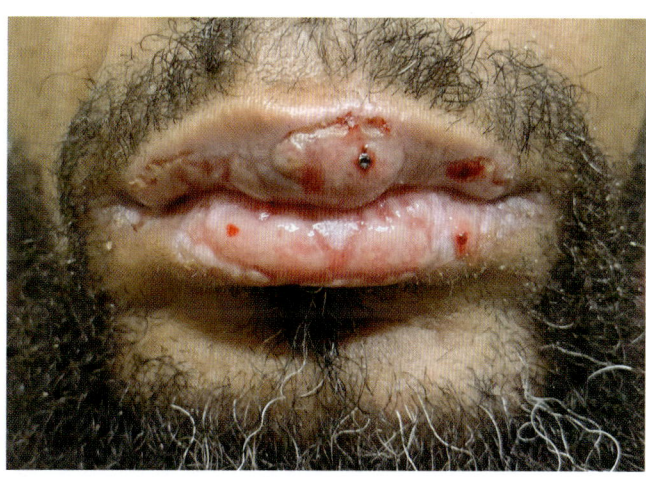

Fig. 6.90 Pembrolizumab-associated lichenoid reaction.

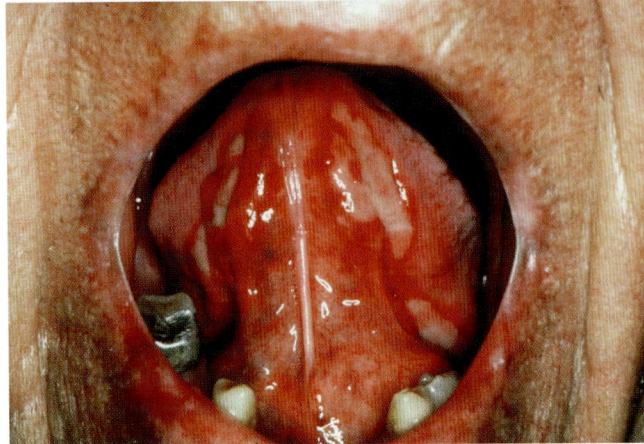

Fig. 6.91 Methotrexate-induced oral ulcers.

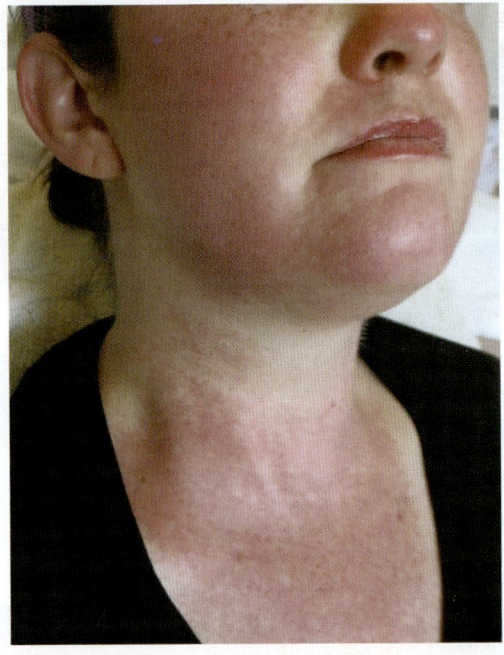

Fig. 6.92 Sunburn recall reaction induced by methotrexate.

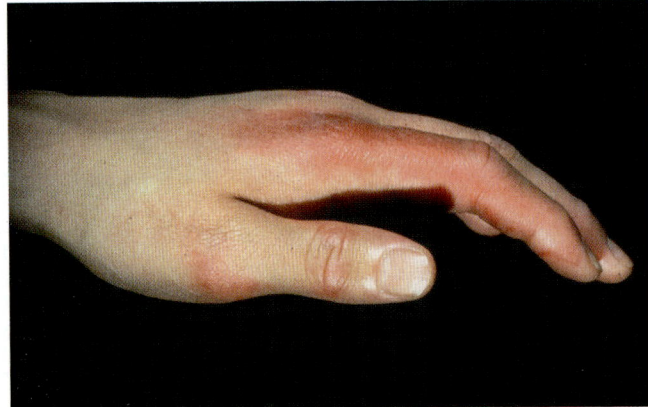

Fig. 6.93 Toxic erythema of chemotherapy.

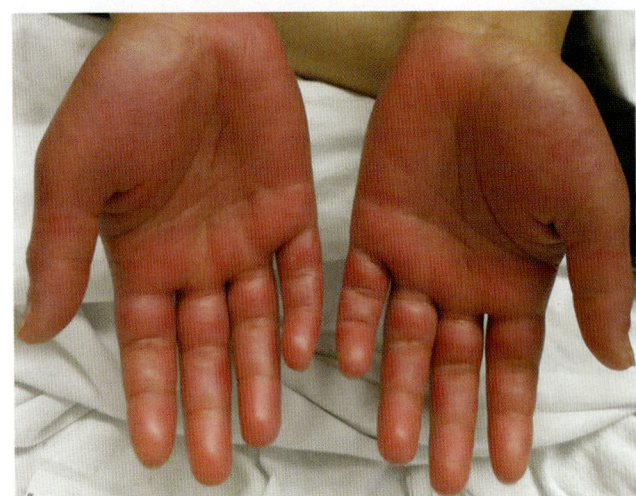

Fig. 6.94 Toxic erythema of chemotherapy.

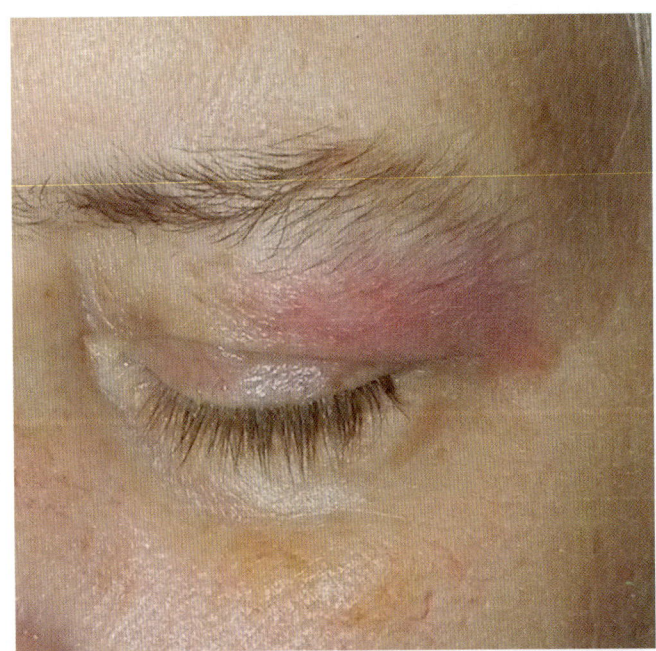

Fig. 6.95 Neutrophilic eccrine hidradenitis. *Courtesy Misha Rosenbach, MD.*

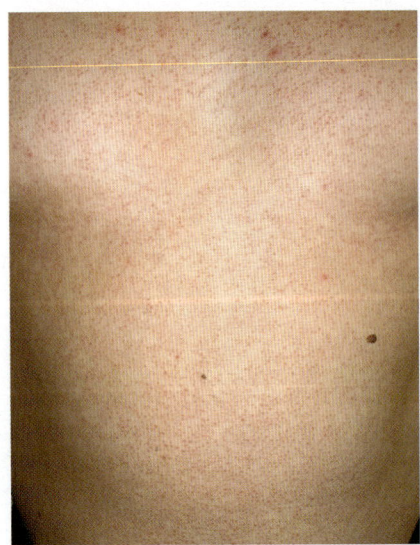

Fig. 6.96 Diffuse keratosis pilaris caused by nilotinib.

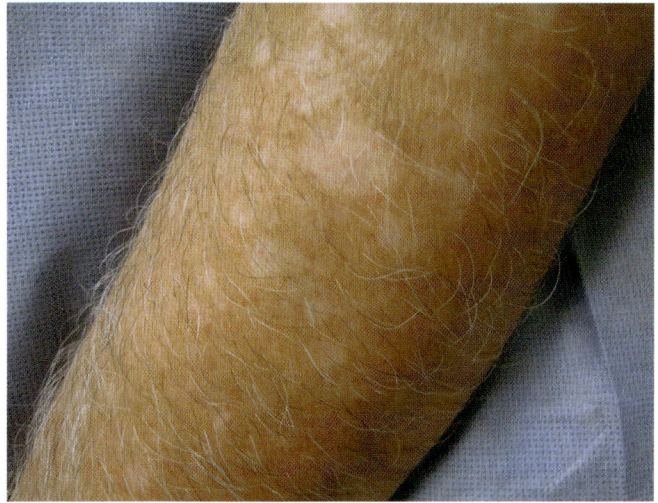

Fig. 6.97 Pembrolizumab-associated vitiligo.

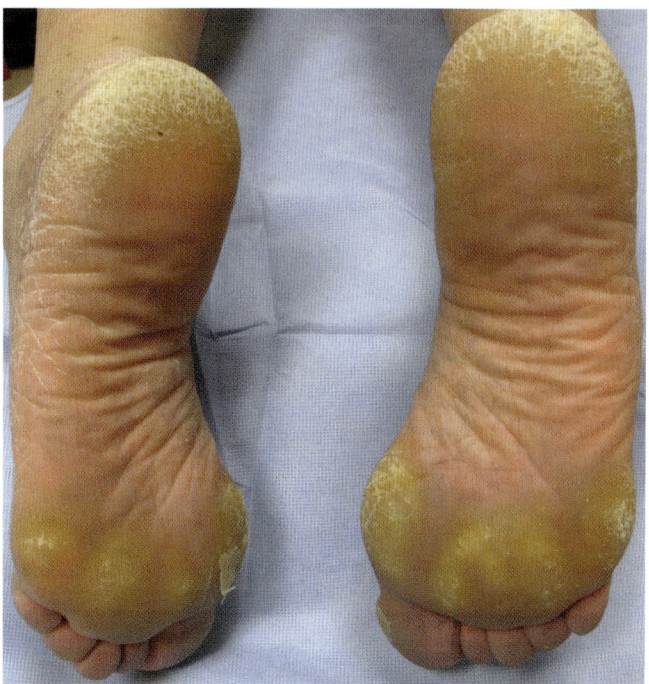

Fig. 6.98 BRAF inhibitor–induced hand–foot reaction. *Courtesy Emily Chu, MD, PhD.*

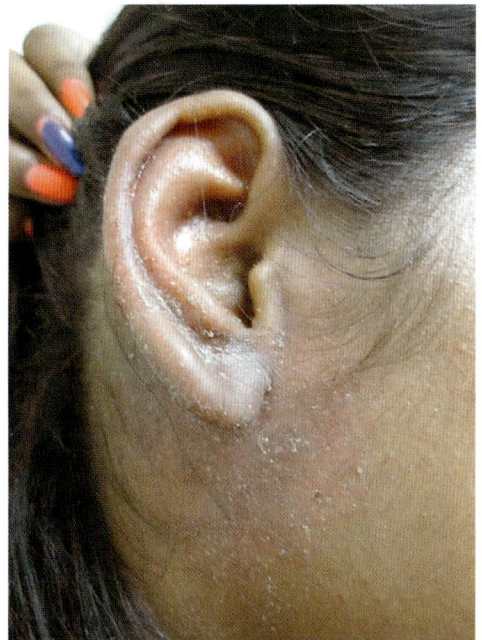

Fig. 6.99 Tumor necrosis factor inhibitor–related psoriasiform reaction.

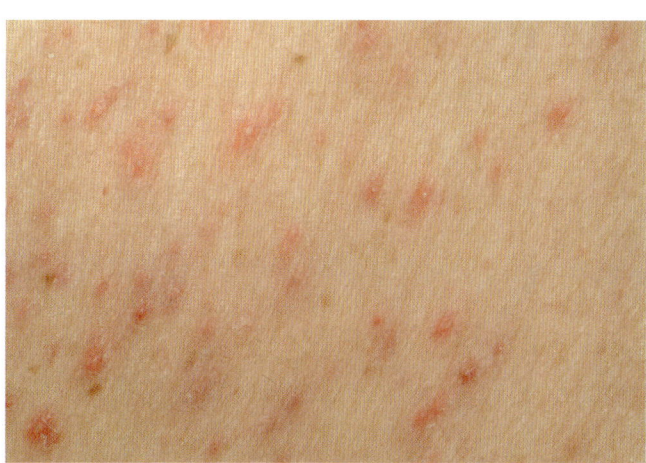

Fig. 6.100 Epidermal growth factor inhibitor–induced acneiform reaction.

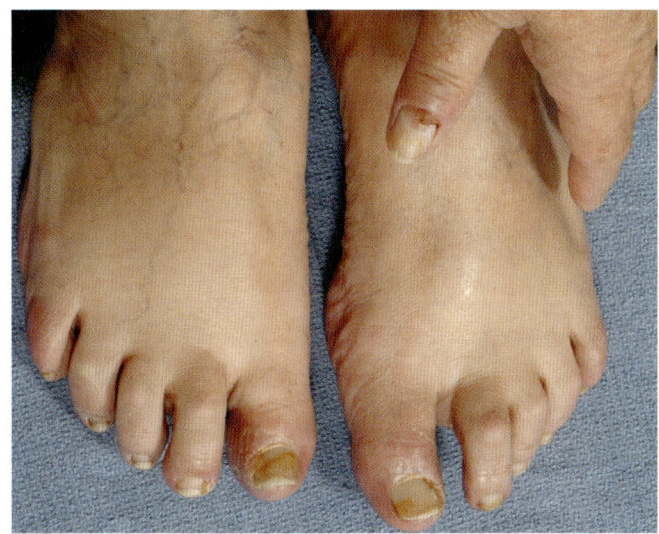

Fig. 6.101 Epidermal growth factor inhibitor–induced paronychia.

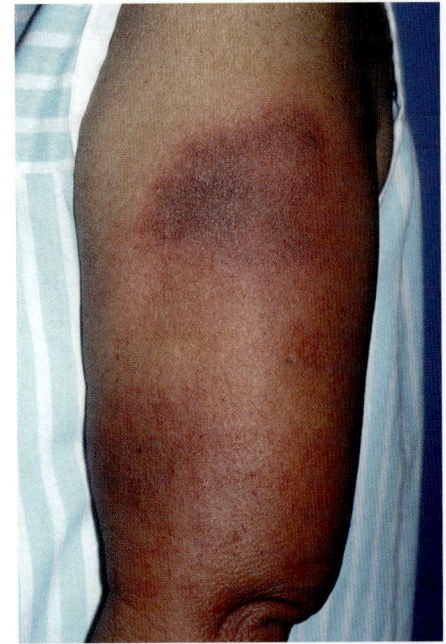

Fig. 6.102 Granulocyte colony-stimulating factor reaction.

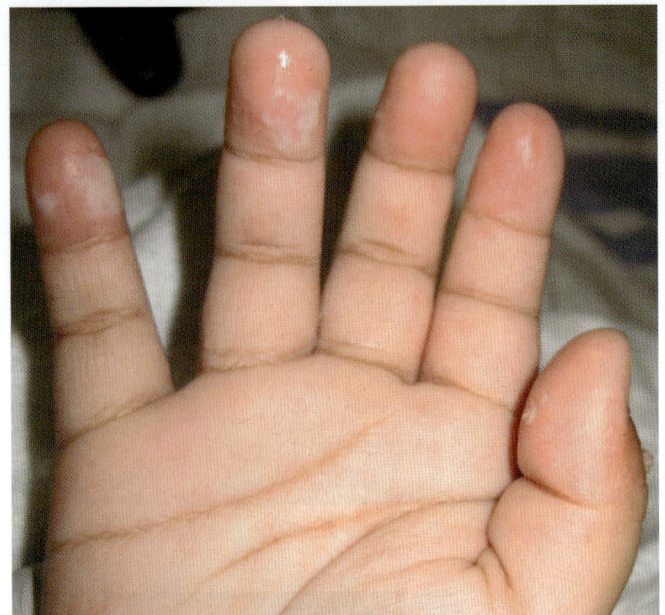

Fig. 6.103 Pink disease (mercury toxicity).

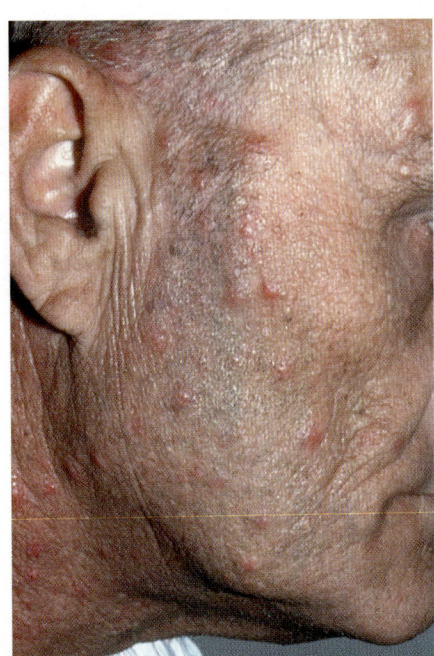

Fig. 6.104 Follicular iododerma.

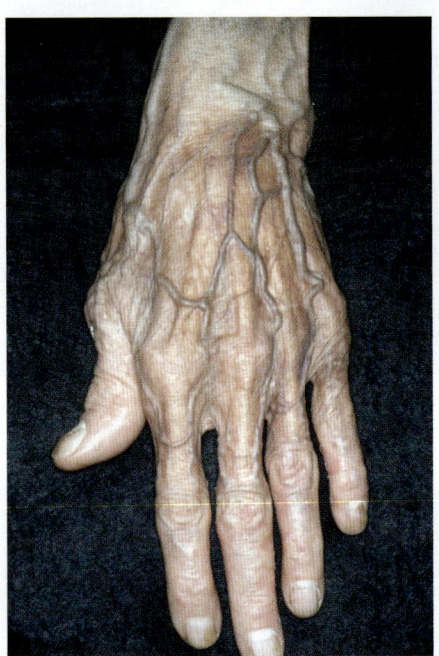

Fig. 6.105 Topical steroid–induced atrophy. *Courtesy Steven Binnick, MD.*

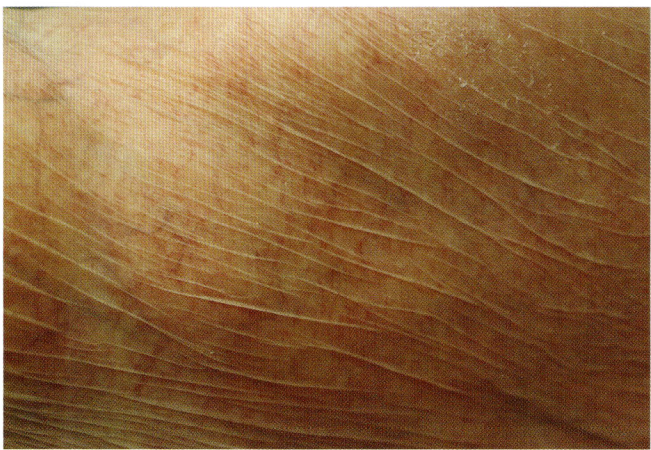

Fig. 6.106 Topical steroid atrophy.

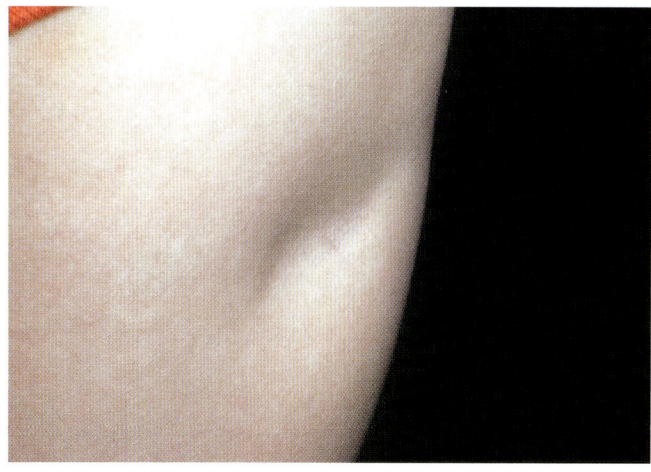

Fig. 6.107 Lipoatrophy after steroid injection. *Courtesy Steven Binnick, MD.*

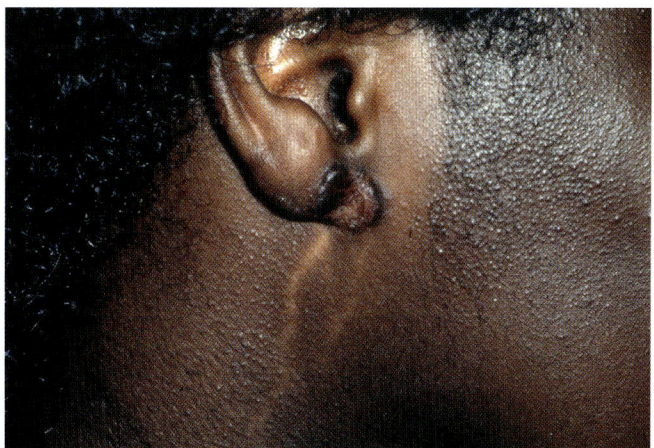

Fig. 6.108 Hypopigmentation after intralesional steroid injection.

Erythema and Urticaria 7

A wide variety of conditions can present with erythema or urticarial lesions. Whereas many conditions such as urticaria and angioedema lack identifiable surface changes, other diagnoses in this chapter have distinctive scaling. Pustules and ulcerations are seen in some cases as a manifestation of intense underlying, often neutrophilic, inflammation.

Many of the erythemas in this portion of the atlas share an annular and polycyclic morphology, including urticaria, erythema annulare centrifugum, and erythema gyratum repens, but only erythema multiforme demonstrates the true fixed target lesion. Noting whether skin findings are migratory or fixed is helpful in distinguishing common urticaria from many other more fixed lesions. Skin testing to demonstrate dermatographism is also helpful as a bedside technique to recapitulate urticaria in a susceptible patient. Ultimately, a skin biopsy may be needed to differentiate reactive neutrophilic dermatoses, such as Sweet syndrome (acute febrile neutrophilic dermatosis), from eosinophilic conditions, such as Wells syndrome (eosinophilic cellulitis). Tissue cultures are often needed when diagnosing pyoderma gangrenosum to rule out infectious etiologies such as bacteria, fungi, or atypical mycobacteria, depending on the clinical setting.

This portion of the atlas features examples of urticaria, urticarial lesions, erythemas, and angioedema.

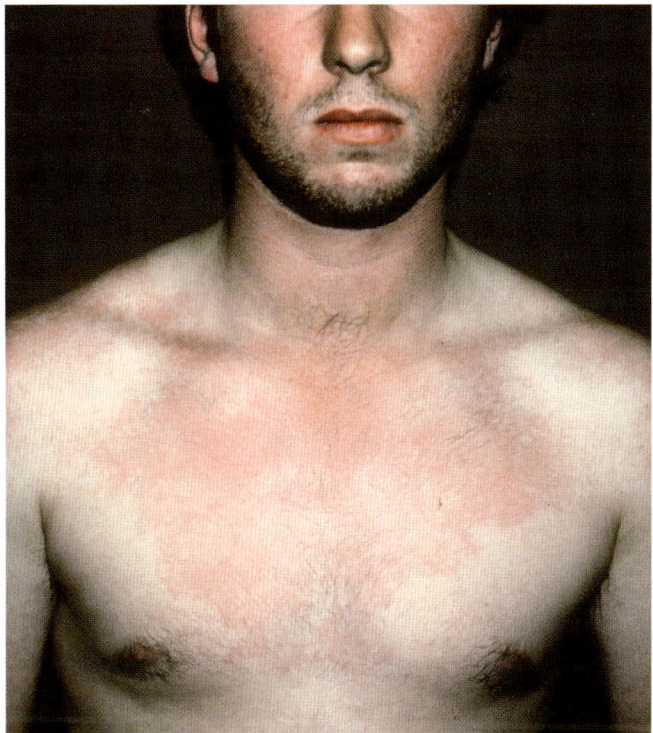

Fig. 7.1 Flushing.

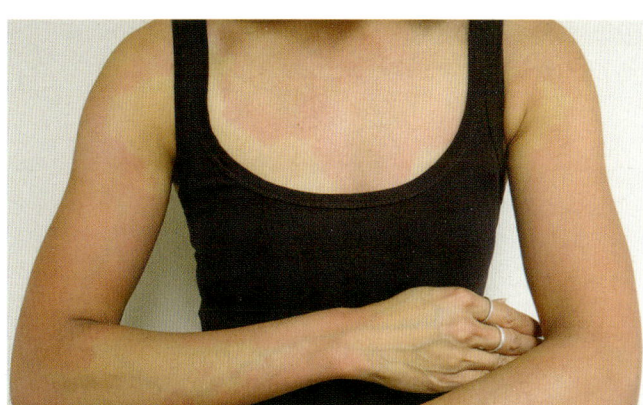

Fig. 7.2 Scombroid poisoning with onset 30 minutes after eating contaminated fish.

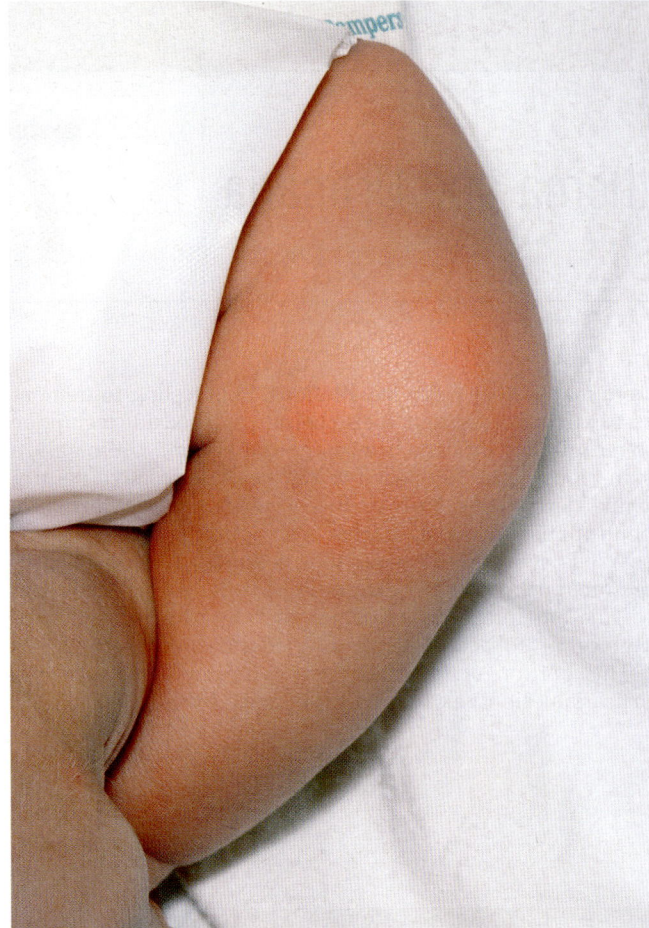

Fig. 7.3 Erythema toxicum neonatorum.

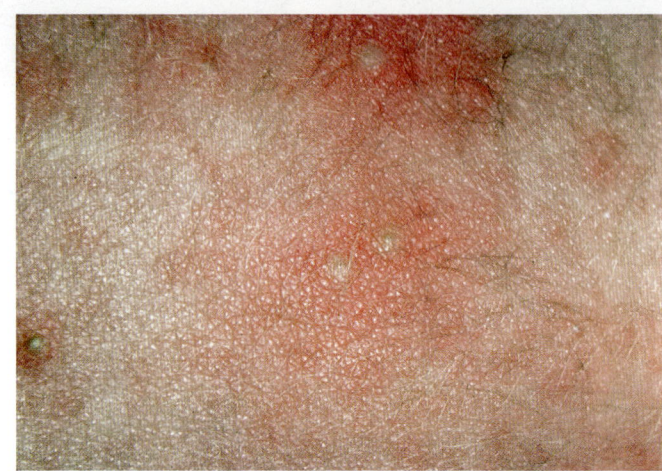

Fig. 7.4 Erythema toxicum neonatorum.

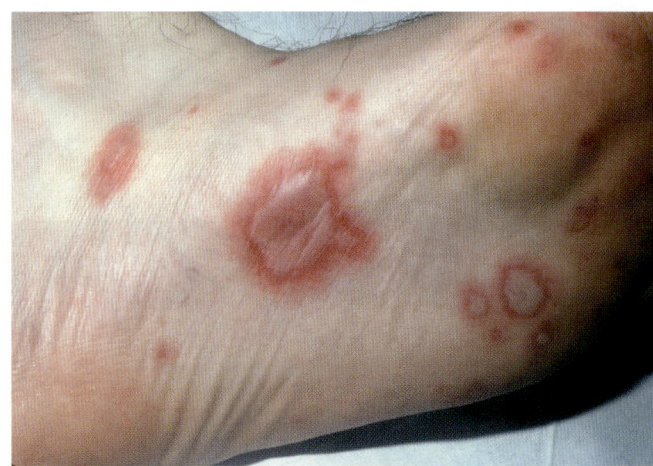

Fig. 7.6 Erythema multiforme. *Courtesy Steven Binnick, MD.*

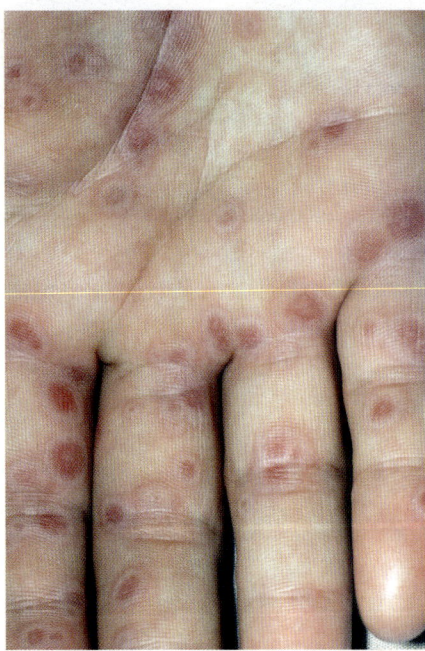

Fig. 7.5 Erythema multiforme. *Courtesy Steven Binnick, MD.*

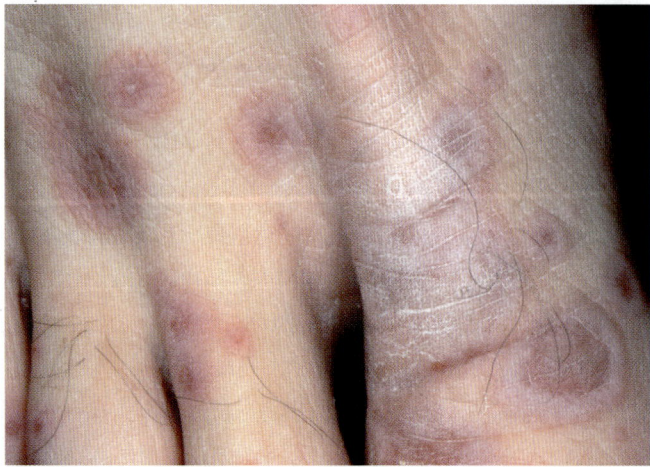

Fig. 7.7 Erythema multiforme secondary to sulfa.

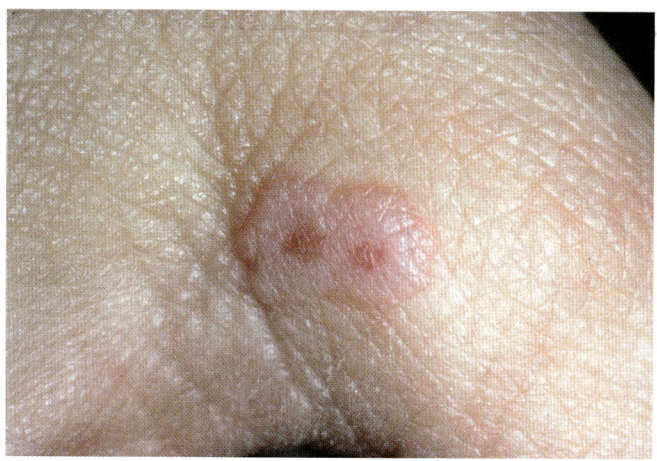

Fig. 7.8 Erythema multiforme. *Courtesy Steven Binnick, MD.*

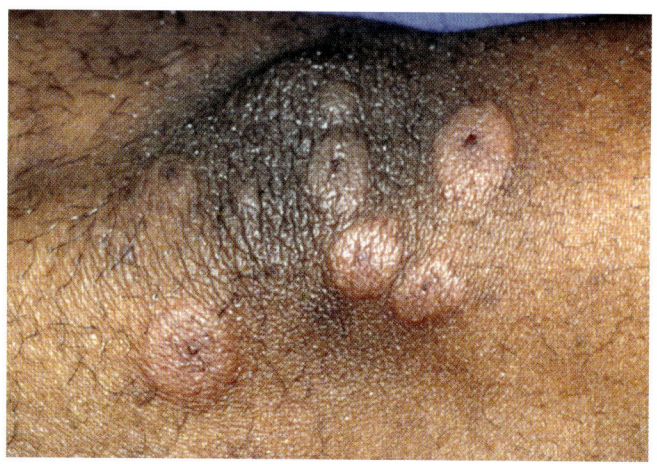

Fig. 7.9 Erythema multiforme.

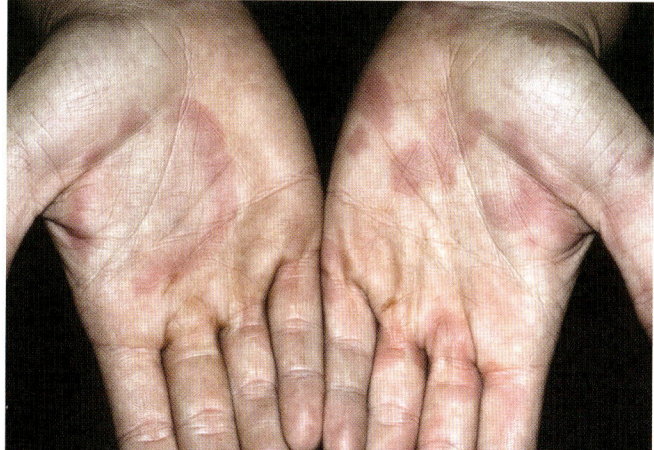

Fig. 7.10 Erythema multiforme.

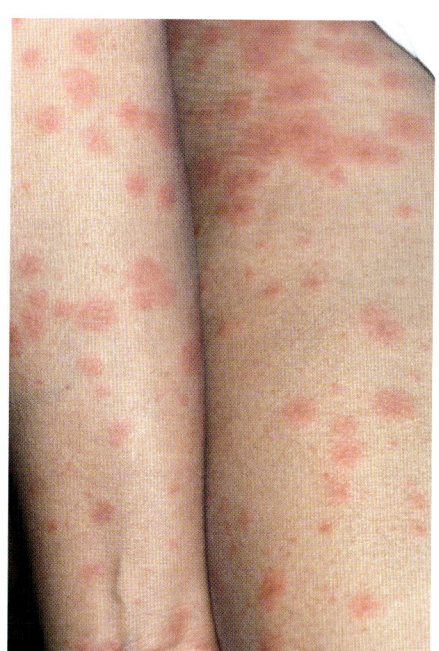

Fig. 7.11 Erythema multiforme. *Courtesy Steven Binnick, MD.*

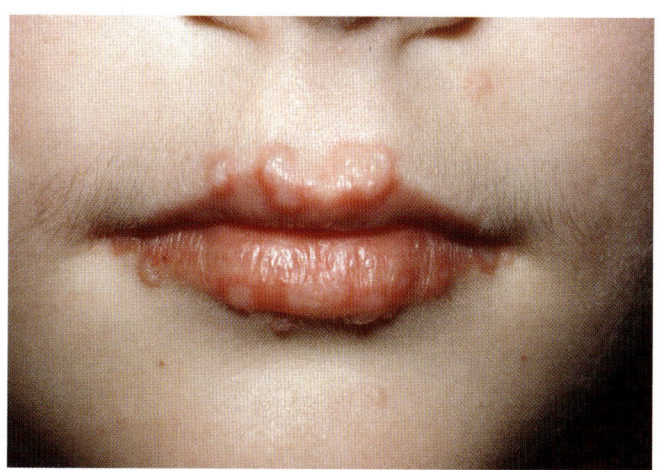

Fig. 7.12 Erythema multiforme. *Courtesy Steven Binnick, MD.*

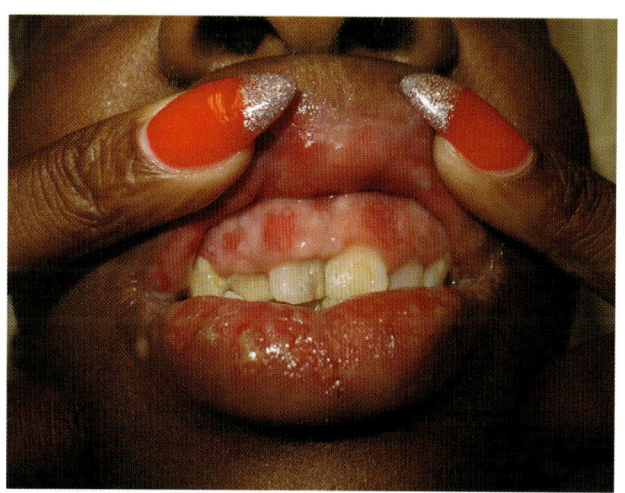

Fig. 7.13 Erythema multiforme.

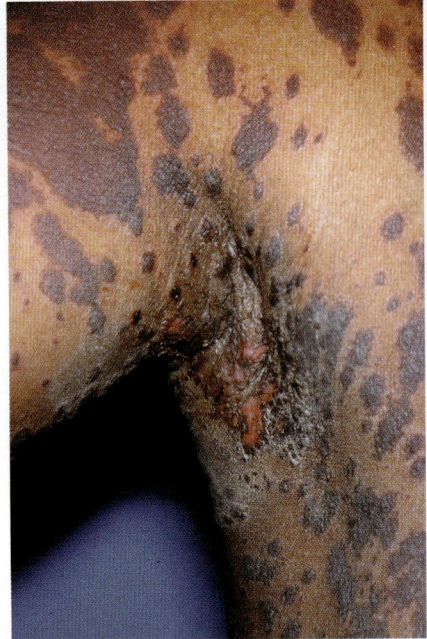

Fig. 7.14 Stevens-Johnson syndrome.

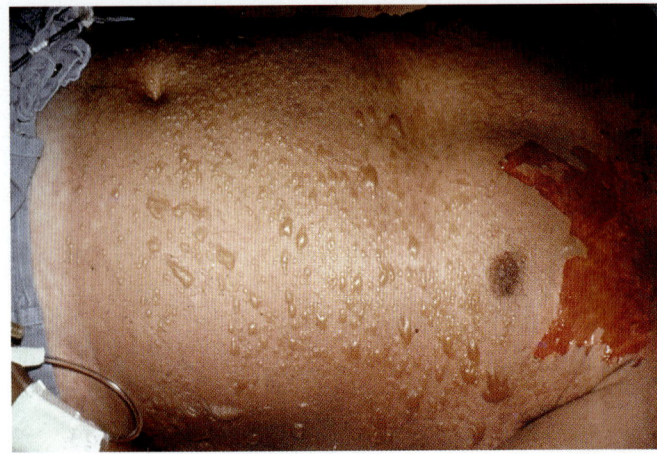

Fig. 7.15 Toxic epidermal necrolysis.

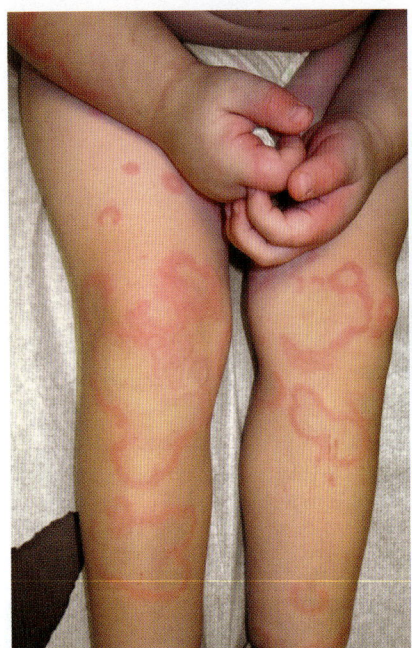

Fig. 7.16 Urticaria multiforme.

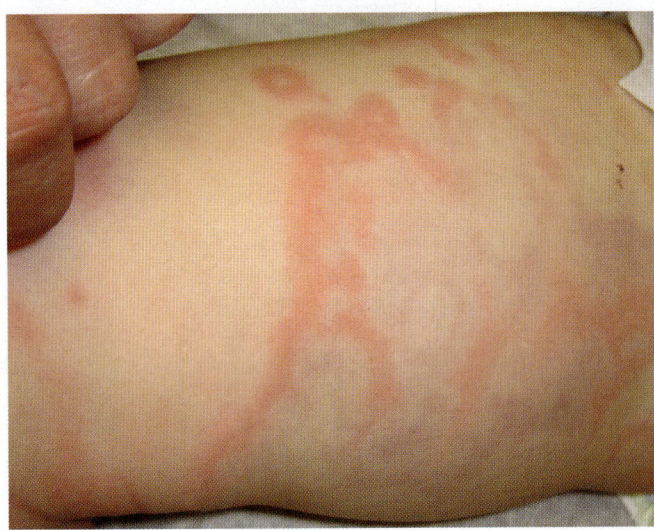

Fig. 7.17 Urticaria multiforme.

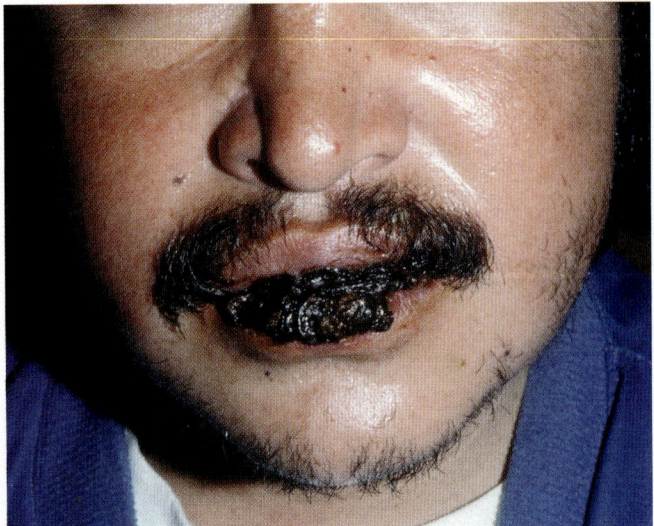

Fig. 7.18 Recurrent oral erythema multiforme.

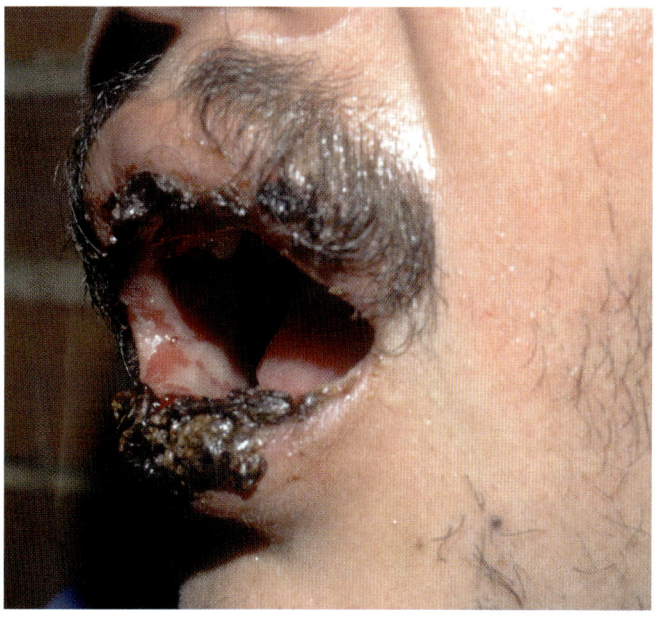

Fig. 7.19 Recurrent oral erythema multiforme.

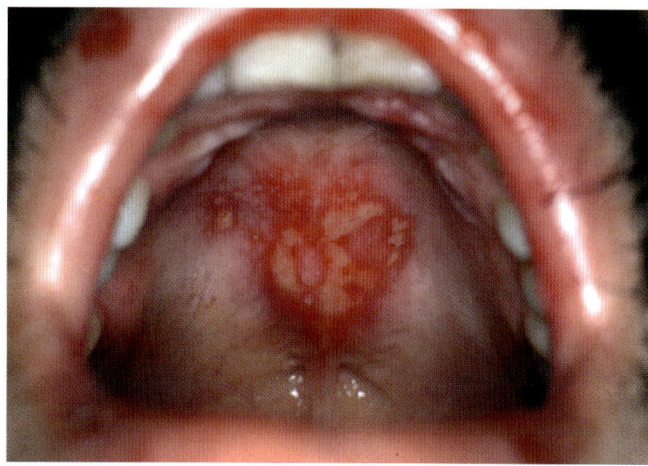

Fig. 7.20 Recurrent oral erythema multiforme. *Courtesy Steven Binnick, MD.*

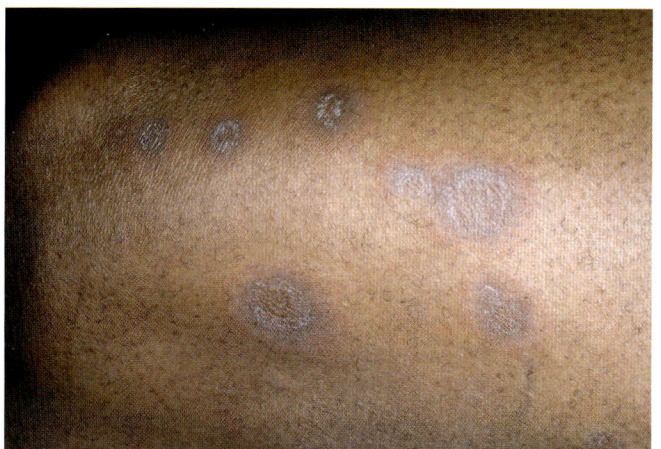

Fig. 7.21 Erythema annulare centrifugum.

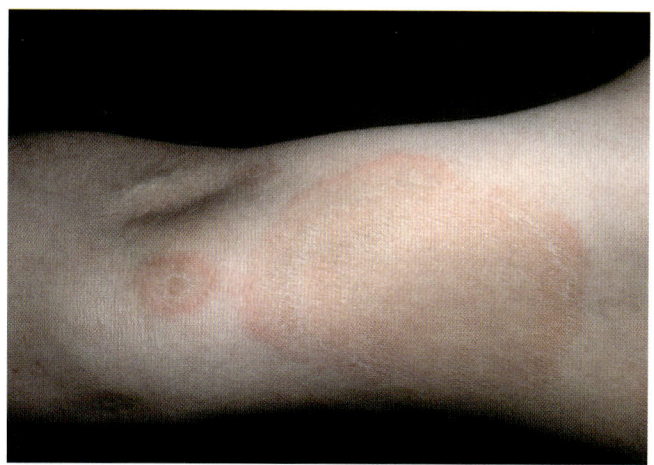

Fig. 7.22 Erythema annulare centrifugum.

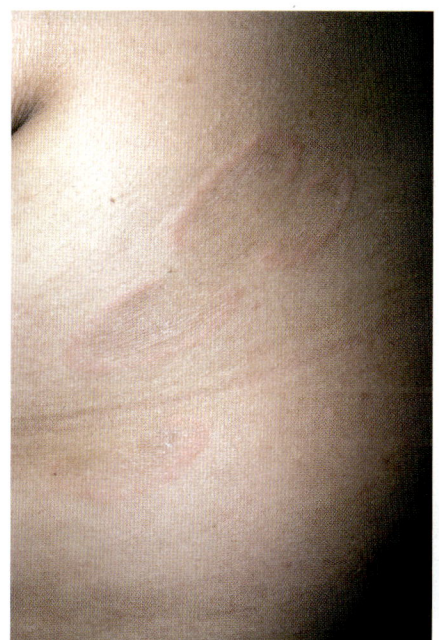

Fig. 7.23 Erythema annulare centrifugum.

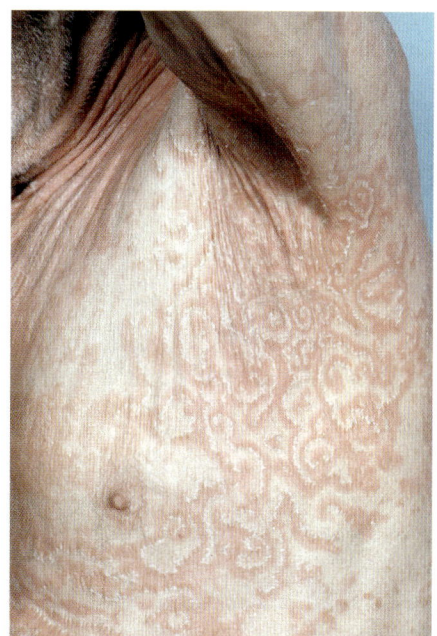

Fig. 7.24 Erythema gyratum repens. *Courtesy Donald Lookingbill, MD.*

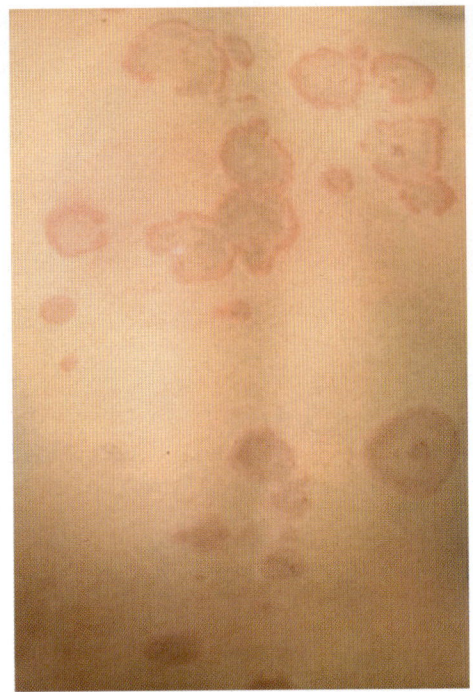

Fig. 7.25 Eosinophilic annular erythema.

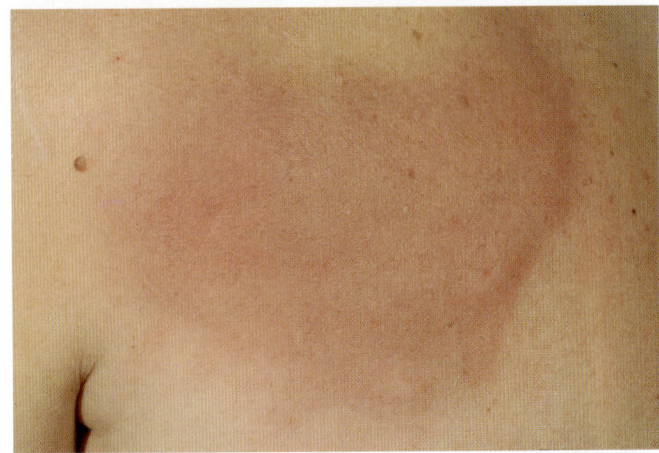

Fig. 7.26 Wells syndrome. *Courtesy Glen Crawford, MD.*

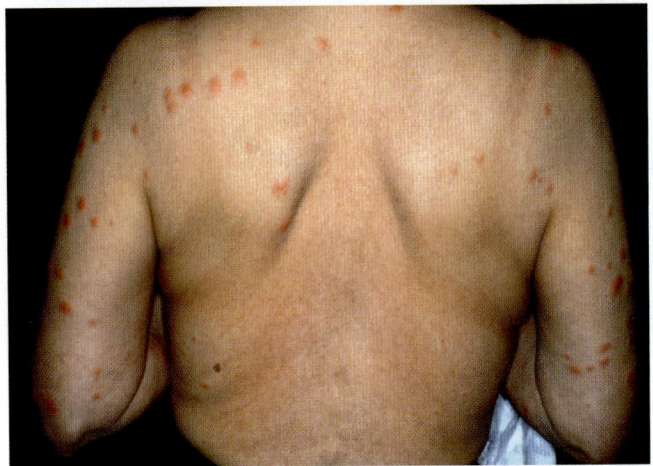

Fig. 7.27 Sweet syndrome.

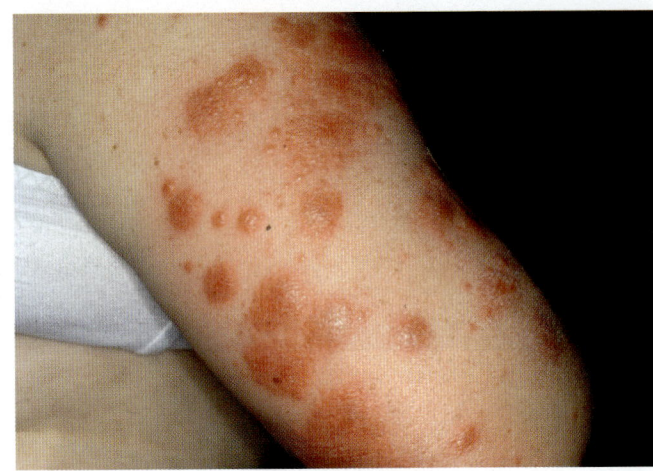

Fig. 7.28 Sweet syndrome in acute myelogenous leukemia.

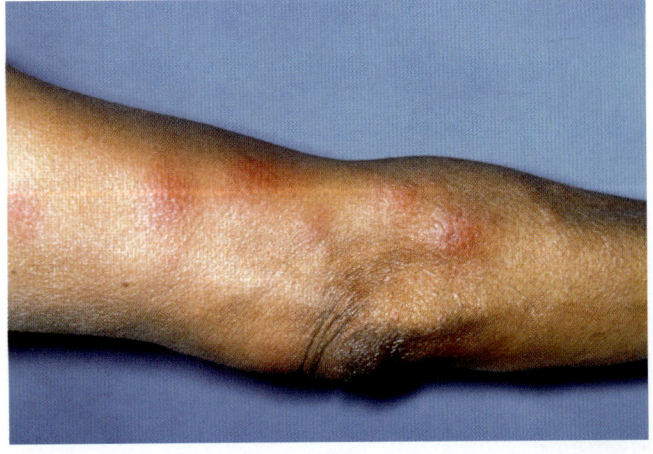

Fig. 7.29 Sweet syndrome.

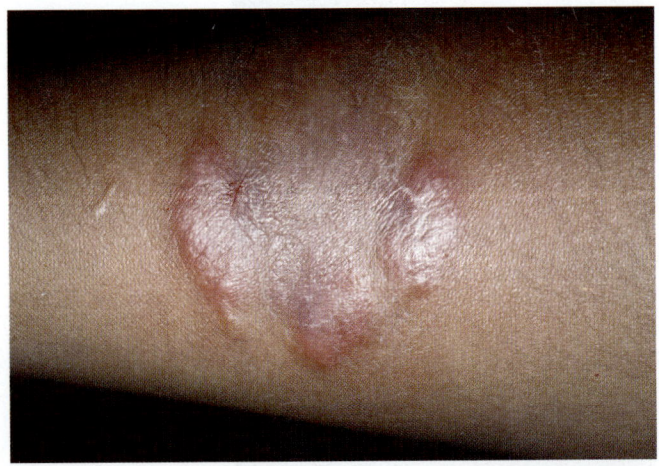

Fig. 7.30 Sweet syndrome.

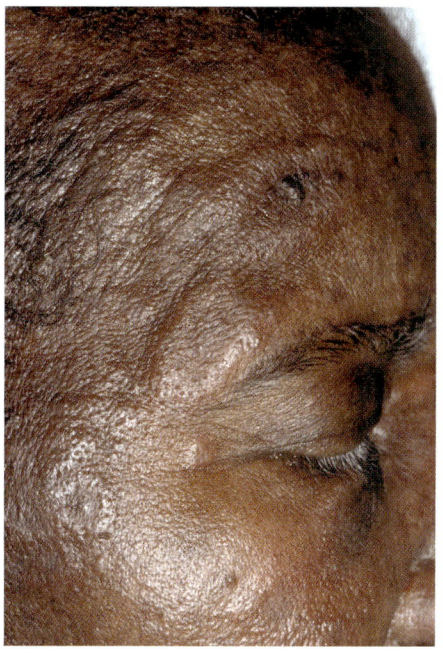

Fig. 7.31 Sweet syndrome.

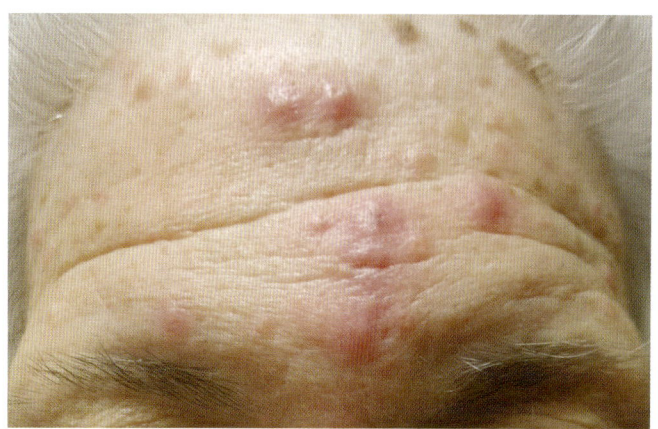

Fig. 7.32 Sweet syndrome.

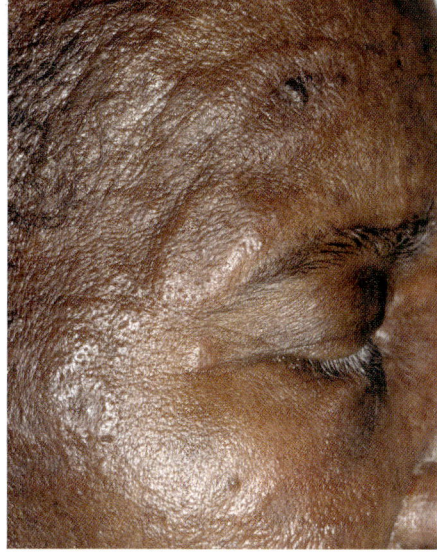

Fig. 7.33 Sweet syndrome in a patient with systemic lupus erythematosus.

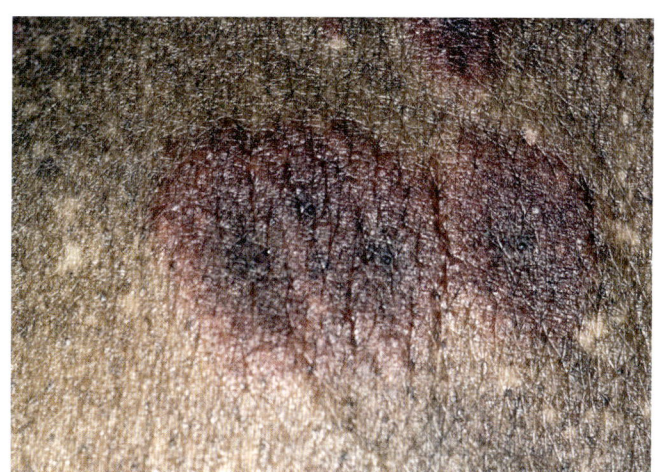

Fig. 7.34 Sweet syndrome in acute myelogenous leukemia.

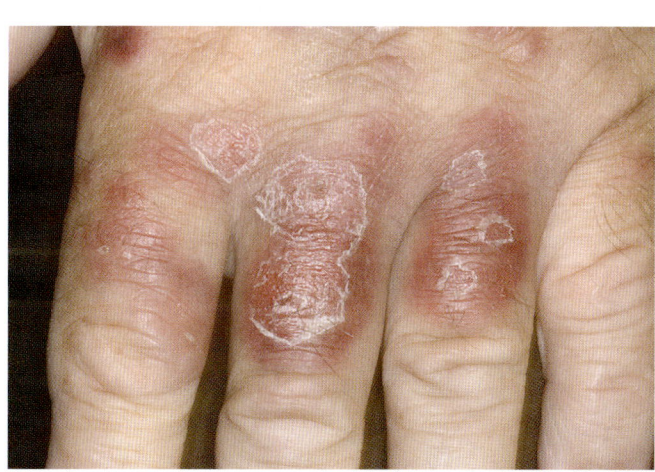

Fig. 7.35 Sweet syndrome in acute leukemia. *Courtesy Misha Rosenbach, MD.*

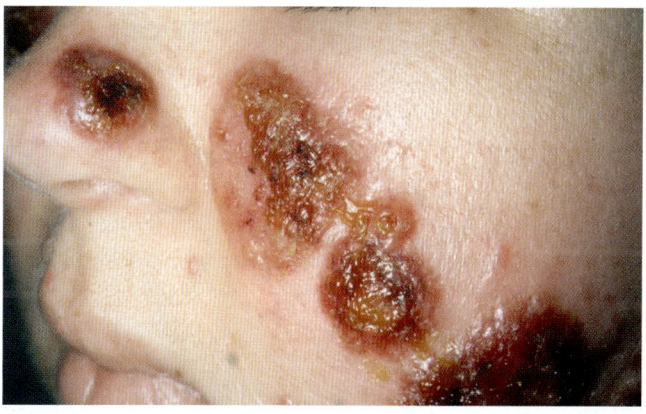

Fig. 7.36 Sweet syndrome in acute leukemia.

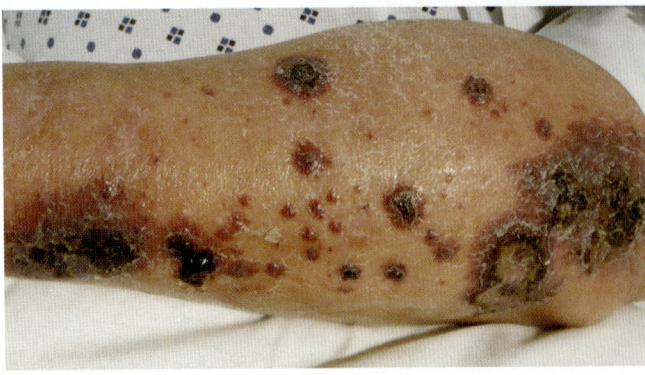

Fig. 7.37 Sweet syndrome in acute leukemia.

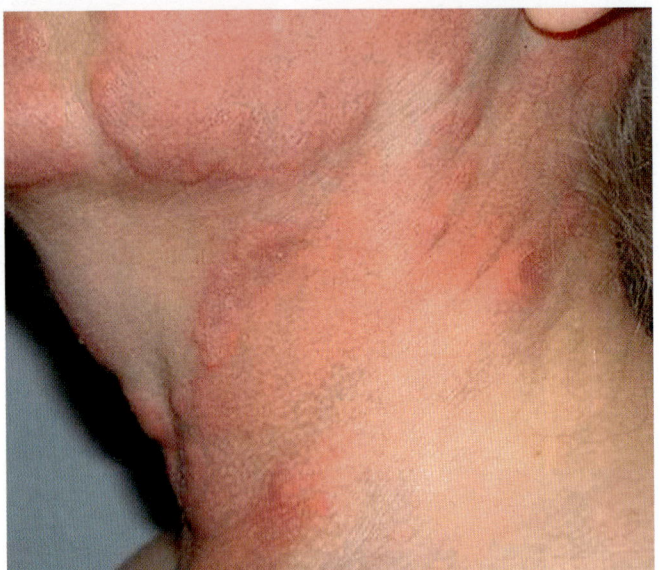

Fig. 7.38 Histiocytoid Sweet syndrome. *Courtesy Misha Rosenbach, MD.*

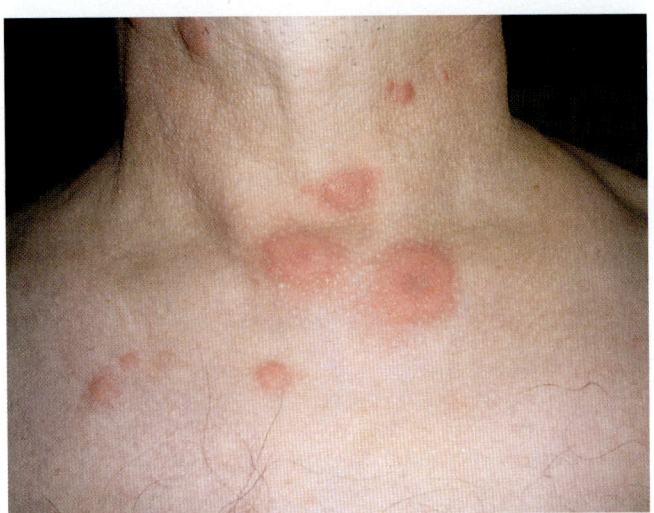

Fig. 7.39 Lymphocytic Sweet syndrome.

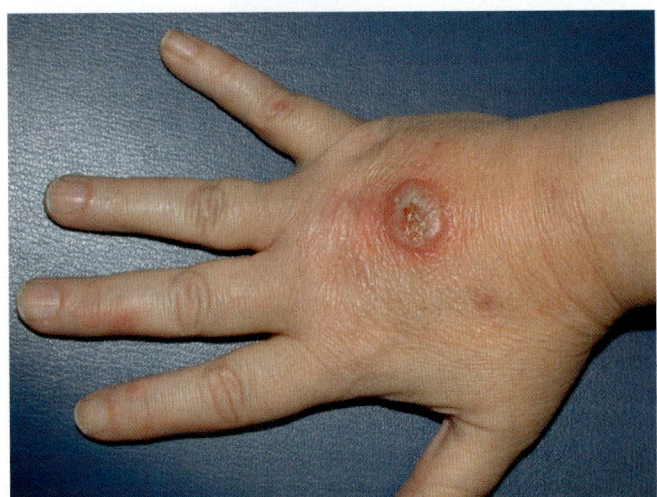

Fig. 7.40 Neutrophilic dermatosis of the dorsal hands.

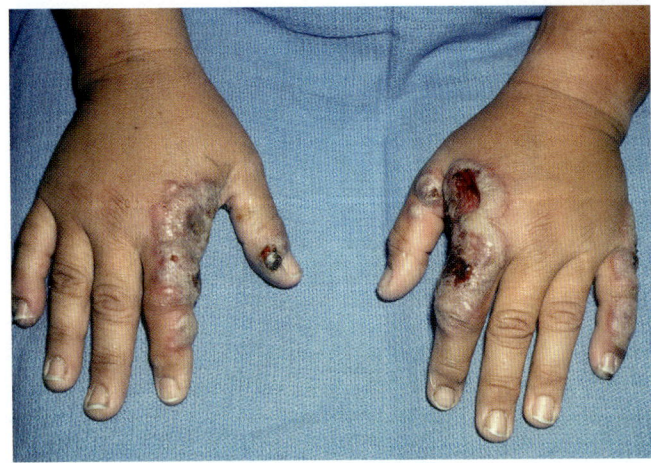

Fig. 7.41 Neutrophilic dermatosis of the dorsal hands.

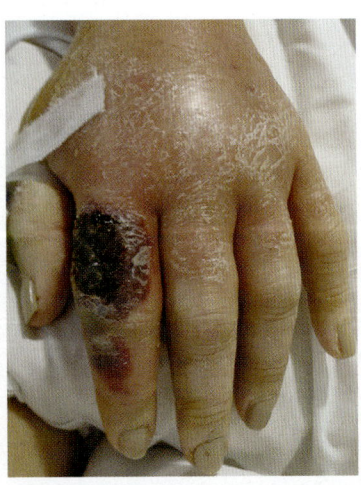

Fig. 7.42 Neutrophilic dermatosis of the dorsal hand.

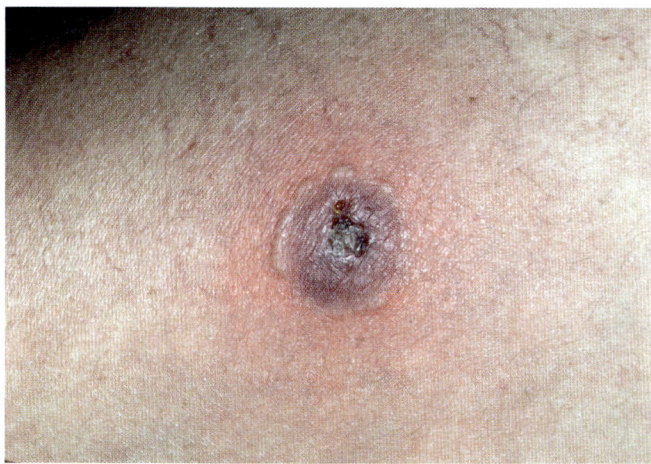

Fig. 7.43 Early pyoderma gangrenosum.

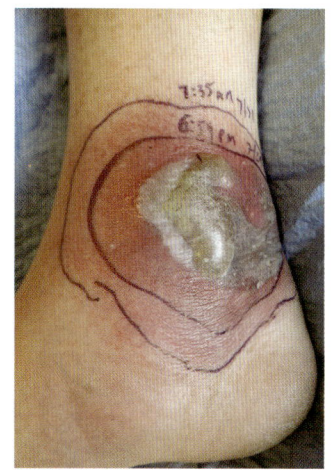

Fig. 7.44 Pyoderma gangrenosum.

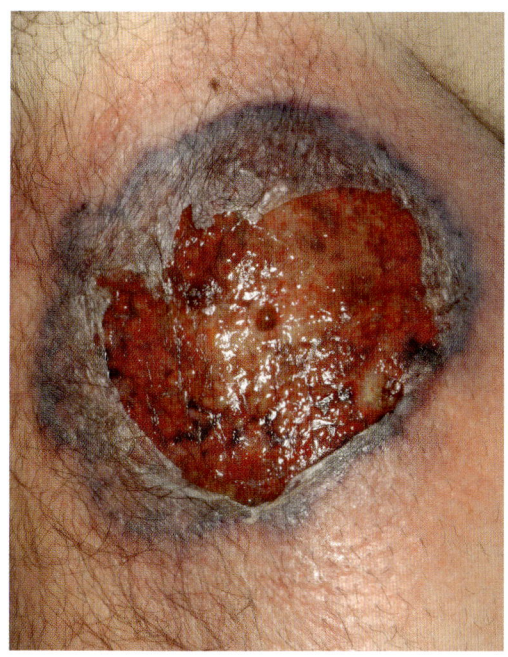

Fig. 7.45 Pyoderma gangrenosum. *Courtesy Misha Rosenbach, MD.*

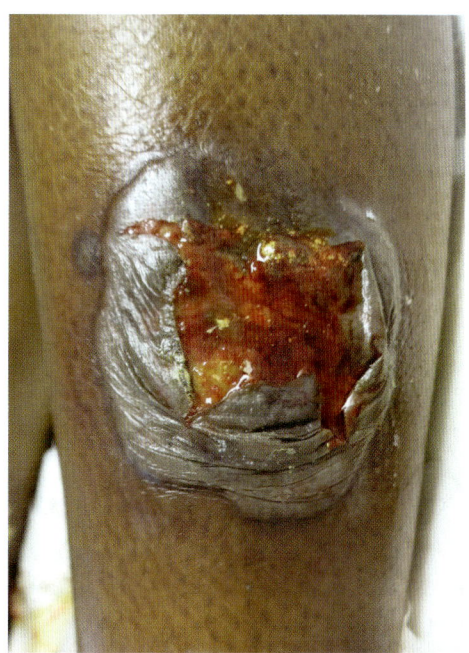

Fig. 7.46 Pyoderma gangrenosum in a patient with granulomatosis with polyangiitis.

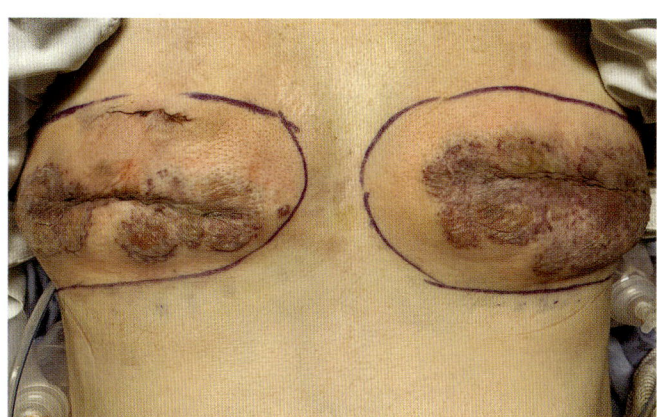

Fig. 7.47 Pyoderma gangrenosum after breast surgery.

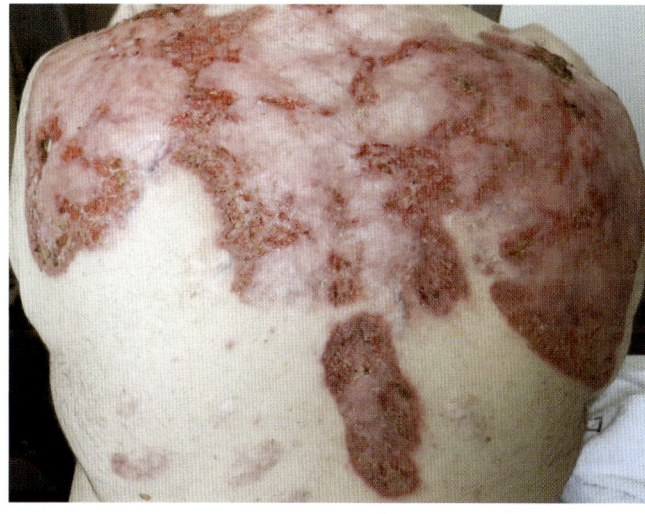

Fig. 7.48 Vegetative pyoderma gangrenosum.

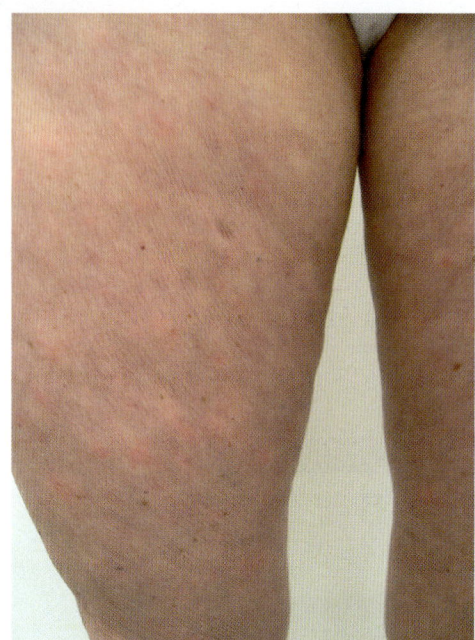

Fig. 7.49 Cryopyrin-associated periodic syndrome (Muckle-Wells syndrome). *Courtesy Karoline Krause, MD.*

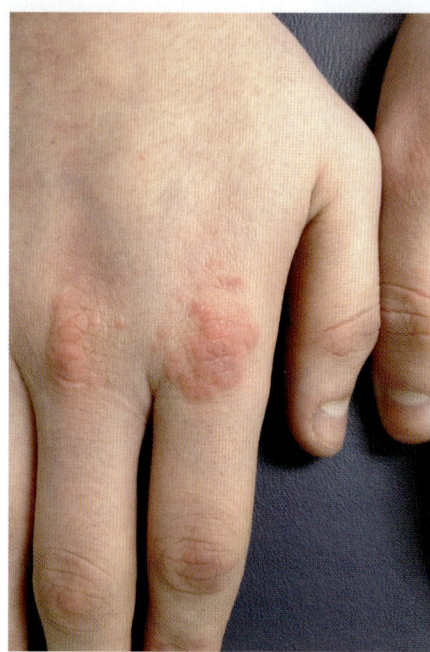

Fig. 7.50 Cryopyrin-associated periodic syndrome with atypical pernio-like lesions.

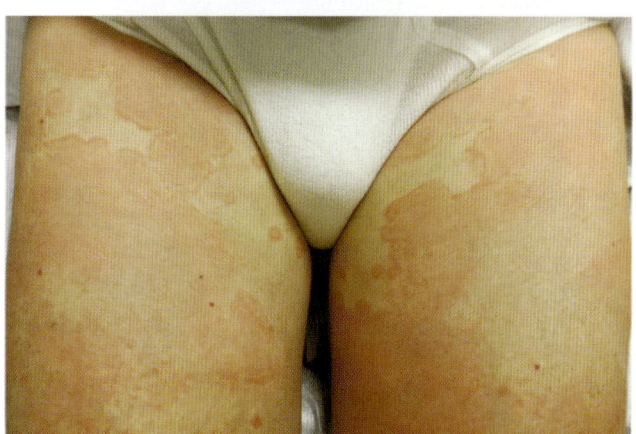

Fig. 7.51 Schnitzler syndrome.

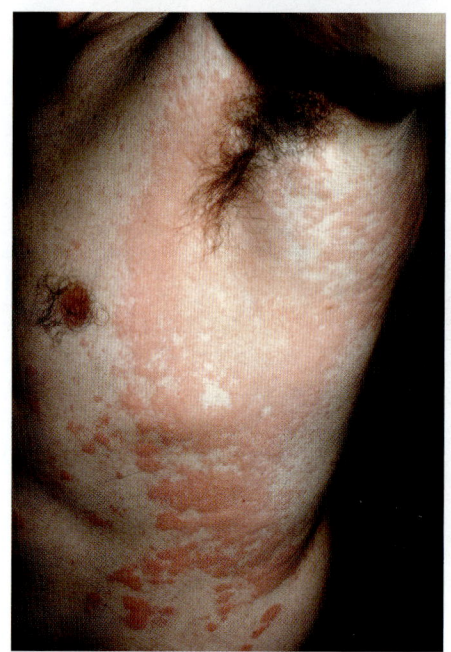

Fig. 7.52 Urticaria.

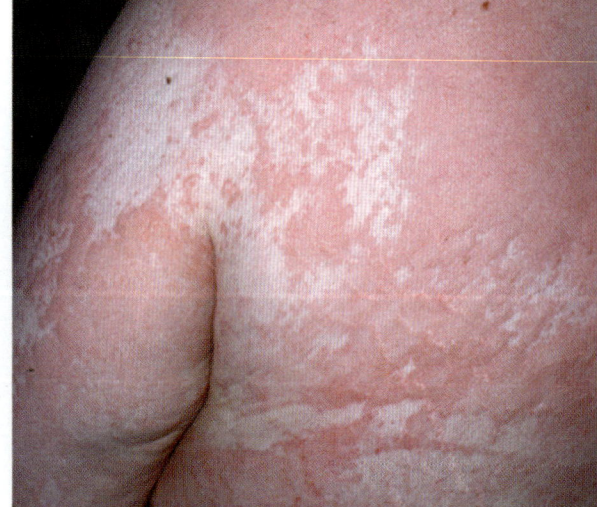

Fig. 7.53 Urticaria. *Courtesy The University of Utah and Oregon Health Sciences University Leonard Swinyer MD image collection.*

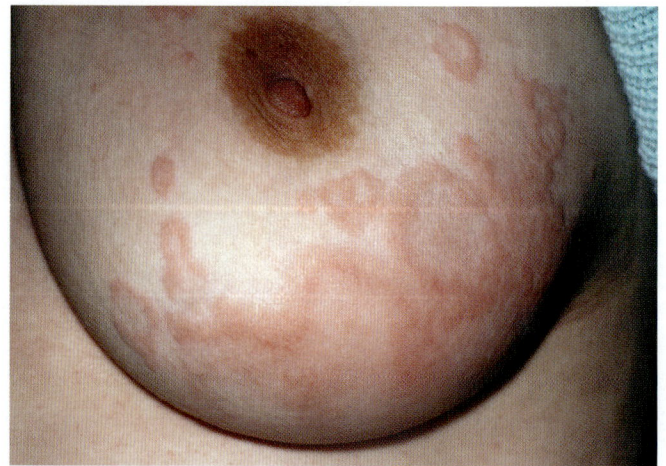

Fig. 7.54 Urticaria. *Courtesy Steven Binnick, MD.*

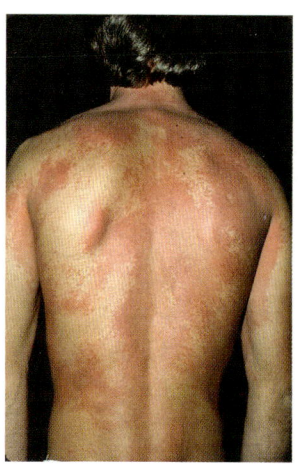

Fig. 7.55 Urticaria. *Courtesy The University of Utah and Oregon Health Sciences University Leonard Swinyer MD image collection.*

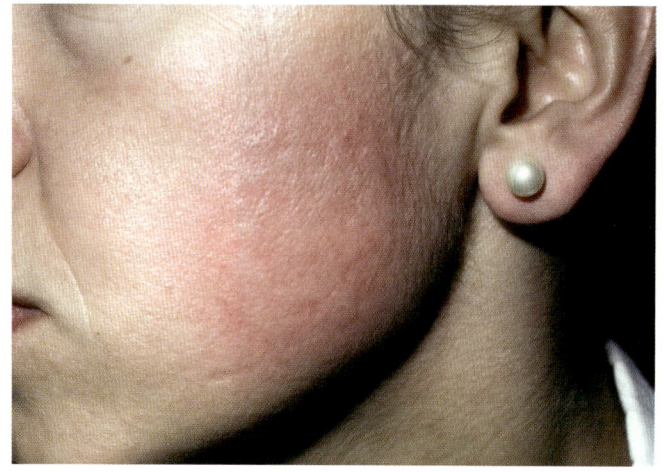

Fig. 7.56 Cold urticaria. *Courtesy Steven Binnick, MD.*

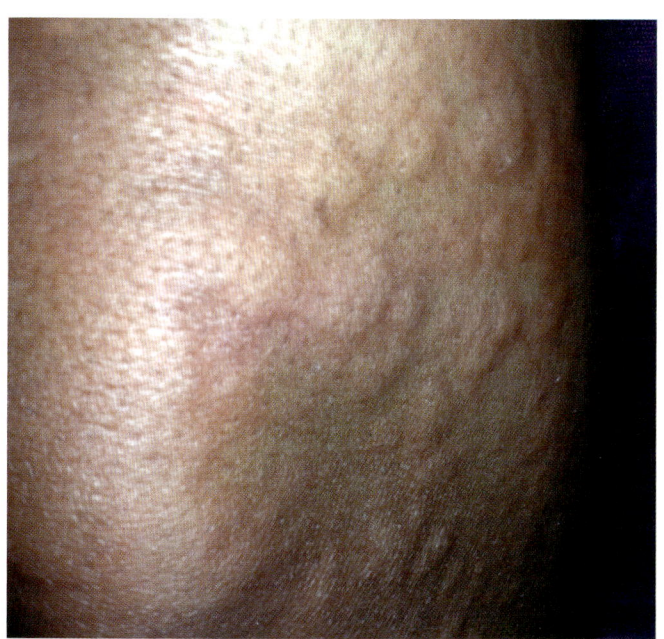

Fig. 7.57 Cold urticaria.

Fig. 7.58 Cold urticaria.

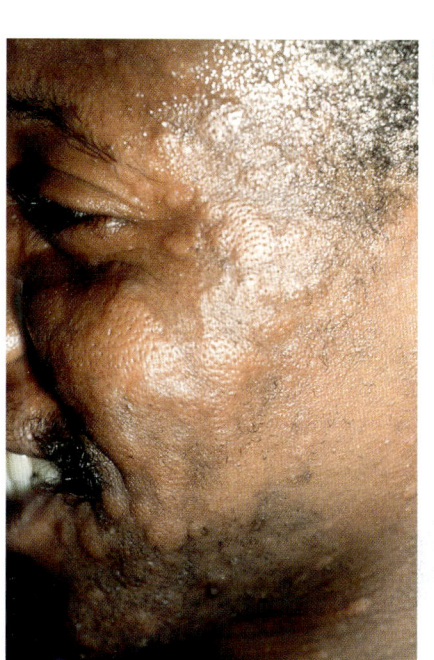

Fig. 7.59 Exercise-induced urticaria.

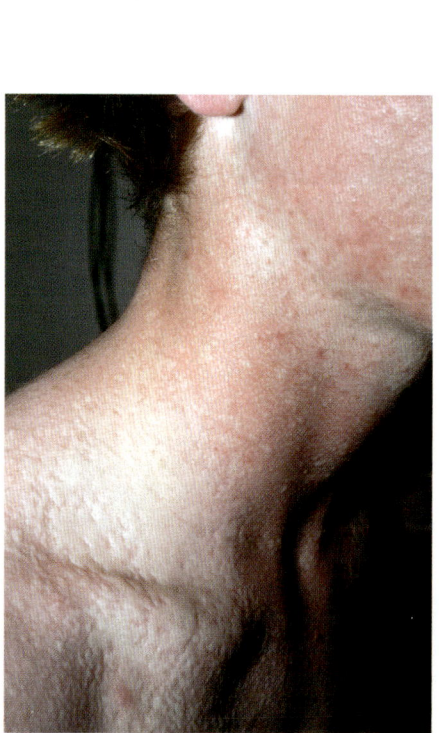

Fig. 7.60 Cholinergic urticaria.

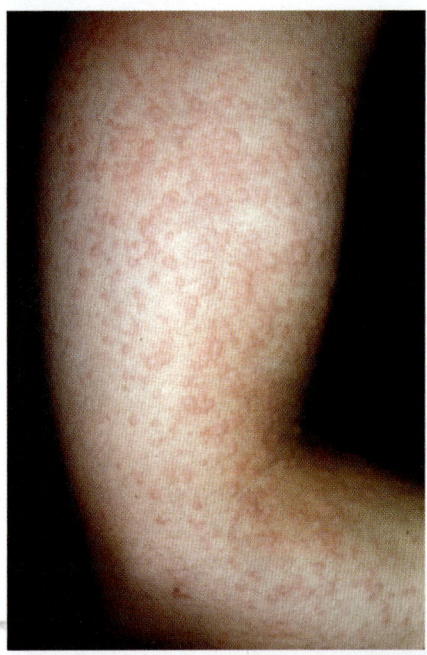

Fig. 7.61 Cholinergic urticaria.

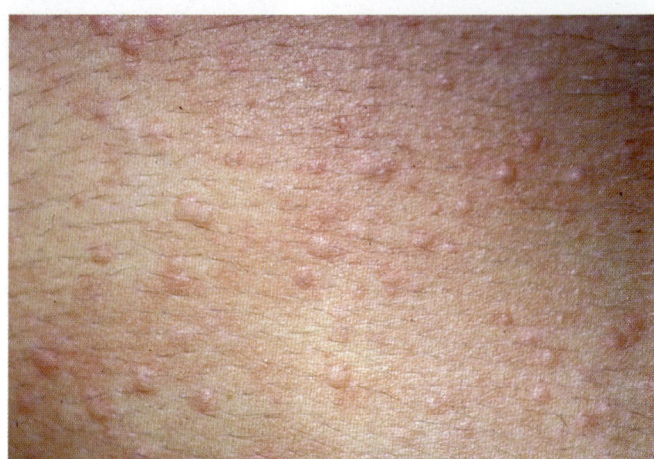

Fig. 7.62 Cholinergic urticaria.

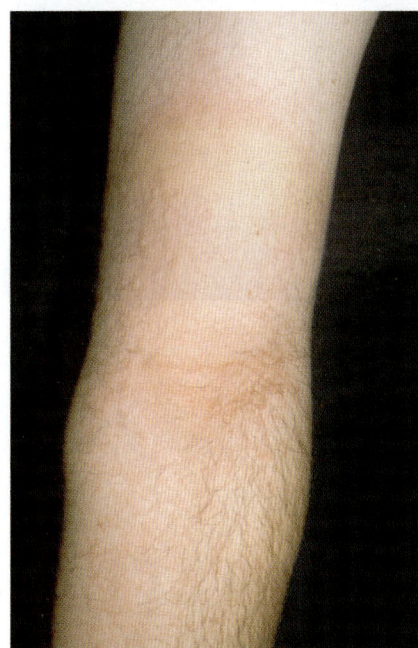

Fig. 7.63 Solar urticaria.

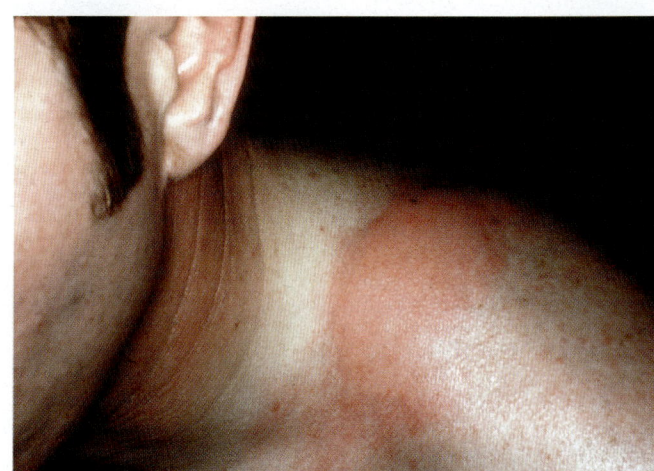

Fig. 7.64 Delayed pressure urticaria.

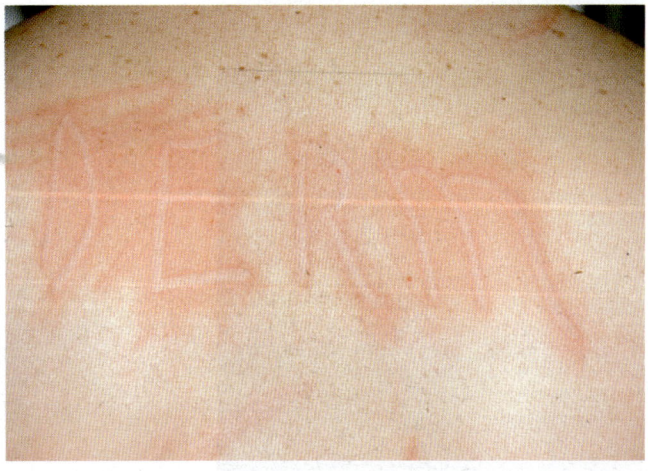

Fig. 7.65 Dermatographism.

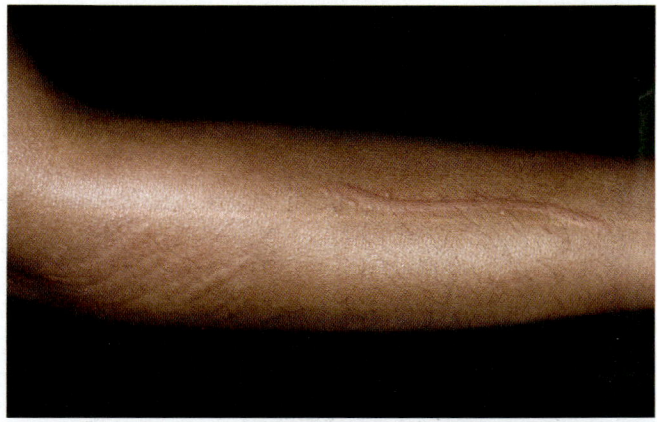

Fig. 7.66 Dermatographism. *Courtesy Curt Samlaska, MD.*

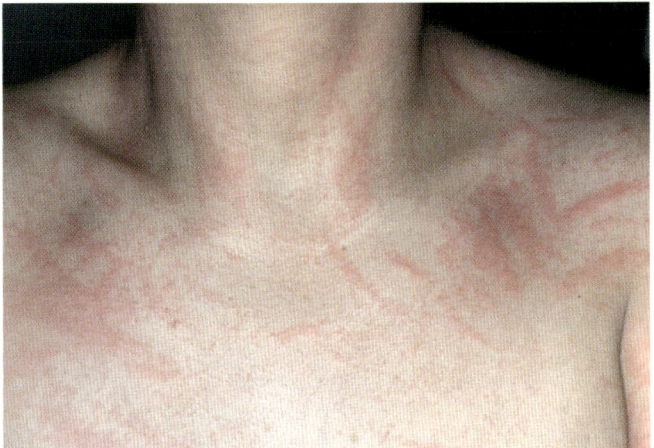

Fig. 7.67 Dermatographism.

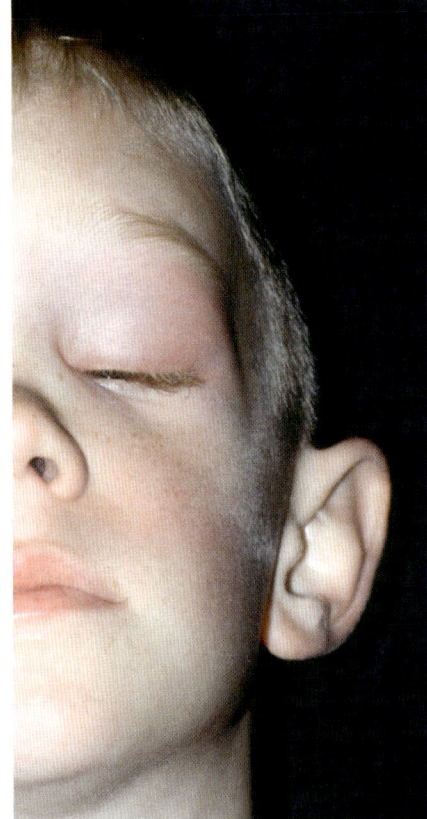

Fig. 7.68 Angioedema.

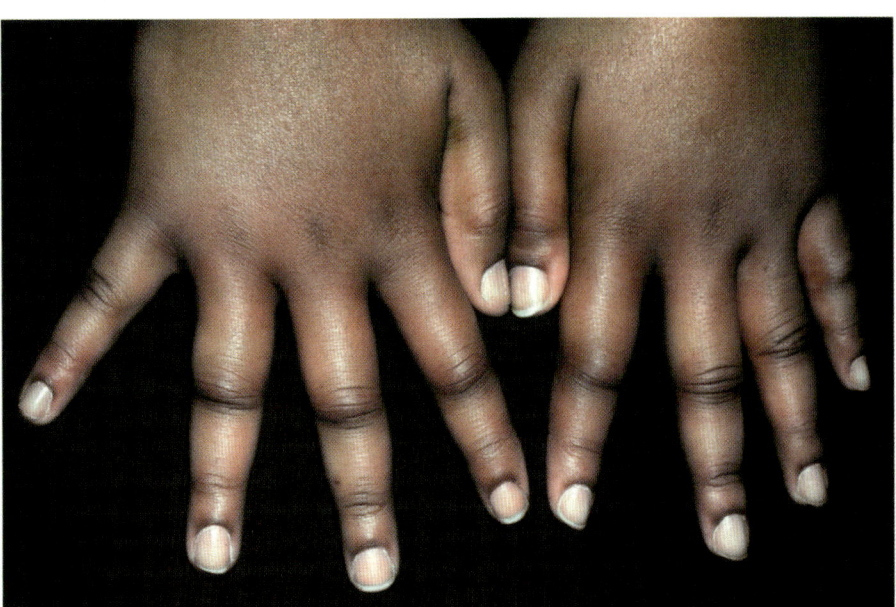

Fig. 7.69 Angioedema. *Courtesy Steven Binnick, MD.*

Connective Tissue Diseases 8

Cutaneous manifestations of connective tissue diseases are important to identify because they can be a clue to an undiagnosed systemic autoimmune disease. Many lesions, such as those seen in systemic lupus erythematosus (SLE) and dermatomyositis (DM), share a notable bright pink or purplish color, likely due to the intense lymphocytic inflammation found at the dermal-epidermal junction. Photosensitivity, as demonstrated best by the malar erythema of SLE and DM, is another shared feature of some connective tissue diseases, and therefore recognizing a photodistributed pattern is again important in this portion of the atlas.

Each subtype of lupus erythematosus has notable physical examination findings, including the scarring and dyspigmentation seen in discoid lupus erythematosus, the annular psoriasiform plaques of subacute cutaneous lupus erythematosus and neonatal lupus erythematosus, and the deeper palpable nodules or depressions of lupus profundus. Classically seen in DM as the heliotrope sign, some patients with DM or SLE will present with purplish patches of the eyelids.

This chapter also includes the spectrum of skin findings seen in localized and systemic scleroderma. Localized scleroderma (morphea) presents with an expanding, indurated, pink or lilac sometimes circinate, plaque that leaves scarlike dyspigmentation centrally and can lead to disfigurement, joint contractures, and skin ulcerations. In contrast, limited and systemic scleroderma present with distinctive cutaneous signs such as matlike telangiectasias, calcinosis cutis, and, in some, a symmetric, progressive, woody edema.

Patients with suspected connective tissue disease deserve a full review of systems and physical examination for rarer mucocutaneous findings, such as mucosal erosions or ulcerations, alopecia, sclerodactyly, nailfold capillary changes, and lymphadenopathy. Skin biopsies are almost always warranted and helpful when gathering information to confirm some of these difficult diagnoses.

This portion of the atlas features the aforementioned and other rarer connective tissue diseases and their multitude of cutaneous stigmata.

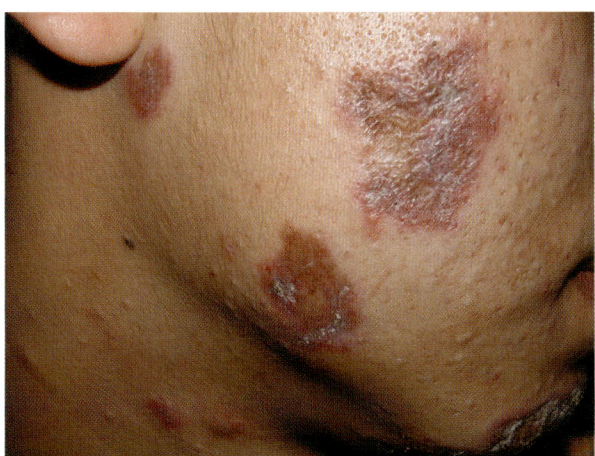

Fig. 8.1 Discoid lupus erythematosus. *Courtesy Chia-Yu Chu, MD, PhD.*

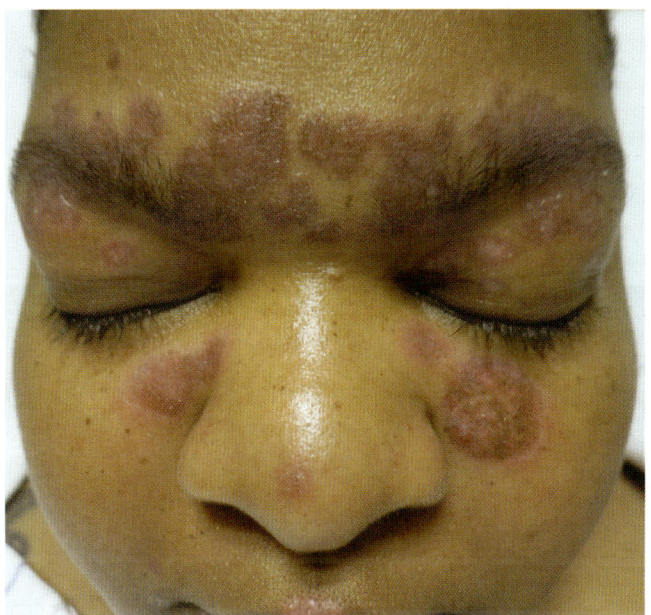

Fig. 8.2 Discoid lupus erythematosus.

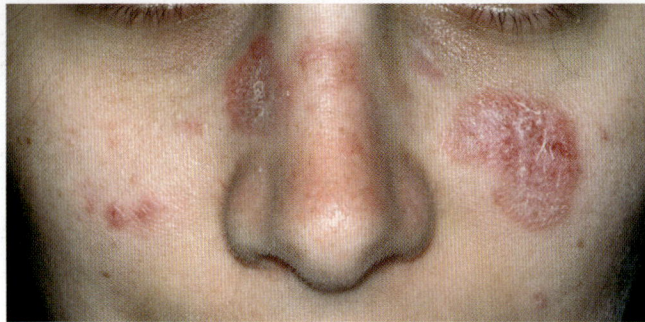

Fig. 8.3 Discoid lupus erythematosus. *Courtesy Steven Binnick, MD.*

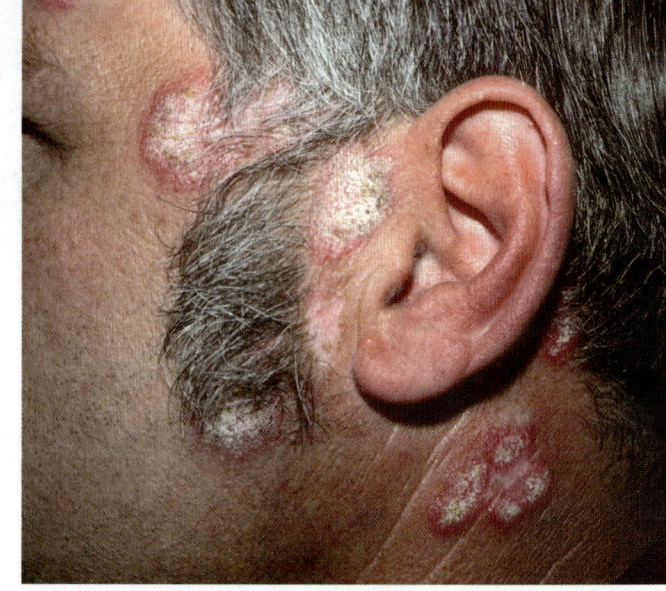

Fig. 8.4 Discoid lupus erythematosus. *Courtesy Steven Binnick, MD.*

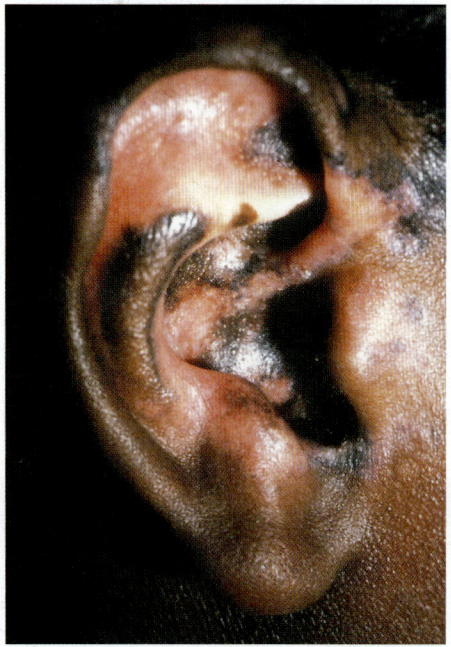

Fig. 8.5 Discoid lupus erythematosus.

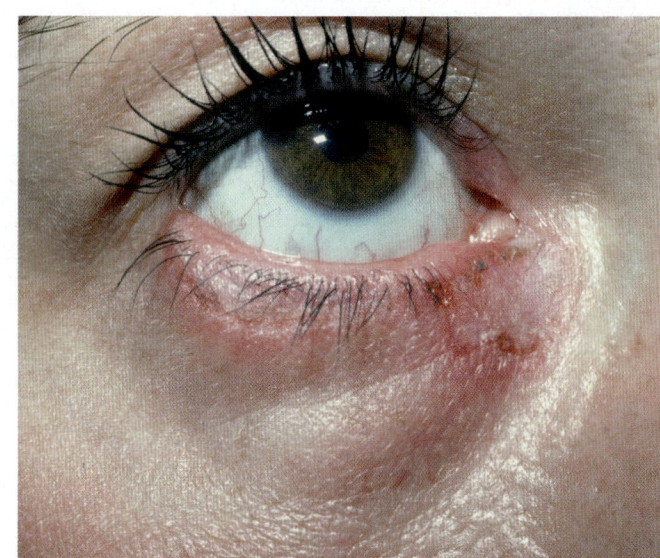

Fig. 8.6 Discoid lupus erythematosus. *Courtesy Steven Binnick, MD.*

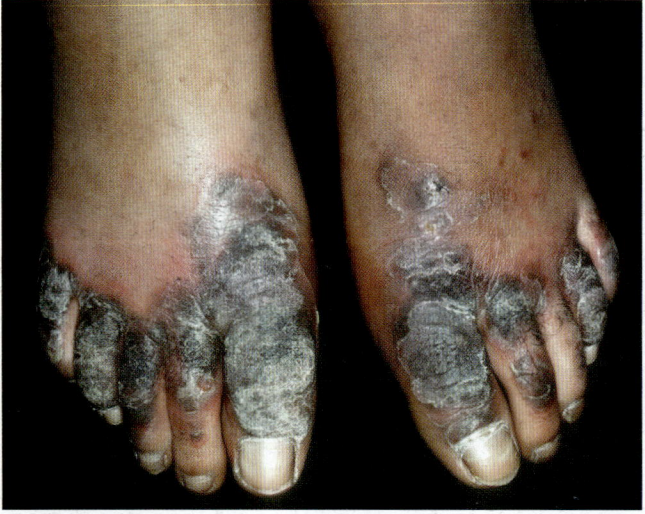

Fig. 8.7 Discoid lupus erythematosus.

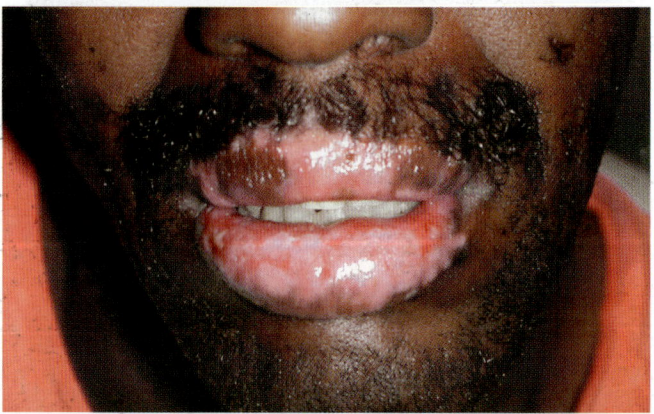

Fig. 8.8 Discoid lupus erythematosus.

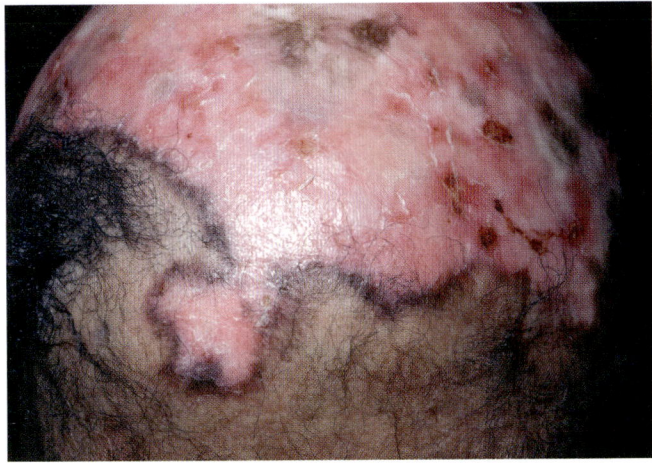

Fig. 8.9 Discoid lupus erythematosus. *Courtesy Steven Binnick, MD.*

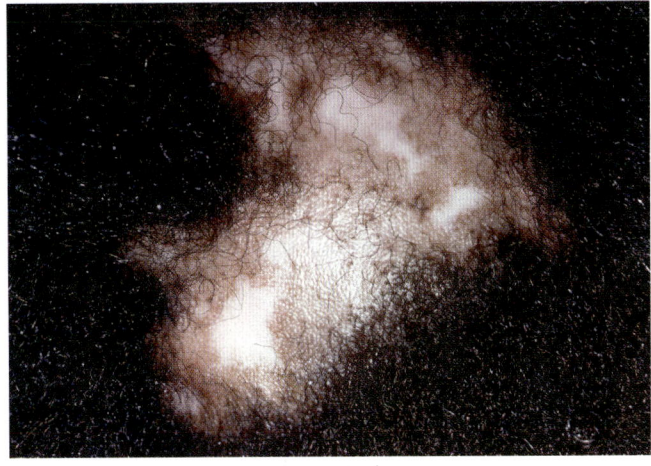

Fig. 8.10 Discoid lupus erythematosus. *Courtesy Steven Binnick, MD.*

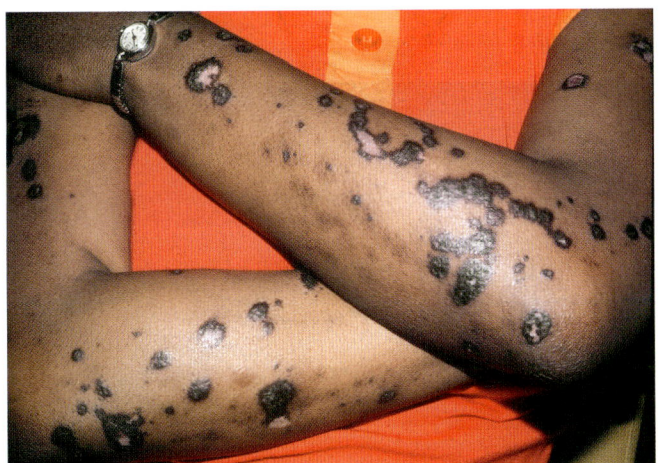

Fig. 8.11 Generalized discoid lupus erythematosus. *Courtesy Steven Binnick, MD.*

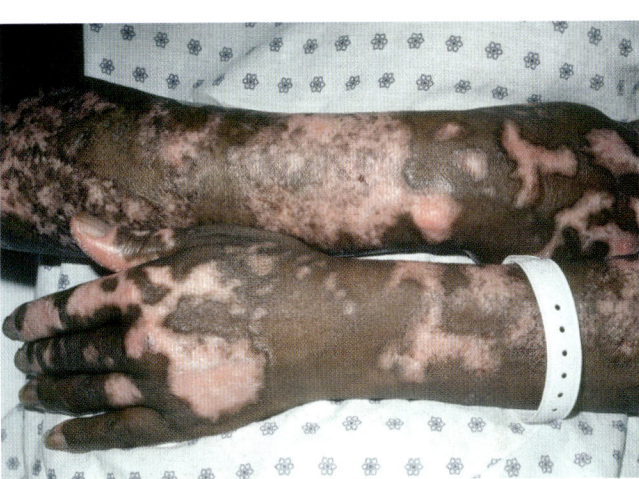

Fig. 8.12 Generalized discoid lupus erythematosus. *Courtesy Steven Binnick, MD.*

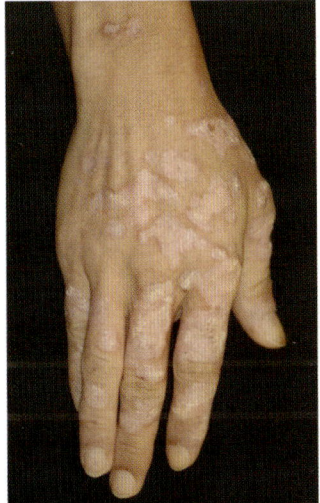

Fig. 8.13 Discoid lupus erythematosus. *Courtesy Kaohsiung Chang Gang Memorial Hospital, Taiwan.*

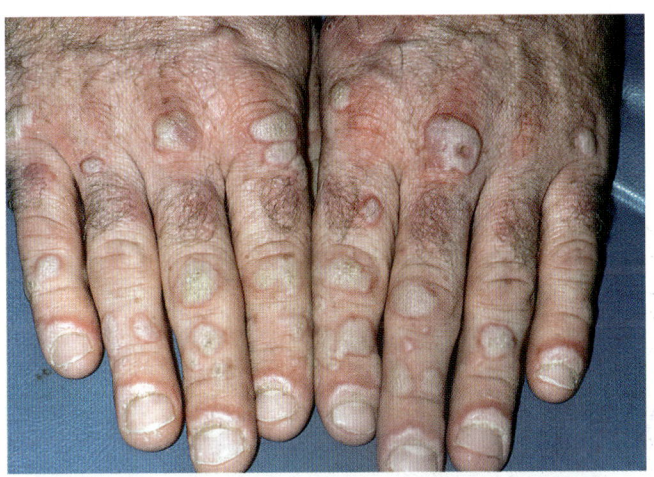

Fig. 8.14 Hypertrophic lupus erythematosus. *Courtesy Steven Binnick, MD.*

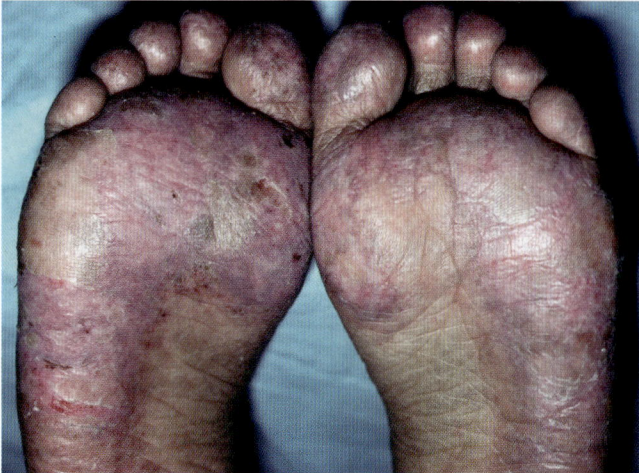

Fig. 8.15 Lichen planus lupus erythematosus overlap. *Courtesy Ken Greer, MD.*

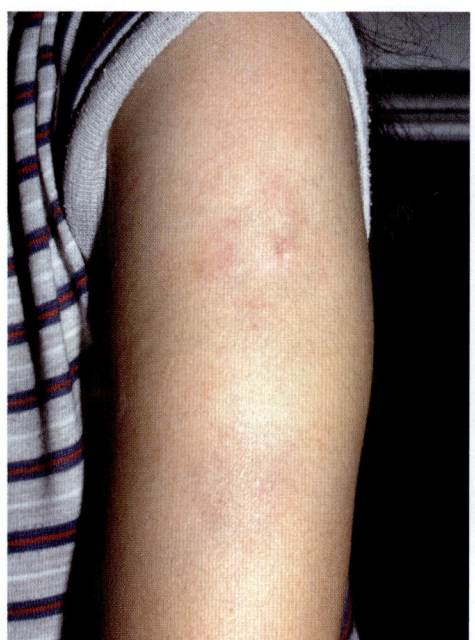

Fig. 8.17 Lupus profundus.

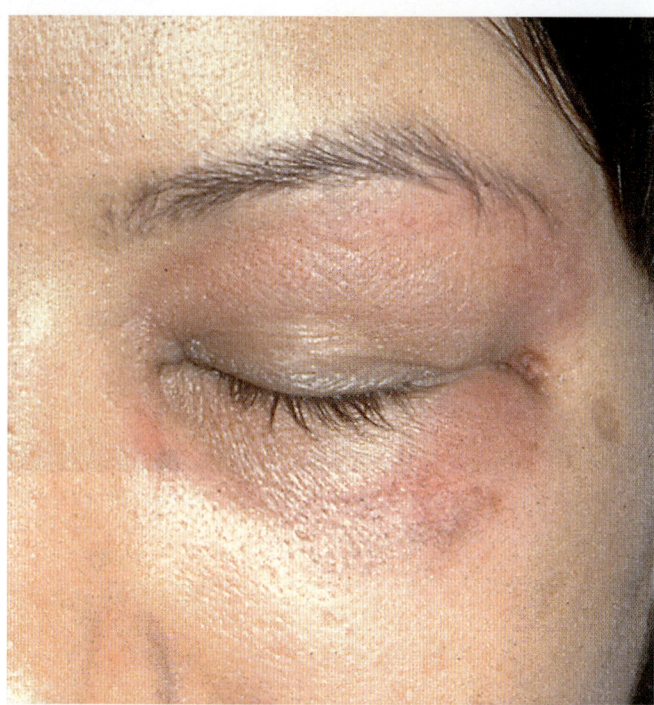

Fig. 8.16 Lupus profundus.

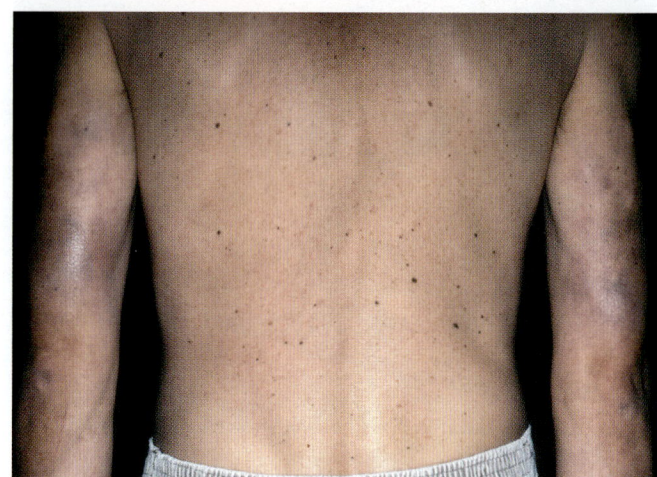

Fig. 8.18 Lupus profundus. *Courtesy Curt Samlaska, MD.*

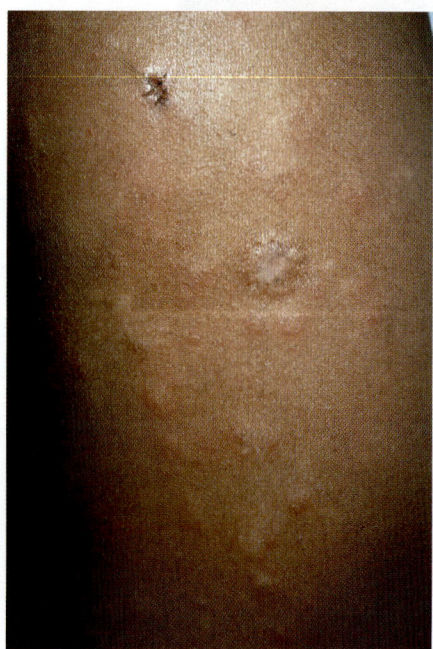

Fig. 8.20 Tumid lupus erythematosus.

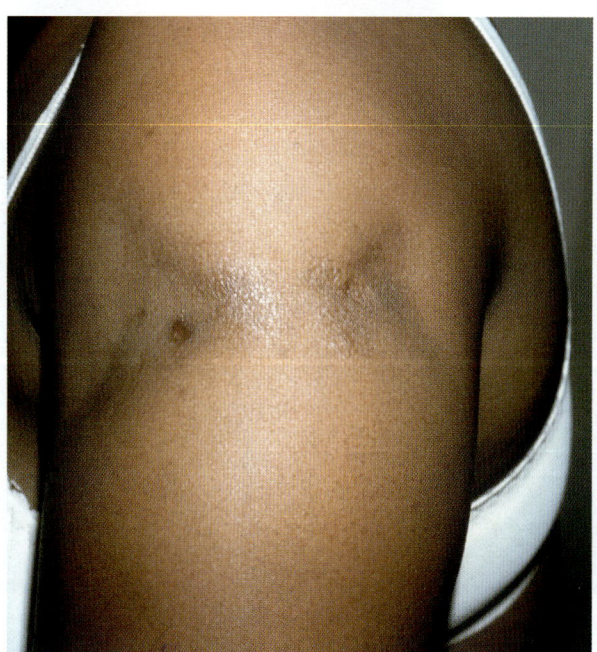

Fig. 8.19 Lupus profundus with resultant atrophy.

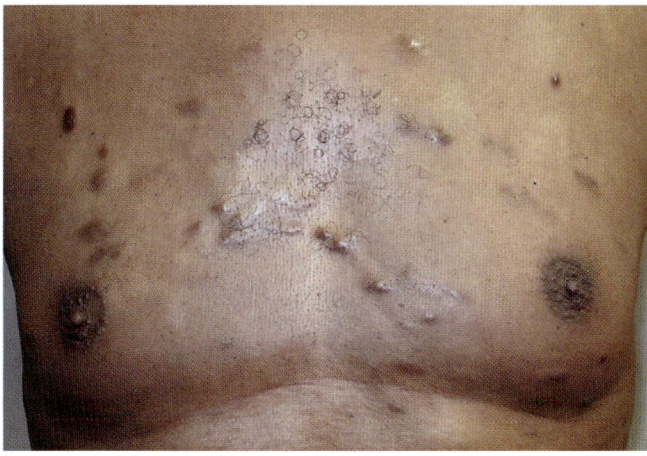

Fig. 8.21 Tumid lupus erythematosus.

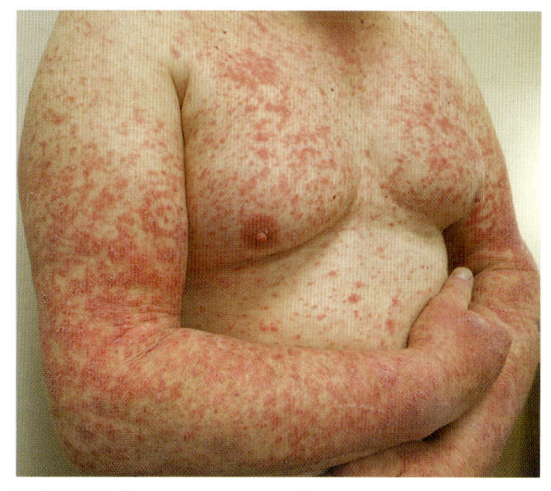

Fig. 8.22 Subacute cutaneous lupus erythematosus secondary to a proton pump inhibitor.

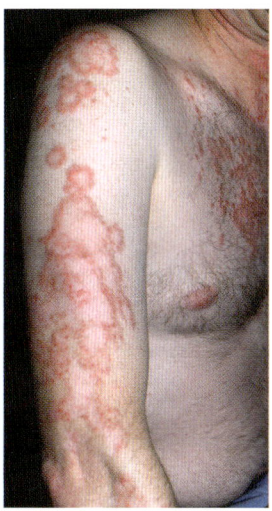

Fig. 8.23 Subacute cutaneous lupus erythematosus. *Courtesy The University of Utah and Oregon Health Sciences University Leonard Swinyer MD image collection.*

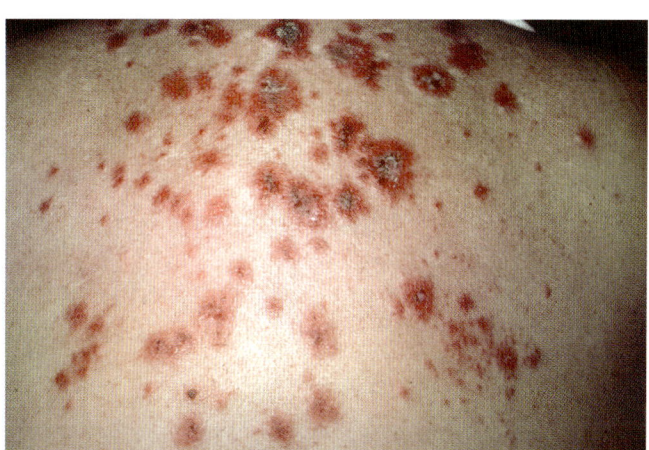

Fig. 8.24 Subacute cutaneous lupus erythematosus.

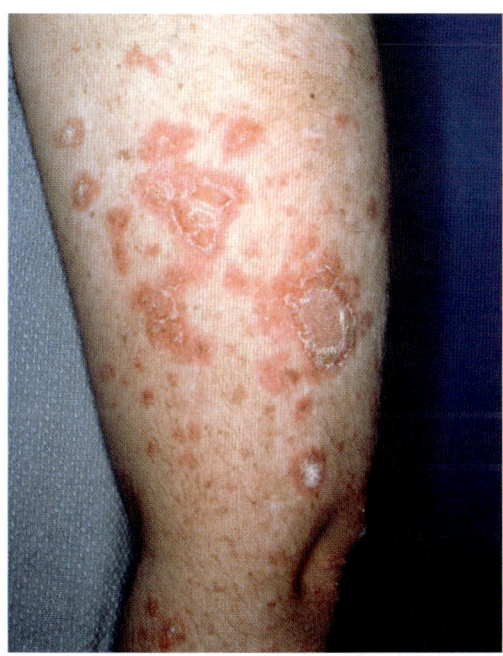

Fig. 8.25 Subacute cutaneous lupus erythematosus.

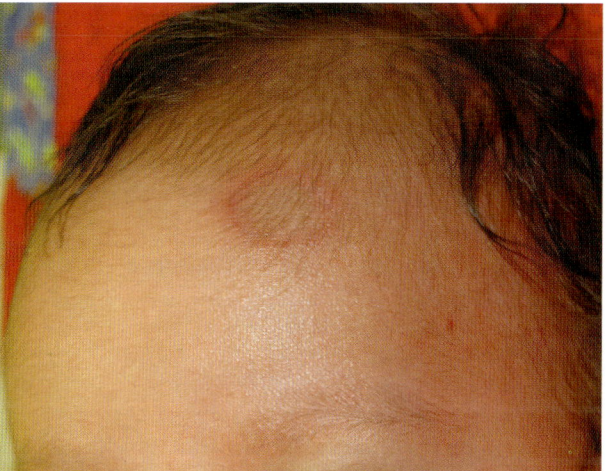

Fig. 8.26 Neonatal lupus erythematosus.

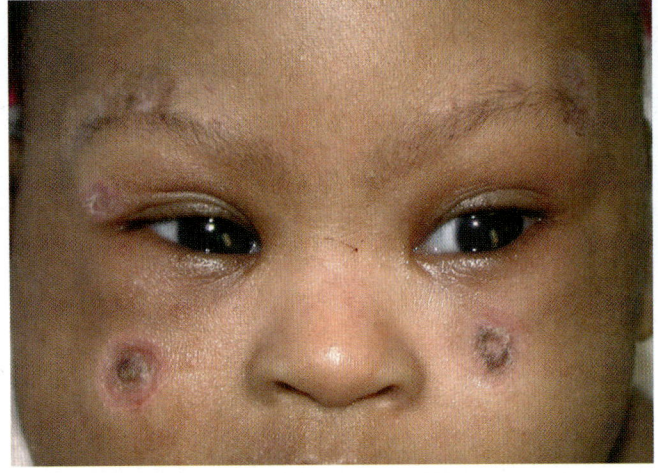

Fig. 8.27 Neonatal lupus erythematosus with scarring.

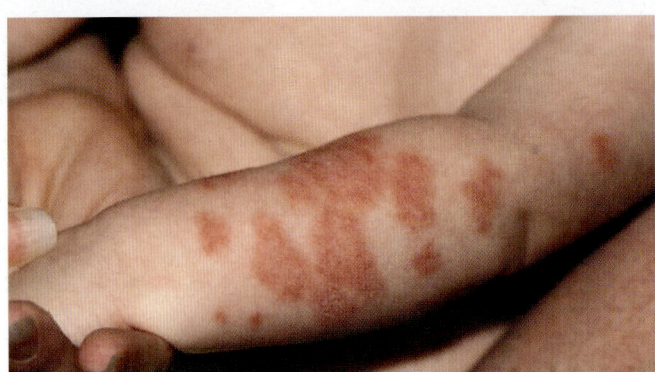

Fig. 8.28 Neonatal lupus erythematosus.

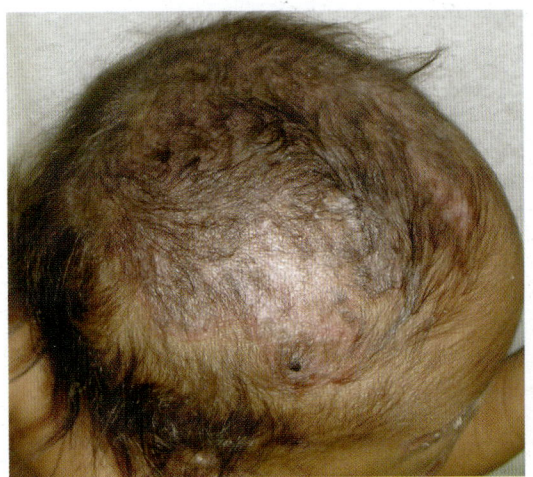

Fig. 8.29 Neonatal lupus erythematosus.

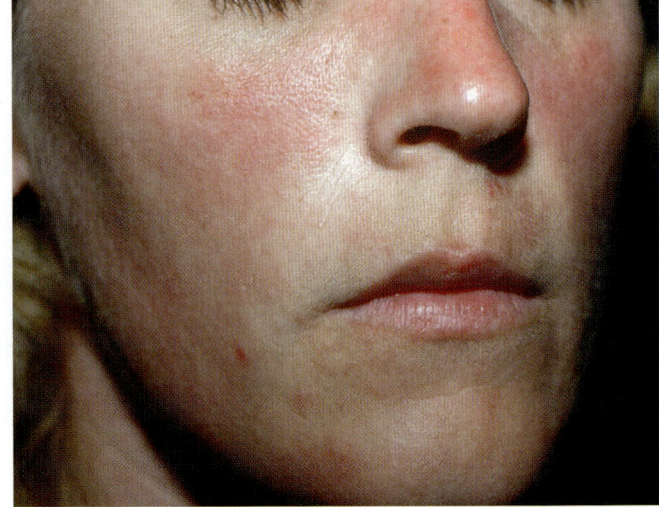

Fig. 8.30 Acute systemic lupus erythematosus.

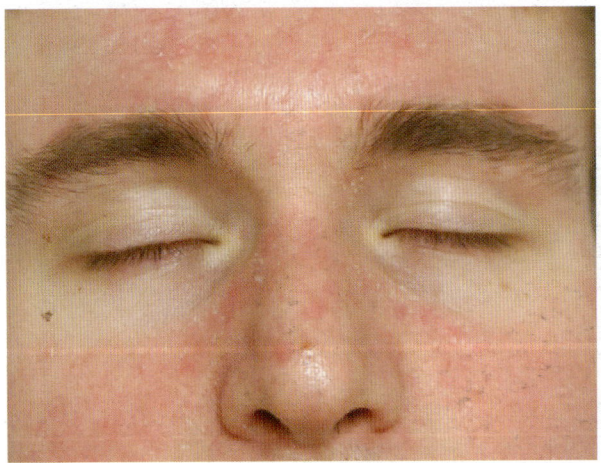

Fig. 8.31 Acute systemic lupus erythematosus.

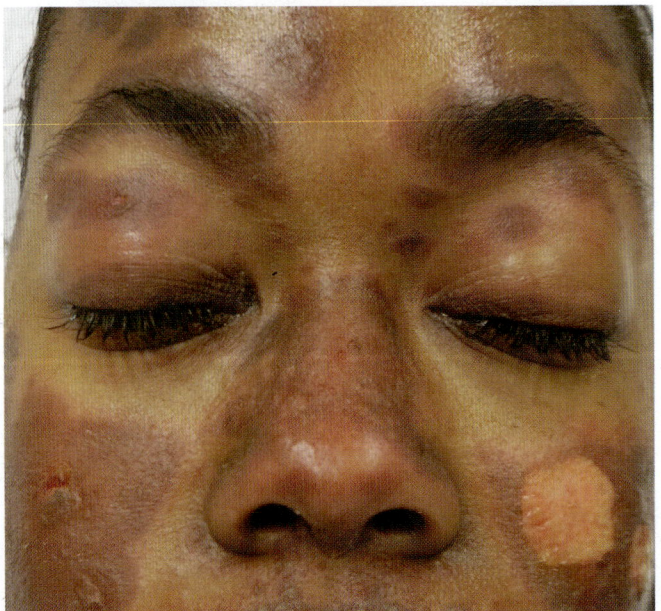

Fig. 8.32 Acute systemic lupus erythematosus.

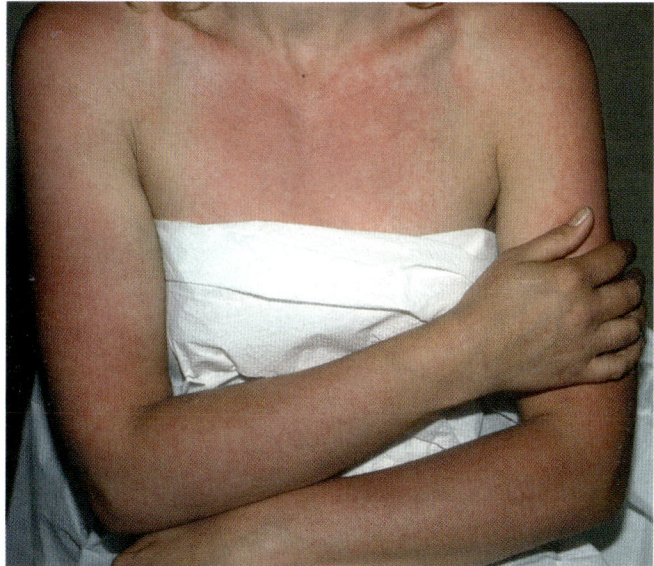

Fig. 8.33 Acute systemic lupus erythematosus.

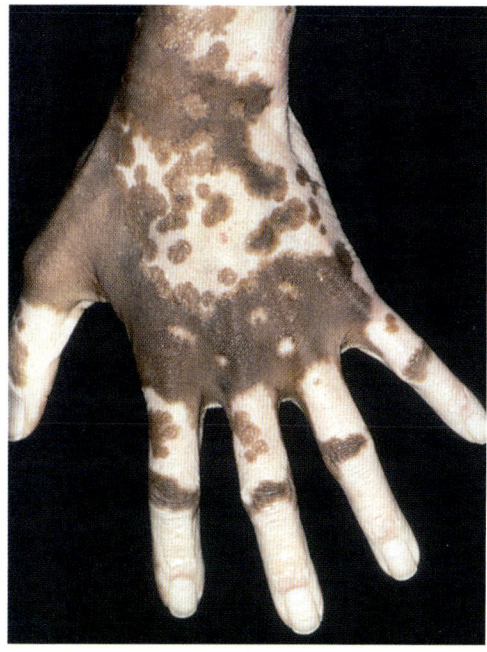

Fig. 8.34 Systemic lupus erythematosus with dyspigmentation. Note sparing over the proximal interphalangeal and metacarpophalangeal joints.

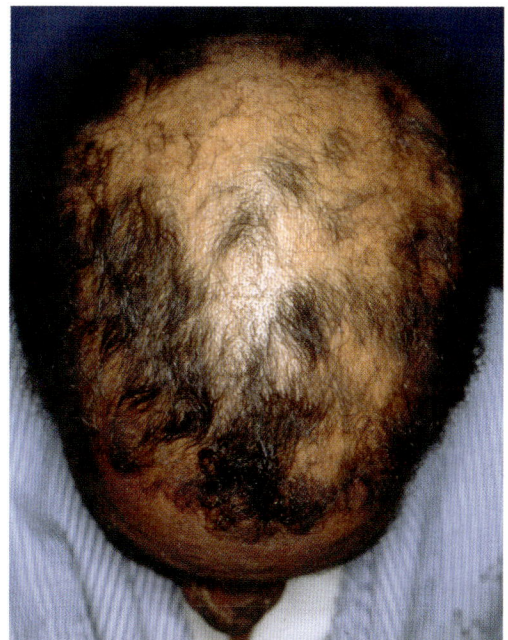

Fig. 8.35 Alopecia in systemic lupus erythematosus.

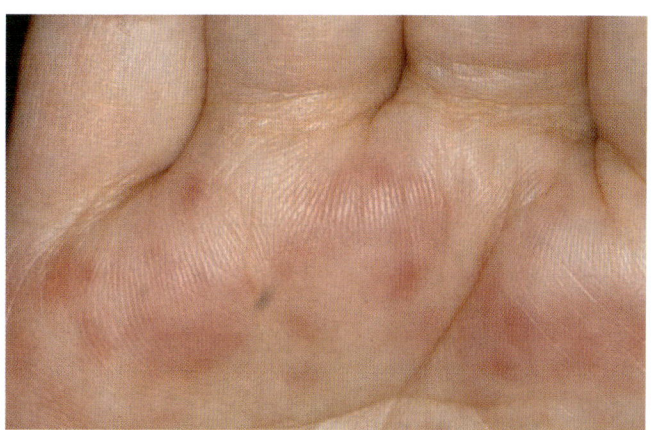

Fig. 8.36 Systemic lupus erythematosus.

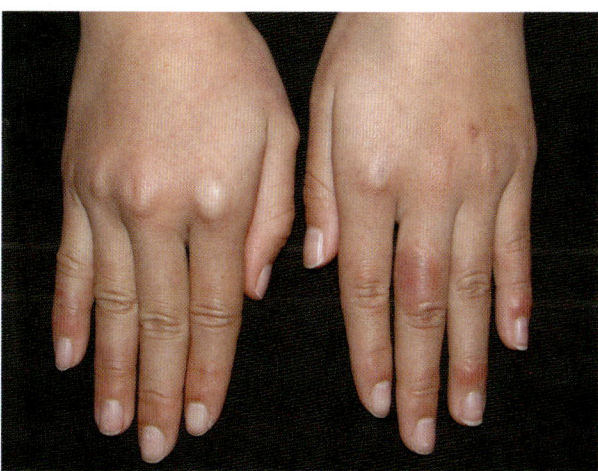

Fig. 8.37 Chilblain systemic lupus erythematosus. *Courtesy Chia-Yu Chu, MD, PhD.*

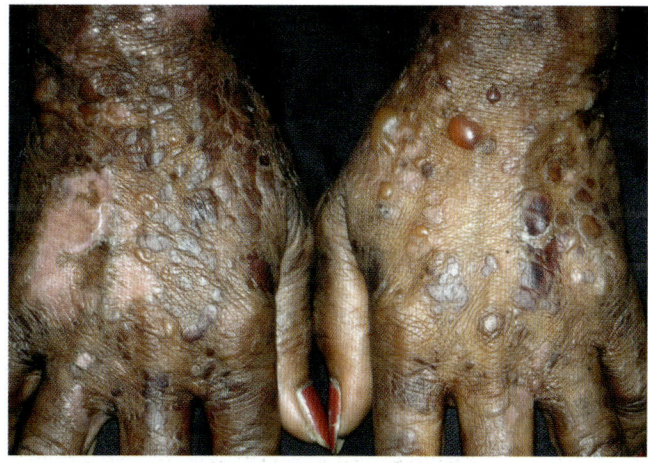

Fig. 8.38 Bullous systemic lupus erythematosus.

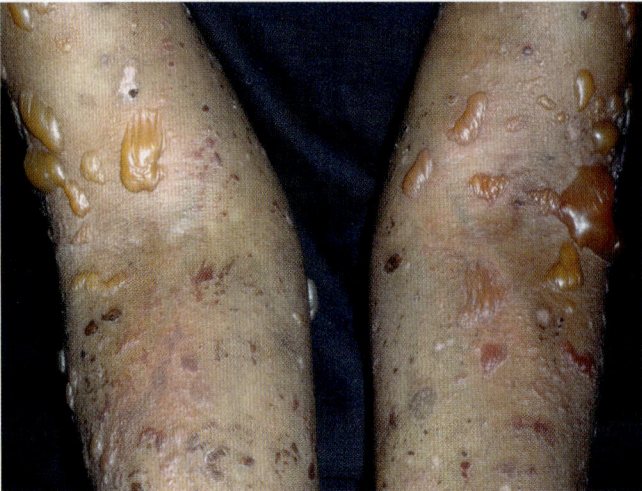

Fig. 8.39 Bullous systemic lupus erythematosus.

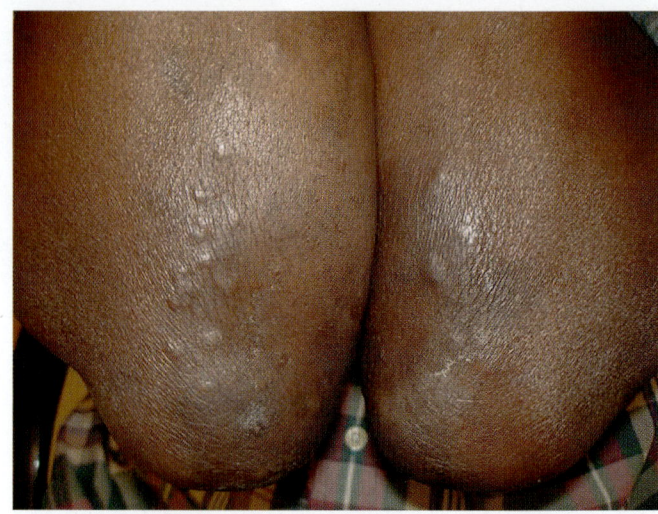

Fig. 8.40 Palisaded neutrophilic granulomatous dermatitis.

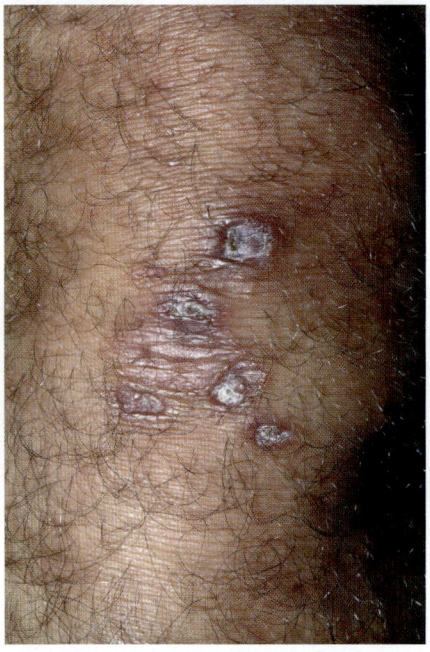

Fig. 8.41 Palisaded neutrophilic granulomatous dermatitis.

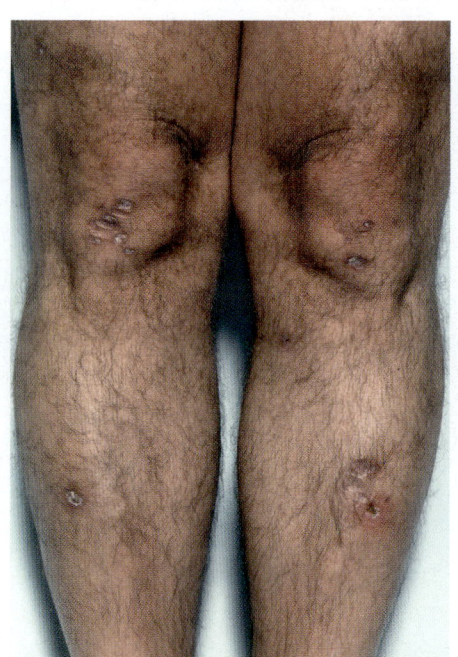

Fig. 8.42 Palisaded neutrophilic granulomatous dermatitis.

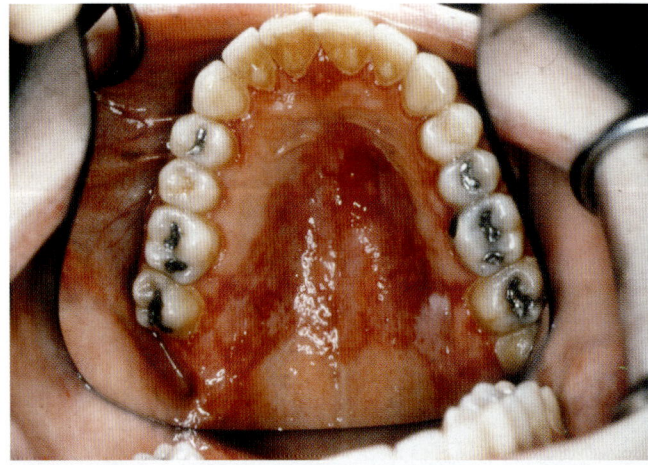

Fig. 8.43 Oral lupus erythematosus.

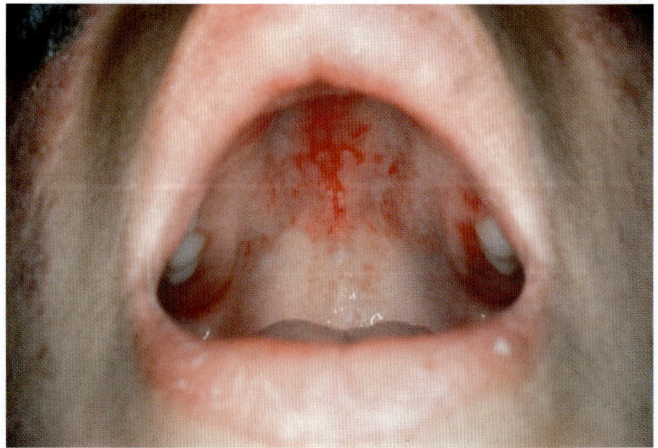

Fig. 8.44 Oral lupus erythematosus.

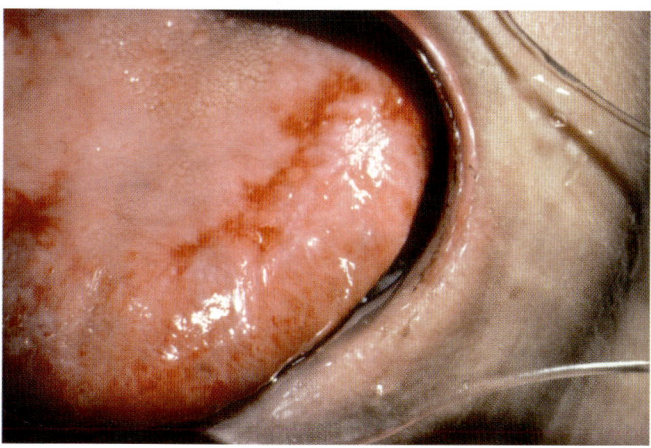

Fig. 8.45 Oral lupus erythematosus.

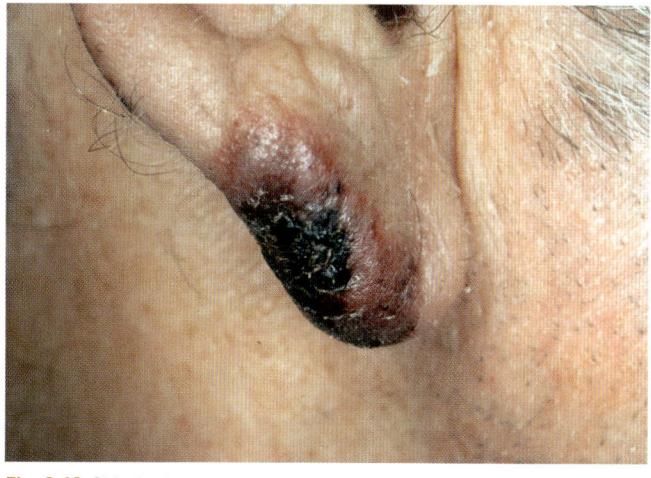

Fig. 8.46 Skin lesions secondary to antiphospholipid antibodies in systemic lupus erythematosus.

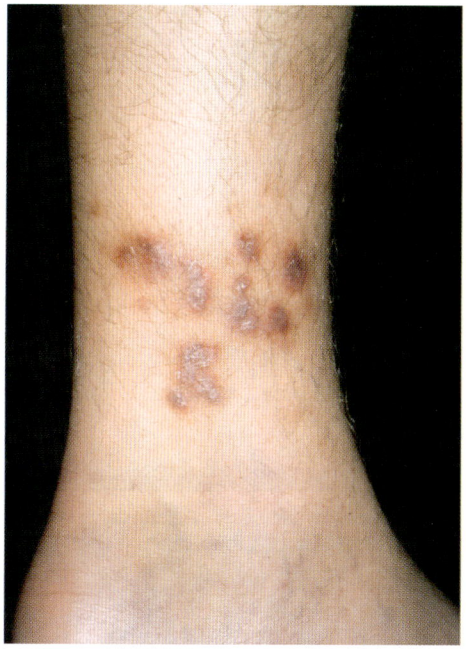

Fig. 8.47 Skin lesions secondary to antiphospholipid antibodies in systemic lupus erythematosus.

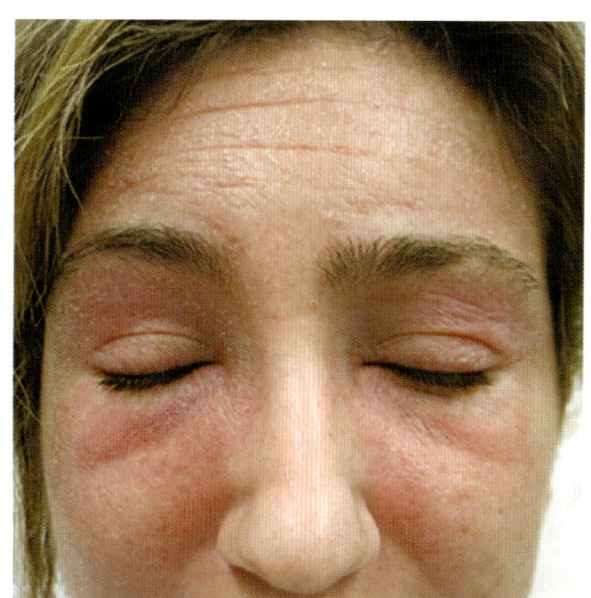

Fig. 8.48 Dermatomyositis, heliotrope.

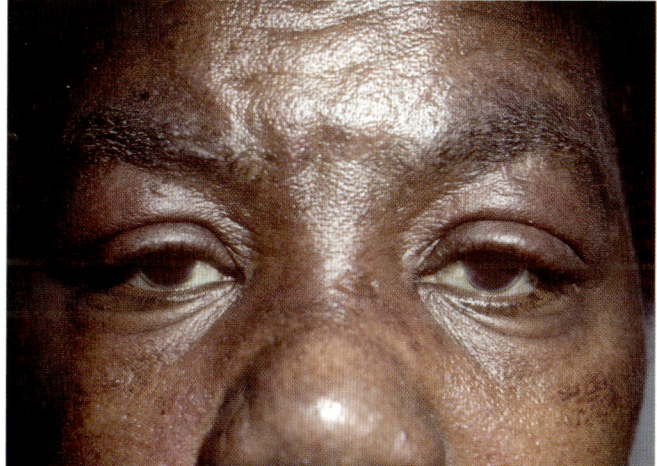

Fig. 8.49 Dermatomyositis, heliotrope. *Courtesy Ken Greer, MD.*

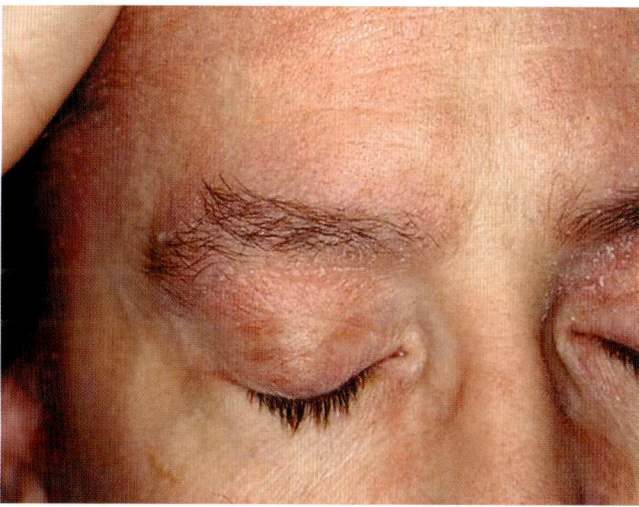

Fig. 8.50 Dermatomyositis, heliotrope.

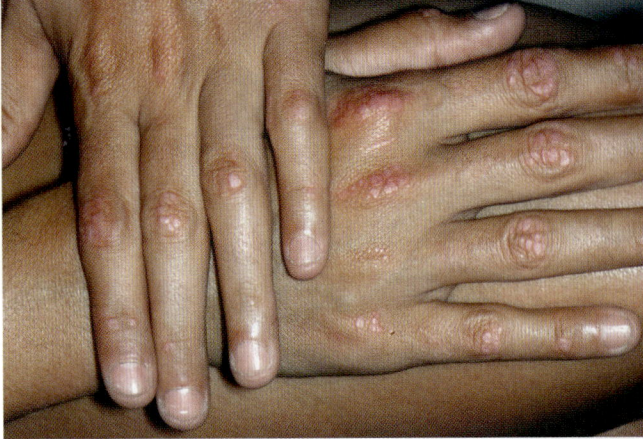

Fig. 8.51 Dermatomyositis, Gottron's papules.

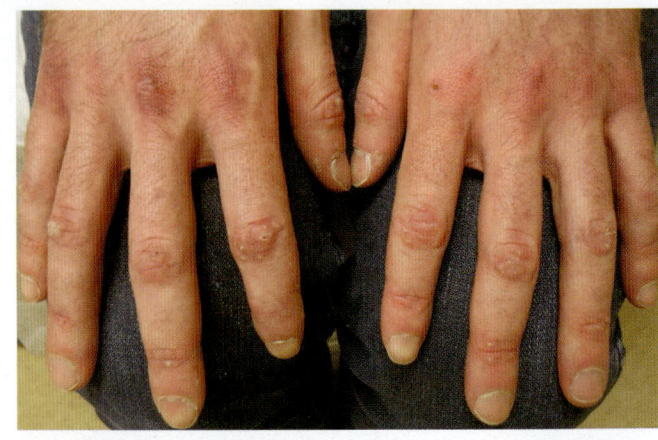

Fig. 8.52 Dermatomyositis, Gottron's papules.

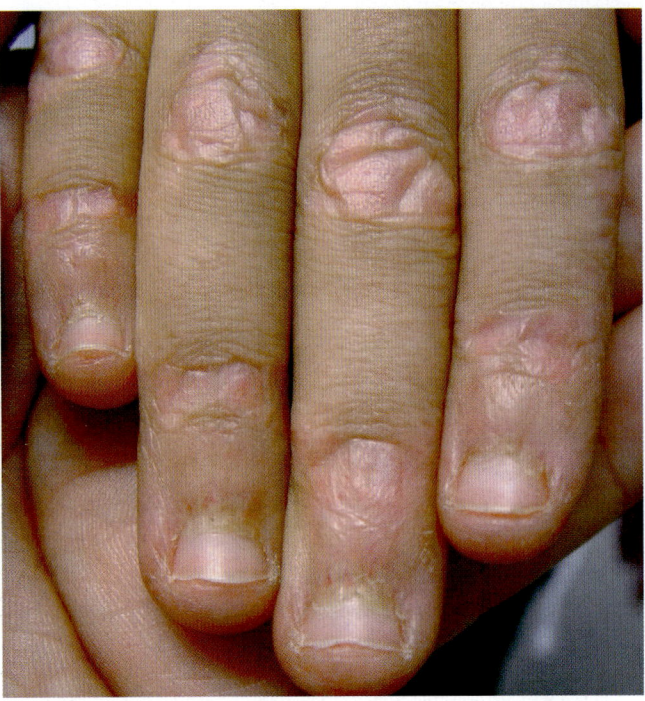

Fig. 8.53 Dermatomyositis, Gottron's papules.

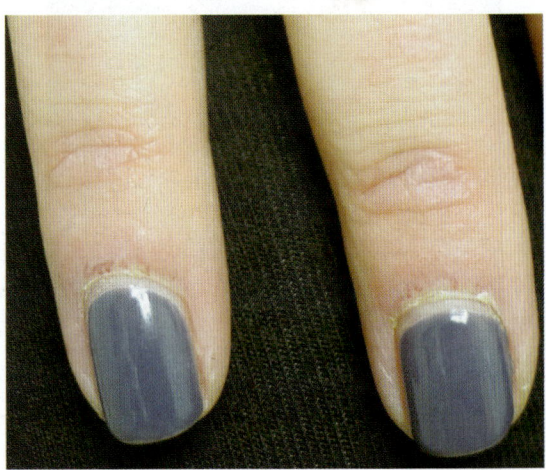

Fig. 8.54 Dermatomyositis, nailfold capillary dilation, Samitz sign, and Gottron's papules.

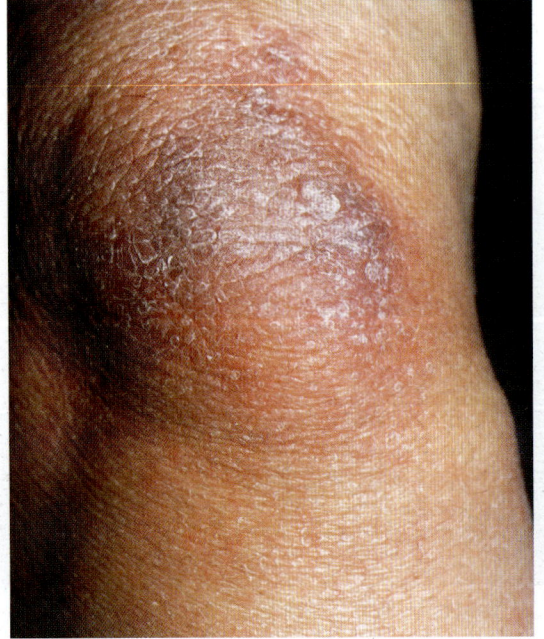

Fig. 8.55 Dermatomyositis, Gottron's sign.

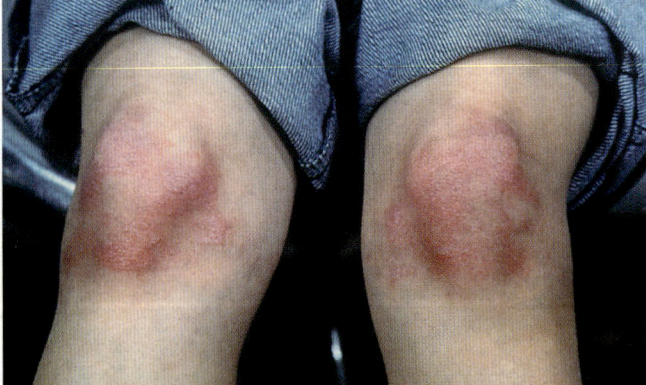

Fig. 8.56 Dermatomyositis, Gottron's sign.

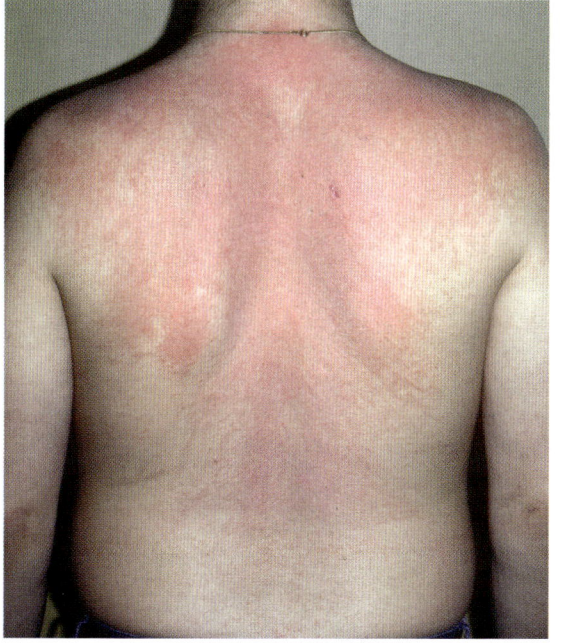

Fig. 8.57 Dermatomyositis, shawl sign. *Courtesy Steven Binnick, MD.*

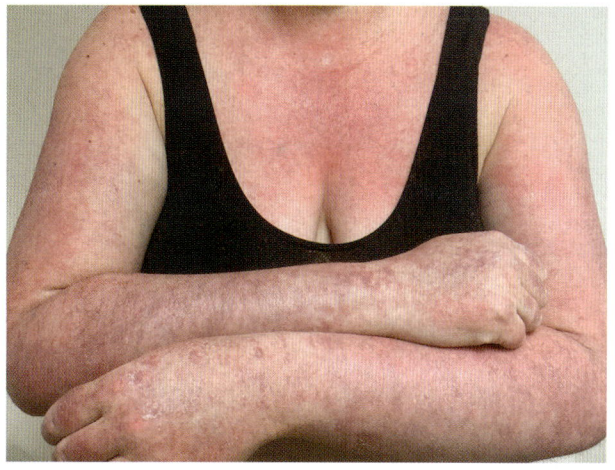

Fig. 8.58 Dermatomyositis, shawl sign.

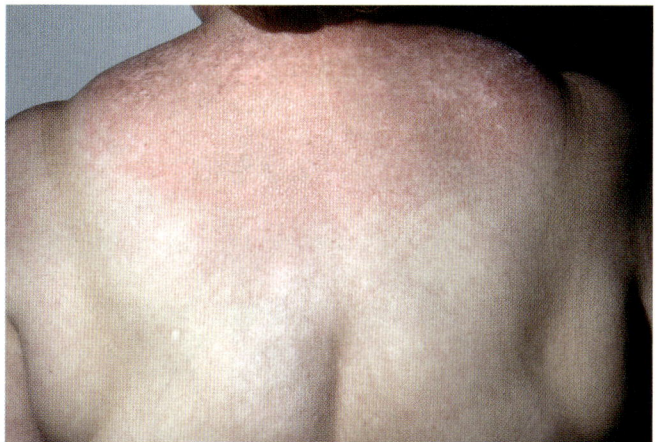

Fig. 8.59 Dermatomyositis, shawl sign.

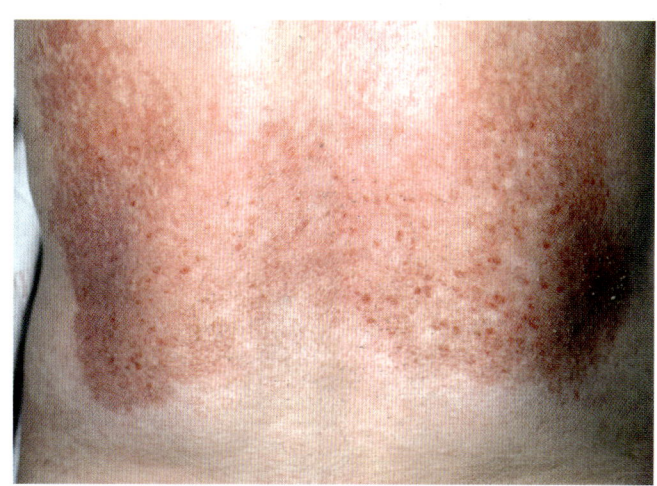

Fig. 8.60 Dermatomyositis.

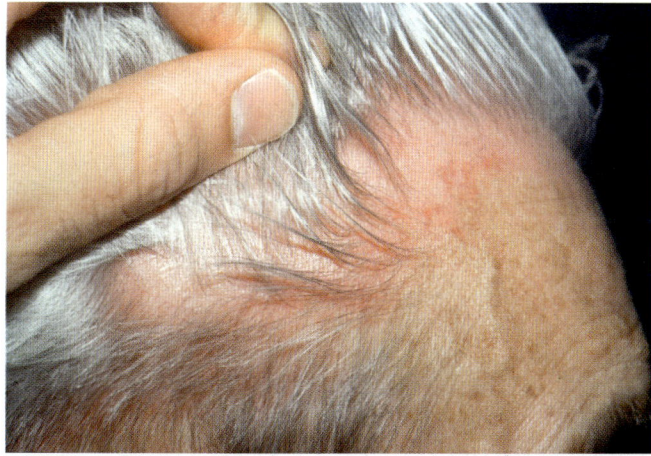

Fig. 8.61 Dermatomyositis.

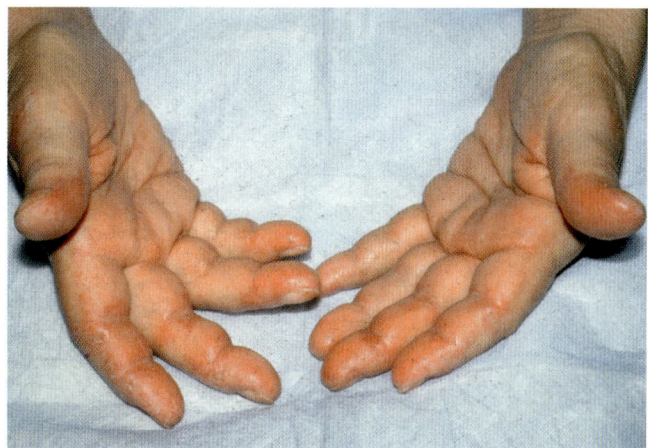

Fig. 8.62 Dermatomyositis, mechanic's hands.

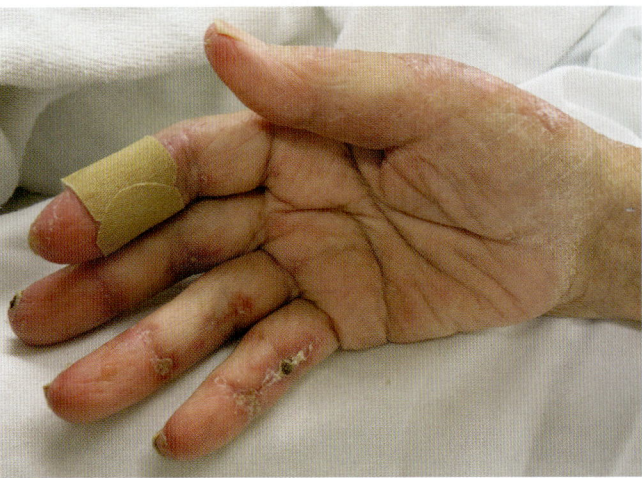

Fig. 8.63 Anti–MDA-5 dermatomyositis with ulcerated inverse Gottron's papules.

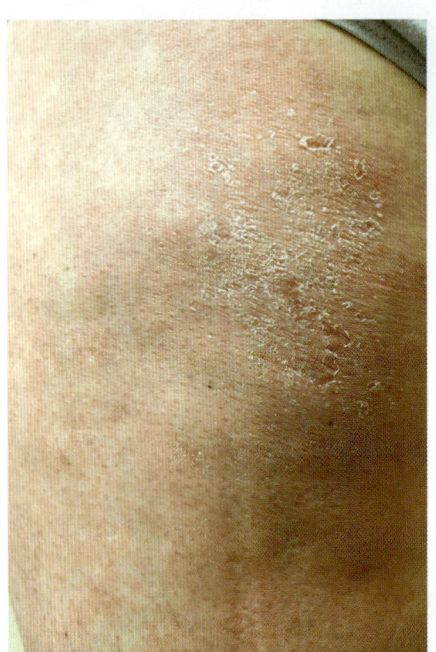

Fig. 8.64 Dermatomyositis on the lateral thigh (holster sign).

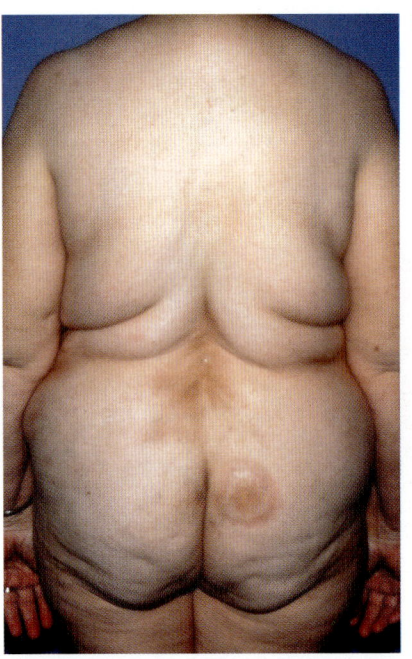

Fig. 8.65 Morphea.

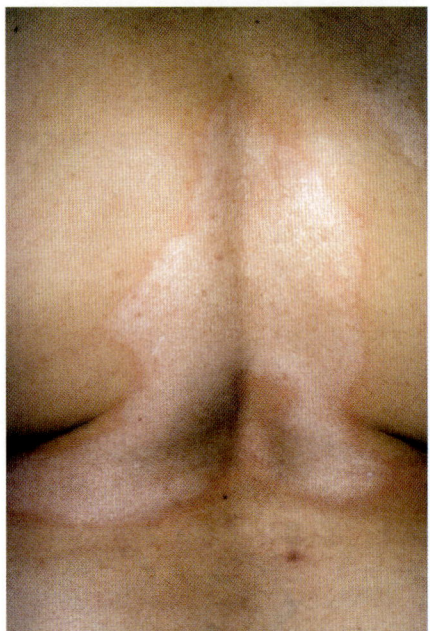

Fig. 8.66 Morphea.

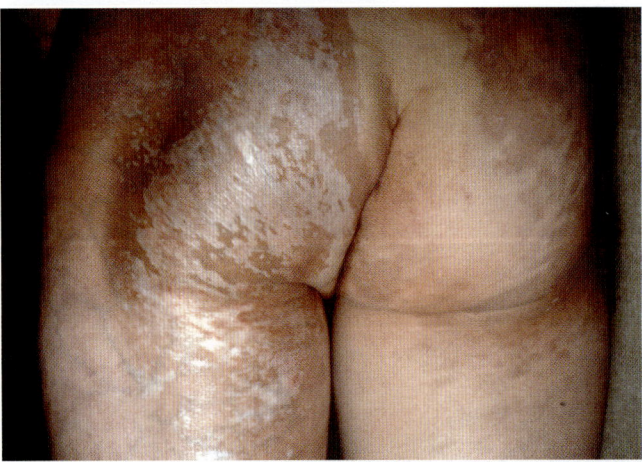

Fig. 8.67 Morphea with lichen sclerosis overlap.

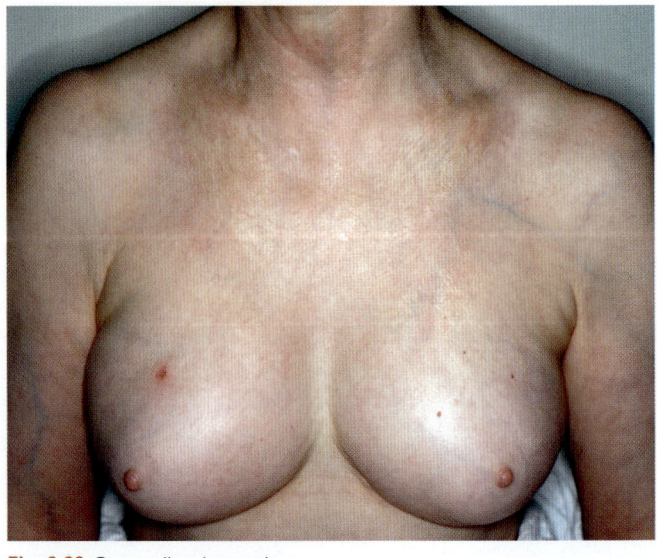

Fig. 8.68 Generalized morphea.

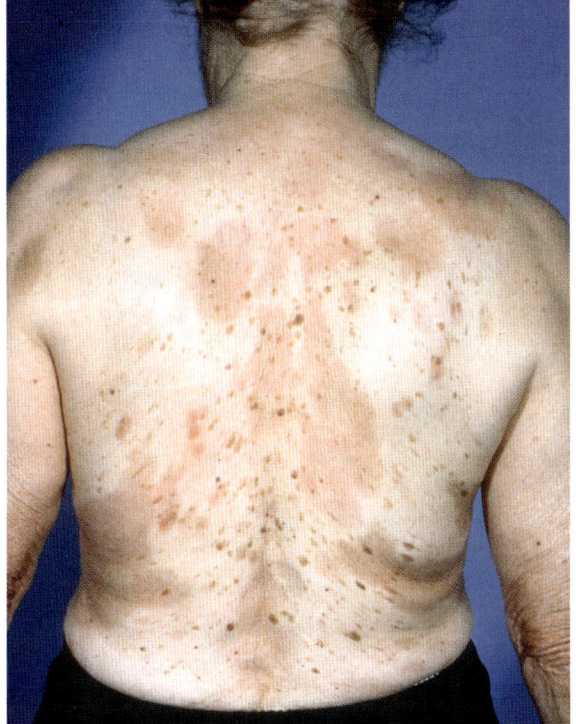

Fig. 8.69 Atrophoderma of Pasini and Pierini.

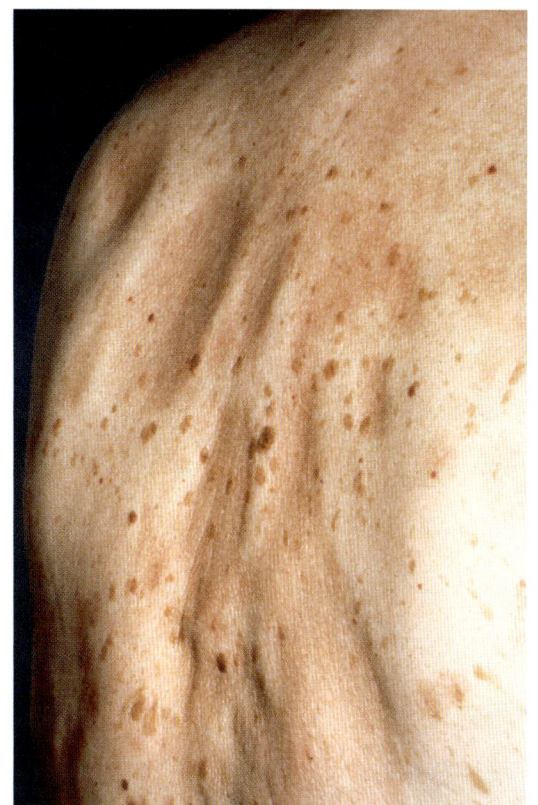

Fig. 8.70 Atrophoderma of Pasini and Pierini.

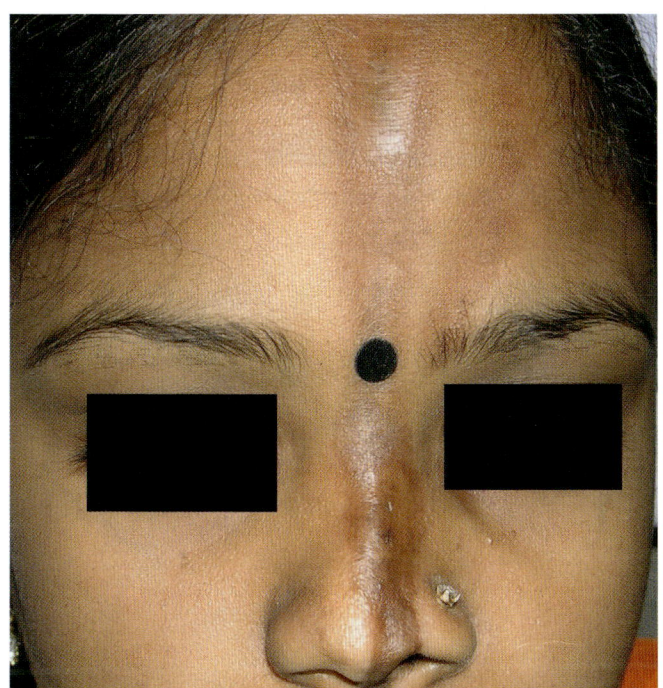

Fig. 8.71 Linear morphea. *Courtesy Debabrata Bandyopadhyay, MD.*

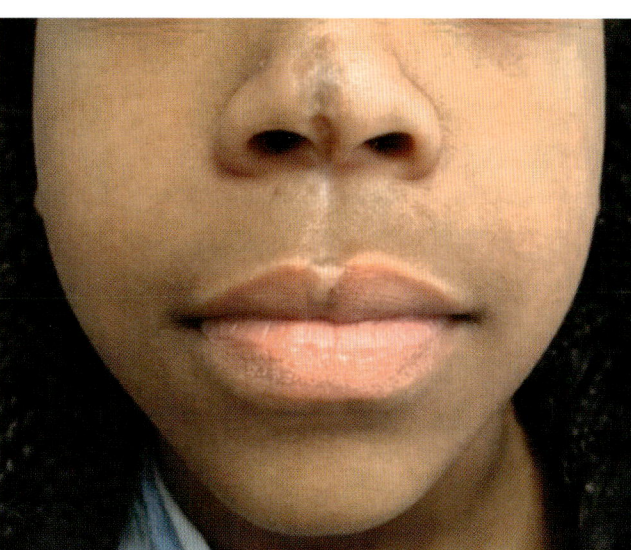

Fig. 8.72 Linear morphea. *Courtesy Lisa Arkin, MD.*

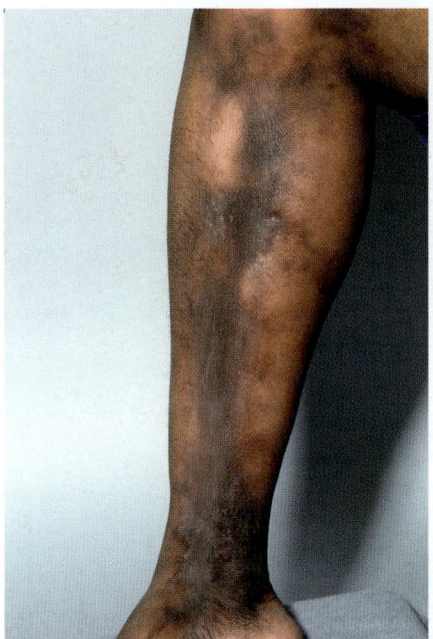

Fig. 8.73 Linear morphea.

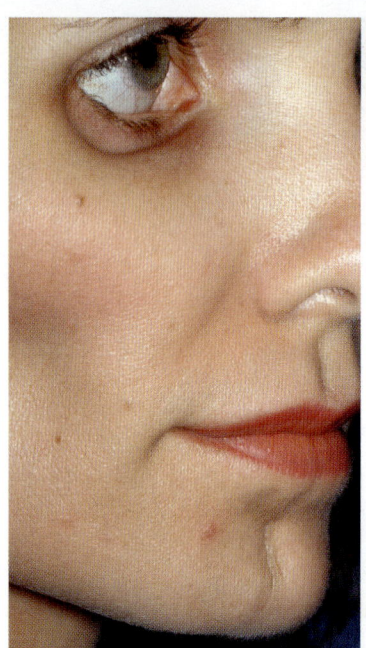

Fig. 8.74 Parry-Romberg syndrome.

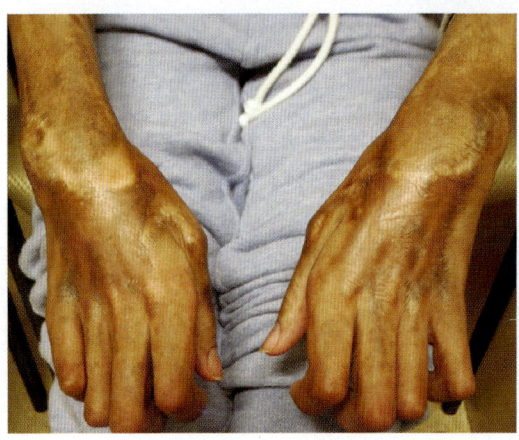

Fig. 8.75 Pansclerotic morphea.

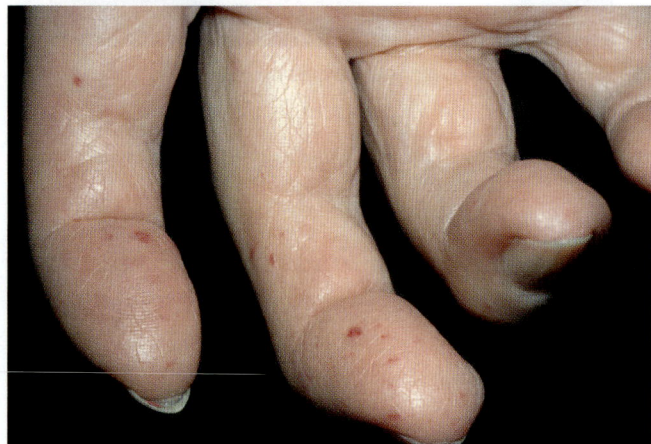

Fig. 8.76 Sclerodactyly and telangiectasias in limited scleroderma, CREST.

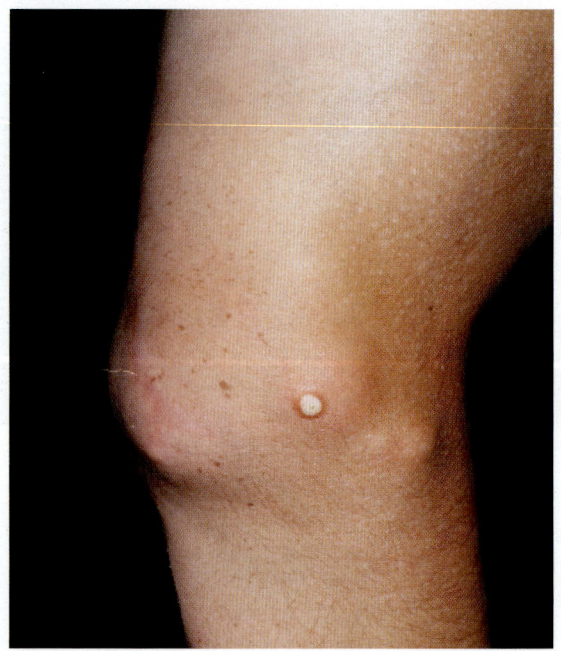

Fig. 8.77 Calcinosis of the knee in a patient with scleroderma.

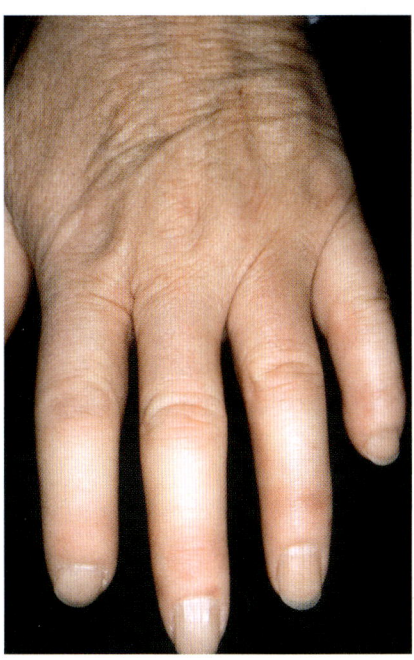

Fig. 8.78 Sclerodactyly in systemic sclerosis.

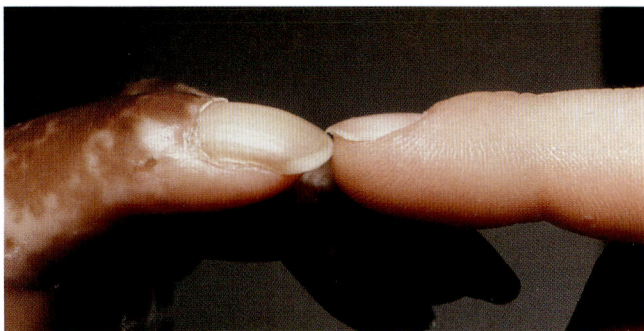

Fig. 8.79 Sclerotic digit (left) versus normal digit (right).

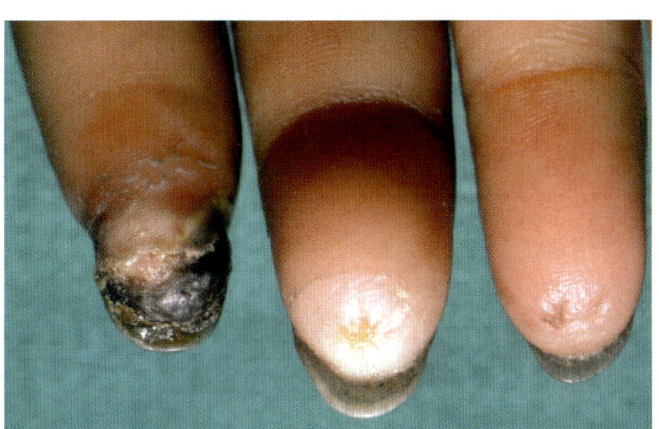

Fig. 8.80 Ulceration in systemic sclerosis.

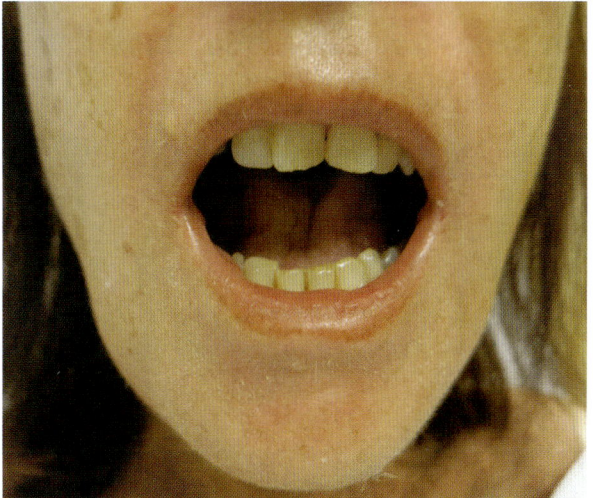

Fig. 8.81 Reduced oral aperture in systemic sclerosis.

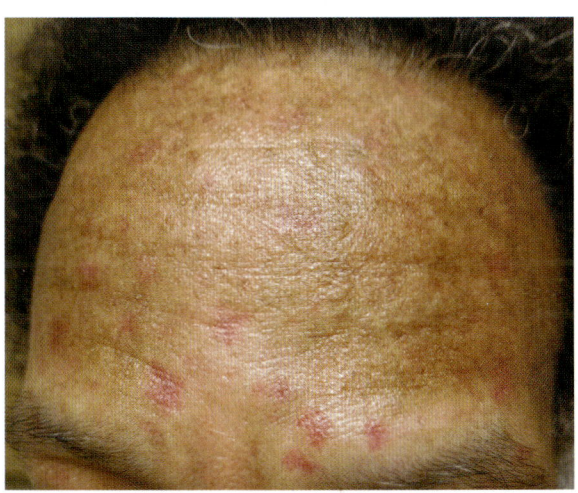

Fig. 8.82 Mat telangiectasias in systemic sclerosis.

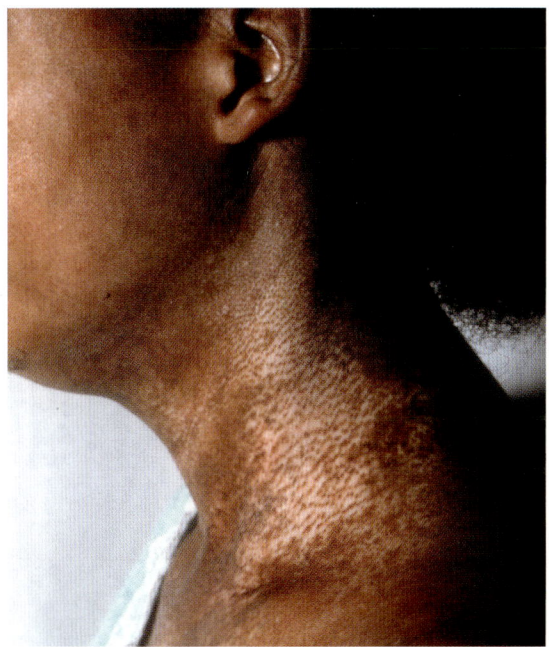

Fig. 8.83 Dyspigmentation in systemic sclerosis.

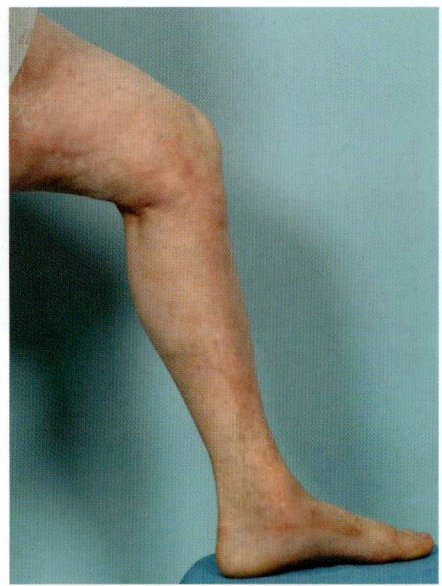

Fig. 8.84 Eosinophilic fasciitis.

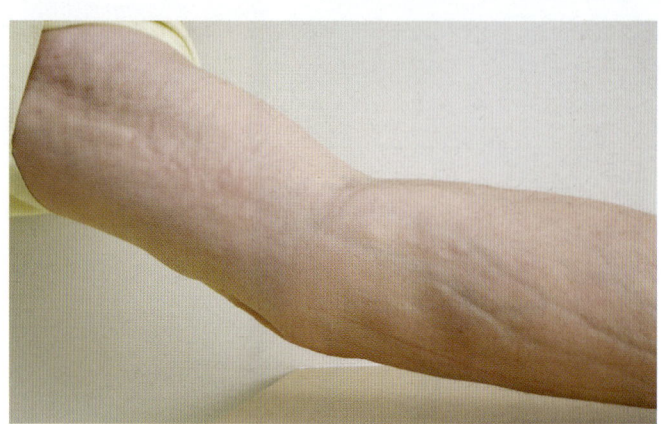

Fig. 8.85 Eosinophilic fasciitis.

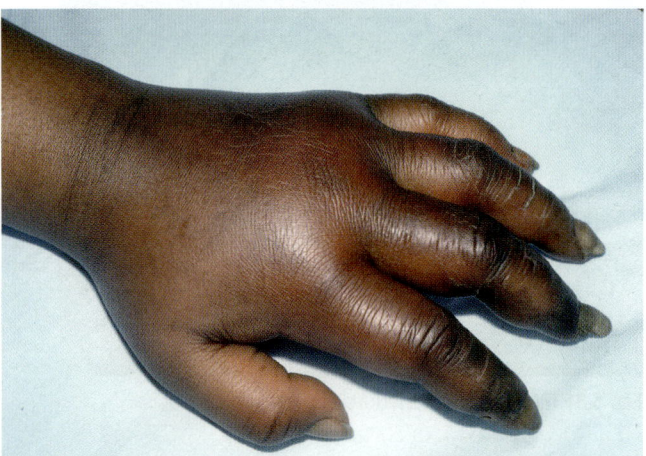

Fig. 8.86 Mixed connective tissue disease. *Courtesy Steven Binnick, MD.*

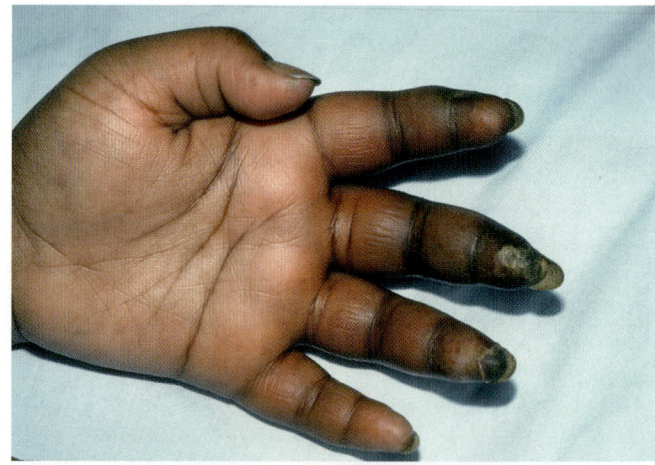

Fig. 8.87 Mixed connective tissue disease. *Courtesy Steven Binnick, MD.*

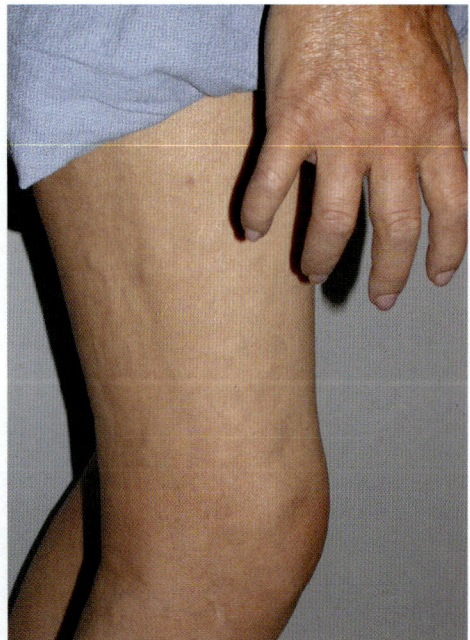

Fig. 8.88 Nephrogenic systemic fibrosis.

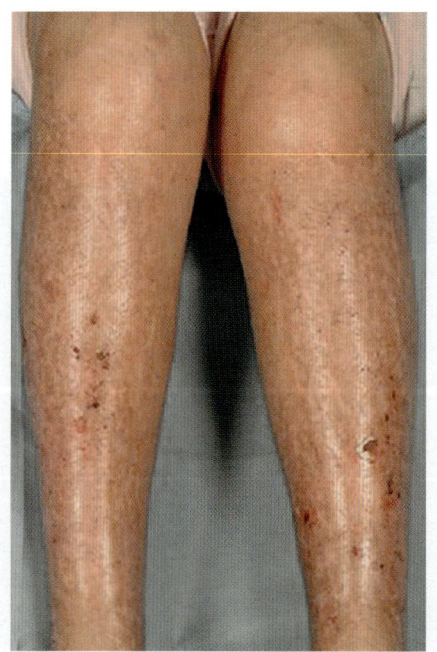

Fig. 8.89 Nephrogenic systemic fibrosis.

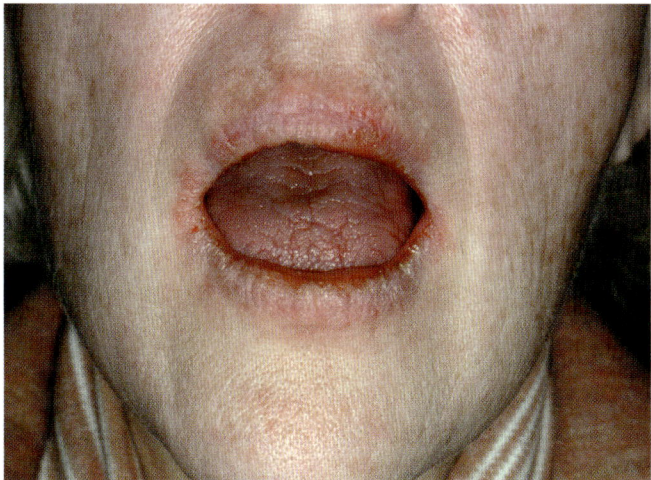

Fig. 8.90 Sjögren syndrome.

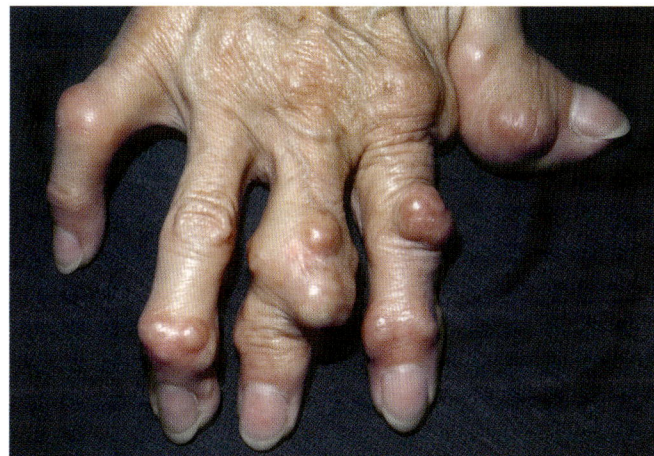

Fig. 8.92 Rheumatoid nodules.

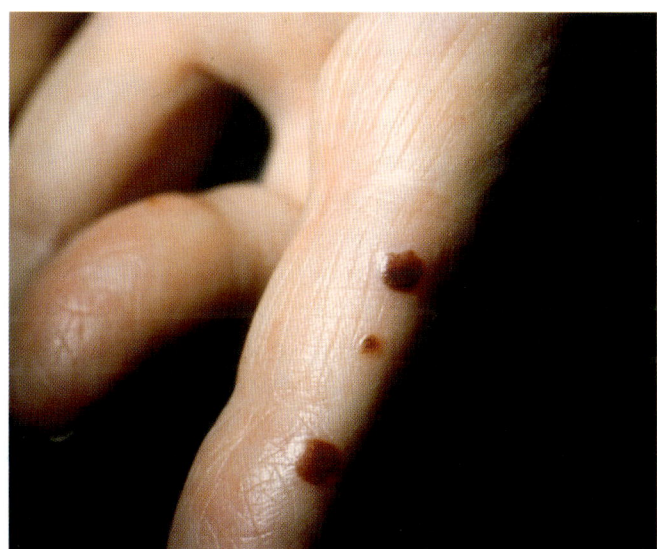

Fig. 8.94 Rheumatoid vasculitis.

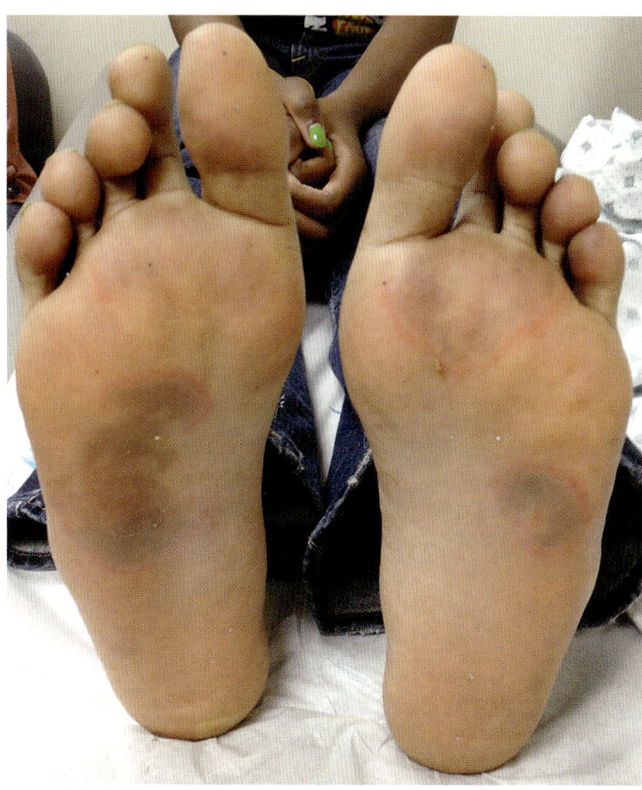

Fig. 8.91 Annular erythema of Sjögren syndrome.

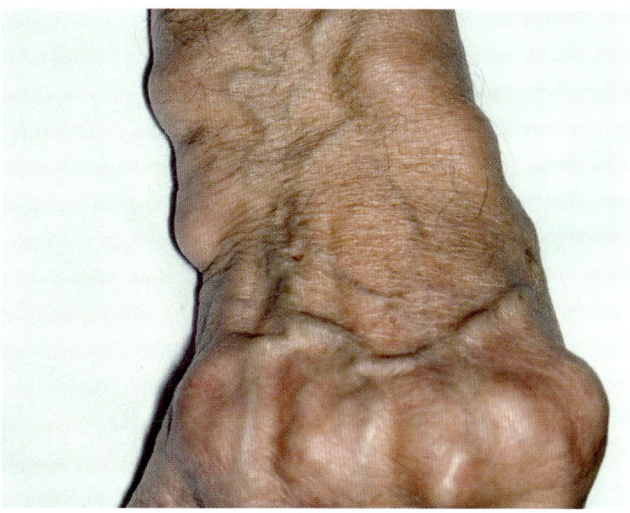

Fig. 8.93 Rheumatoid nodules.

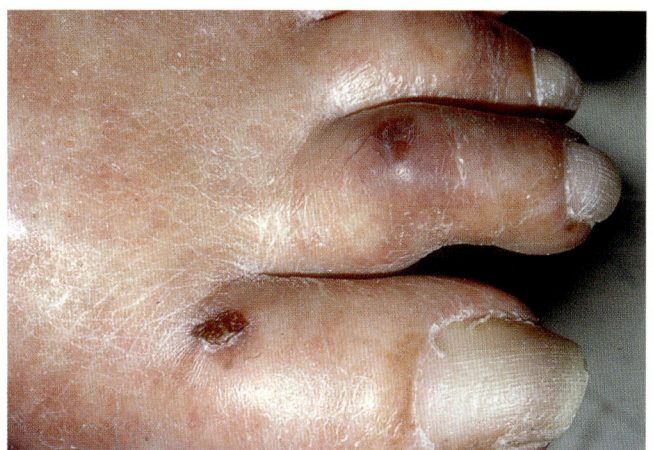

Fig. 8.95 Rheumatoid vasculitis.

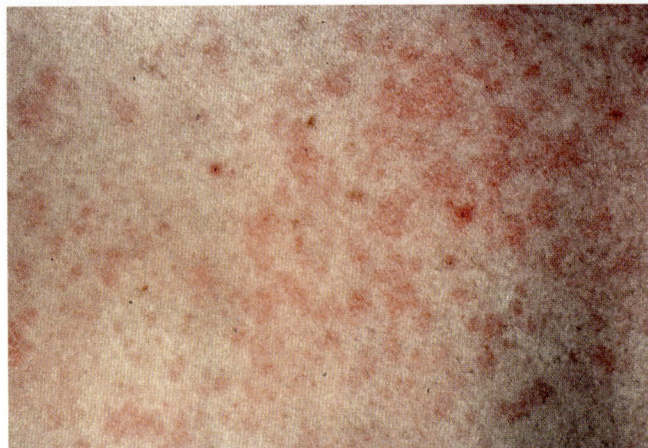

Fig. 8.96 Still's disease.

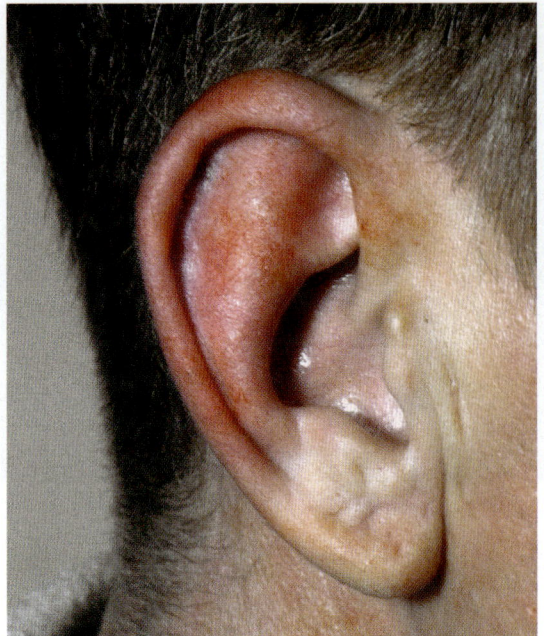

Fig. 8.97 Relapsing polychondritis.

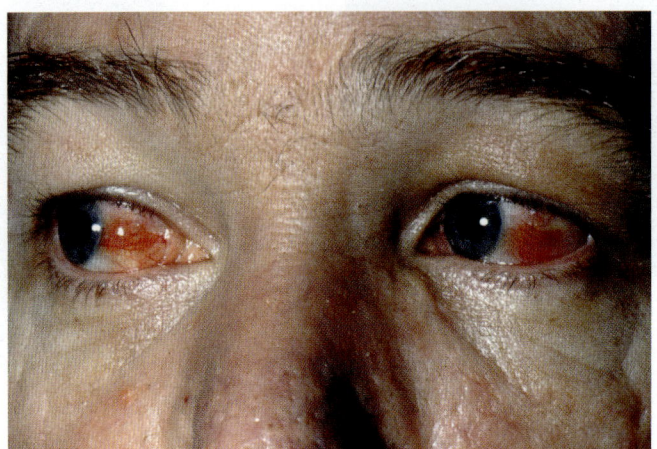

Fig. 8.98 Relapsing polychondritis.

Mucinoses 9

Localized cutaneous mucin deposition results in translucent pale to erythematous papules, as in digital myxoid cysts or focal cutaneous mucinosis. Papular mucinosis related to plasma cell dyscrasia with paraproteinemia causes papules with a distinct tendency to form linear arrays. Histologically, mucin is less apparent than an increase in fibroblasts and ropey collagen. This translates to induration of the skin over time, leading to a clinical appearance resembling systemic sclerosis.

Myxedema results in subtle dermal mucin deposition often manifesting below the eyes, whereas pretibial myxedema can produce dramatic deposition within the skin of the dorsal foot as well as the pretibial region. Stasis-induced mucinosis can produce a similar appearance, but the mucin is confined to the upper dermis rather than affecting the full thickness of the dermis as is seen in thyroid disease.

Follicular mucinosis can occur as erythematous, indurated, hairless plaques in benign alopecia mucinosa, as well as in the setting of mycosis fungoides. Dilated follicular orifices can give the appearance of comedones (blackheads), and sticky gelatinous material may be extruded from the lesions. This portion of the atlas will guide you through the various clinical presentations associated with mucinosis.

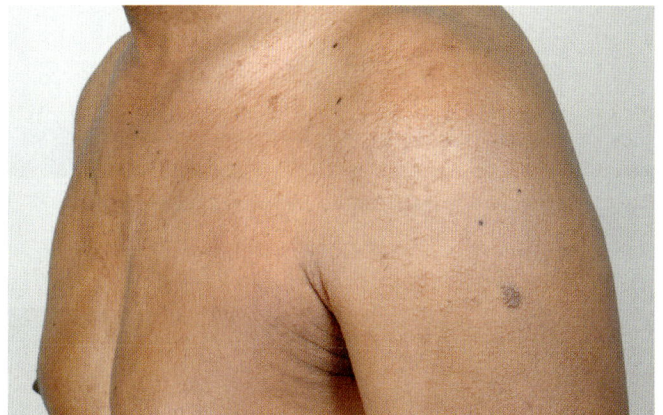

Fig. 9.1 Early scleromyxedema.

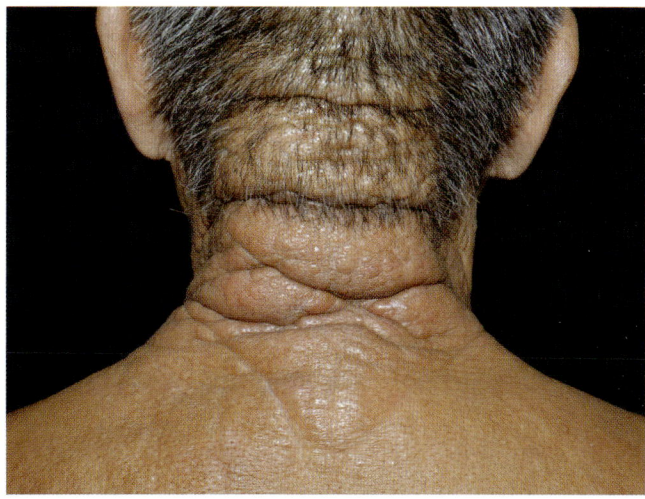

Fig. 9.2 Scleromyxedema. *Courtesy National Cheng Kung University, Taiwan.*

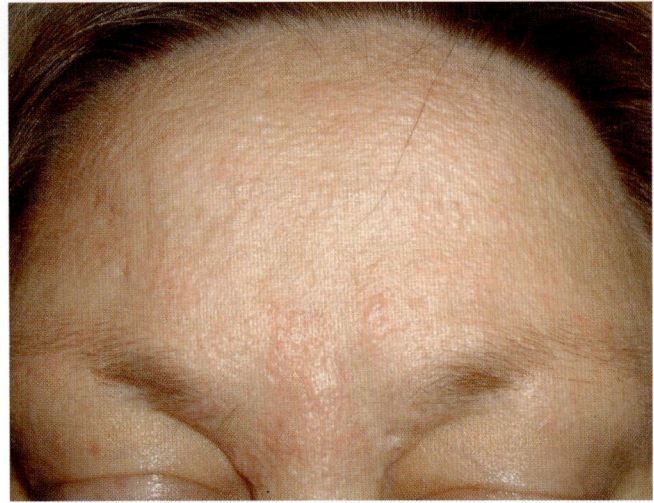

Fig. 9.3 Scleromyxedema. *Courtesy Robert Lee, MD.*

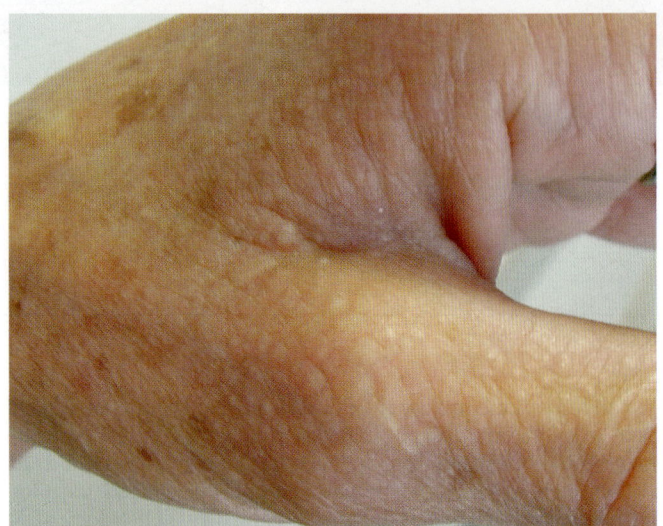

Fig. 9.4 Scleromyxedema.

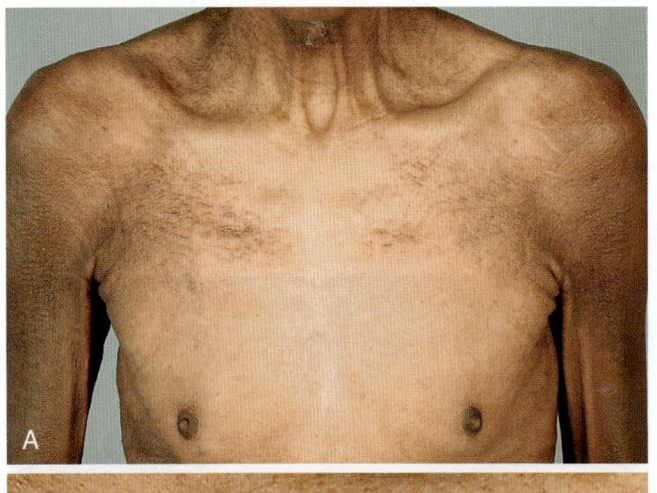

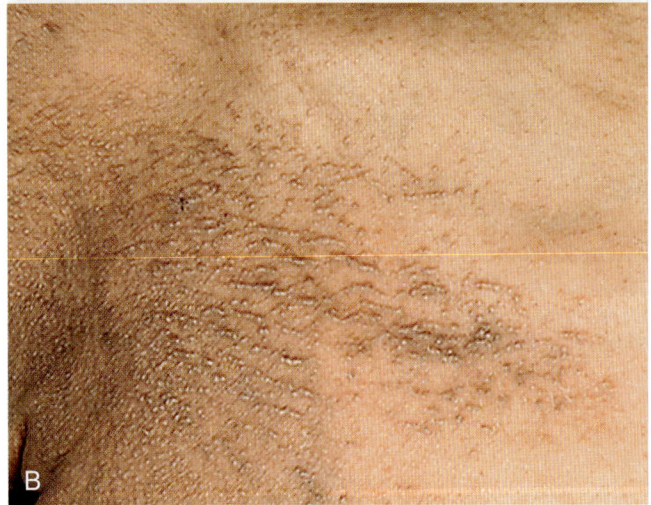

Fig. 9.5 (A) Scleromyxedema. (B) Scleromyxedema. *Courtesy Douglas Pugliese, MD.*

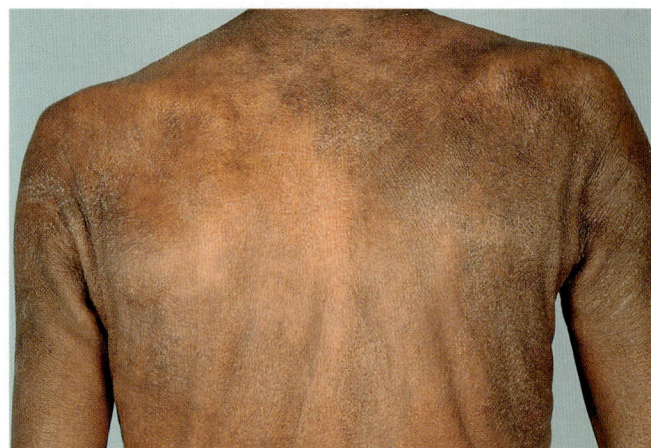

Fig. 9.6 Scleromyxedema. *Courtesy Douglas Pugliese, MD.*

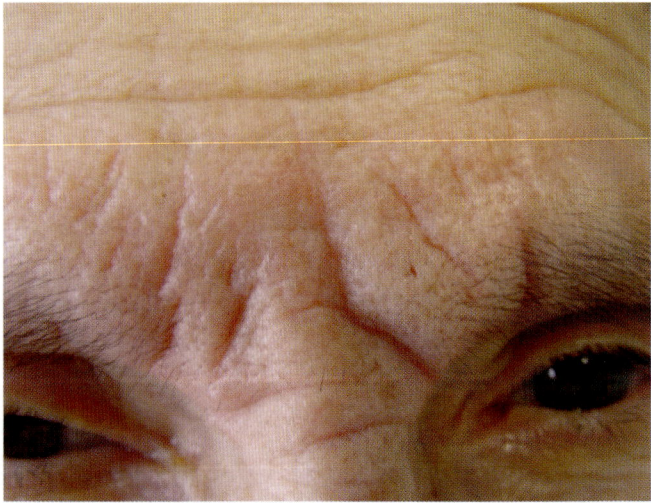

Fig. 9.7 Scleromyxedema. *Courtesy Rui Tavares Bello, MD.*

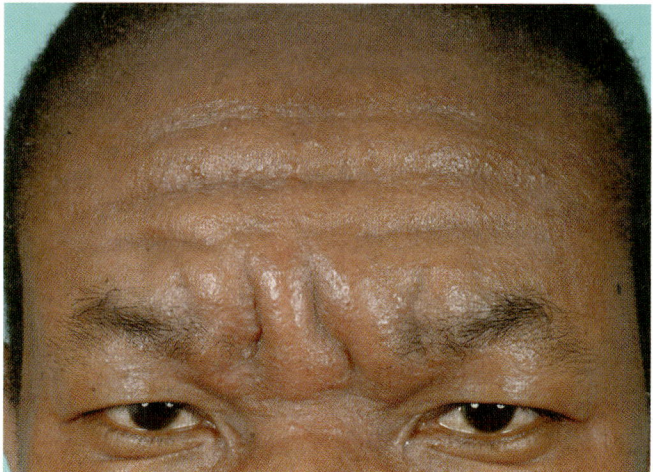

Fig. 9.8 Scleromyxedema. *Courtesy Douglas Pugliese, MD.*

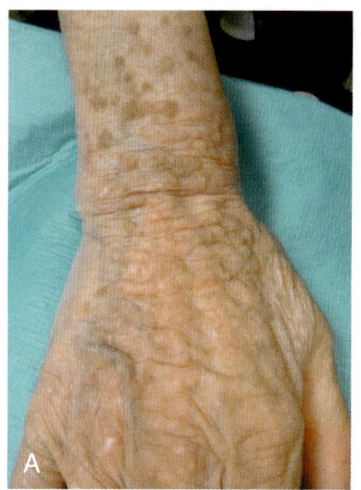

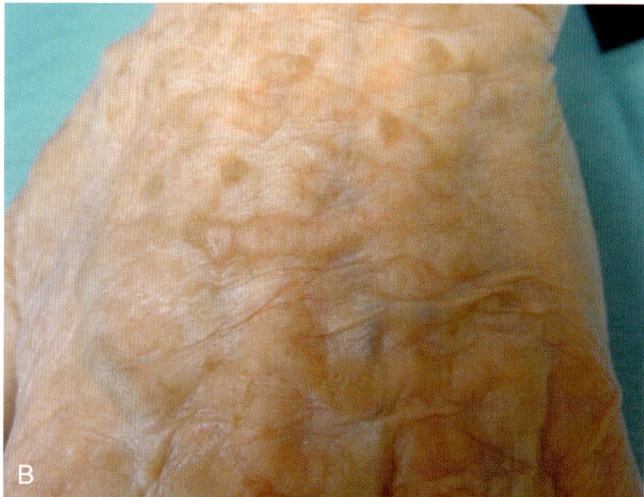

Fig. 9.9 (A) Acral persistent papular mucinosis. (B) Acral persistent papular mucinosis. *Courtesy Juliana Choi, MD, and Iris K. Aronson, MD.*

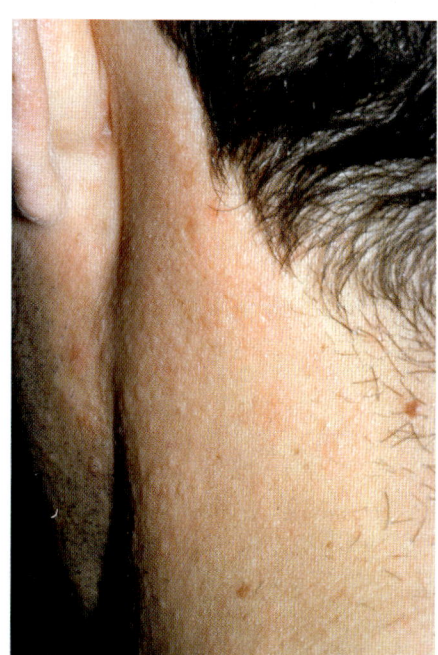

Fig. 9.10 Mucinous papules in an HIV-positive patient.

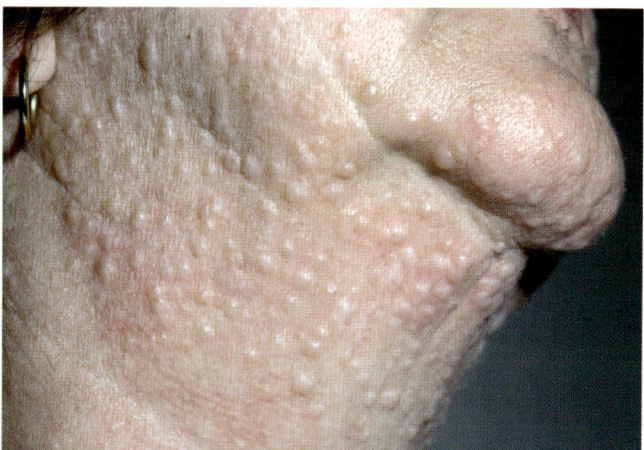

Fig. 9.11 Self-healing papular mucinosis.

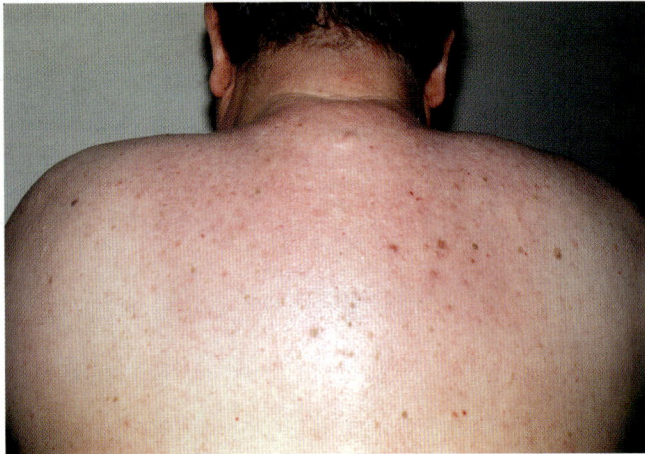

Fig. 9.12 Scleredema. *Courtesy Steven Binnick, MD.*

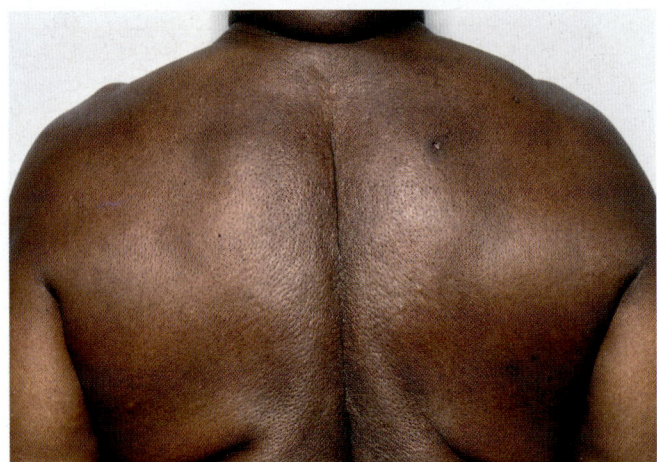

Fig. 9.13 Scleredema.

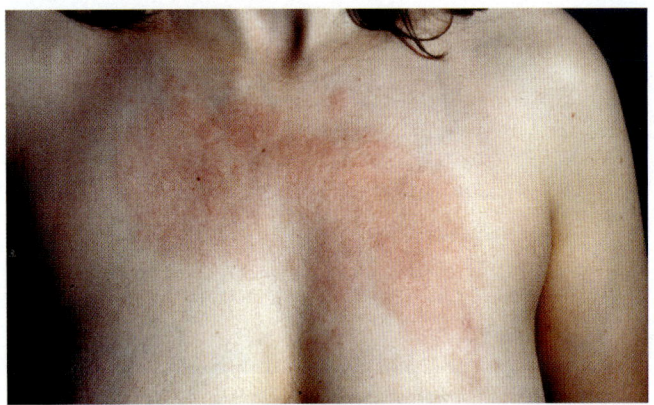

Fig. 9.14 Reticular erythematous mucinosis.

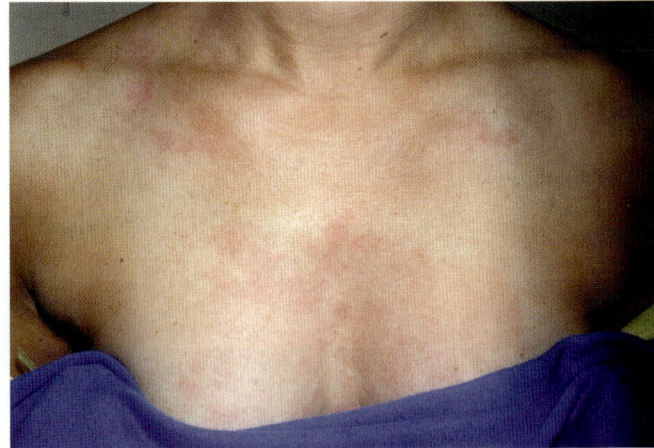

Fig. 9.15 Reticular erythematous mucinosis.

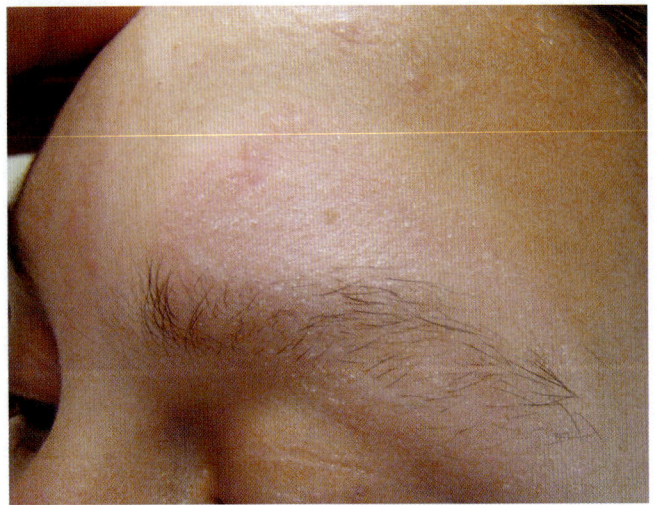

Fig. 9.16 Benign follicular mucinosis. *Courtesy Rui Tavares Bello, MD.*

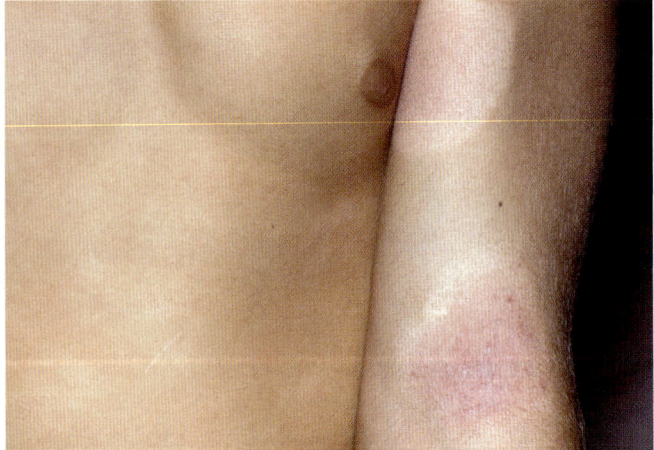

Fig. 9.17 Benign follicular mucinosis. *Courtesy Steven Binnick, MD.*

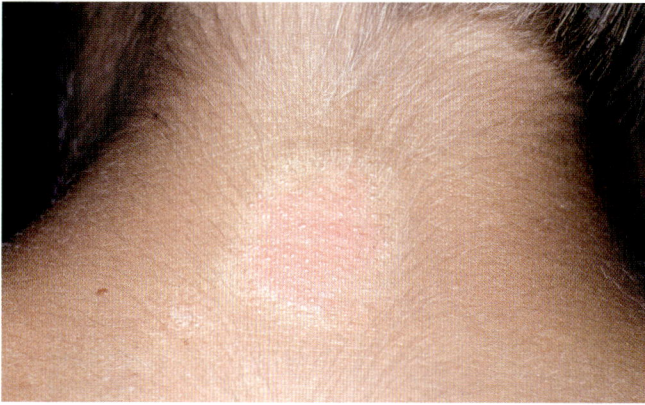

Fig. 9.18 Benign follicular mucinosis. *Courtesy Steven Binnick, MD.*

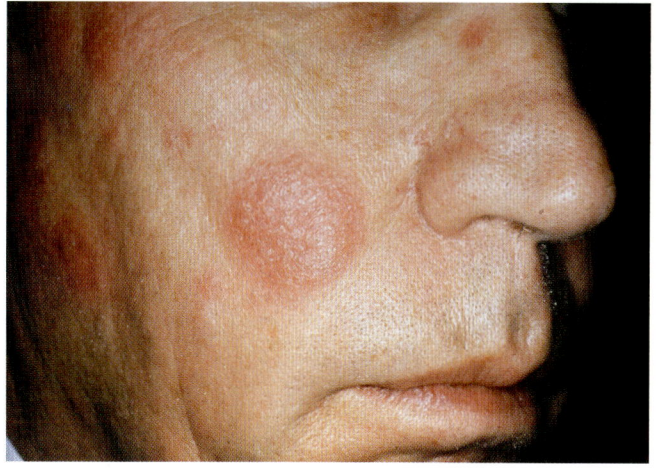

Fig. 9.19 Benign follicular mucinosis. *Courtesy Scott Norton, MD.*

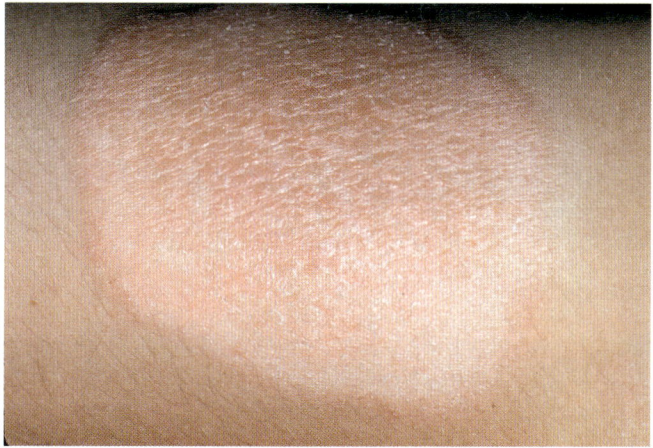

Fig. 9.20 Benign follicular mucinosis. *Courtesy Steven Binnick, MD.*

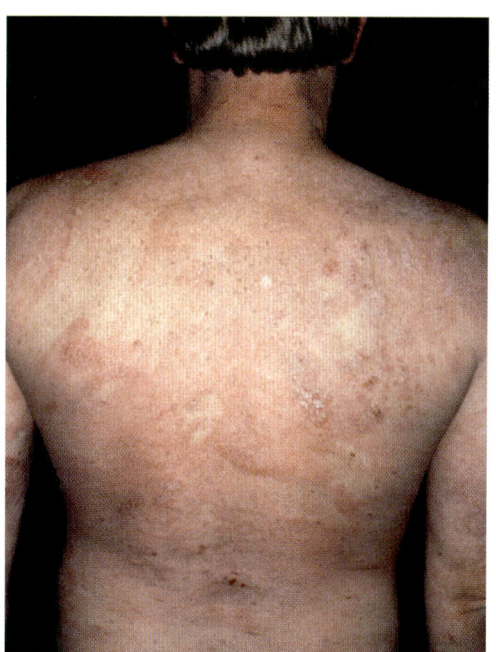

Fig. 9.21 Follicular mucinosis associated with mycosis fungoides.

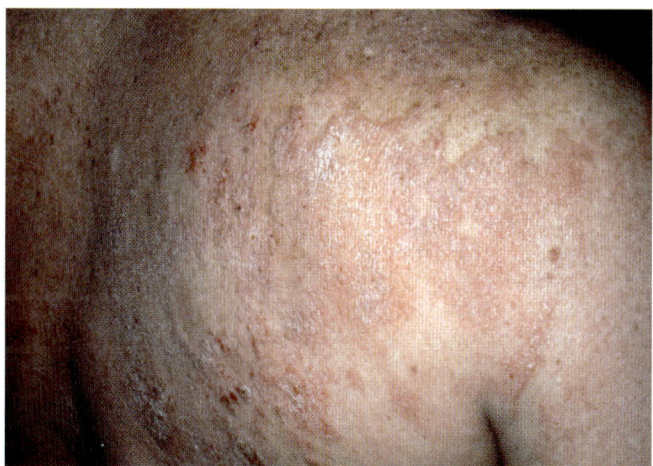

Fig. 9.22 Follicular mucinosis associated with mycosis fungoides.

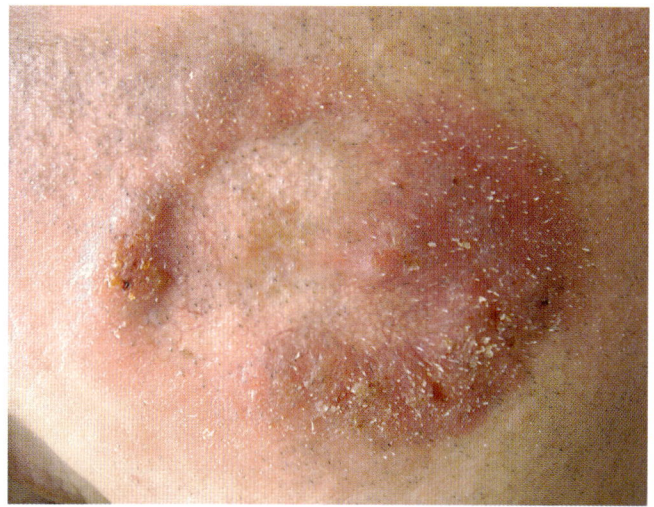

Fig. 9.23 Follicular mucinosis associated with mycosis fungoides. *Courtesy Ellen Kim, MD.*

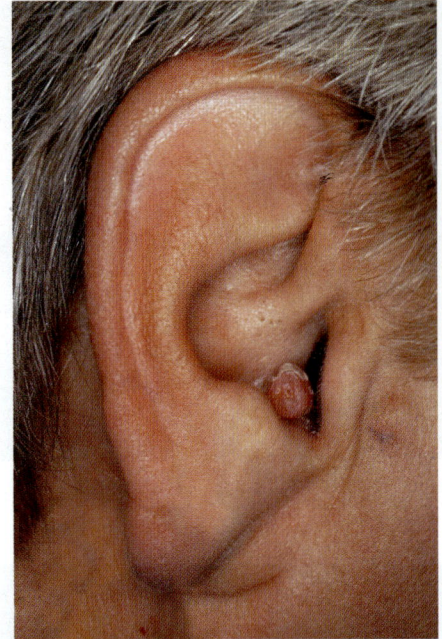

Fig. 9.24 Focal cutaneous mucinosis.

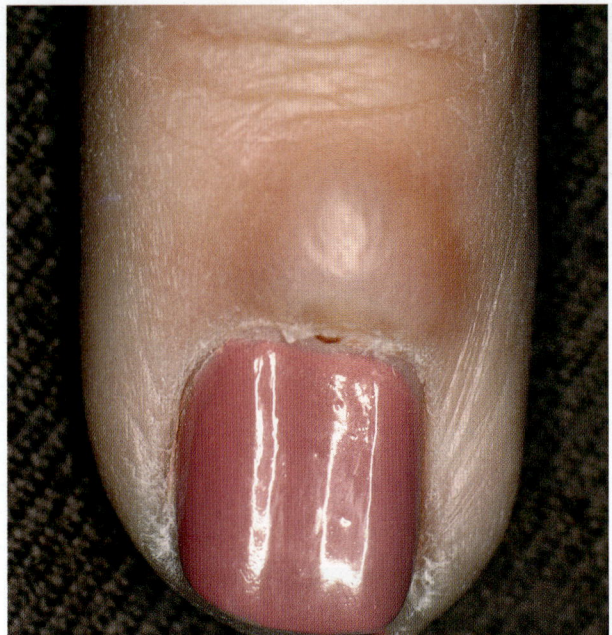

Fig. 9.25 Myxoid cyst. Note nail deformity. *Courtesy Steven Binnick, MD.*

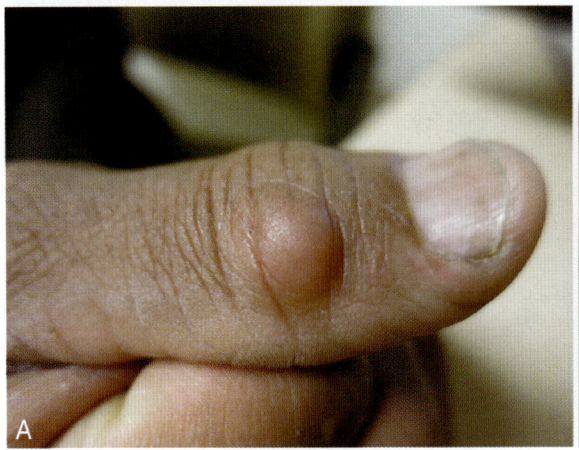
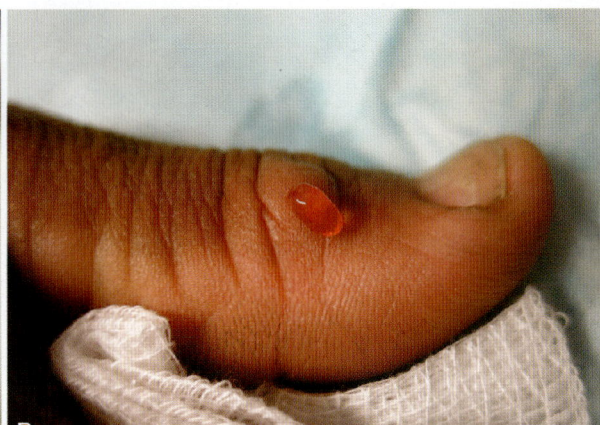

Fig. 9.26 (A) Myxoid cyst. (B) After expression of mucin.

Seborrheic Dermatitis, Psoriasis, Recalcitrant Palmoplantar Eruptions, Pustular Dermatitis, and Erythroderma

10

The primary lesion of a papulosquamous disorder is a papule with scale, but because patients often present later in the course of disease, the primary lesions may not be visible, and the physician may observe scaly plaques, patches, postinflammatory change, or diffuse redness and scaling (erythroderma).

Seborrheic dermatitis may involve the eyebrows, nasolabial and melolabial folds, scalp, ears, retroauricular regions, central chest, and axillae. The scale often exhibits a yellow hue, most likely related to carotenoids within the serum crusts. This is in stark contrast to the silvery white scale of typical plaque psoriasis. Plaque psoriasis lacks spongiosis (and the yellow carotenoids that are dissolved in the aqueous phase of tissue fluids). Several forms of psoriasis exhibit spongiosis and can sometimes have a slightly yellow appearance to the scale. These include guttate, inverse, acral, and erythrodermic forms of psoriasis. Even in these forms, frankly yellow scale and honey crusts are rare.

Erythroderma presents with generalized erythema and scaling. Edema may be present, especially involving the face and extremities, and patients may suffer chills as a result of loss of body heat. Older patients may exhibit signs of high-output cardiac failure. This portion of the atlas will guide you through the various clinical manifestations of seborrheic dermatitis, psoriasis, and related disorders.

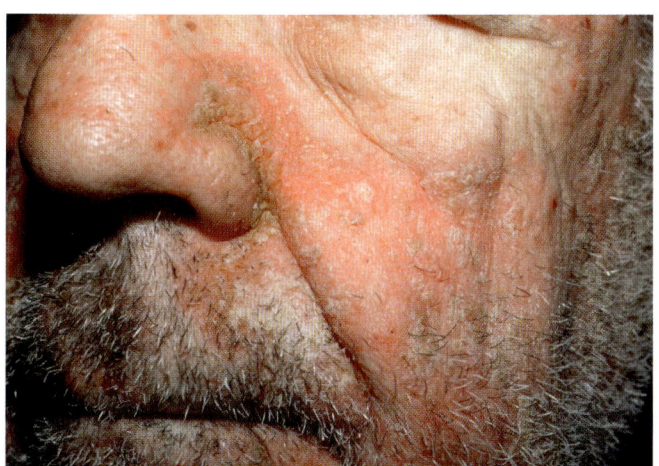

Fig. 10.1 Seborrheic dermatitis.

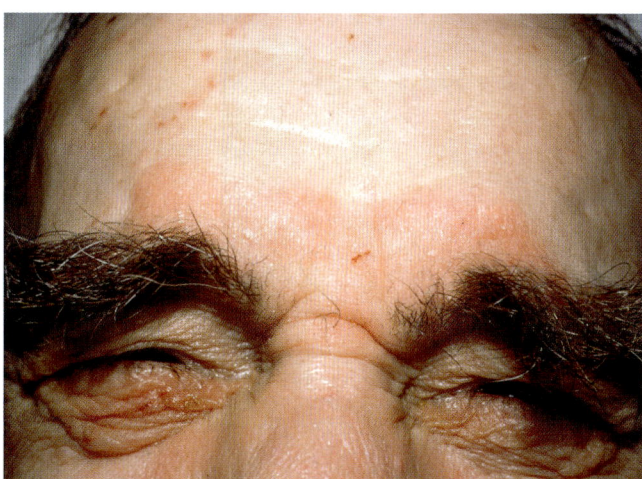

Fig. 10.2 Seborrheic dermatitis.

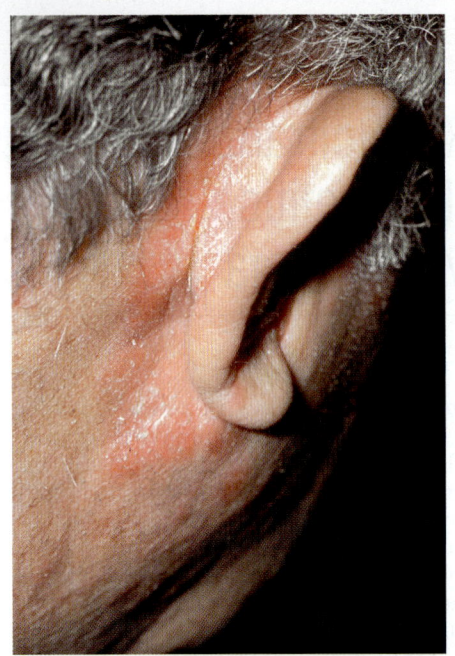

Fig. 10.3 Seborrheic dermatitis.

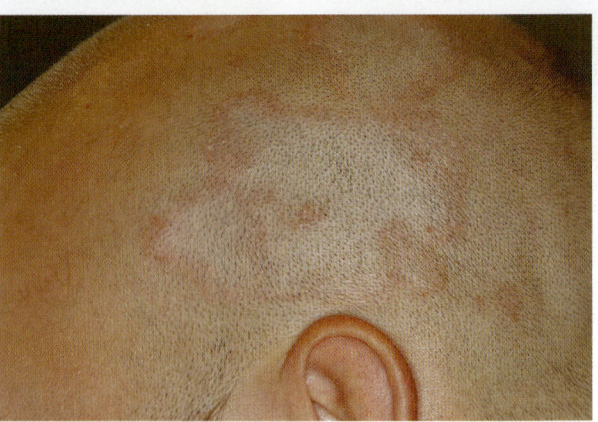

Fig. 10.4 Seborrheic dermatitis.

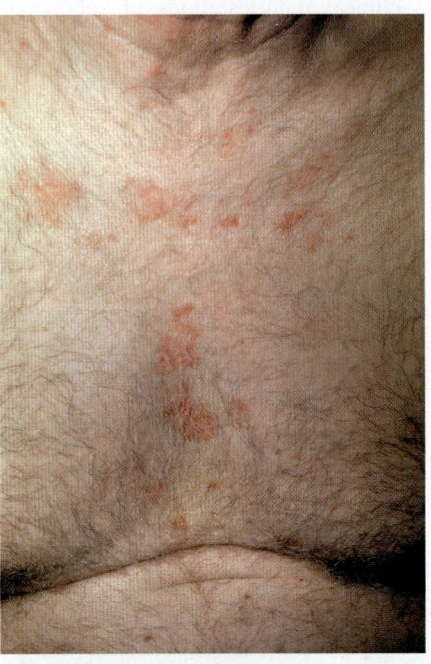

Fig. 10.5 Seborrheic dermatitis. *Courtesy Steven Binnick, MD.*

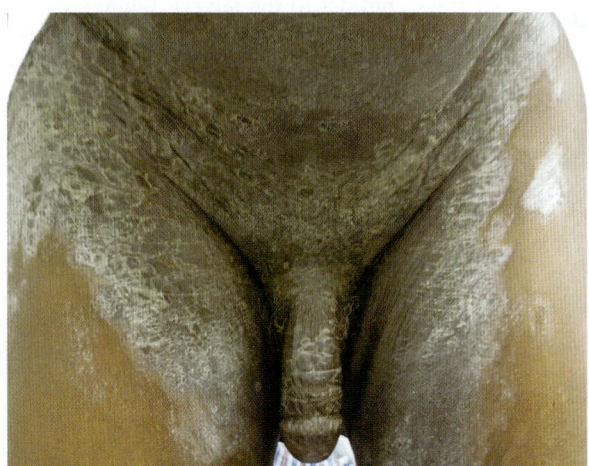

Fig. 10.6 Seborrheic dermatitis in an HIV-positive patient.

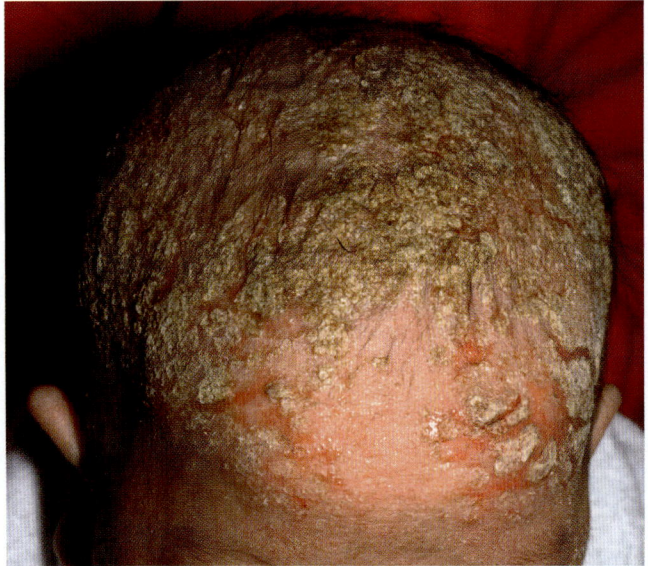

Fig. 10.7 Cradle cap.

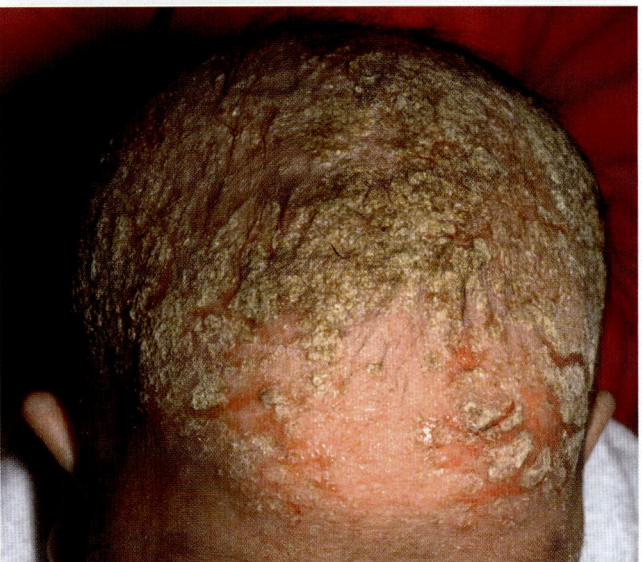

Fig. 10.8 Seborrheic dermatitis with hyperpigmentation in an African American patient.

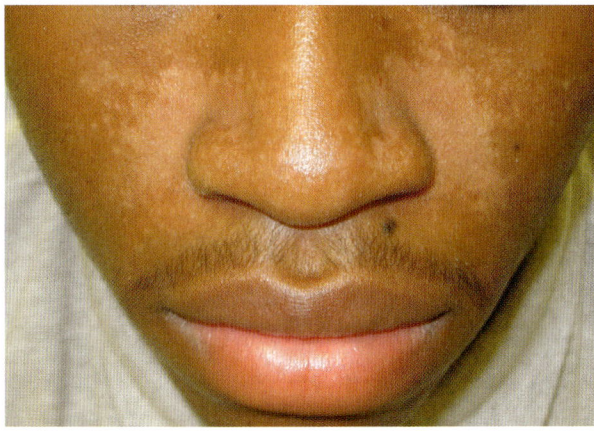

Fig. 10.9 Seborrheic dermatitis with hypopigmentation in an African American patient.

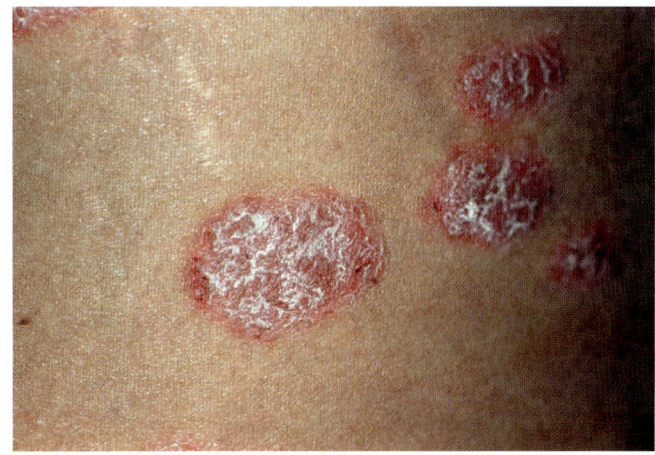

Fig. 10.10 Psoriasis.

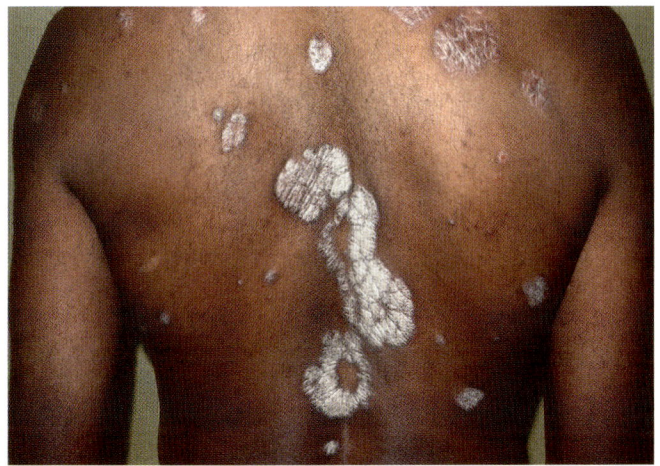

Fig. 10.11 Psoriasis.

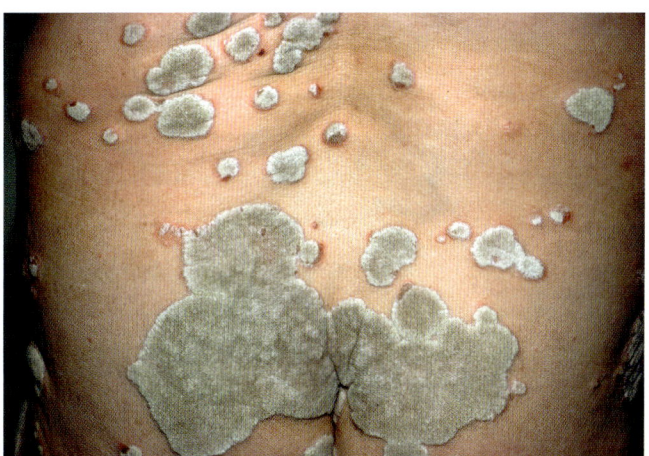

Fig. 10.12 Psoriasis.

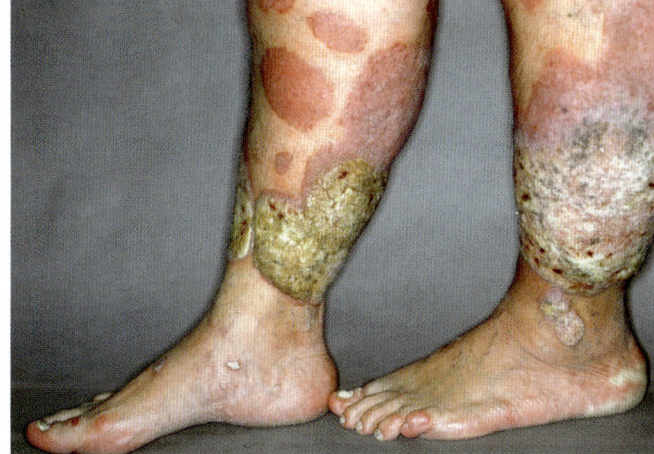

Fig. 10.13 Psoriasis.

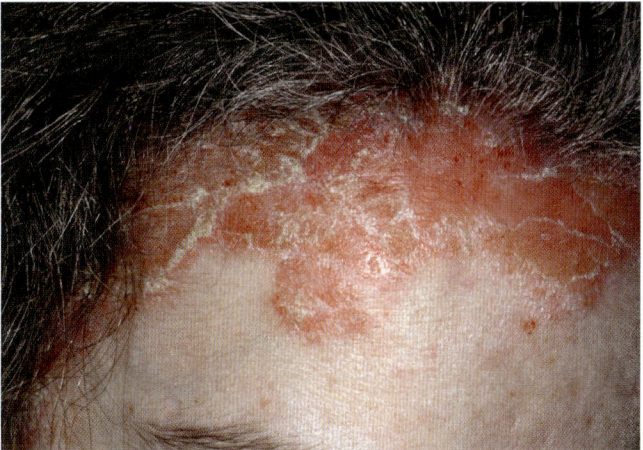

Fig. 10.14 Psoriasis.

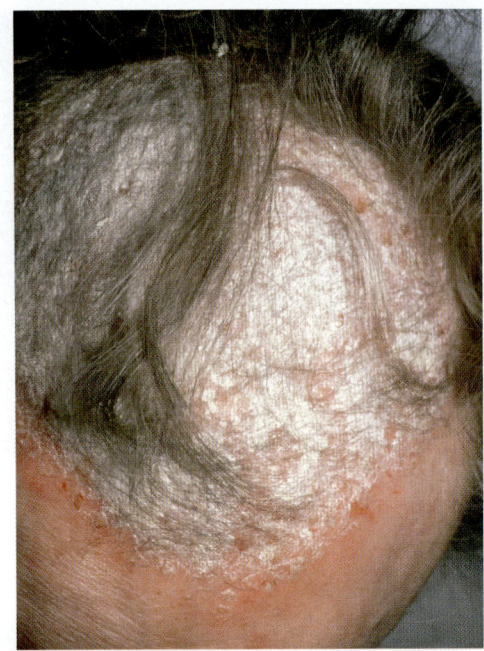

Fig. 10.15 Psoriasis.

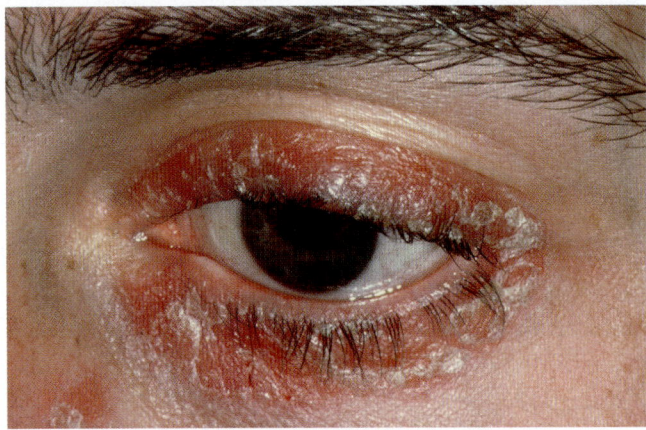

Fig. 10.17 Psoriasis.

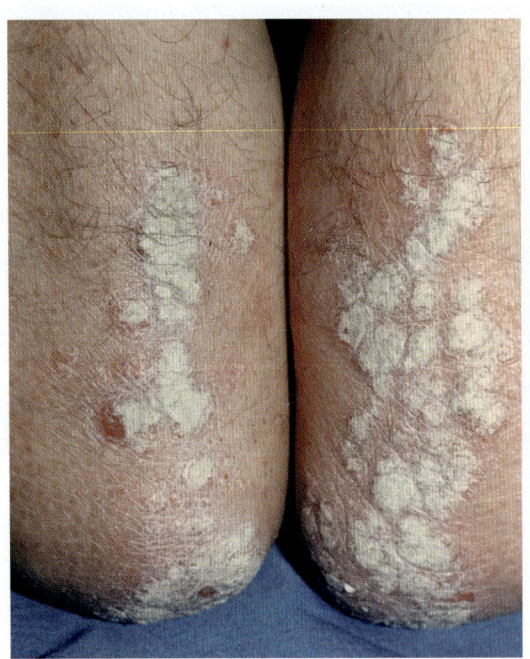

Fig. 10.19 Psoriasis.

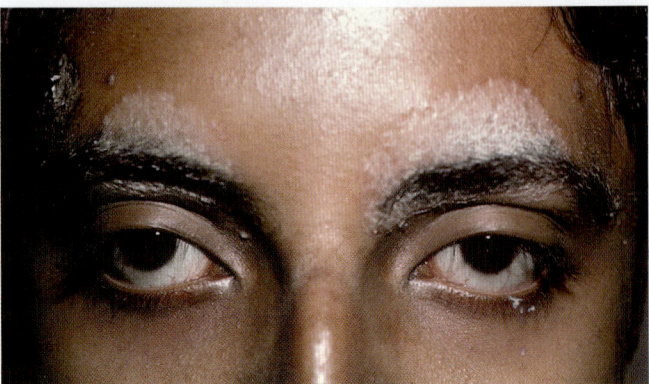

Fig. 10.16 Psoriasis.

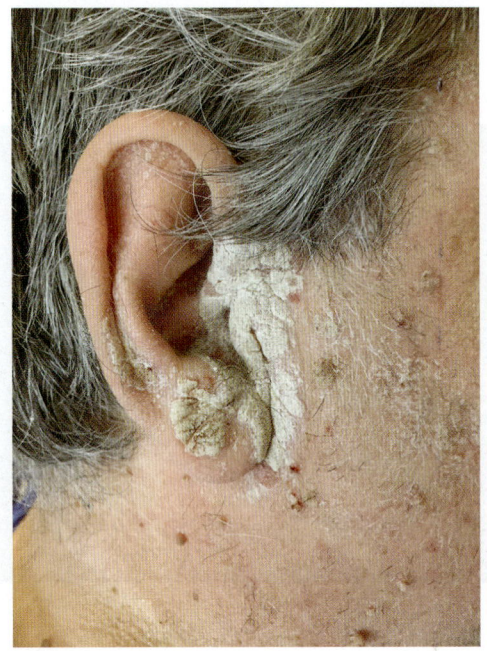

Fig. 10.18 Psoriasis.

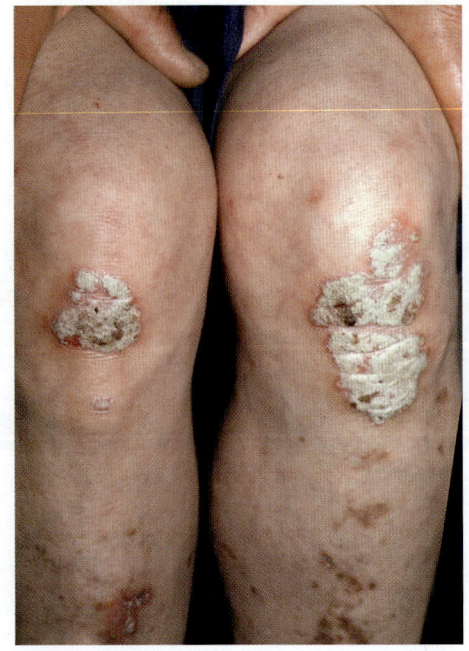

Fig. 10.20 Psoriasis.

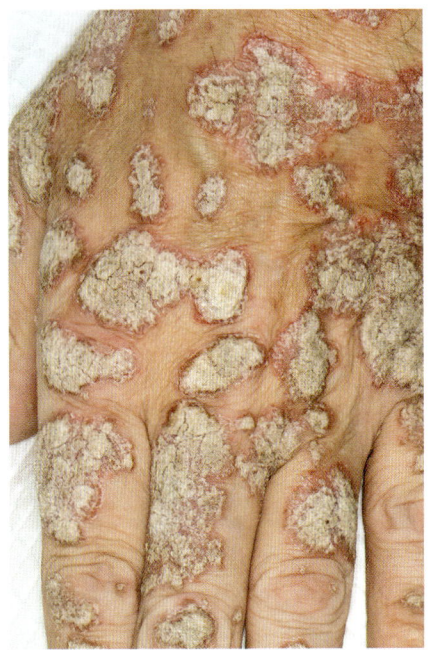

Fig. 10.21 Psoriasis.

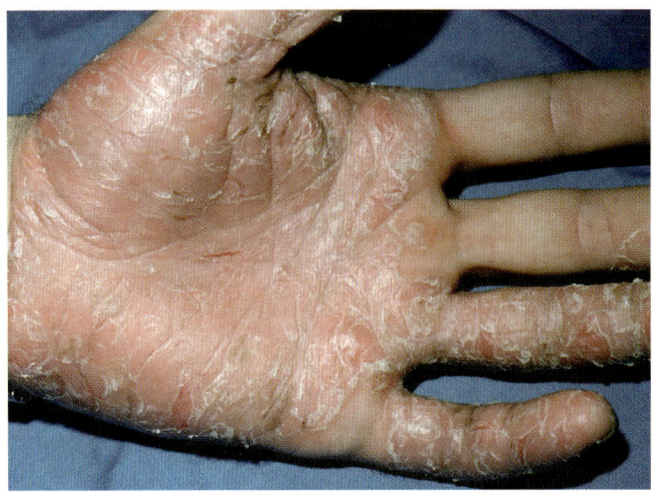

Fig. 10.22 Psoriasis.

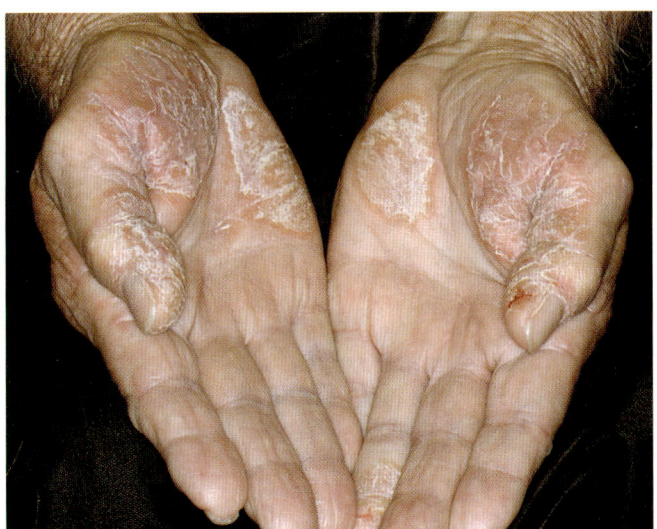

Fig. 10.23 Psoriasis.

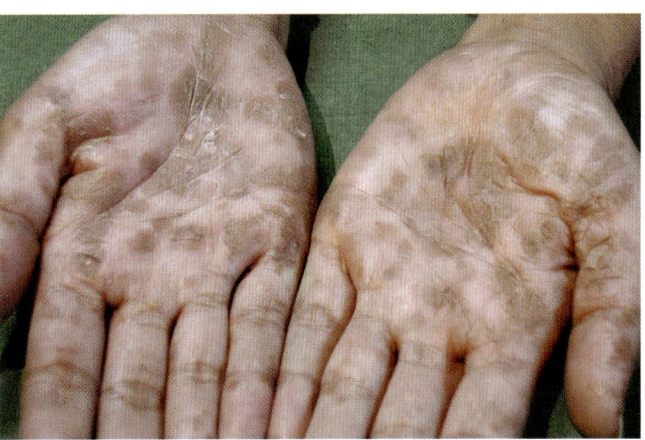

Fig. 10.24 Psoriasis. *Courtesy Shyam Verma, MBBS, DVD.*

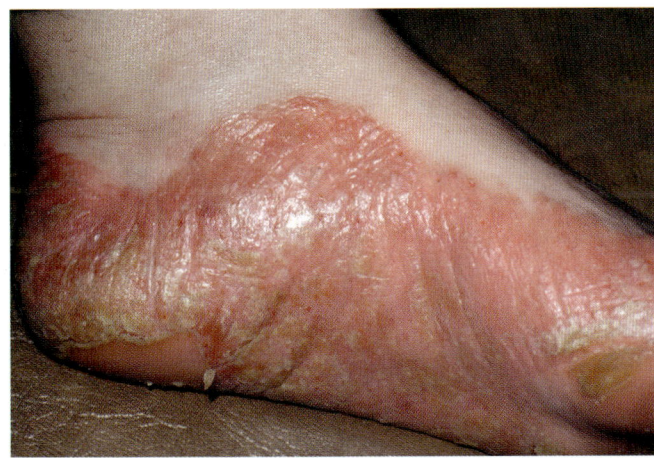

Fig. 10.25 Psoriasis. *Courtesy Steven Binnick, MD.*

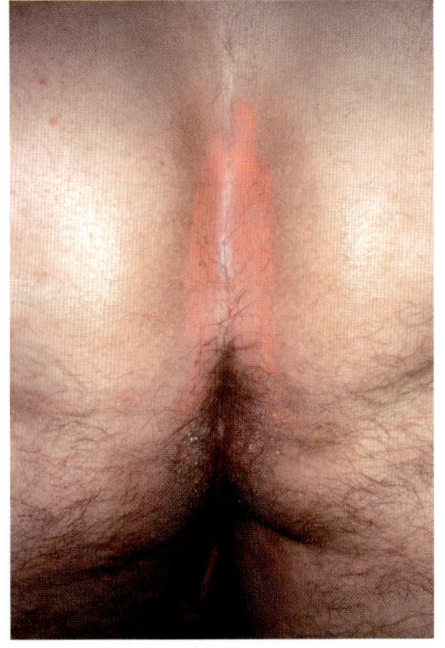

Fig. 10.26 Psoriasis.

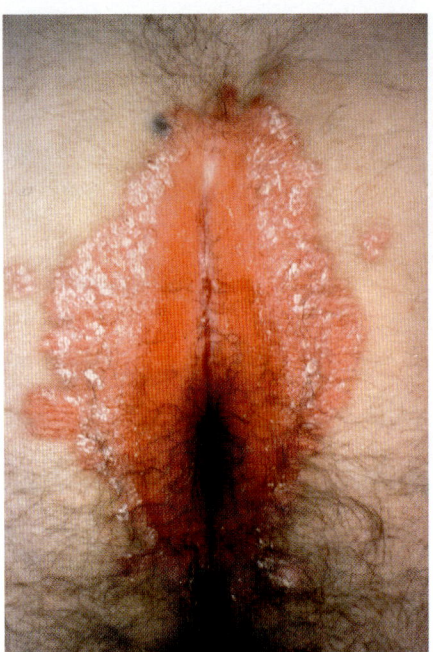

Fig. 10.27 Psoriasis.

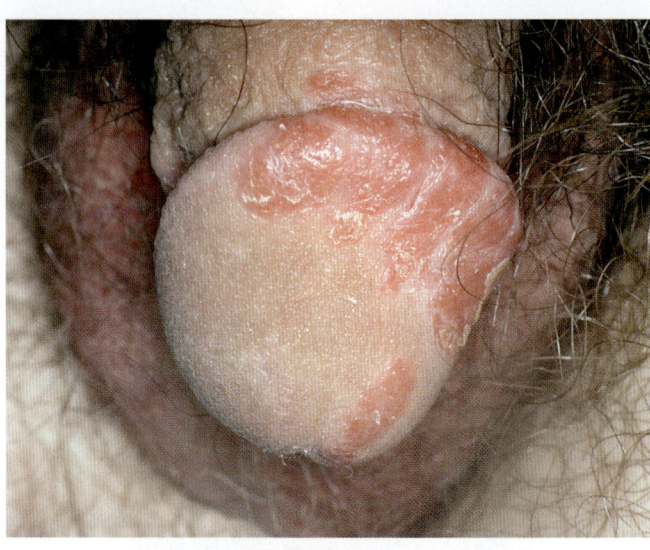

Fig. 10.28 Psoriasis. *Courtesy Steven Binnick, MD.*

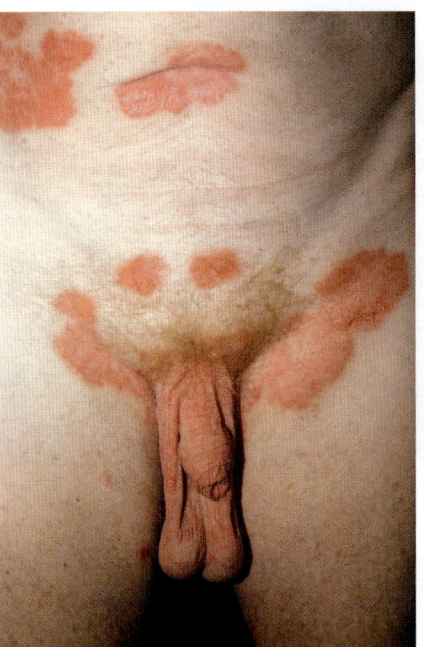

Fig. 10.29 Psoriasis. *Courtesy Steven Binnick, MD.*

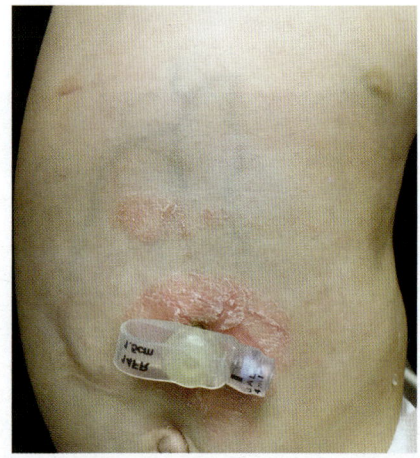

Fig. 10.30 Psoriasis at the site of a G-tube (Koebner phenomenon).

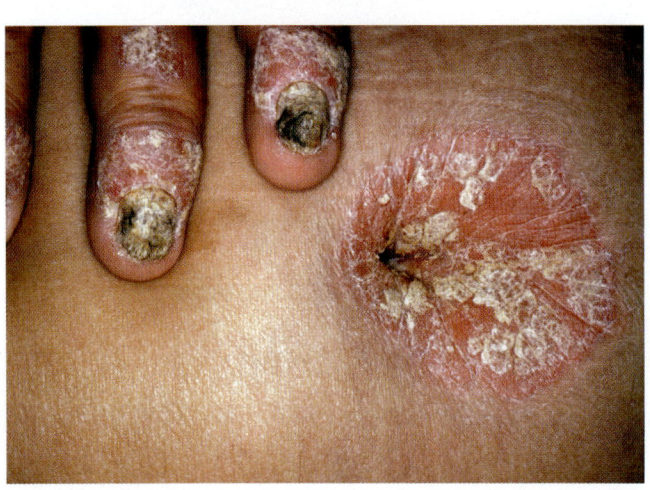

Fig. 10.31 Psoriasis.

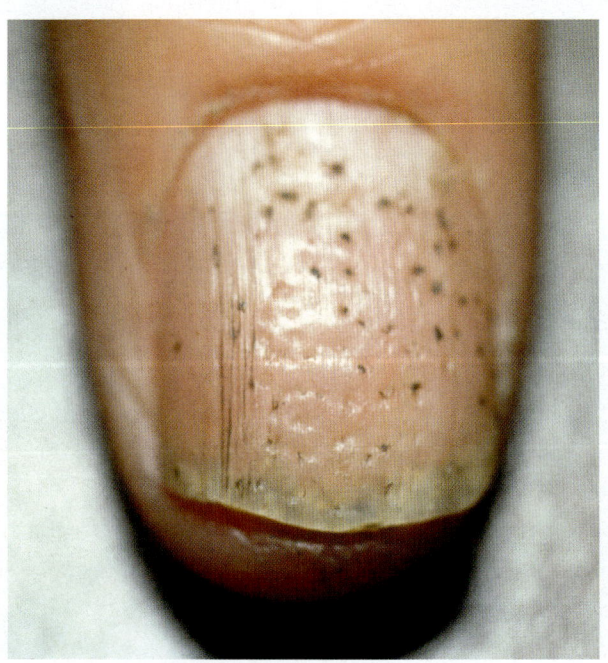

Fig. 10.32 Nail pitting in psoriasis.

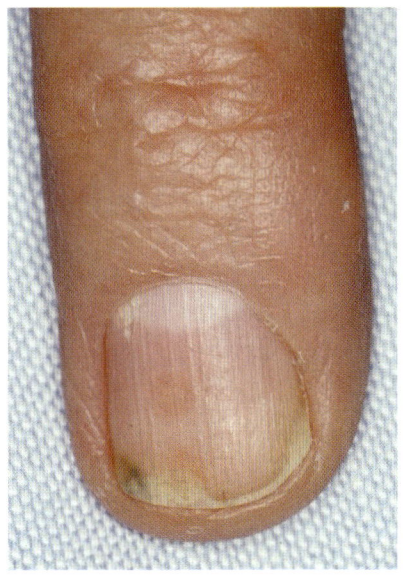

Fig. 10.33 Oil spot and subungual hyperkeratosis in nail psoriasis.

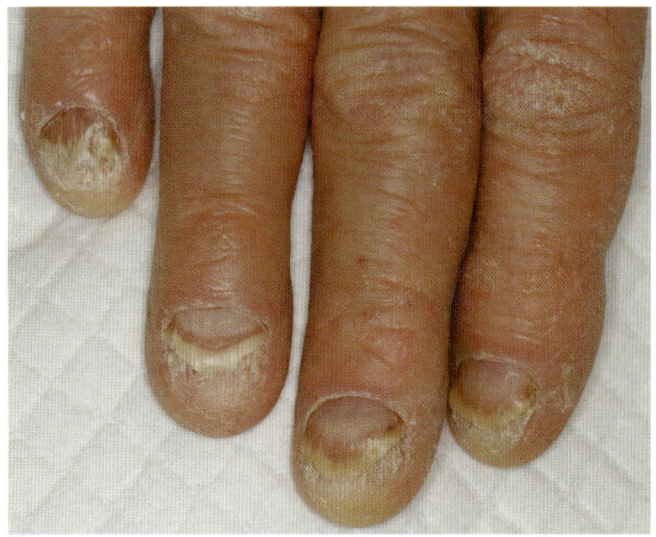

Fig. 10.34 Nail psoriasis.

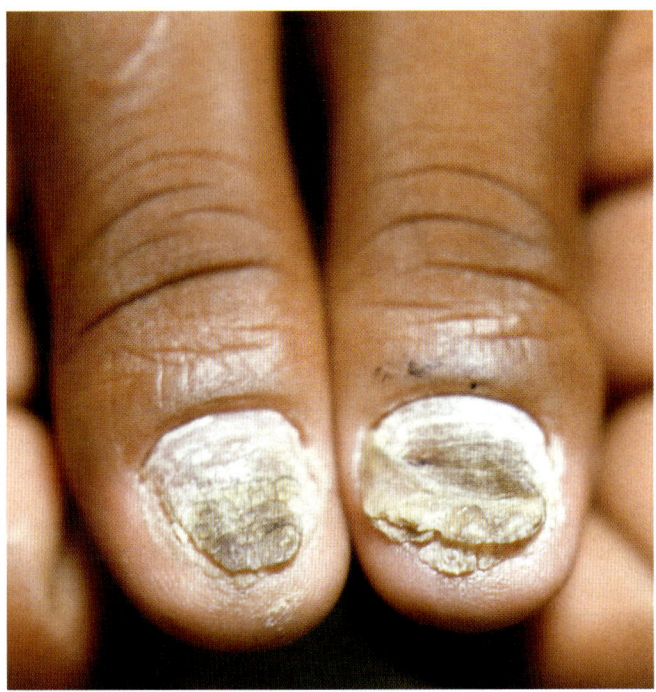

Fig. 10.35 Nail psoriasis.

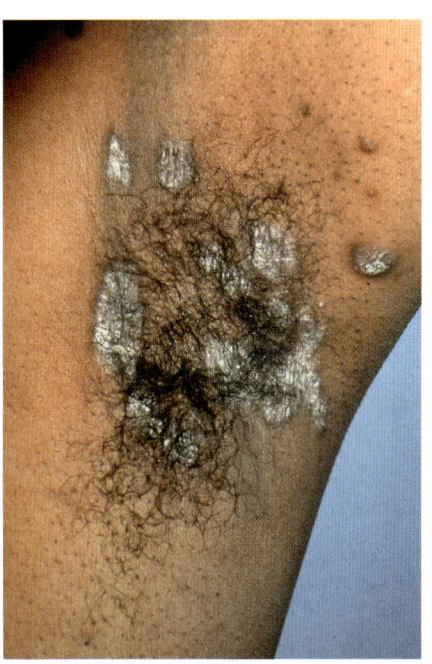

Fig. 10.36 Inverse psoriasis.

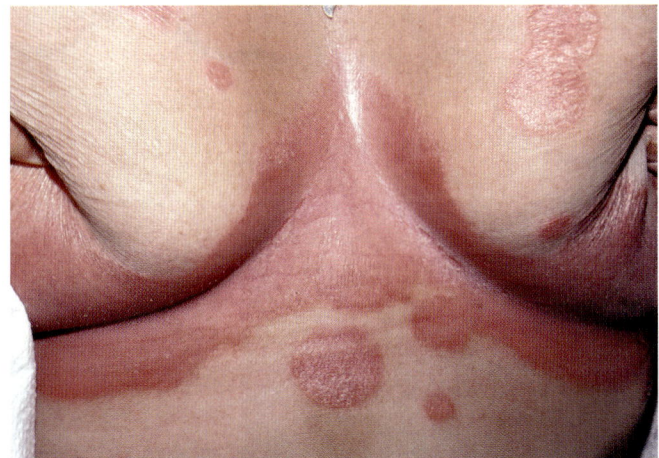

Fig. 10.37 Inverse psoriasis. *Courtesy Steven Binnick, MD.*

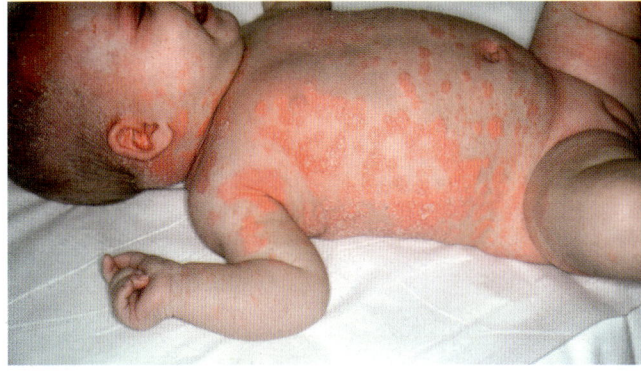

Fig. 10.38 Infantile psoriasis.

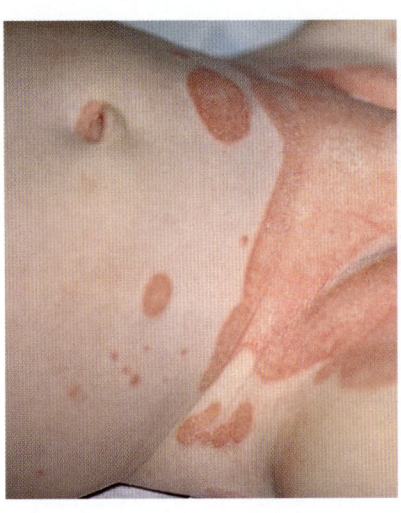

Fig. 10.39 Infantile psoriasis. *Courtesy Paul Honig, MD.*

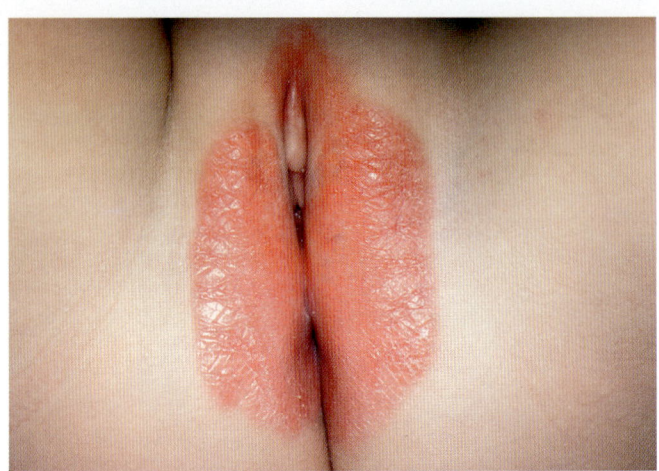

Fig. 10.40 Infantile psoriasis.

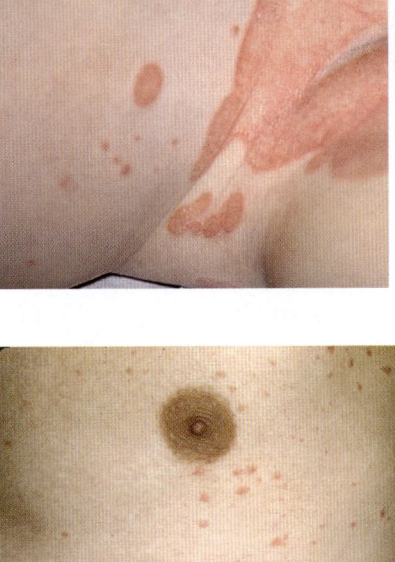

Fig. 10.41 Guttate psoriasis. *Courtesy The University of Utah and Oregon Health Sciences University Leonard Swinyer MD image collection.*

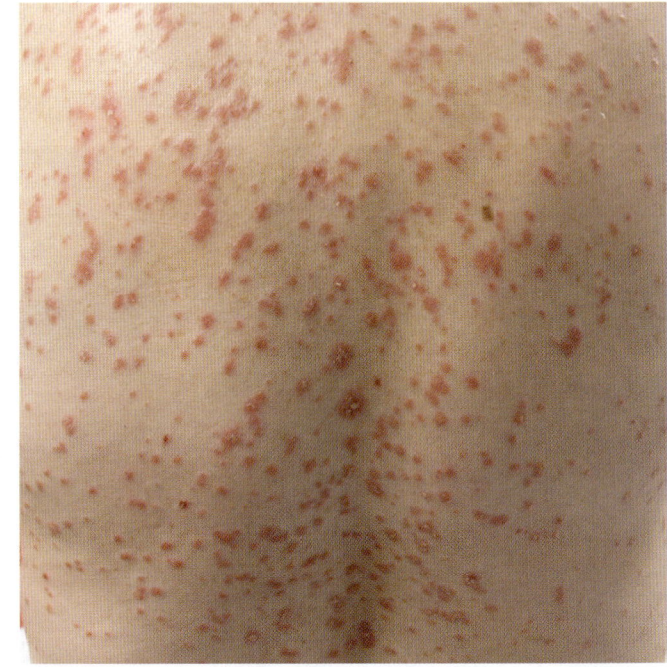

Fig. 10.42 Guttate psoriasis.

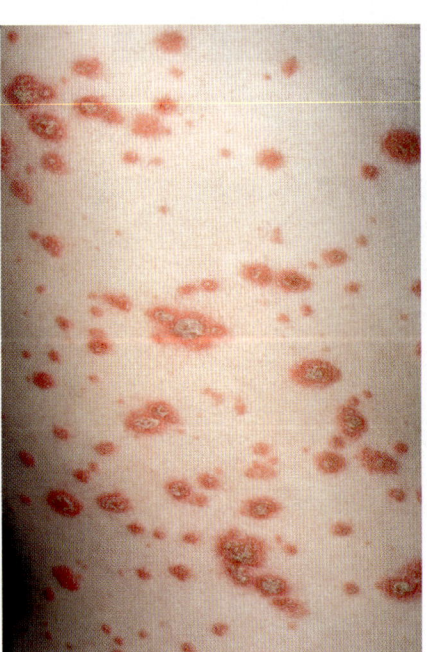

Fig. 10.43 Guttate psoriasis.

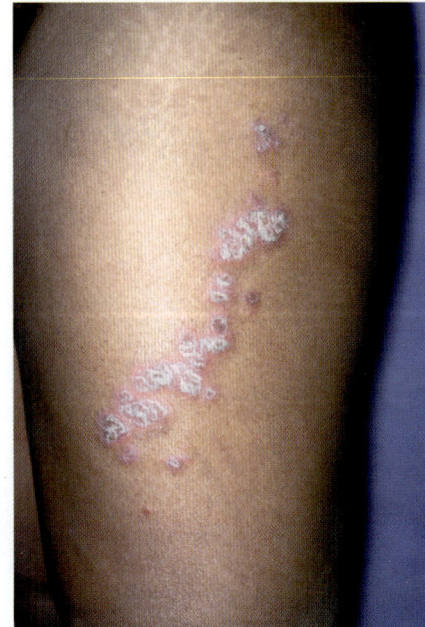

Fig. 10.44 Linear psoriasis.

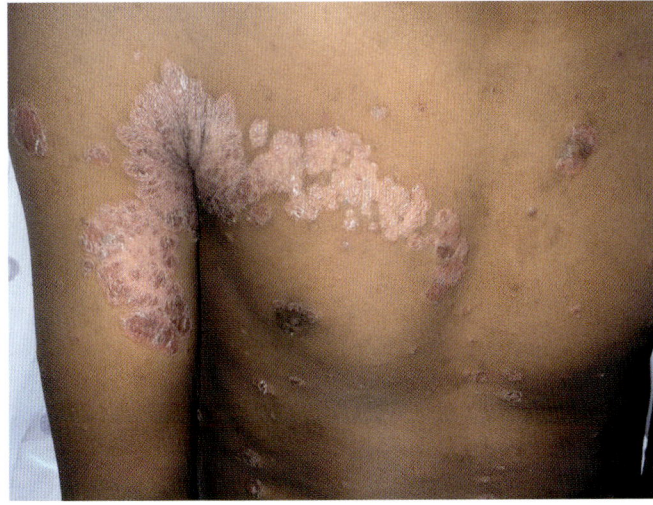

Fig. 10.45 Psoriasis after zoster in an HIV-infected patient. *Courtesy Vikash Oza, MD.*

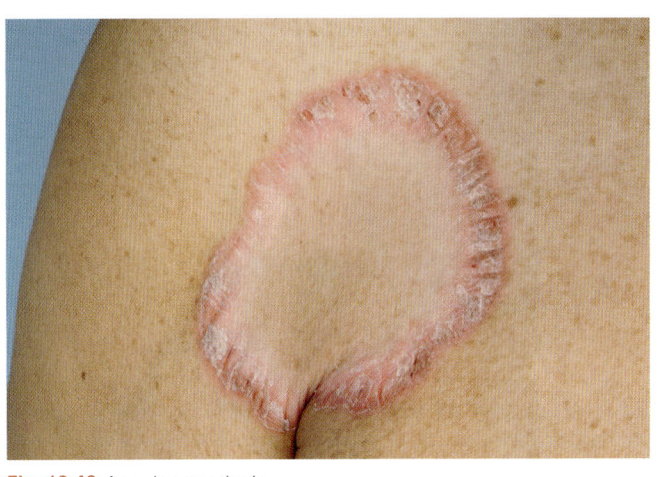

Fig. 10.46 Annular psoriasis.

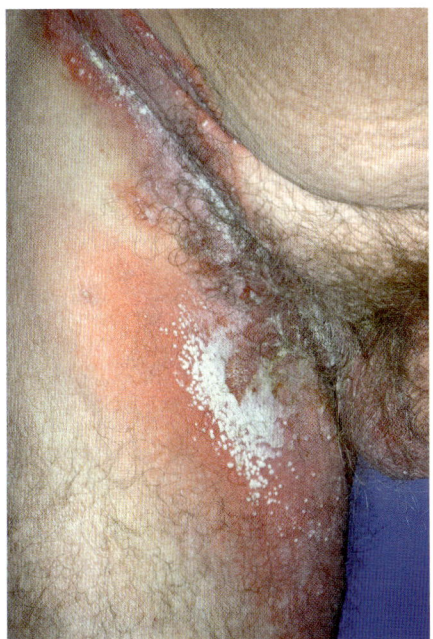

Fig. 10.47 Pustular psoriasis.

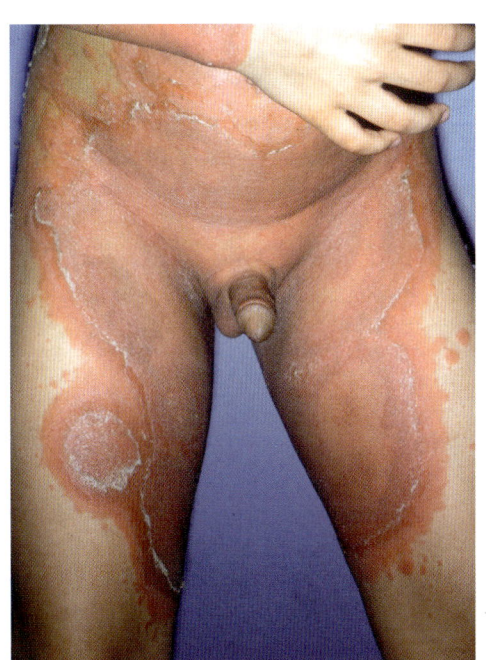

Fig. 10.48 Pustular psoriasis.

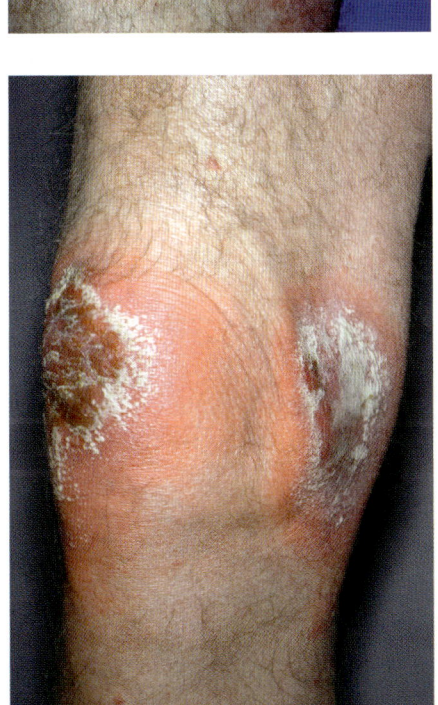

Fig. 10.49 Pustular psoriasis.

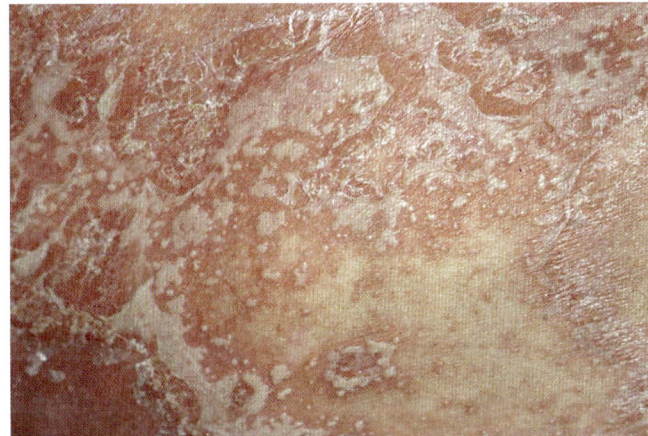

Fig. 10.50 Pustular psoriasis.

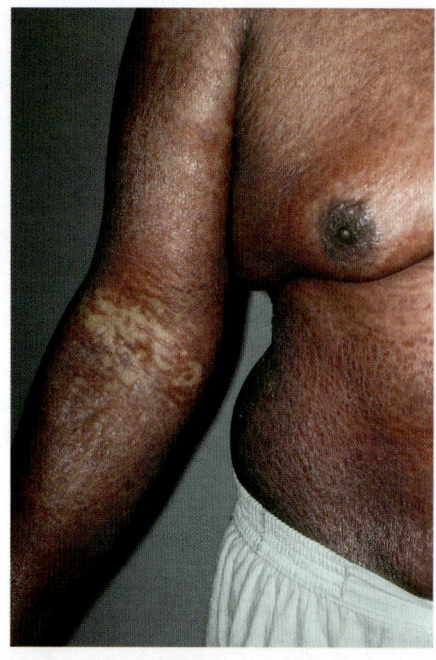

Fig. 10.51 Erythrodermic psoriasis.

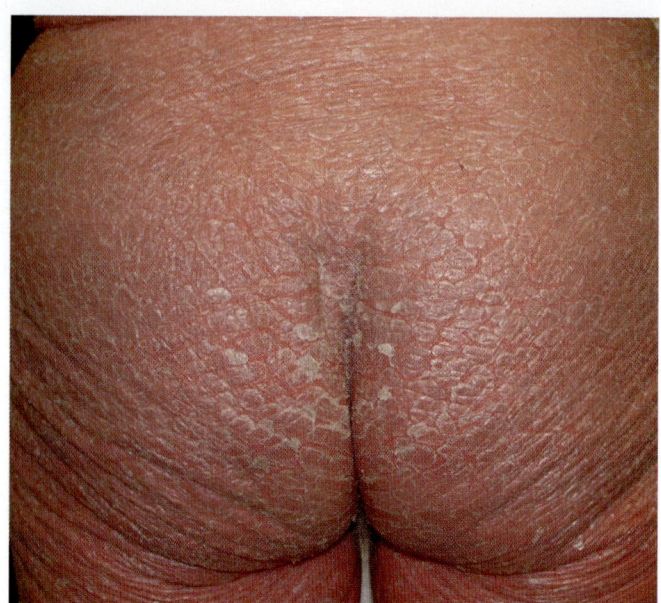

Fig. 10.52 Erythrodermic psoriasis.

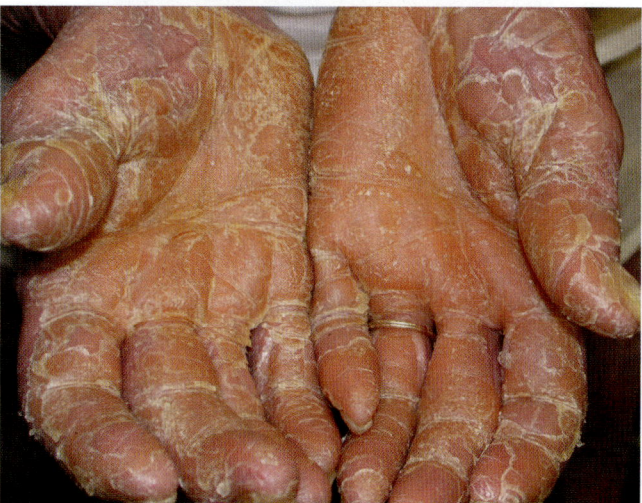

Fig. 10.53 Hands in erythrodermic psoriasis.

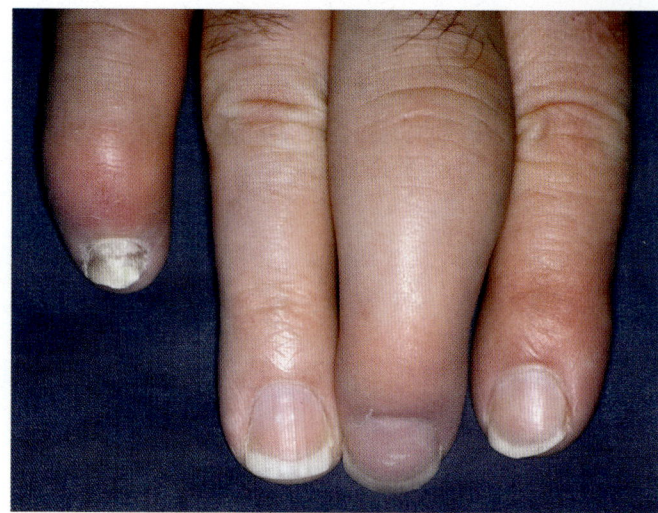

Fig. 10.54 Psoriatic arthritis. *Courtesy Steven Binnick, MD.*

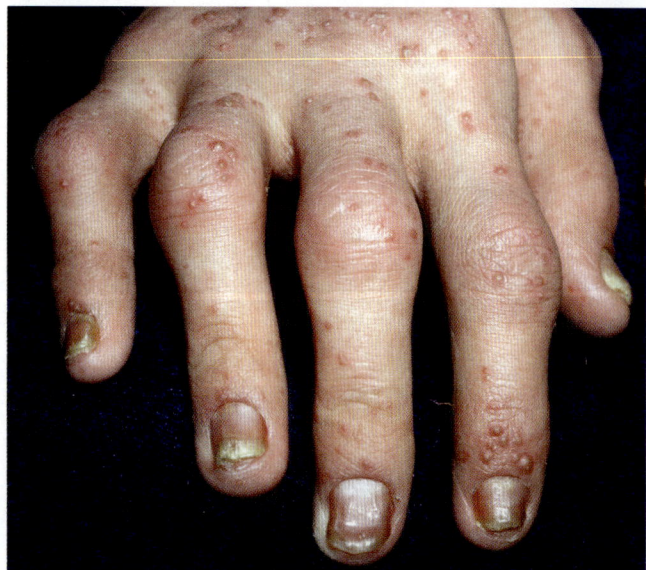

Fig. 10.55 Psoriatic arthritis.

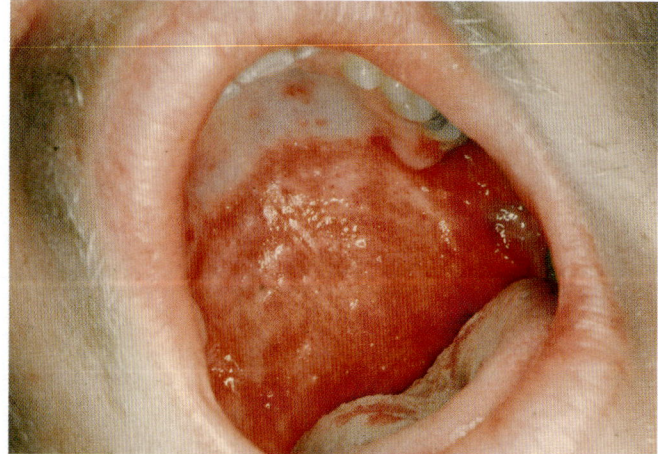

Fig. 10.56 Reactive arthritis with oral erythema.

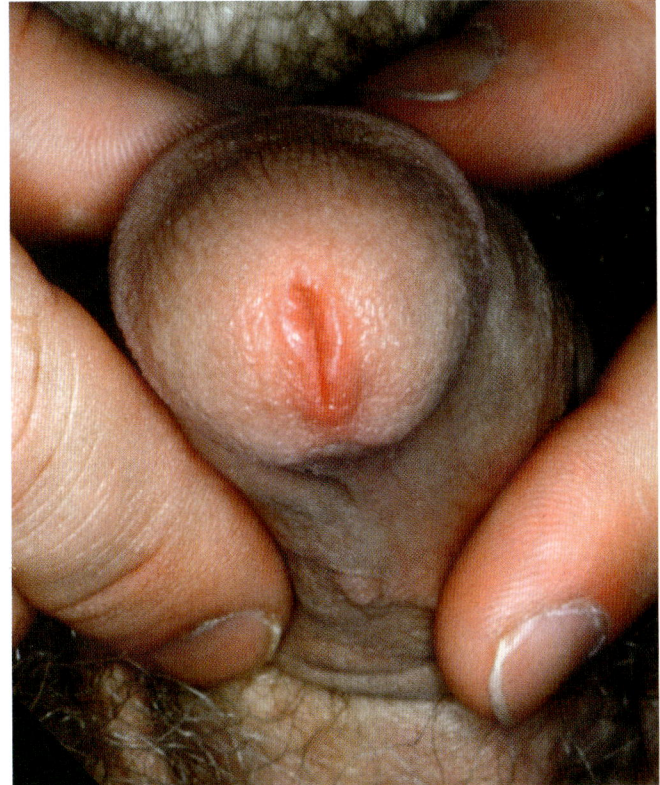

Fig. 10.57 Reactive arthritis with urethral inflammation.

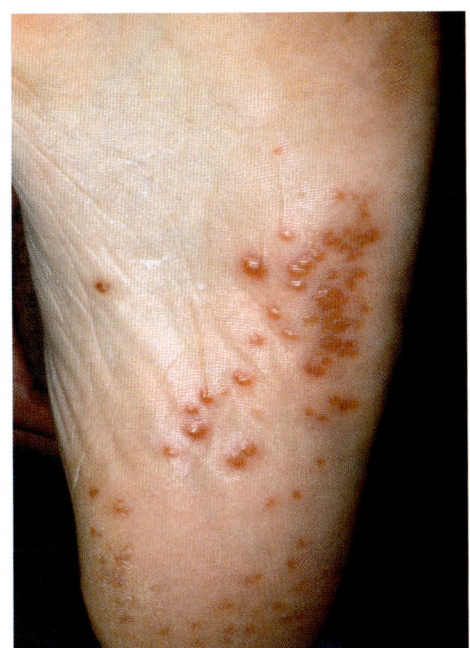

Fig. 10.59 Reactive arthritis.

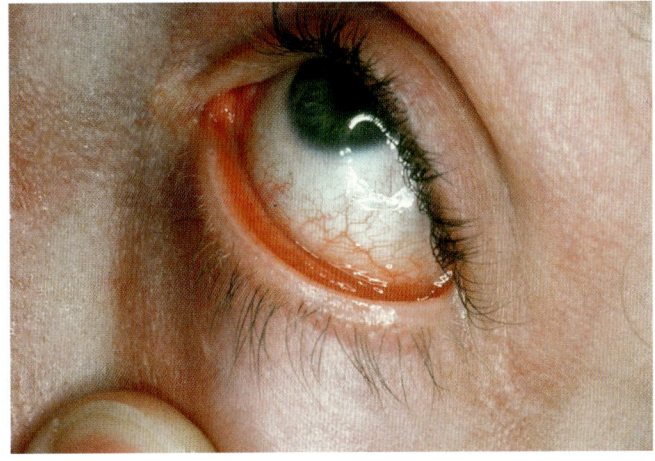

Fig. 10.58 Reactive arthritis with conjunctival erythema.

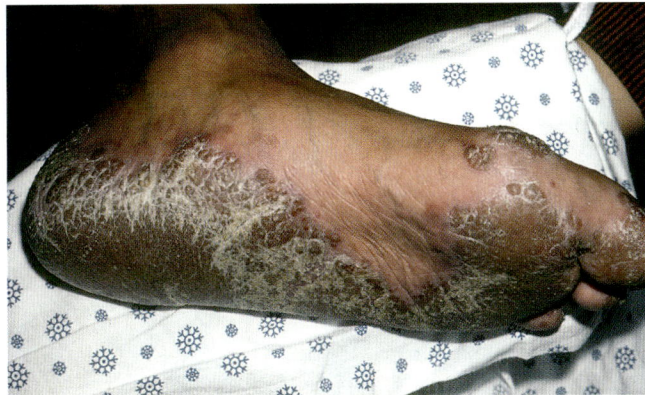

Fig. 10.60 Reactive arthritis.

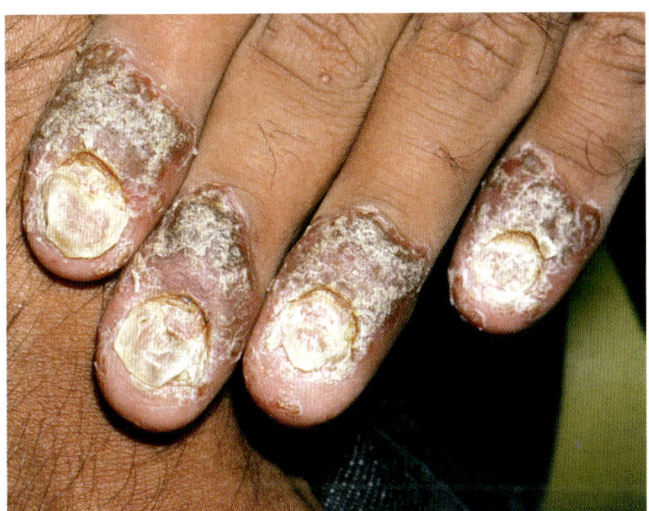

Fig. 10.61 Reactive arthritis.

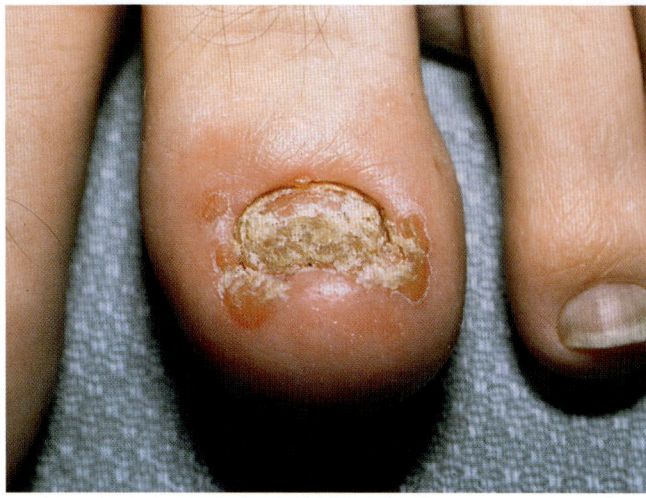

Fig. 10.62 Reactive arthritis.

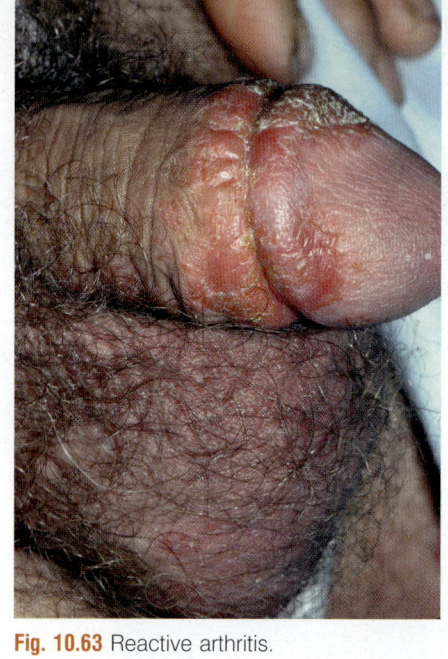

Fig. 10.63 Reactive arthritis.

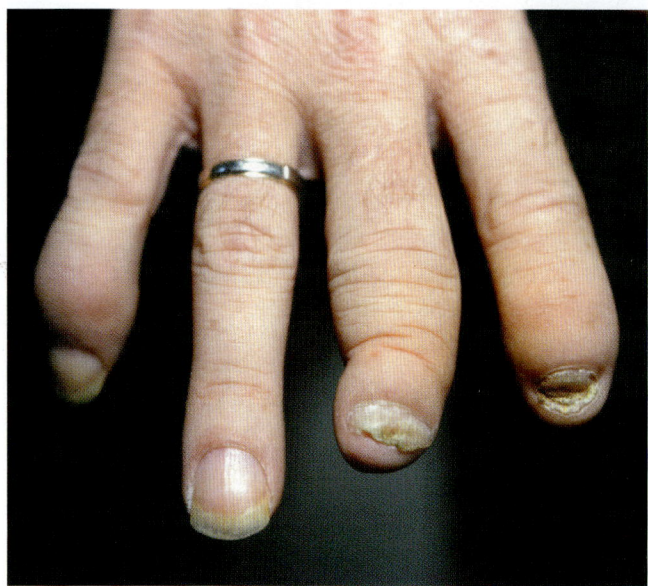

Fig. 10.64 Reactive arthritis.

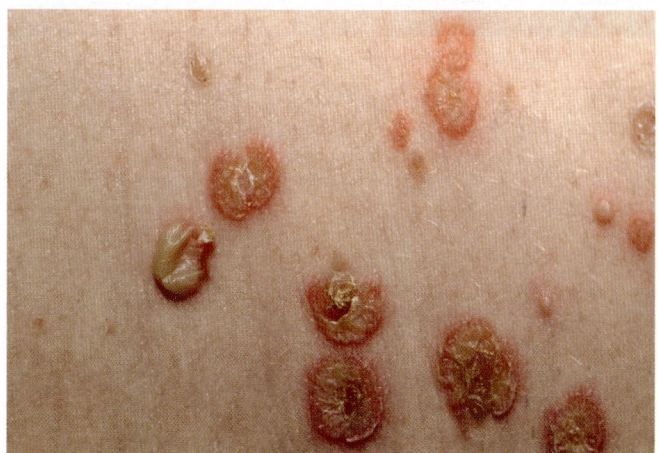

Fig. 10.65 Subcorneal pustular dermatosis. *Courtesy Steven Binnick, MD.*

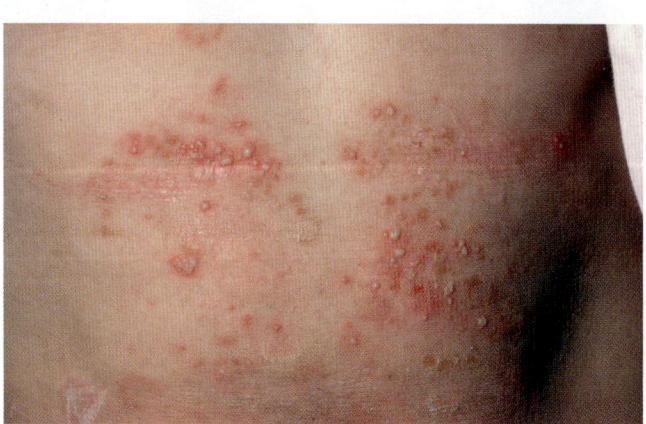

Fig. 10.66 Subcorneal pustular dermatosis.

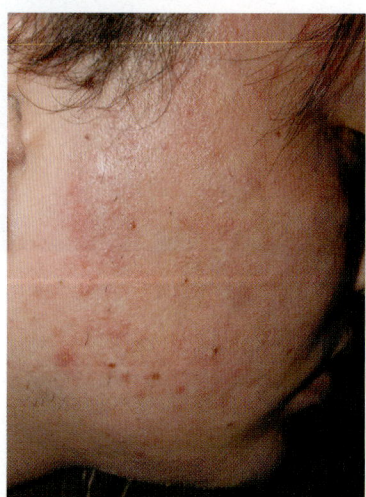

Fig. 10.67 Eosinophilic pustular folliculitis of Ofuji. *Courtesy Chia-Yu Chu, MD, PhD.*

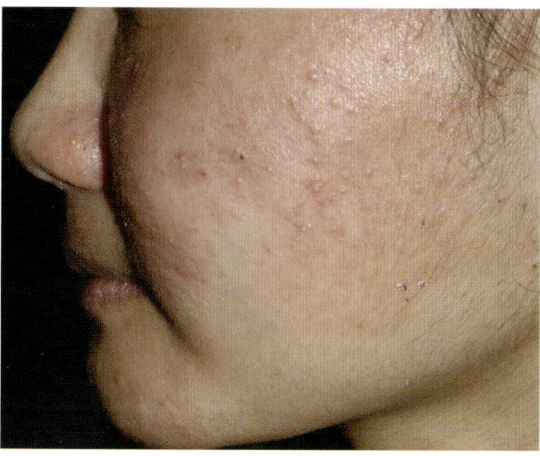

Fig. 10.68 Eosinophilic pustular folliculitis. *Courtesy Vasanop Vachiramon, MD.*

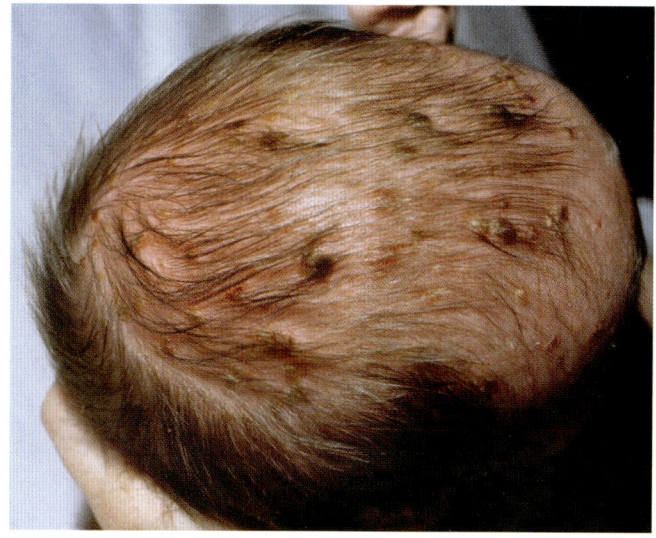

Fig. 10.69 Pediatric eosinophilic pustular folliculitis. *Courtesy Paul Honig, MD.*

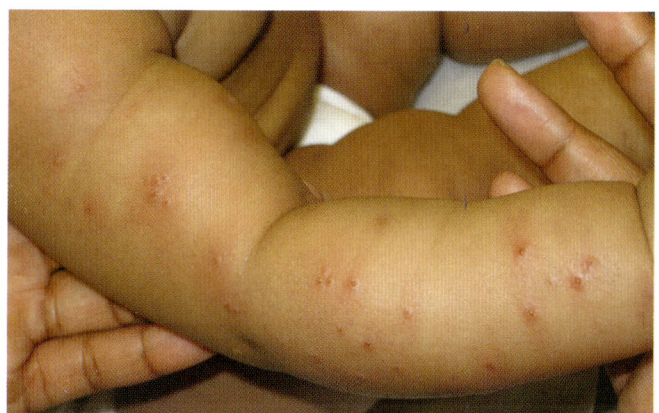

Fig. 10.70 Eosinophilic pustular folliculitis.

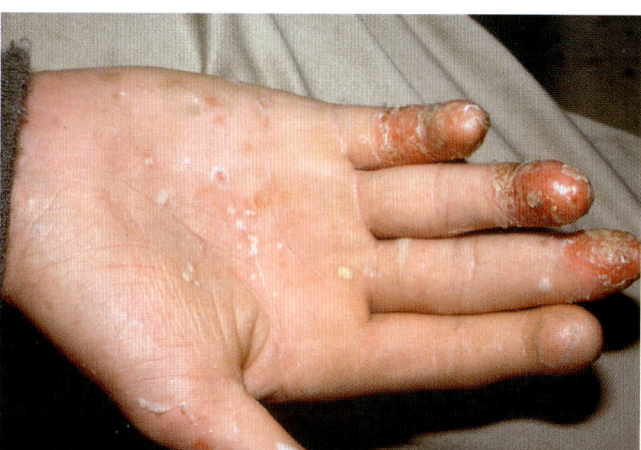

Fig. 10.71 Acrodermatitis continua.

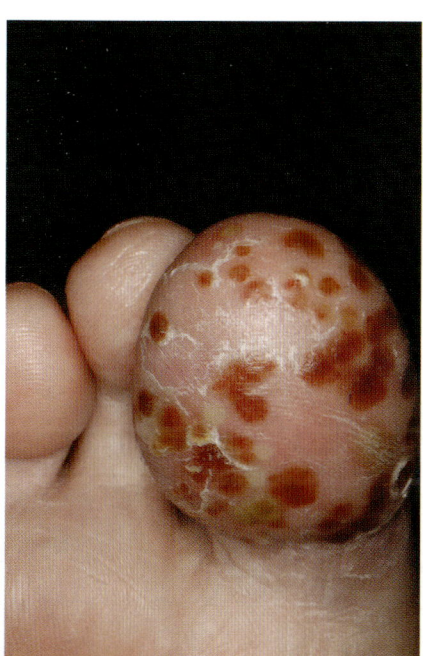

Fig. 10.72 Acrodermatitis continua.

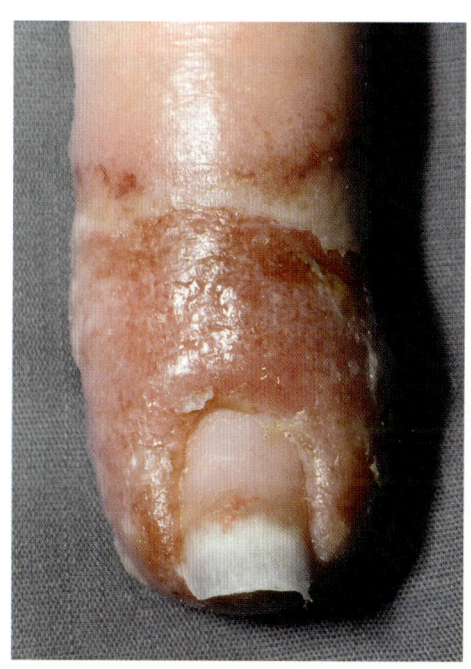

Fig. 10.73 Acrodermatitis continua. *Courtesy Steven Binnick, MD.*

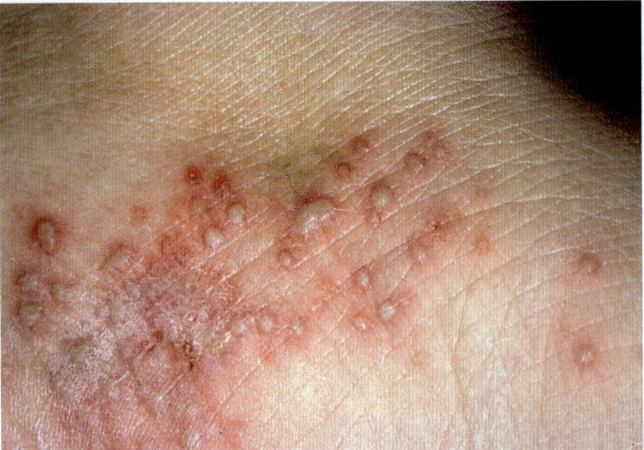

Fig. 10.74 Recurrent palmoplantar pustulosis.

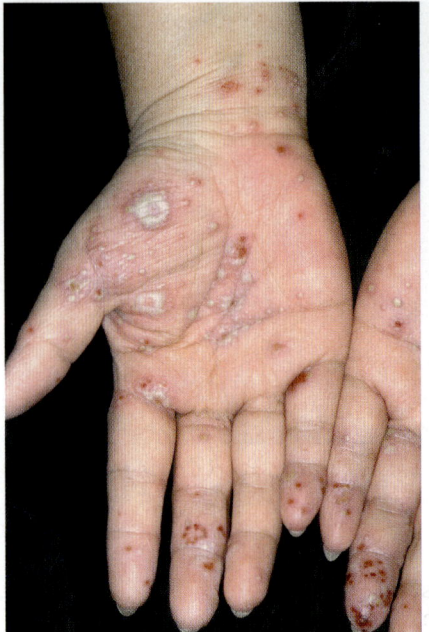

Fig. 10.75 Palmoplantar pustulosis.

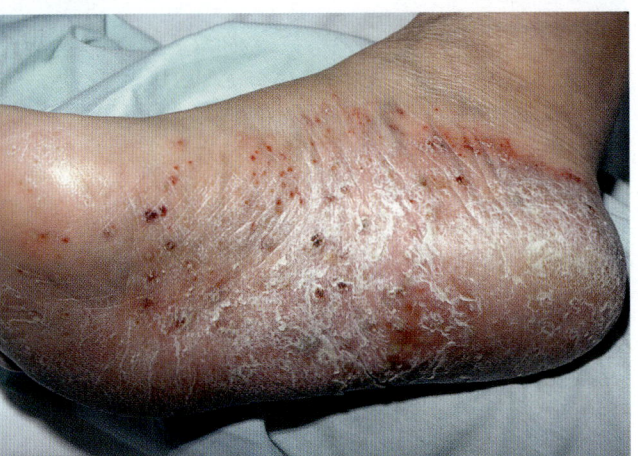

Fig. 10.76 Palmoplantar pustulosis. *Courtesy Steven Binnick, MD.*

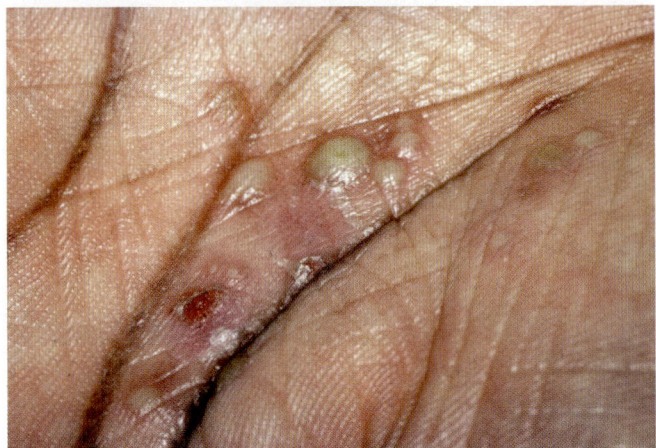

Fig. 10.77 Palmoplantar pustulosis.

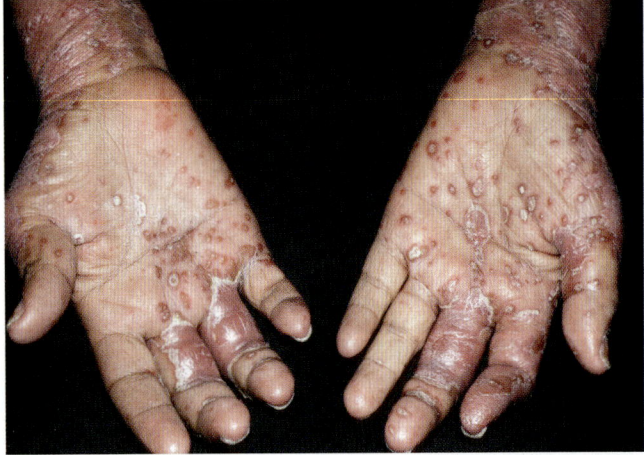

Fig. 10.78 Palmoplantar pustulosis.

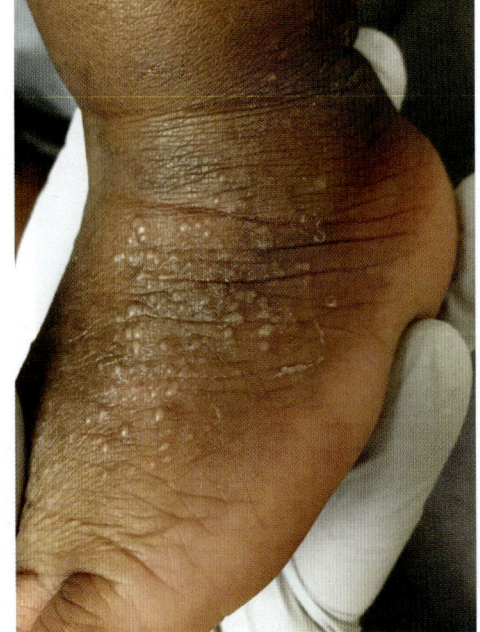

Fig. 10.79 Acropustulosis of infancy.

Pityriasis Rosea, Pityriasis Rubra Pilaris, and Other Papulosquamous and Hyperkeratotic Diseases

11

Pityriasis rosea presents with erythematous macules that develop a delicate central silver scale. As the lesions evolve, they assume an oval configuration often best observed on the back and flanks. The scale becomes a peripheral collarette as the lesions evolve. Histologically, erythrocyte extravasation is characteristic, and clinically purpuric lesions may occasionally be noted. In patients with darker skin, the lesions of pityriasis rosea may assume a papular appearance. A more characteristic oval character is often evident on the upper flank near the axillary vault and can be helpful in confirming the diagnosis.

Pityriasis rubra pilaris (PRP) may present with classic nutmeg-grater, spiky, keratotic papules involving the dorsal digits, or may present with more subtle erythema and scale involving the hands, face, and scalp. Evolution can be rapid, and the patient can assume the appearance of erythroderma with characteristic islands of sparing. The eruptions often have a distinctly orange appearance, especially on the palms. Juvenile forms of PRP can present with nummular arrays of spiky papules or with hyperkeratotic plaques involving the extensors in a pattern reminiscent of psoriasis. Discrete keratotic follicular papules are often present at the periphery and are helpful in establishing the correct diagnosis without the need for biopsy. This portion of the atlas will guide you through the various clinical presentations of these disorders.

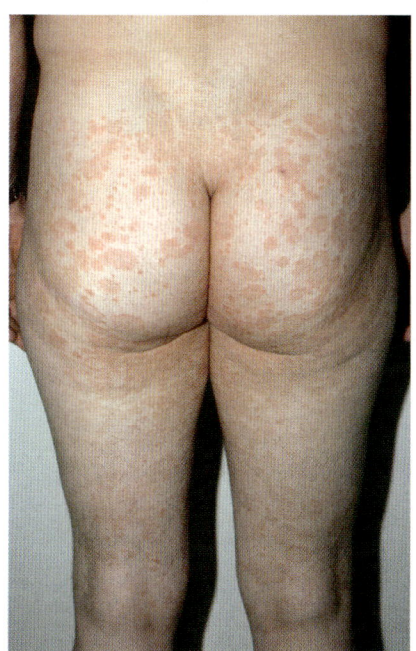

Fig. 11.1 Small plaque parapsoriasis.

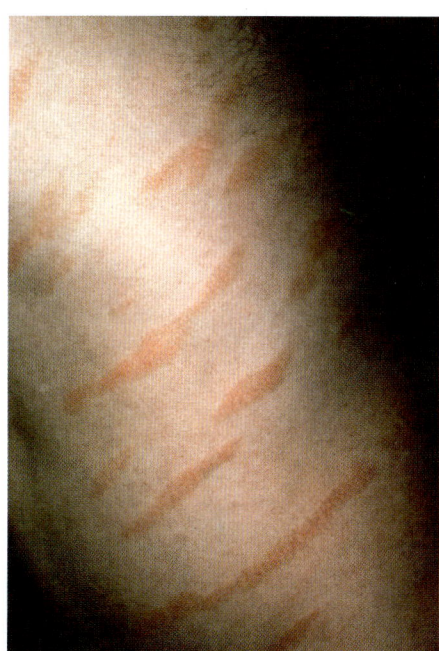

Fig. 11.2 Digitate parapsoriasis.

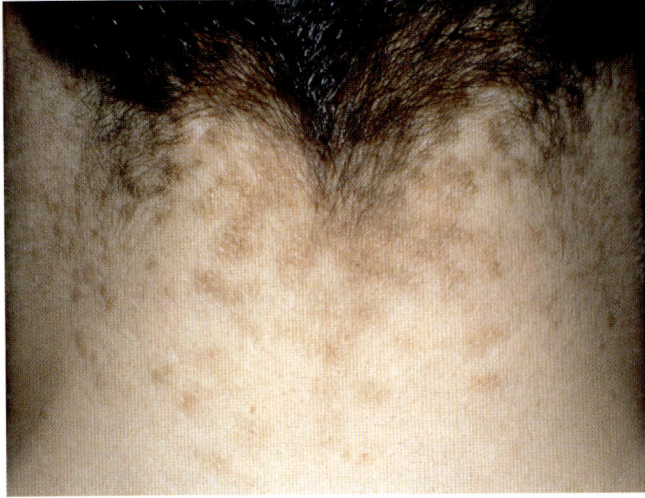

Fig. 11.3 Confluent and reticulated papillomatosis.

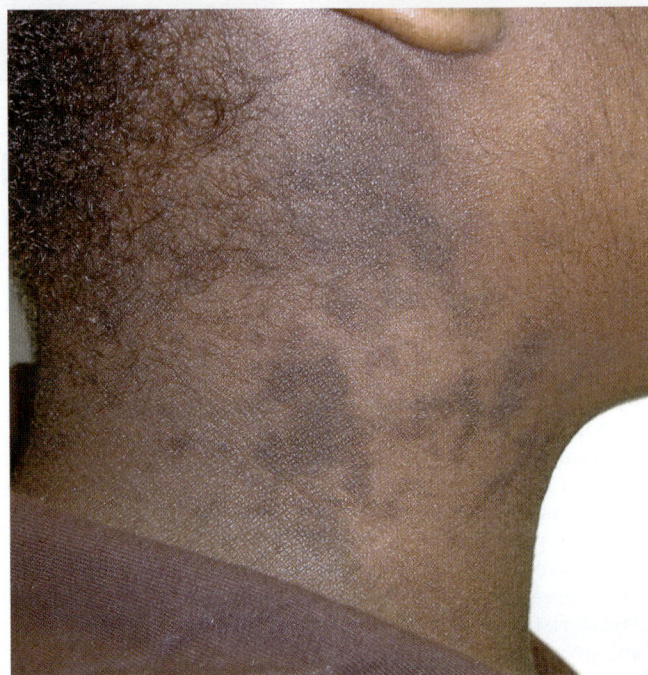

Fig. 11.4 Confluent and reticulated papillomatosis.

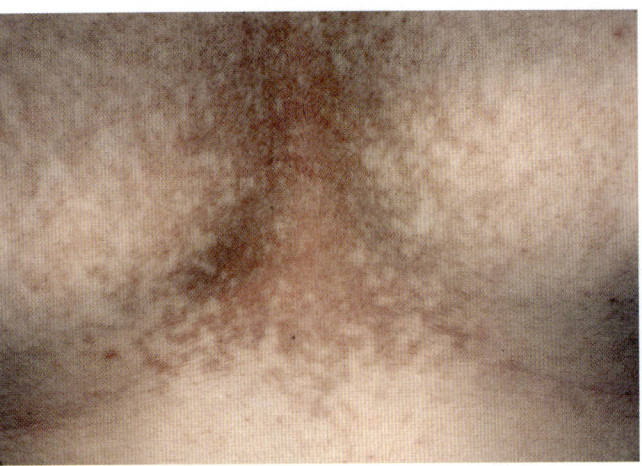

Fig. 11.5 Confluent and reticulated papillomatosis. *Courtesy Steven Binnick, MD.*

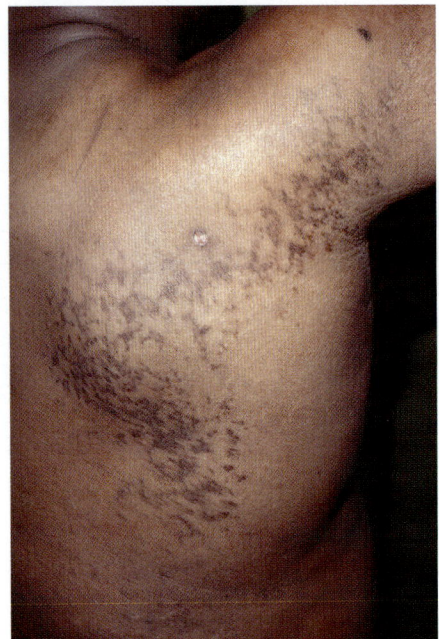

Fig. 11.6 Confluent and reticulated papillomatosis.

Fig. 11.7 Confluent and reticulated papillomatosis.

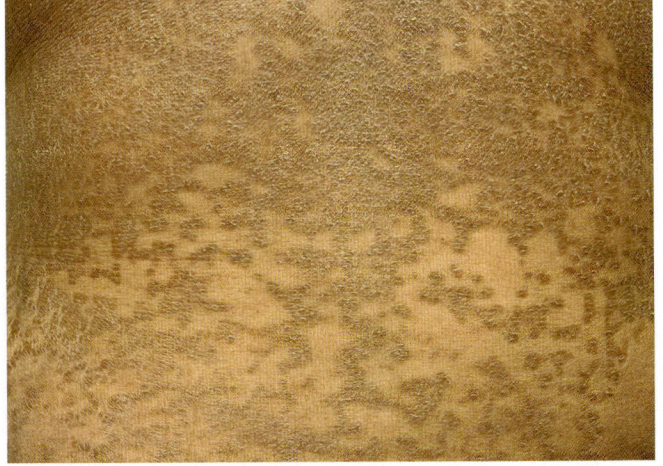

Fig. 11.8 Confluent and reticulated papillomatosis.

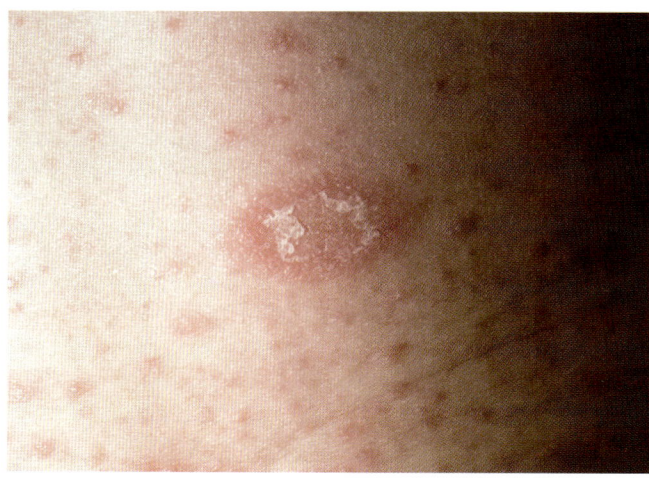

Fig. 11.9 Pityriasis rosea herald patch. *Courtesy Steven Binnick, MD.*

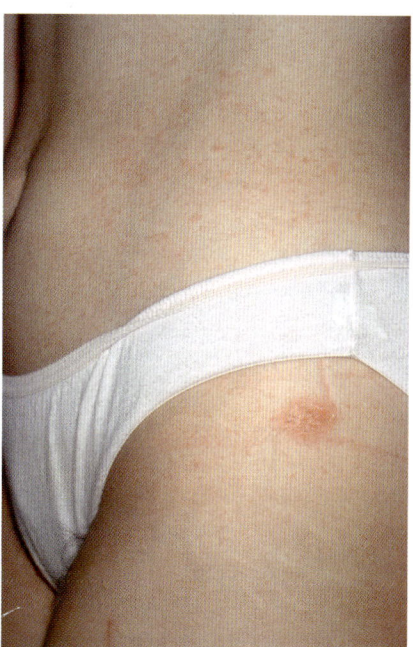

Fig. 11.10 Pityriasis rosea herald patch.

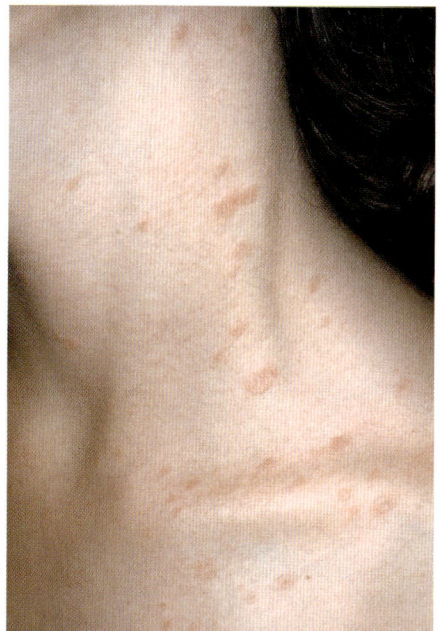

Fig. 11.11 Pityriasis rosea.

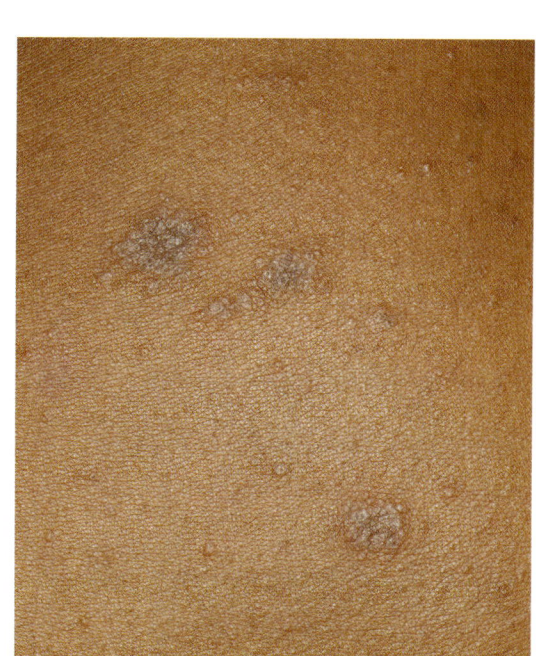

Fig. 11.12 Pityriasis rosea.

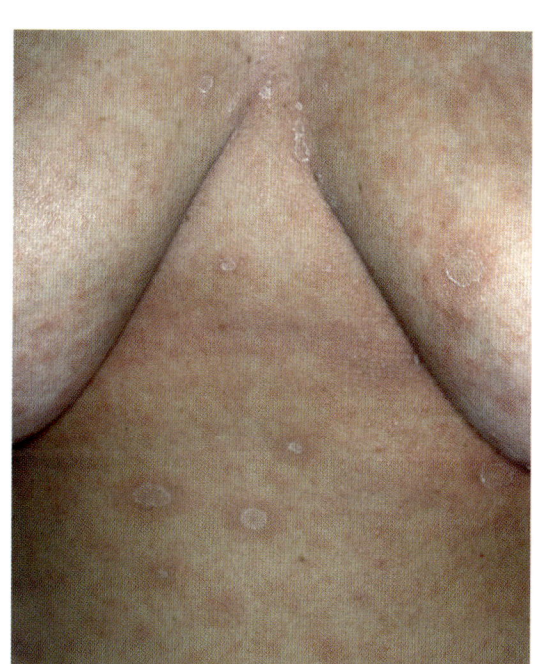

Fig. 11.13 Pityriasis rosea.

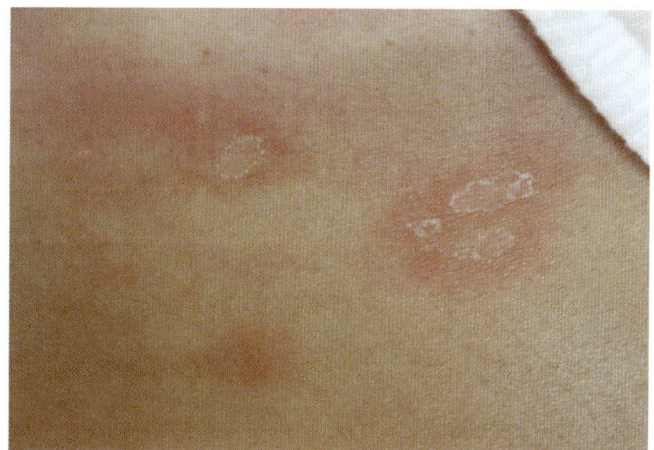

Fig. 11.14 Pityriasis rosea.

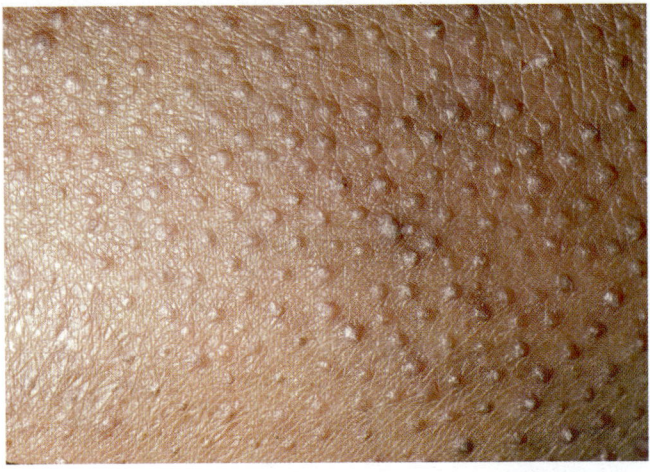

Fig. 11.15 Pityriasis rubra pilaris with early follicular hyperkeratosis.

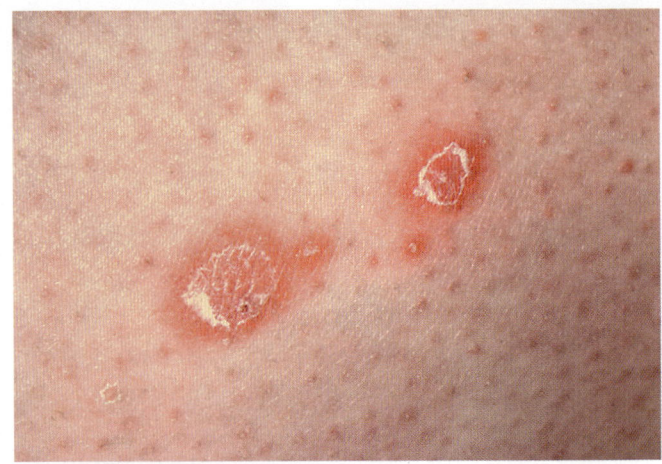

Fig. 11.16 Pityriasis rubra pilaris. *Courtesy Steven Binnick, MD.*

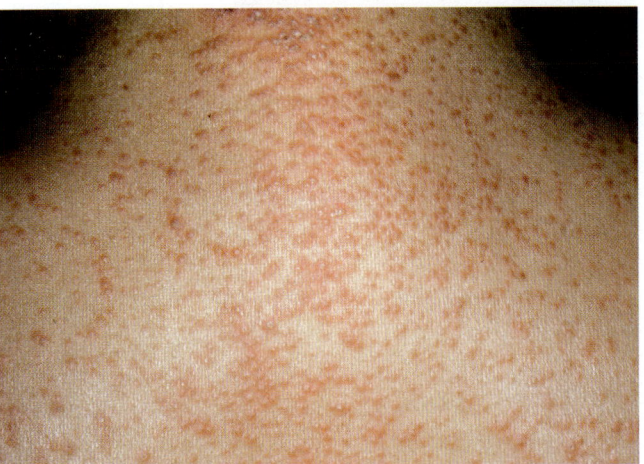

Fig. 11.17 Pityriasis rubra pilaris.

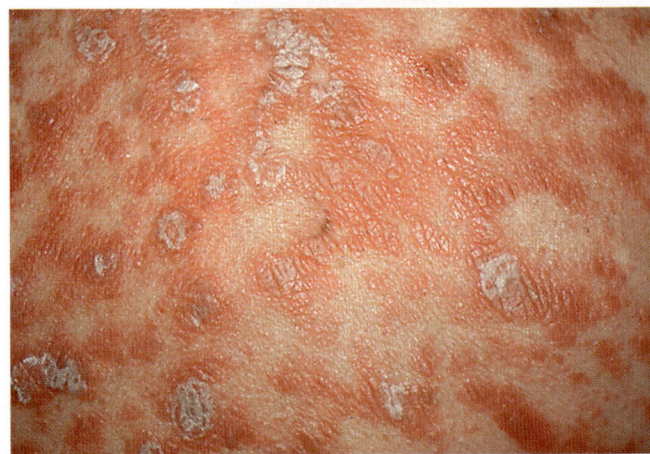

Fig. 11.18 Pityriasis rubra pilaris.

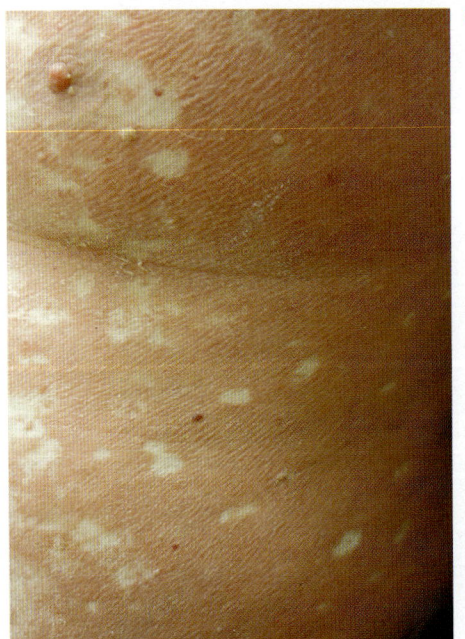

Fig. 11.19 Pityriasis rubra pilaris.

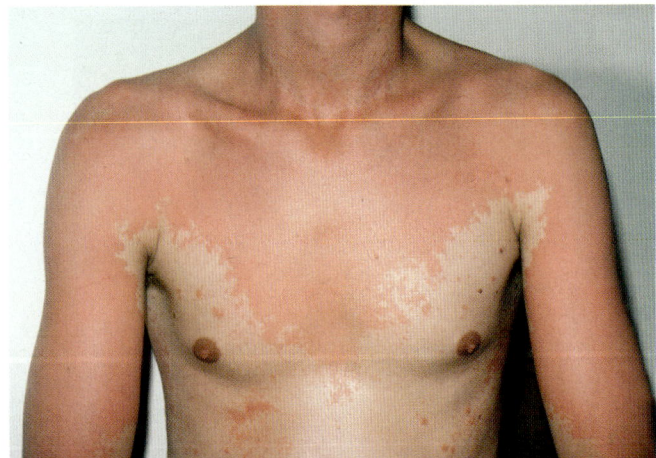

Fig. 11.20 Pityriasis rubra pilaris.

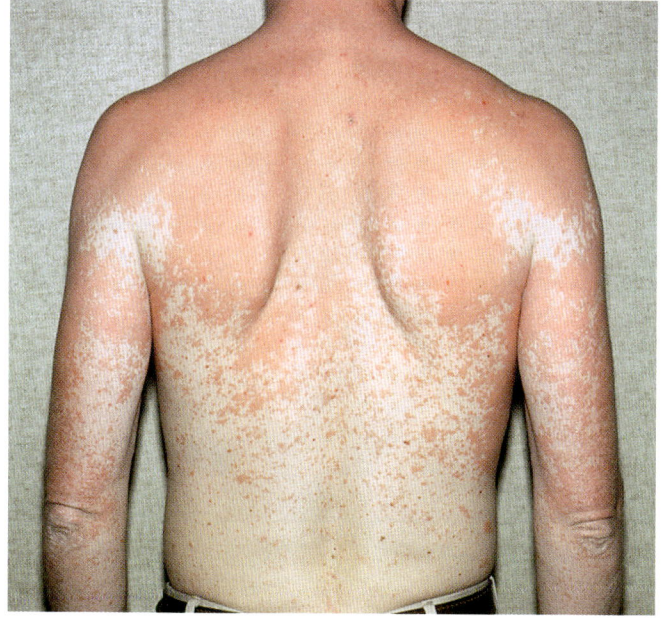

Fig. 11.21 Pityriasis rubra pilaris. *Courtesy Steven Binnick, MD.*

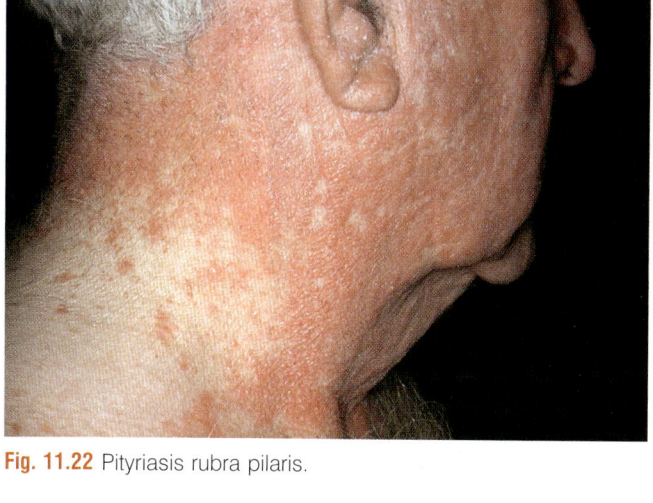

Fig. 11.22 Pityriasis rubra pilaris.

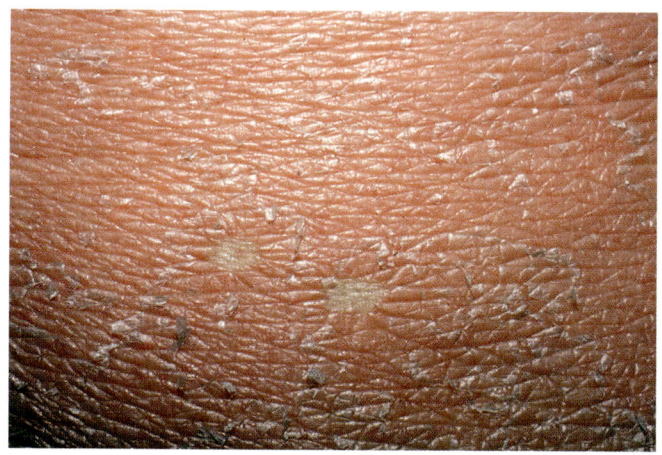

Fig. 11.23 Pityriasis rubra pilaris.

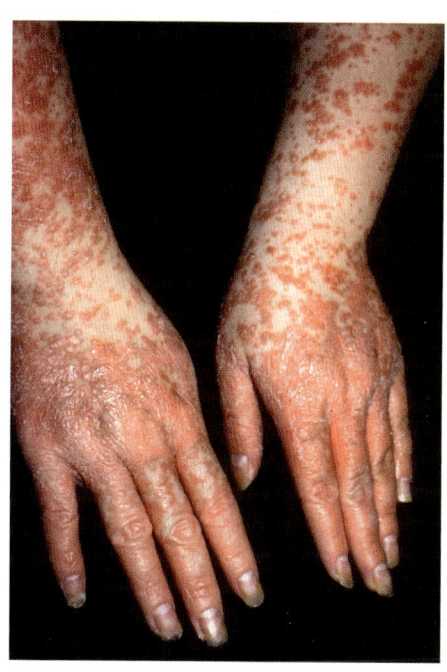

Fig. 11.24 Pityriasis rubra pilaris.

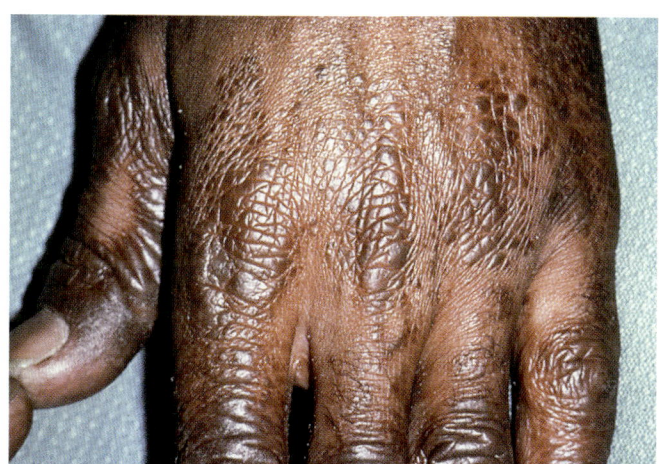

Fig. 11.25 Pityriasis rubra pilaris.

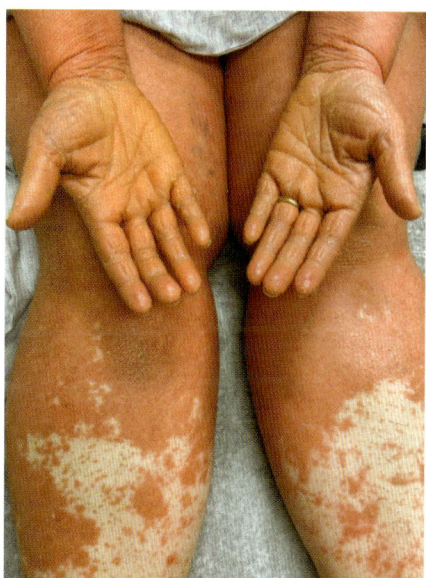

Fig. 11.26 Pityriasis rubra pilaris.

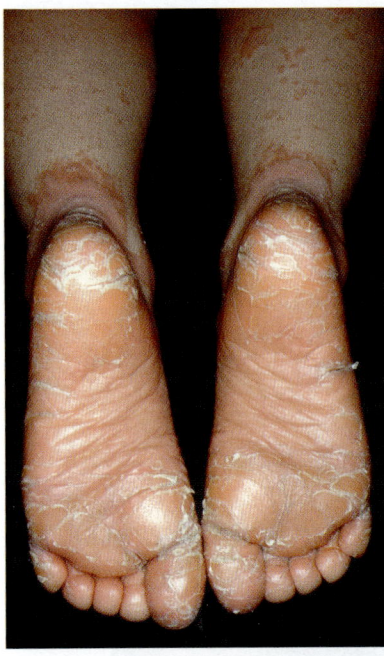

Fig. 11.27 Pityriasis rubra pilaris.

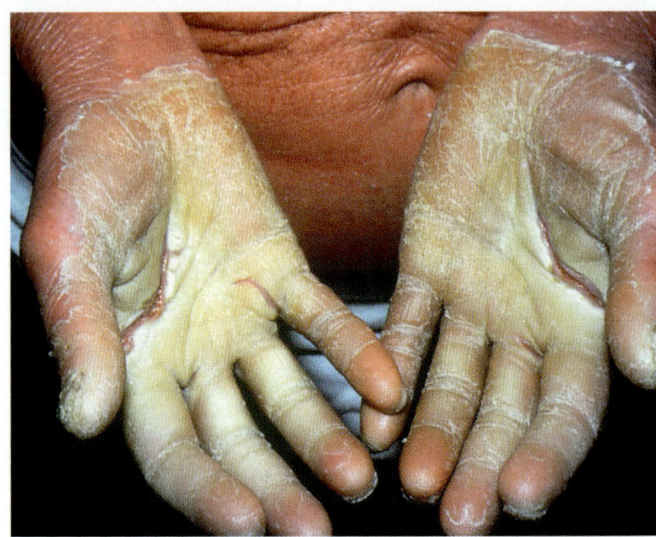

Fig. 11.28 Pityriasis rubra pilaris. *Courtesy Steven Binnick, MD.*

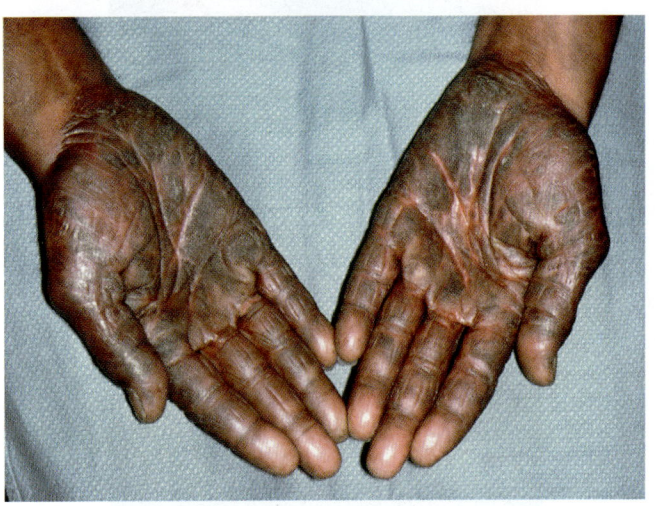

Fig. 11.29 Pityriasis rubra pilaris.

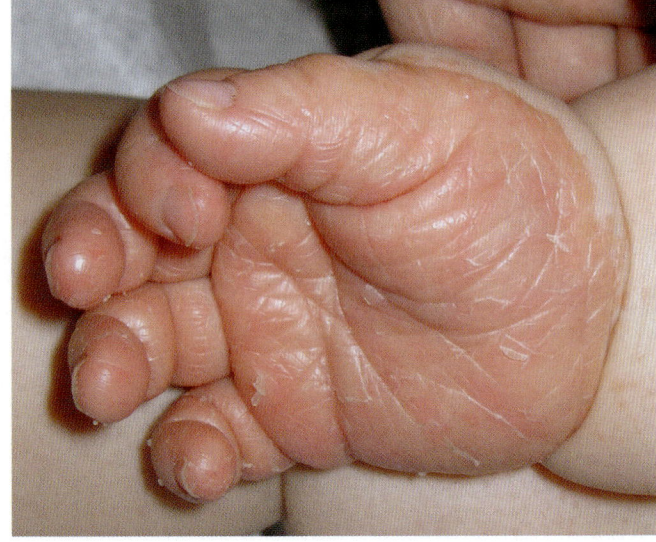

Fig. 11.30 Childhood pityriasis rubra pilaris.

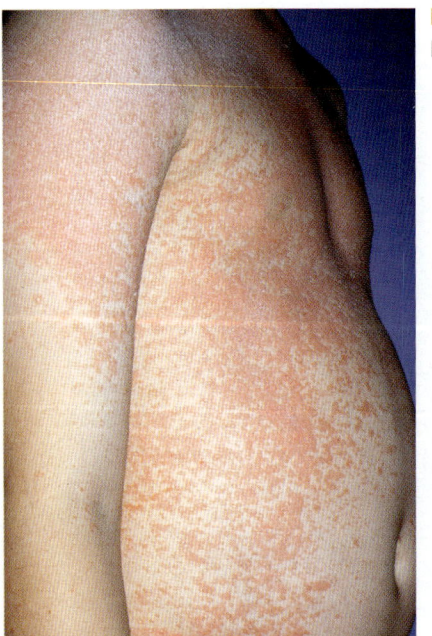

Fig. 11.31 Childhood pityriasis rubra pilaris.

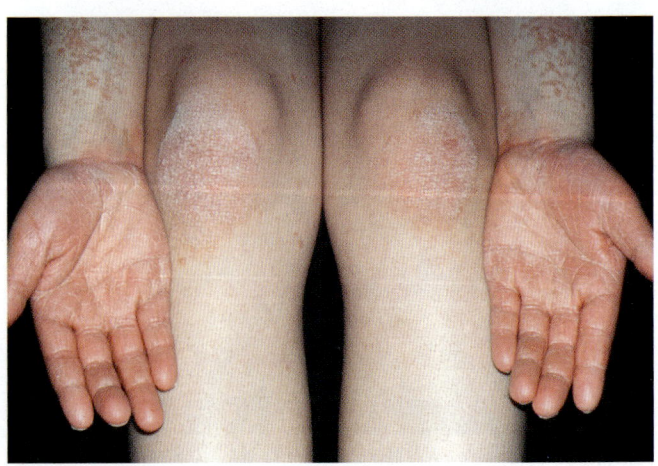

Fig. 11.32 Childhood pityriasis rubra pilaris.

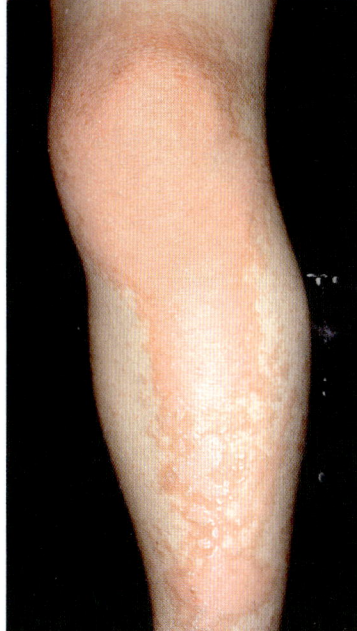

Fig. 11.33 Circumscribed juvenile pityriasis rubra pilaris.

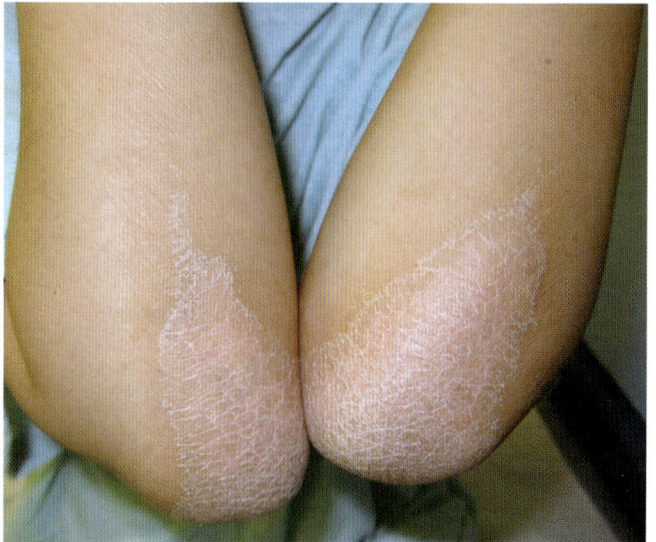

Fig. 11.34 Circumscribed juvenile pityriasis rubra pilaris.

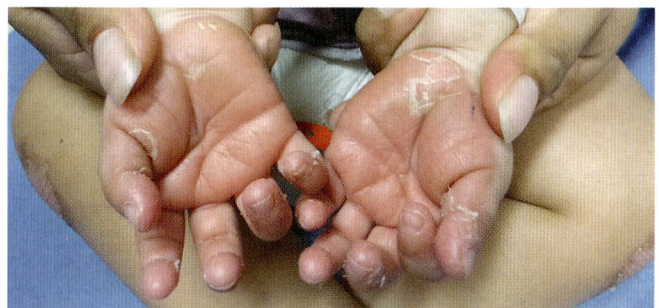

Fig. 11.35 Circumscribed juvenile pityriasis rubra pilaris.

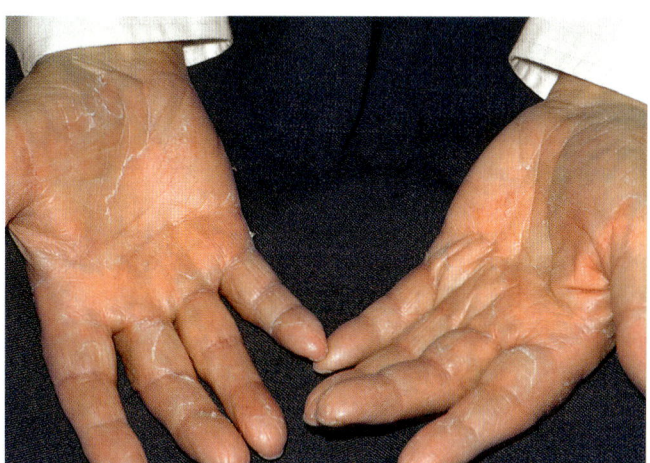

Fig. 11.36 Keratolysis exfoliativa.

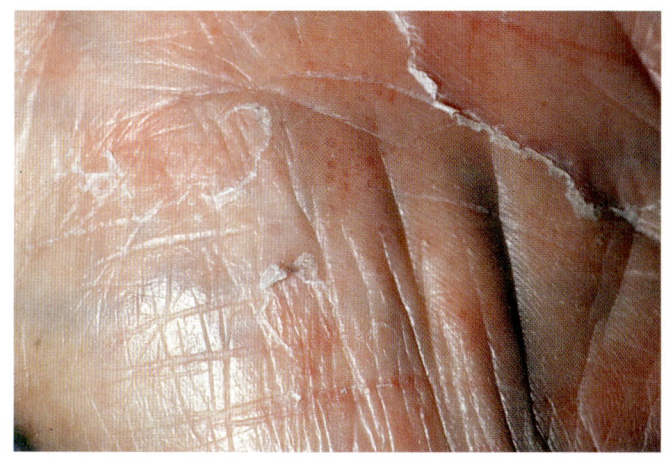

Fig. 11.37 Keratolysis exfoliativa.

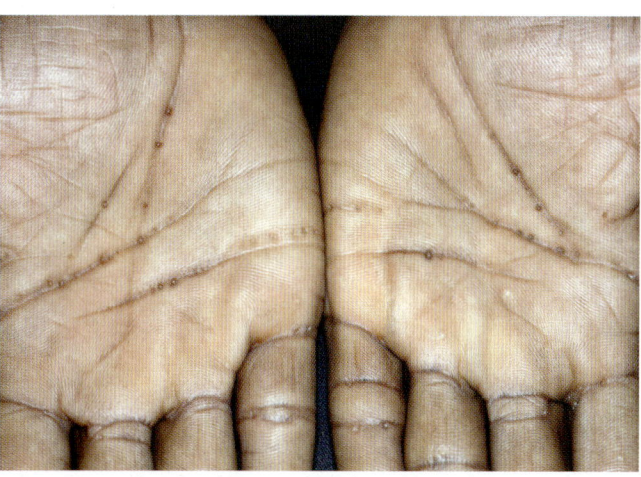

Fig. 11.38 Keratosis punctata of the palmar creases.

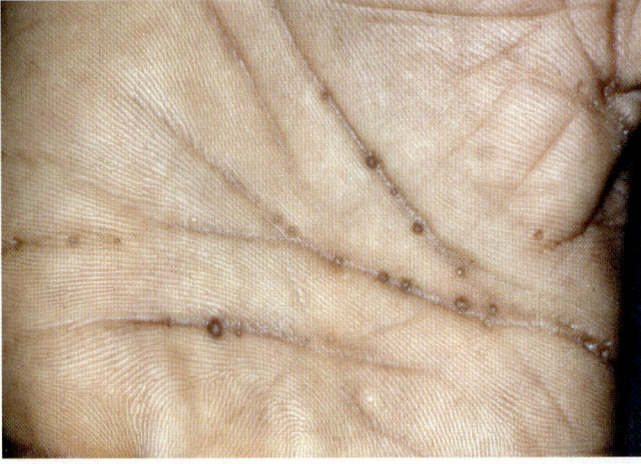

Fig. 11.39 Keratosis punctata of the palmar creases.

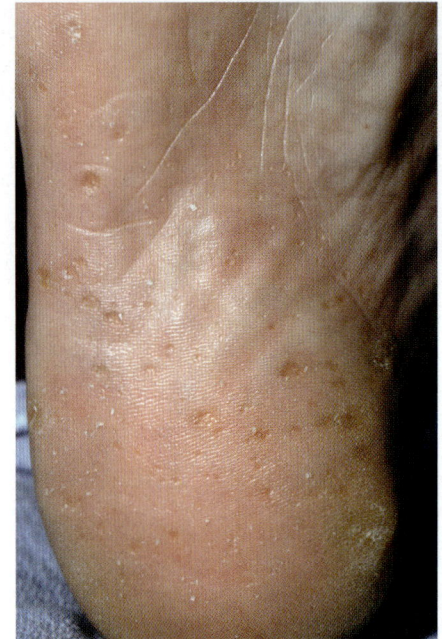

Fig. 11.40 Punctate keratoderma.

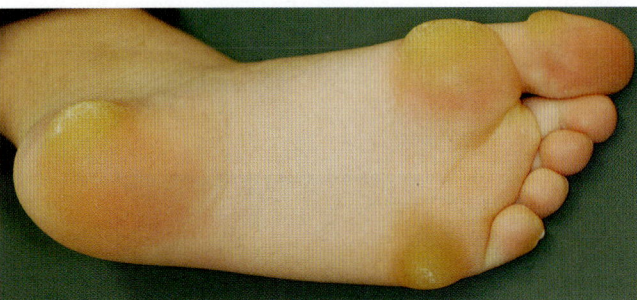

Fig. 11.41 Focal palmoplantar keratoderma.

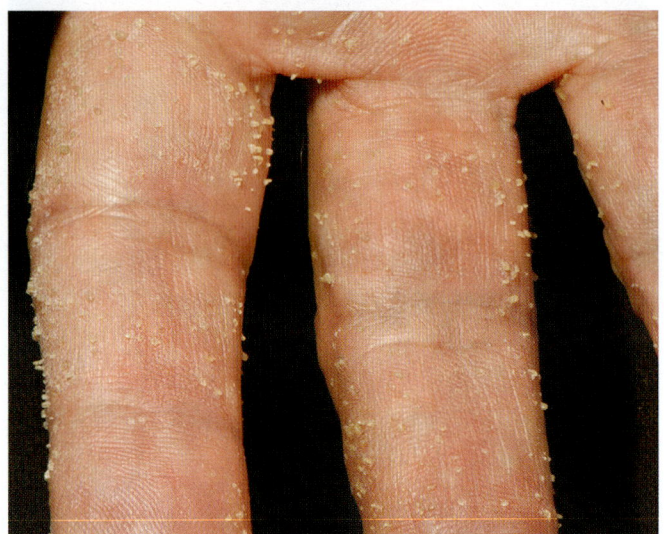

Fig. 11.43 Punctate palmoplantar keratoderma. *Courtesy Curt Samlaska, MD.*

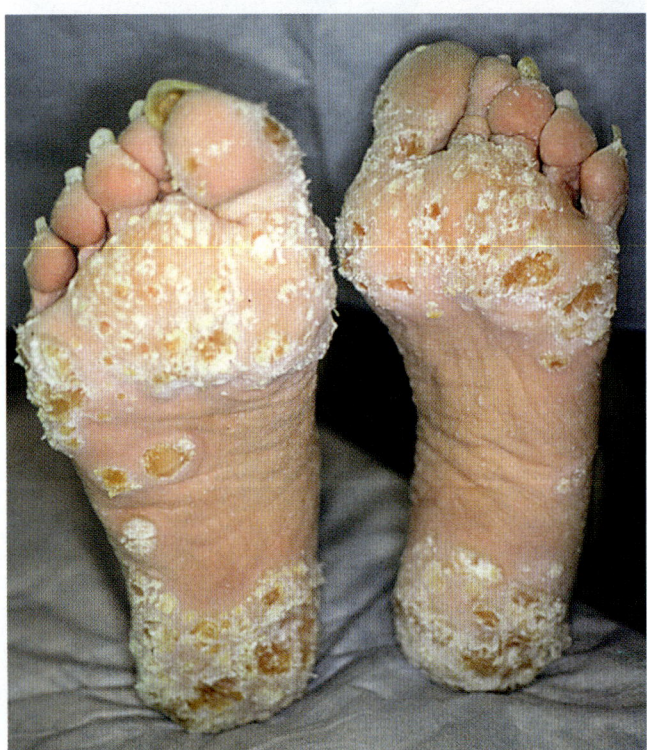

Fig. 11.42 Punctate keratoderma.

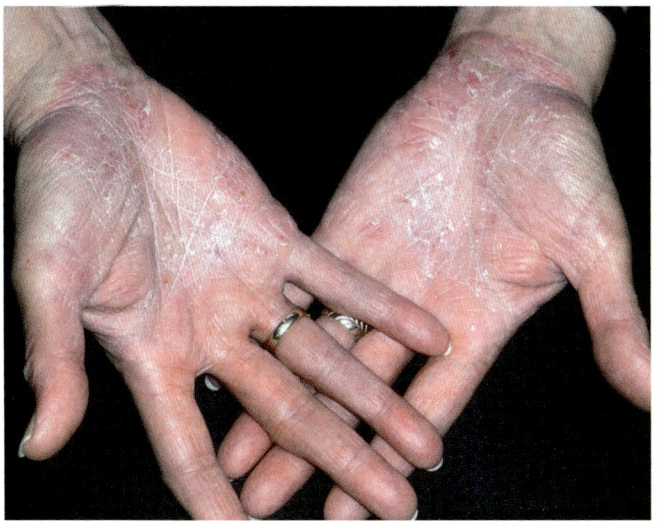

Fig. 11.44 Keratoderma climactericum.

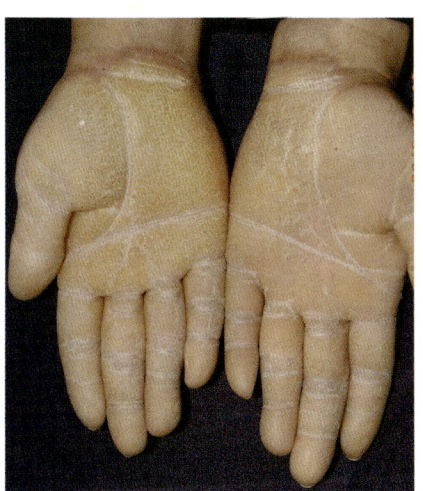

Fig. 11.46 Diffuse hyperkeratosis of the palms, Unna-Thost. *Courtesy National Cheng Kung University, Taiwan.*

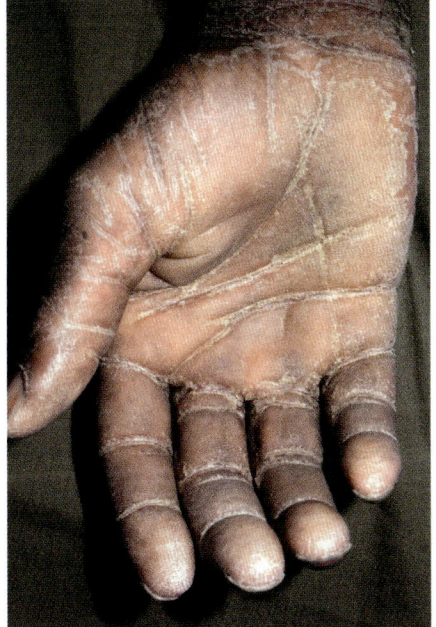

Fig. 11.48 Tylosis with lung cancer.

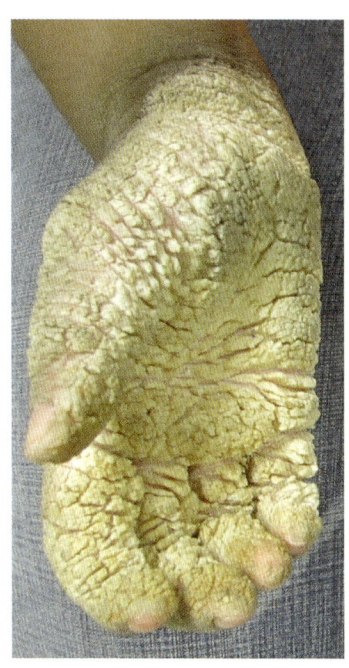

Fig. 11.45 Ichthyosis hystrix of Curth-Macklin with keratin 1 mutation.

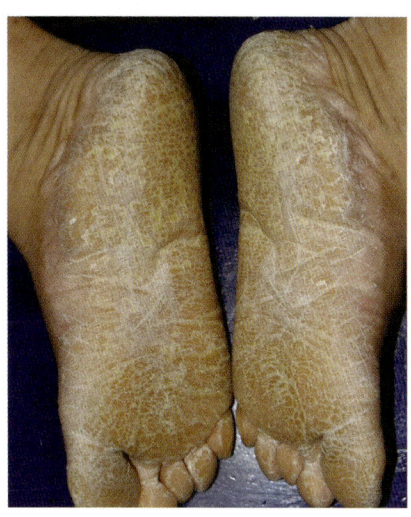

Fig. 11.47 Diffuse hyperkeratosis of the soles, Unna-Thost. *Courtesy National Cheng Kung, University, Taiwan.*

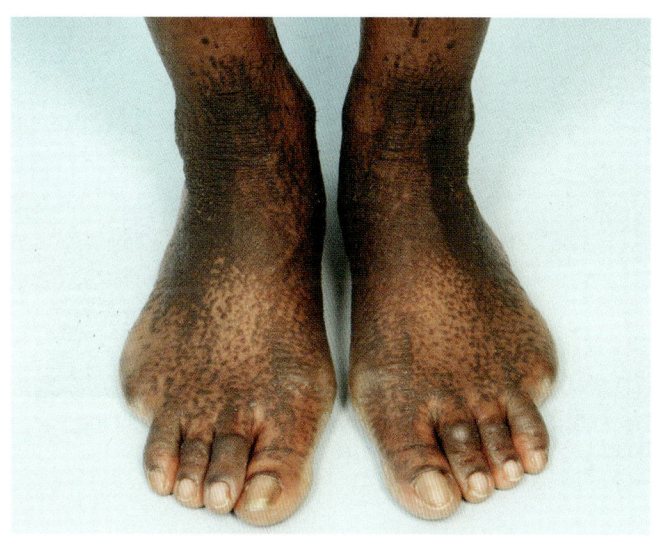

Fig. 11.49 Mutilating keratoderma of Vohwinkel.

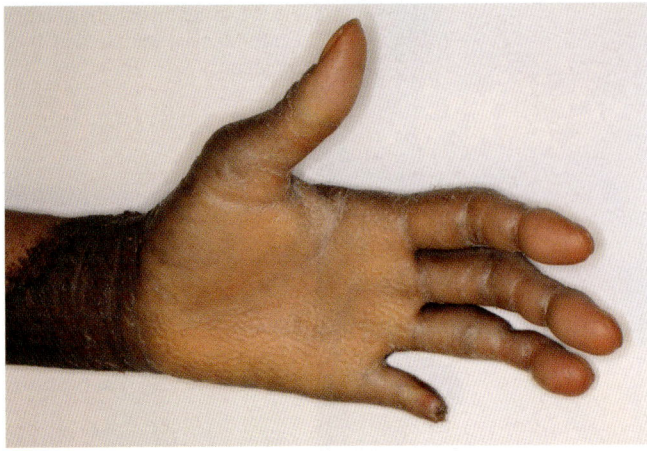

Fig. 11:50 Mutilating keratoderma of Vohwinkel.

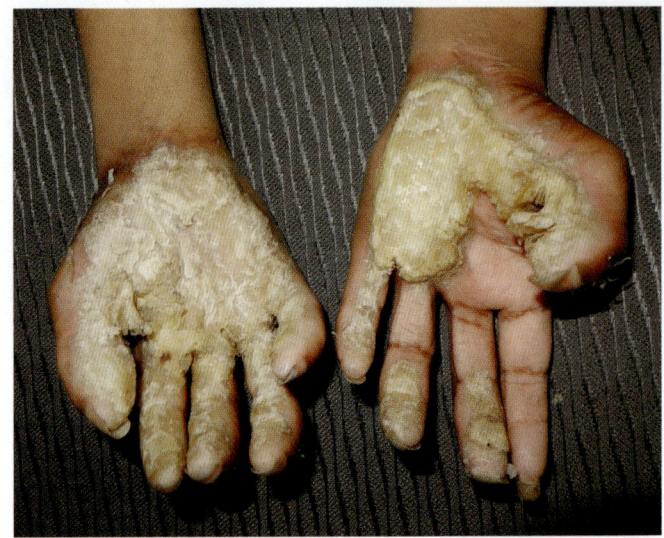

Fig. 11.51 Olmsted syndrome. *Courtesy Debabrata Bandyopadhyay.*

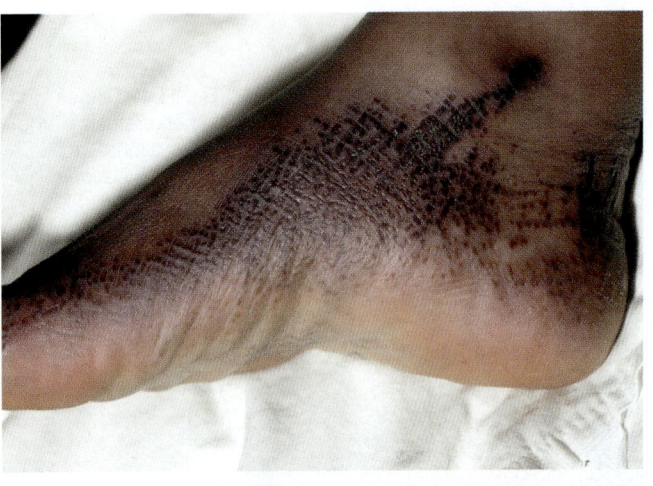

Fig. 11.52 Acrokeratoelastoidosis.

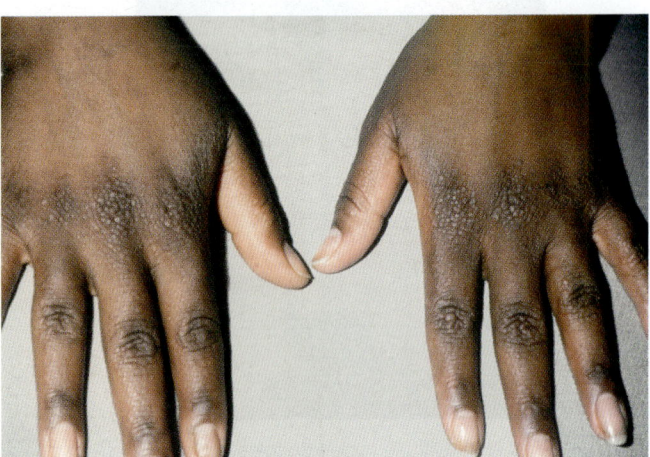

Fig. 11.53 Acrokeratoelastoidosis.

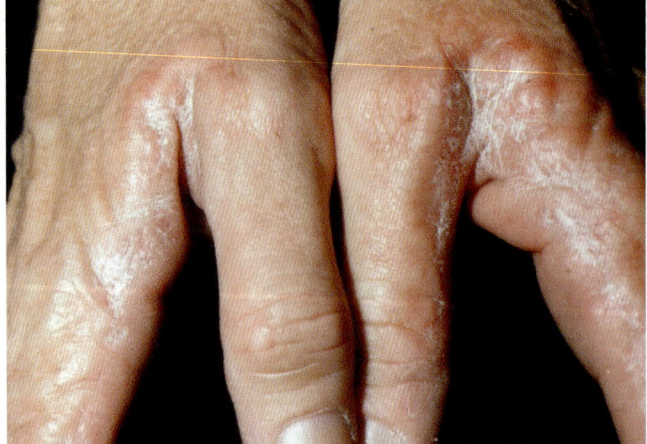

Fig. 11.54 Collagenous and elastotic marginal plaques of the hands.

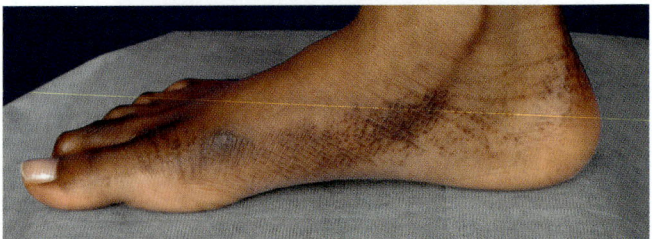

Fig. 11.55 Focal acral hyperkeratosis.

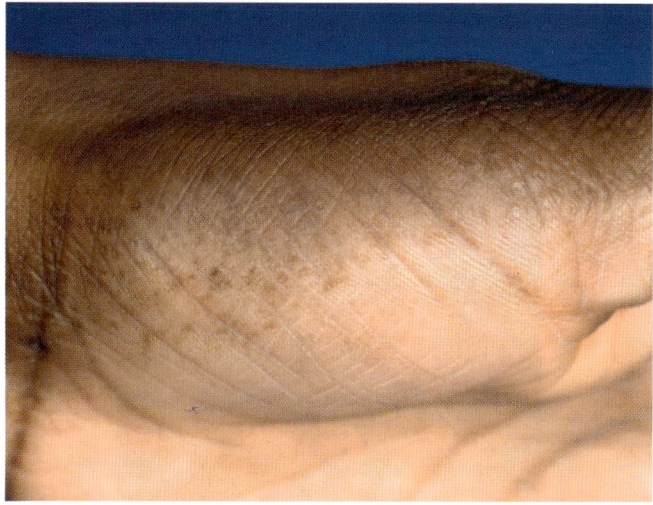

Fig. 11.56 Focal acral hyperkeratosis.

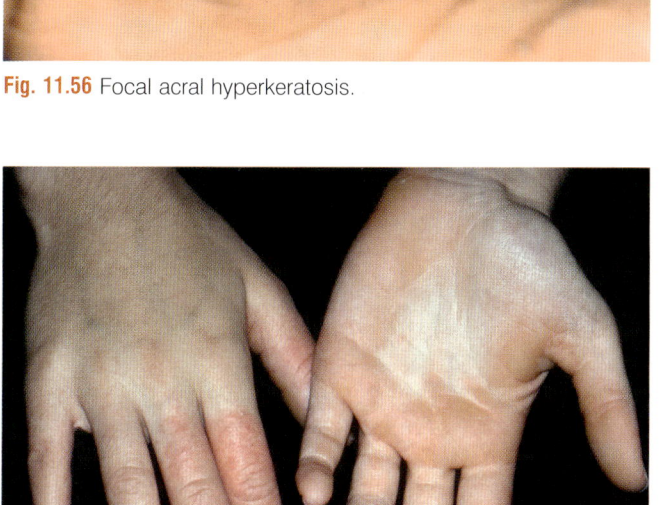

Fig. 11.58 Mal de Meleda. *Courtesy Curt Samlaska, MD.*

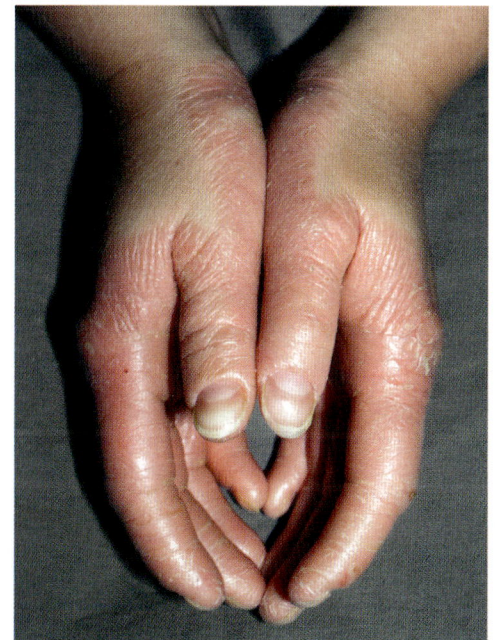

Fig. 11.60 Papillon-Lefevre syndrome. *Courtesy Ken Greer, MD.*

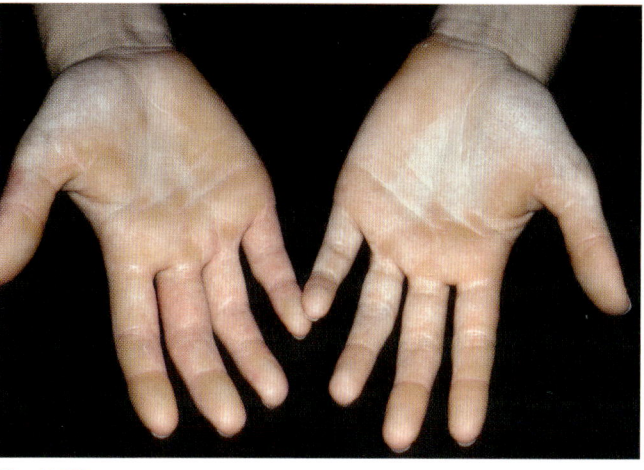

Fig. 11.57 Mal de Meleda. *Courtesy Curt Samlaska, MD.*

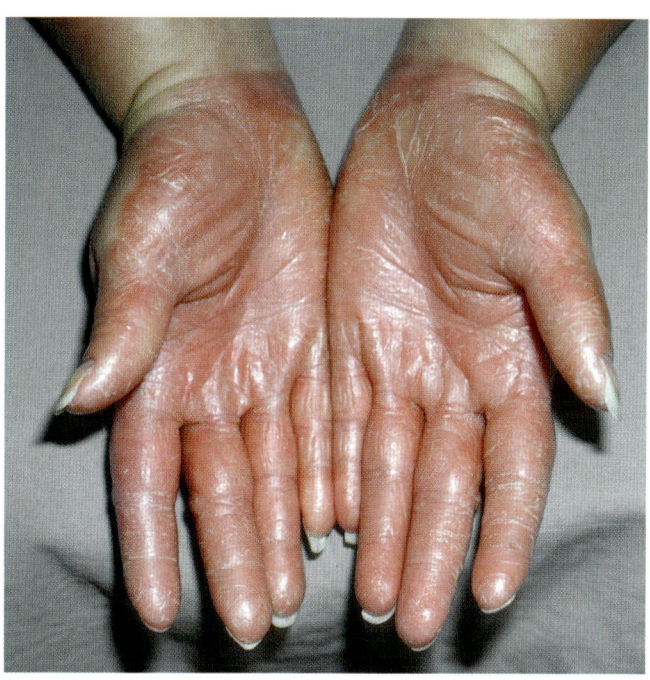

Fig. 11.59 Papillon-Lefevre syndrome. *Courtesy Ken Greer, MD.*

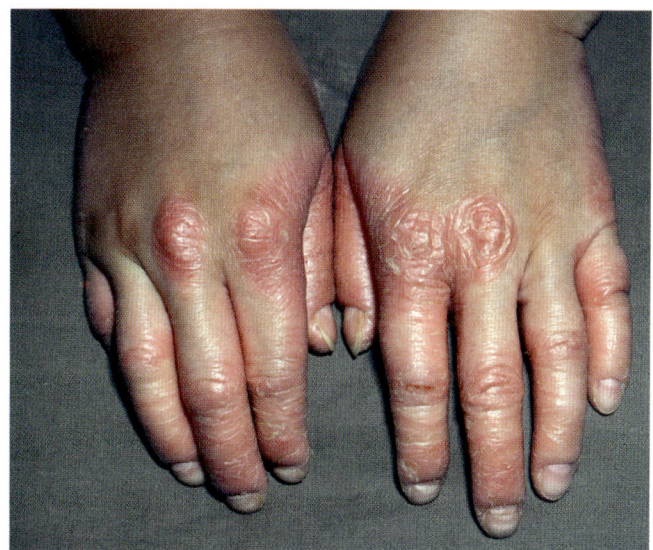

Fig. 11.61 Papillon-Lefevre syndrome. *Courtesy Ken Greer, MD.*

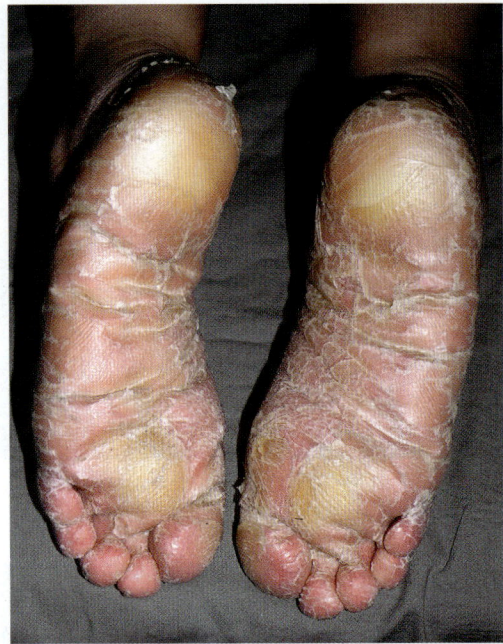

Fig. 11.62 Papillon-Lefevre syndrome. *Courtesy Ken Greer, MD.*

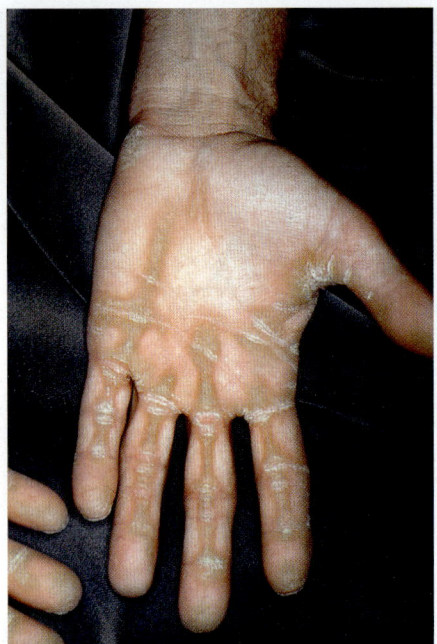

Fig. 11.63 Striate keratoderma.

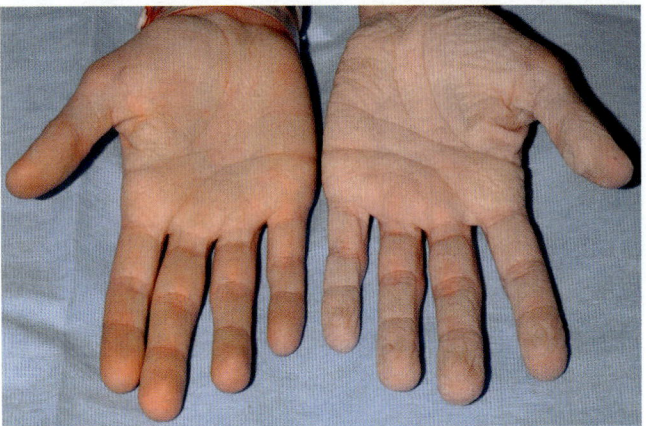

Fig. 11.64 Aquagenic wrinkling after immersing patient's left hand in water. First published in Katz KA, Yan AC, Turner ML: Aquagenic wrinkling of the palms in patients with cystic fibrosis homozygous for the delta F508 CFTR mutation. *Arch Dermatol* 2005;141: 621-624.

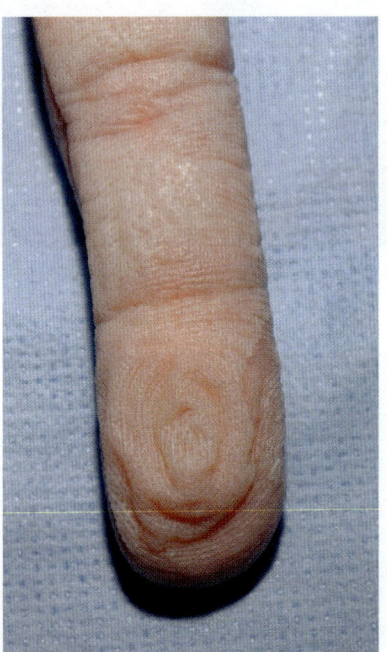

Fig. 11.65 Aquagenic wrinkling after immersing the patient's left hand in water. First published in Katz KA, Yan AC, Turner ML: Aquagenic wrinkling of the palms in patients with cystic fibrosis homozygous for the delta F508 CFTR mutation. *Arch Dermatol* 2005;141: 621–624.

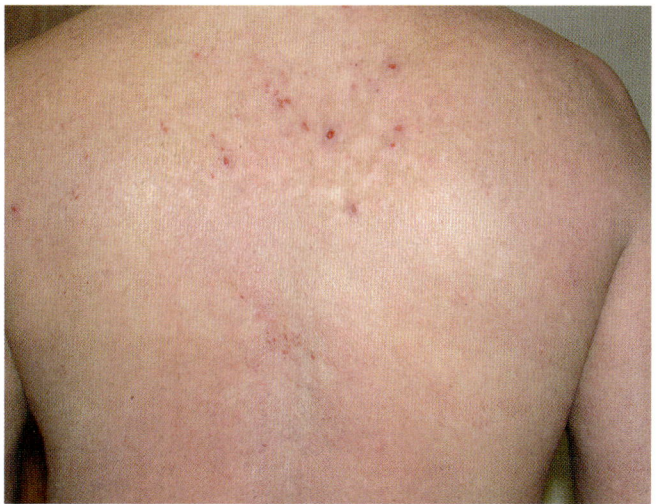

Fig. 11.66 Erythroderma from atopic dermatitis.

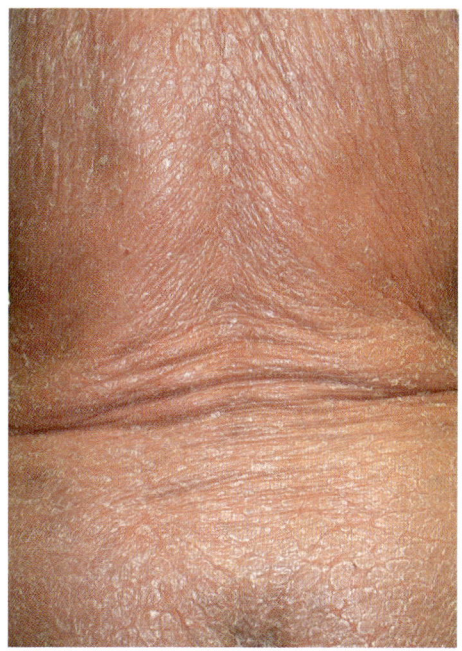

Fig. 11.67 Psoriatic erythroderma.

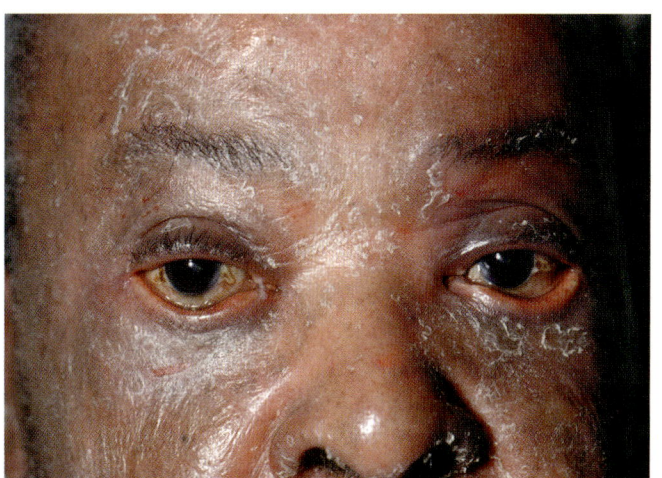

Fig. 11.68 Psoriatic erythroderma.

Lichen Planus and Related Conditions 12

Lichen planus (LP) and other lichenoid eruptions tend to create characteristic primary lesions and patterns. The pruritic, purple, polygonal, flat-topped papules of LP can appear unmistakably shiny as they reflect light back at the keen diagnostician. These papules can be widespread and coalesce into plaques and streaks that demonstrate the Koebner phenomenon as another clue to the diagnosis. A thorough physical examination can reveal white lacy leukoplakia of the oral mucosa, annular lesions of the genitalia, or a variety of nail changes from ridging to pterygium formation. Lichen planus pigmentosus/actinicus is an often photodistributed LP variant that demonstrates more distinctive hyperpigmentation.

Lichen nitidus and lichen striatus are lichenoid conditions that are more common in children. With its almost pinpoint, shiny, flat-topped papules, lichen nitidus can appear slightly hypopigmented against darker skin. As in LP, papules can demonstrate the Koebner phenomenon and be either localized or widespread. Lichen striatus presents with a characteristically curvilinear plaque most commonly on the extremities of a child; however, lesions can be seen on the trunk and, rarely, the face. The eruption follows the lines of Blaschko and can involve the nail with longitudinal dystrophy. In the later phase, a hypopigmented or hyperpigmented patch will remain on the skin temporarily as a sign of the recently resolved plaque of lichen striatus.

Lichen sclerosus most commonly involves the genitalia, with a higher incidence in females. Genital lichen sclerosus classically presents with atrophic white patches that can appear wrinkled and erosive, and can obliterate and scar normal anatomic landmarks. In some patients, the presence of bruising can be misdiagnosed as trauma from sexual abuse, highlighting the importance of a careful physical examination with consideration of skin biopsy in unclear cases. Extragenital lichen sclerosus can present with atrophic white papules and macules, often on the trunk.

Skin biopsy can be diagnostic in many lichenoid conditions, demonstrating the typical bandlike inflammation at the dermal-epidermal junction, along with more specific differentiating features depending on the specific eruption. This portion of the atlas features many images to help clinically distinguish lichen planus and its many related conditions.

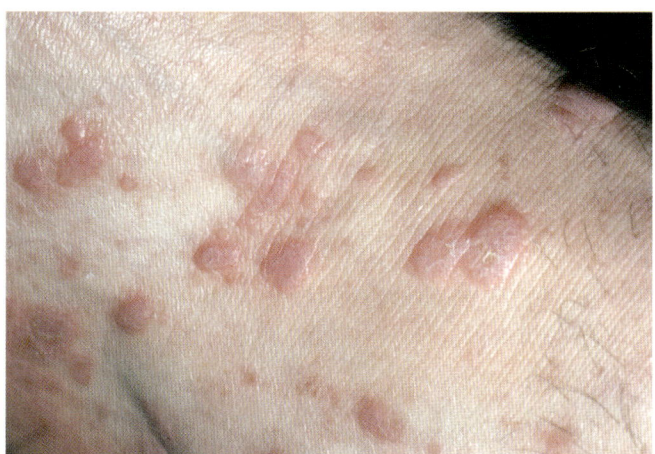

Fig. 12.1 Lichen planus. *Courtesy Steven Binnick, MD.*

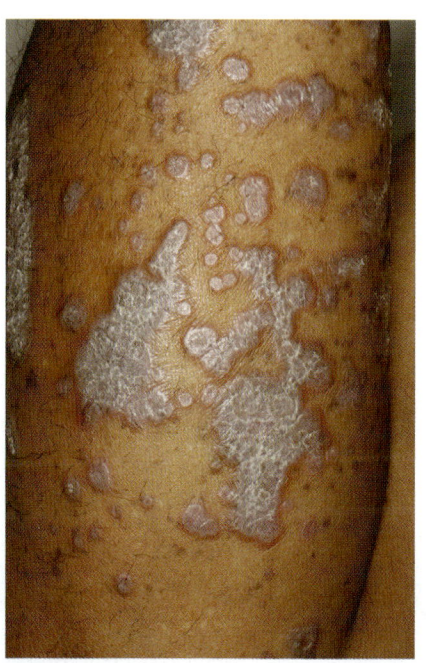

Fig. 12.2 Lichen planus.

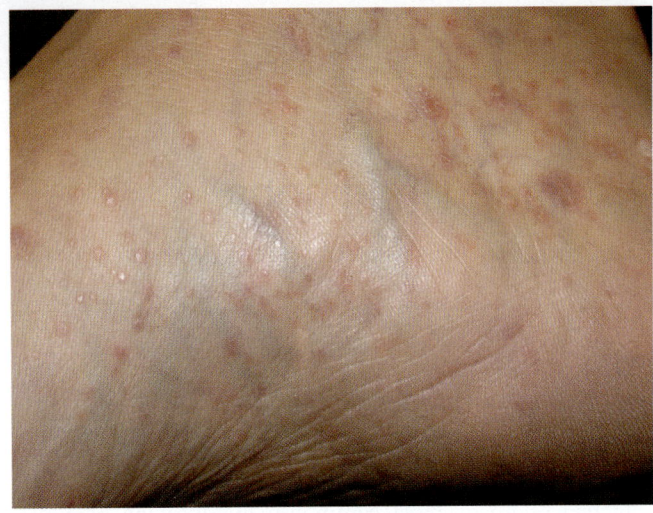

Fig. 12.3 Lichen planus.

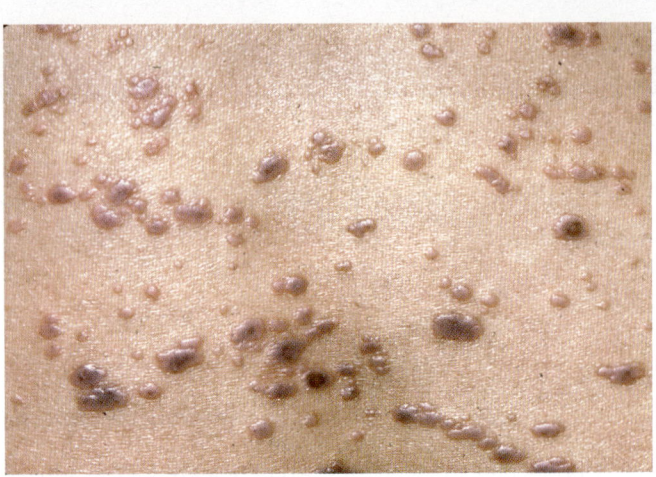

Fig. 12.4 Lichen planus.

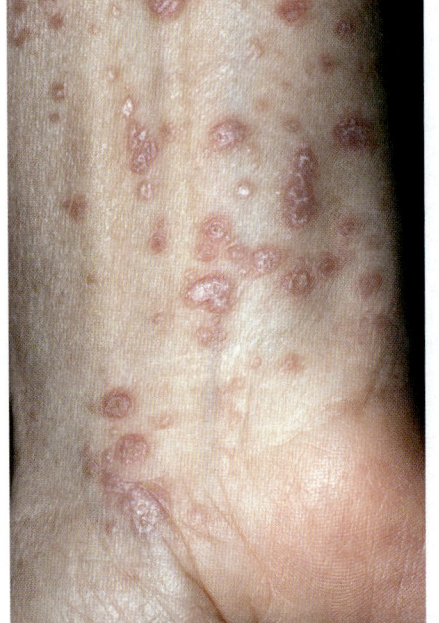

Fig. 12.5 Lichen planus. *Courtesy Steven Binnick, MD.*

Fig. 12.6 Lichen planus.

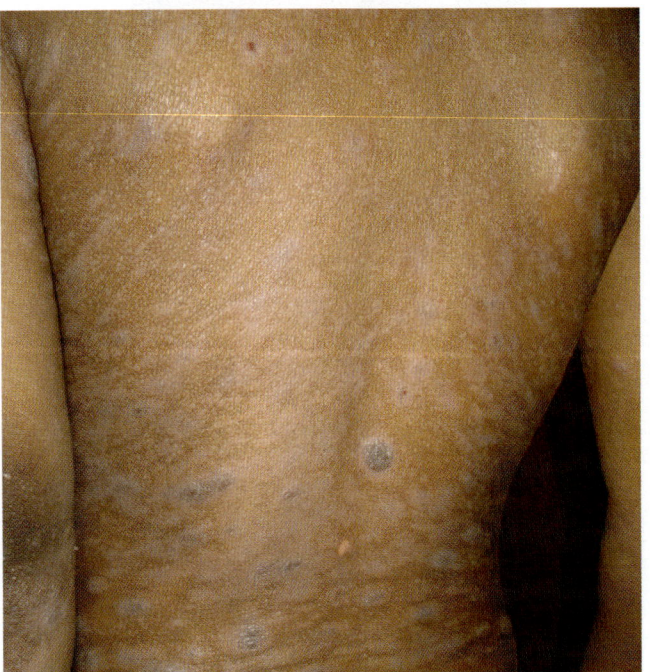

Fig. 12.8 Lichen planus.

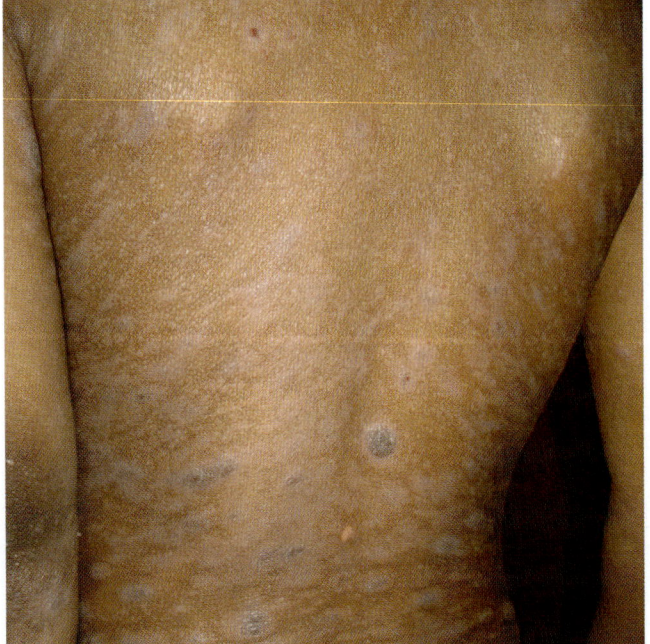

Fig. 12.7 Lichen planus.

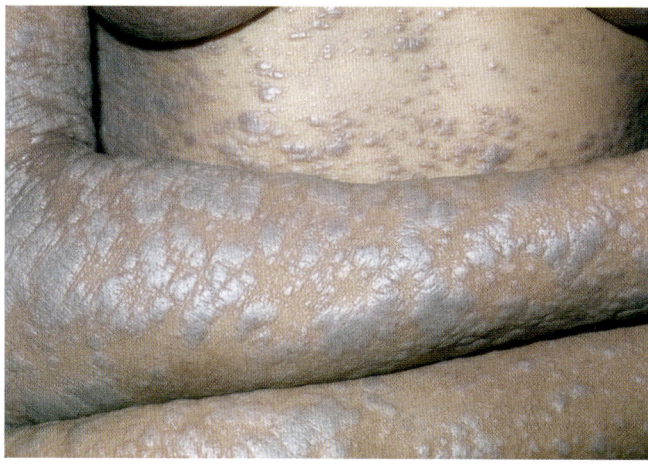

Fig. 12.9 Lichen planus. *Courtesy Steven Binnick, MD.*

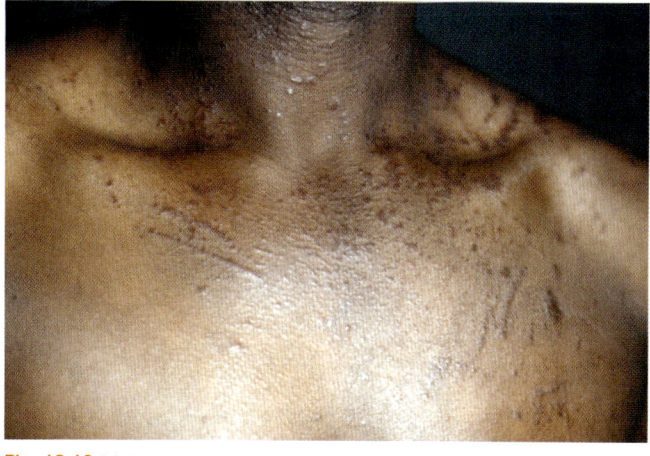

Fig. 12.10 Lichen planus. Note Koebner phenomenon.

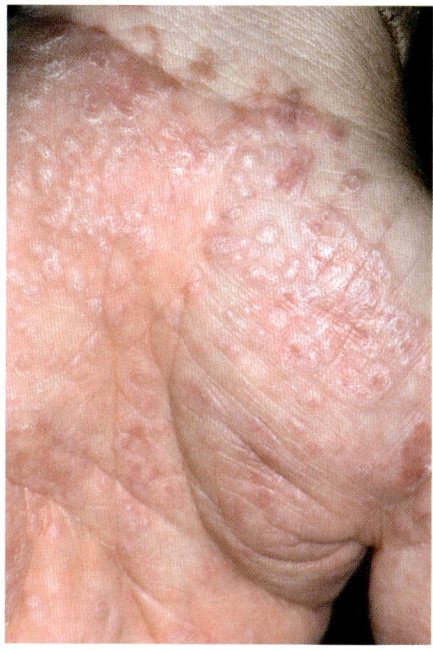

Fig. 12.11 Lichen planus. *Courtesy Steven Binnick, MD.*

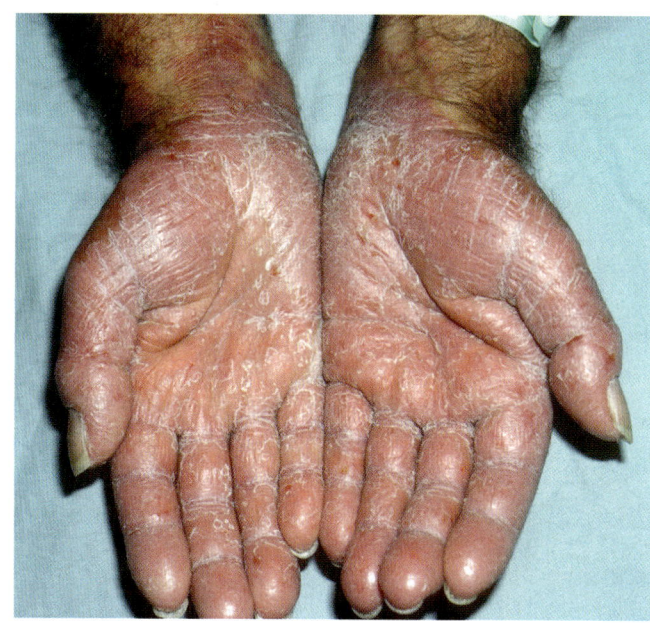

Fig. 12.12 Lichen planus. *Courtesy Ken Greer, MD.*

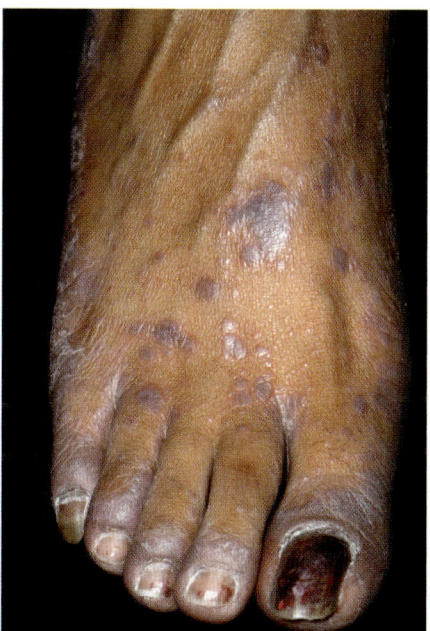

Fig. 12.13 Lichen planus.

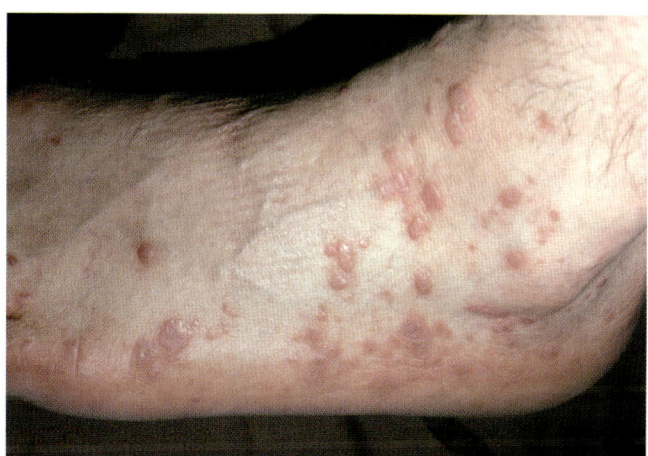

Fig. 12.14 Lichen planus.

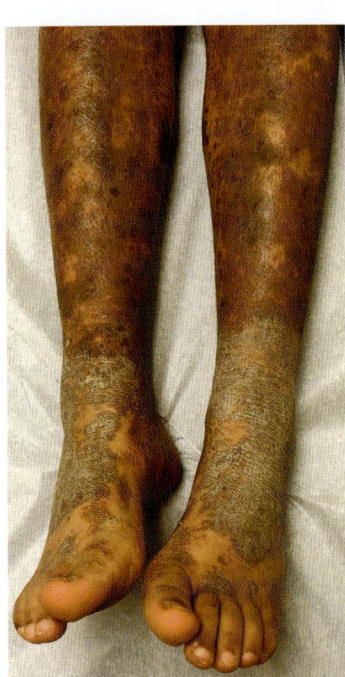

Fig. 12.15 Lichen planus with hyperpigmentation.

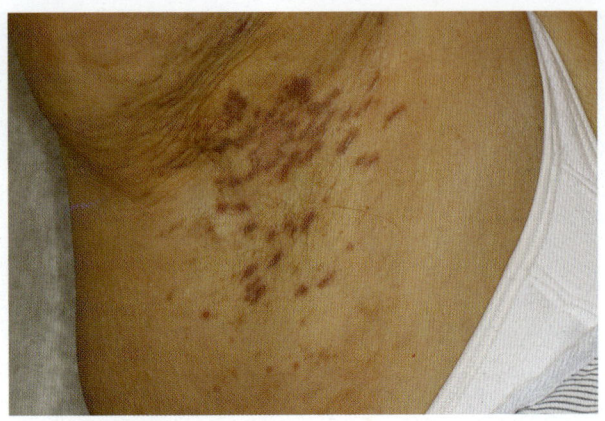

Fig. 12.16 Inverse lichen planus.

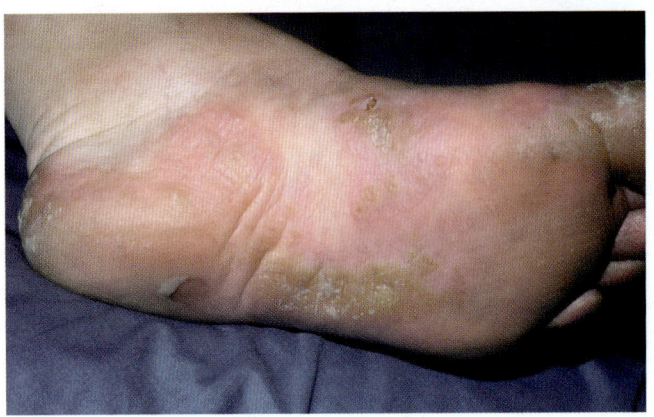

Fig. 12.17 Lichen planus. *Courtesy Steven Binnick, MD.*

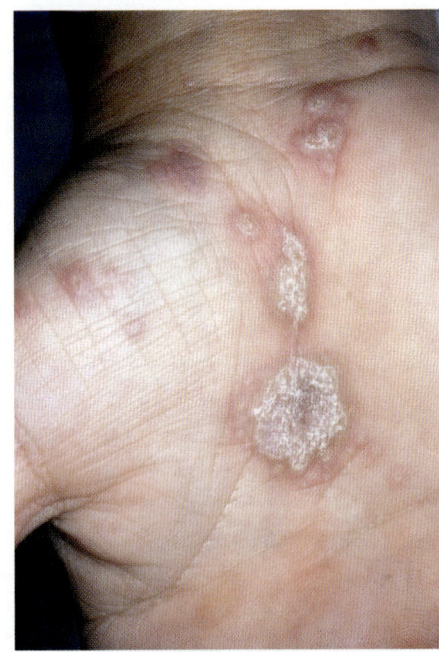

Fig. 12.18 Lichen planus.

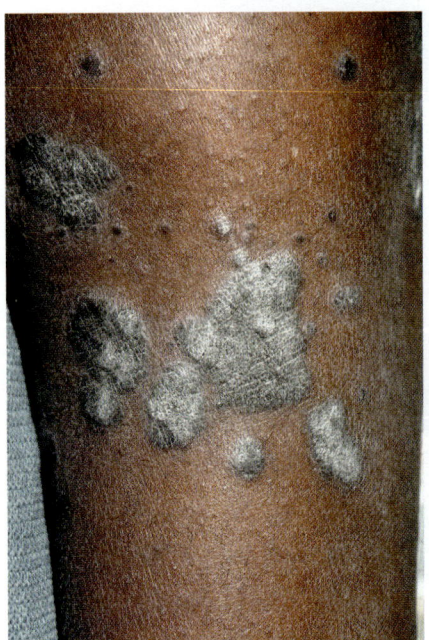

Fig. 12.19 Hypertrophic lichen planus.

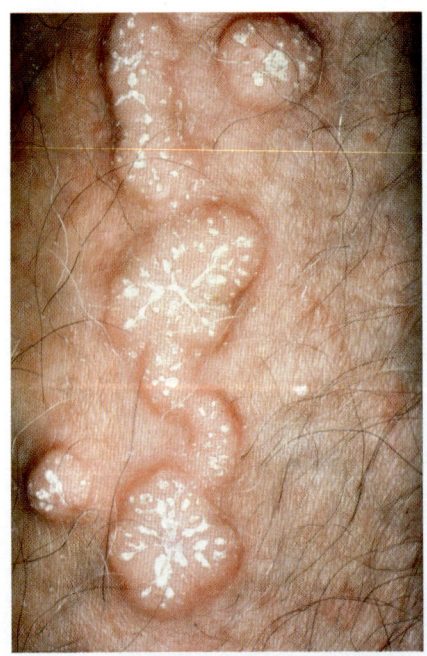

Fig. 12.20 Hypertrophic lichen planus.

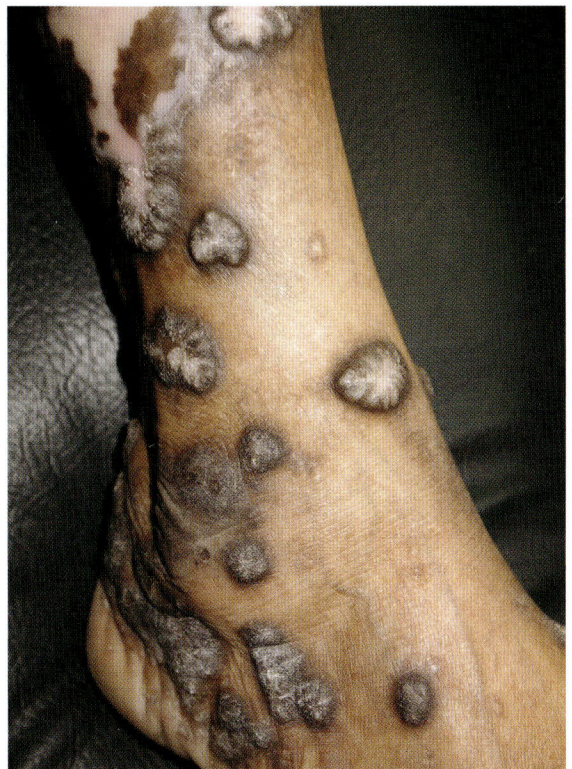

Fig. 12.21 Hypertrophic lichen planus. *Courtesy Debabrata Bandyopadhyay, MD.*

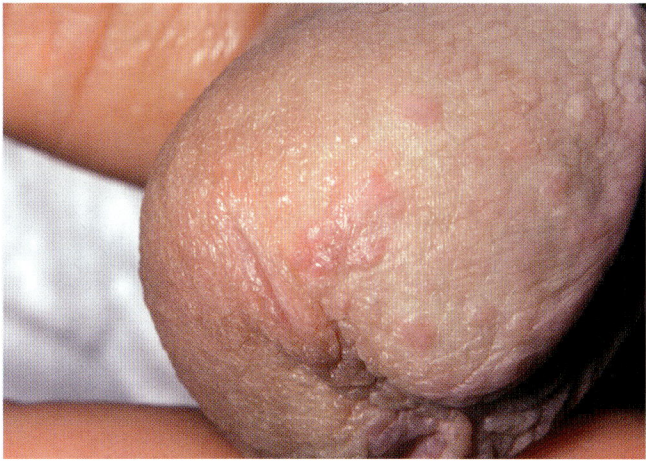

Fig. 12.22 Lichen planus, glans penis.

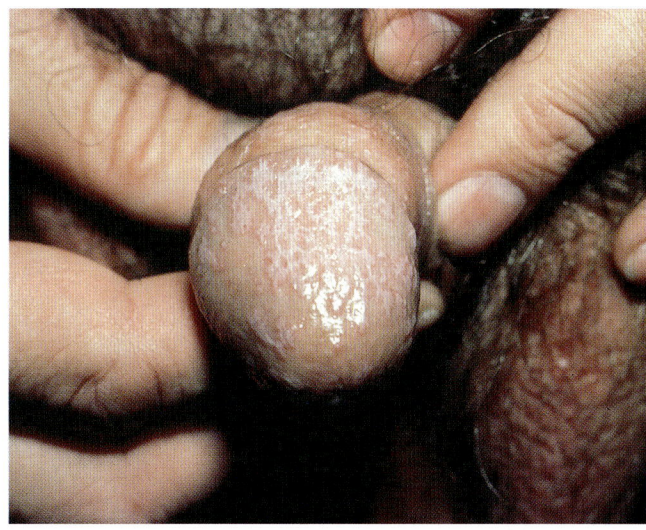

Fig. 12.24 Lichen planus.

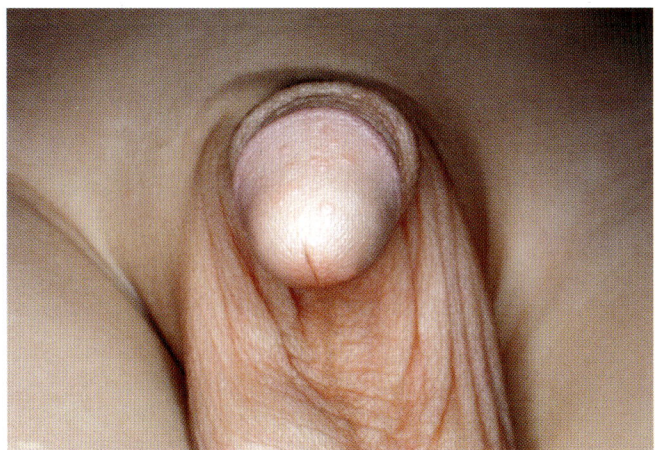

Fig. 12.23 Lichen planus.

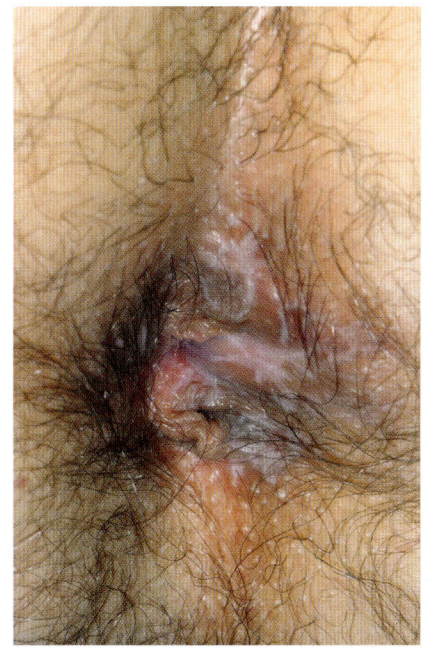

Fig. 12.25 Lichen planus.

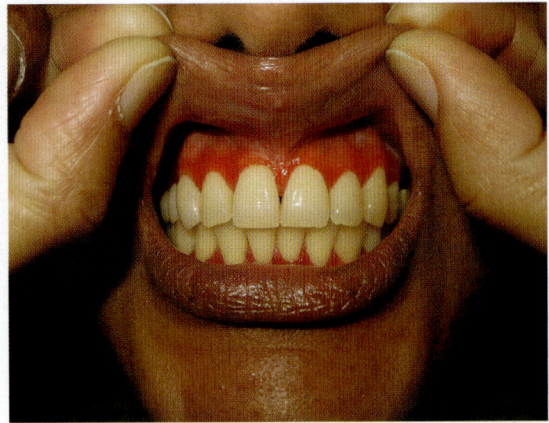

Fig. 12.26 Desquamative gingivitis caused by lichen planus.

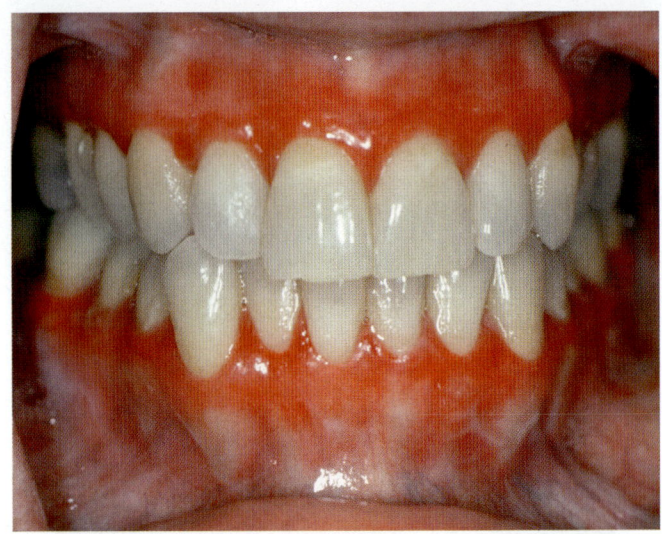

Fig. 12.27 Vulvovaginal-gingival syndrome.

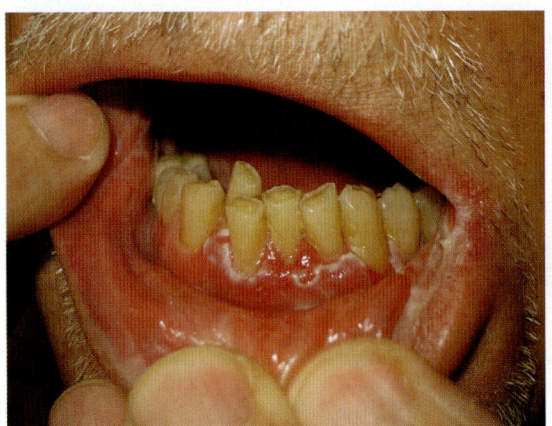

Fig. 12.28 Oral lichen planus.

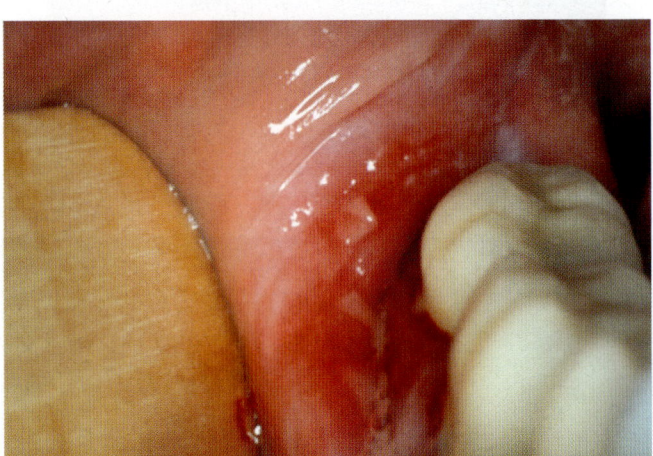

Fig. 12.29 Oral lichen planus.

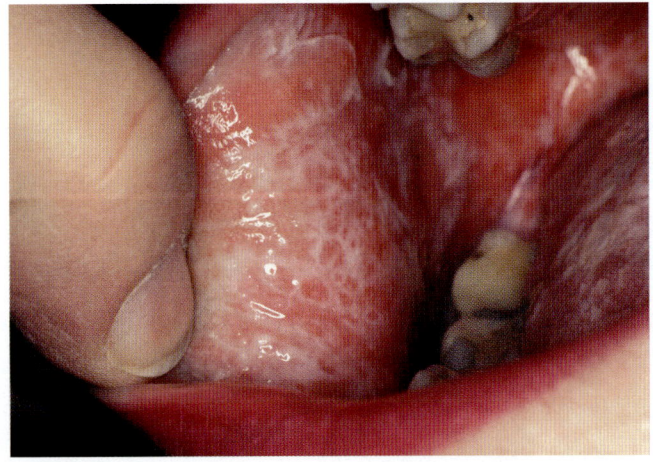

Fig. 12.30 Oral lichen planus.

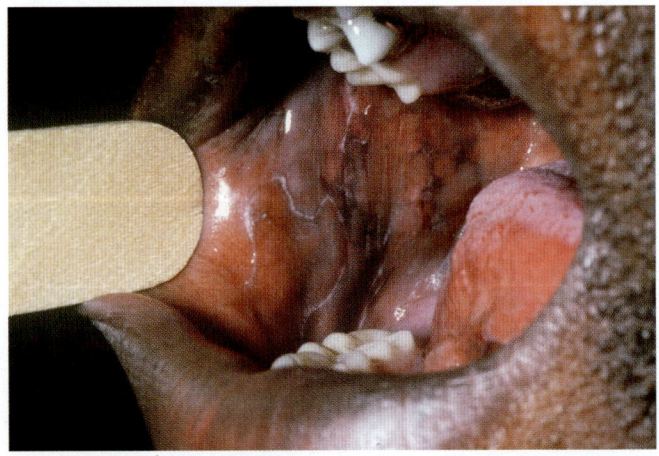

Fig. 12.31 Oral lichen planus.

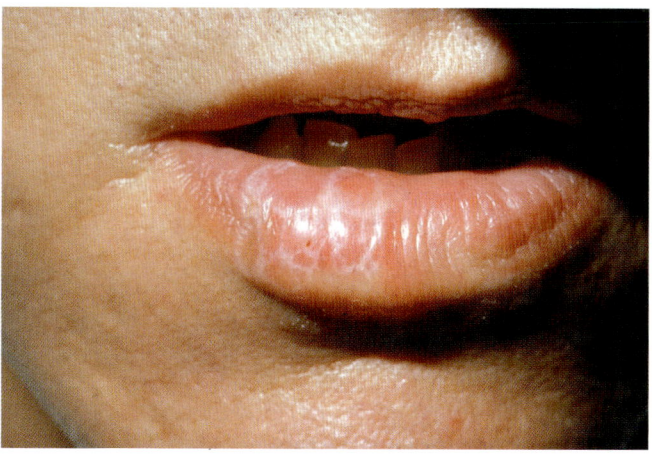

Fig. 12.32 Lip lichen planus. *Courtesy Steven Binnick, MD.*

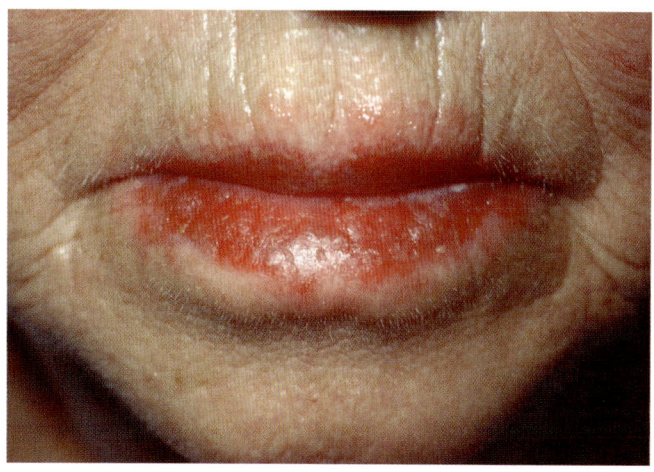

Fig. 12.33 Erosive lichen planus. *Courtesy Steven Binnick, MD.*

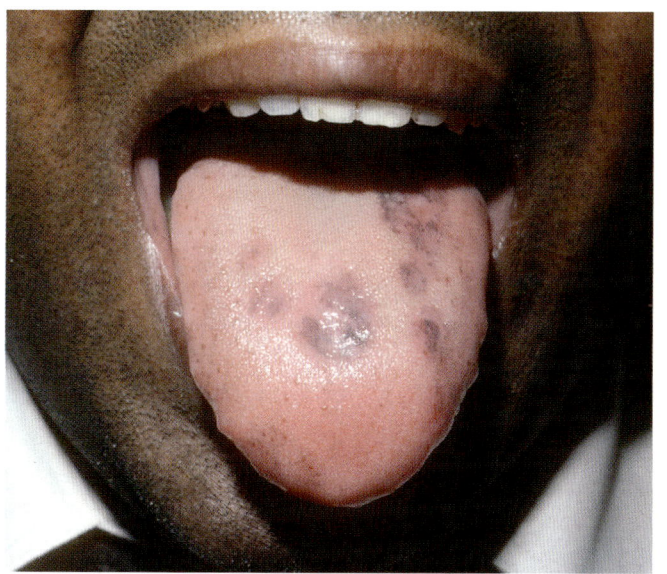

Fig. 12.34 Lichen planus.

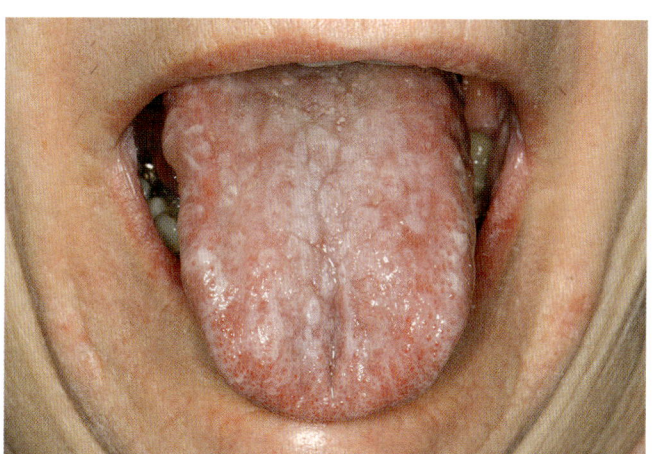

Fig. 12.35 Lichen planus.

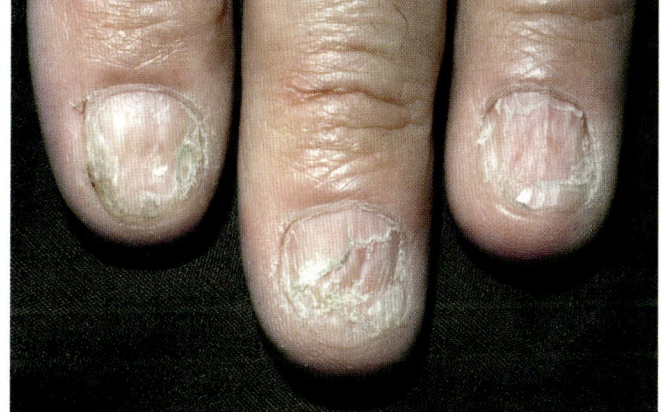

Fig. 12.36 Lichen planus of the nails.

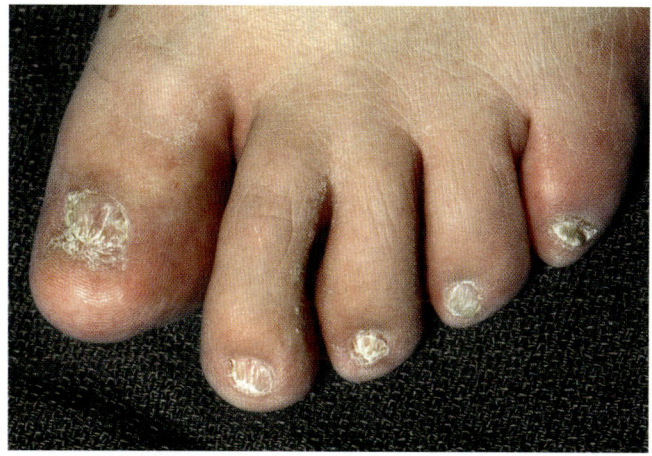

Fig. 12.37 Lichen planus of the nails.

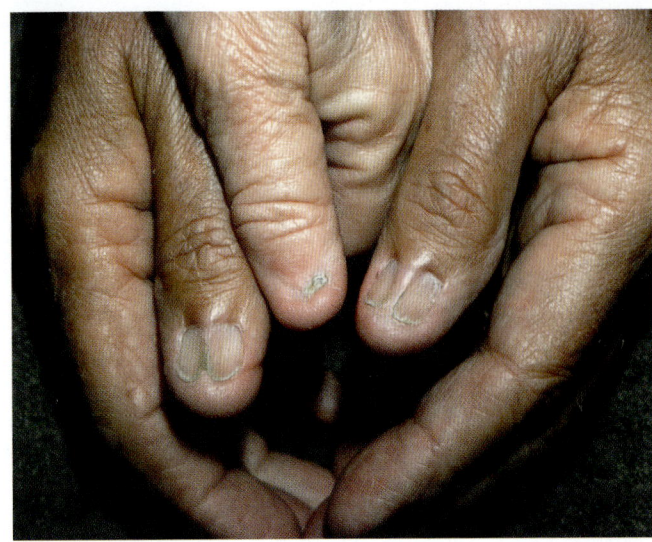

Fig. 12.38 Lichen planus of the nails.

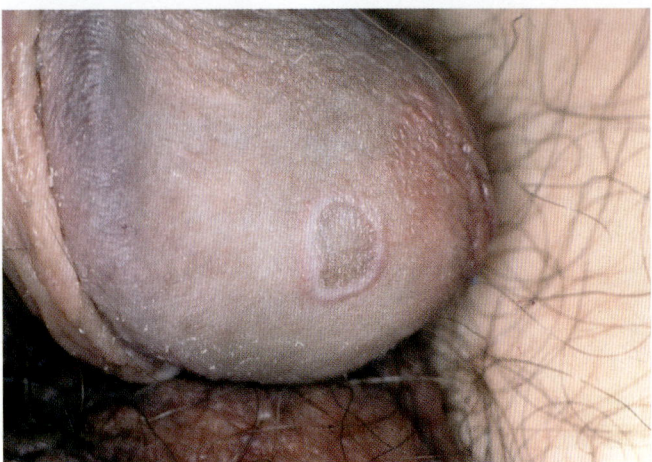

Fig. 12.39 Annular lichen planus. *Courtesy Steven Binnick, MD.*

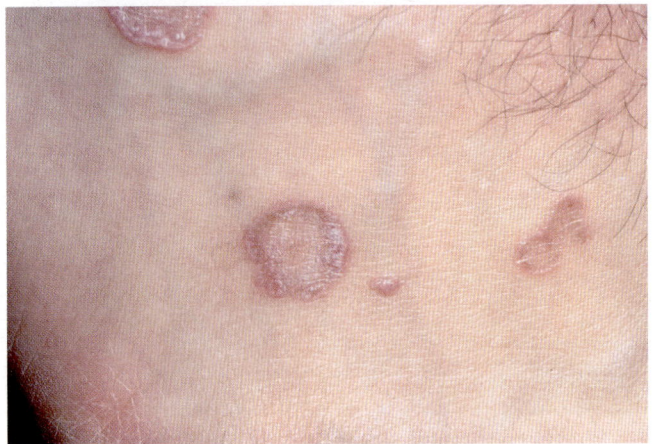

Fig. 12.40 Annular lichen planus.

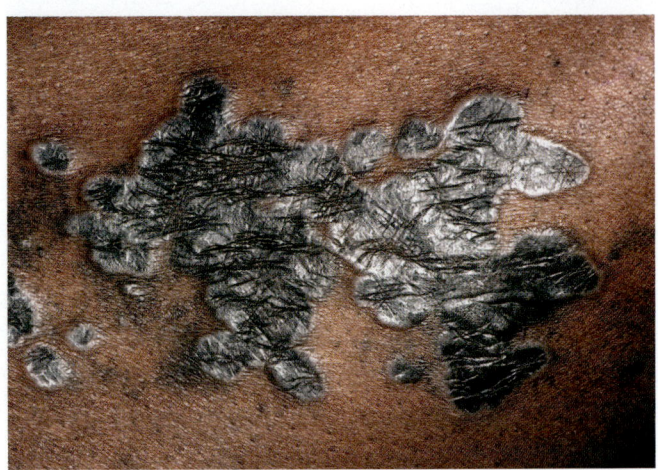

Fig. 12.41 Annular lichen planus.

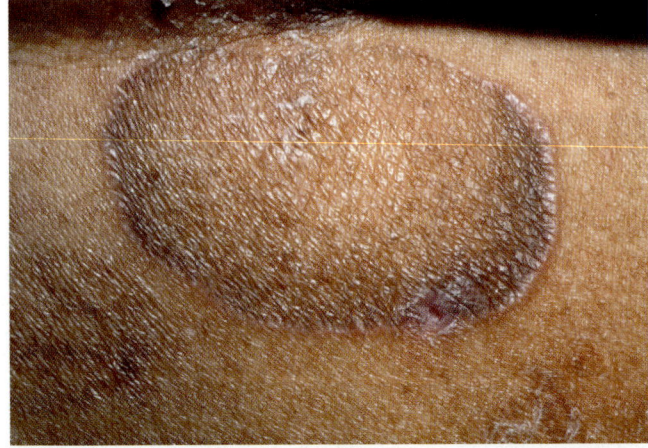

Fig. 12.42 Annular lichen planus.

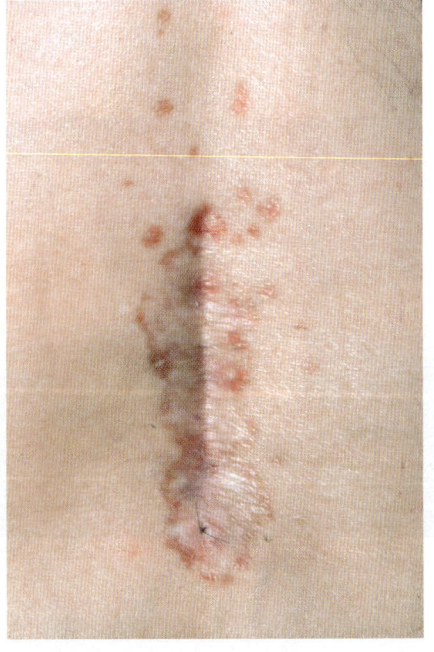

Fig. 12.43 Atrophic lichen planus.

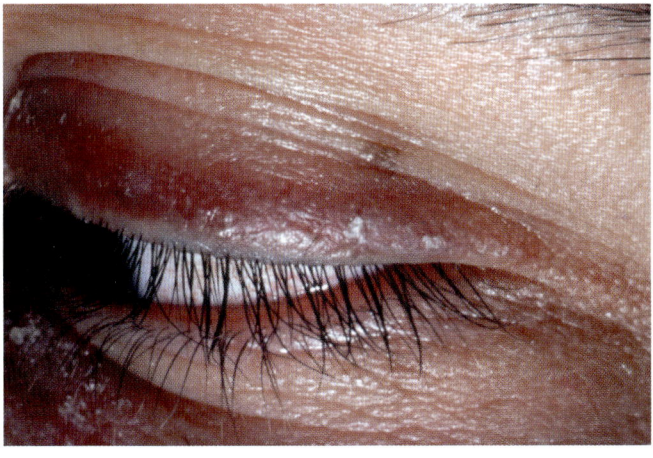

Fig. 12.44 Eyelid lichen planus.

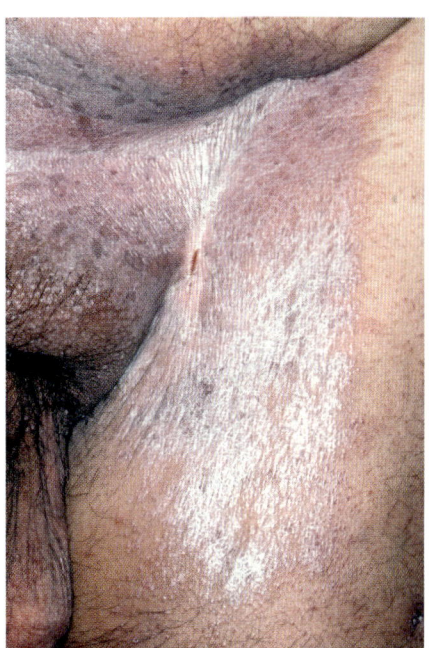

Fig. 12.45 Lichen planus after radiation therapy.

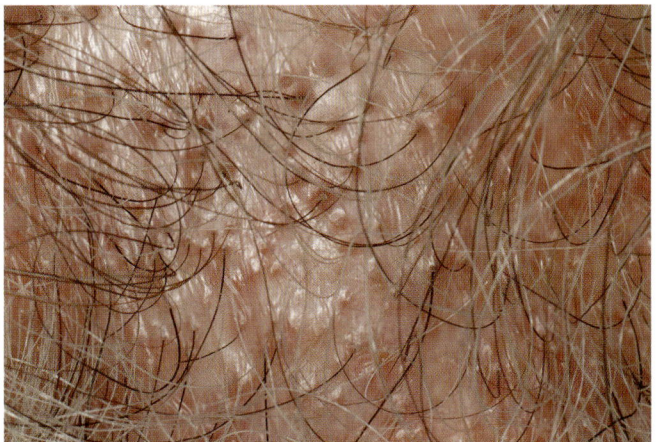

Fig. 12.46 Lichen planopilaris.

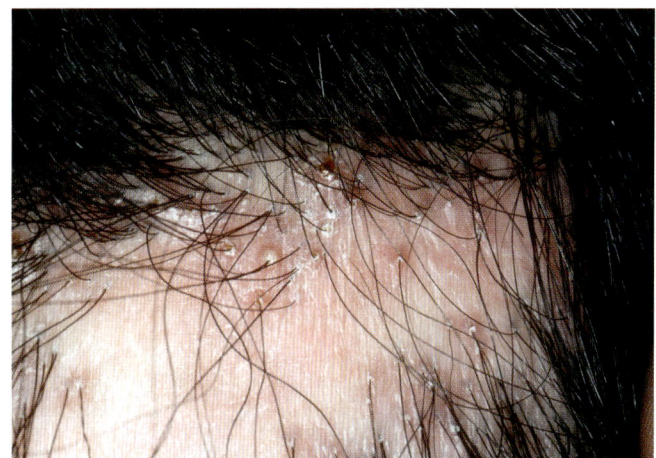

Fig. 12.47 Lichen planopilaris.

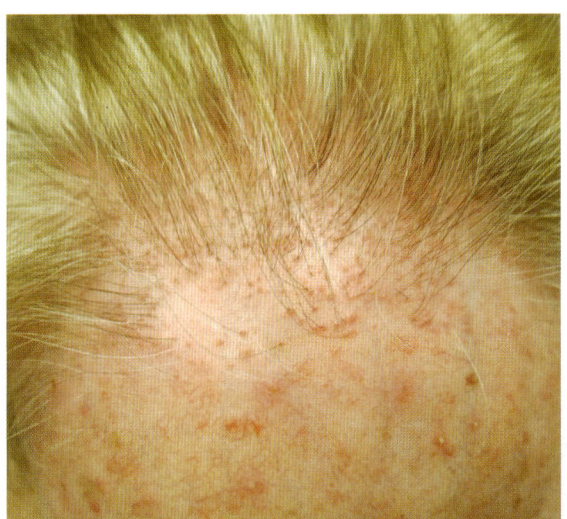

Fig. 12.48 Frontal fibrosing alopecia.

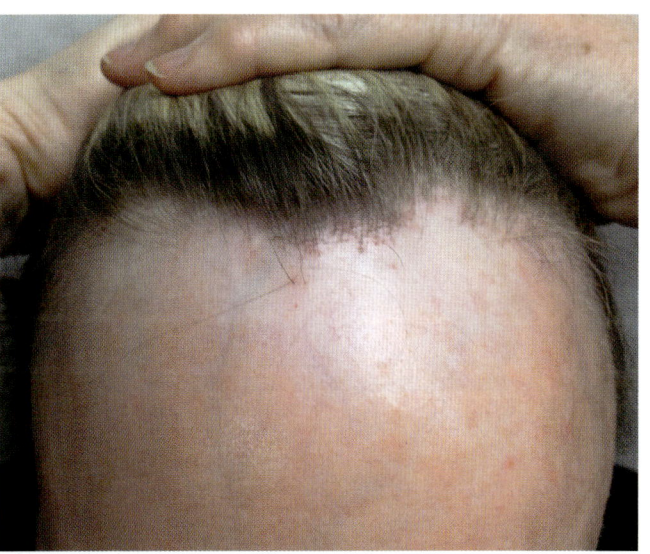

Fig. 12.49 Frontal fibrosing alopecia. *Courtesy Len Sperling, MD.*

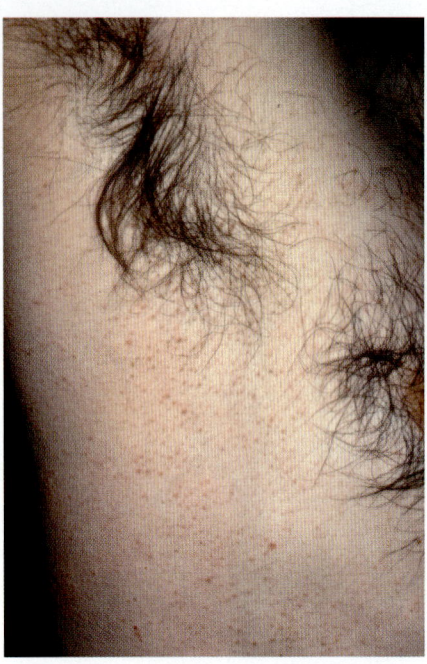

Fig. 12.50 Graham-Little-Piccardi syndrome nonscarring hair loss of the trunk.

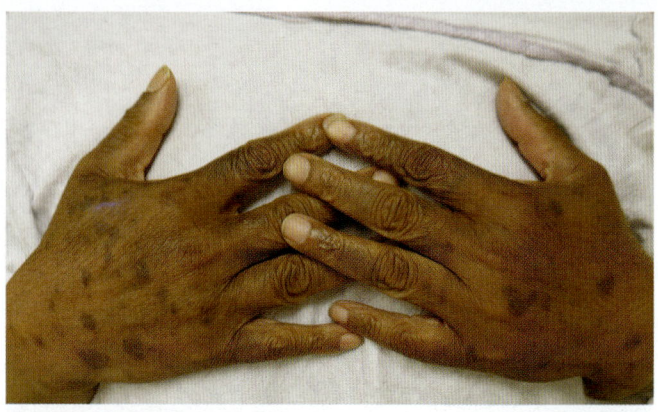

Fig. 12.51 Lichen planus pigmentosus.

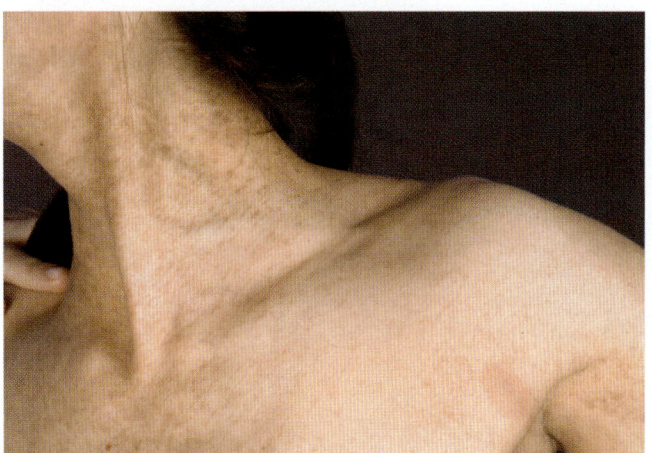

Fig. 12.52 Lichen planus pigmentosa.

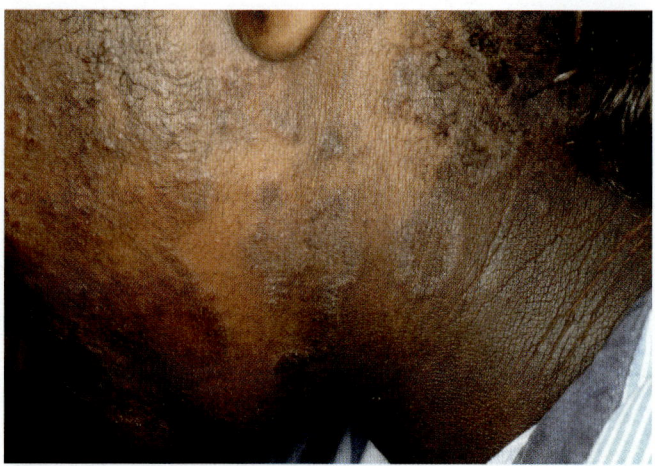

Fig. 12.53 Lichen planus actinicus. *Courtesy Steven Binnick, MD.*

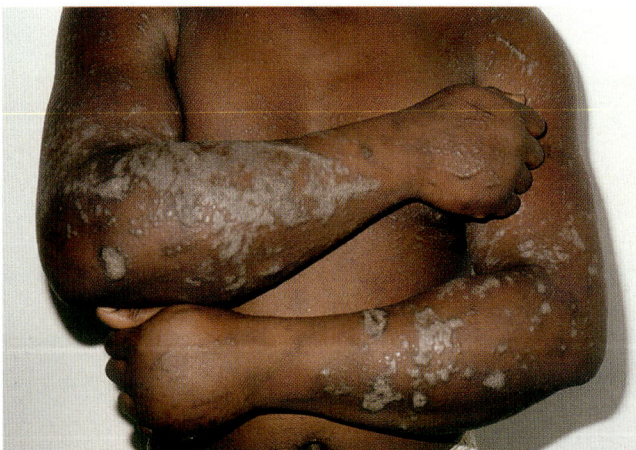

Fig. 12.54 Lichen planus actinicus.

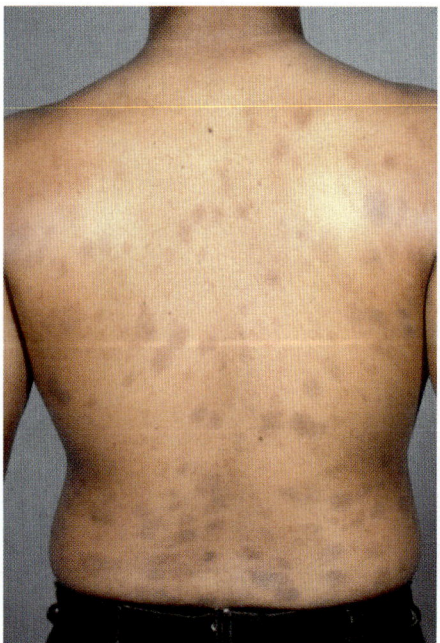

Fig. 12.55 Erythema dyschromicum perstans.

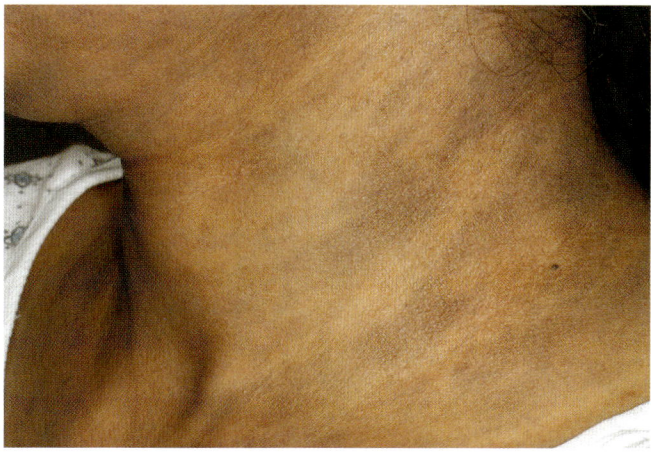

Fig. 12.56 Erythema dyschromicum perstans.

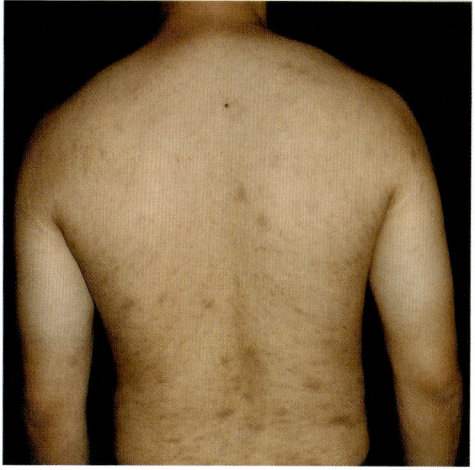

Fig. 12.57 Idiopathic macular hyperpigmentation. *Courtesy National Cheng Kung University, Taiwan.*

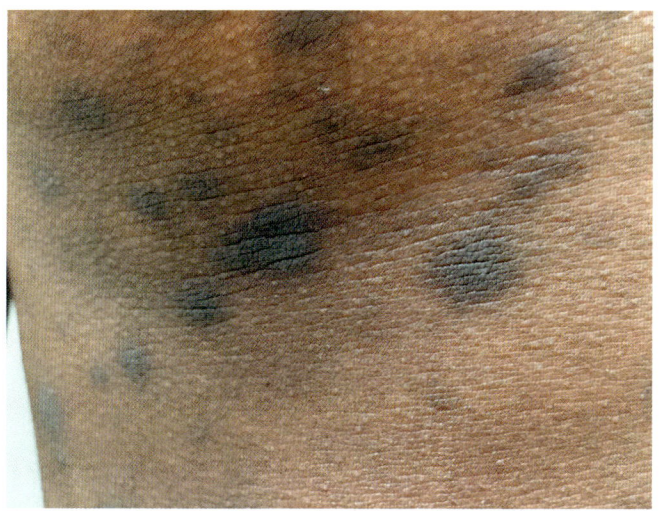

Fig. 12.58 Idiopathic eruptive macular hyperpigmentation with papillomatosis. *Courtesy Dr. Ang Chia Chun.*

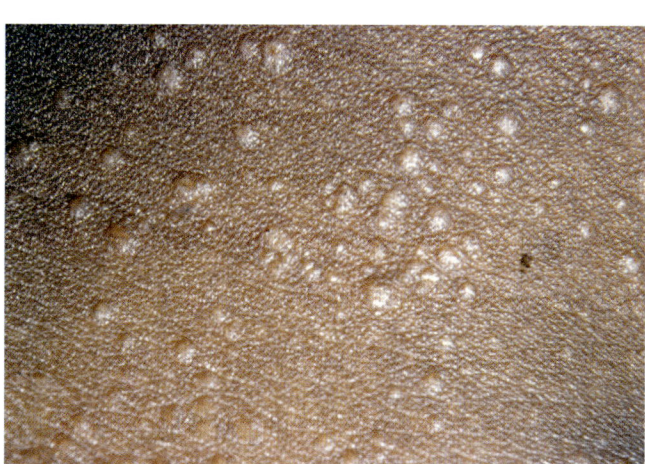

Fig. 12.59 Lichen nitidus.

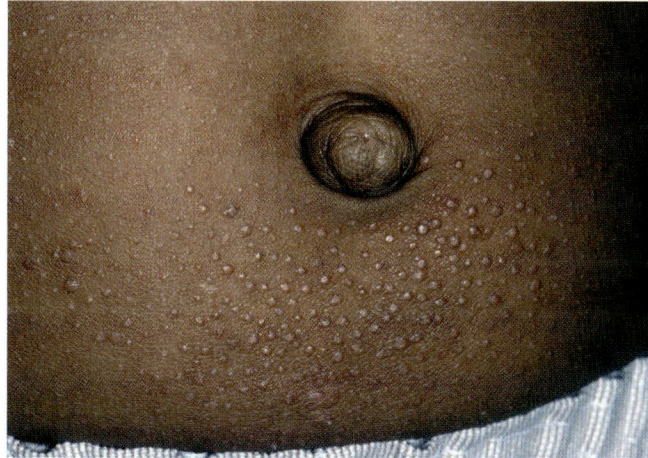

Fig. 12.60 Lichen nitidus.

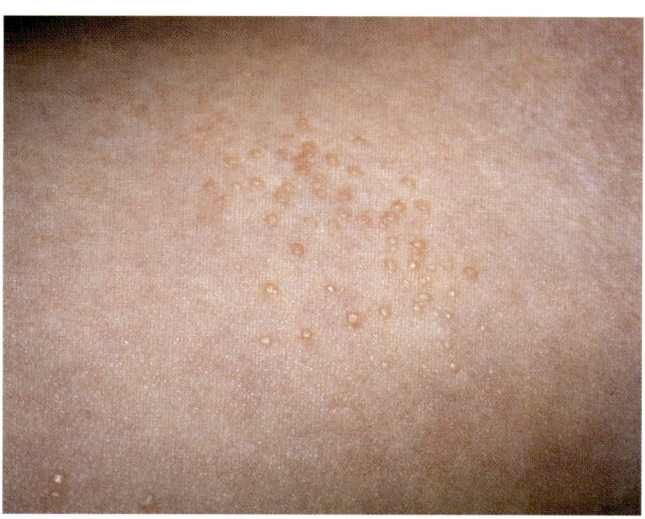

Fig. 12.61 Lichen nitidus.

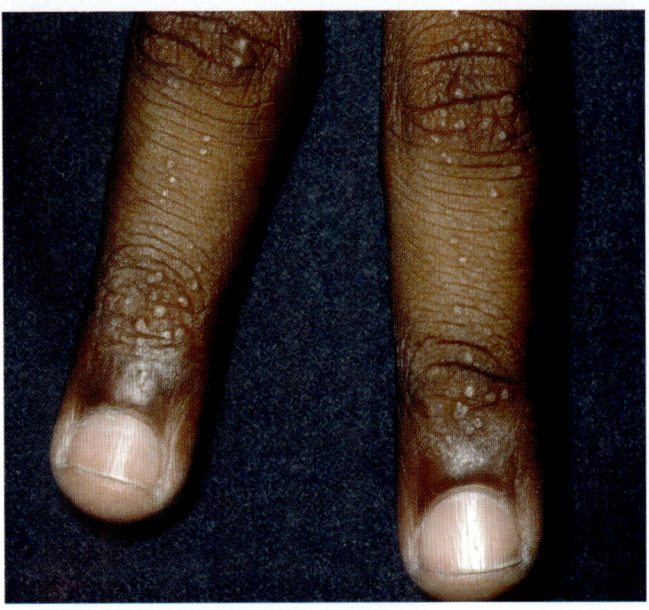

Fig. 12.62 Lichen nitidus.

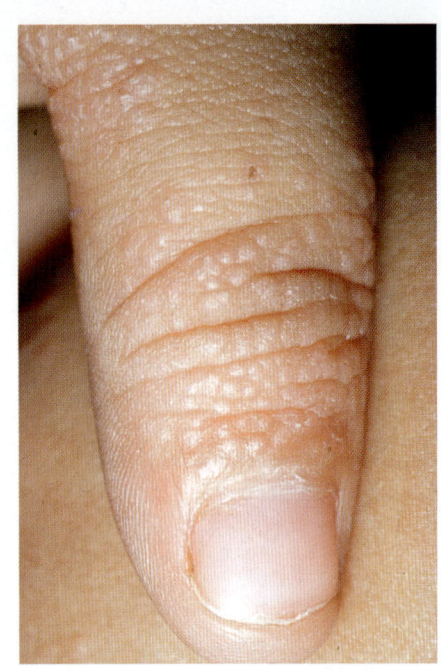

Fig. 12.63 Lichen nitidus. *Courtesy Curt Samlaska, MD.*

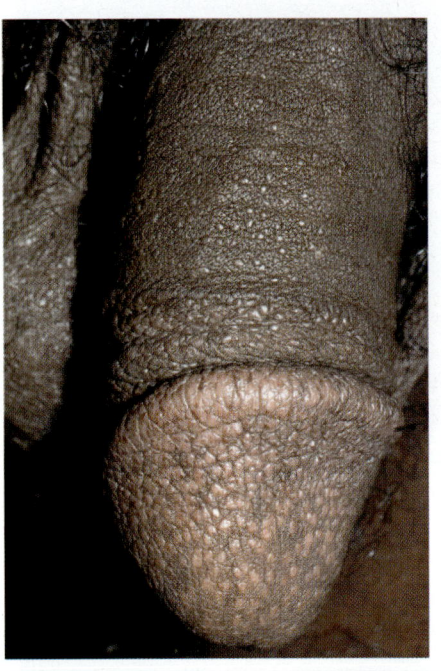

Fig. 12.64 Lichen nitidus. *Courtesy Curt Samlaska, MD.*

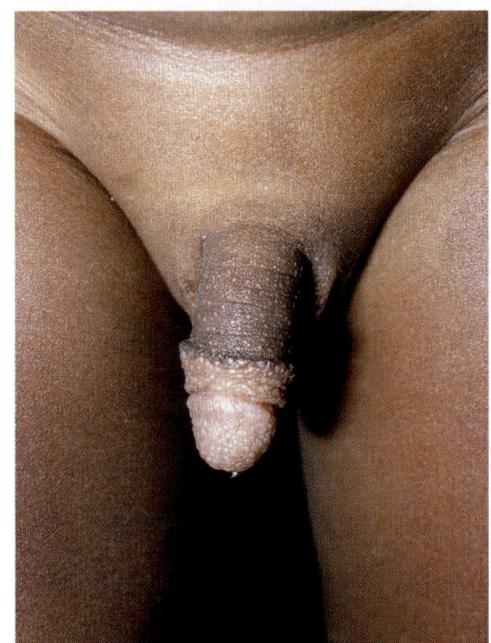

Fig. 12.65 Lichen nitidus.

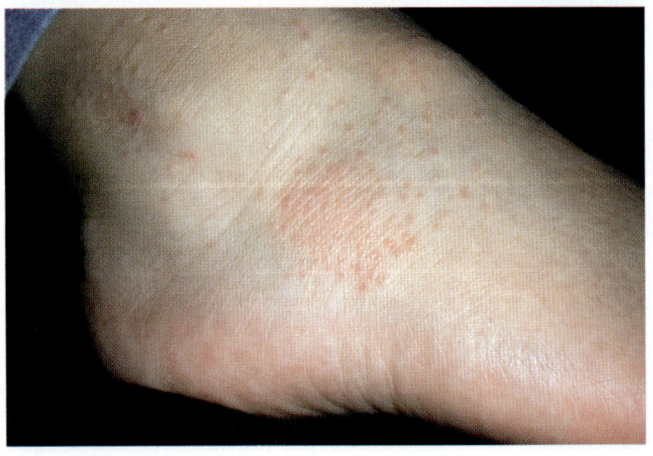

Fig. 12.66 Lichen nitidus.

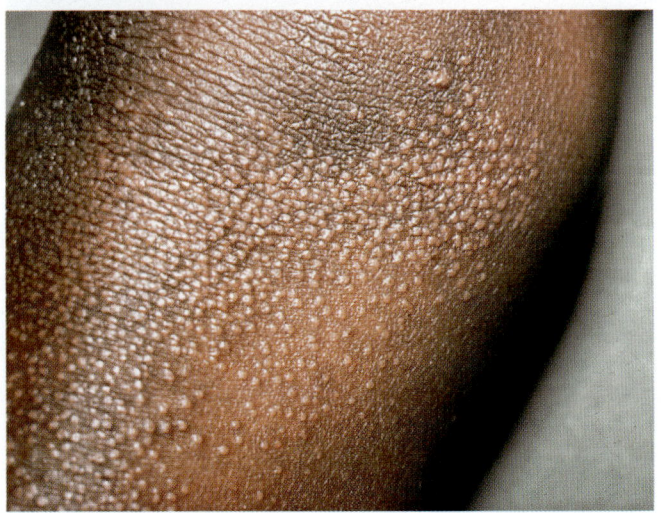

Fig. 12.67 Lichen nitidus.

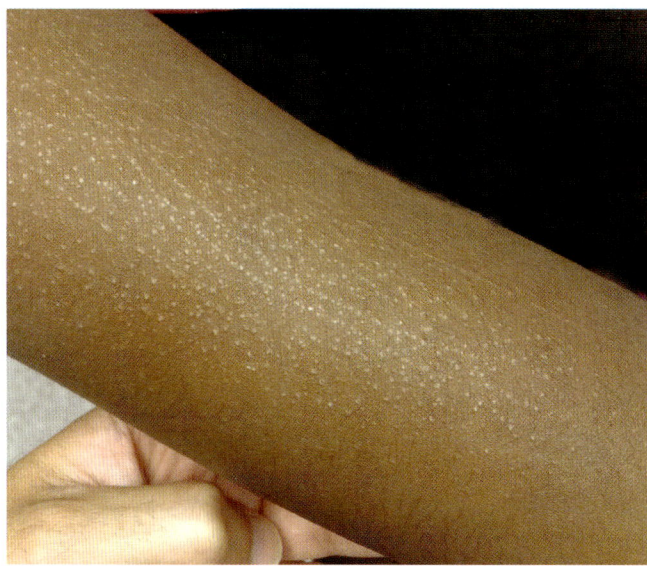

Fig. 12.68 Lichen nitidus. *Courtesy Omar Noor, MD.*

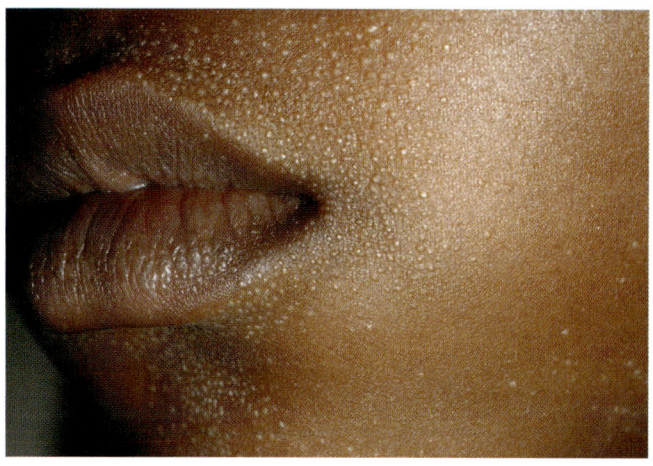

Fig. 12.69 Lichen nitidus.

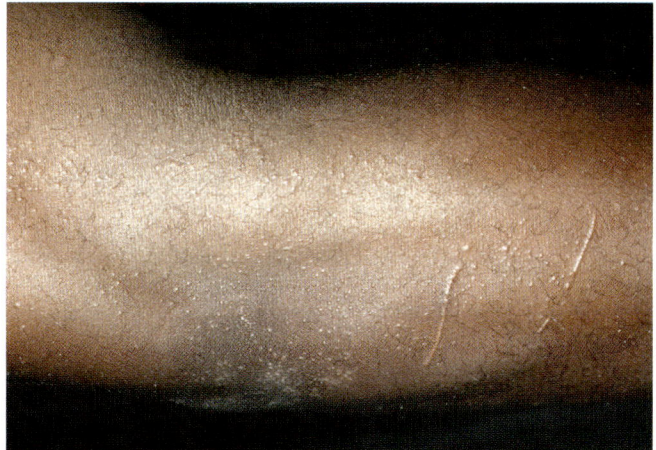

Fig. 12.70 Lichen nitidus. Note Koebner phenomenon. *Courtesy Curt Samlaska, MD.*

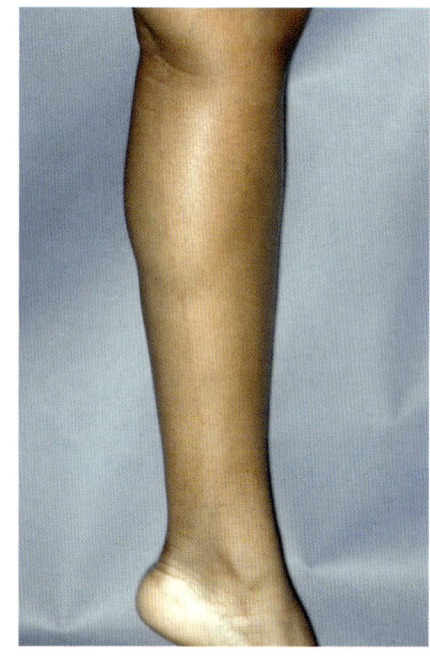

Fig. 12.71 Lichen striatus.

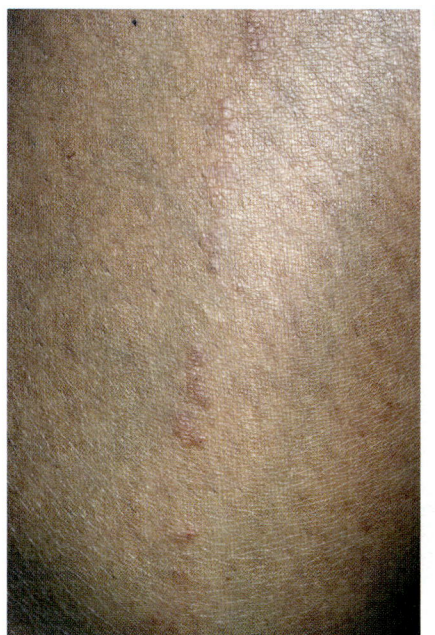

Fig. 12.72 Lichen striatus.

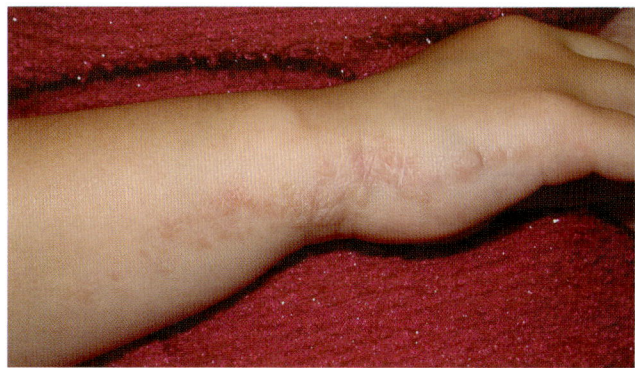

Fig. 12.73 Lichen striatus.

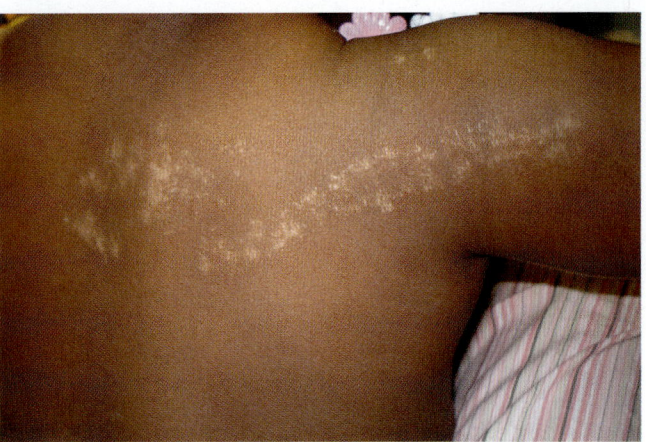

Fig. 12.74 Lichen striatus.

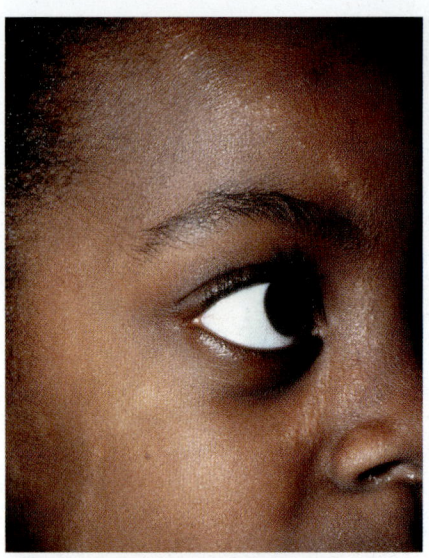

Fig. 12.75 Lichen striatus.

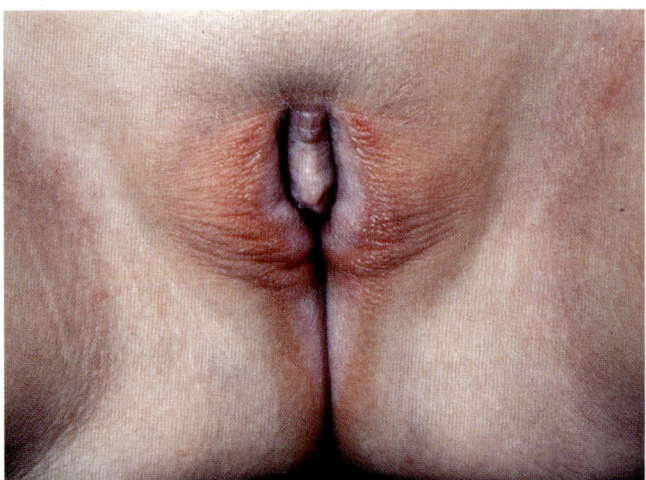

Fig. 12.76 Lichen sclerosus et atrophicus.

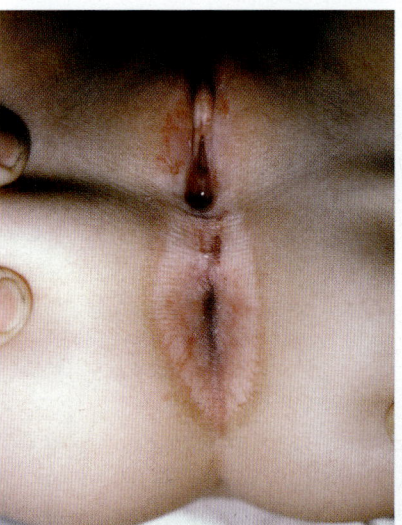

Fig. 12.77 Lichen sclerosus et atrophicus.

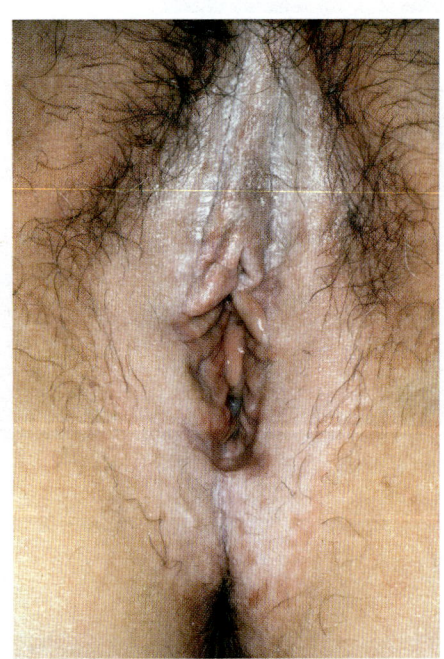

Fig. 12.78 Lichen sclerosus et atrophicus. *Courtesy Ken Greer, MD.*

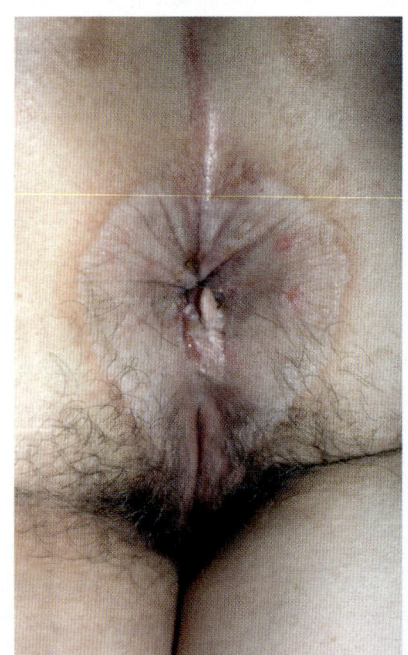

Fig. 12.79 Lichen sclerosus et atrophicus. *Courtesy Steven Binnick, MD.*

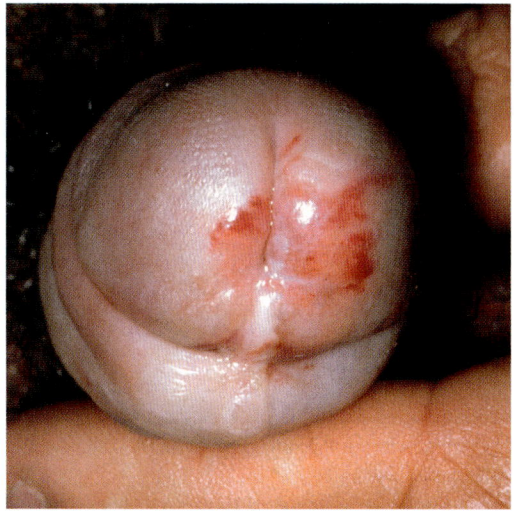

Fig. 12.80 Lichen sclerosus et atrophicus, with hemorrhage secondary to atrophy and trauma.

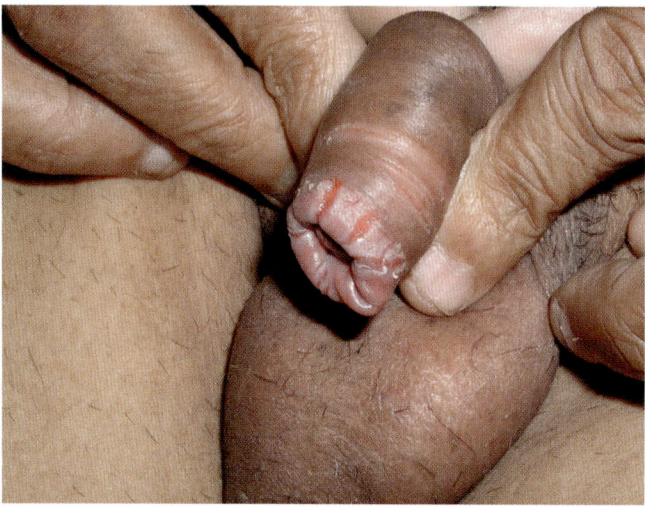

Fig. 12.81 Lichen sclerosus et atrophicus. *Courtesy Shyam Verma, MBBS, DVD.*

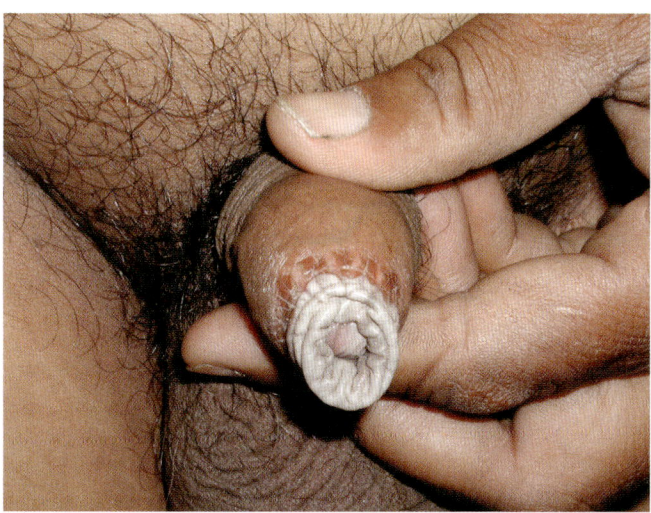

Fig. 12.82 Lichen sclerosus et atrophicus. *Courtesy Shyam Verma, MBBS, DVD.*

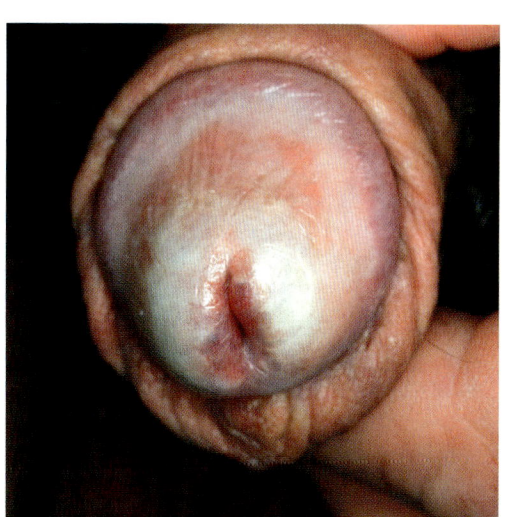

Fig. 12.83 Lichen sclerosus et atrophicus.

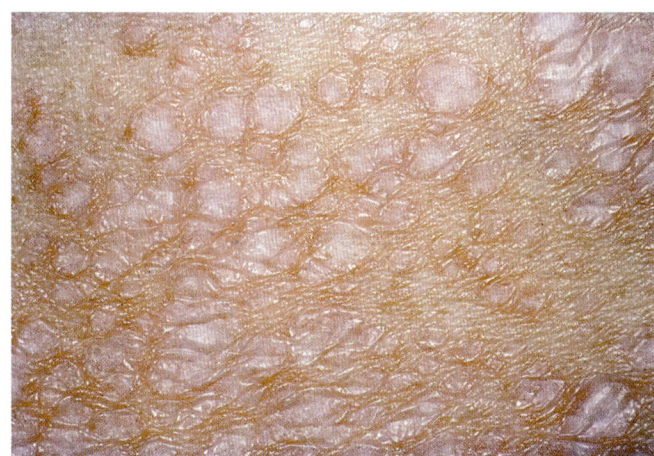

Fig. 12.84 Lichen sclerosus et atrophicus.

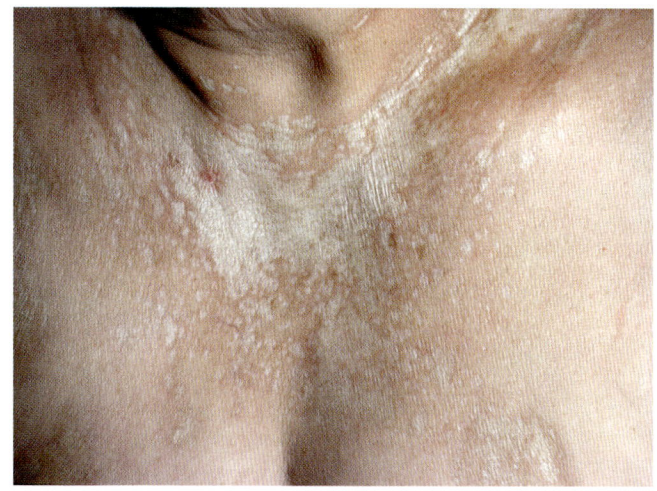

Fig. 12.85 Lichen sclerosus et atrophicus.

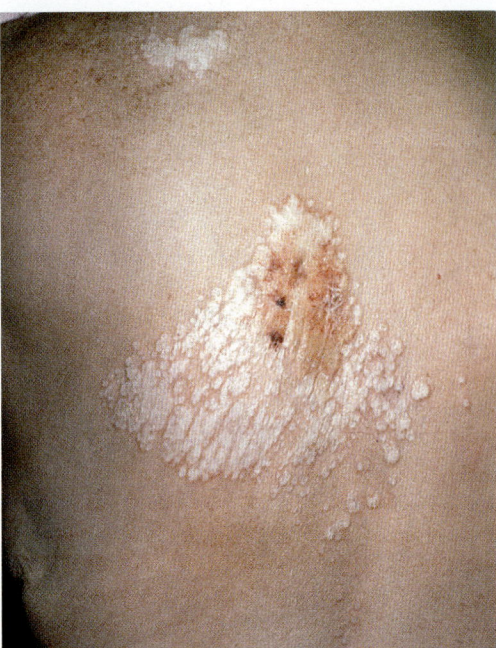

Fig. 12.86 Lichen sclerosus et atrophicus, with hemorrhage secondary to atrophy and trauma.

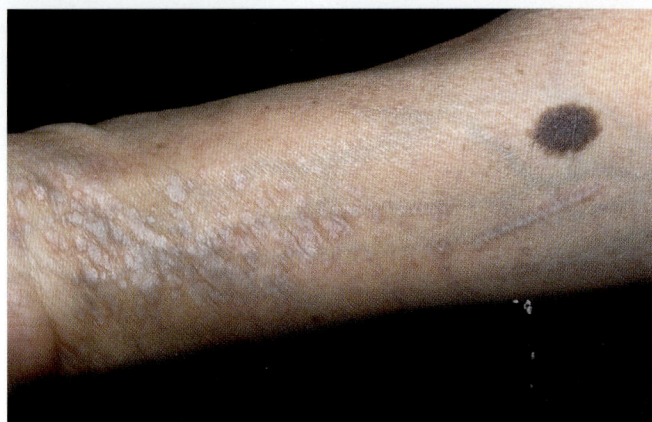

Fig. 12.87 Lichen sclerosus et atrophicus. *Note Koebner phenomena.*

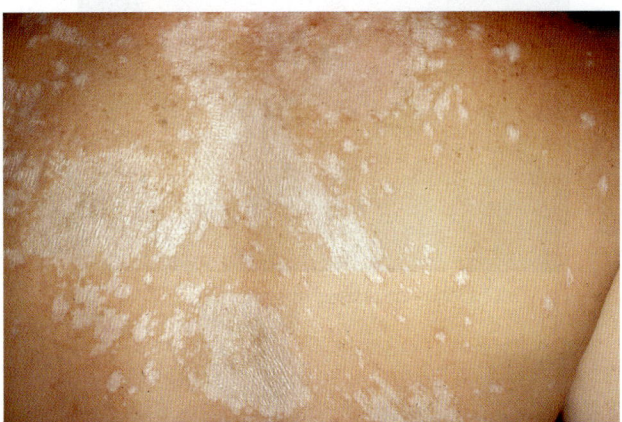

Fig. 12.88 Lichen sclerosus et atrophicus.

Acne 13

Typical acne is so commonplace that its comedones, papules, and pustules are immediately recognizable. There exist, however, a wide spectrum of acne lesions, acneiform eruptions, and rosacea that are exhibited here to assist the deciphering medical provider.

The earliest lesions of acne are open and closed comedones that are often first present on the forehead of adolescent patients. Papules, pustules, nodules, cysts, and scarring can also be seen in the typical acne-prone anatomic regions of the face, upper back, chest, shoulders, and upper arms. The most severe form of acne, acne fulminans, is characterized by joint pains, painful nodulocystic lesions, and even fevers. Other acneiform eruptions include the scarring follicular pustules of acne keloidalis nuchae, the more monomorphous pustular eruption of corticosteroid-induced acne, and the pustules and nodules of gram-negative folliculitis.

In neonates, the transient micropustular eruption on the head and neck that has been historically known as *neonatal acne* has now been renamed *neonatal cephalic pustulosis* due to its lack of comedones, nodules, or scarring. Infantile acne, in contrast, occurs mostly on the cheeks of infants and toddlers and is a true subset of acne with its comedones, papules, pustules, nodules, and potential scarring. Finally, periorificial dermatitis is a distinctive acneiform eruption notable for papules and pustules located around the mouth, nose, and eyes of children and younger adults.

Hidradenitis suppurativa is also included in this chapter with its chronic inflammatory abscesses, nodules, and sinus tract formation in the axillae, inframammary folds, inguinal folds, and gluteal cleft.

Rosacea is also highlighted here to allow for direct comparison with acne. Flushing, erythema, and fine telangiectasias seen on the convex surfaces of the face define the erythrotelangiectatic subtype of rosacea, whereas the papules, pustules, and in some cases nodules are present in the papulopustular and glandular forms.

Most conditions in this chapter will depend on clinical findings to arrive at a diagnosis, but in some cases a skin biopsy or bacterial culture will be useful. This portion of the atlas features examples of important clinical findings to recognize in patients with acne and the many acneiform eruptions.

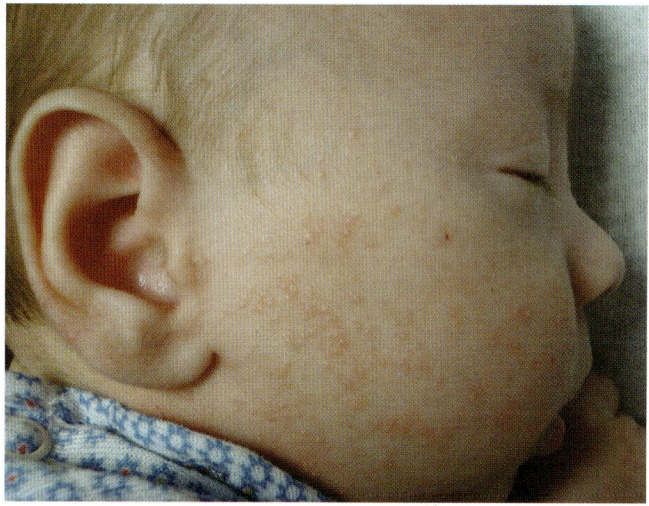

Fig. 13.2 Neonatal cephalic pustulosis (neonatal acne).

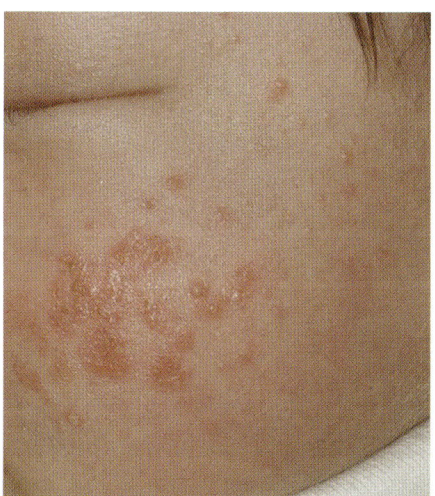

Fig. 13.1 Neonatal cephalic pustulosis (neonatal acne). *Courtesy National Cheng Kung University, Taiwan.*

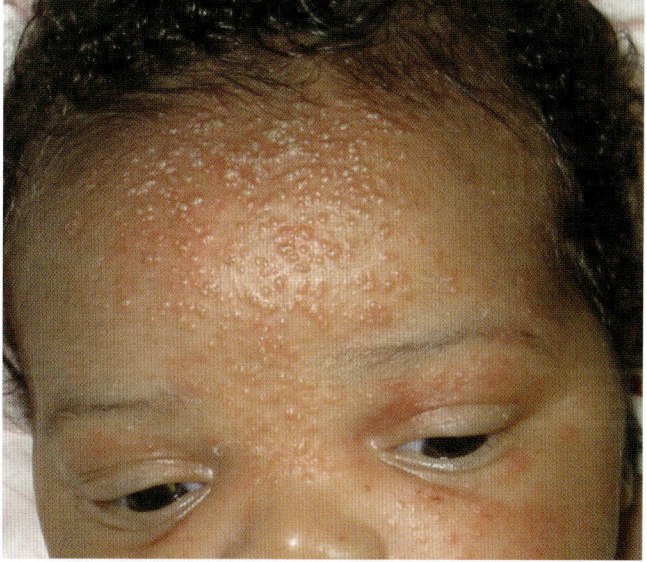

Fig. 13.3 Neonatal cephalic pustulosis (neonatal acne).

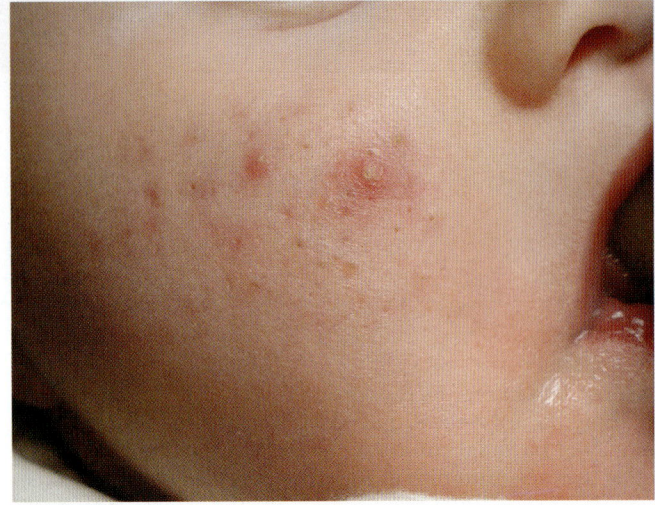

Fig. 13.4 Infantile acne.

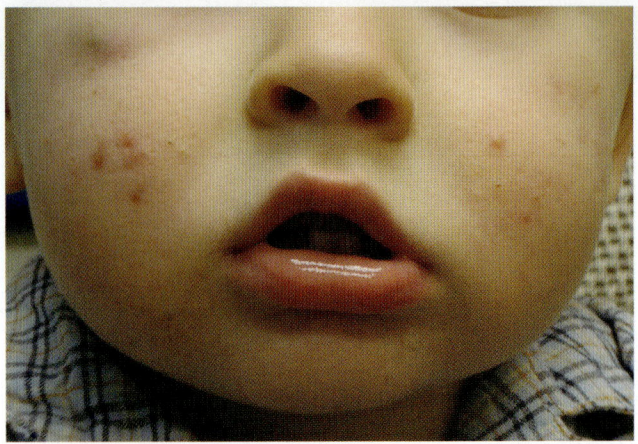

Fig. 13.5 Infantile acne.

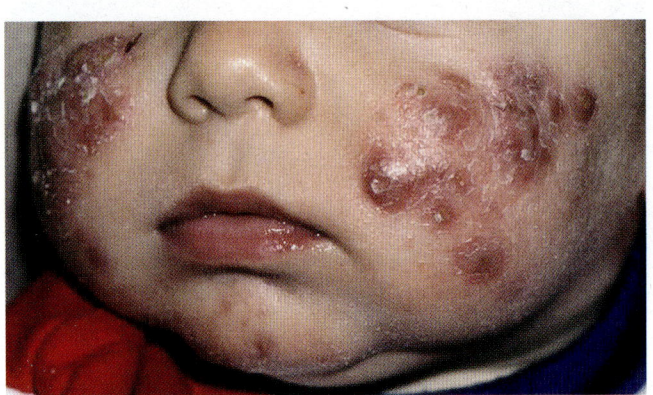

Fig. 13.6 Severe infantile acne.

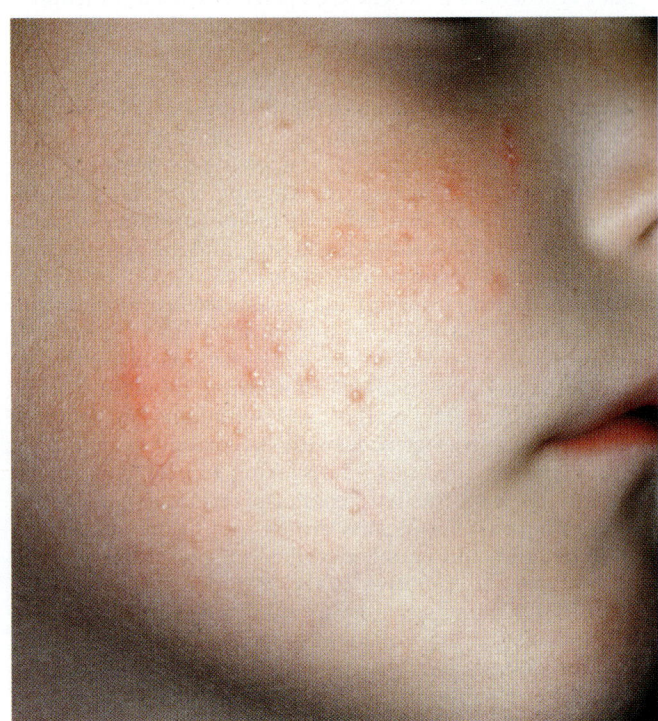

Fig. 13.7 Childhood acne.

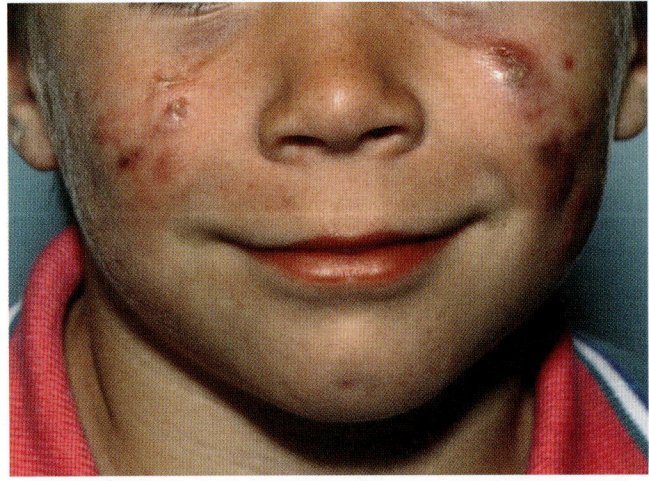

Fig. 13.8 Childhood acne.

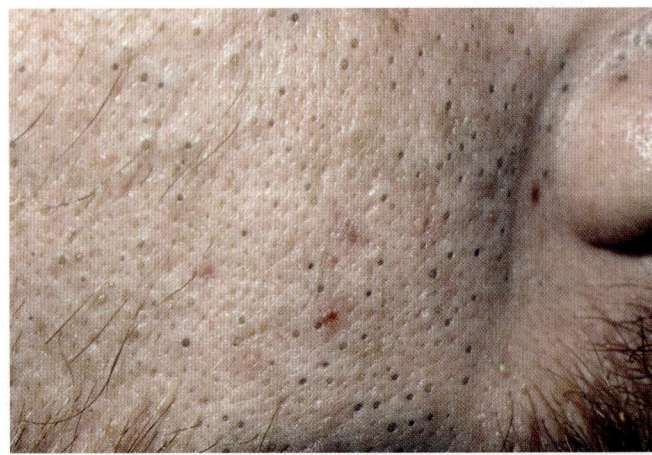

Fig. 13.9 Open comedones. *Courtesy Steven Binnick, MD.*

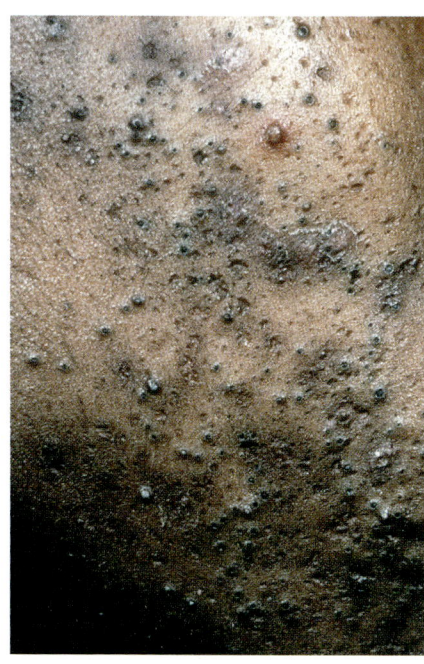

Fig. 13.10 Open comedones.

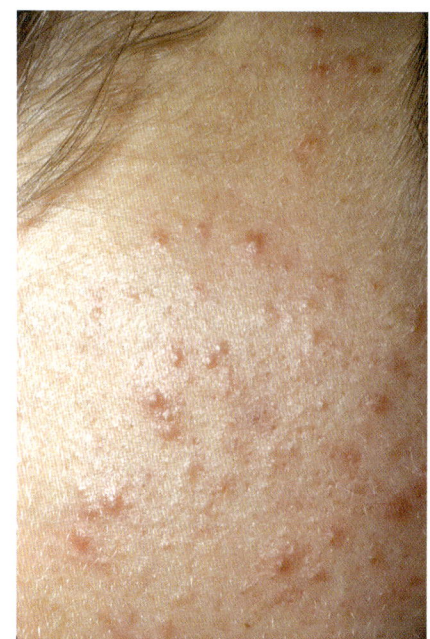

Fig. 13.11 Closed comedones.

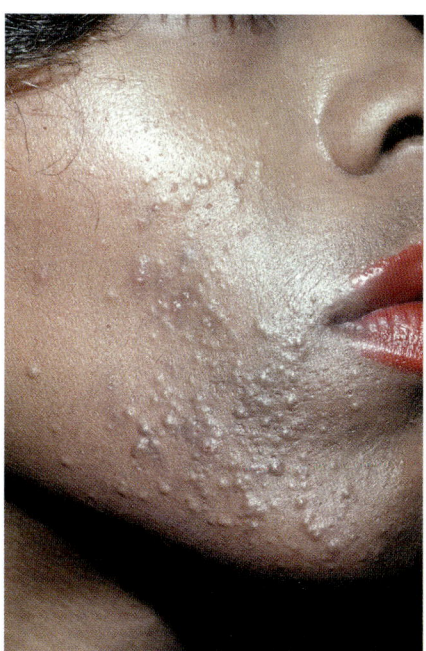

Fig. 13.12 Closed comedones.

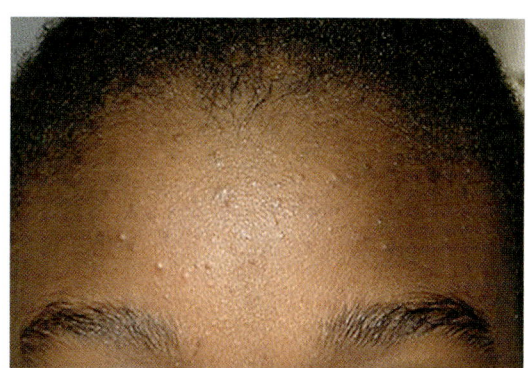

Fig. 13.13 Preadolescent acne.

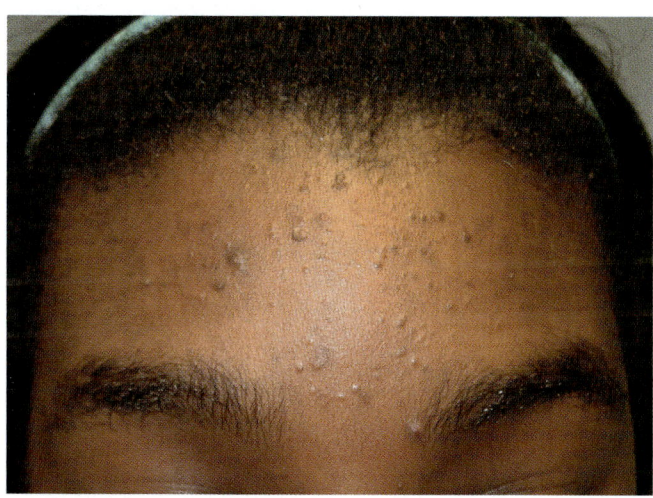

Fig. 13.14 Preadolescent acne.

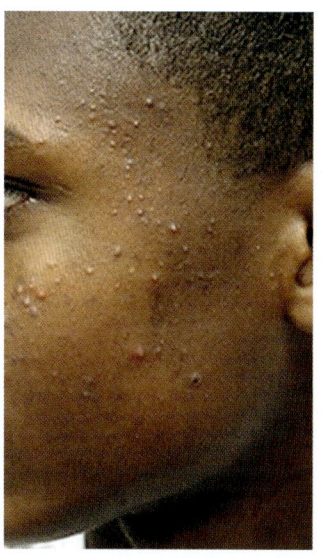

Fig. 13.15 Mild to moderate acne.

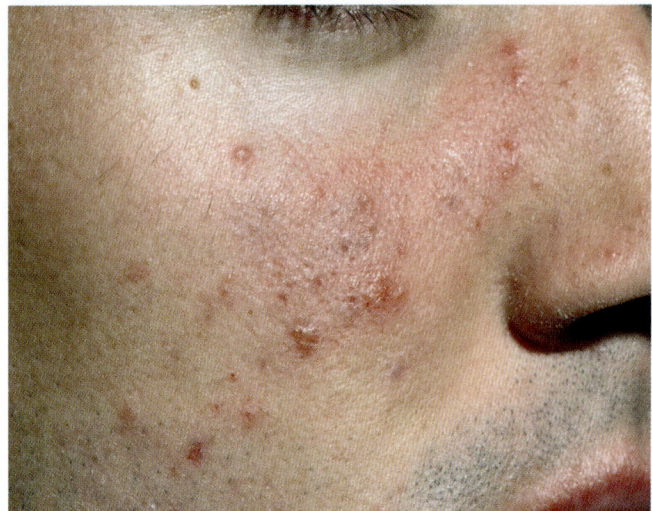
Fig. 13.16 Mild to moderate acne.

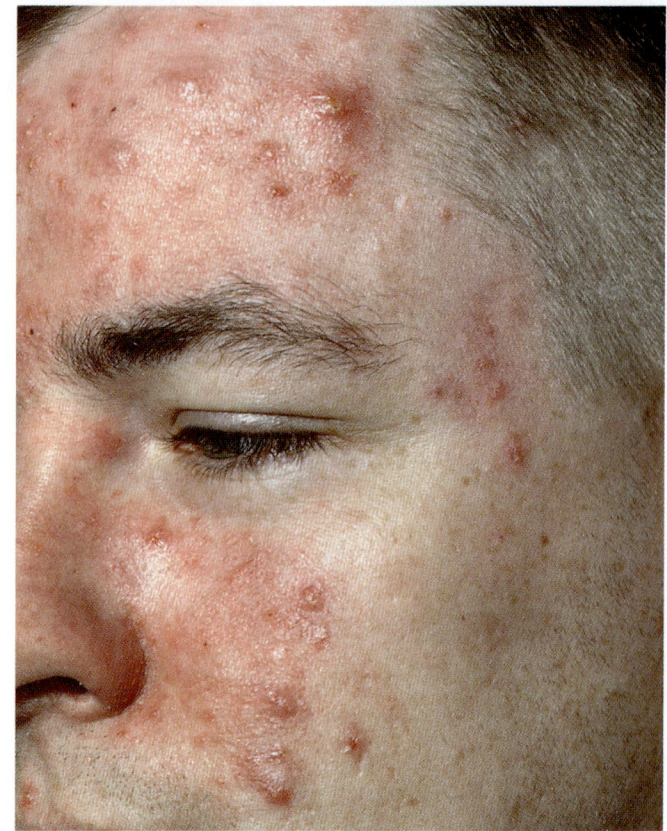
Fig. 13.17 Moderate to severe acne.

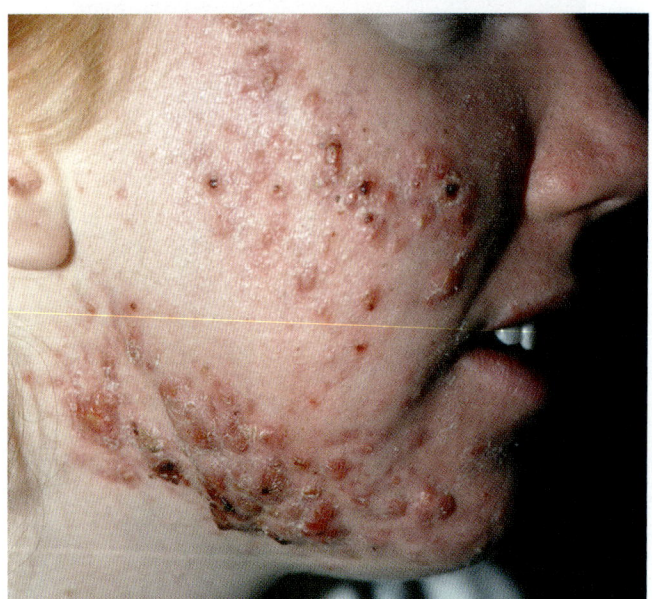
Fig. 13.18 Severe acne.

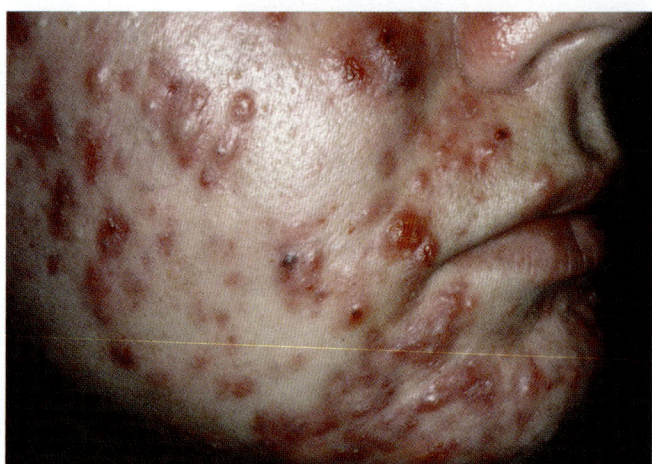
Fig. 13.19 Severe acne.

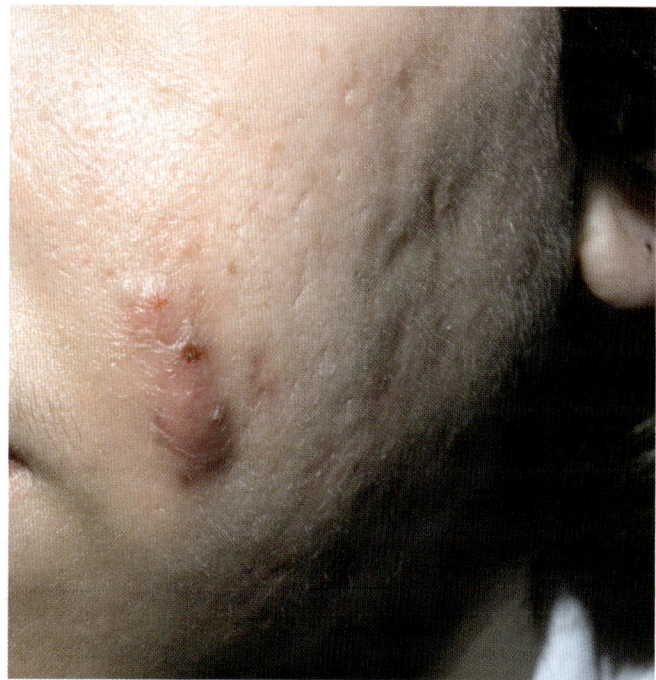

Fig. 13.20 Acne cyst with scarring. *Courtesy Steven Binnick, MD.*

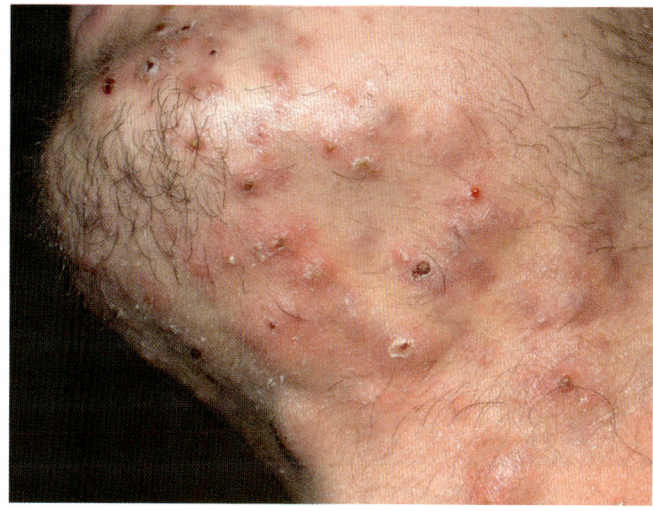

Fig. 13.21 Severe acne.

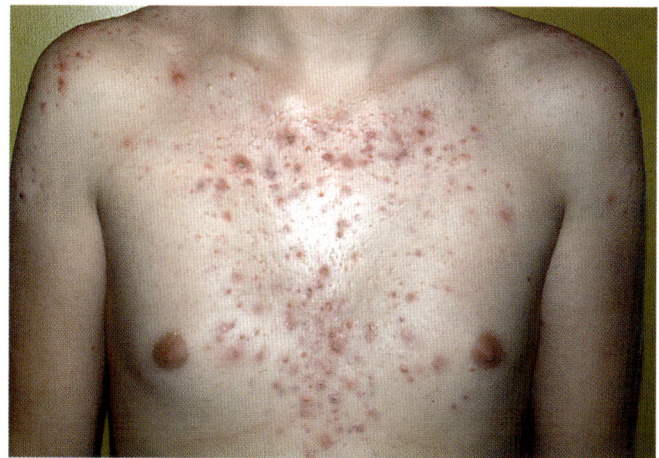

Fig. 13.22 Severe truncal acne. *Courtesy Steven Binnick, MD.*

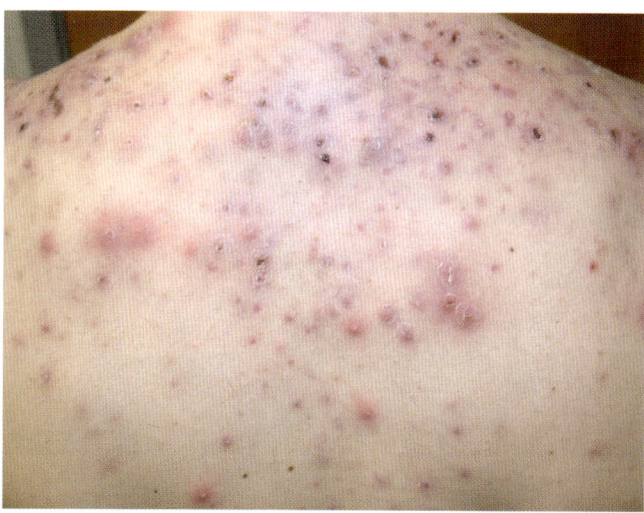

Fig. 13.23 Severe truncal acne.

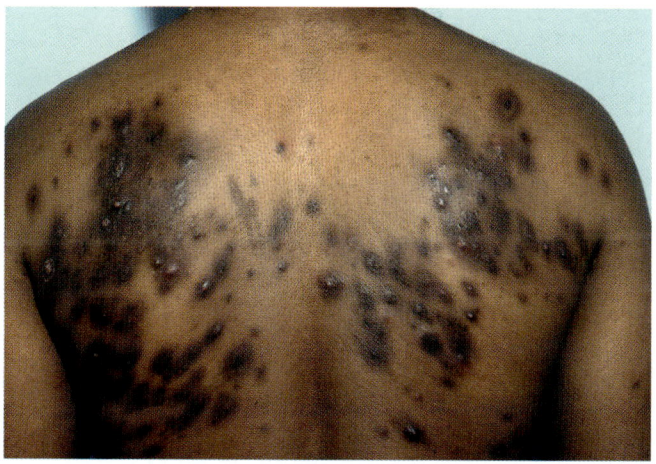

Fig. 13.24 Severe truncal acne with hyperpigmentation.

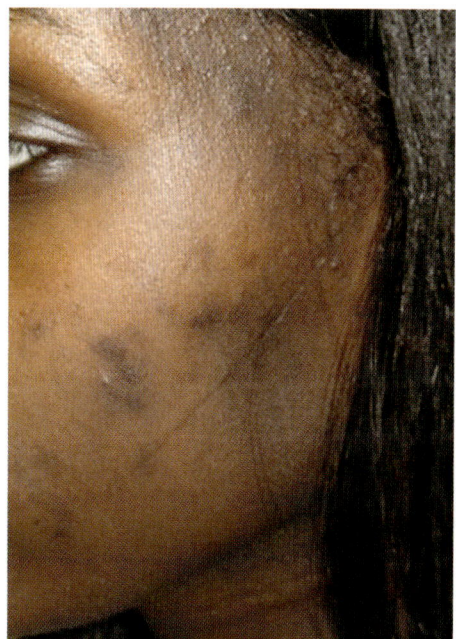

Fig. 13.25 Acne with hyperpigmentation.

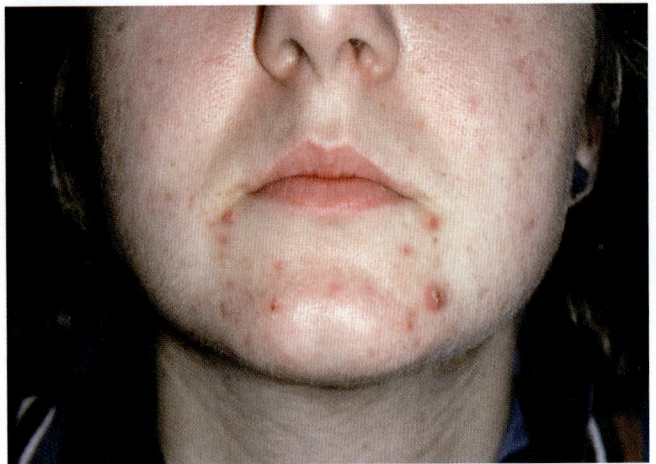

Fig. 13.26 Woman with lower face acne.

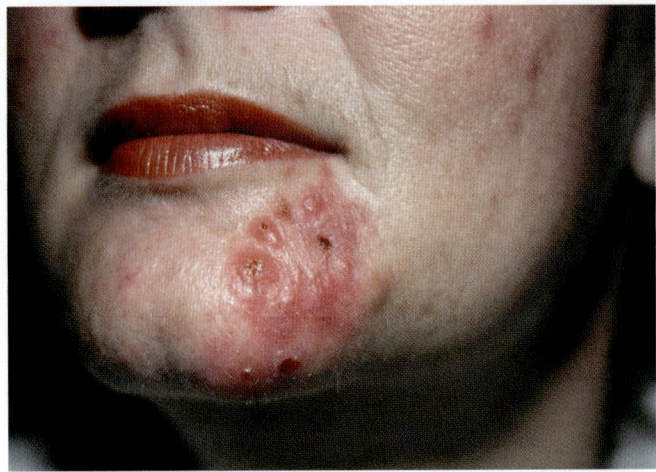

Fig. 13.27 Woman with lower face acne.

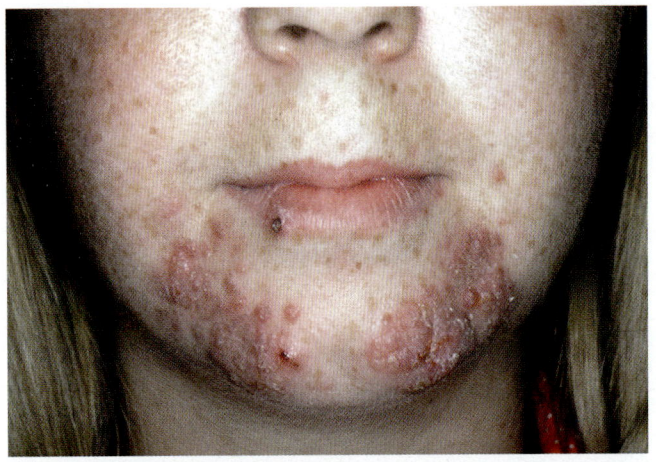

Fig. 13.28 Woman with lower face acne.

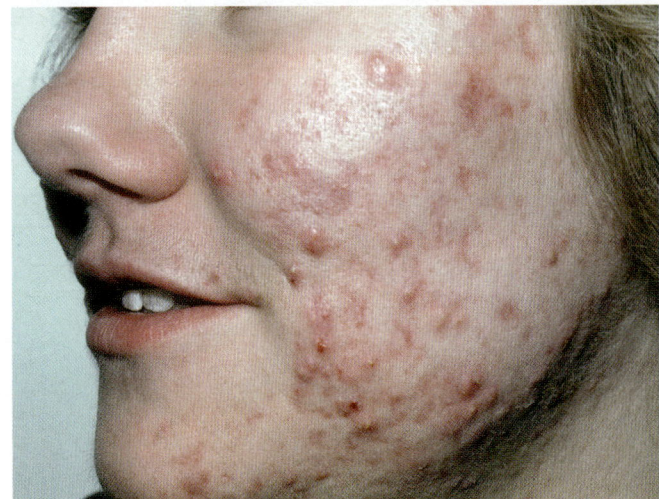

Fig. 13.29 Acne in a woman with 21-hydroxylase deficiency. *Courtesy Steven Binnick, MD.*

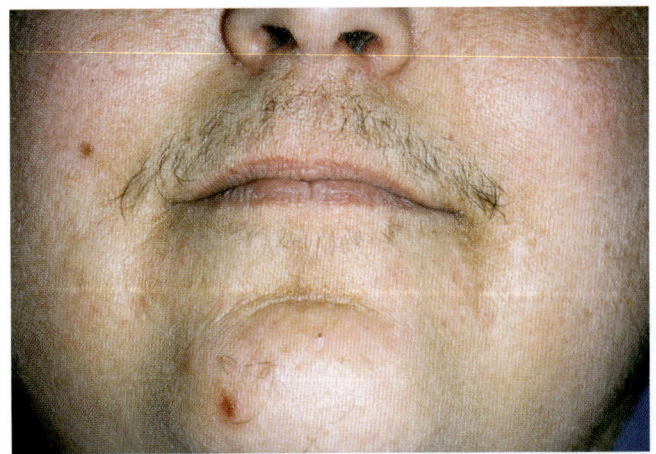

Fig. 13.30 Acne and hirsutism in a woman with Cushing disease.

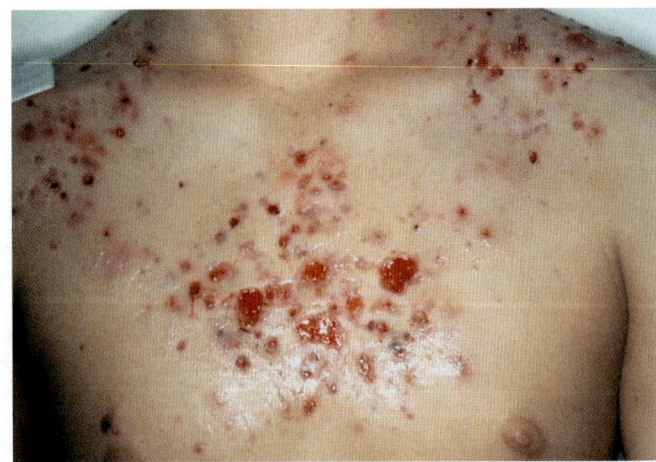

Fig. 13.31 Acne fulminans.

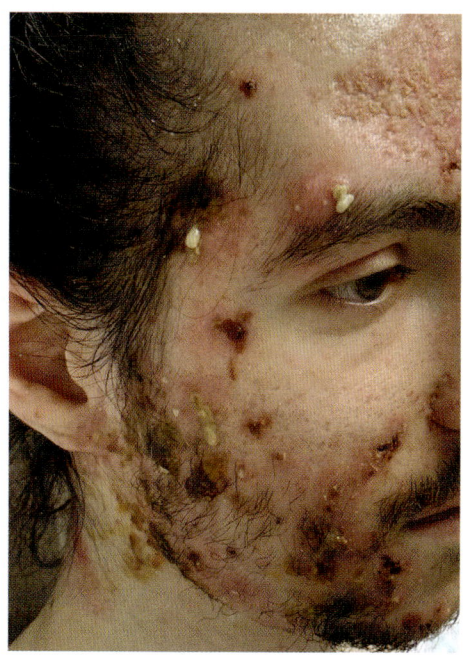

Fig. 13.32 Acne fulminans.

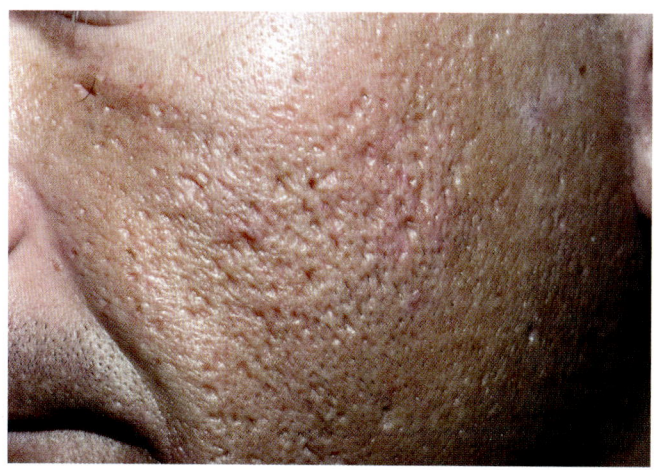

Fig. 13.33 Acne scarring. *Courtesy Steven Binnick, MD.*

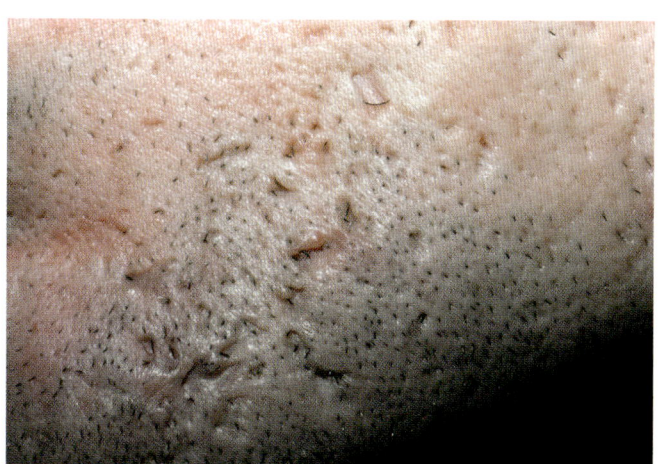

Fig. 13.34 Acne scarring. *Courtesy Steven Binnick, MD.*

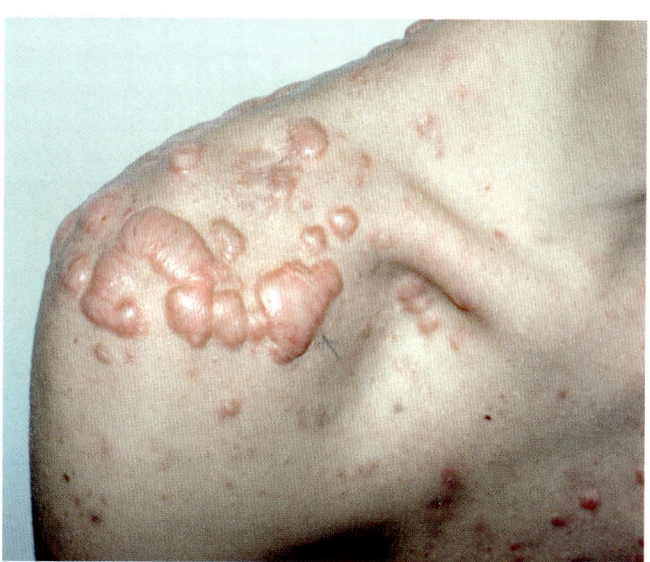

Fig. 13.35 Keloids resulting from acne. *Courtesy Steven Binnick, MD.*

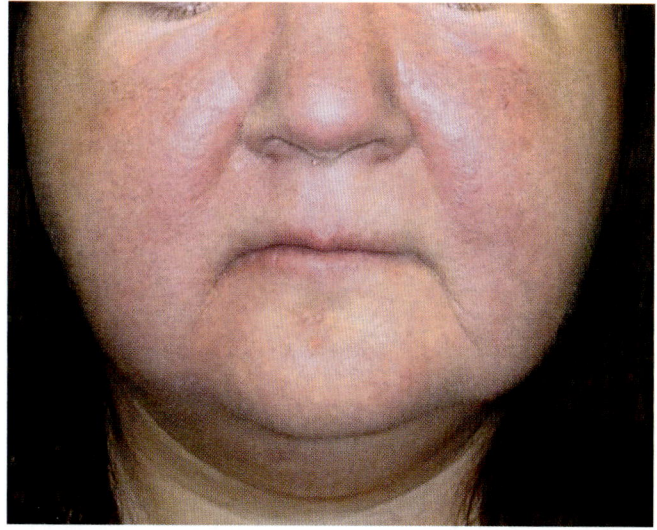

Fig. 13.36 Solid facial edema.

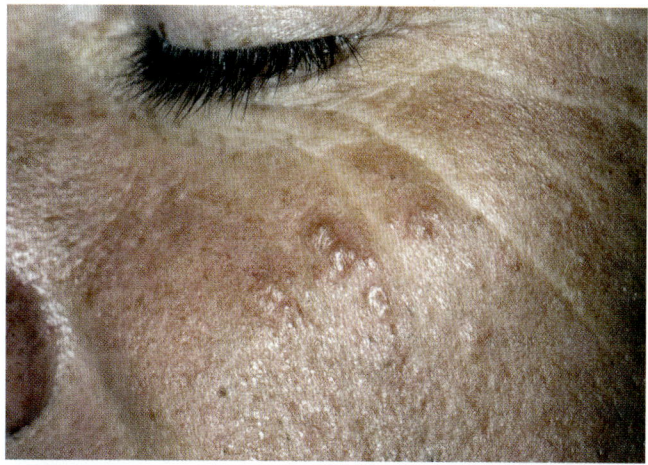

Fig. 13.37 Osteoma cutis.

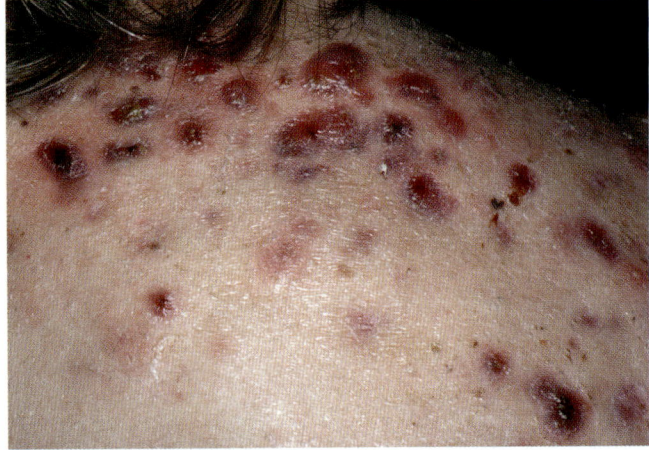

Fig. 13.38 Granulation tissue in a patient taking isotretinoin. *Courtesy Steven Binnick, MD.*

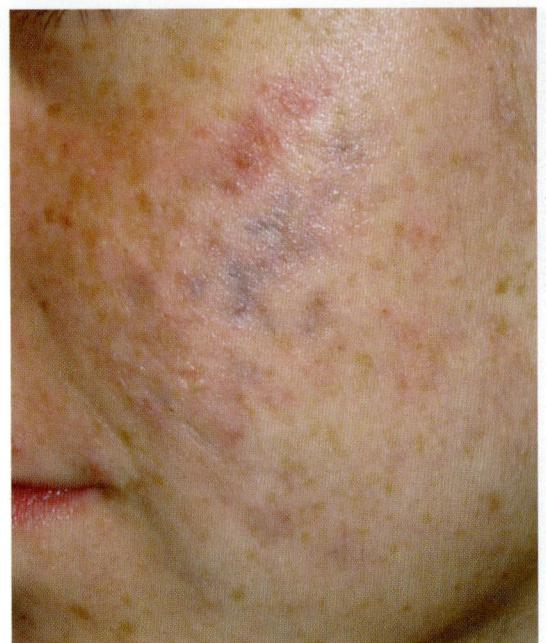

Fig. 13.39 Minocycline pigmentation in a patient with acne.

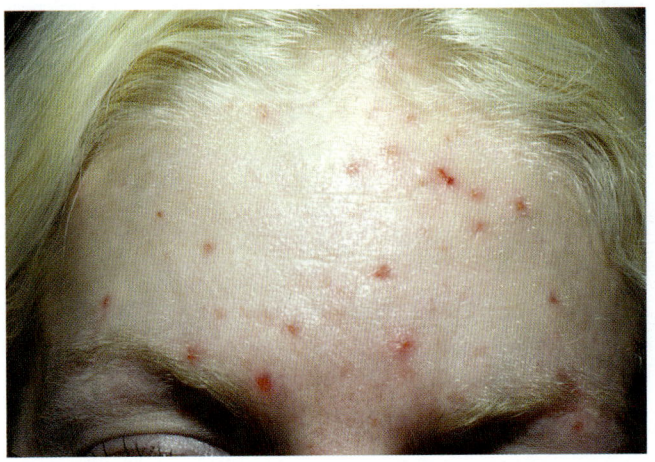

Fig. 13.40 Acne excoriée. *Courtesy The University of Utah and Oregon Health Sciences University Leonard Swinyer MD image collection.*

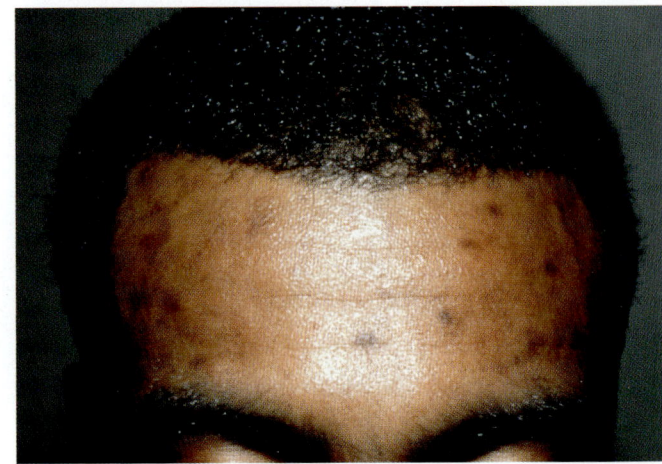

Fig. 13.41 Acne mechanica.

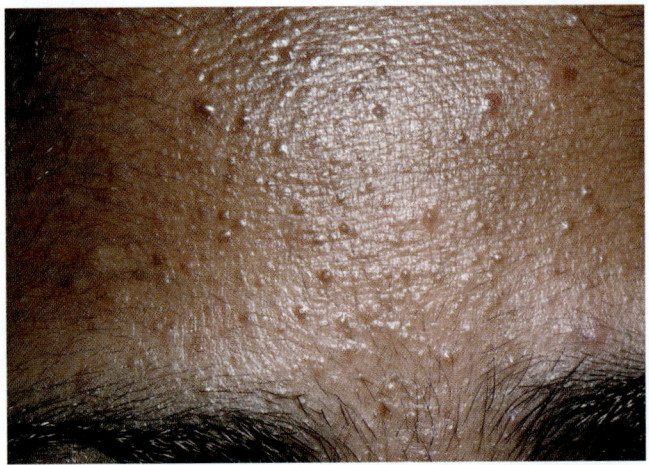

Fig. 13.42 Pomade acne.

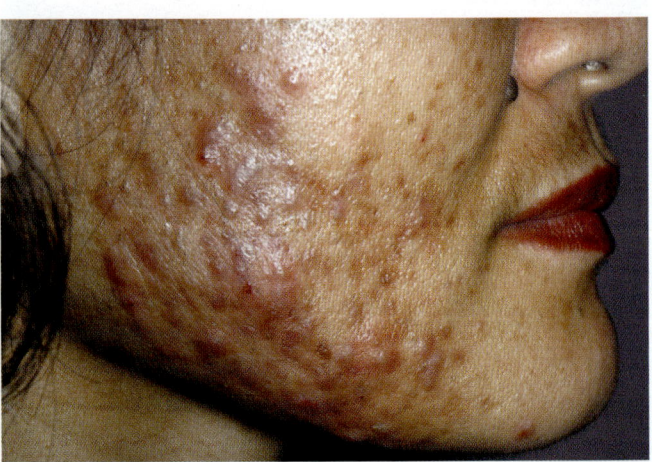

Fig. 13.43 Acne cosmetica.

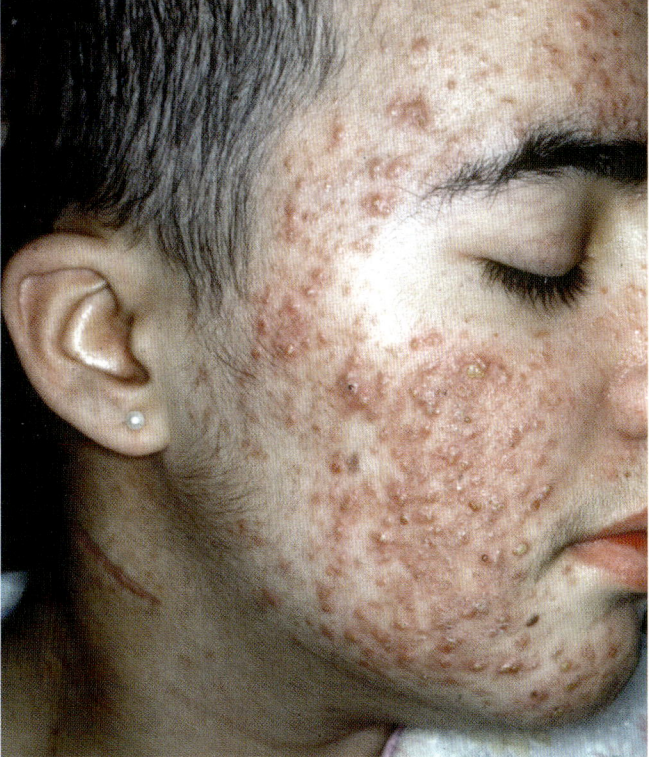

Fig. 13.44 Steroid-induced acne in patient taking oral steroids after neurosurgery.

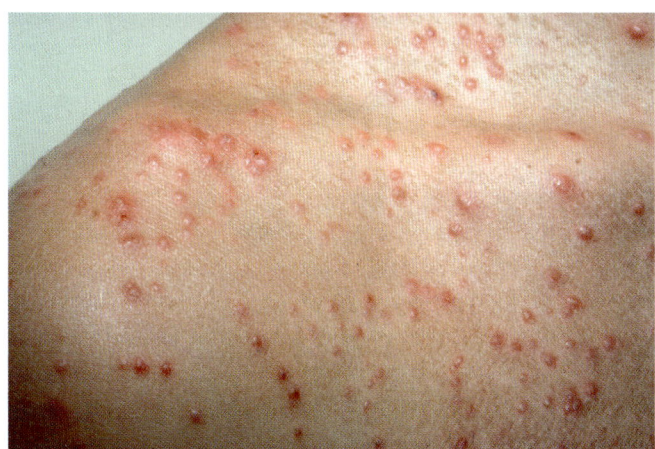

Fig. 13.46 Steroid-induced acne.

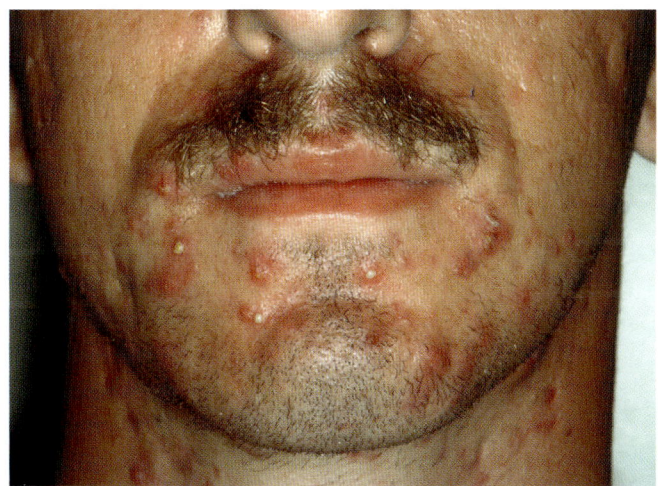

Fig. 13.48 Gram-negative folliculitis.

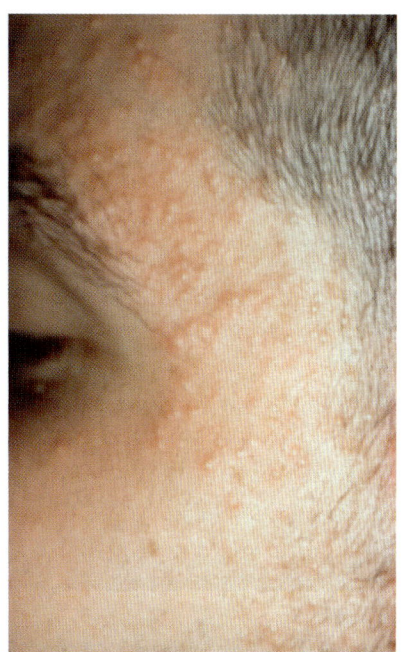

Fig. 13.45 Steroid-induced acne.

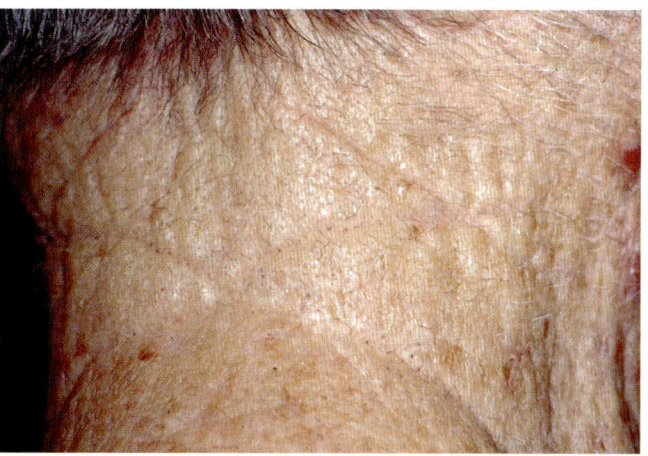

Fig. 13.47 Chloracne.

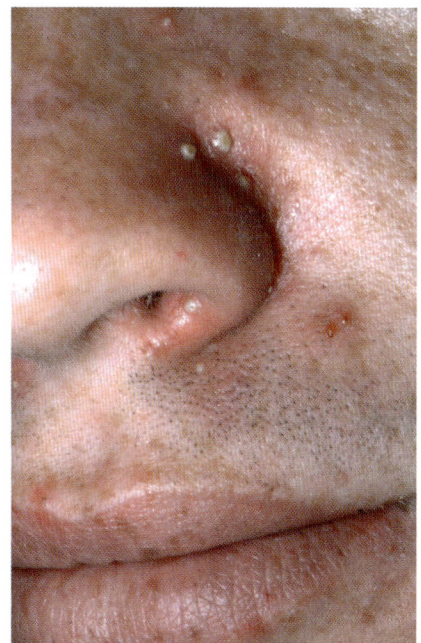

Fig. 13.49 Gram-negative folliculitis.

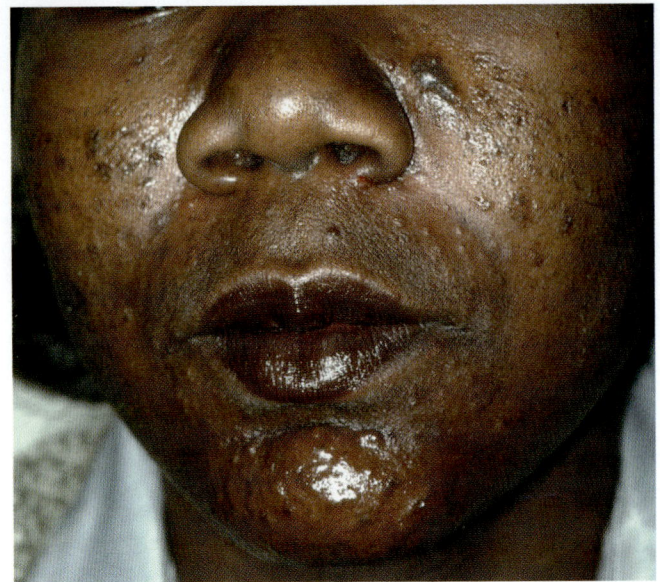

Fig. 13.50 Gram-negative folliculitis.

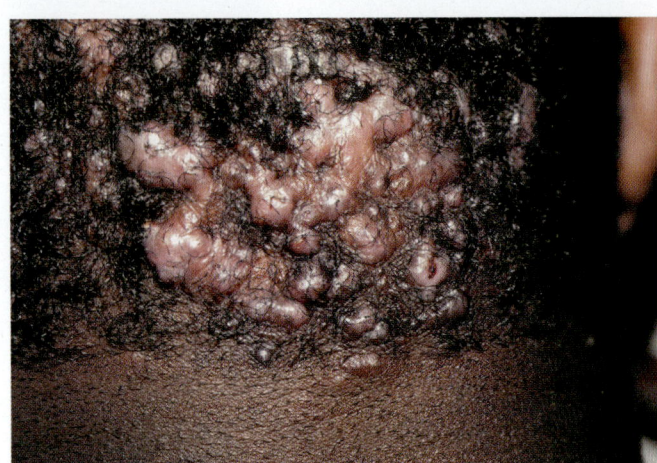

Fig. 13.51 Acne keloidalis. *Courtesy Steven Binnick, MD.*

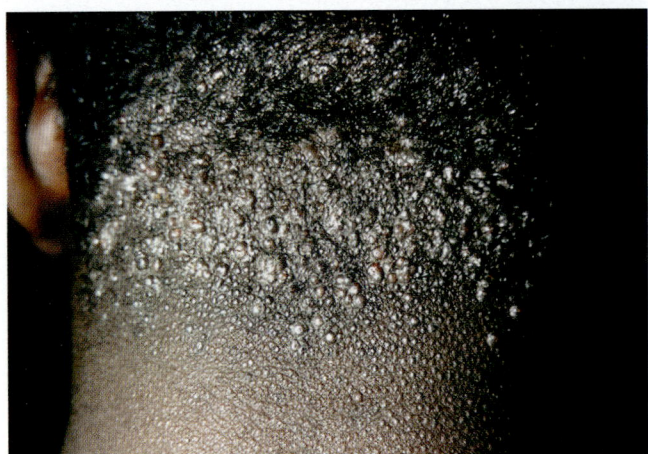

Fig. 13.52 Acne keloidalis.

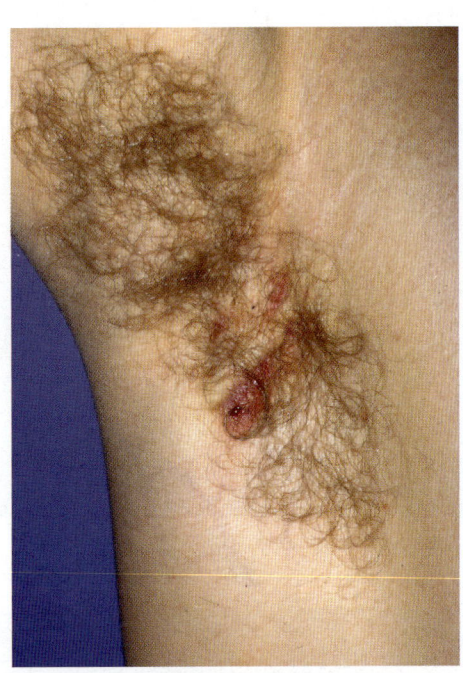

Fig. 13.53 Hidradenitis suppurativa.

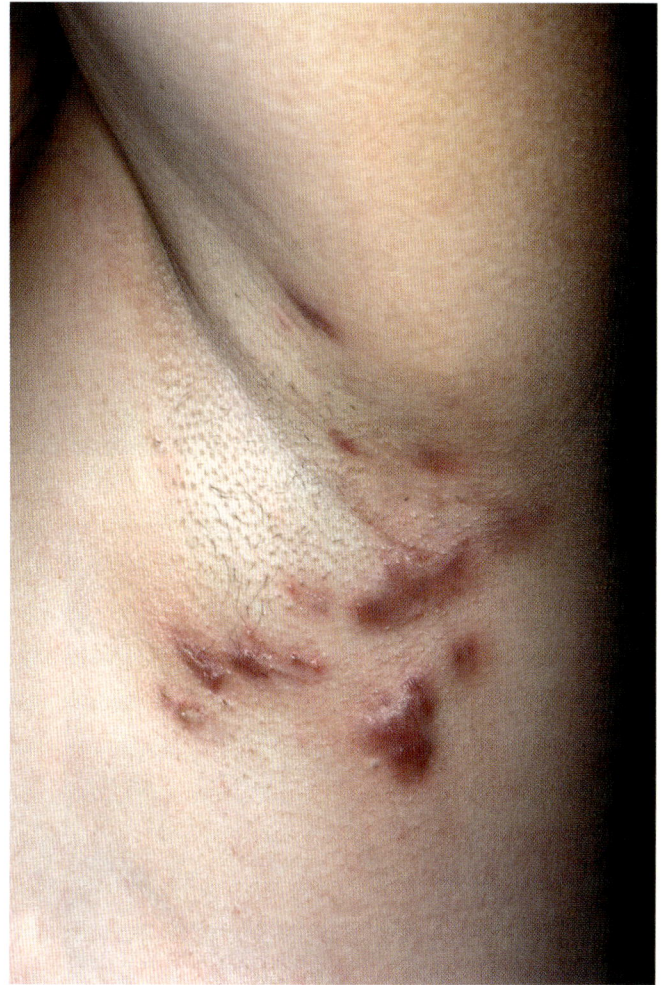

Fig. 13.54 Hidradenitis suppurativa.

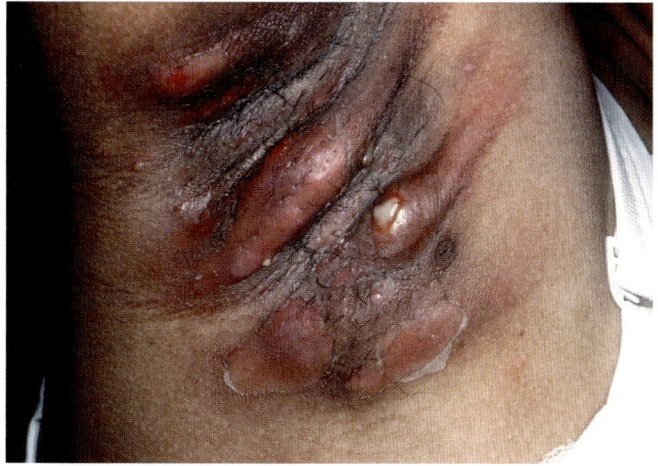

Fig. 13.56 Hidradenitis suppurativa.

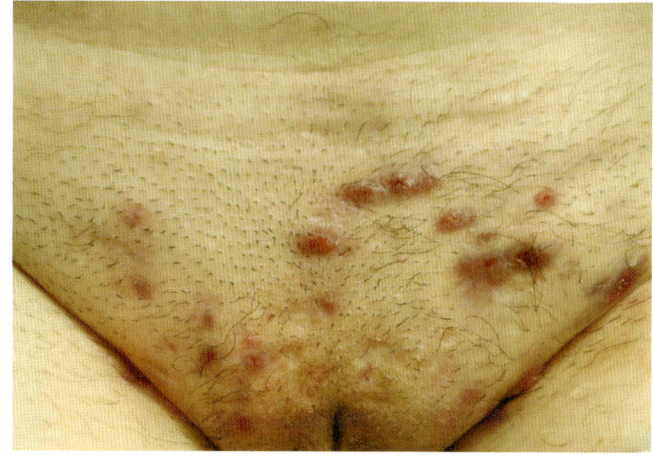

Fig. 13.55 Hidradenitis suppurativa.

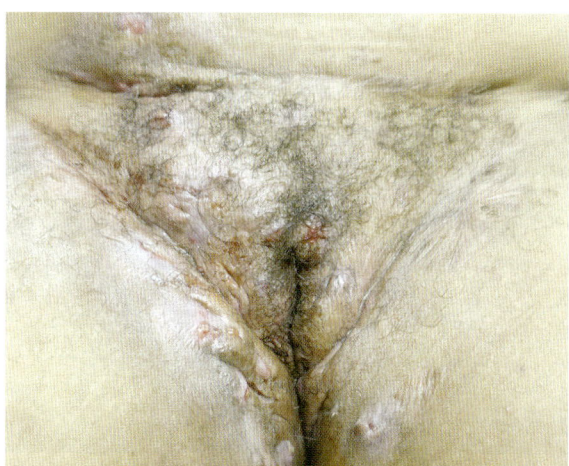

Fig. 13.57 Hidradenitis suppurativa.

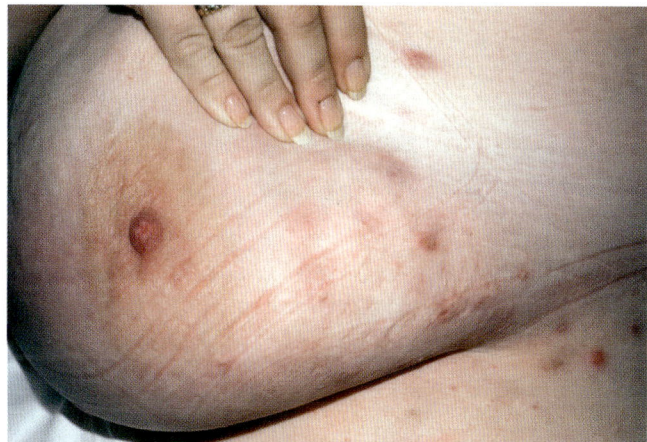

Fig. 13.58 Hidradenitis suppurativa.

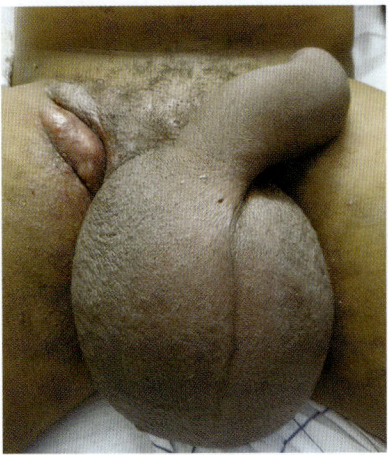

Fig. 13.59 Genital lymphedema complicating hidradenitis suppurativa.

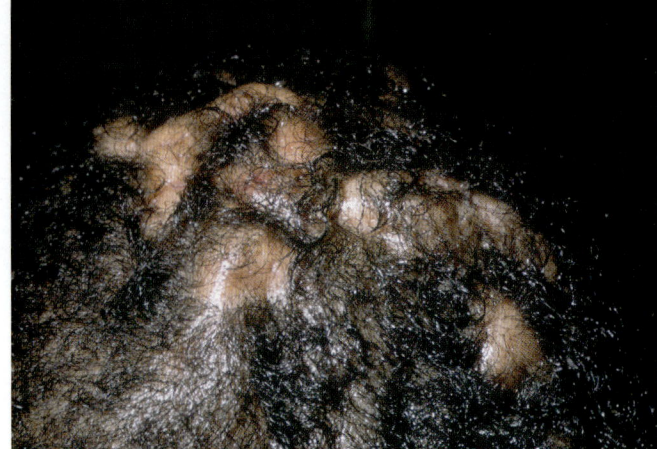

Fig. 13.60 Dissecting cellulitis of the scalp.

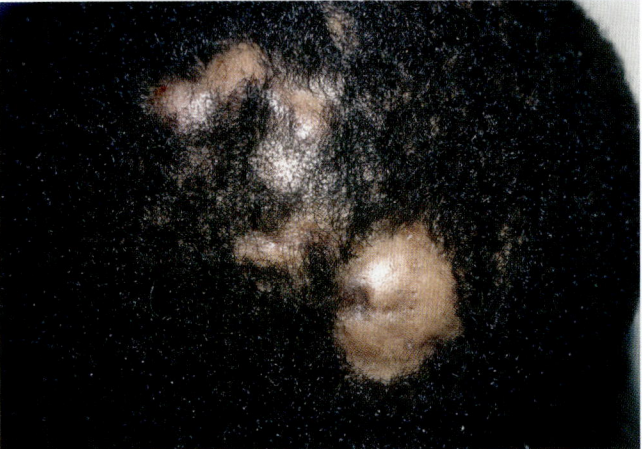

Fig. 13.61 Dissecting cellulitis of the scalp.

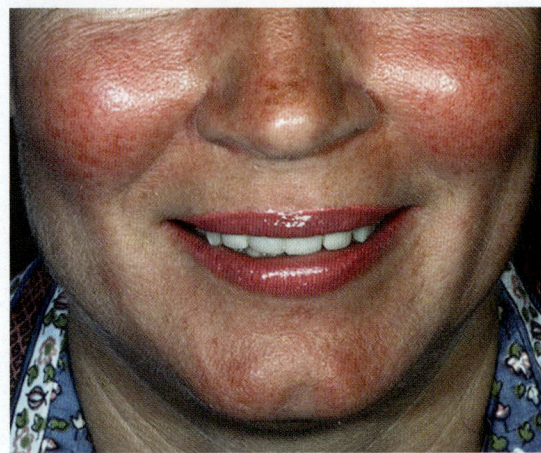

Fig. 13.62 Rosacea with erythema. *Courtesy The University of Utah and Oregon Health Sciences University Leonard Swinyer MD image collection.*

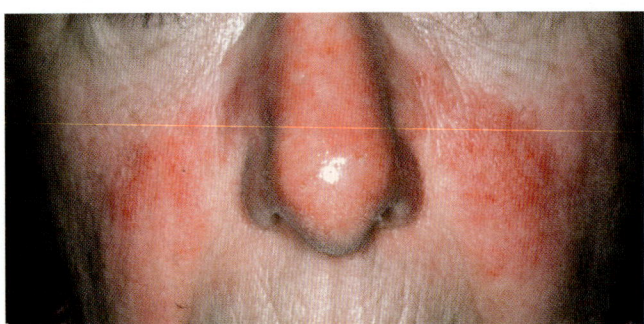

Fig. 13.63 Erythematotelangiectatic rosacea.

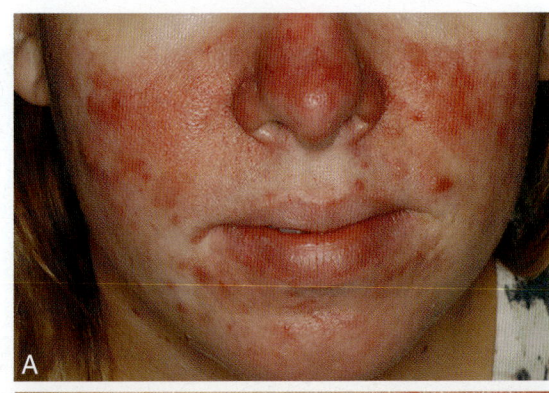
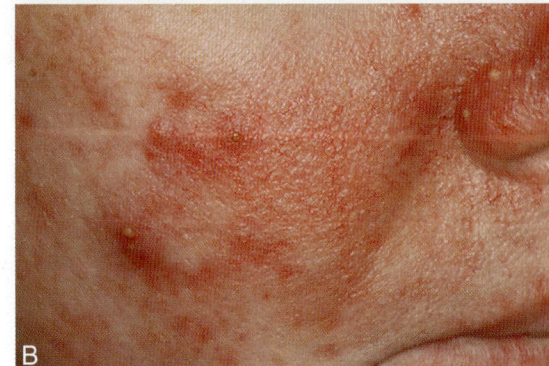

Fig. 13.64 (A) and (B) Rosacea with erythema, papules, and pustules.

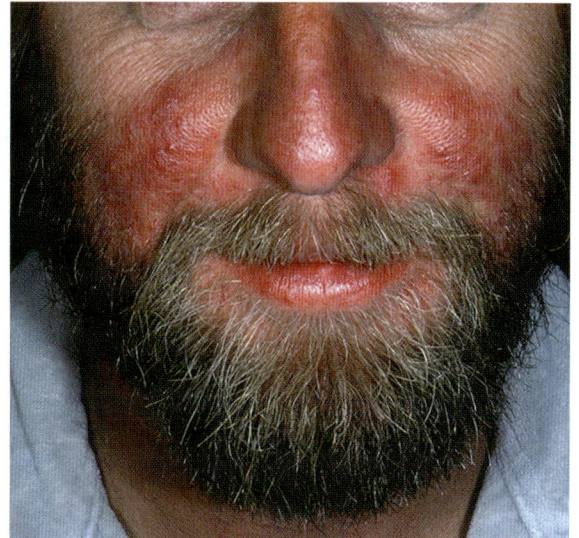

Fig. 13.65 Rosacea. Note the periocular sparing. *Courtesy The University of Utah and Oregon Health Sciences University Leonard Swinyer MD image collection.*

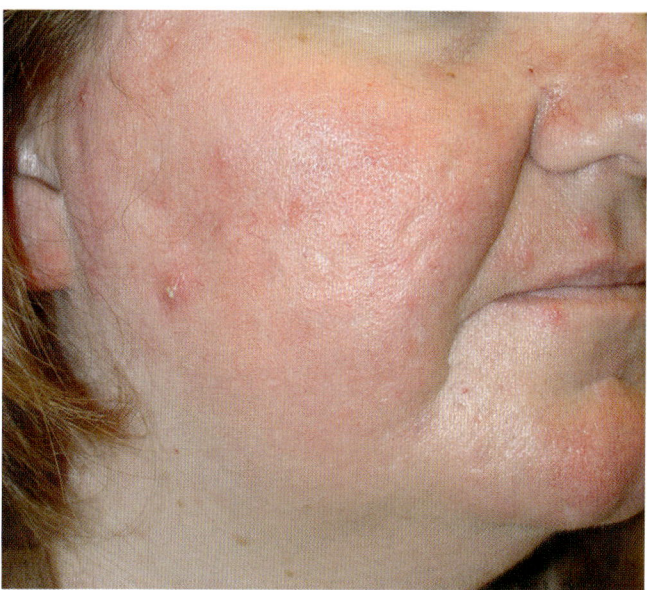

Fig. 13.66 Glandular rosacea.

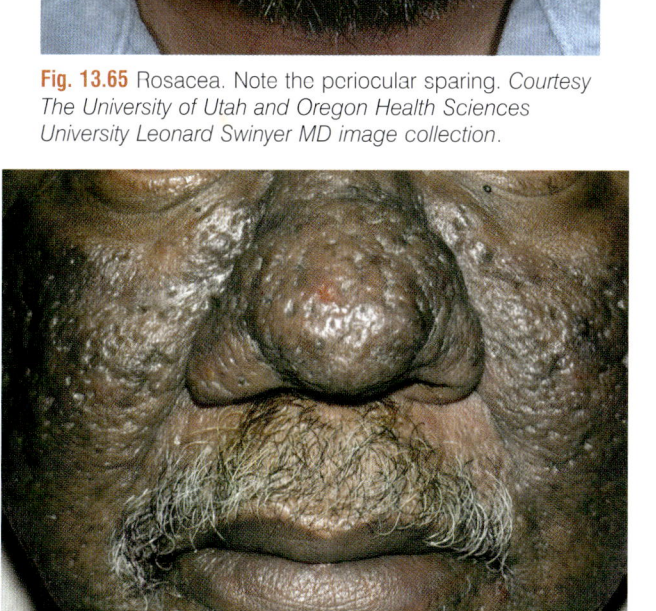

Fig. 13.67 Glandular rosacea with rhinophyma.

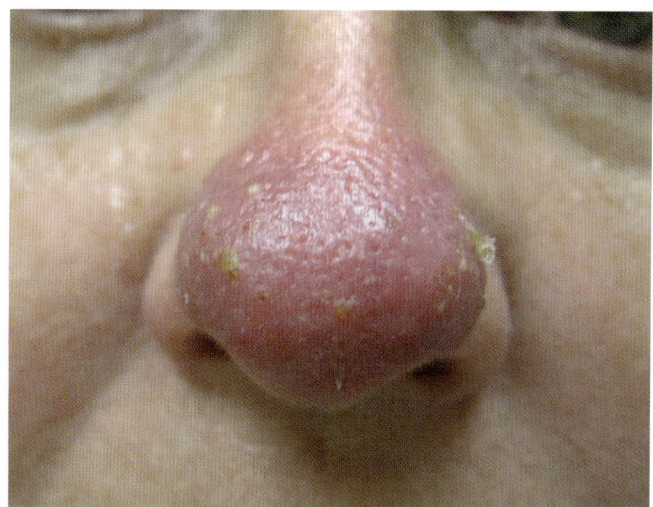

Fig. 13.68 Glandular rosacea with rhinophyma.

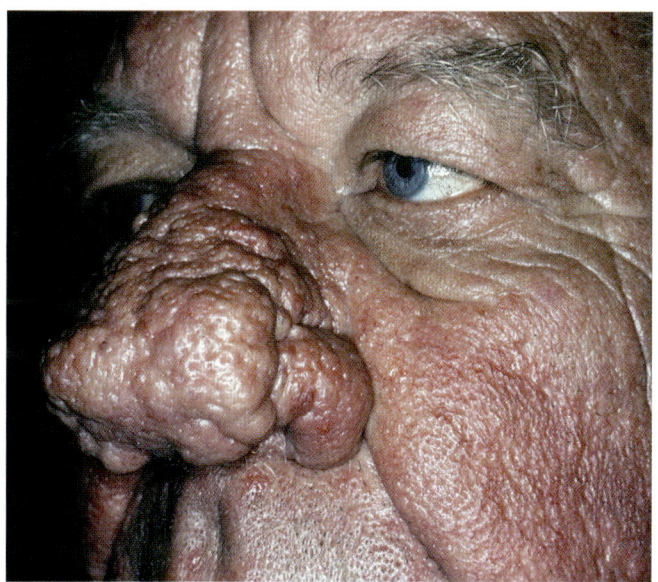

Fig. 13.69 Glandular rosacea with rhinophyma.

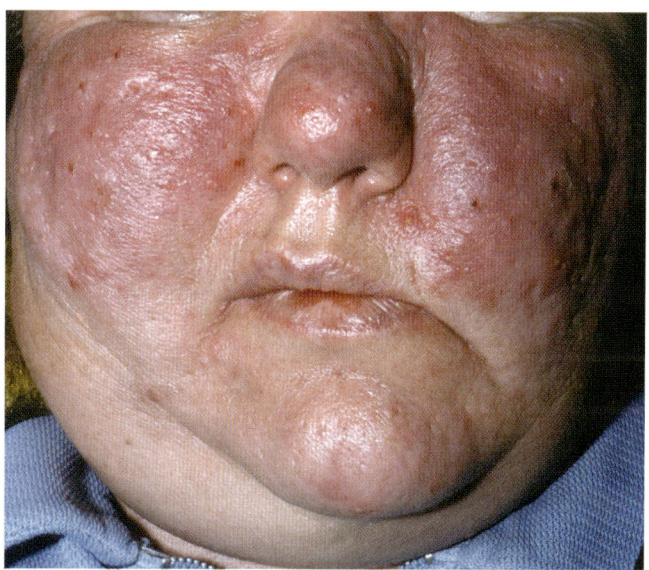

Fig. 13.70 Edema in severe rosacea. *Courtesy The University of Utah and Oregon Health Sciences University Leonard Swinyer MD image collection.*

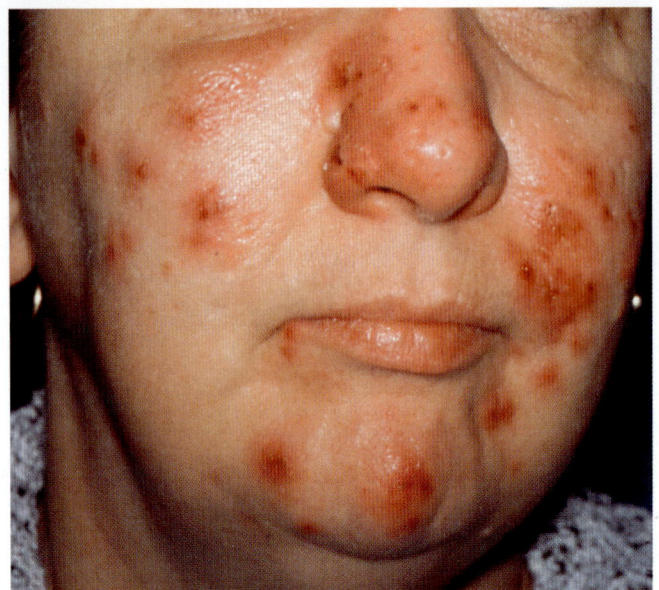

Fig. 13.71 Pyoderma faciale.

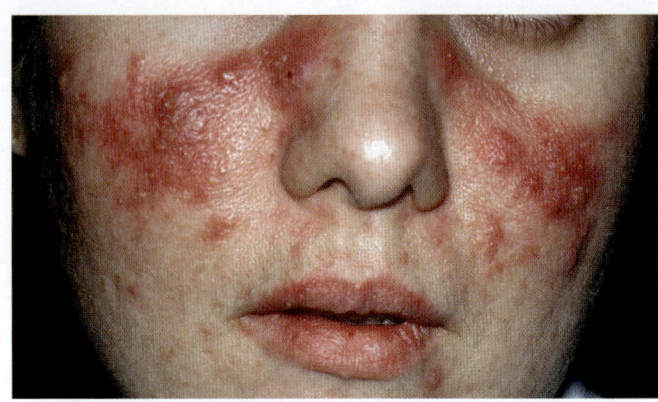

Fig. 13.72 Pyoderma faciale. *Courtesy Steven Binnick, MD.*

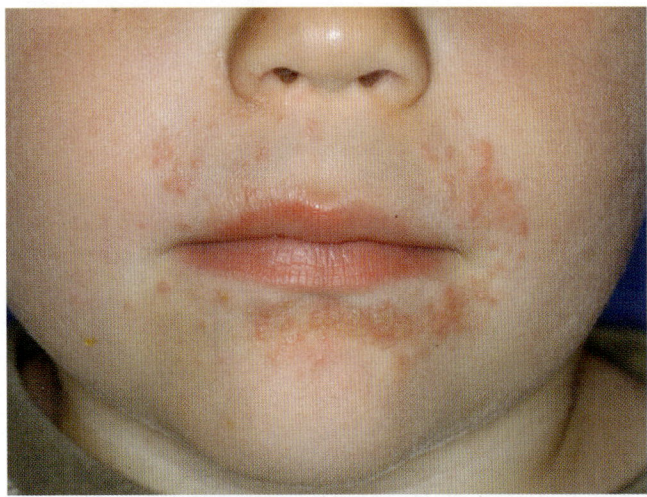

Fig. 13.73 Perioral dermatitis.

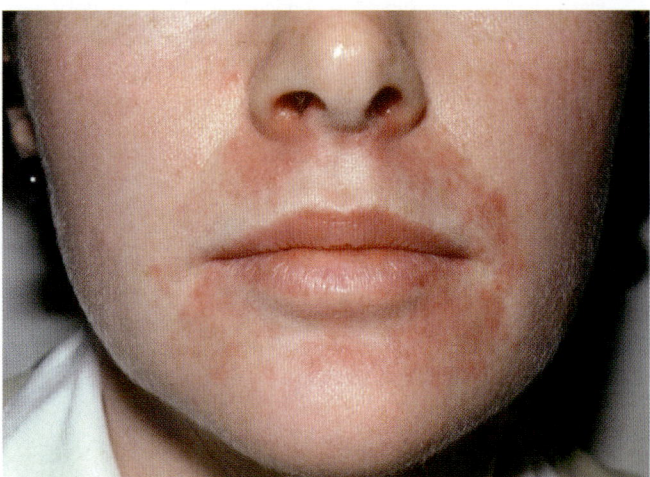

Fig. 13.74 Perioral dermatitis. *Courtesy Steven Binnick, MD.*

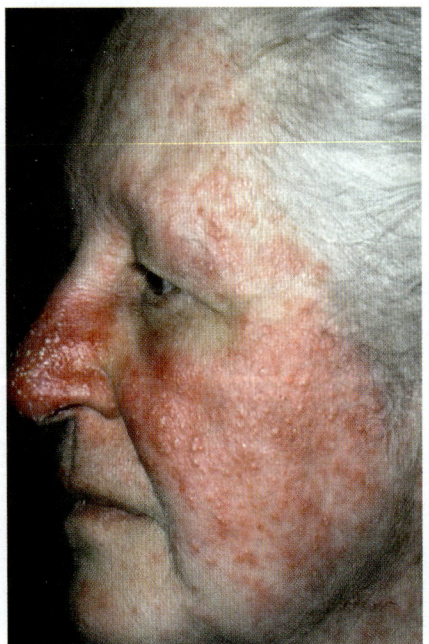

Fig. 13.75 Rosacea induced by topical steroids.

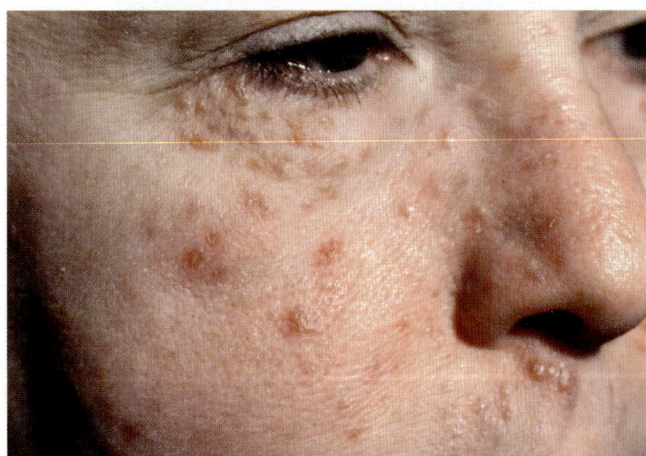

Fig. 13.76 Granulomatous facial dermatitis.

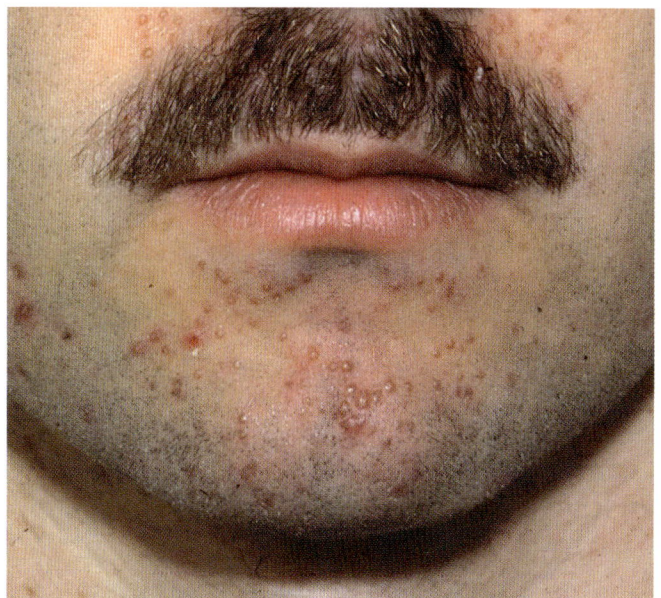

Fig. 13.77 Granulomatous facial dermatitis.

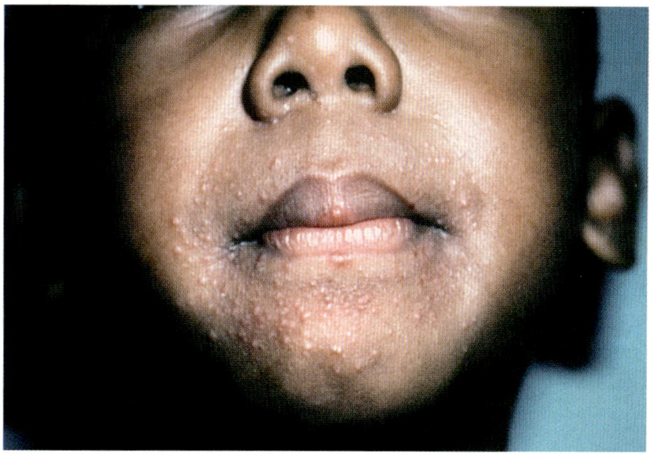

Fig. 13.78 Granulomatous facial dermatitis. *Courtesy Ken Greer, MD.*

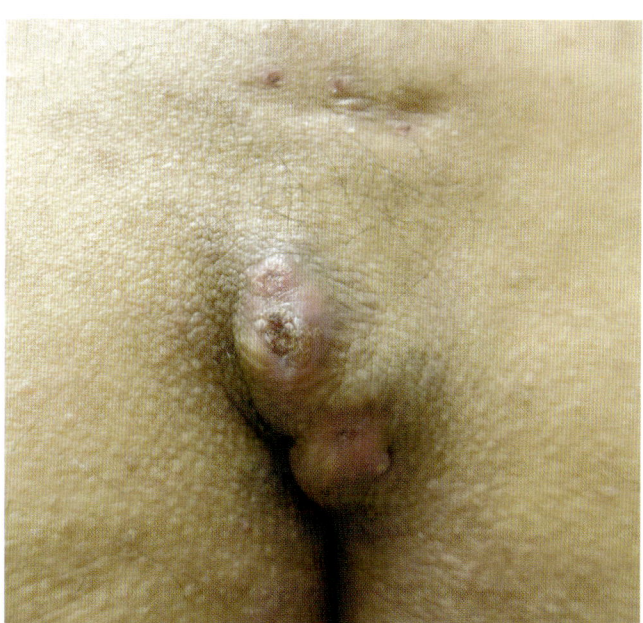

Fig. 13.79 Pilonidal cyst

Bacterial Infections 14

Bacterial infections create a multitude of skin lesions, from pustules, to necrotic nodules, to ulcers. These infections range from the superficial crusted erosions of impetigo to the systemic purpuric plaques of meningococcemia. This chapter categorizes these bacterial conditions into gram positive, gram negative, and others, including rickettsial diseases.

Recognizing the signs of bacterial infections is critical because most conditions will require treatment, whether topical or systemic. Staphylococcal skin infections can present with pustules, crusting, furuncles, or bullae in the case of bullous impetigo. Toxin-mediated conditions, such as staphylococcal scalded skin syndrome or toxic shock syndrome, will manifest as sunburn-like transient erythema accentuated in the folds. Streptococcal infections can present with pustules and crusting, as well as the firm painful erythematous plaques of cellulitis or erysipelas, or the ulcerative lesions in the case of ecthyma.

The anatomic locations involved can be a clue to which bacterial infections are most likely, such as in blistering distal dactylitis, perianal streptococcal infections, intertrigo, or gram-negative toe web infections.

Certain bacterial infections, along with deep fungal infections and atypical mycobacteria, should be included on the list of causes when evaluating a patient with isolated or multifocal necrotic dusky papules, nodules, ulcers, and eschars. This differential diagnosis is especially important in the setting of an immunocompromised host. These bacterial infections can include disseminated diseases from more common opportunistic organisms such as pseudomonas and those rarer conditions such as tularemia or anthrax.

Lastly, more distinctive conditions are included, such as the petechial exanthem of Rocky Mountain spotted fever, angiomatous papules of bacillary angiomatosis, and the expanding annular plaques of erythema migrans seen in Lyme disease.

Depending on the infections suspected, the workup for these conditions can include surface cultures, tissue cultures, and skin biopsy samples with subsequent special stains. This portion of the atlas contains images of common, uncommon, superficial, and disseminated bacterial infections and their many manifestations in the skin.

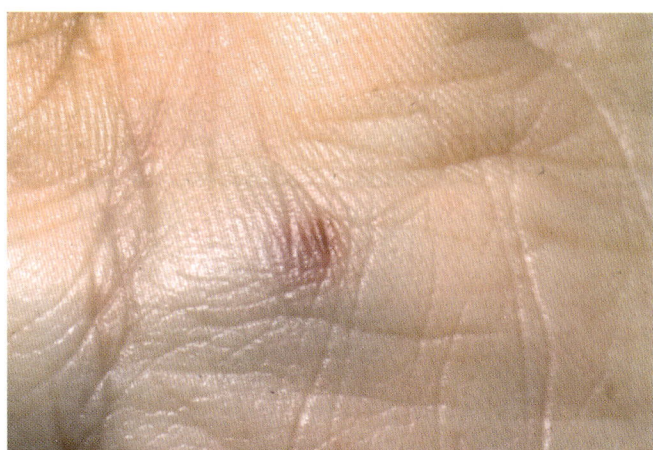

Fig. 14.1 Janeway spot in staphylococcal endocarditis. *Courtesy Curt Samlaska, MD.*

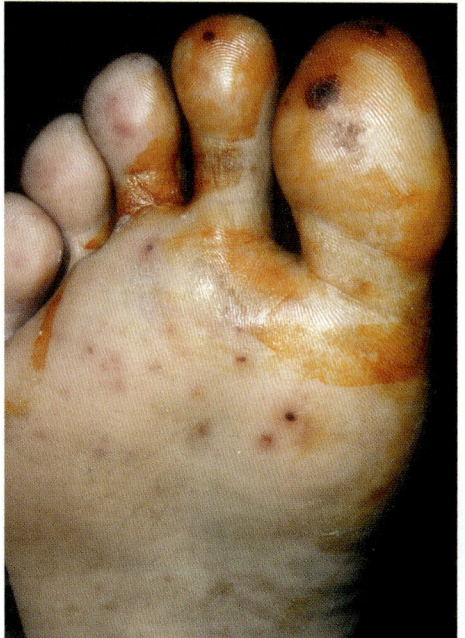

Fig. 14.2 Staphylococcal emboli from an infected iliac aneurysm. *Courtesy Curt Samlaska, MD.*

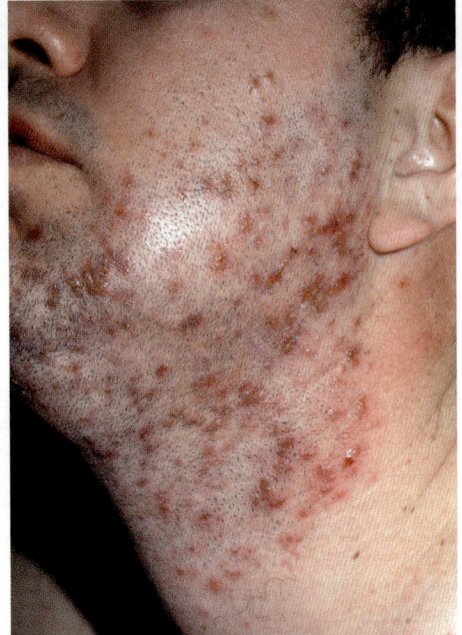

Fig. 14.3 Sycosis barbae. *Courtesy Steven Binnick, MD.*

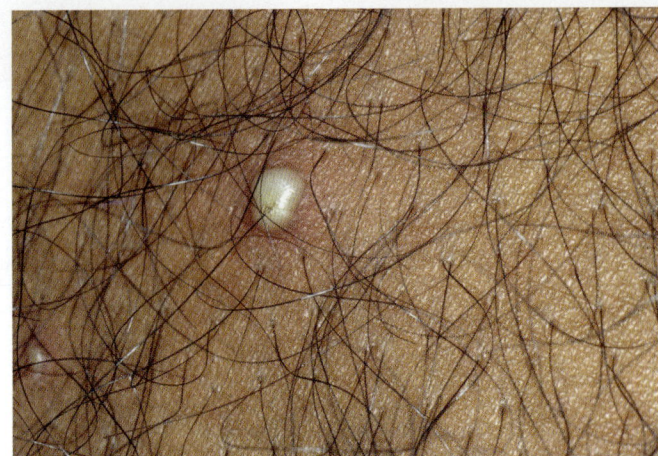

Fig. 14.4 Staphylococcal folliculitis.

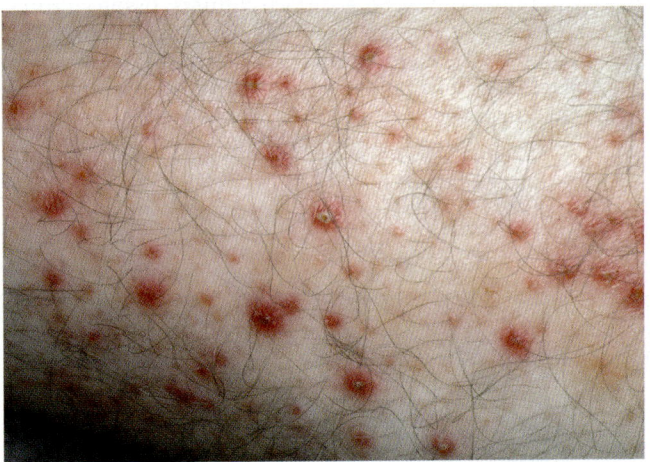

Fig. 14.5 Staphylococcal folliculitis.

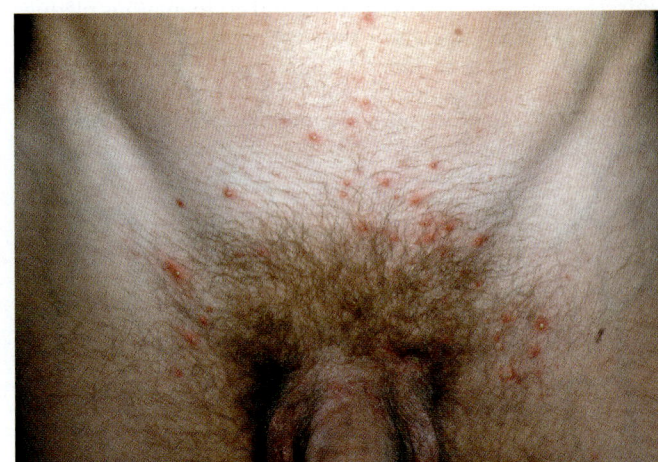

Fig. 14.6 Staphylococcal folliculitis.

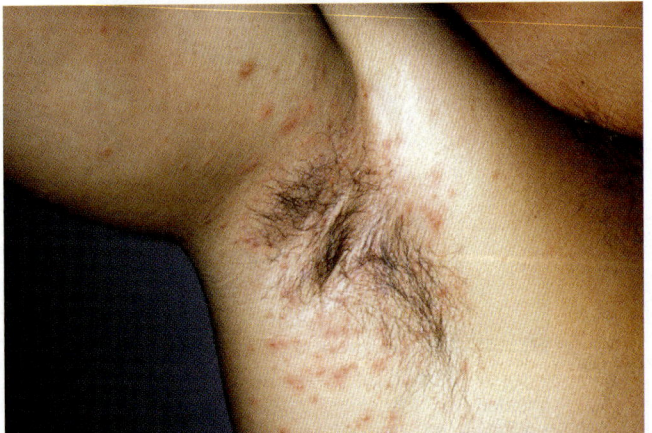

Fig. 14.7 Staphylococcal folliculitis.

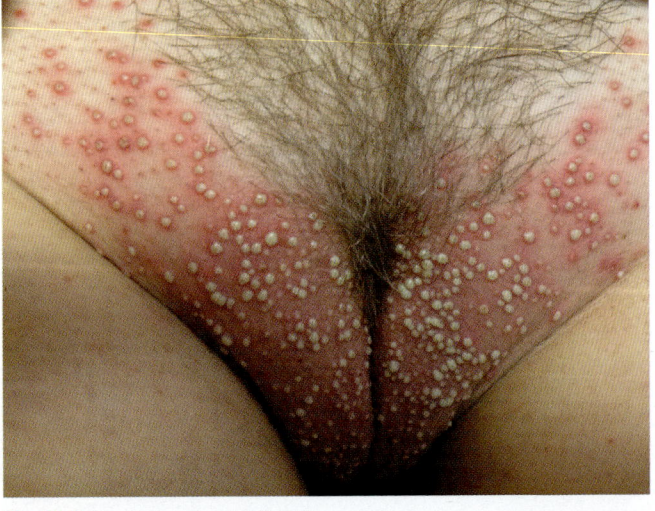

Fig. 14.8 Staphylococcal folliculitis.

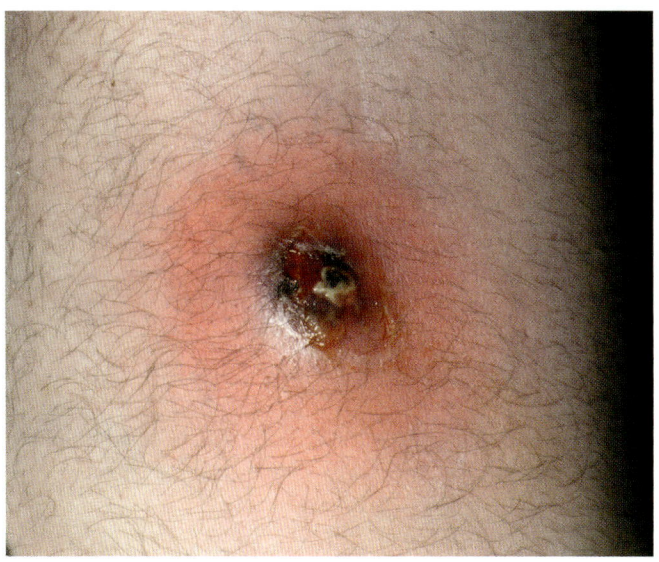

Fig. 14.9 Staphylococcal abscess. *Courtesy Steven Binnick, MD.*

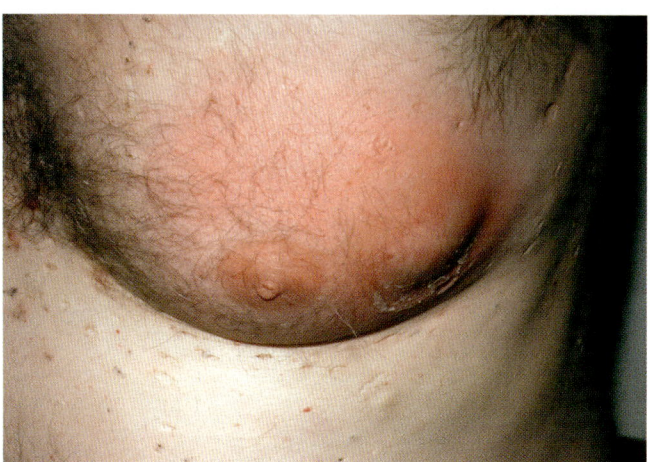

Fig. 14.10 Staphylococcal abscess. *Courtesy Steven Binnick, MD.*

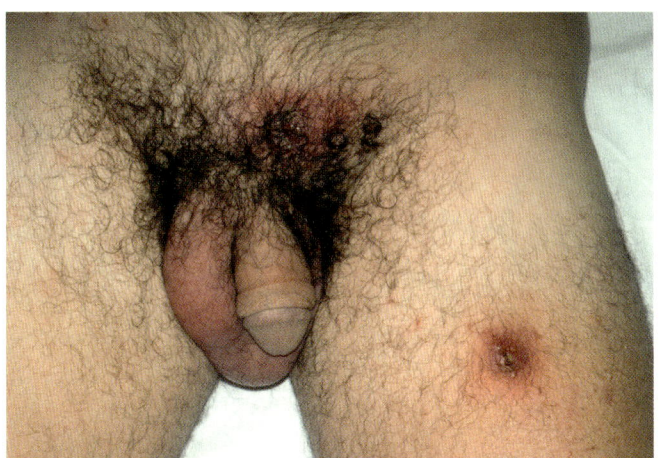

Fig. 14.11 Staphylococcal abscess.

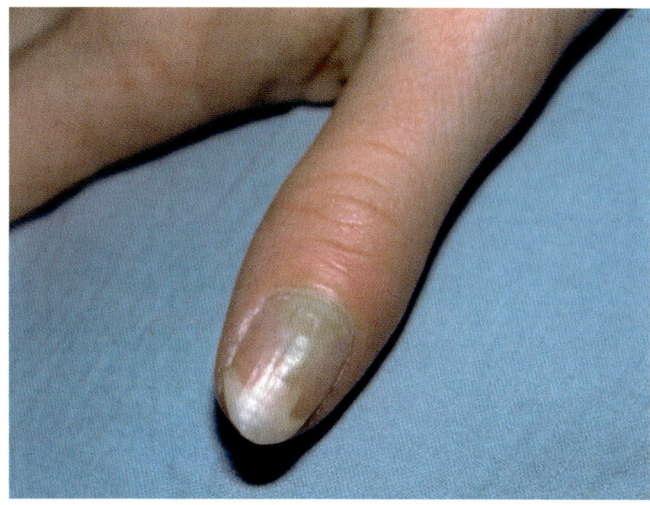

Fig. 14.12 Subungual staphylococcal abscess. *Courtesy Ken Greer, MD.*

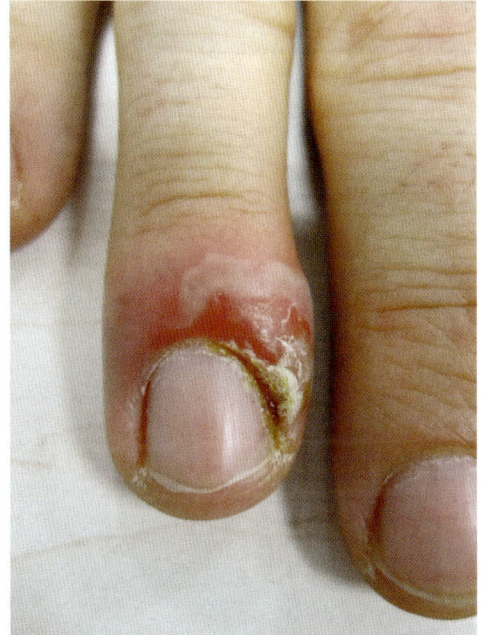

Fig. 14.13 Acute paronychia.

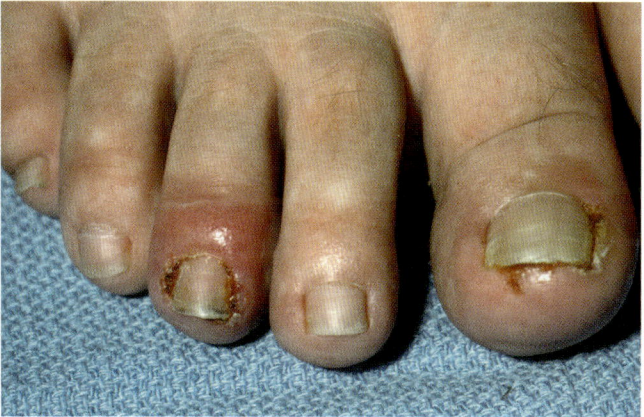

Fig. 14.14 Acute paronychia.

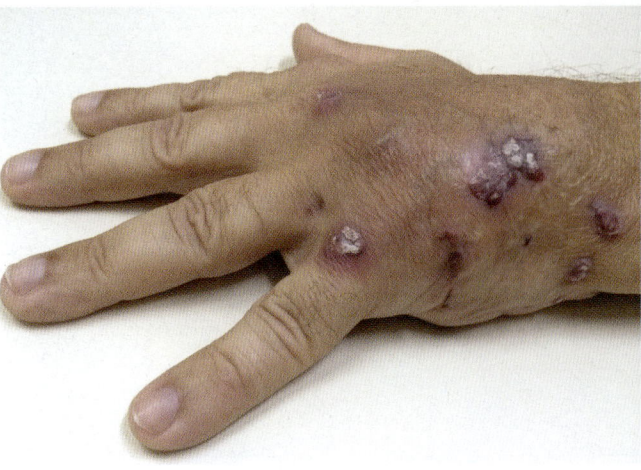

Fig. 14.15 Botryomycosis. *Courtesy Dermatology Division, University of Campinas, Brazil.*

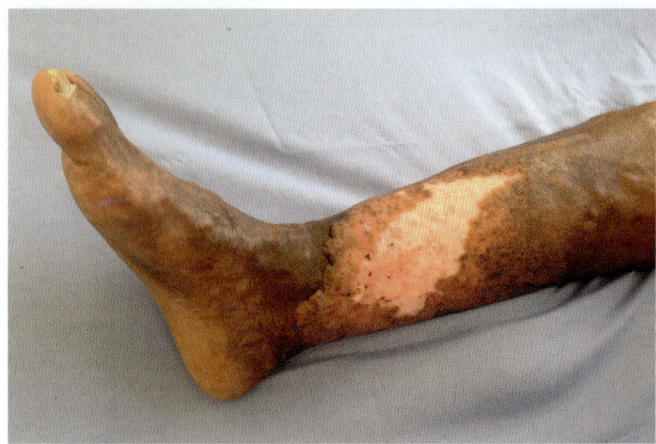

Fig. 14.16 Botryomycosis. *Courtesy Tatiana C. P. Cordeiro de Andrade, MD.*

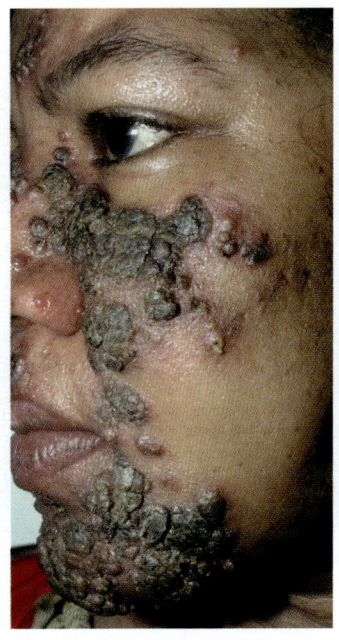

Fig. 14.17 Vegetating pyoderma.

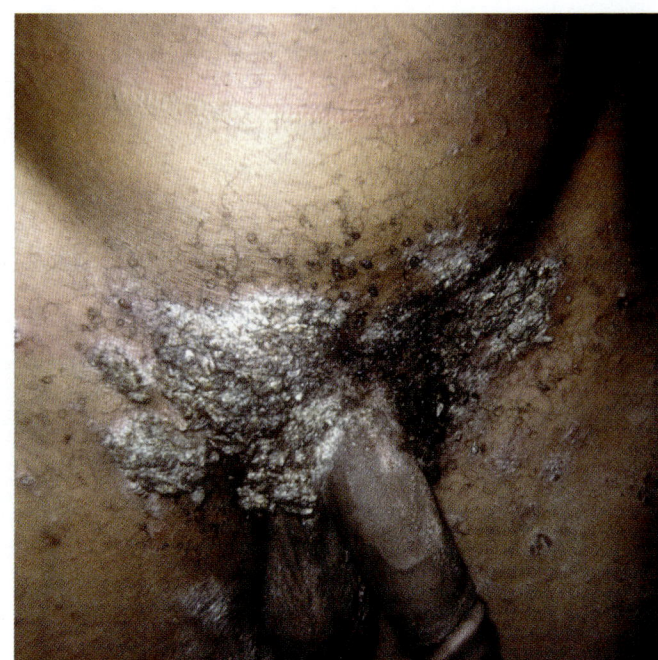

Fig. 14.18 Vegetating pyoderma.

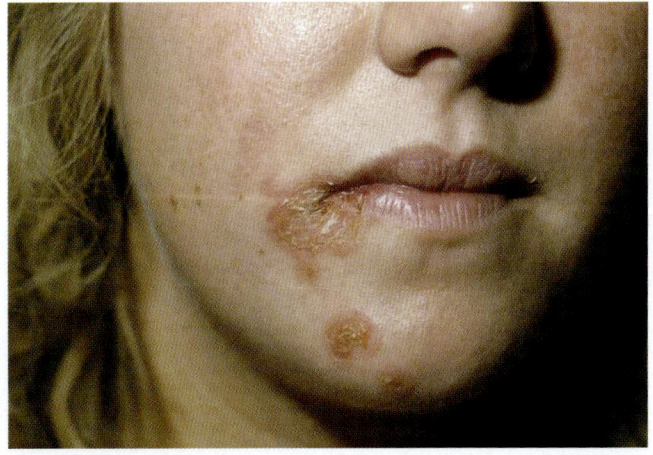

Fig. 14.19 Impetigo.

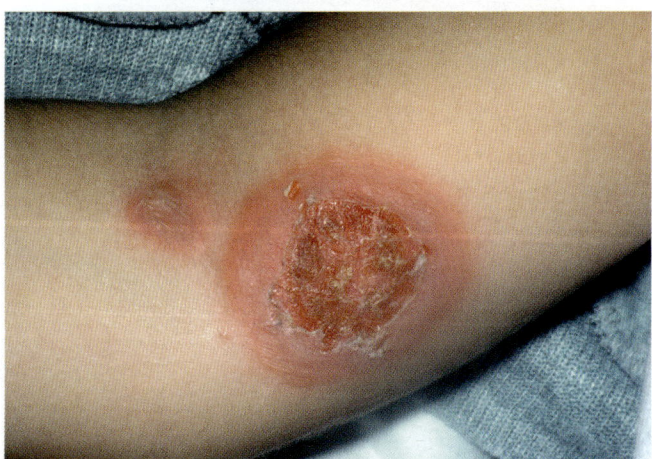

Fig. 14.20 Impetigo. *Courtesy Steven Binnick, MD.*

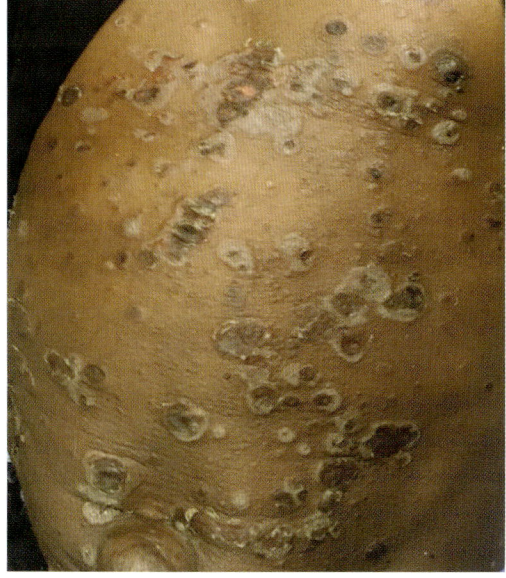

Fig. 14.21 Bullous impetigo.

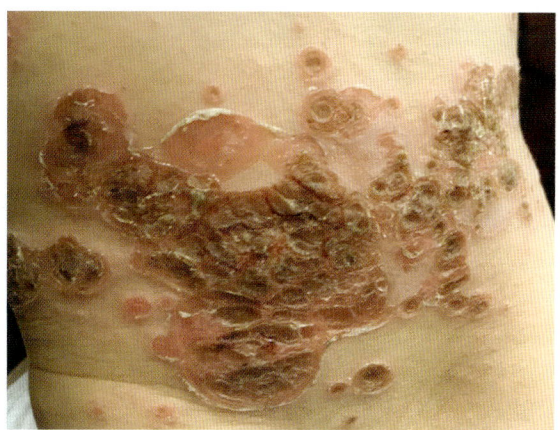

Fig. 14.22 Bullous impetigo, back.

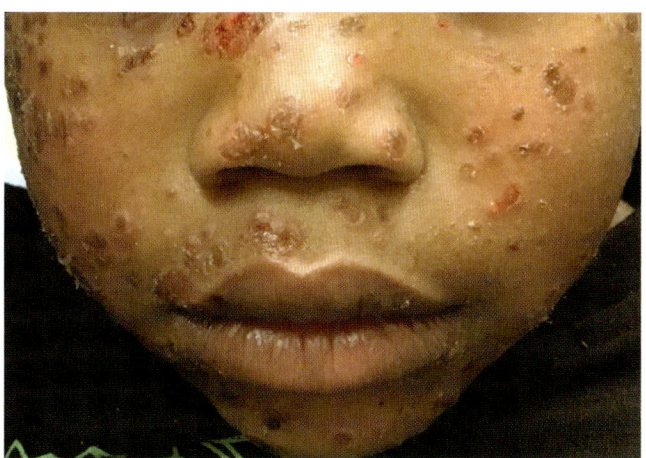

Fig. 14.23 Bullous impetigo.

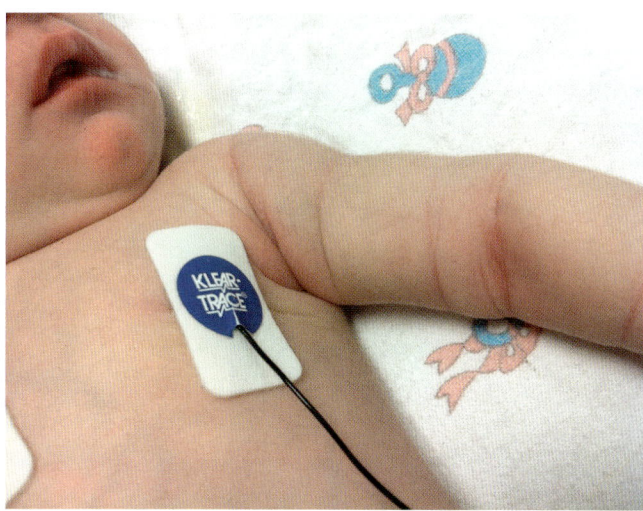

Fig. 14.24 Early staphylococcal scalded skin syndrome. Note erythema accentuated in folds.

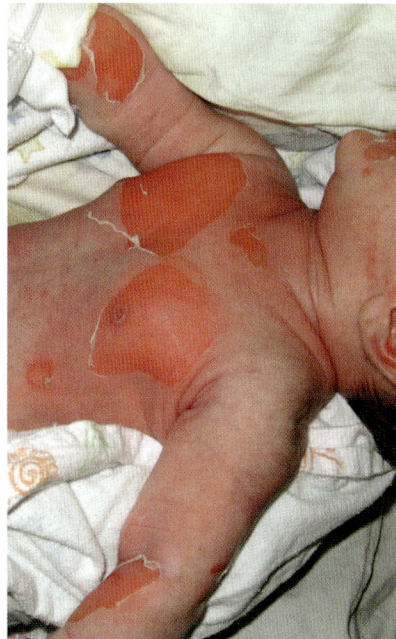

Fig. 14.26 Staphylococcal scalded skin syndrome.

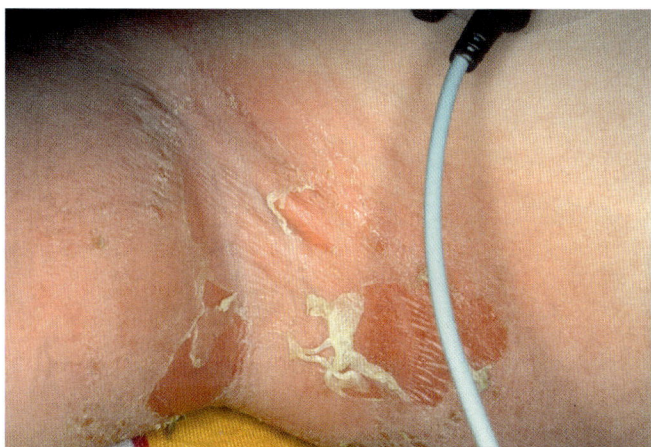

Fig. 14.25 Staphylococcal scalded skin syndrome.

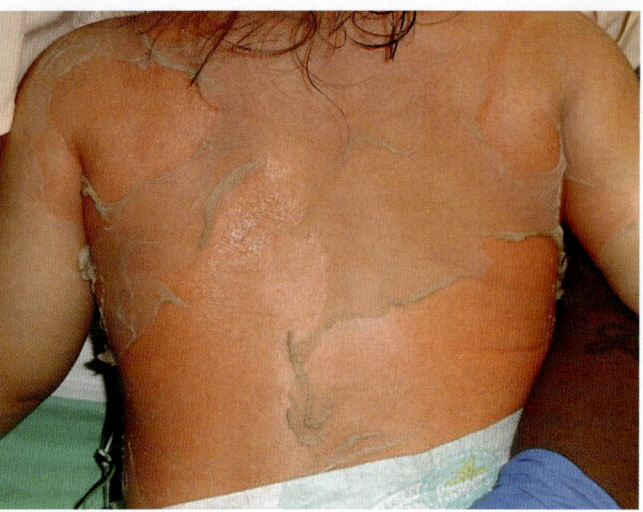

Fig. 14.27 Staphylococcal scalded skin syndrome.

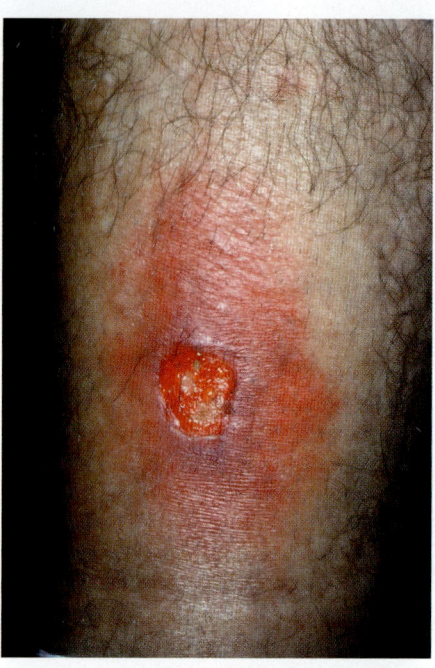

Fig. 14.28 Ecthyma.

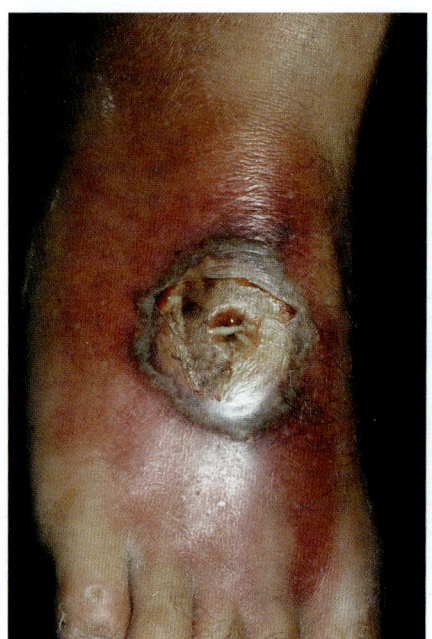

Fig. 14.29 Ecthyma. *Courtesy Curt Samlaska, MD.*

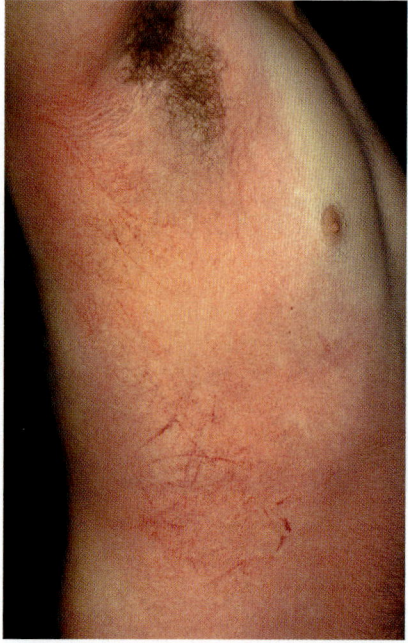

Fig. 14.30 Scarlet fever.

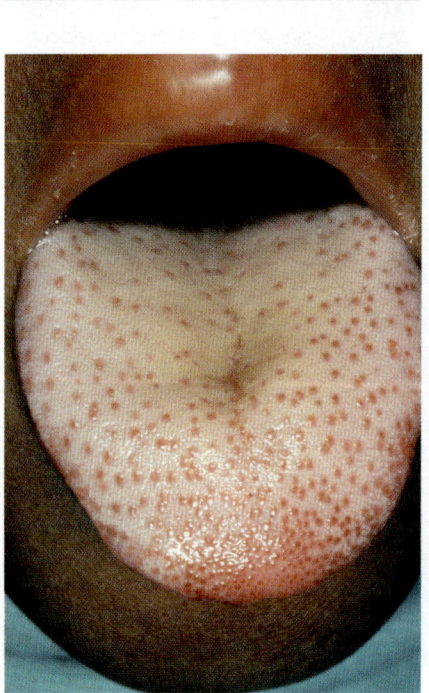

Fig. 14.31 Strawberry tongue.

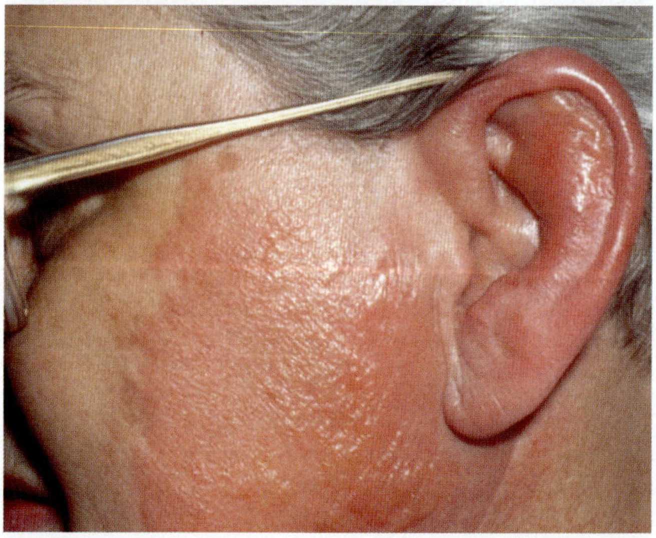

Fig. 14.32 Erysipelas.

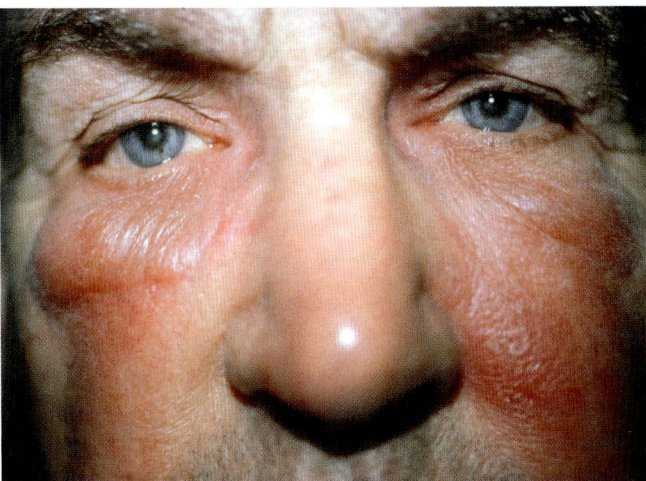

Fig. 14.33 Erysipelas.

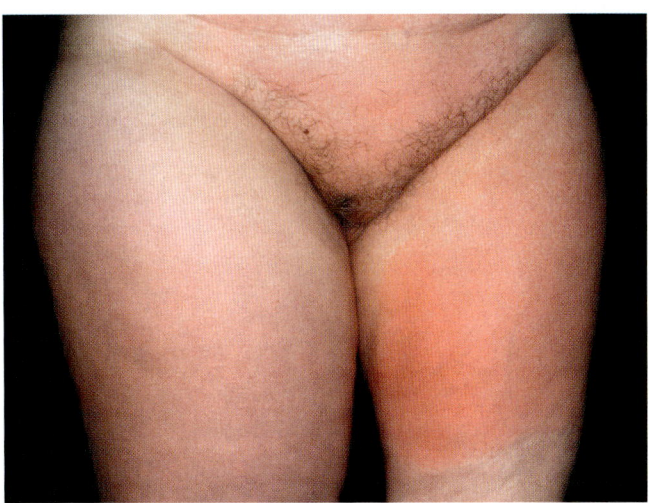

Fig. 14.34 Erysipelas. *Courtesy Steven Binnick, MD.*

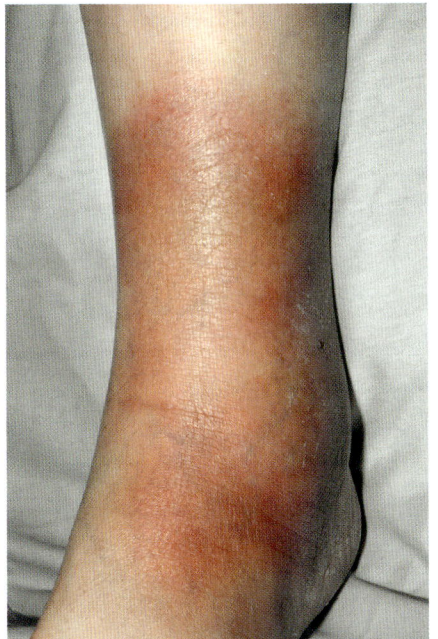

Fig. 14.35 Cellulitis. *Courtesy Steven Binnick, MD.*

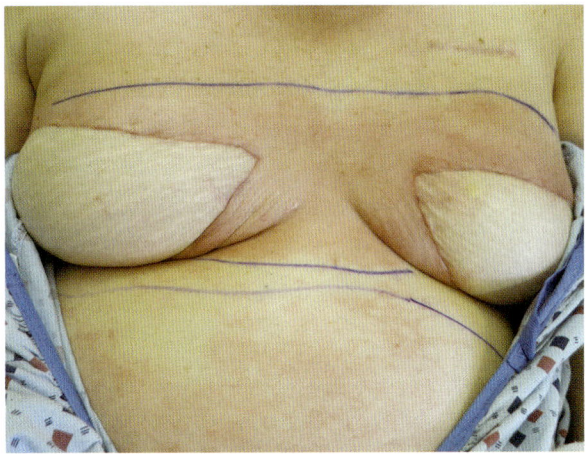

Fig. 14.36 Cellulitis after mastectomy and breast reconstruction (note sparing of areas with different lymphatic drainage).

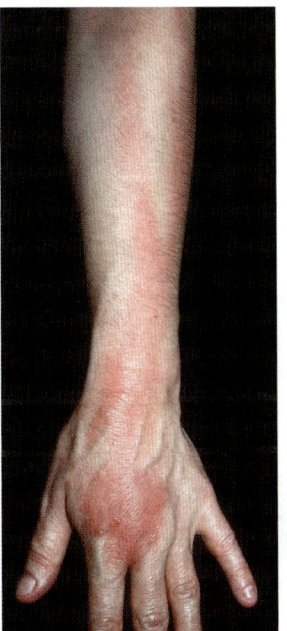

Fig. 14.37 Lymphangitis. *Courtesy The University of Utah and Oregon Health Sciences University Leonard Swinyer MD image collection.*

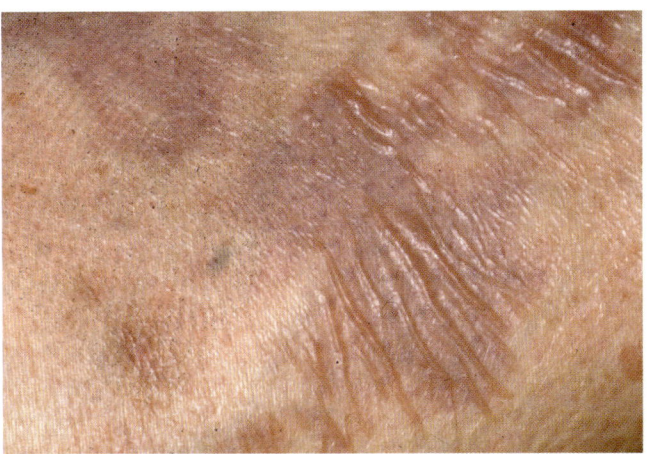

Fig. 14.38 Early necrotizing fasciitis.

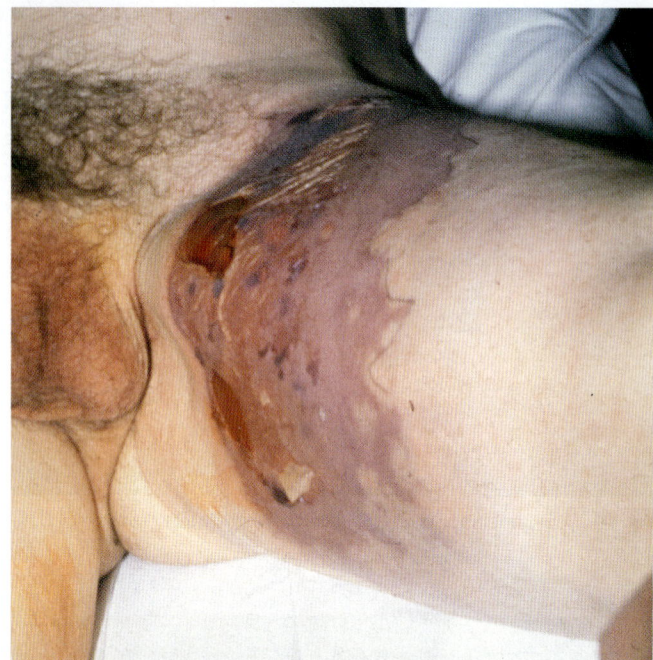

Fig. 14.39 Necrotizing fasciitis.

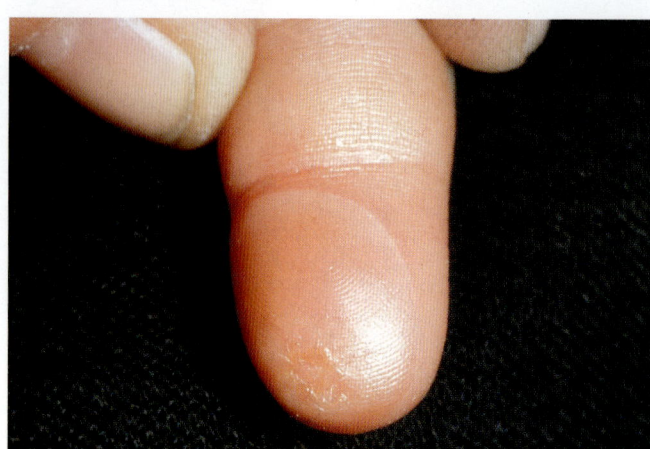

Fig. 14.40 Blistering dactylitis.

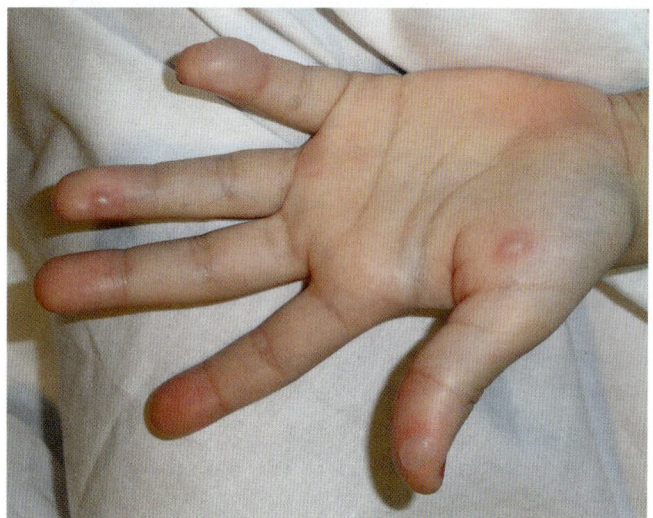

Fig. 14.41 Blistering dactylitis. *Courtesy Scott Norton, MD.*

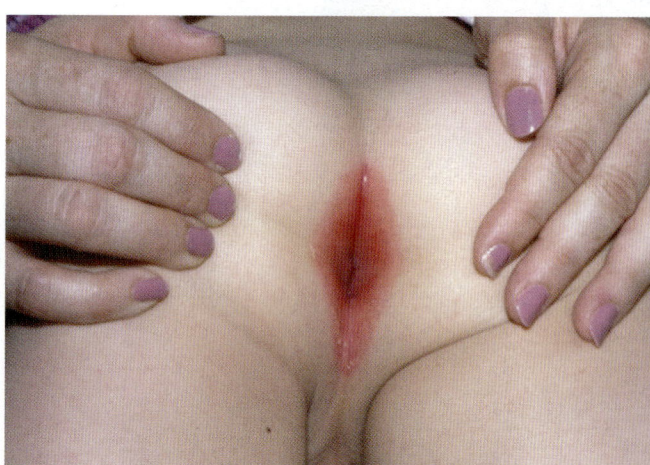

Fig. 14.42 Perianal streptococcal infection.

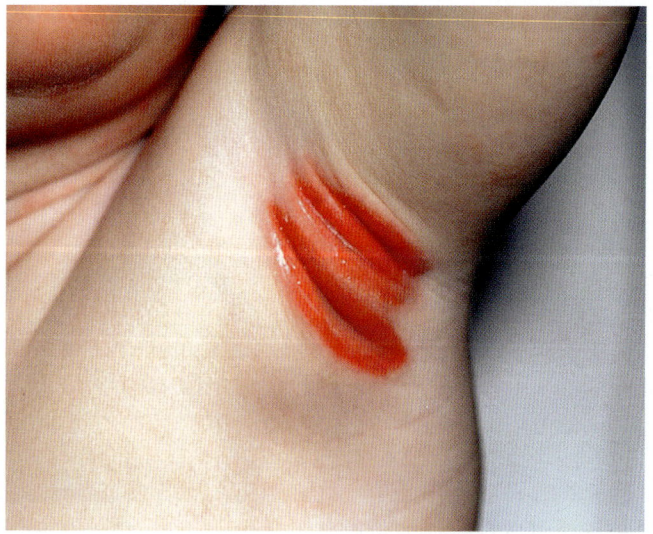

Fig. 14.43 Streptococcal intertrigo. *Courtesy Paul Honig, MD.*

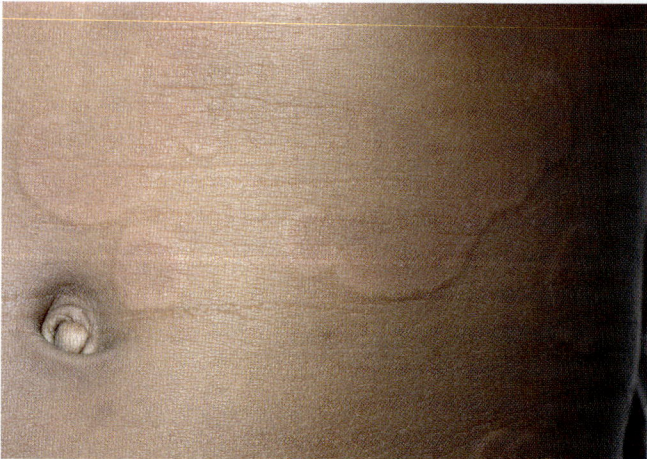

Fig. 14.44 Erythema marginatum. *Courtesy Steven Binnick, MD.*

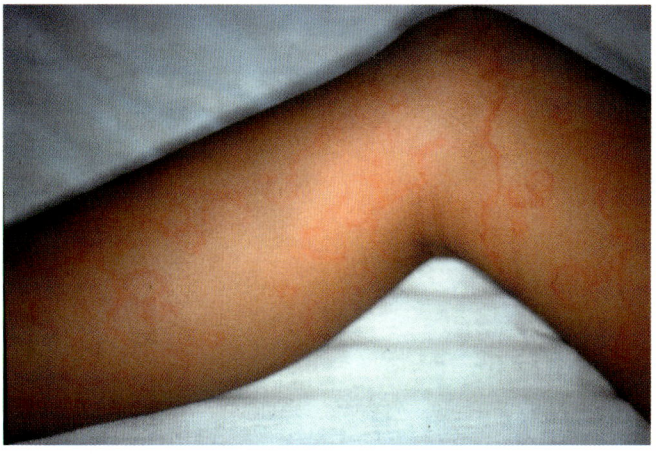

Fig. 14.45 Erythema marginatum.

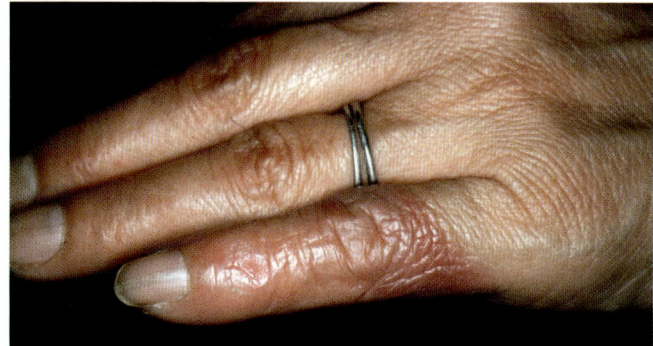

Fig. 14.46 Erysipeloid. *Courtesy Steven Binnick, MD.*

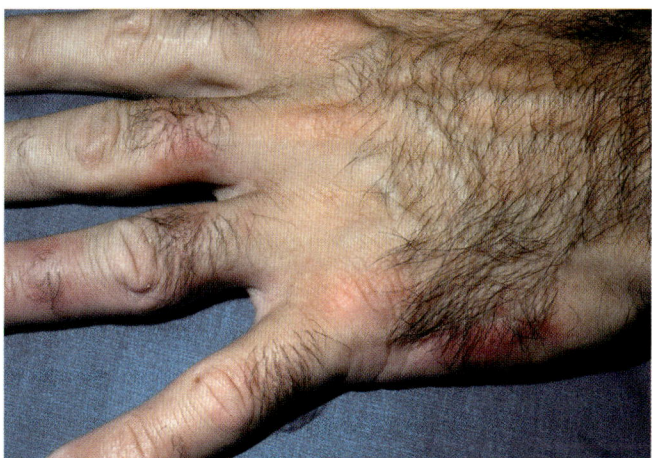

Fig. 14.47 Erysipeloid.

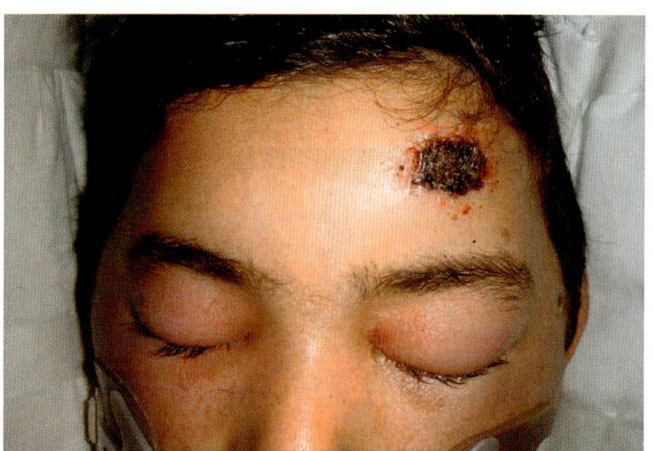

Fig. 14.48 Anthrax with severe edema. *Courtesy Steve Krivda, MD.*

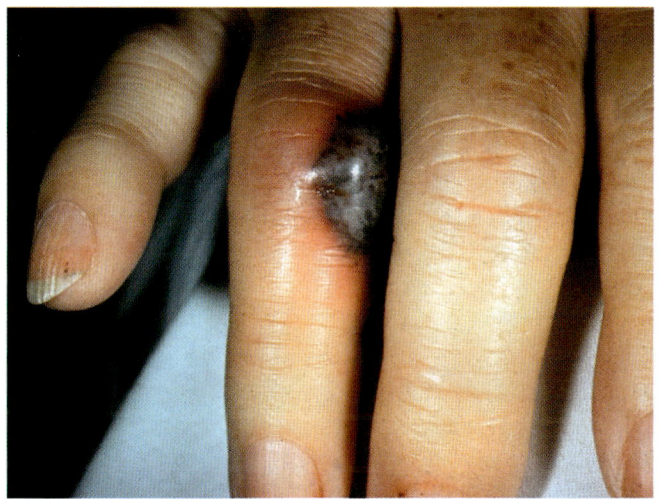

Fig. 14.49 Cutaneous diphtheria.

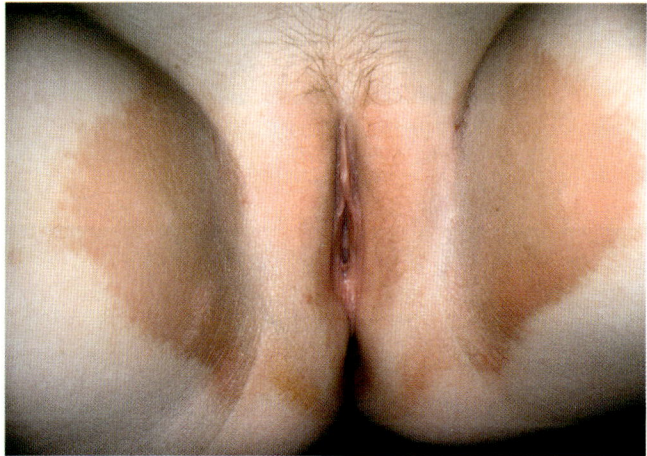

Fig. 14.50 Erythrasma. *Courtesy Steven Binnick, MD.*

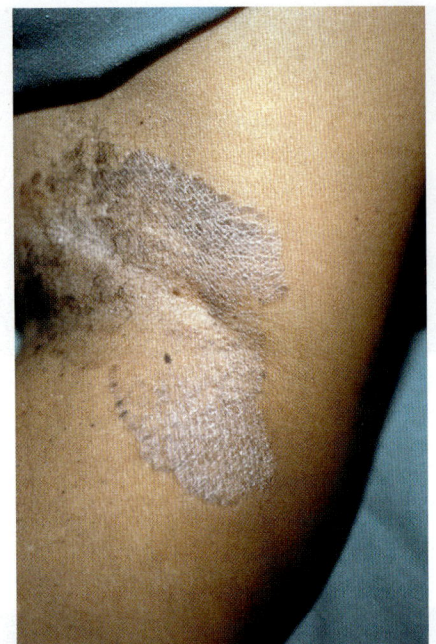

Fig. 14.51 Erythrasma.

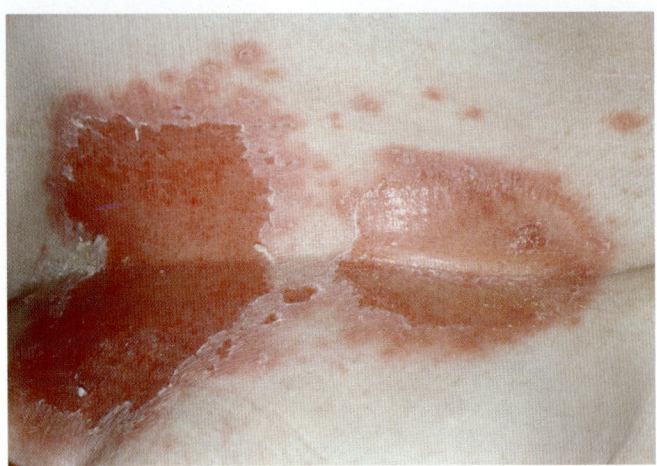

Fig. 14.52 Intertrigo.

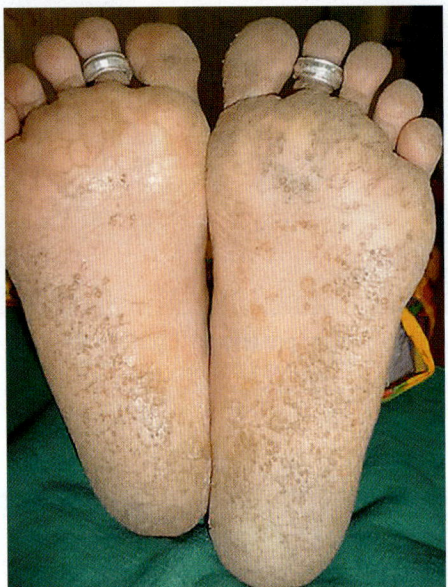

Fig. 14.53 Pitted keratolysis. *Courtesy Shyam Verma, MBBS, DVD.*

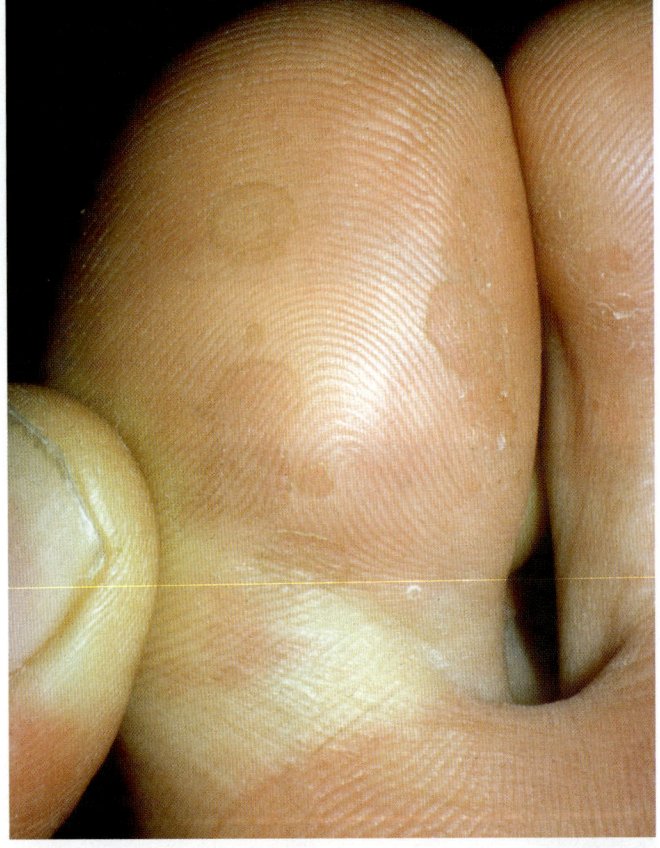

Fig. 14.54 Pitted keratolysis.

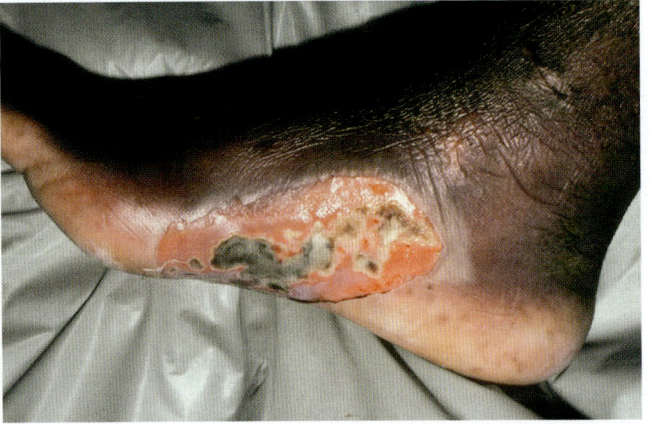

Fig. 14.55 Clostridial ulcer. *Courtesy Steven Binnick, MD.*

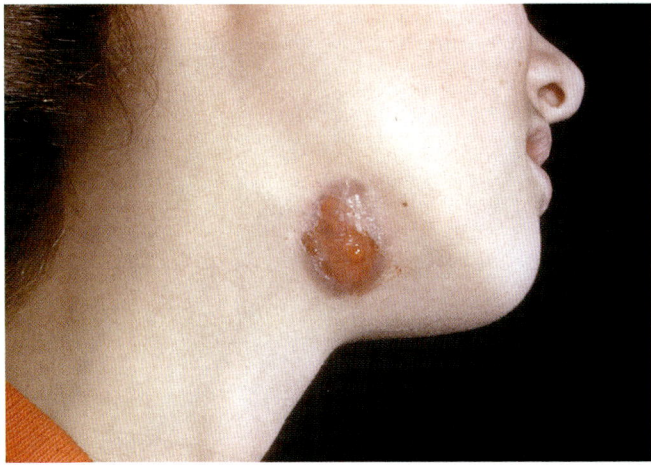

Fig. 14.56 Actinomycosis. *Courtesy Steven Binnick, MD.*

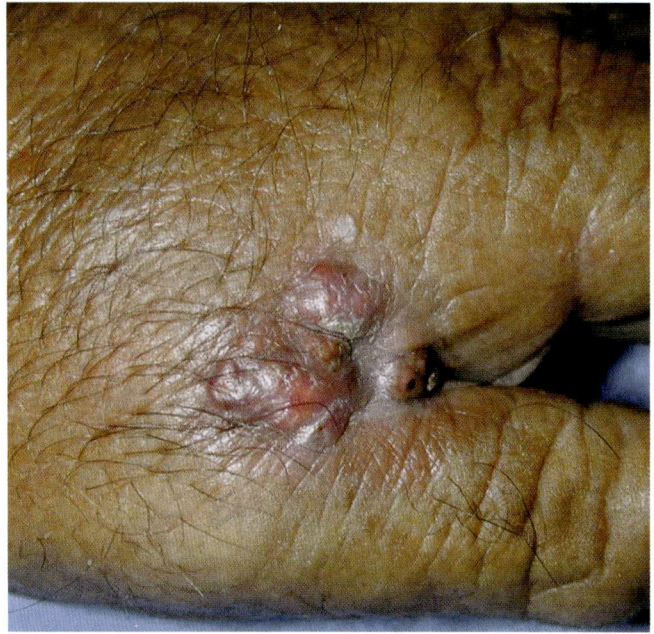

Fig. 14.57 Actinomycosis. *Courtesy Dermatology Division, University of Campinas, Brazil.*

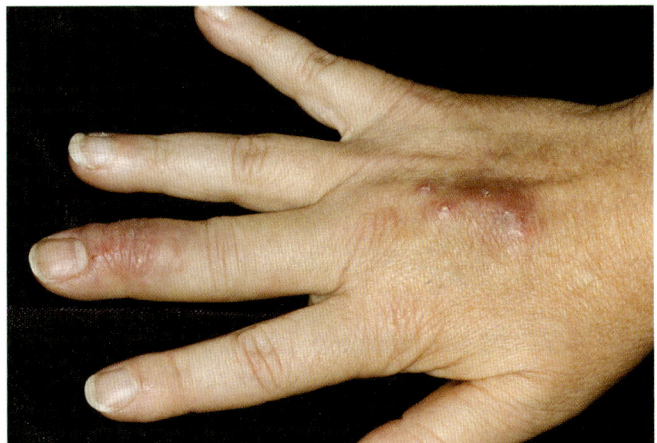

Fig. 14.58 Nocardia with sporotrichoid spread.

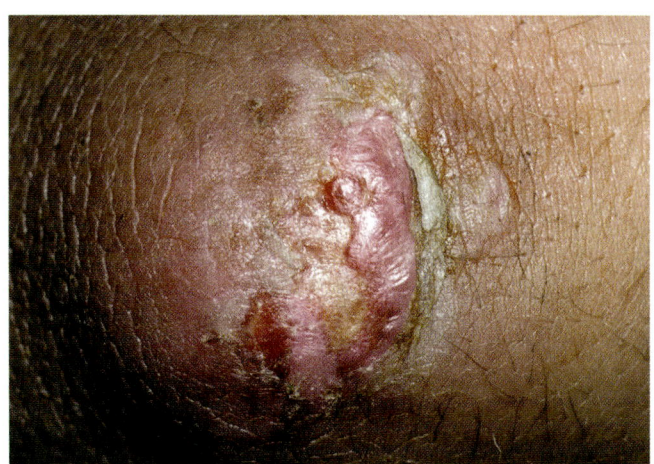

Fig. 14.59 Nocardia. *Courtesy Curt Samlaska, MD.*

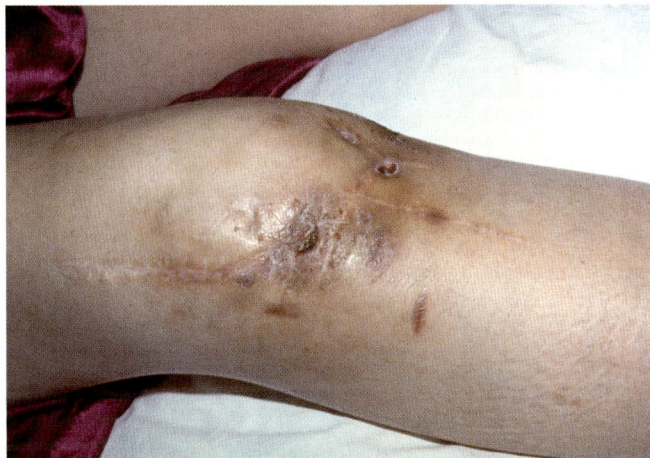

Fig. 14.60 Nocardia.

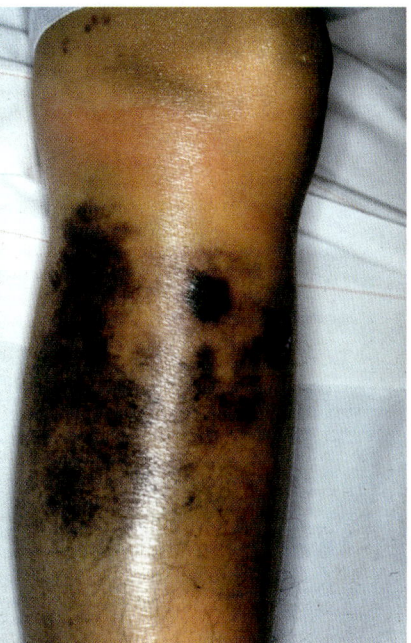

Fig. 14.61 Ecthyma gangrenosum.

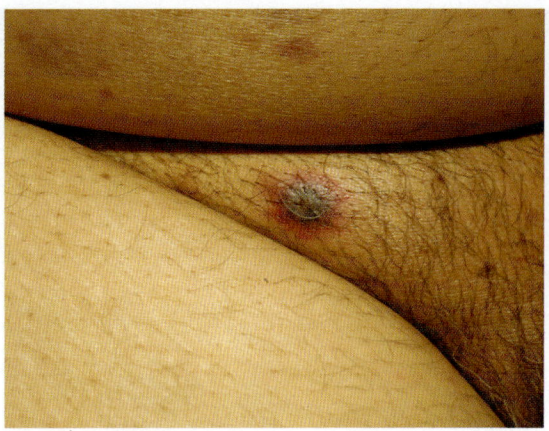

Fig. 14.62 Ecthyma gangrenosum (disseminated *Pseudomonas*).

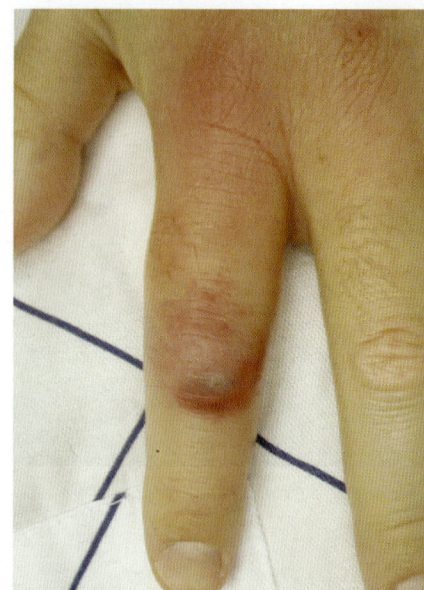

Fig. 14.63 Ecthyma gangrenosum (primary inoculation of *Pseudomonas* spp.).

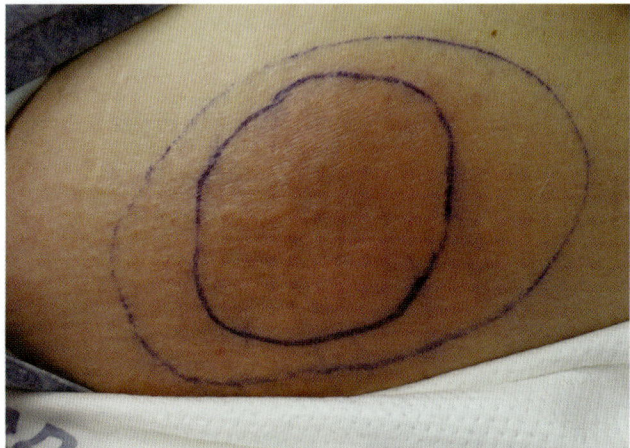

Fig. 14.64 Disseminated *Stenotrophomonas* infection.

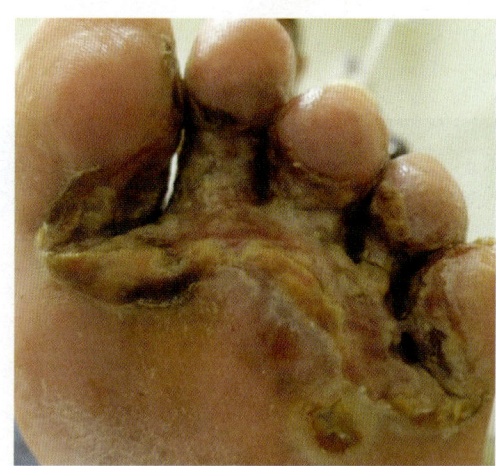

Fig. 14.65 Gram-negative toe web infection (*Pseudomonas* spp.).

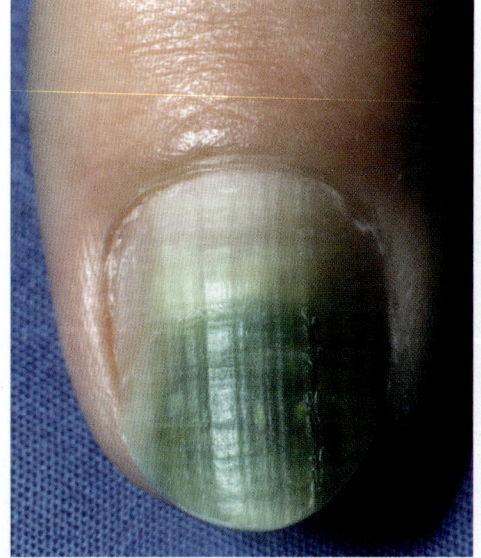

Fig. 14.66 Green nail secondary to *Pseudomonas* infection. *Courtesy Steven Binnick, MD.*

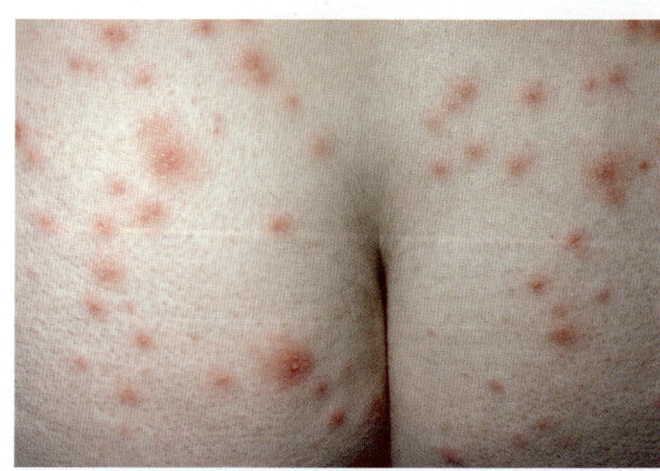

Fig. 14.67 Hot tub folliculitis. *Courtesy Steven Binnick, MD.*

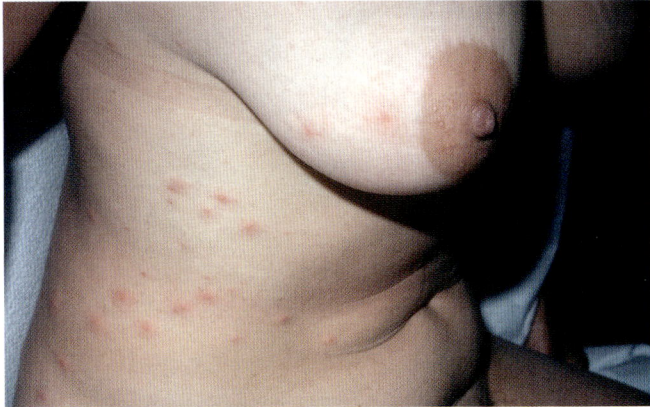

Fig. 14.68 Hot tub folliculitis. *Courtesy Steven Binnick, MD.*

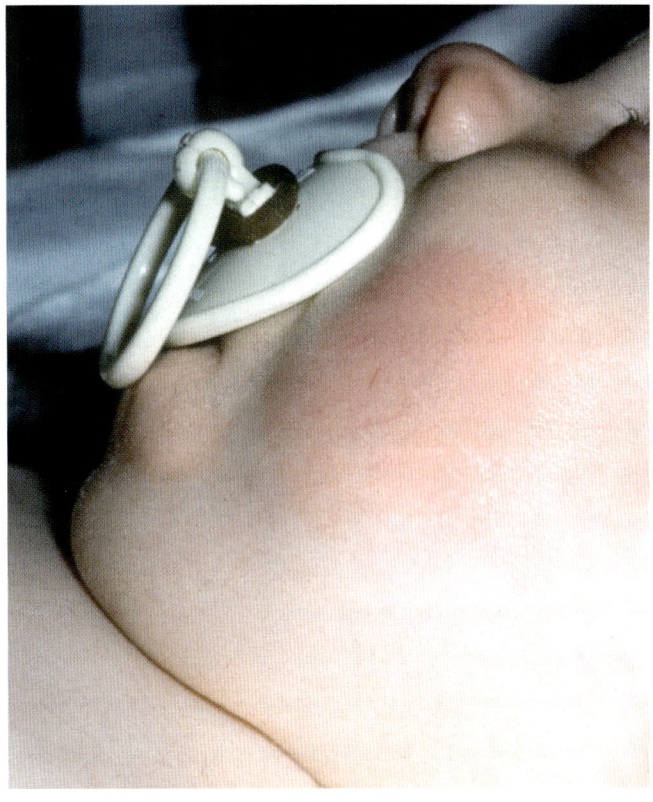

Fig. 14.69 *Haemophilus influenzae* cellulitis.

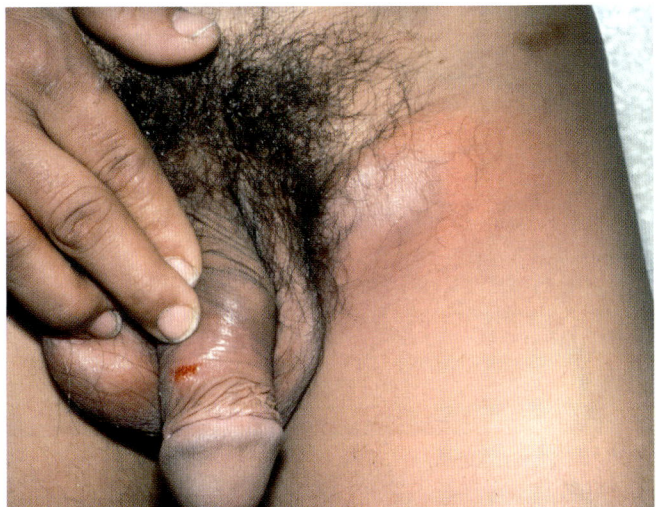

Fig. 14.70 Chancroid.

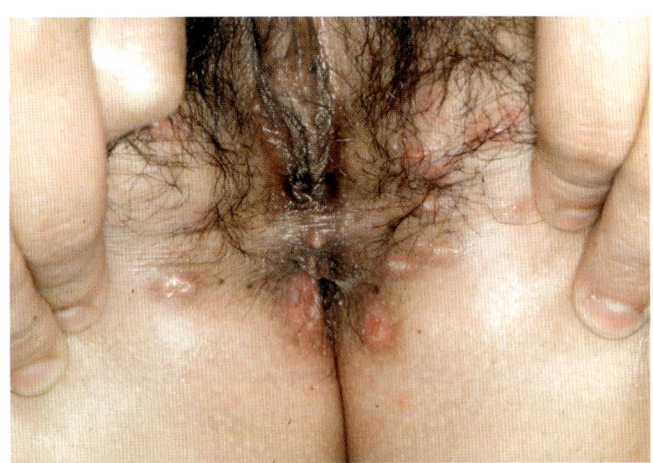

Fig. 14.71 Chancroid.

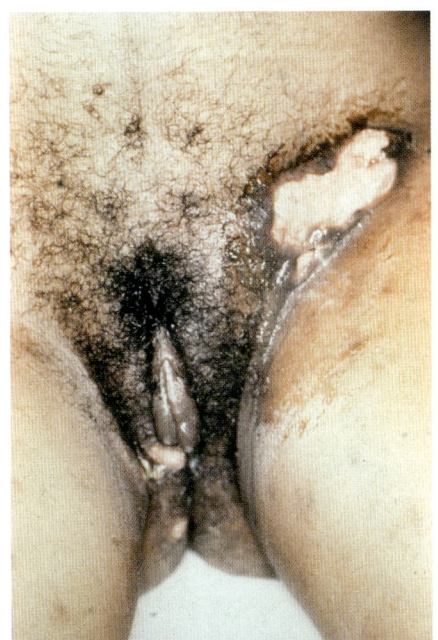

Fig. 14.72 Chancroid. *Courtesy Scott Norton, MD.*

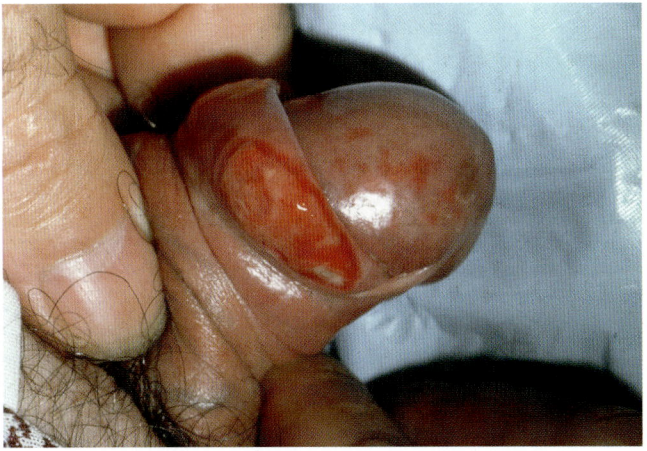

Fig. 14.73 Granuloma inguinale.

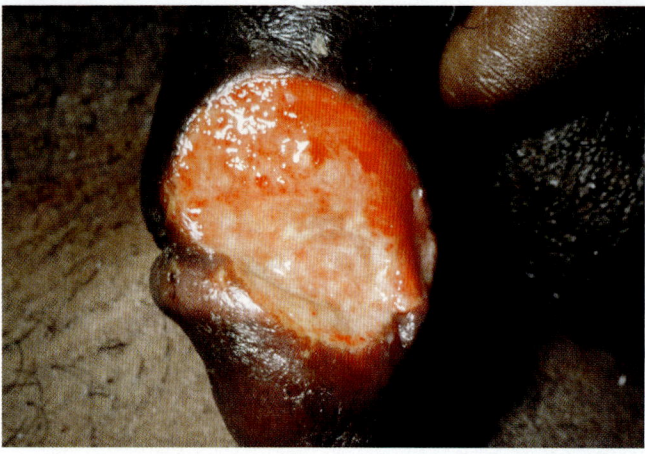

Fig. 14.74 Granuloma inguinale.

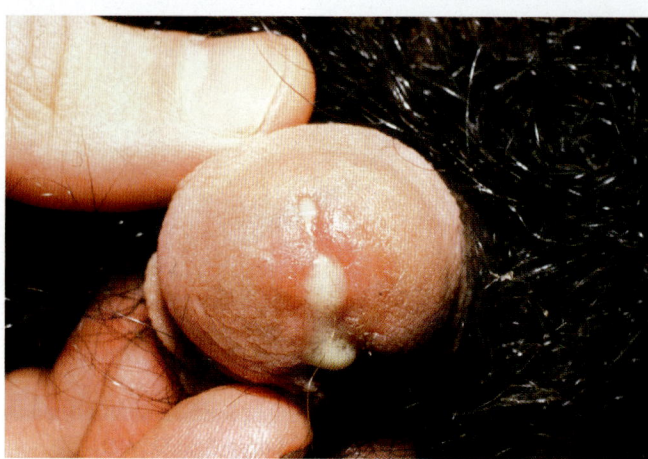

Fig. 14.75 Gonococcal infection.

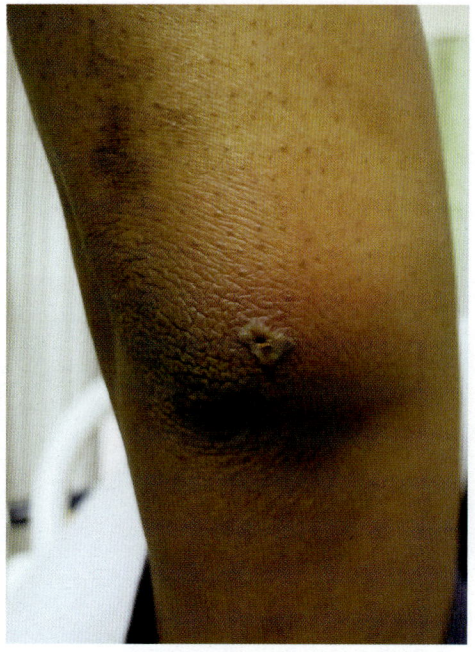

Fig. 14.76 Gonococcemia.

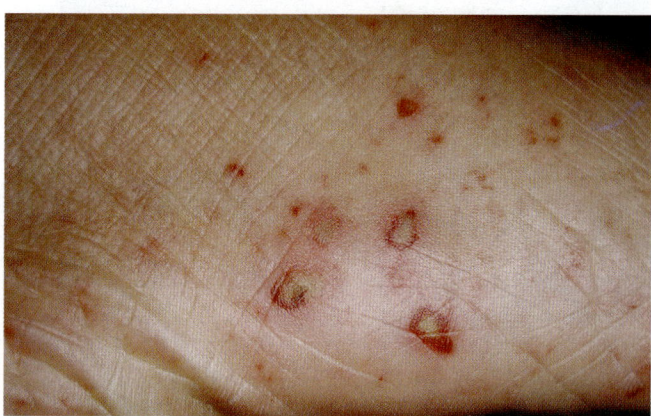

Fig. 14.77 Gonococcemia. *Courtesy National Cheng Kung University, Taiwan.*

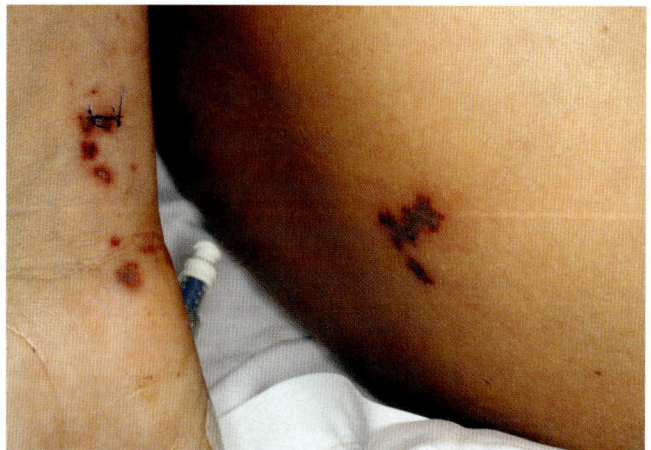

Fig. 14.78 Meningococcemia. *Courtesy Scott Norton, MD.*

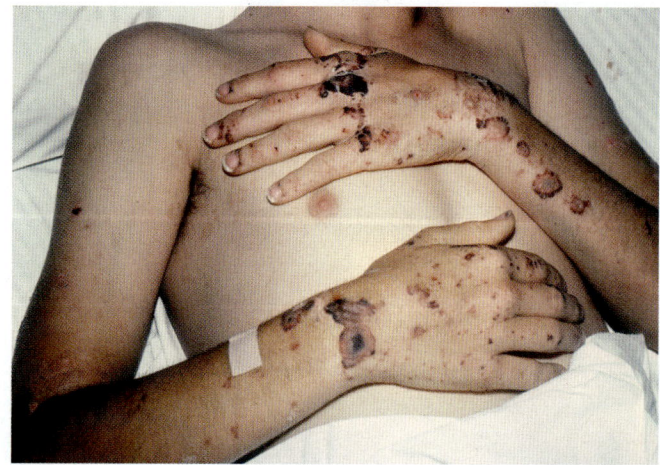

Fig. 14.79 Meningococcemia.

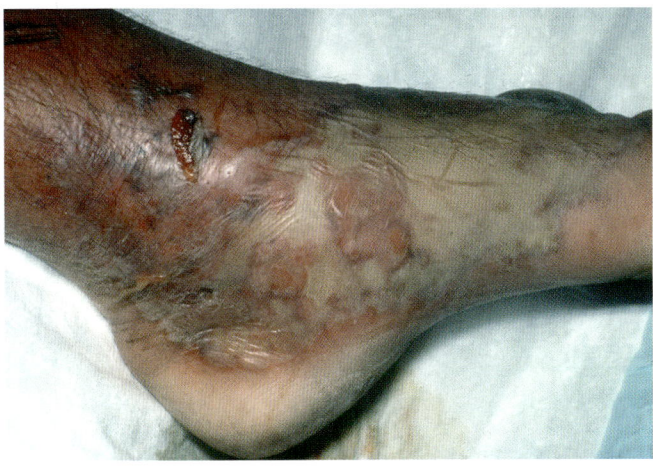

Fig. 14.80 *Vibrio vulnificus* infection. *Courtesy Curt Samlaska, MD.*

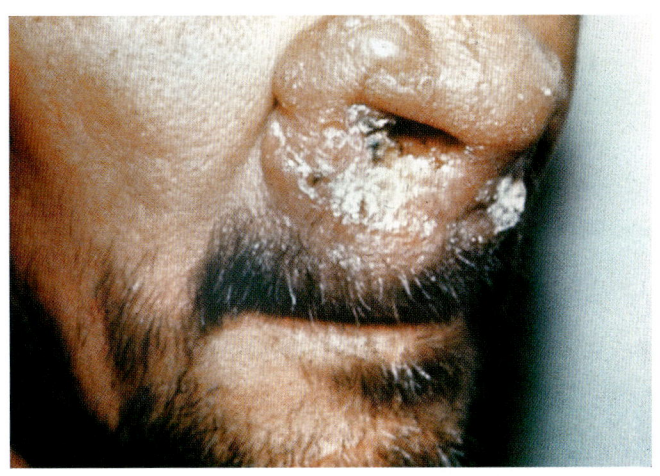

Fig. 14.81 Rhinoscleroma. *Courtesy Steven Binnick, MD.*

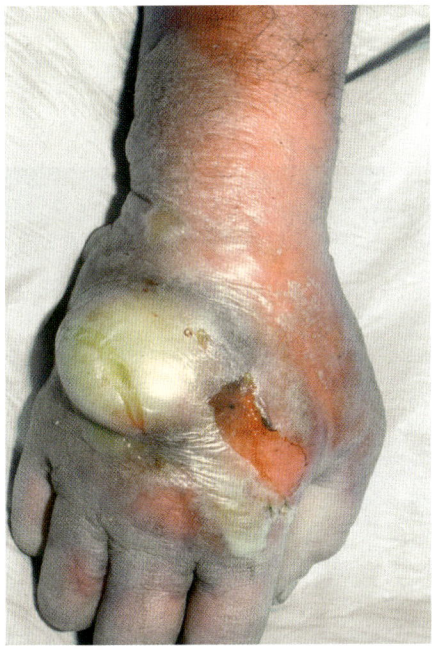

Fig. 14.82 Infected human bite. *Courtesy Steven Binnick, MD.*

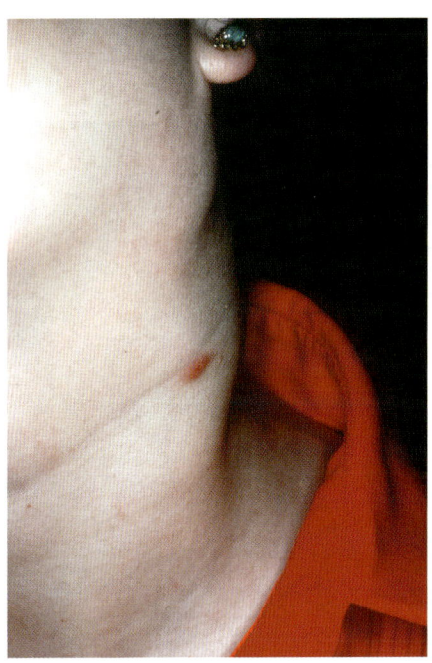

Fig. 14.83 Cat scratch disease.

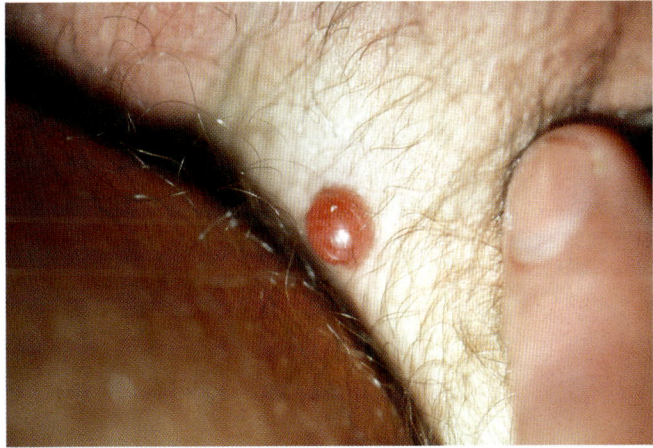

Fig. 14.84 Bacillary angiomatosis.

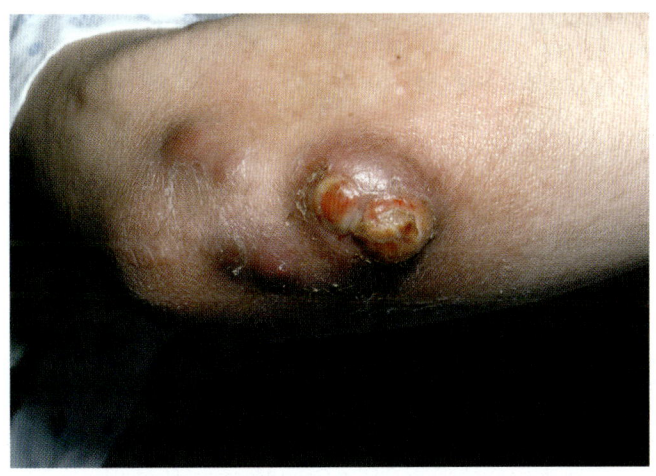

Fig. 14.85 Bacillary angiomatosis.

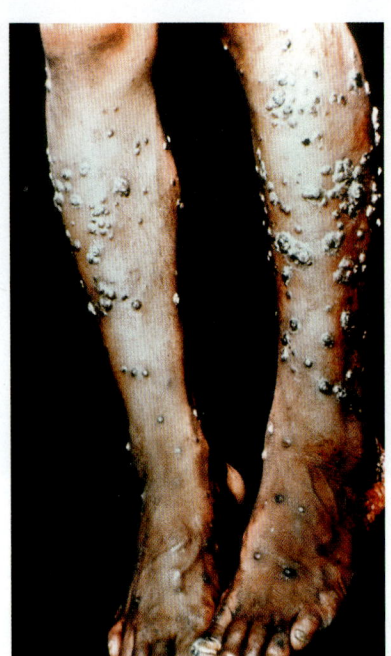

Fig. 14.86 Verruga peruana. *Courtesy Steven Binnick, MD.*

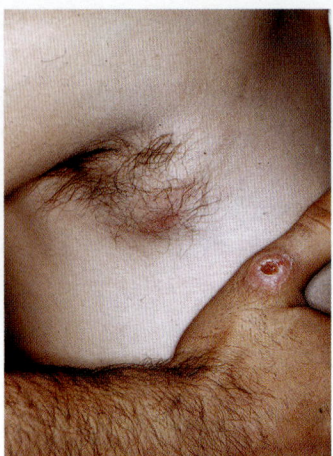

Fig. 14.87 Tularemia, ulceroglandular. *Courtesy The University of Utah and Oregon Health Sciences University Leonard Swinyer MD image collection.*

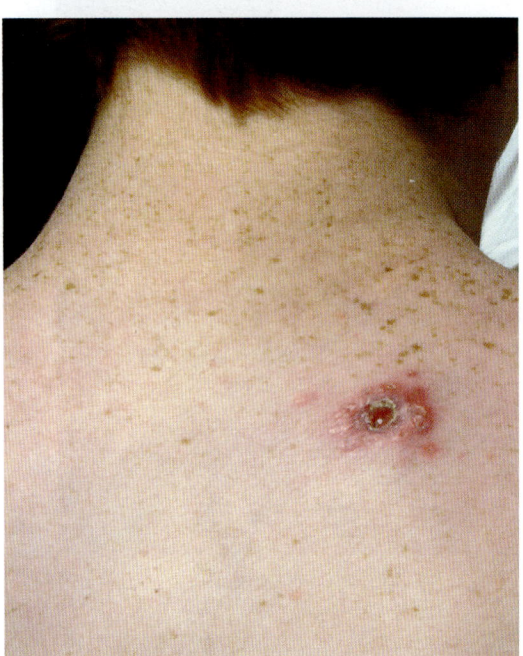

Fig. 14.88 Tularemia. *Courtesy Stephen D. Hess, MD, PhD.*

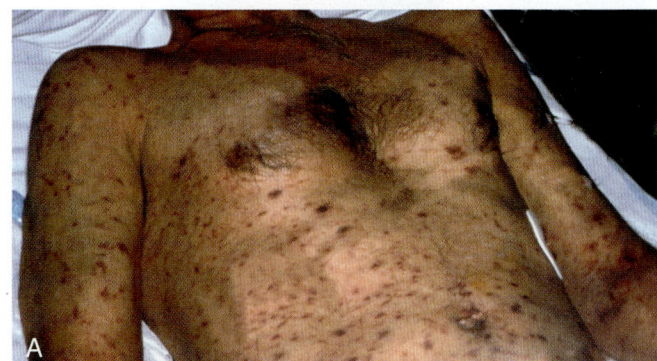

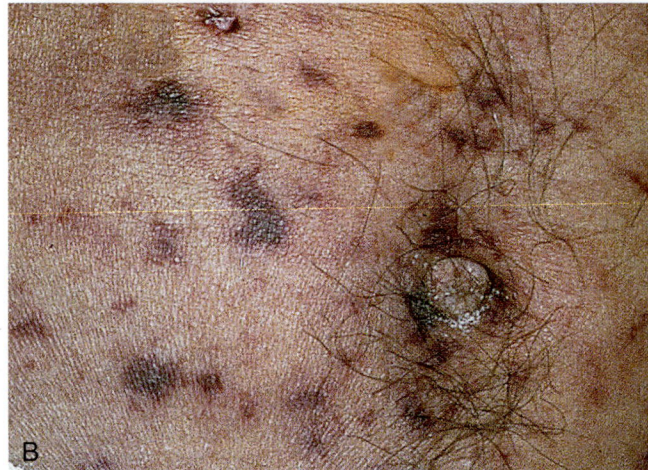

Fig. 14.89 (A) and (B) Epidemic typhus. *Courtesy Richard De Villez, MD.*

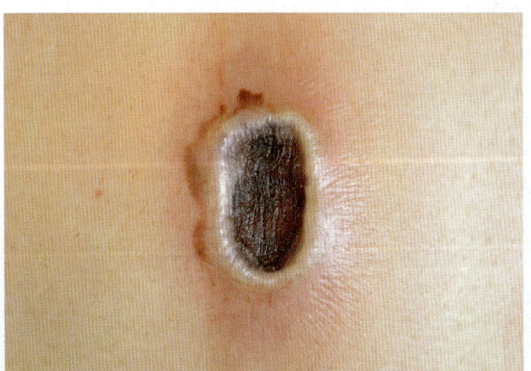

Fig. 14.90 Scrub typhus (tsutsugamushi fever). *Courtesy Kaohsiung Chang Gang Memorial Hospital, Taiwan.*

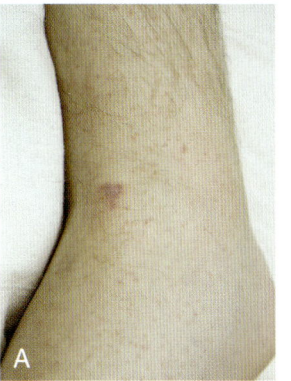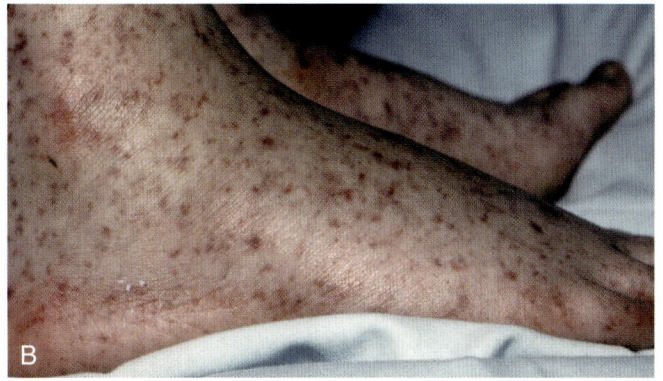

Fig. 14.91 (A) Rocky Mountain spotted fever. (B) Rocky Mountain spotted fever, *Courtesy Paul Honig, MD.*

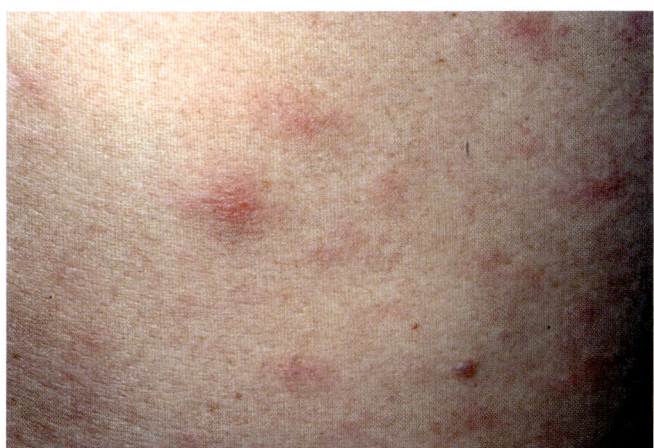

Fig. 14.92 Boutonneuse fever.

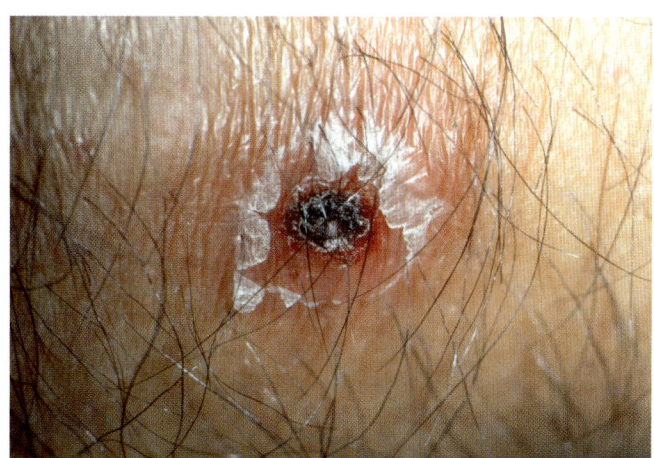

Fig. 14.93 Tache noire.

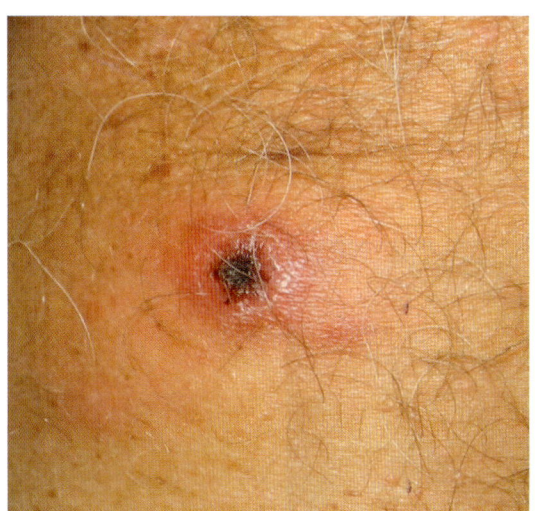

Fig. 14.94 Rickettsial pox.

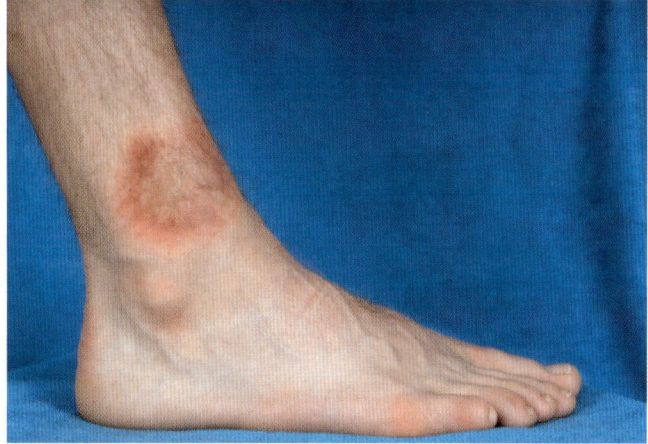

Fig. 14.95 Lyme disease (erythema chronicum migrans).

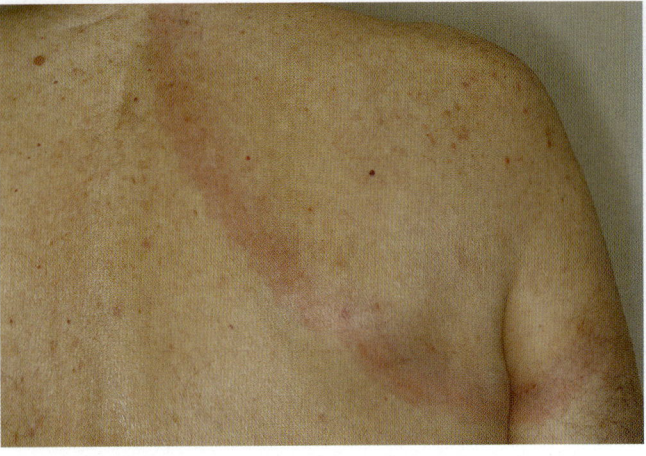

Fig. 14.96 Lyme disease (erythema chronicum migrans)

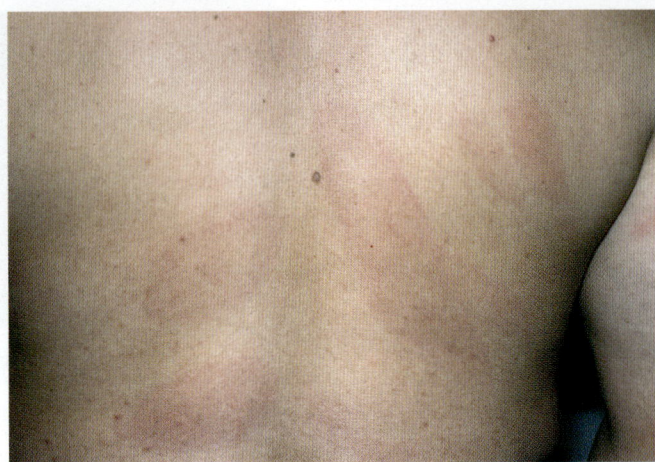

Fig. 14.97 Disseminated Lyme disease (multiple erythema migrans lesions). *Courtesy Steven Binnick, MD.*

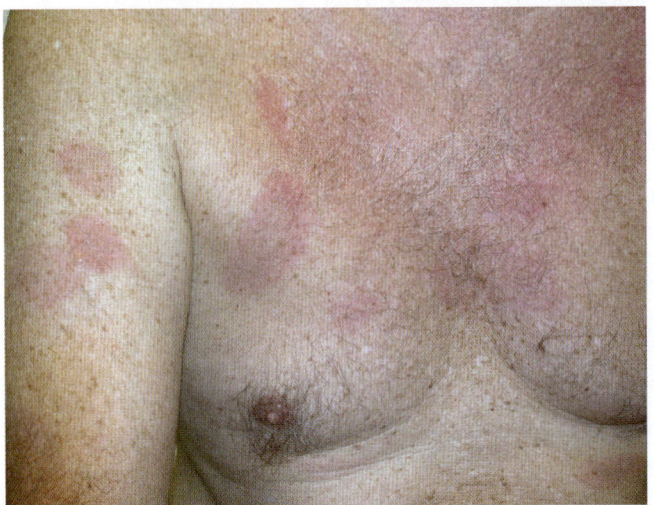

Fig. 14.98 Disseminated Lyme disease (multiple erythema migrans lesions).

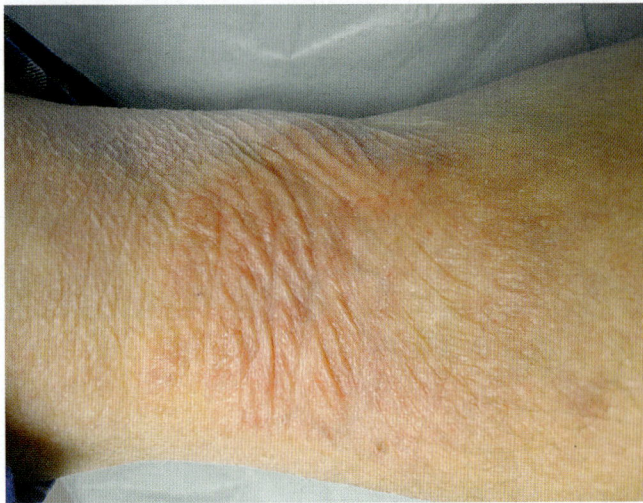

Fig. 14.99 Acrodermatitis chronica atrophicans. *Courtesy Jisun Cha, MD, Rutgers-Robert Wood Johnson Medical School.*

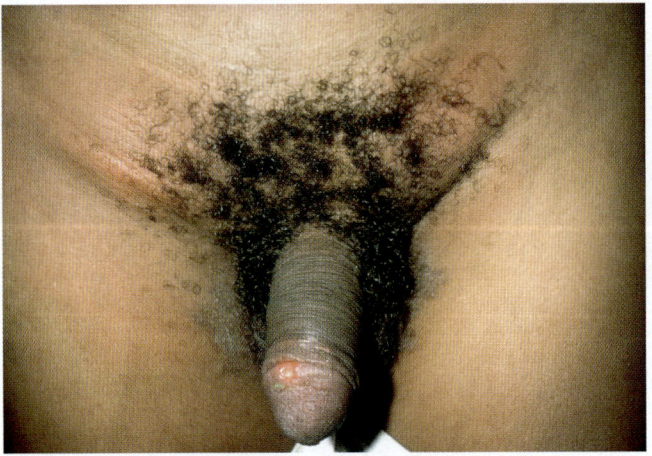

Fig. 14.100 Lymphogranuloma venereum.

Diseases Resulting From Fungi and Yeasts | 15

Fungi and yeasts can cause both superficial and deep infections in the skin with a great variation in clinical findings. In healthy hosts, commensal organisms such as candida remain superficial, whereas in the setting of an immunocompromised host they can be opportunistic, disseminated, and in some, lethal. Being familiar with both the common and uncommon fungi and yeasts and how they can present in the skin is important to allow for early diagnosis and treatment.

Dermatophyte infections in the skin are common, often pruritic, and almost always demonstrate persistent erythema and scaling of the affected regions. Tinea capitis can present with alopecia, broken hairs, localized or diffuse, fine scalp scaling, pustules, or painful boggy plaques with reactive cervical or occipital lymphadenopathy. Tinea, like other fungi and yeasts, tends to involve moist anatomic locations such as the body folds (axillae and groin) and the nail folds. Tinea corporis and faciei classically display the telltale annular or arcuate expanding patches or thin plaques with prominent scale at the leading edges. Appreciating this annularity can be difficult in some anatomic sites that are more convex or complicated such as around the ears or nose. Similarly difficult is when topical corticosteroids are used inadvertently on cutaneous dermatophyte infections resulting in a misleading clinical appearance with less scaling and erythema.

Candidal infections in the skin are also diverse, resulting in oral leukoplakia (thrush); the fissuring and erythema of the oral commissures known as *angular cheilitis*; chronic paronychia; itching, erythema and white discharge of candidal vulvovaginitis; and the beefy red, erosive intertrigo of the folds with surrounding satellite pustules seen commonly in the diaper region of infants. In newborns, congenital candidiasis can take on multiple forms, including a widespread miliaria-like eruption, pustules, or erosions that are most likely self-limited in full-term patients, but can disseminate in those born prematurely.

Deep fungal and mold infections include those regional organisms that infect otherwise well patients, such as *Histoplasmosis* and *Coccidiomycosis*, and those opportunistic and ubiquitous pathogens such as *Fusarium*, *Aspergillosis*, and the zygomycoses. Although many of these fungi and molds can present with nonspecific skin lesions, including abscesses, ulcers, verrucous or hyperkeratotic plaques, or nodules with central crusts or eschars, some more specific eruptions are also seen with these infections. These more specific eruptions can be a clue to the underlying immune status of the patient, including erythema nodosum seen more commonly in immunocompetent patients with coccidiomycosis or histoplasmosis versus the disseminated molluscum-like papules seen more in immunocompromised patients with these same infections.

This portion of the atlas portrays the myriad of skin findings due to fungi and yeasts and how their appearance can vary depending on the underlying immune status of the host patient.

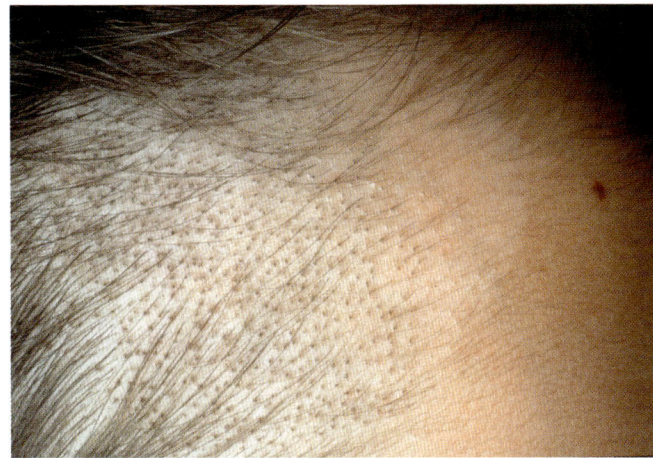

Fig. 15.1 Tinea capitis.

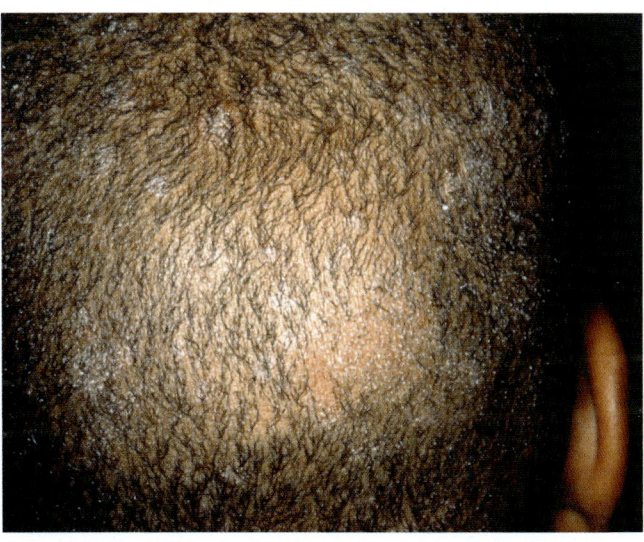

Fig. 15.2 Tinea capitis.

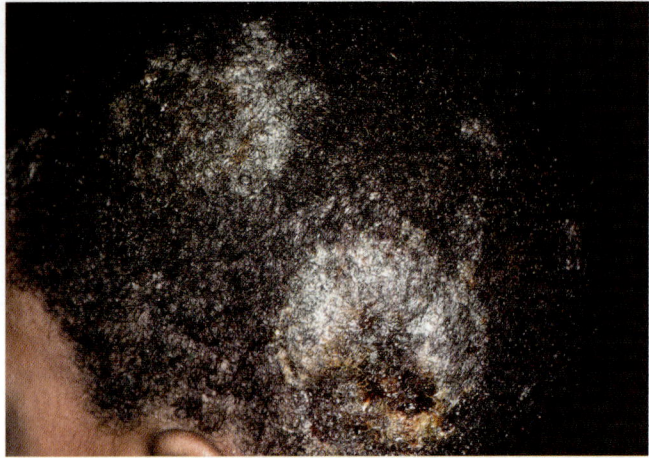

Fig. 15.3 Kerion. *Courtesy Steven Binnick, MD.*

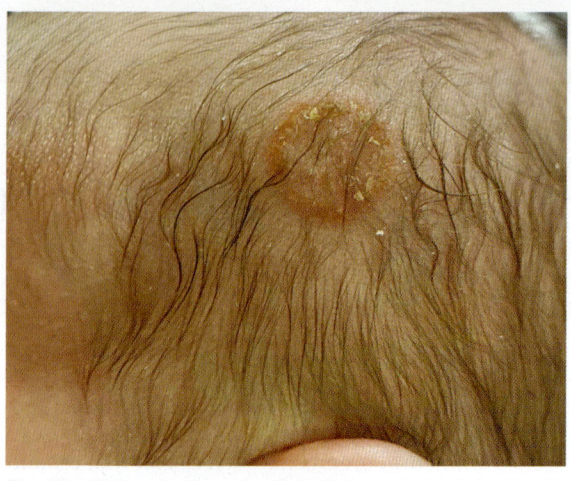

Fig. 15.4 Tinea capitis caused by *Microsporum* infection in a neonate.

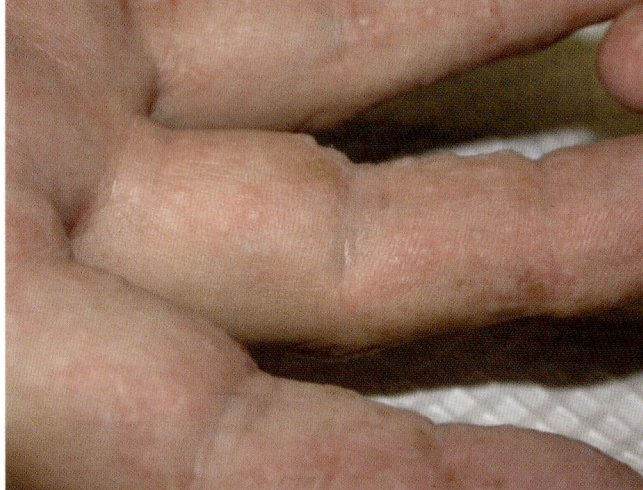

Fig. 15.5 Id reaction.

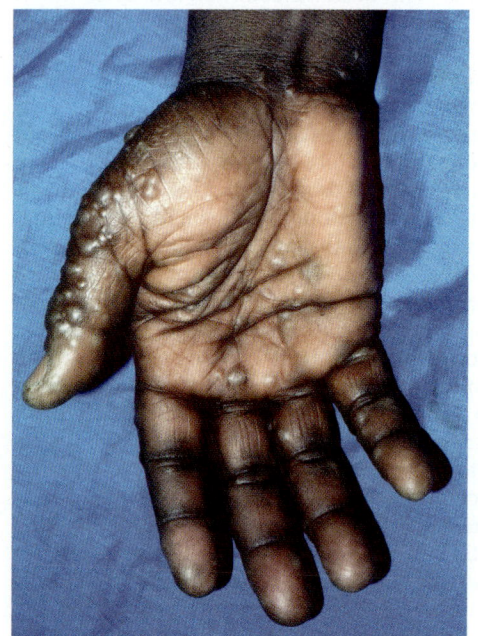

Fig. 15.6 Id reaction.

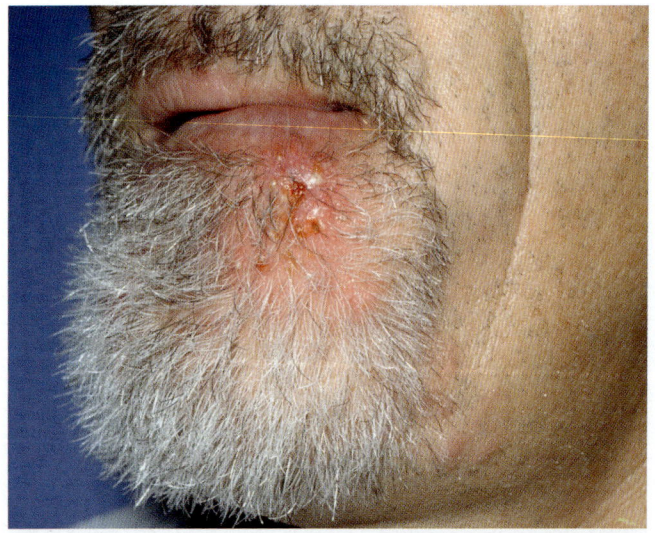

Fig. 15.7 Tinea barbae.

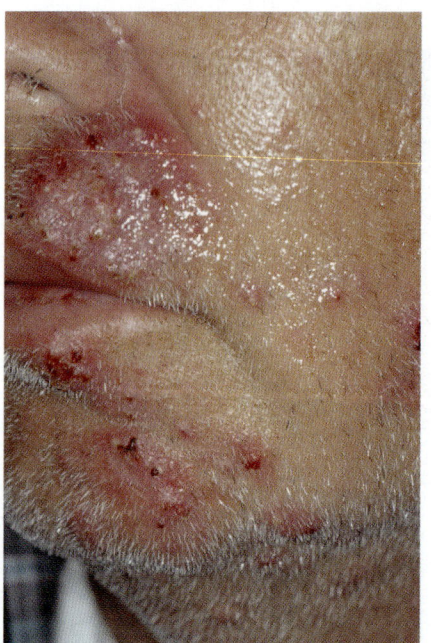

Fig. 15.8 Tinea barbae.

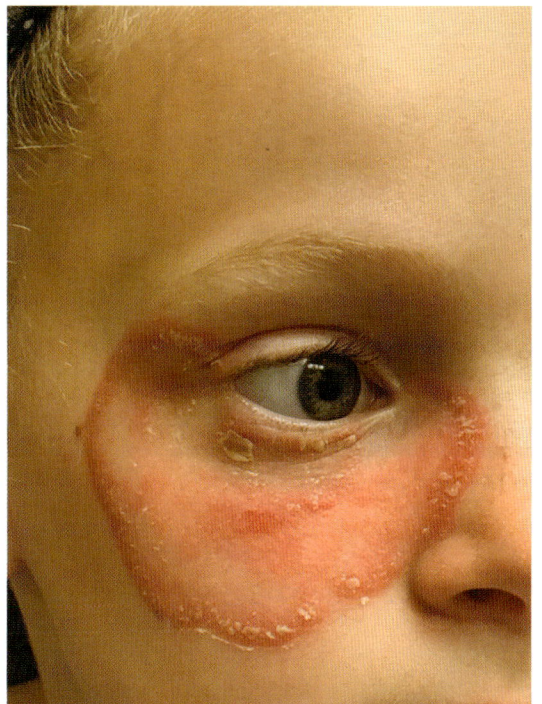

Fig. 15.9 Tinea faciei.

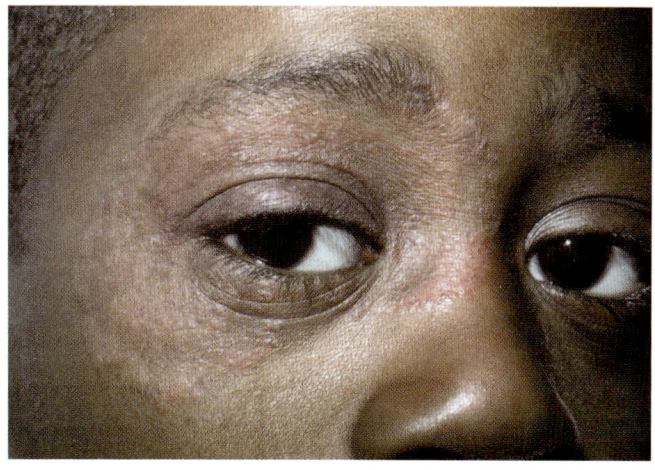

Fig. 15.10 Tinea faciei. *Courtesy Steven Binnick, MD.*

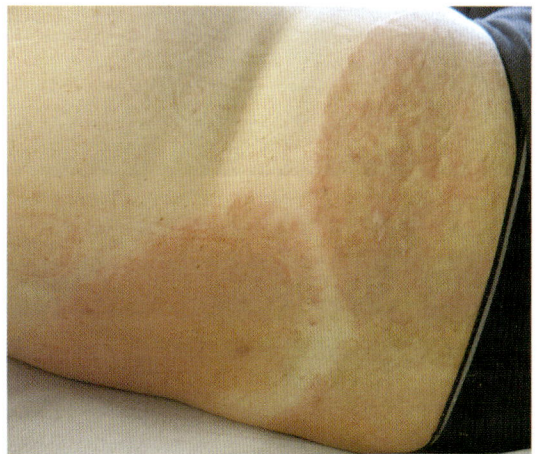

Fig. 15.11 Tinea corporis.

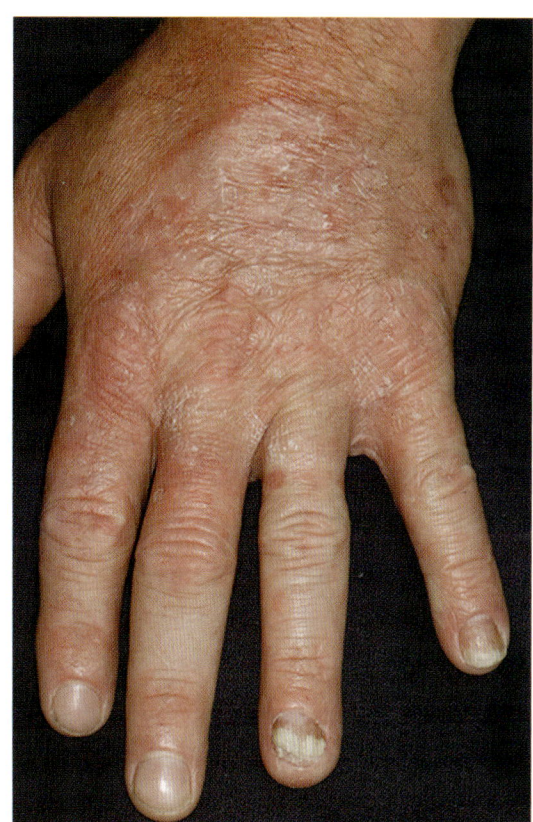

Fig. 15.12 Tinea manuum and onychomycosis.

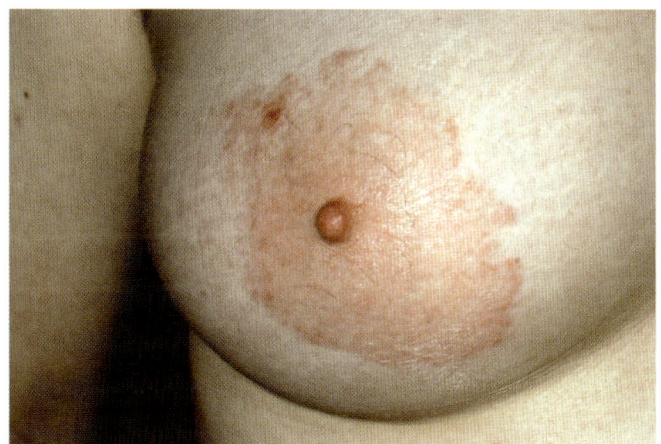

Fig. 15.13 Tinea corporis.

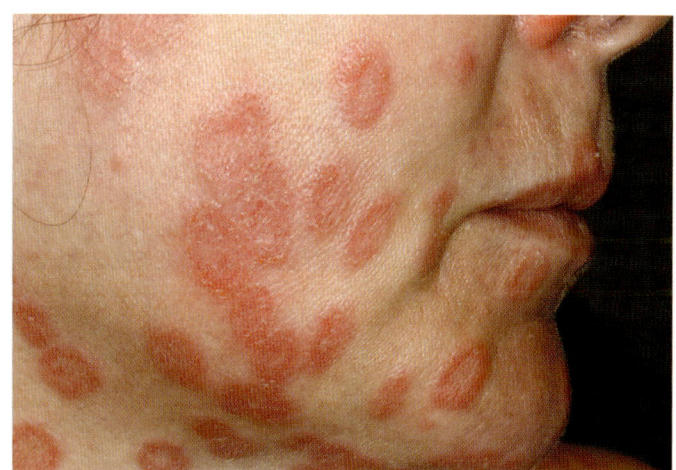

Fig. 15.14 Tinea faciei caused by *Microsporum canis* from a kitten.

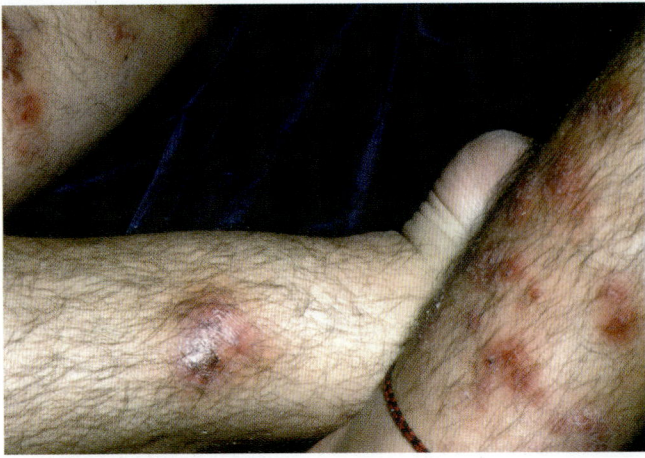

Fig. 15.15 Majocchi granuloma.

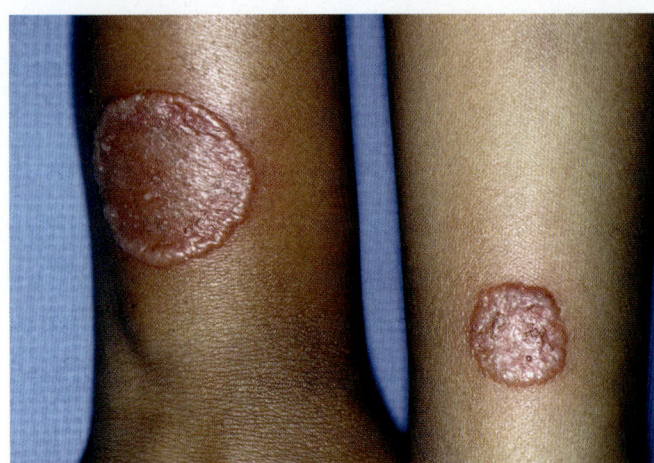

Fig. 15.16 Majocchi granuloma.

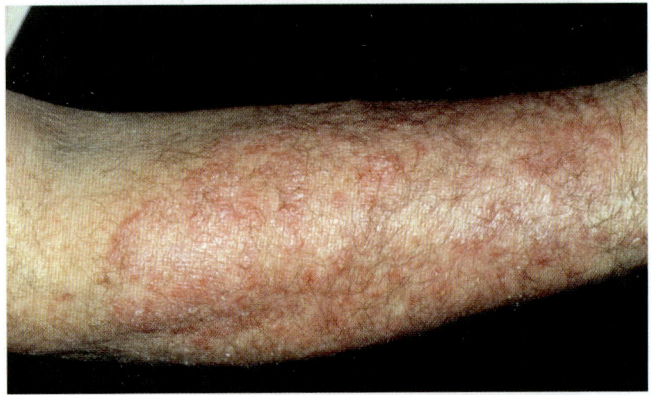

Fig. 15.17 Majocchi granuloma.

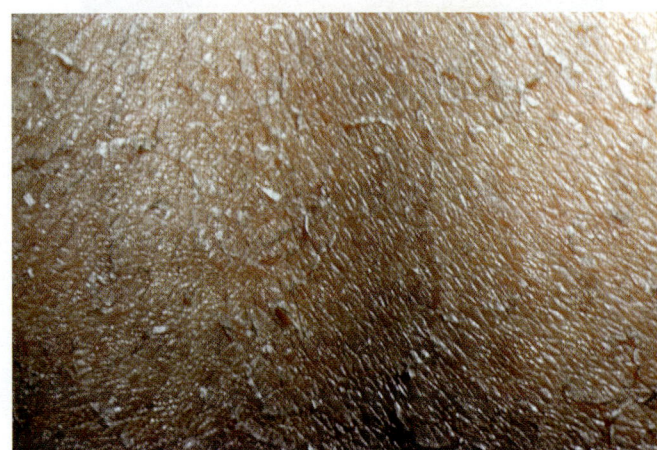

Fig. 15.18 Tinea imbricata.

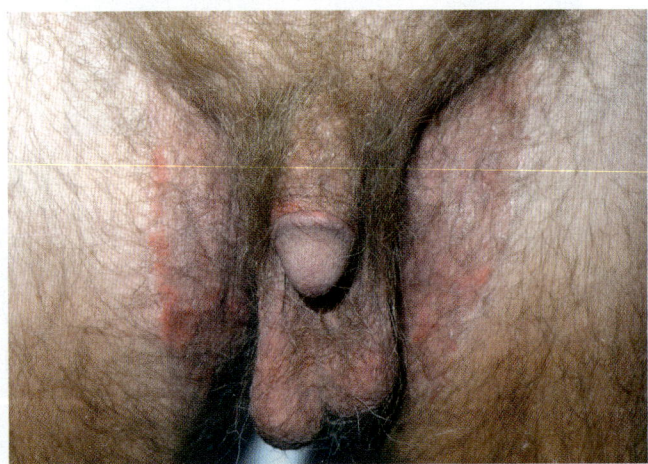

Fig. 15.19 Tinea cruris.

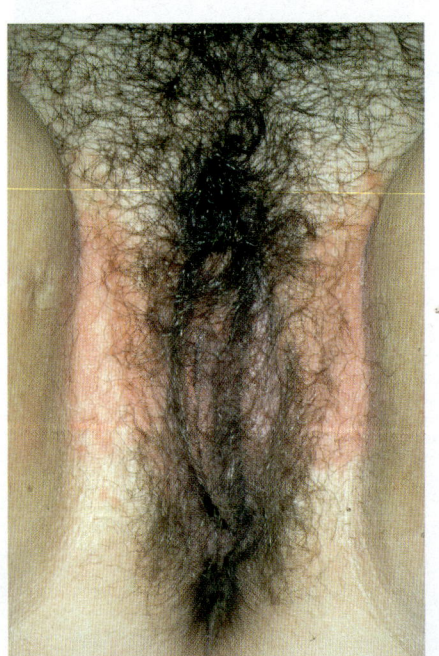

Fig. 15.20 Tinea cruris.

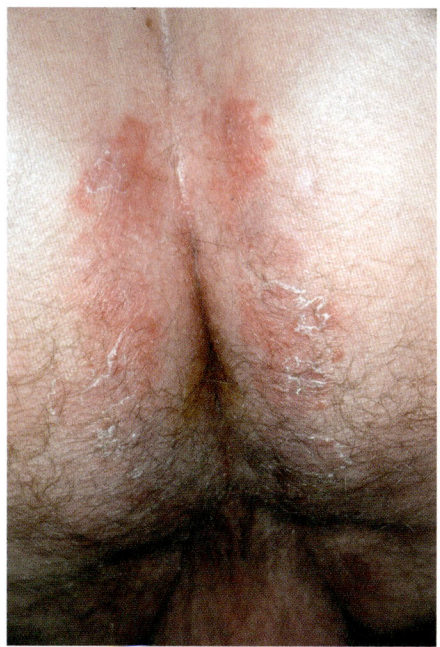

Fig. 15.21 Perianal tinea.

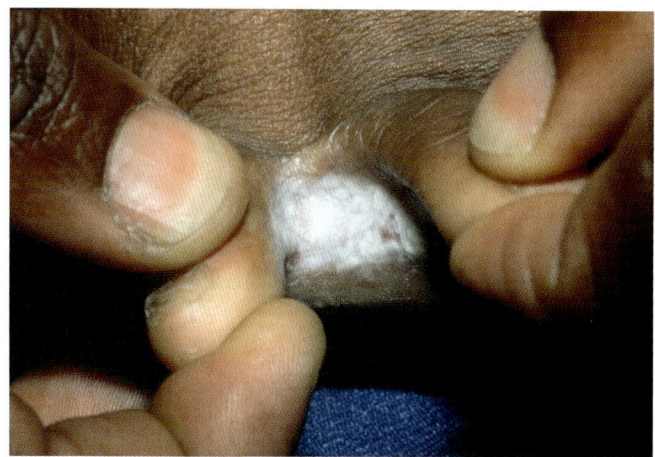

Fig. 15.22 Interdigital tinea.

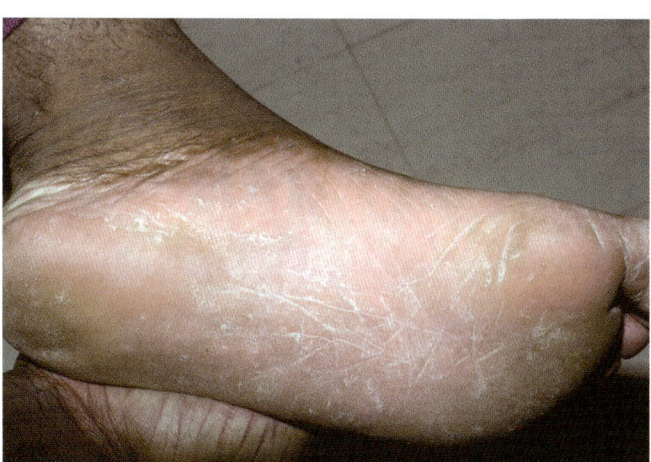

Fig. 15.23 Tinea pedis. *Courtesy Steven Binnick, MD.*

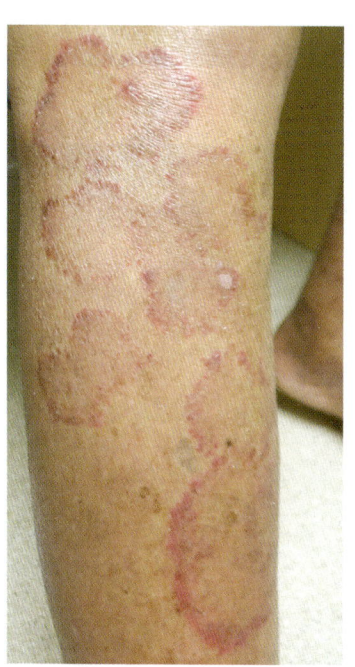

Fig. 15.24 Tinea corporis.

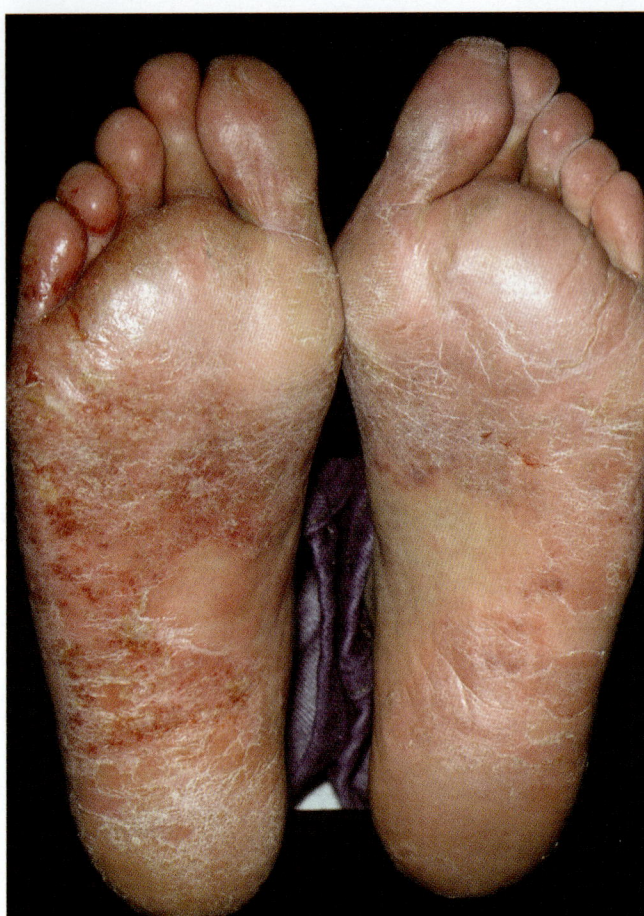

Fig. 15.25 Tinea pedis.

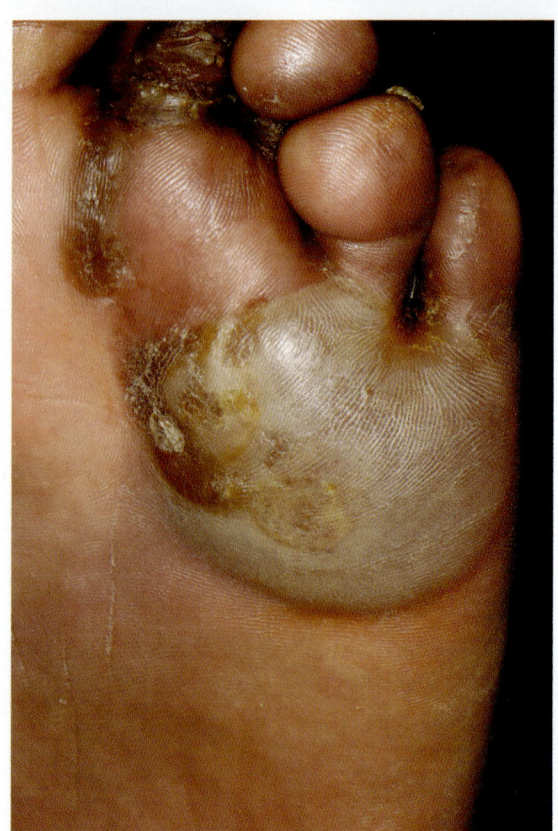

Fig. 15.26 Bullous tinea.

Fig. 15.27 Bullous tinea pedis.

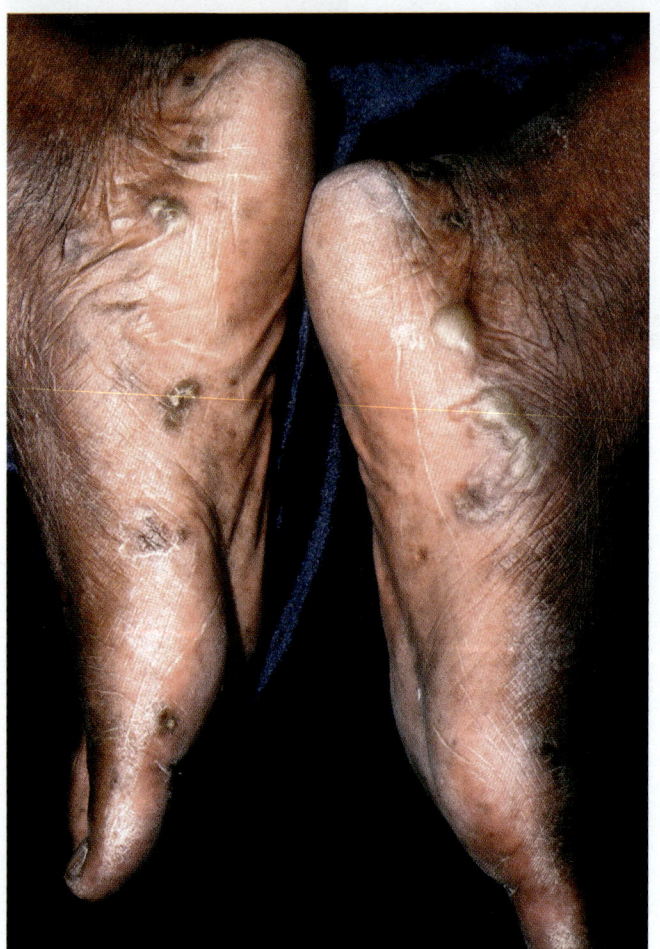

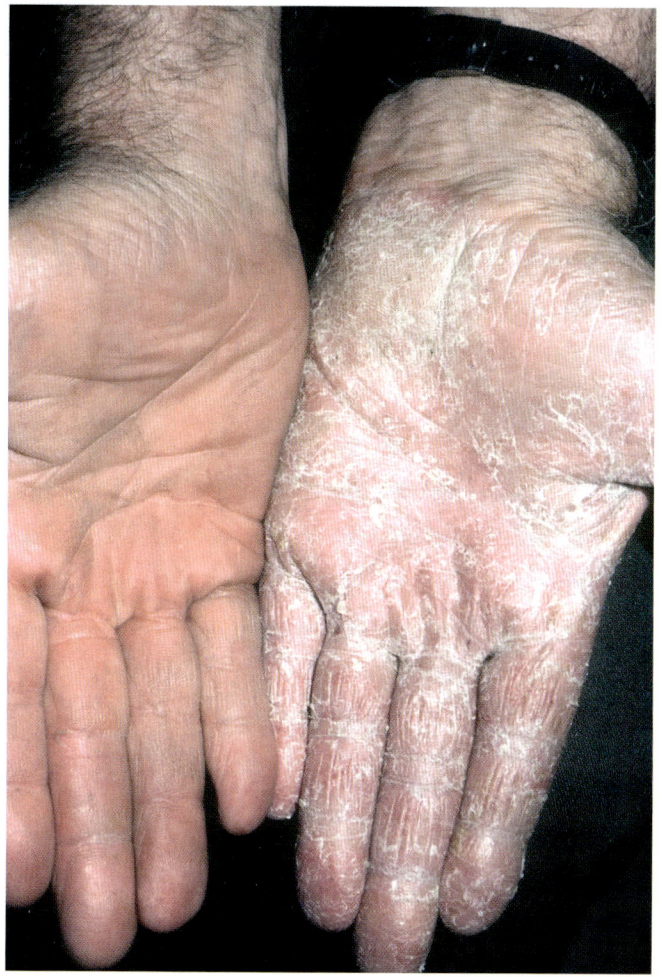

Fig. 15.28 One-hand involvement with tinea. Patient had both feet involved. *Courtesy Steven Binnick, MD.*

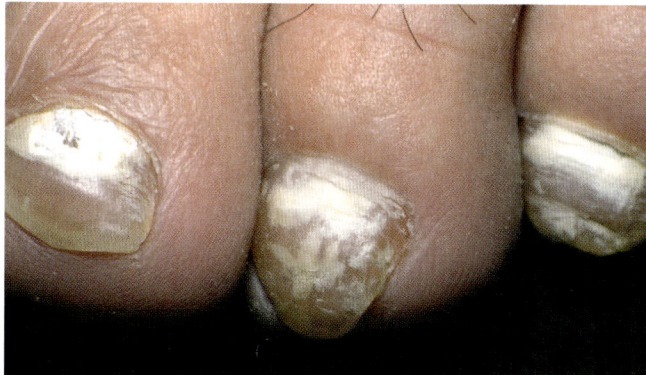

Fig. 15.30 Onychomycosis.

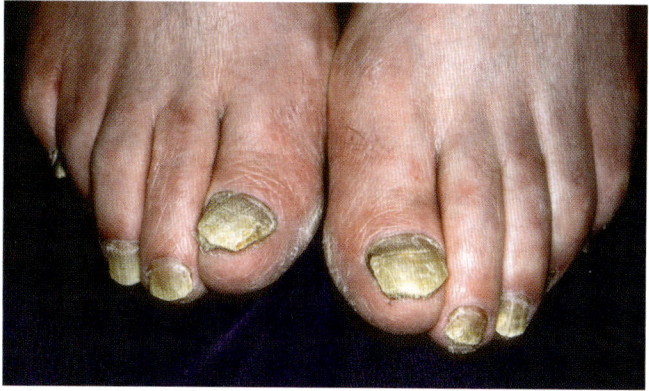

Fig. 15.29 Onychomycosis.

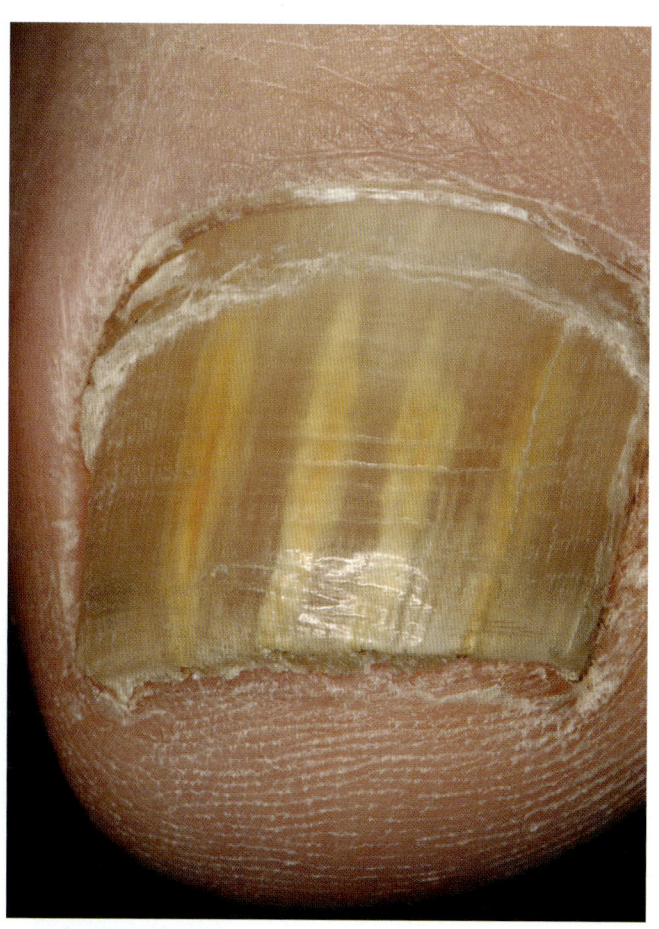

Fig. 15.31 Dermatophytoma.

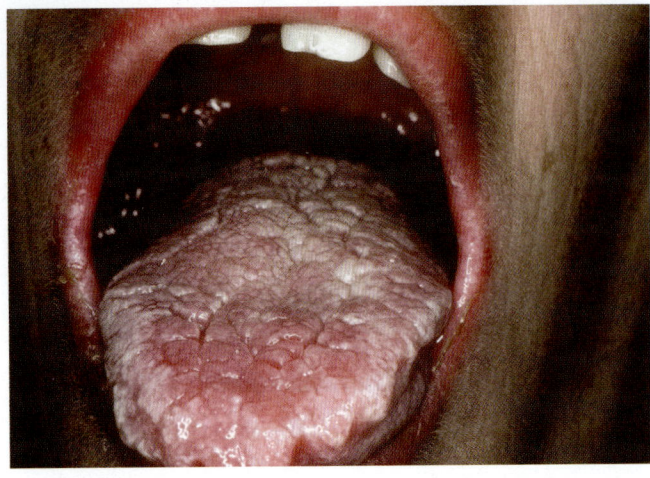

Fig. 15.32 Thrush in chronic mucocutaneous candidiasis.

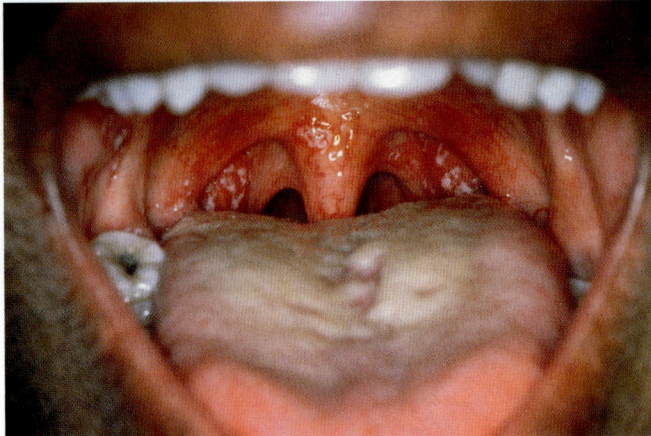

Fig. 15.33 Oral candidiasis in an HIV-infected patient.

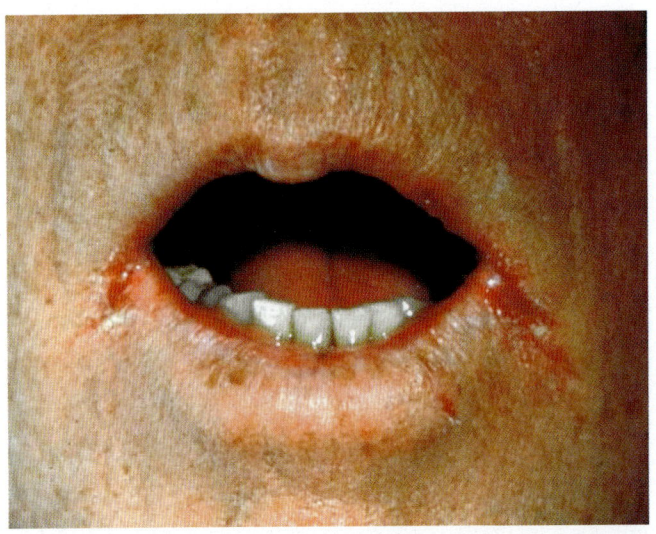

Fig. 15.34 Perlèche.

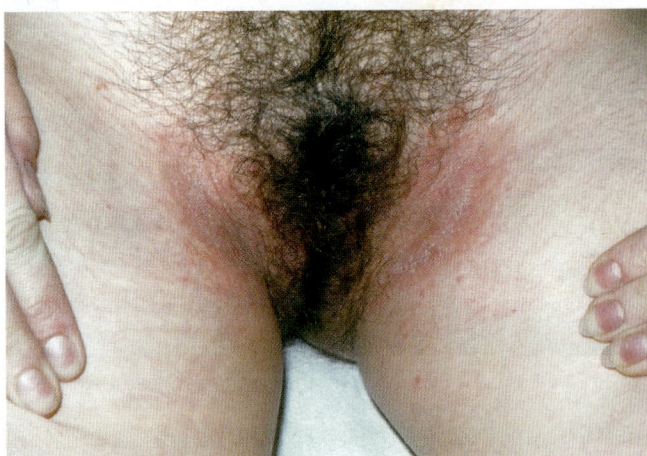

Fig. 15.35 Candidiasis. *Courtesy Steven Binnick, MD.*

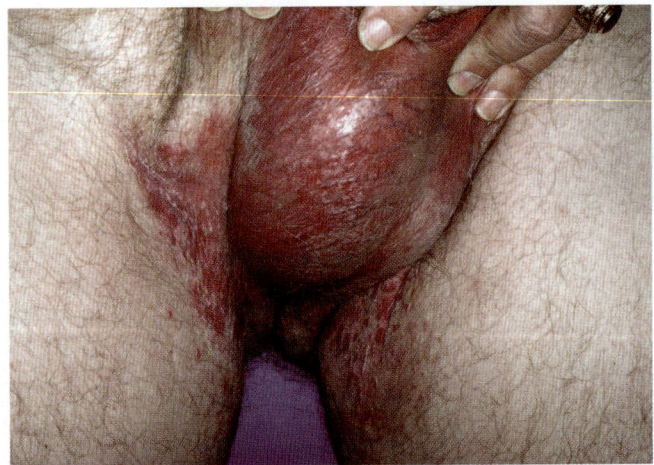

Fig. 15.36 Candidiasis. *Courtesy Curt Samlaska, MD.*

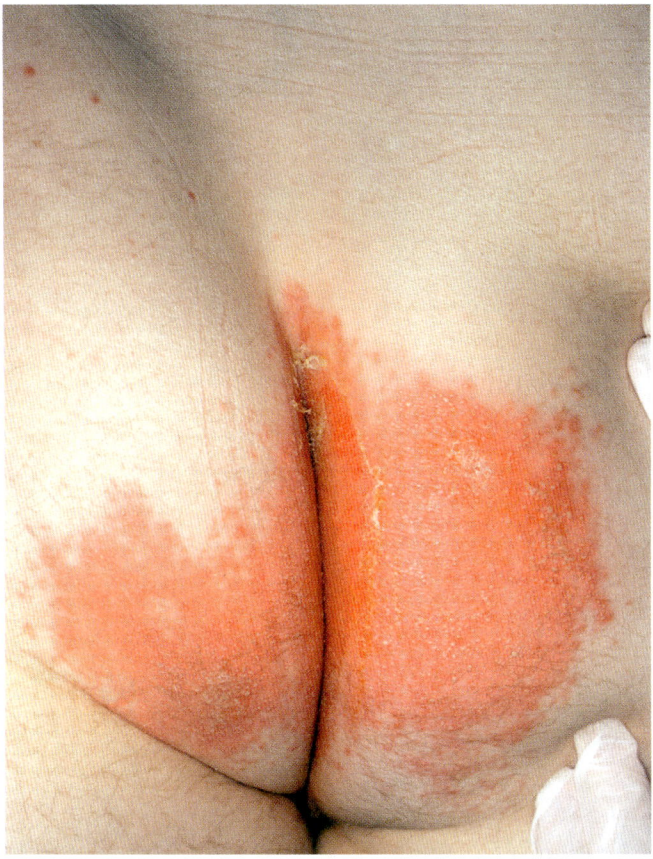

Fig. 15.37 Candidiasis. *Courtesy Curt Samlaska, MD.*

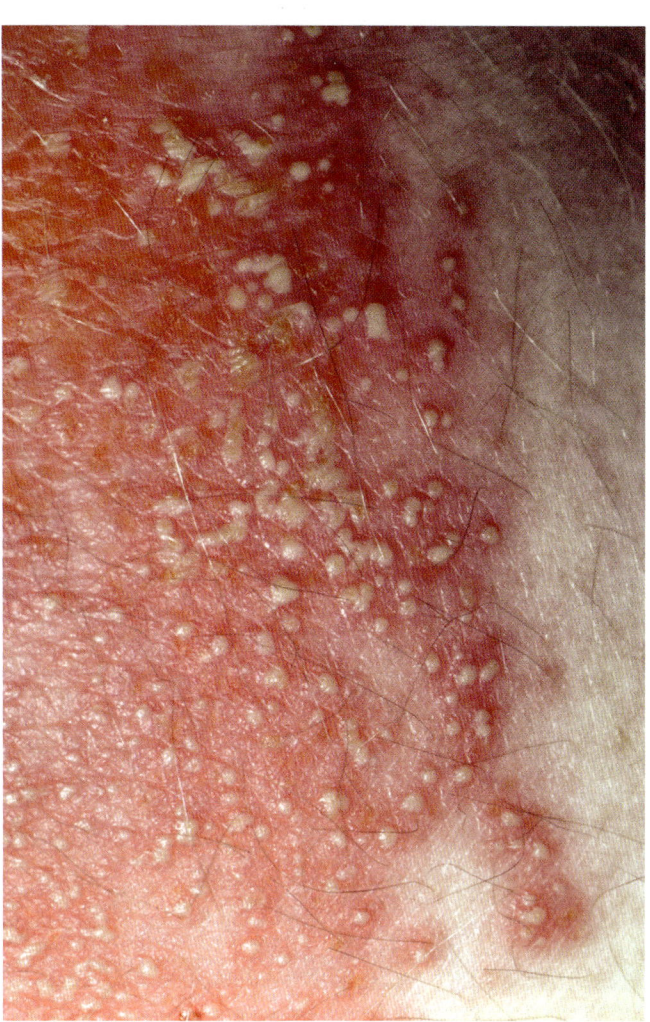

Fig. 15.38 Candidiasis. *Courtesy Curt Samlaska, MD.*

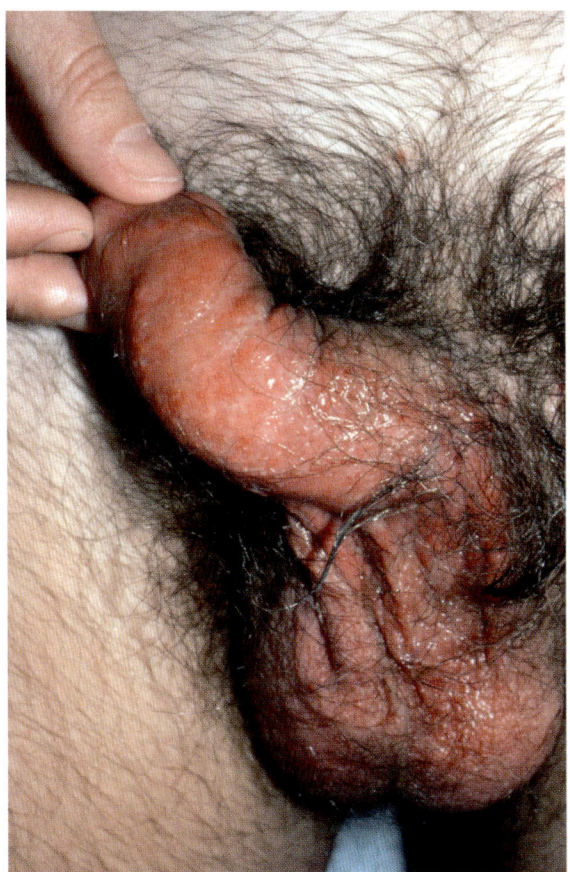

Fig. 15.39 Candidiasis. *Courtesy Curt Samlaska, MD.*

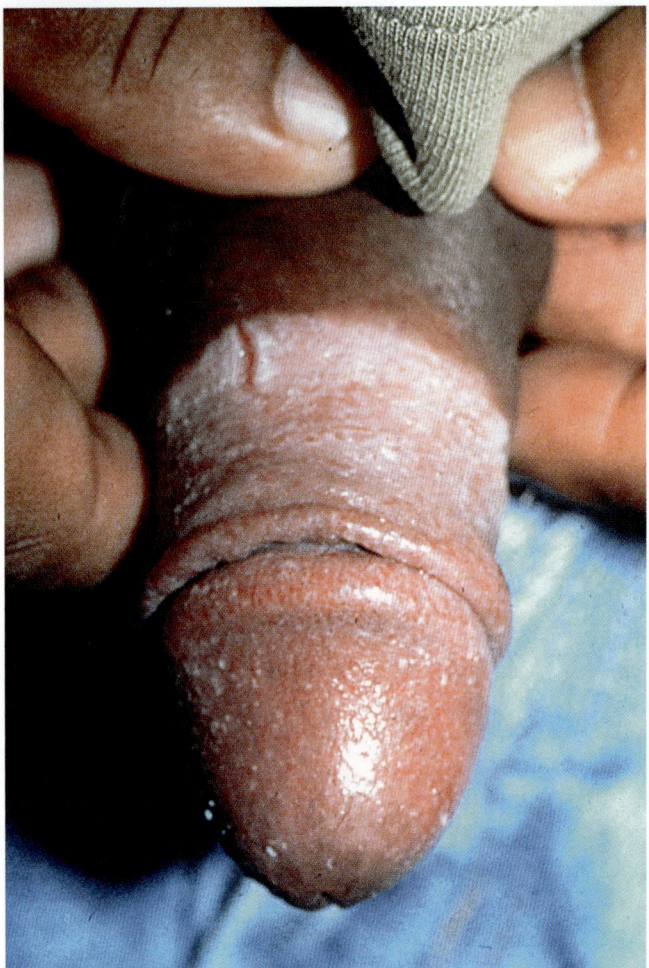

Fig. 15.40 Candidiasis.

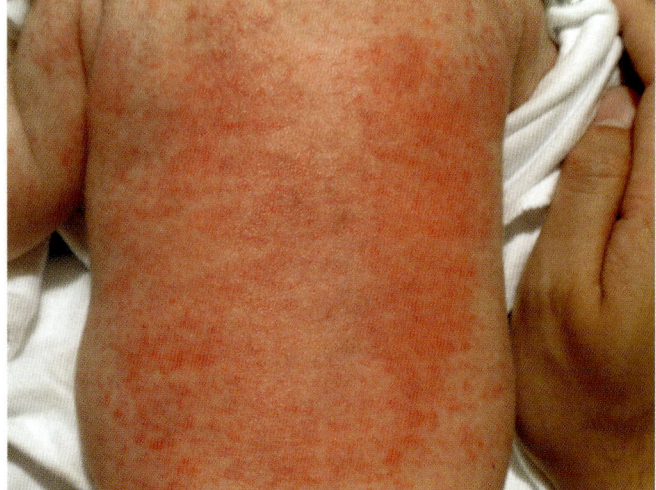

Fig. 15.42 Congenital candidiasis.

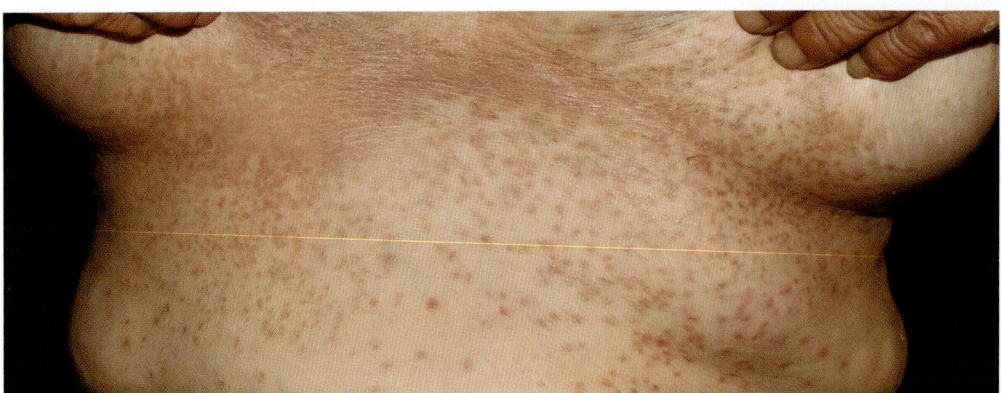

Fig. 15.41 Candidiasis. *Courtesy National Cheng Kung University, Taiwan.*

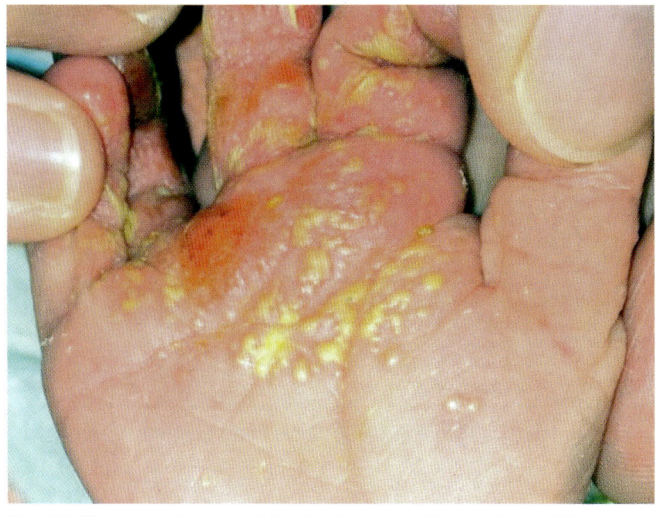

Fig. 15.43 Congenital candidiasis. *Courtesy Vikash Oza, MD.*

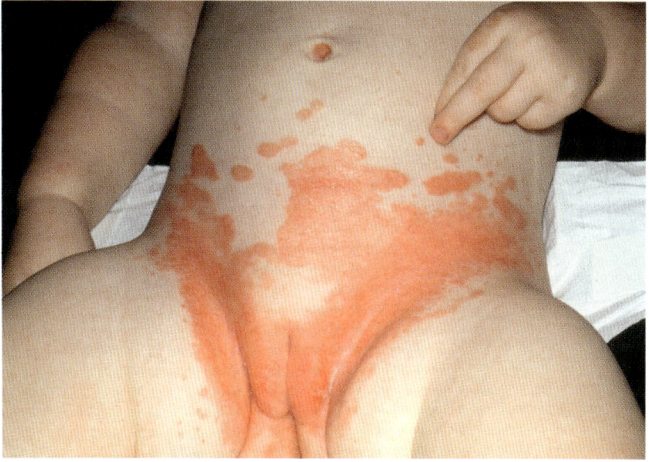

Fig. 15.44 Candidiasis. *Courtesy Curt Samlaska, MD.*

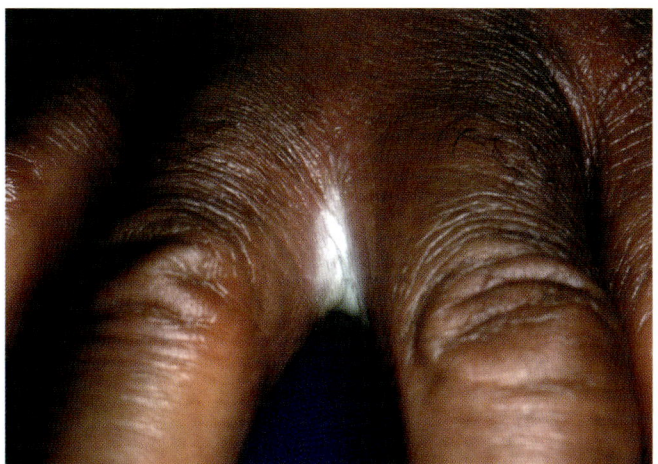

Fig. 15.45 Erosio interdigitalis blastomycetica.

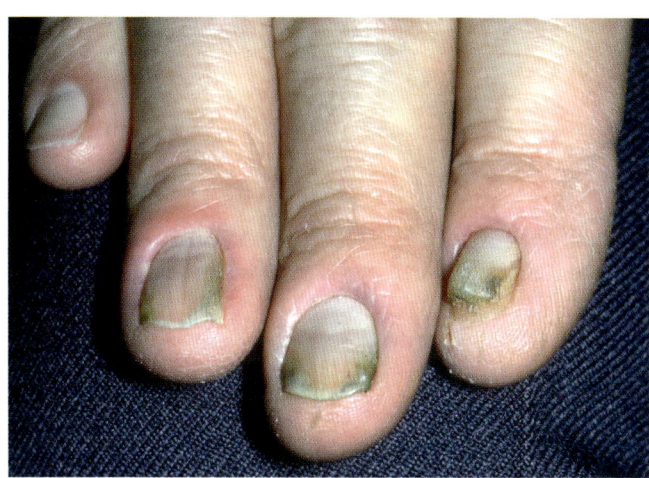

Fig. 15.46 Chronic paronychia.

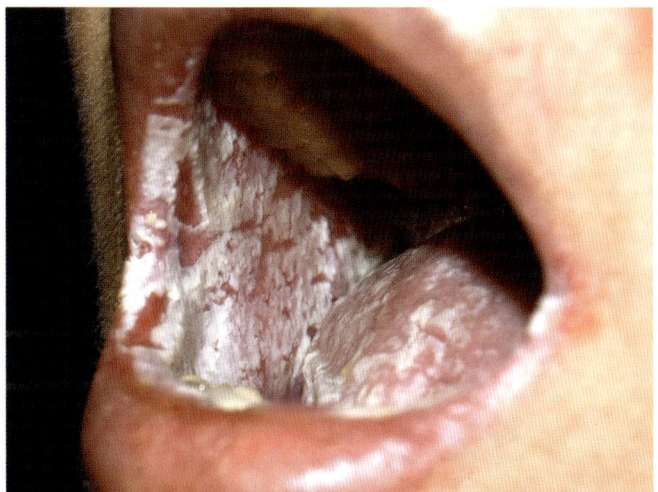

Fig. 15.47 Chronic mucocutaneous candidiasis. *Courtesy National Cheng Kung University, Taiwan.*

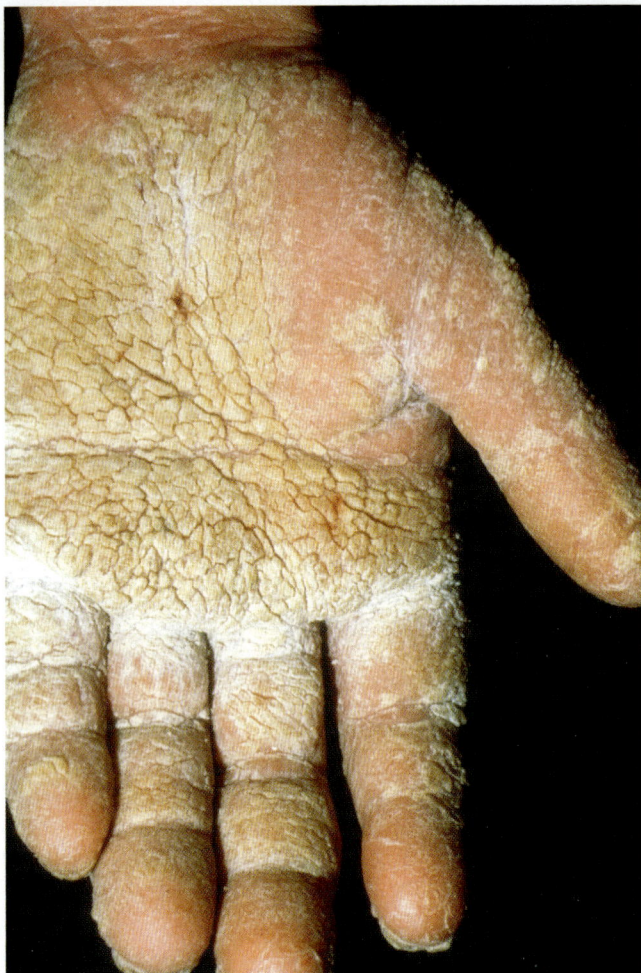

Fig. 15.48 Chronic mucocutaneous candidiasis.

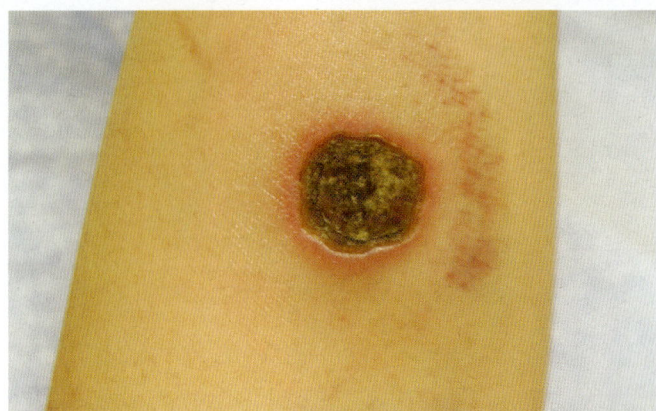

Fig. 15.49 Invasive *Candida parapsilosis* in an immunosuppressed patient.

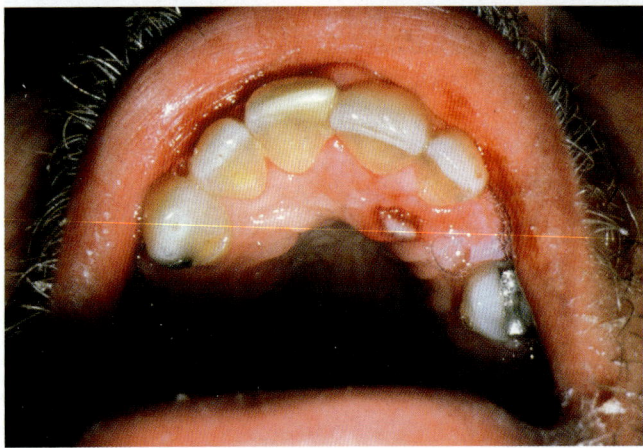

Fig. 15.50 Candidal sepsis.

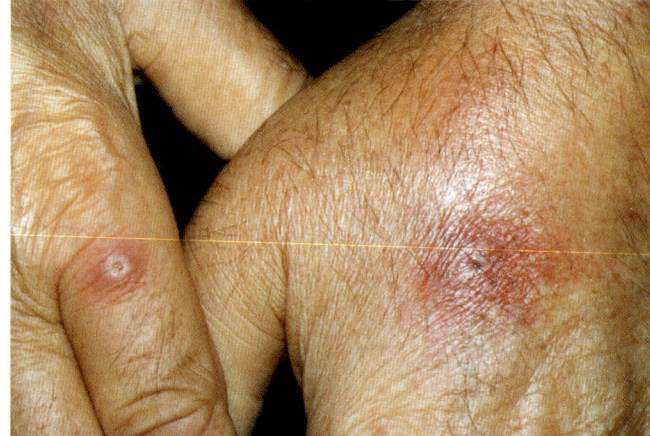

Fig. 15.51 Candidal sepsis.

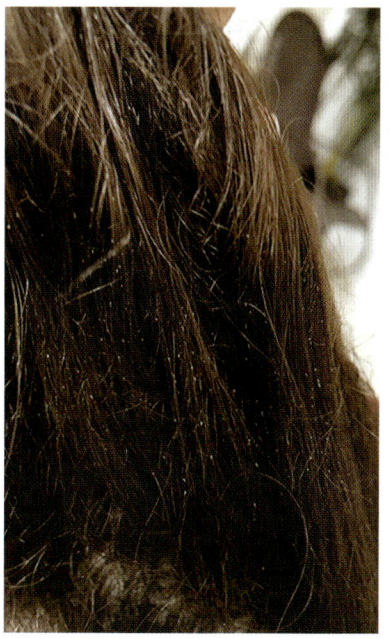

Fig. 15.52 White piedra.

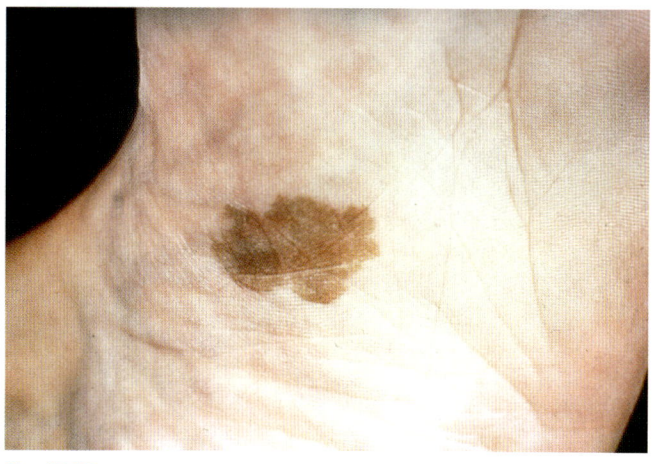

Fig. 15.53 Tinea nigra.

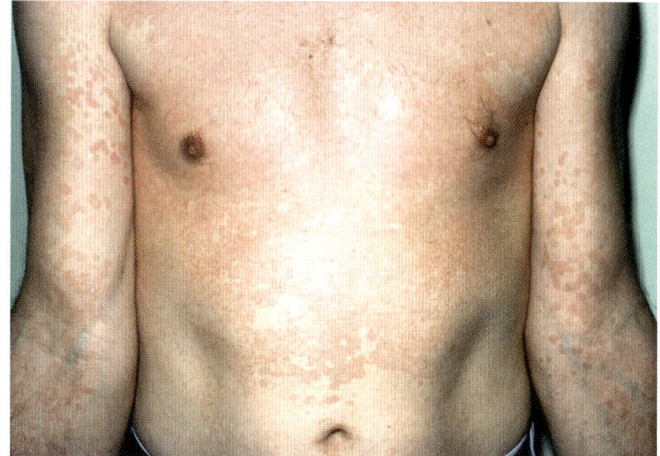

Fig. 15.54 Tinea versicolor.

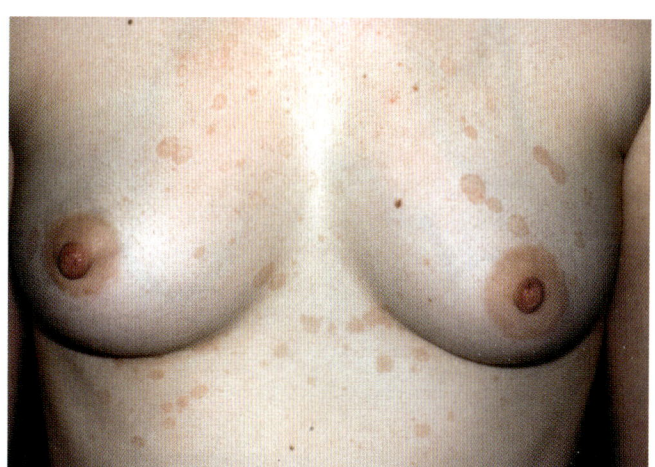

Fig. 15.55 Tinea versicolor. *Courtesy Steven Binnick, MD.*

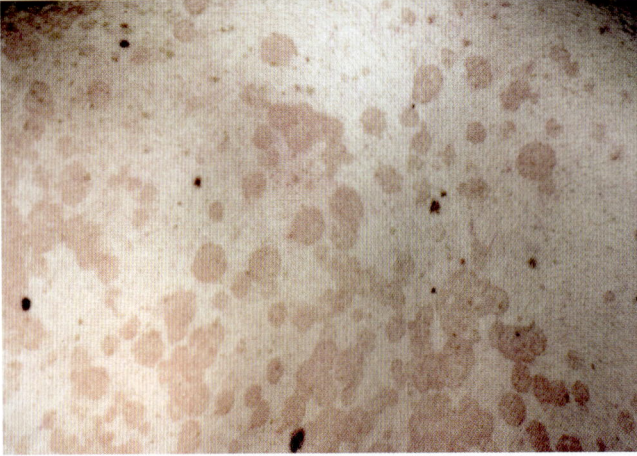

Fig. 15.56 Tinea versicolor. *Courtesy Steven Binnick, MD.*

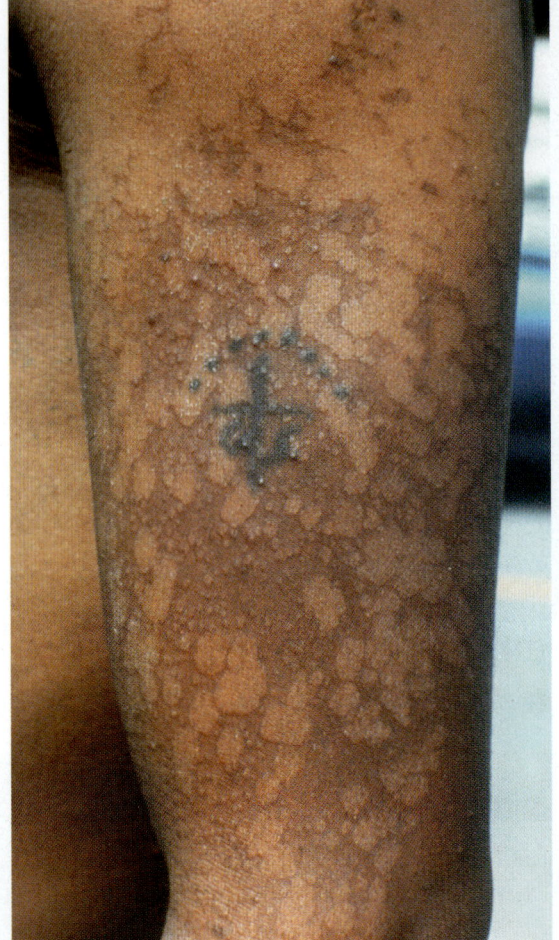

Fig. 15.57 Tinea versicolor.

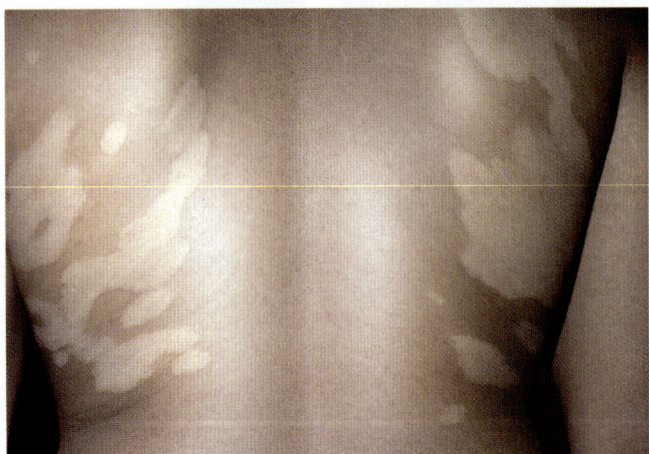

Fig. 15.58 Tinea versicolor. *Courtesy Steven Binnick, MD.*

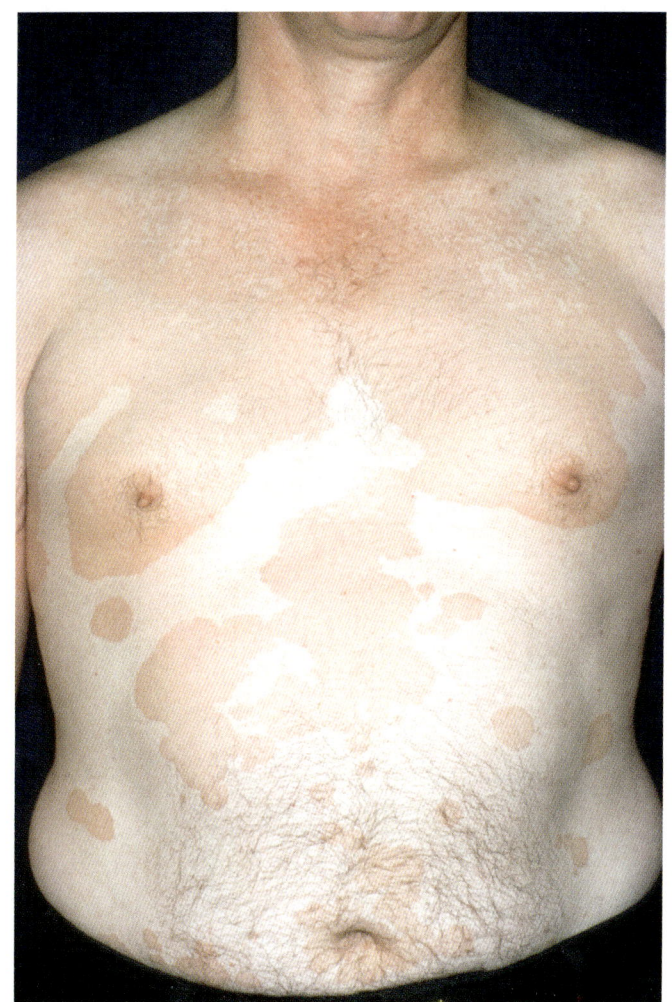

Fig. 15.59 Tinea versicolor.

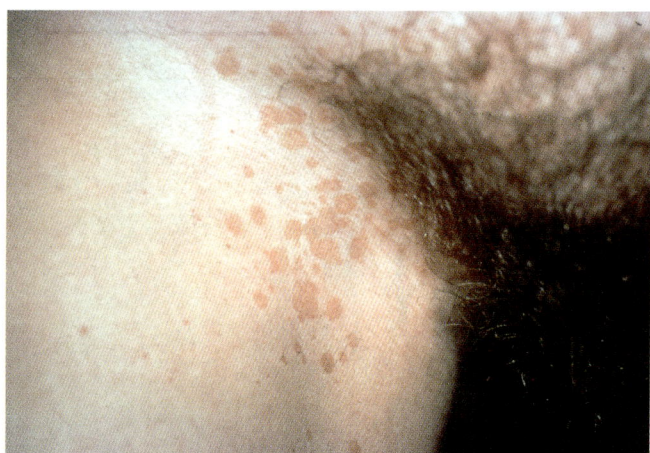

Fig. 15.60 Tinea versicolor.

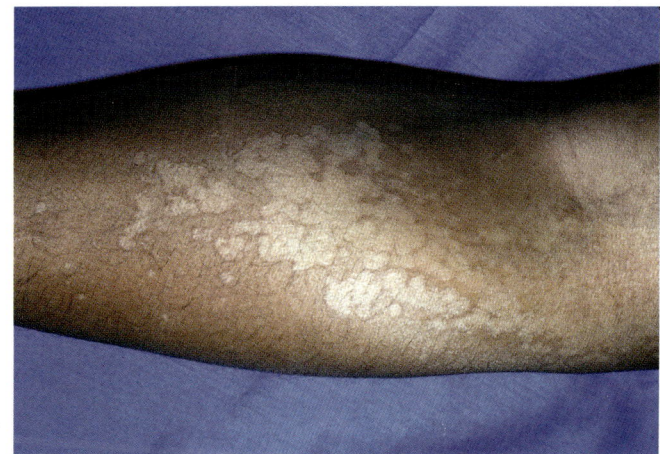

Fig. 15.61 Tinea versicolor. *Courtesy Steven Binnick, MD.*

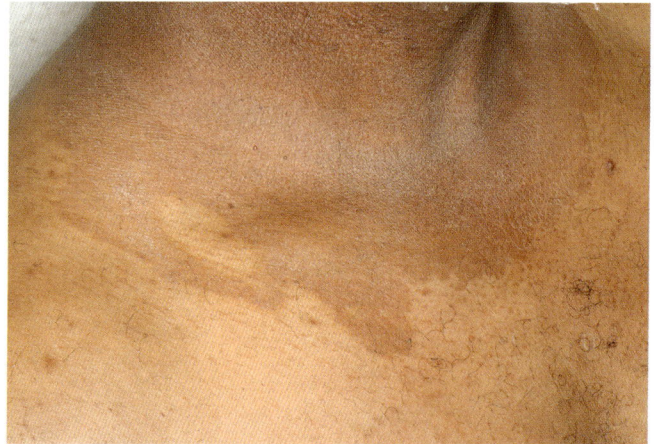

Fig. 15.62 Tinea versicolor.

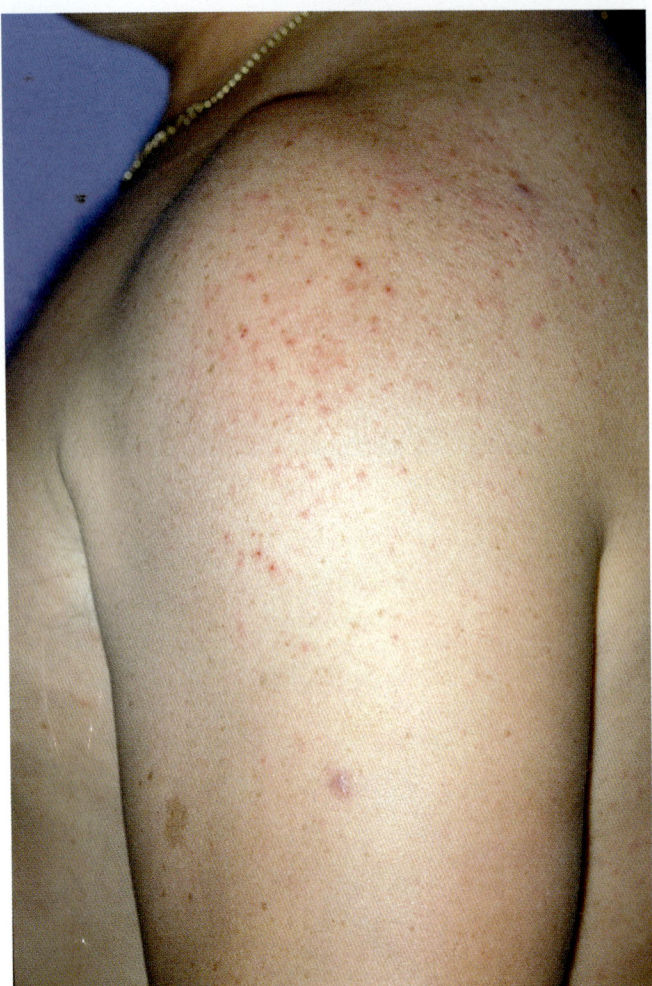

Fig. 15.63 Pityrosporum folliculitis.

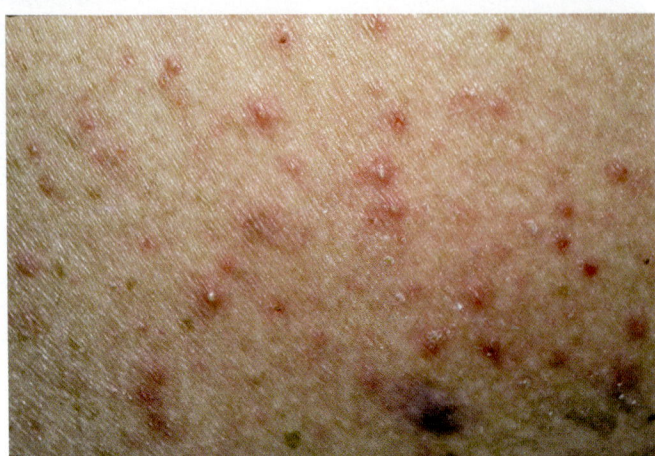

Fig. 15.64 Pityrosporum folliculitis.

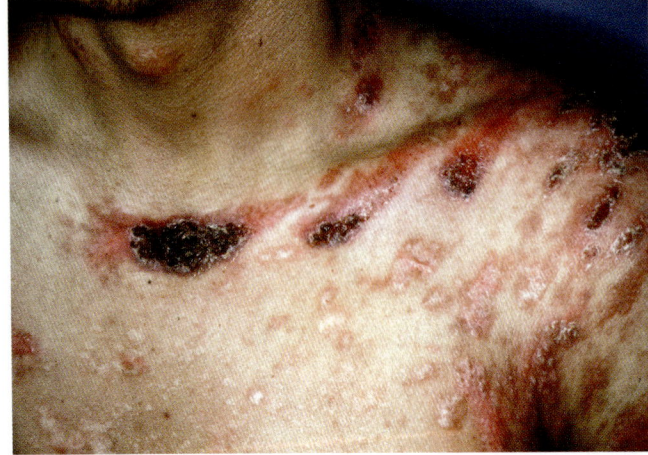

Fig. 15.65 Coccidioidomycosis.

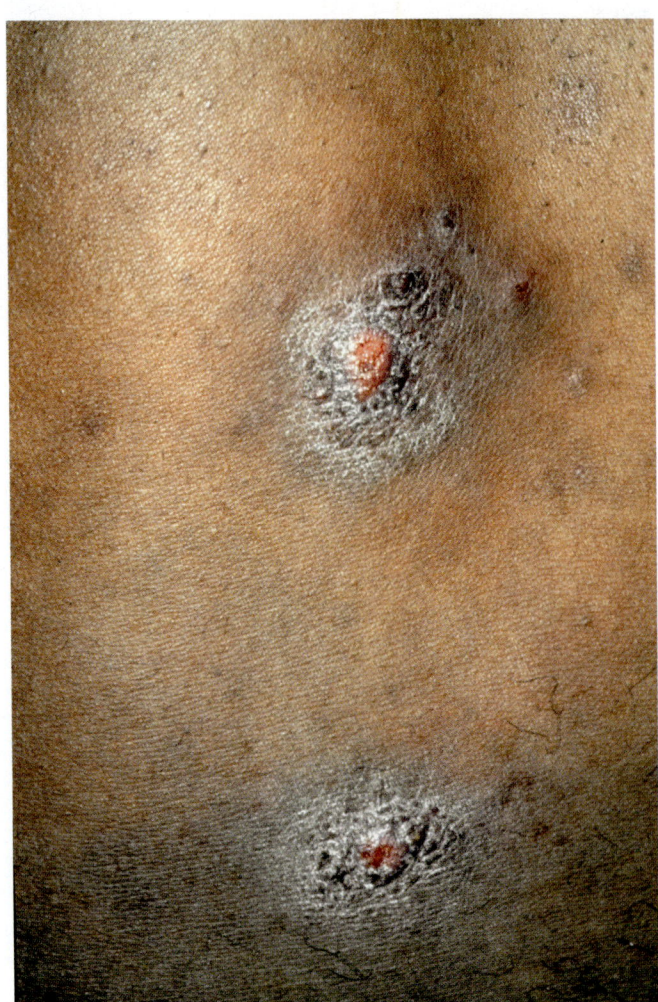

Fig. 15.66 Coccidioidomycosis.

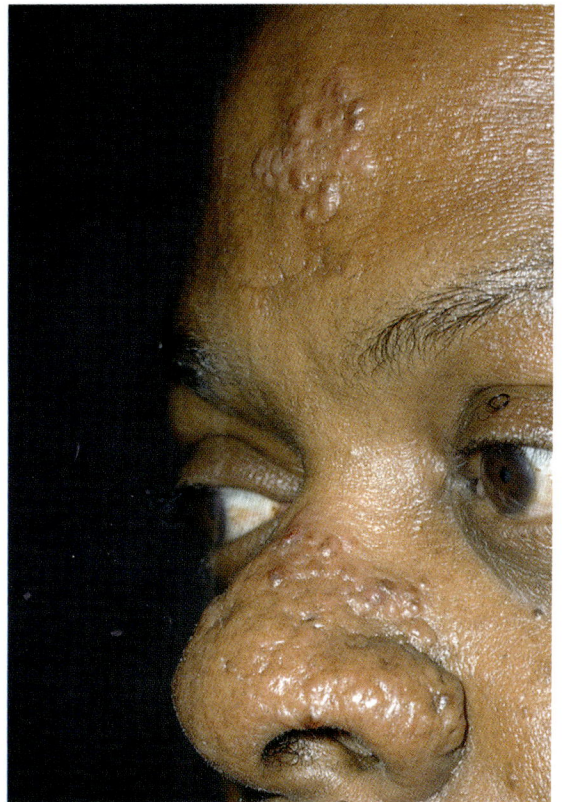

Fig. 15.67 Coccidioidomycosis. *Courtesy Curt Samlaska, MD.*

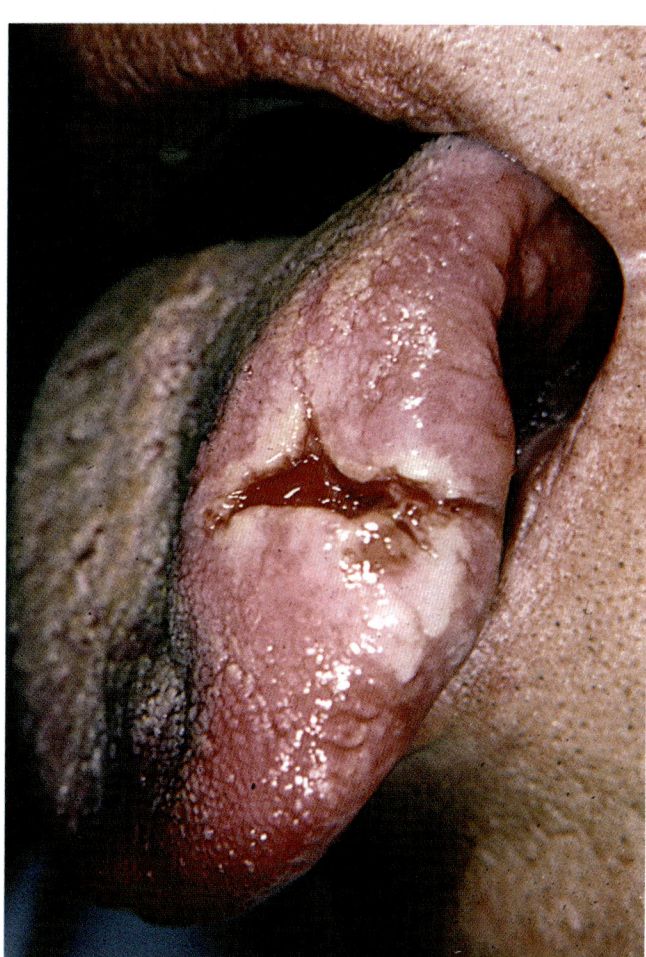

Fig. 15.68 Histoplasmosis. *Courtesy Steven Binnick, MD.*

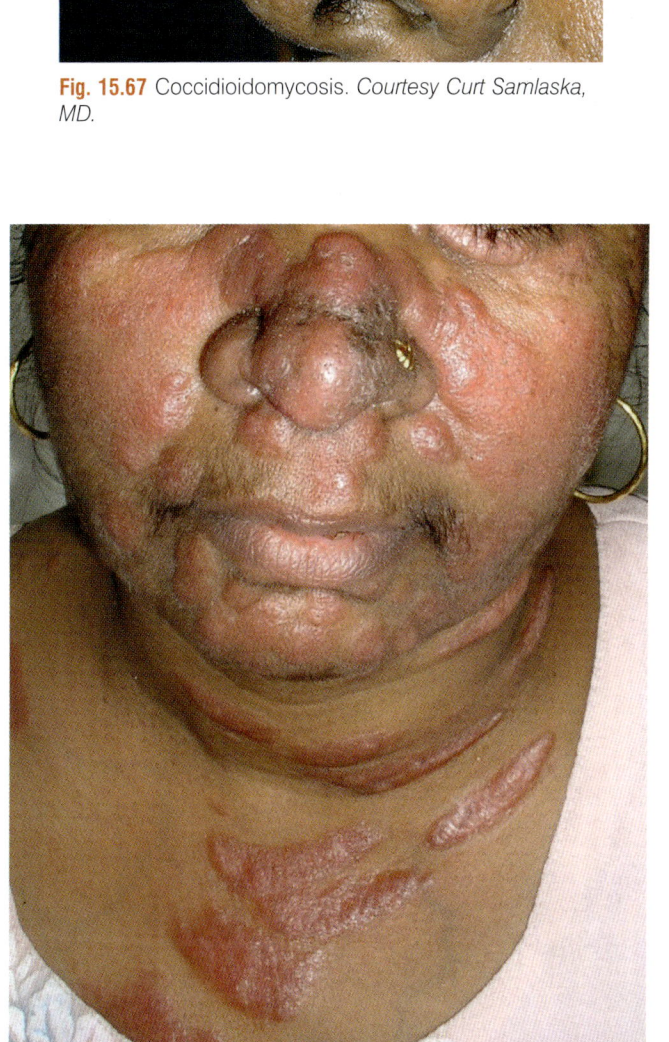

Fig. 15.69 Histoplasmosis. *Courtesy Shyam Verma, MBBS, DVD.*

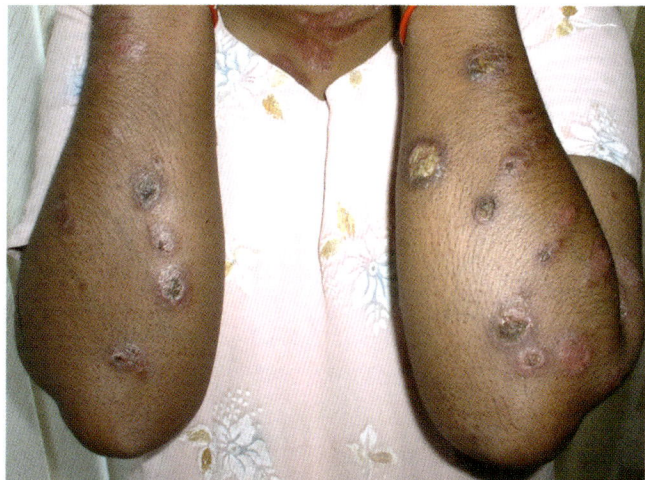

Fig. 15.70 Histoplasmosis. *Courtesy Shyam Verma, MBBS, DVD.*

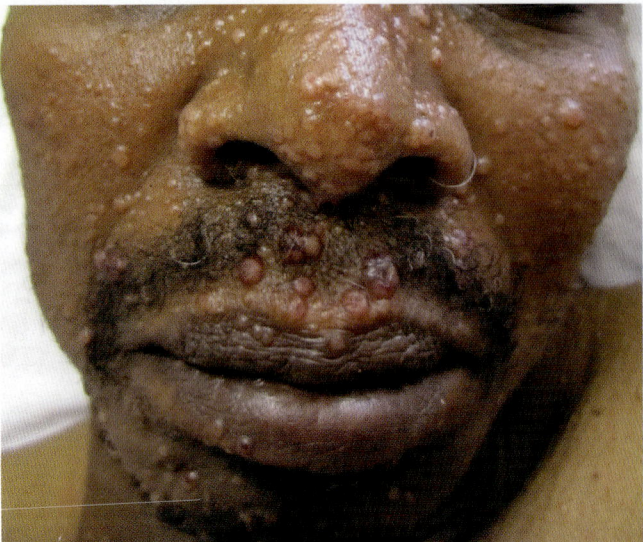

Fig. 15.71 Cryptococcal infection in an HIV-infected patient. *Courtesy Michelle Weir, MD.*

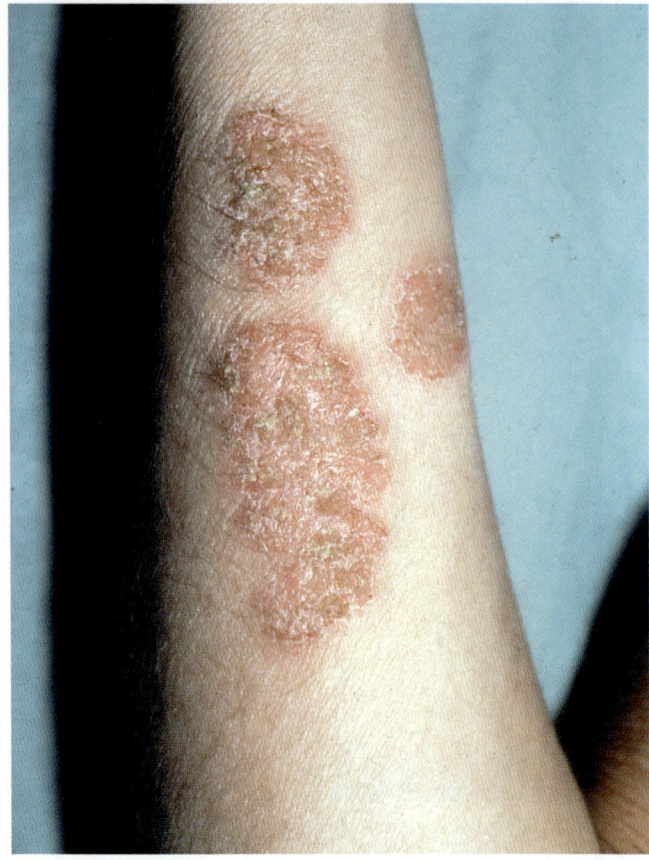

Fig. 15.72 Cryptococcal infection.

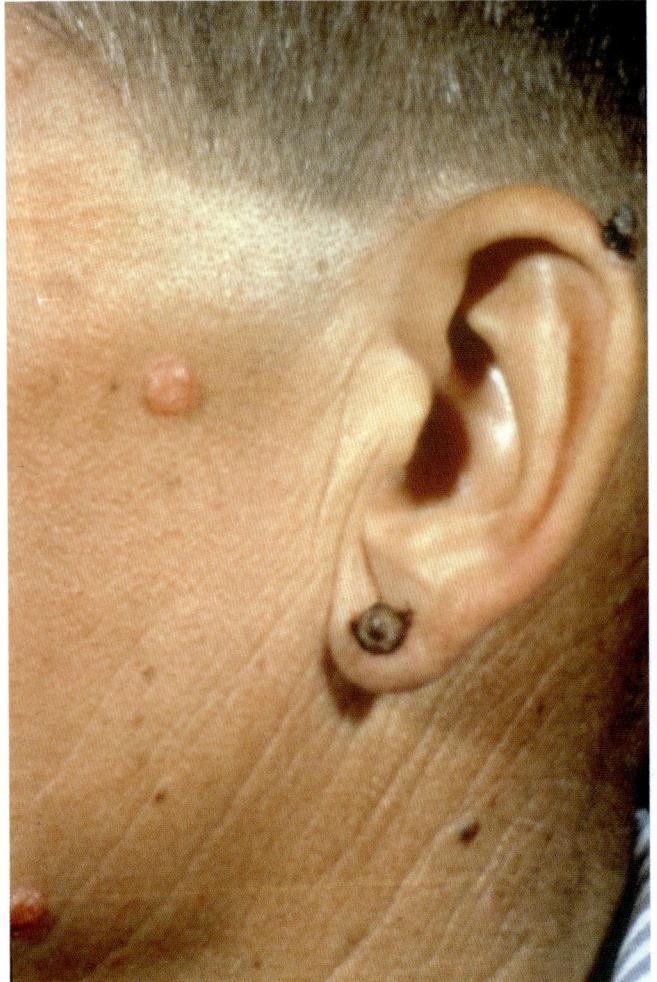

Fig. 15.73 Cryptococcal infection.

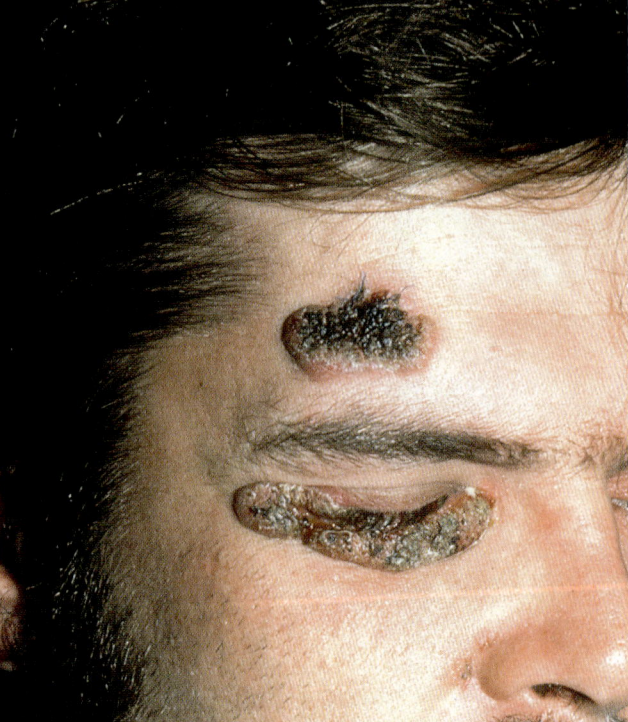

Fig. 15.74 North American blastomycosis.

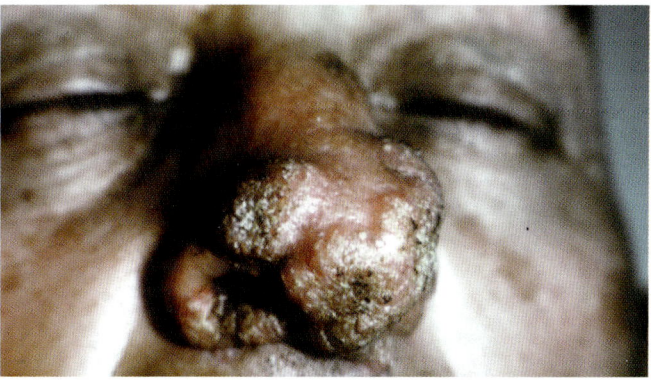

Fig. 15.75 North American blastomycosis.

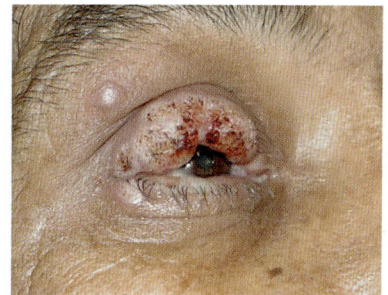

Fig. 15.76 Paracoccidioidomycosis. *Courtesy Lauro de Souza Lima Institute, Brazil.*

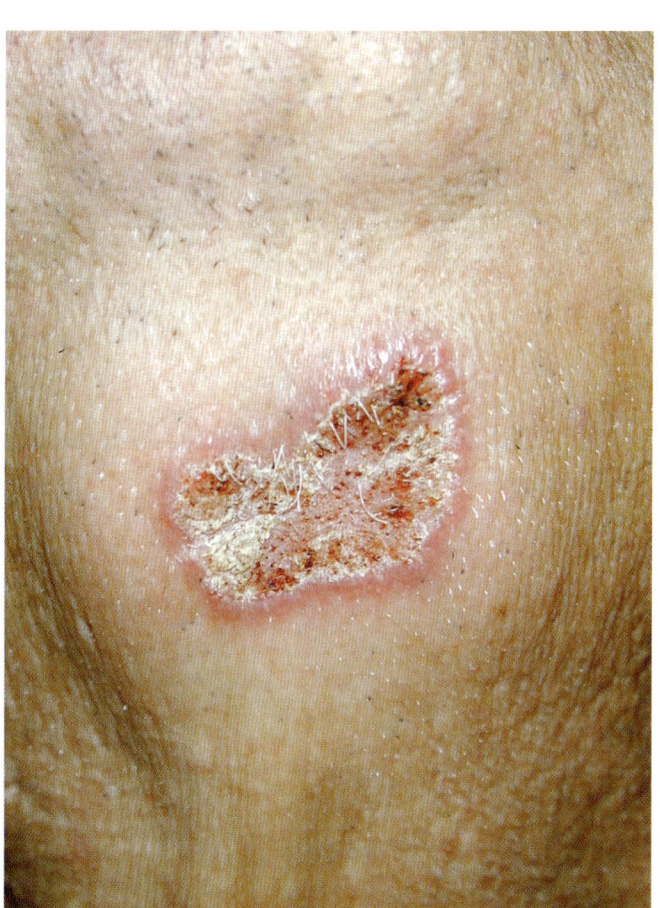

Fig. 15.77 Paracoccidioidomycosis. *Courtesy Lauro de Souza Lima Institute, Brazil.*

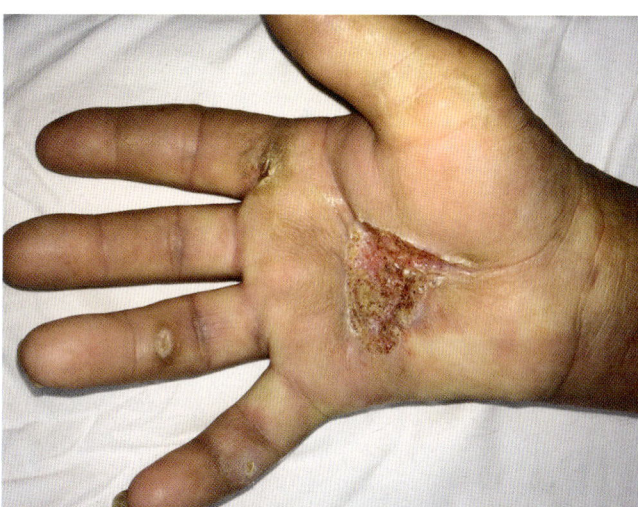

Fig. 15.78 Paracoccidiomycosis. *Courtesy Tatiana C. P. Cordeiro de Andrade, MD.*

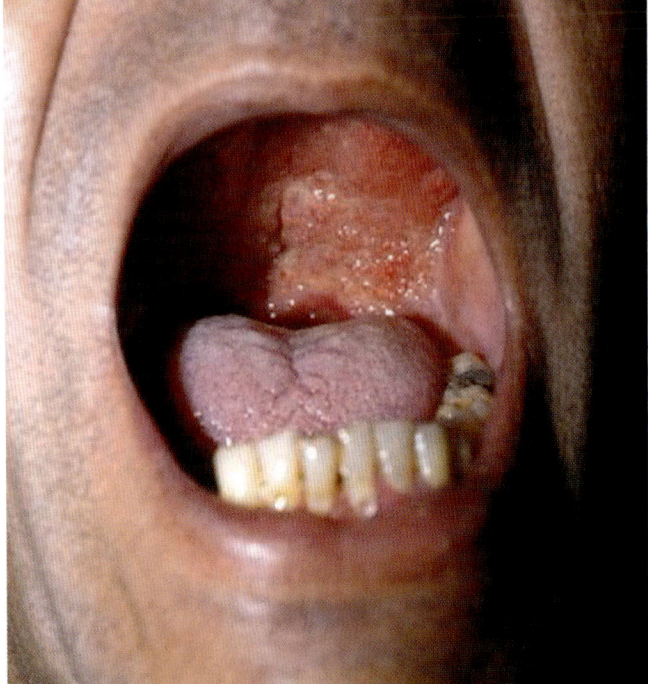

Fig. 15.79 Paracoccidioidomycosis. *Courtesy Lauro de Souza Lima Institute, Brazil.*

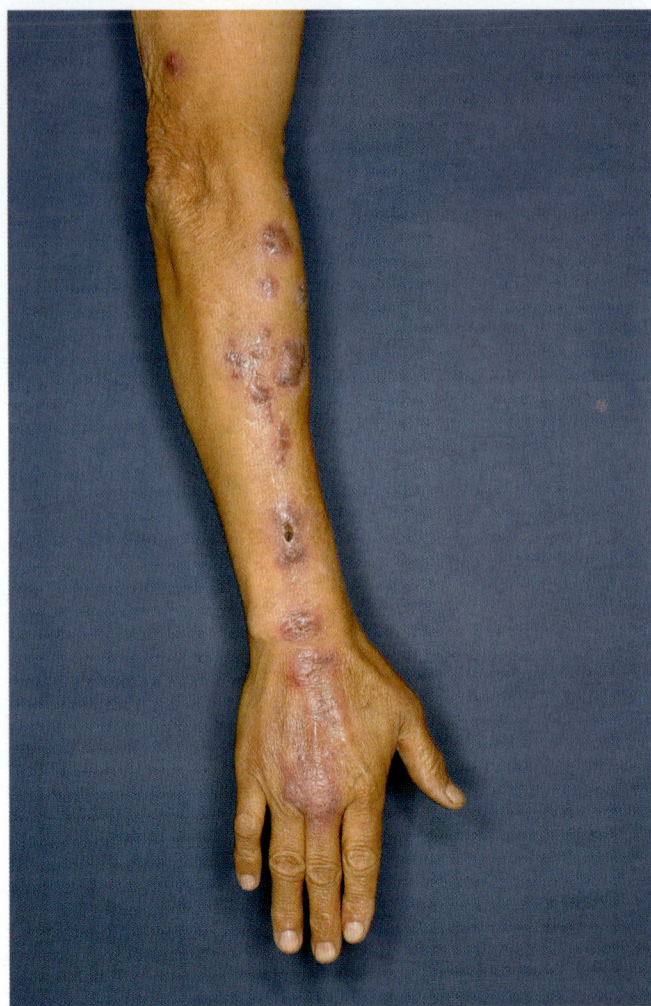

Fig. 15.80 Sporotrichosis. *Courtesy Lauro de Souza Lima Institute, Brazil.*

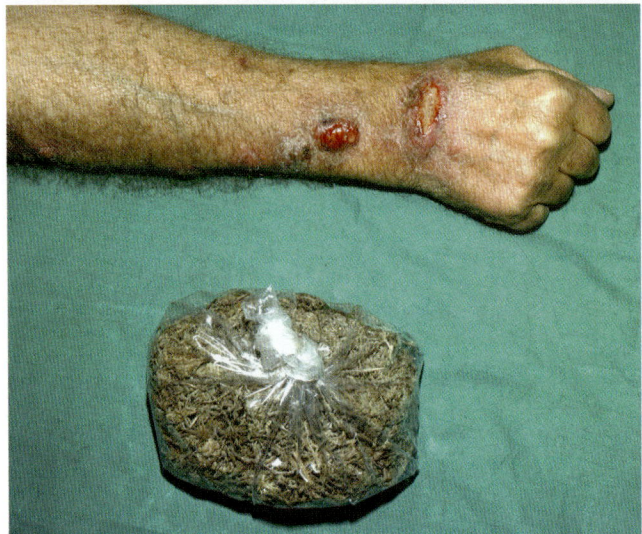

Fig. 15.81 Patient with sporotrichosis from sphagnum moss (bag). *Courtesy The University of Utah and Oregon Health Sciences University Leonard Swinyer MD image collection.*

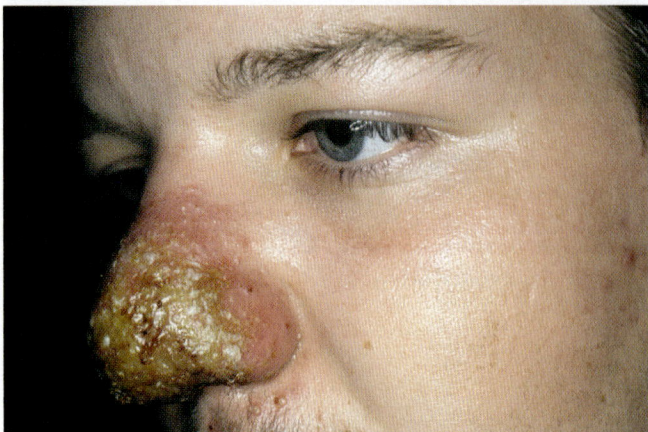

Fig. 15.82 Fixed cutaneous sporotrichosis. *Courtesy Scott Norton, MD.*

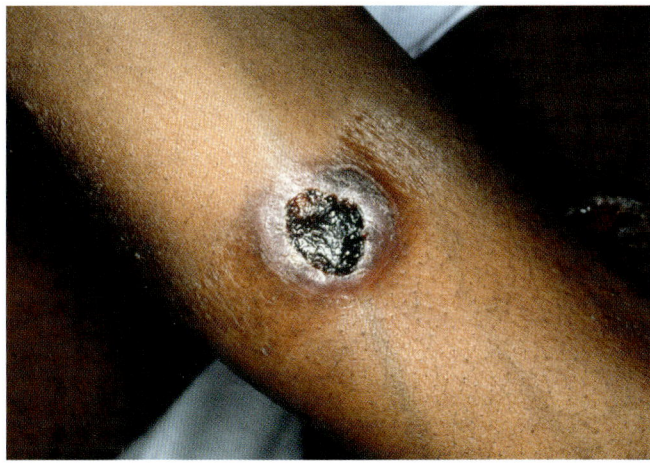

Fig. 15.83 Disseminated sporotrichosis. *Courtesy Scott Norton, MD.*

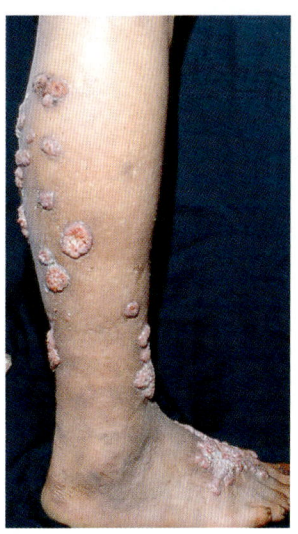

Fig. 15.84 Chromomycosis. *Courtesy Department of Dermatology, University of Campinas, Brazil.*

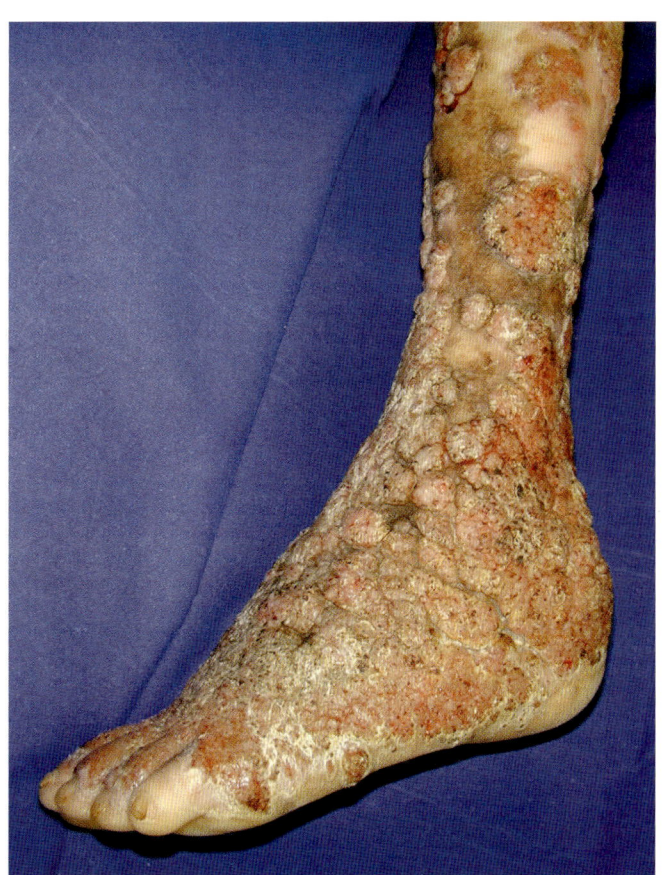

Fig. 15.85 Chromomycosis. *Courtesy Lauro de Souza Lima Institute, Brazil.*

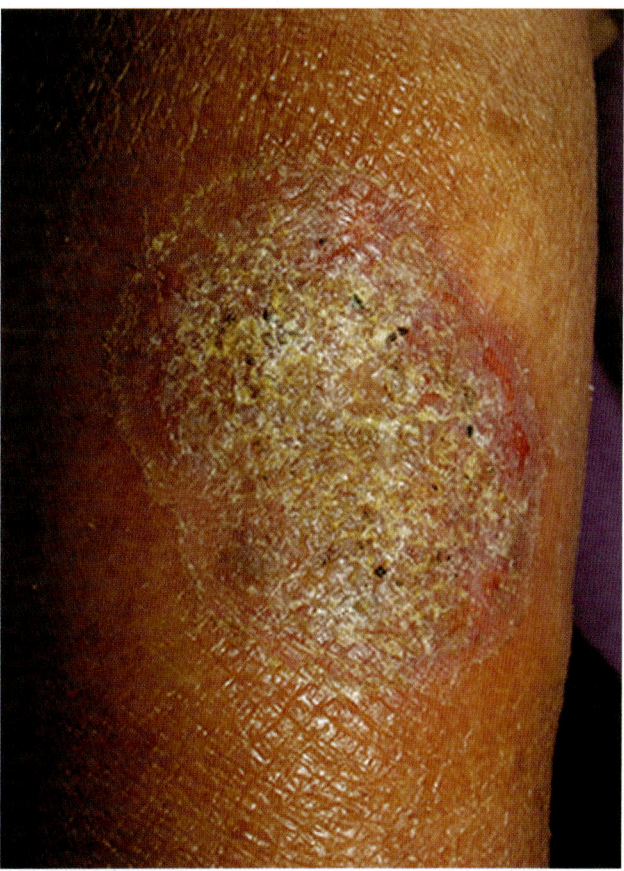

Fig. 15.86 Chromomycosis. *Courtesy Vasanop Vachiramon, MD.*

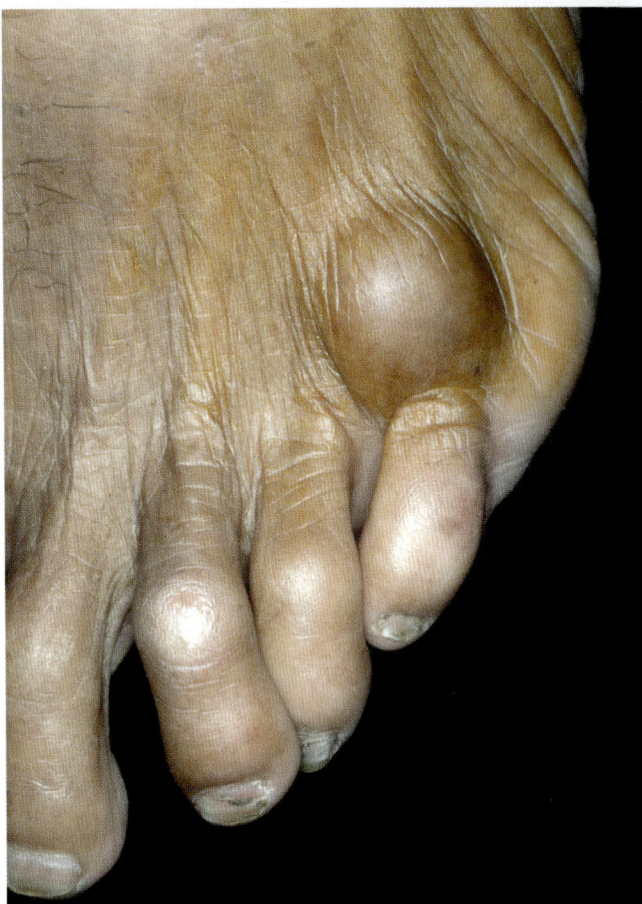

Fig. 15.87 Phaeohyphomycosis. *Courtesy Scott Norton, MD.*

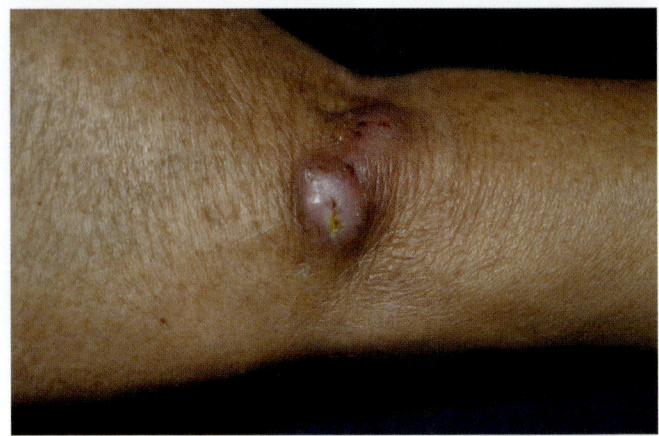

Fig. 15.88 Phaeohyphomycosis. *Courtesy National Cheng Kung University, Taiwan.*

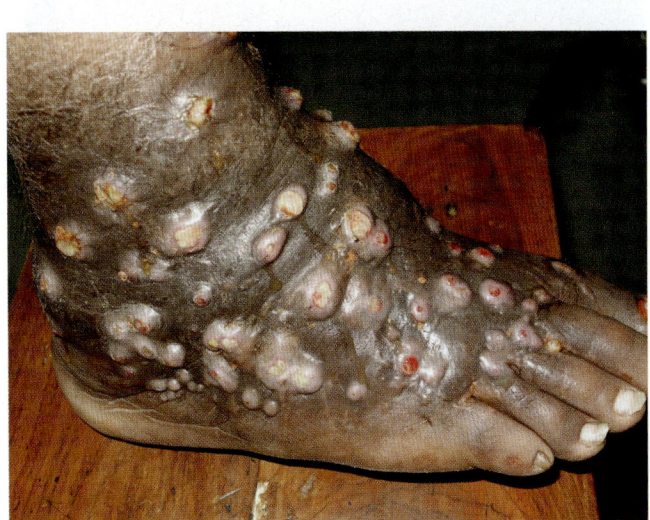

Fig. 15.89 Mycetoma. *Courtesy Debabrata Bandyopadhyay, MD.*

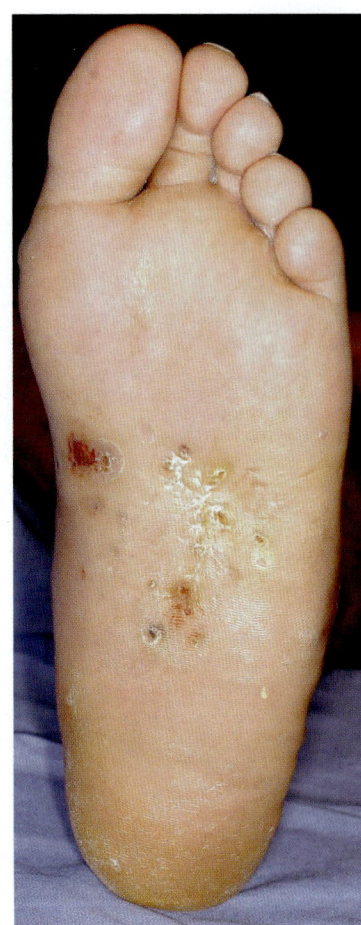

Fig. 15.90 Mycetoma. *Courtesy Lauro de Souza Lima Institute, Brazil.*

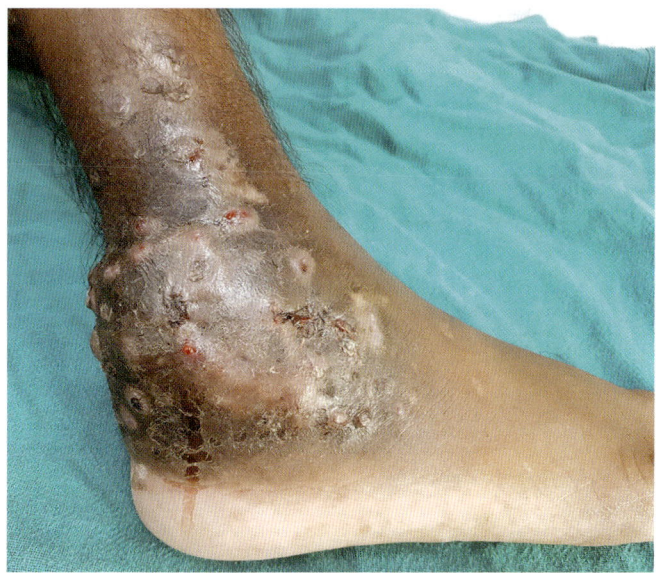

Fig. 15.91 Mycetoma. *Courtesy Archana Singal, MD.*

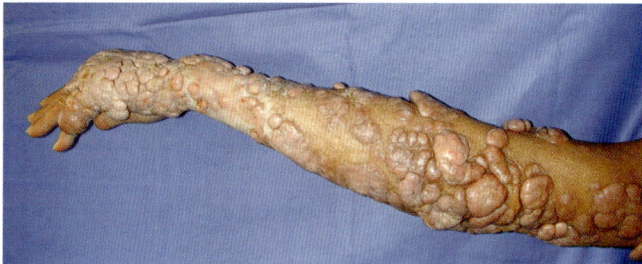

Fig. 15.92 Lobomycosis. *Courtesy Lauro de Souza Lima Institute, Brazil.*

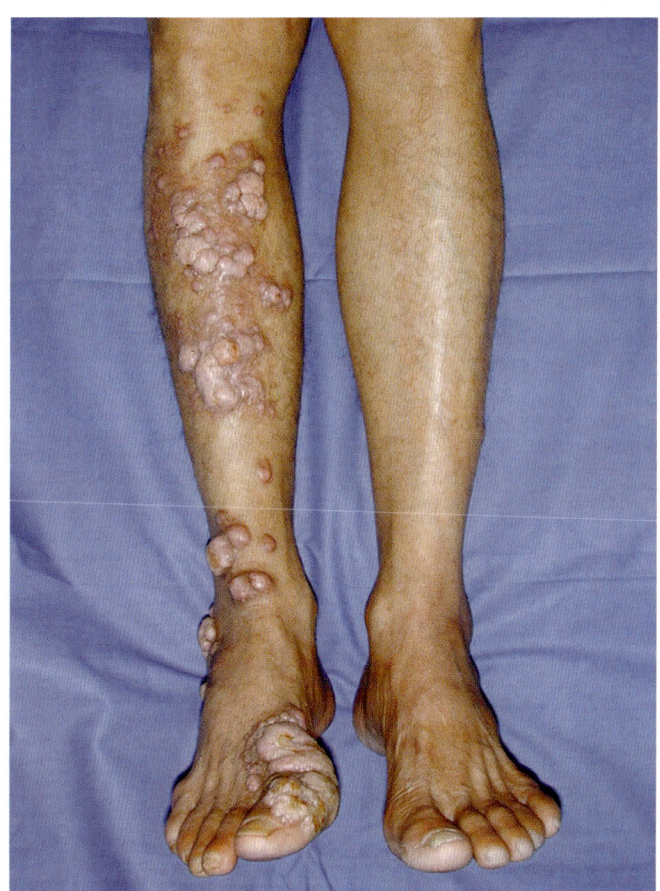

Fig. 15.93 Lobomycosis. *Courtesy Lauro de Souza Lima Institute, Brazil.*

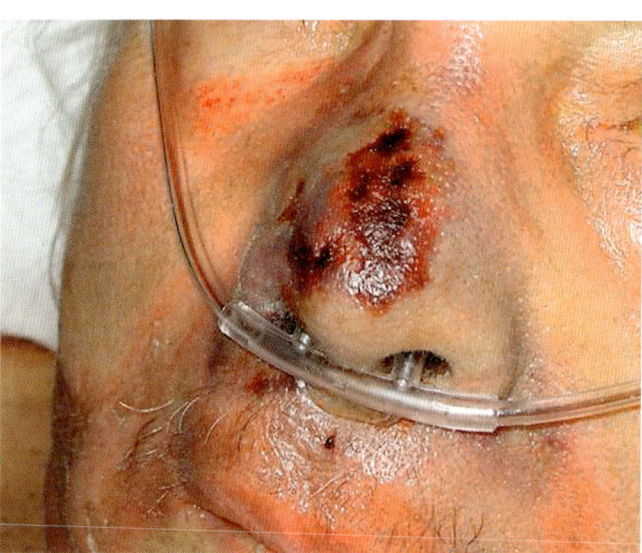

Fig. 15.94 Mucormycosis.

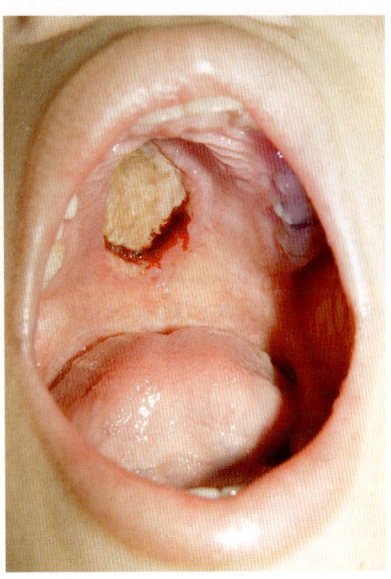

Fig. 15.95 Mucormycosis. *Courtesy National Cheng Kung University, Taiwan.*

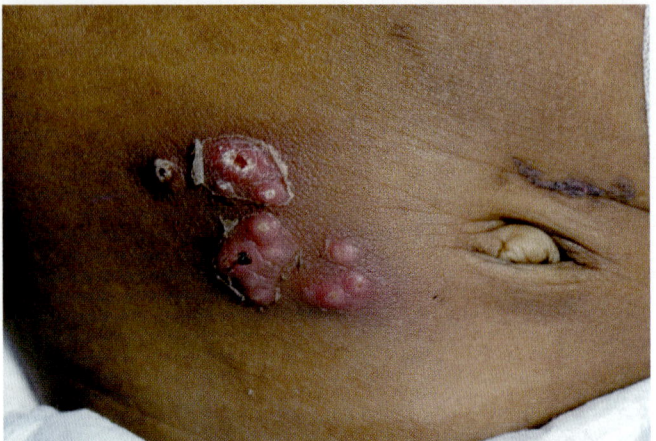

Fig. 15.96 *Rhizopus* infection.

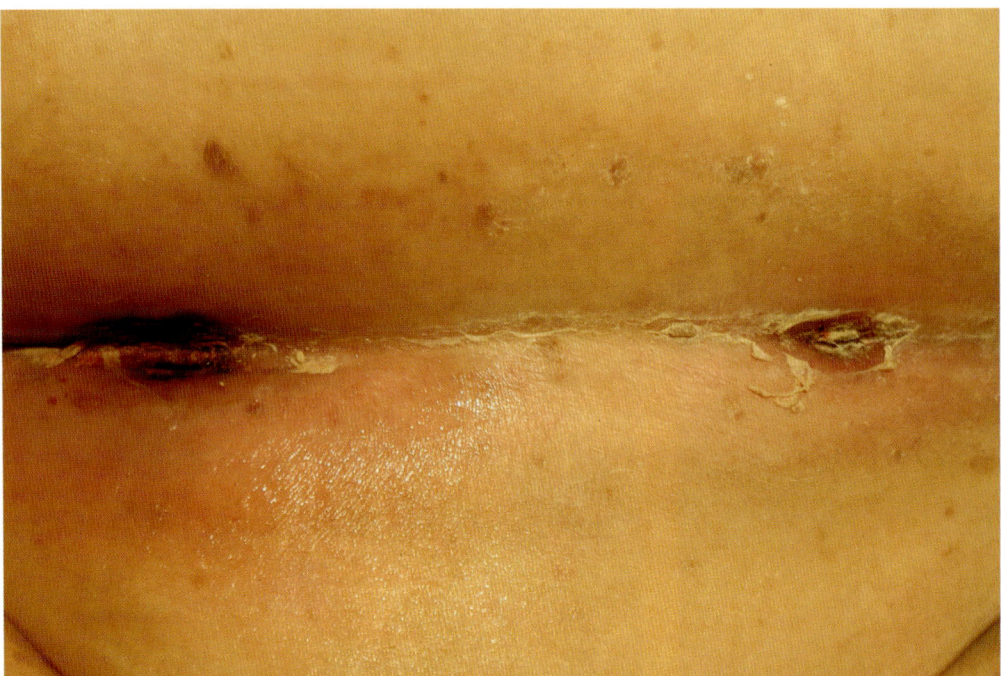

Fig. 15.97 *Fusarium* infection in a leukemic patient.

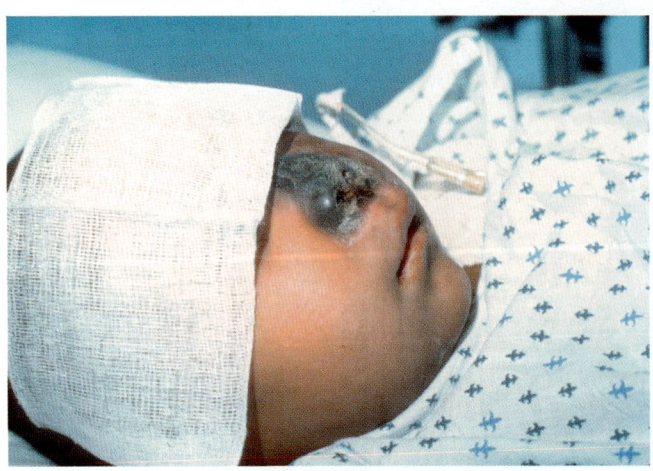

Fig. 15.98 *Aspergillus* infection in a patient with leukemia.

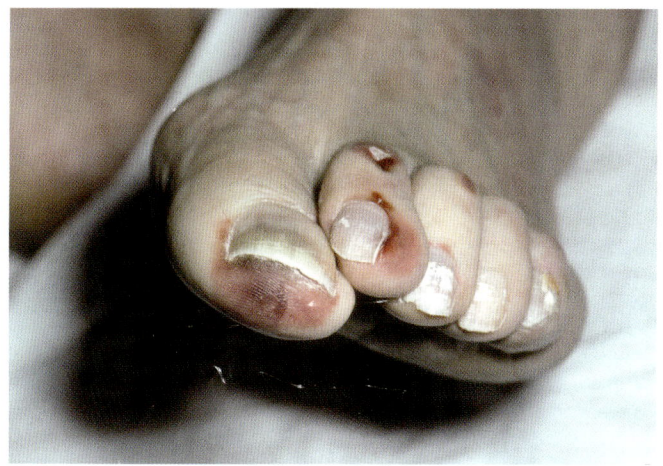

Fig. 15.99 *Aspergillus* infection in a patient with leukemia.

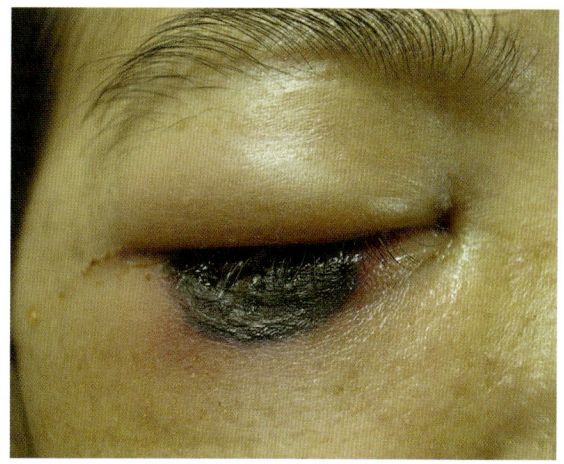

Fig. 15.100 Aspergillosis. *Courtesy Yung-Tsu Cho, MD.*

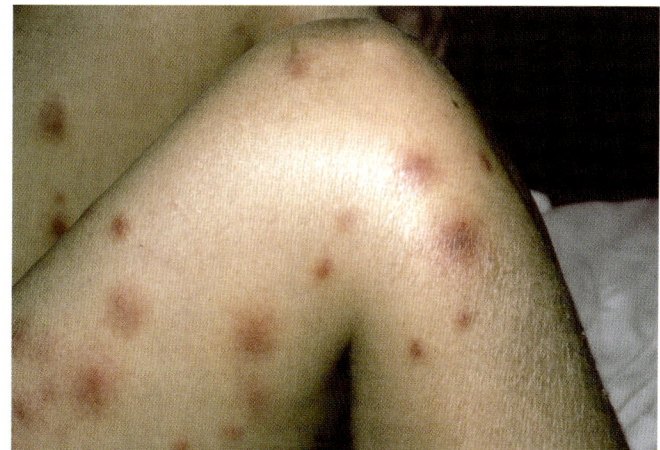

Fig. 15.101 *Aspergillus* infection in a patient with leukemia.

Mycobacterial Diseases 16

Tuberculosis (TB) and atypical mycobacterial infections can be difficult to diagnose clinically and require a high index of suspicion and familiarity with their manifestations in the skin.

Tuberculosis is more prevalent in the developing countries, especially those with particularly high rates of human immunodeficiency virus (HIV)–positive populations. The classification system of cutaneous TB depends on how the infection was acquired, and these four forms include many different cutaneous lesions. Examples of these four categories include 1) verrucous papules or plaques of primary inoculation TB (TB verrucosa cutis); 2) masses and nodules with possible suppuration and ulceration overlying infected lymph nodes representing endogenous, contiguous spread; 3) widespread macules, papules, pustules, nodules, or purpura seen in miliary TB from hematogenous spread; and 4) persistent nodules of the posterior lower calf representing a lobular panniculitis known as *erythema induratum*, a form of a tuberculid. These cutaneous manifestations of TB, along with the many other specific and nonspecific findings, should prompt testing including skin biopsy, tissue culture, screening with blood testing if available such as QuantiFERON-Gold, tuberculin skin testing, and in some, a chest x-ray.

Atypical mycobacterial infections can occur in immunocompetent hosts after trauma, surgery, or exposures to organisms in specific locations such as fish tanks (*Mycobacterium marinum*) or pedicure spas (*Mycobacterium fortuitum*). Immunocompromised individuals are at risk of developing infections with atypical mycobacteria such as the *Mycobacterium avium-intracellulare* as seen in patients infected with HIV. Despite the great variety of atypical mycobacterial organisms, the clinical findings tend to be similar and nonspecific, including papules, pustules, nodules, and ulcers. They can be localized or widespread depending on the cause, exposure, and underlying immune status of the patient. Tissue culture with antibiotic sensitivity testing is helpful, but can take several weeks to be completed.

This chapter of the atlas catalogs the many cutaneous findings seen in patients with both TB and nontuberculous mycobacterial infections.

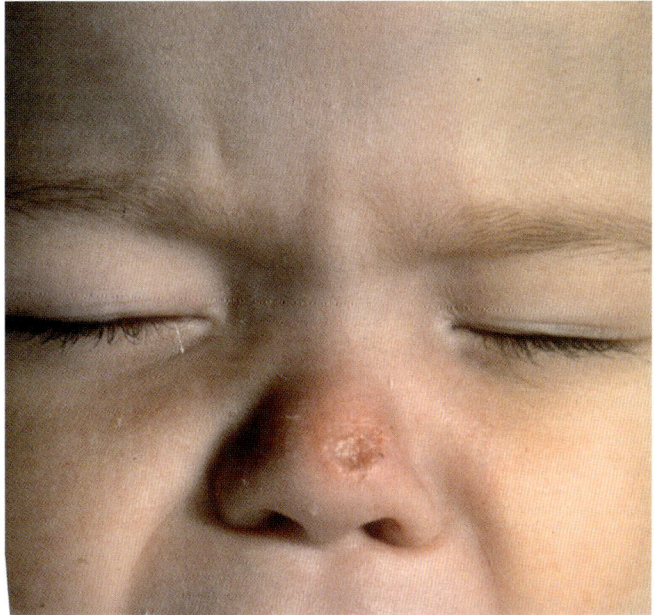

Fig. 16.1 Primary inoculation tuberculosis.

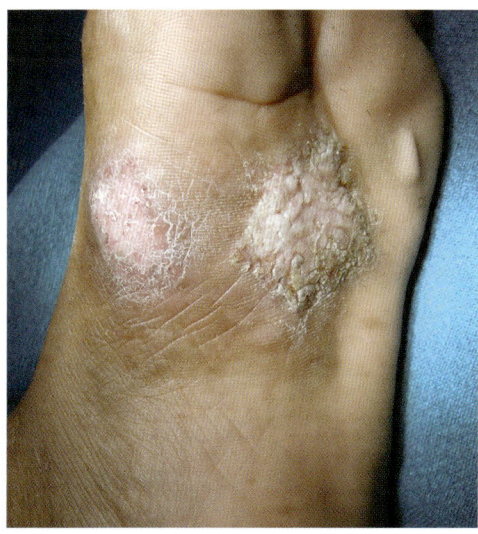

Fig. 16.2 Tuberculosis verrucosa cutis. *Courtesy Archana Singal, MD.*

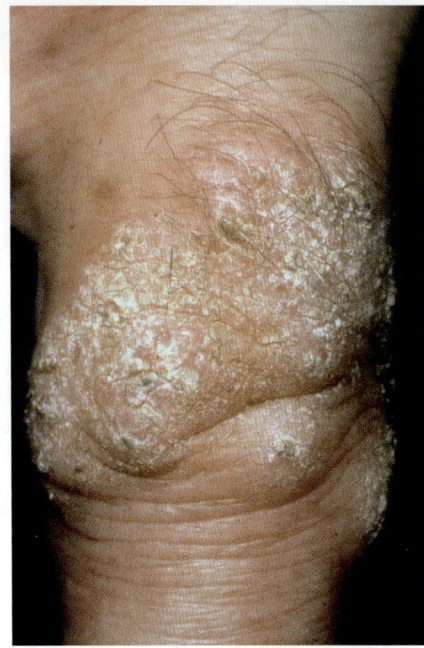

Fig. 16.3 Tuberculosis verrucosa cutis.

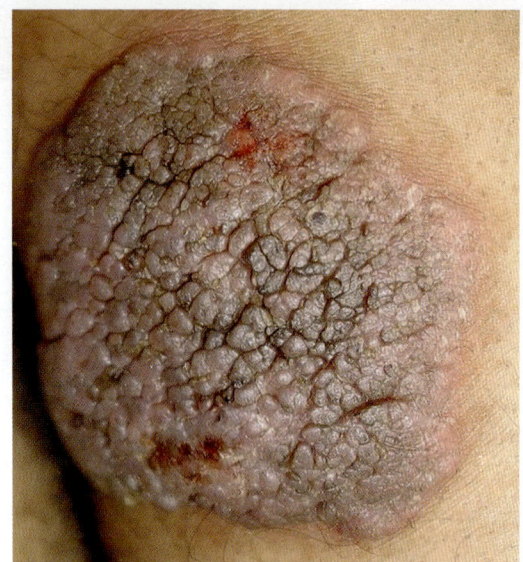

Fig. 16.4 Tuberculosis verrucosa cutis. *Courtesy Shyam Verma, MBBS, DVD.*

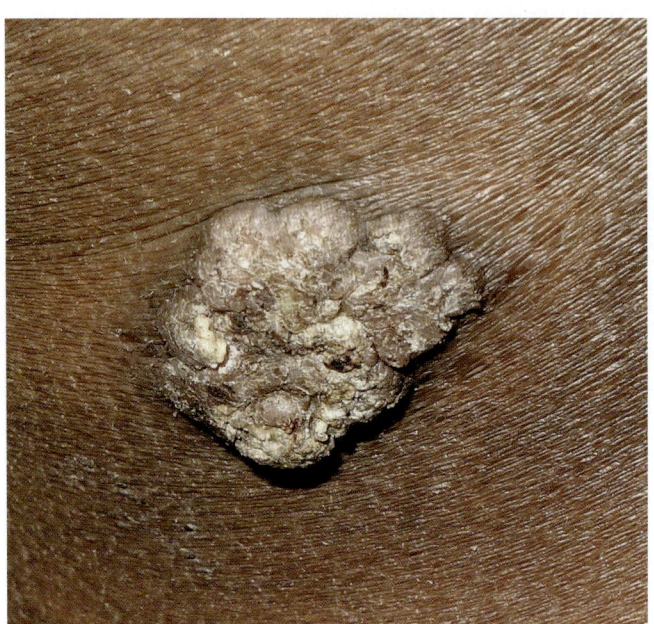

Fig. 16.5 Tuberculosis verrucosa cutis. *Courtesy Debabrata Bandyopadhyay, MD.*

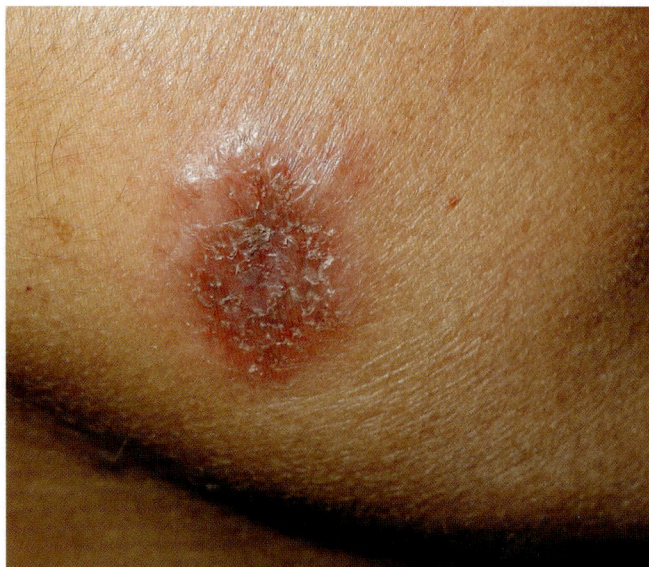

Fig. 16.6 Lupus vulgaris. *Courtesy Debabrata Bandyopadhyay, MD.*

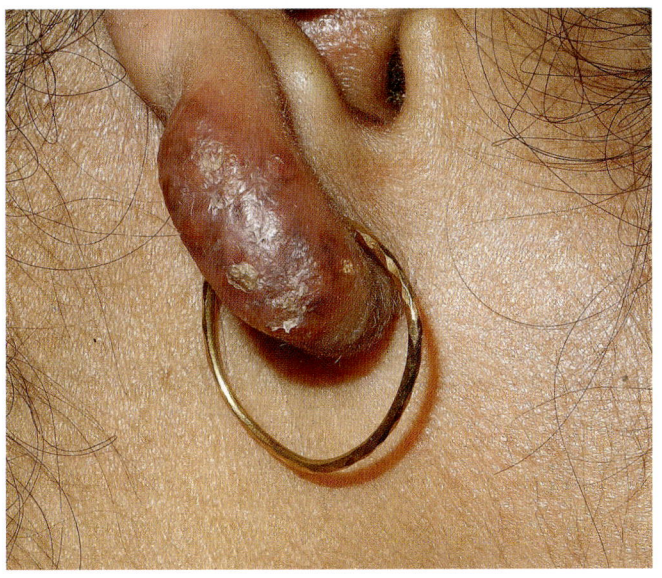

Fig. 16.7 Lupus vulgaris. *Courtesy Debabrata Bandyopadhyay.*

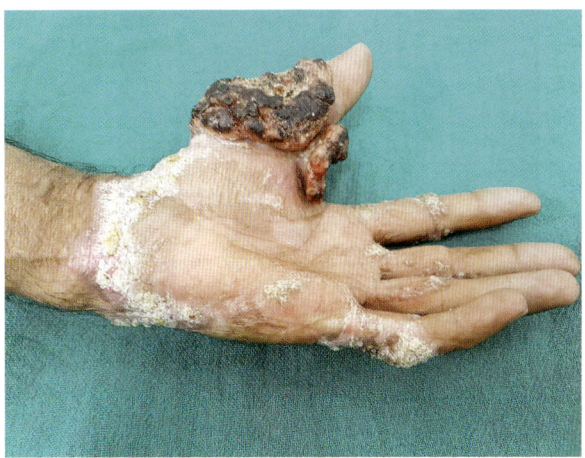

Fig. 16.8 Lupus vulgaris with a squamous cell carcinoma complicating a long-standing lesion. *Courtesy Archana Singal, MD.*

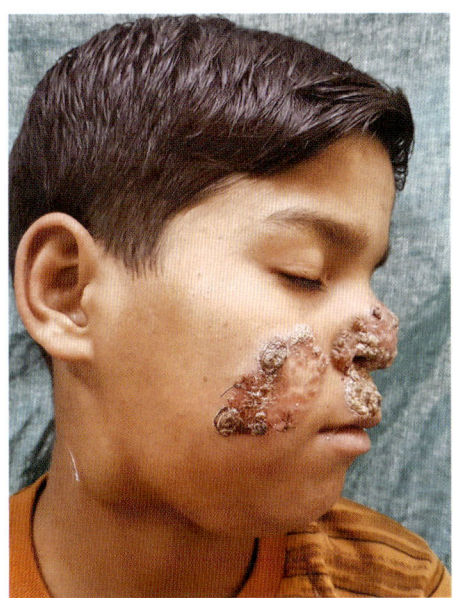

Fig. 16.9 Lupus vulgaris. *Courtesy Archana Singal, MD.*

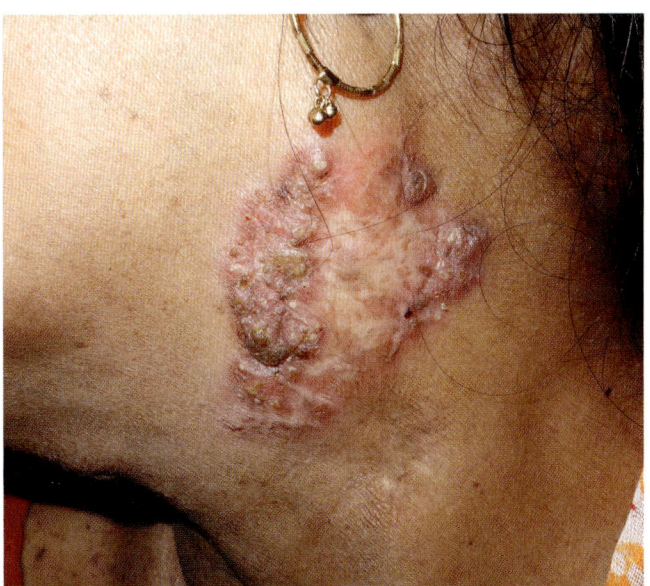

Fig. 16.10 Lupus vulgaris. *Courtesy Debabrata Bandyopadhyay, MD.*

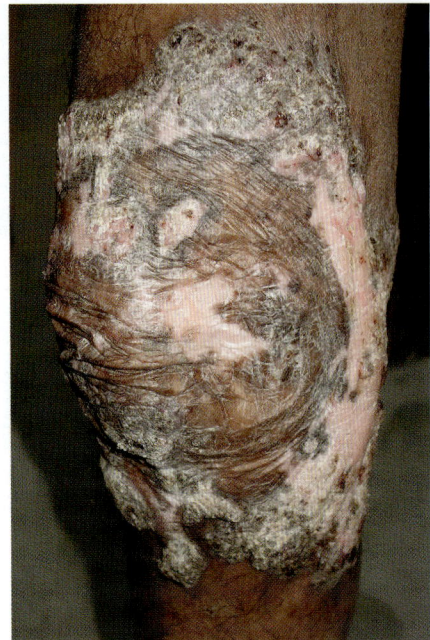

Fig. 16.11 Lupus vulgaris. *Courtesy Debabrata Bandyopadhyay, MD.*

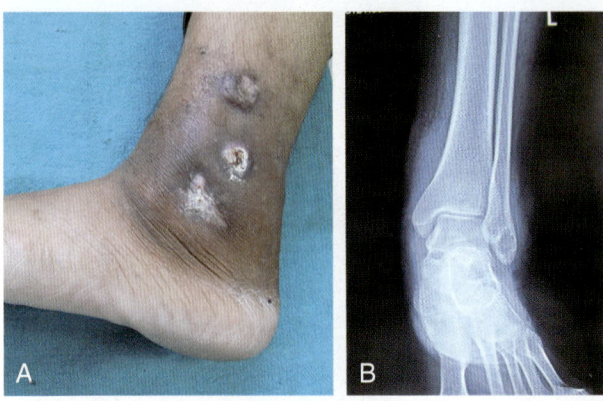

Fig. 16.12 Photograph (A) and radiograph (B) of scrofuloderma from underlying tuberculous bony involvement. *Courtesy Archana Singal, MD.*

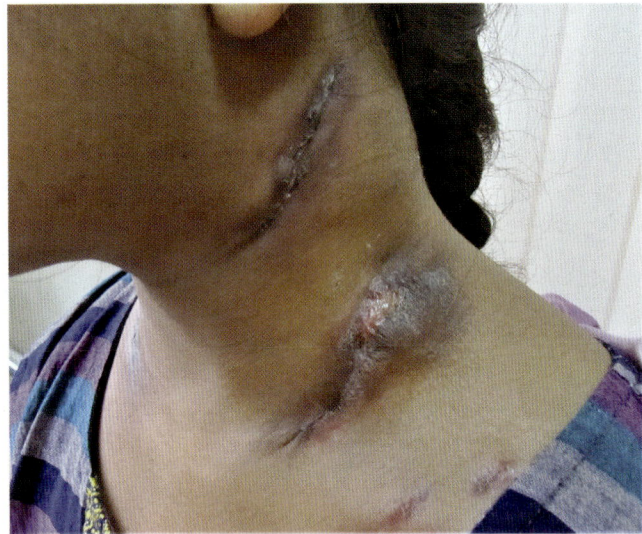

Fig. 16.13 Scrofuloderma. *Courtesy Archana Singal, MD.*

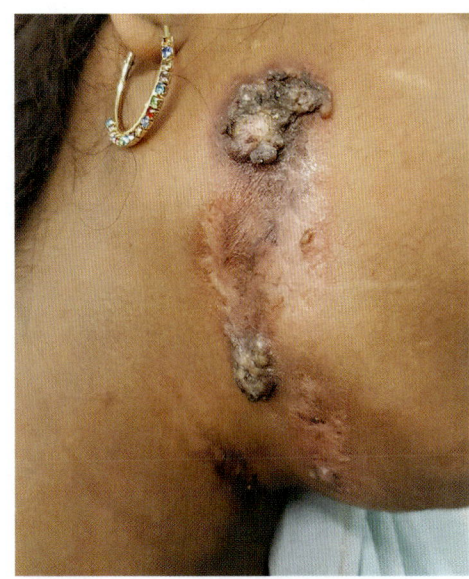

Fig. 16.14 Scrofuloderma. *Courtesy Archana Singal, MD.*

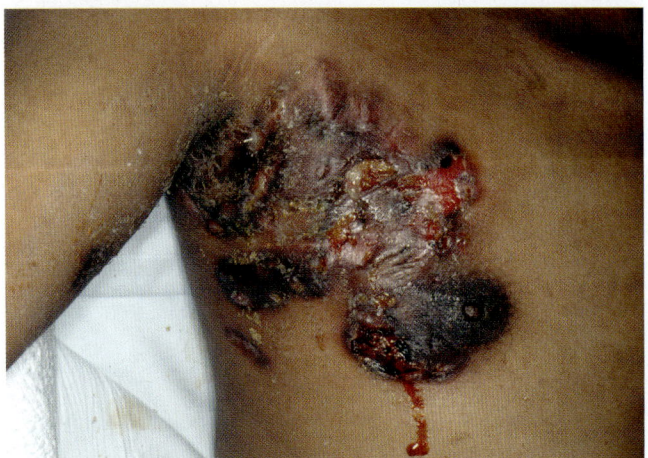

Fig. 16.15 Scrofuloderma. *Courtesy Scott Norton, MD.*

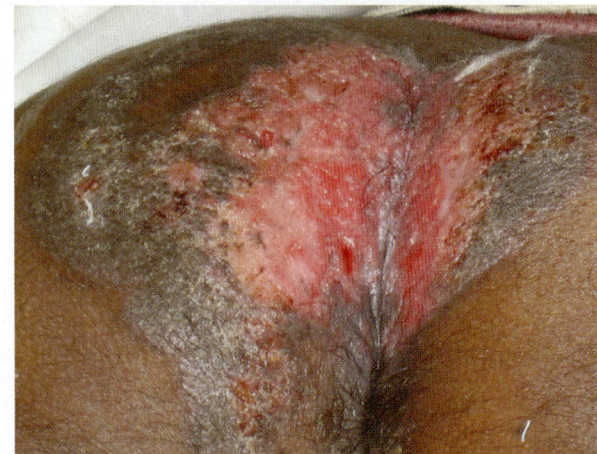

Fig. 16.16 Orificial tuberculosis. *Courtesy Archana Singal, MD.*

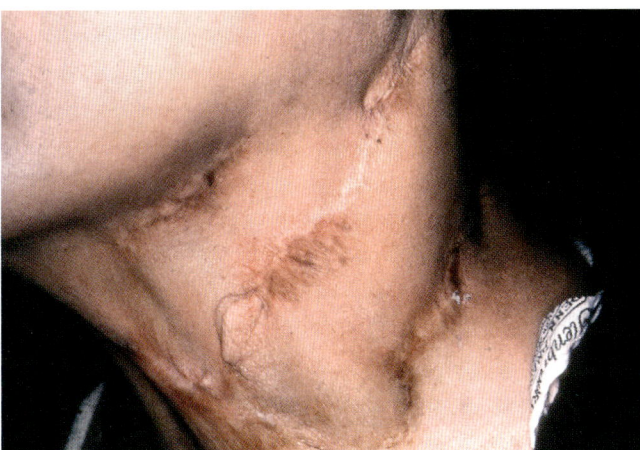

Fig. 16.17 Linear scarring after scrofuloderma.

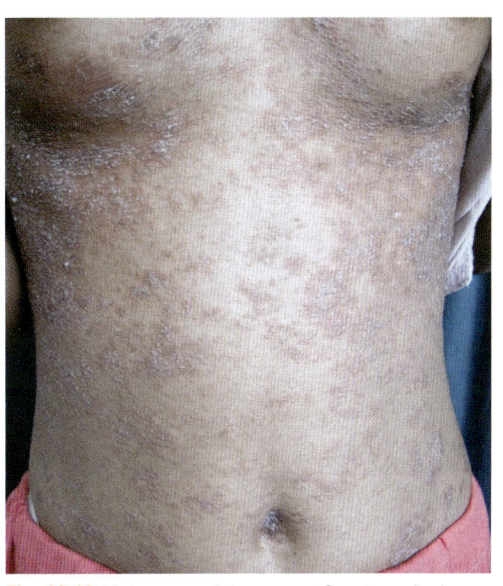

Fig. 16.18 Lichen scrofulosorum. *Courtesy Archana Singal, MD.*

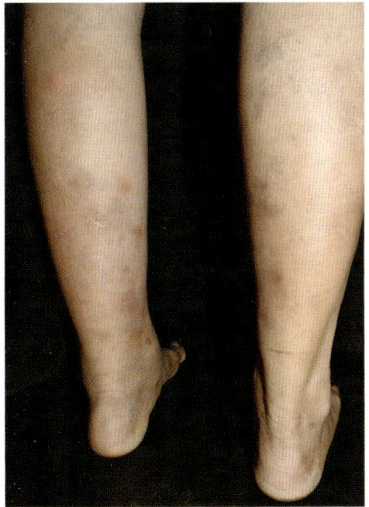

Fig. 16.19 Erythema induratum. *Courtesy National Taiwan University Hospital.*

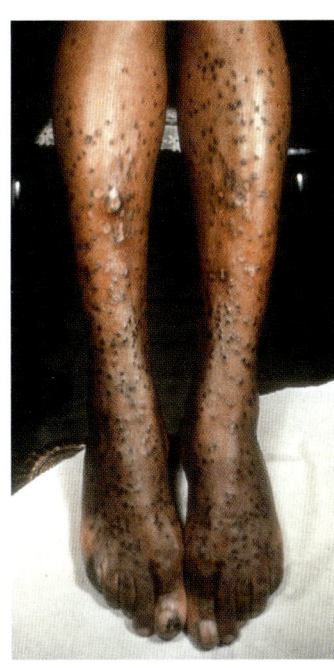

Fig. 16.20 Papulonecrotic tuberculid. *Courtesy James Steger, MD.*

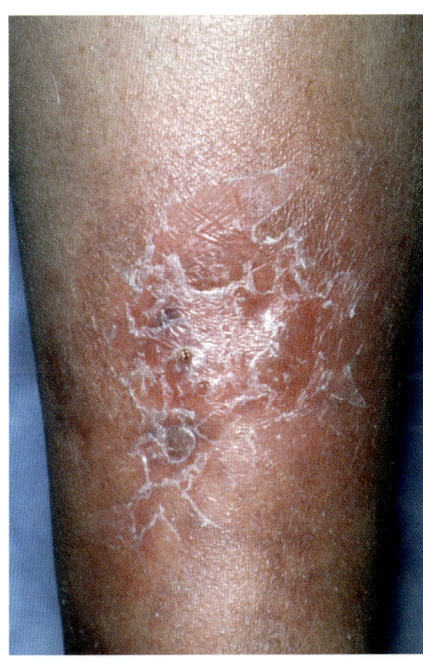

Fig. 16.21 Erythema induratum.

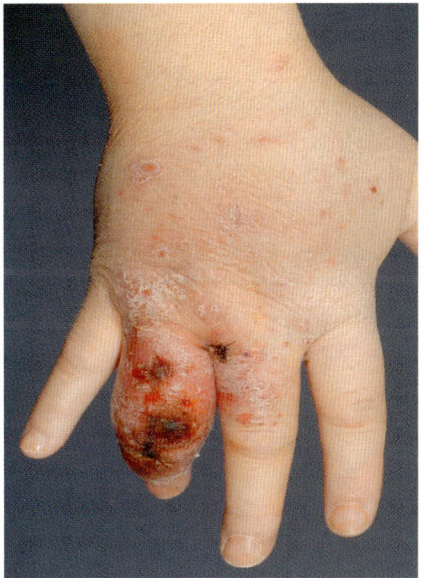

Fig. 16.22 *Mycobacterium marinum* infection in an immunocompromised patient.

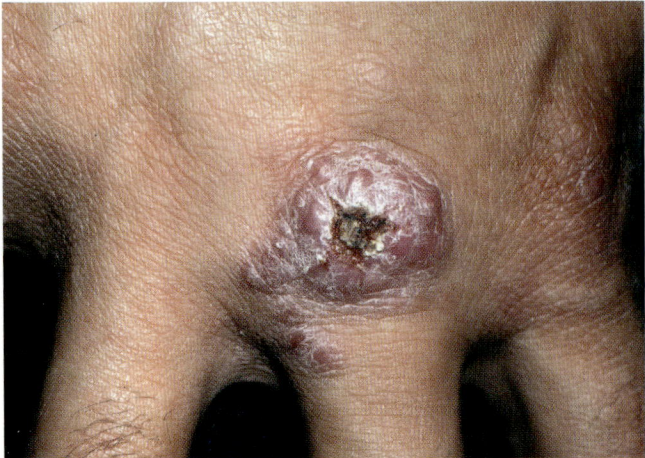

Fig. 16.23 *Mycobacterium marinum* infection. *Courtesy Steven Binnick, MD.*

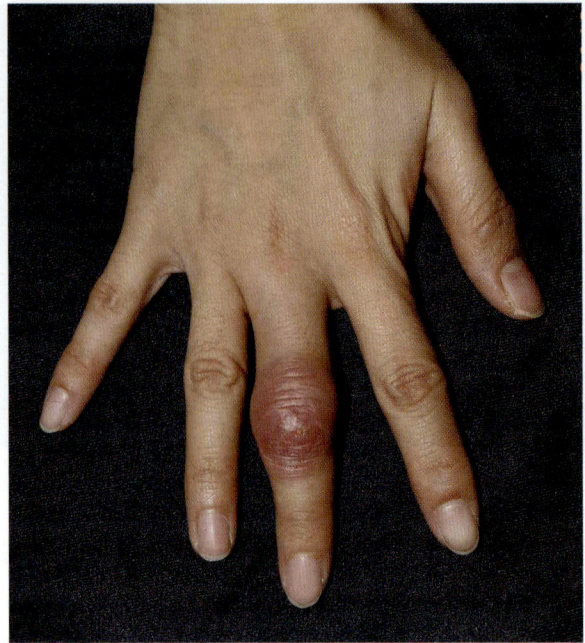

Fig. 16.24 *Mycobacterium marinum* infection. *Courtesy National Cheng Kung University, Taiwan.*

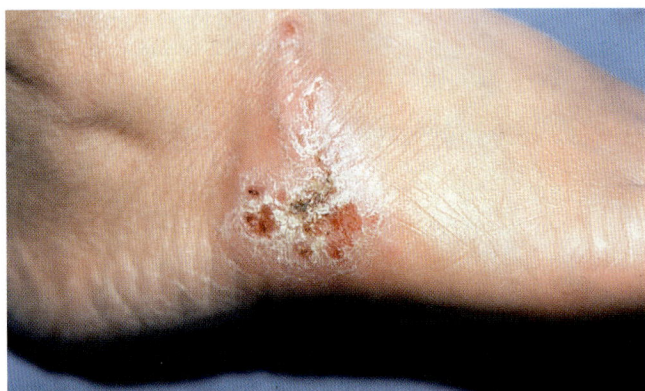

Fig. 16.25 *Mycobacterium marinum* infection. *Courtesy Edward C. Oldfield, III, MD.*

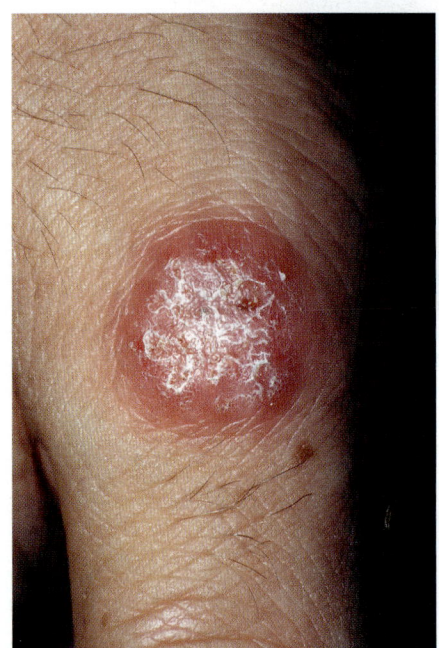

Fig. 16.26 *Mycobacterium marinum* infection in a sporotrichoid pattern. *Courtesy Dr. Steven Binnick, MD.*

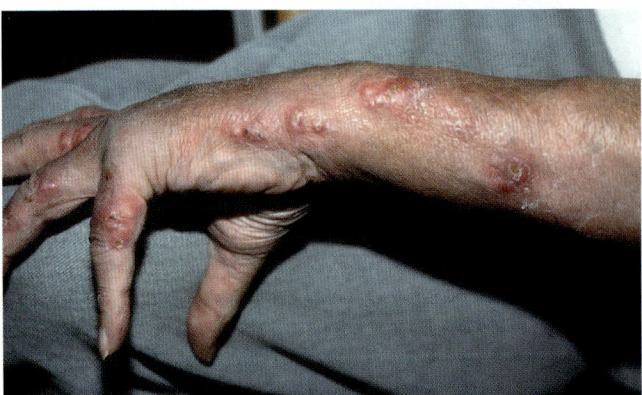

Fig. 16.27 *Mycobacterium marinum* infection in a sporotrichoid pattern.

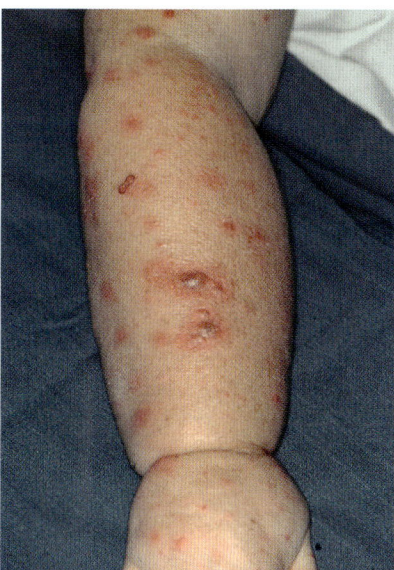

Fig. 16.28 *Mycobacterium marinum* infection in a sporotrichoid pattern.

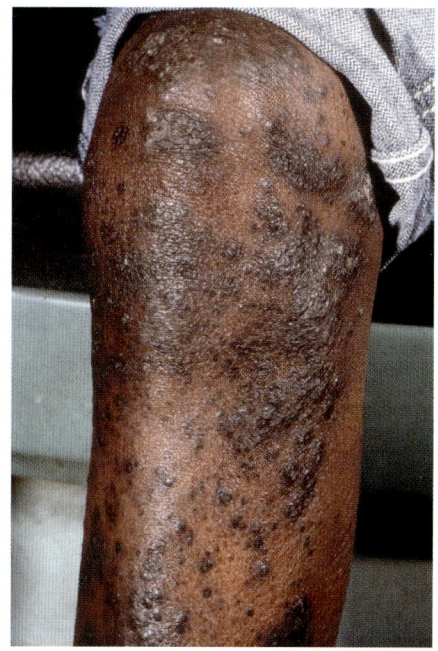

Fig. 16.29 Disseminated *Mycobacterium marinum* infection in a patient with lupus. Minocycline pigmentation is present. *Courtesy Curt Samlaska, MD.*

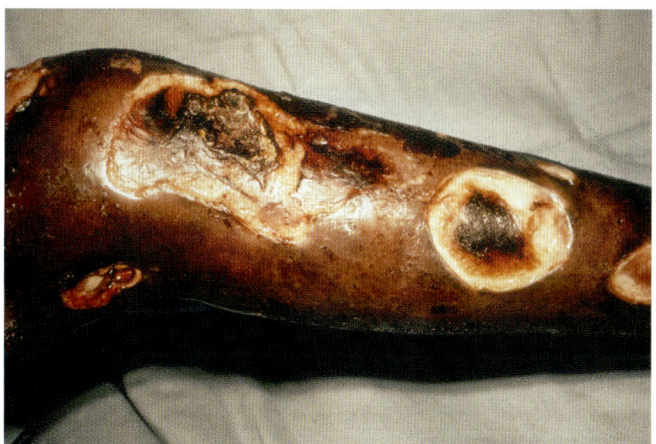

Fig. 16.30 Buruli ulcer. *Courtesy Scott Norton, MD.*

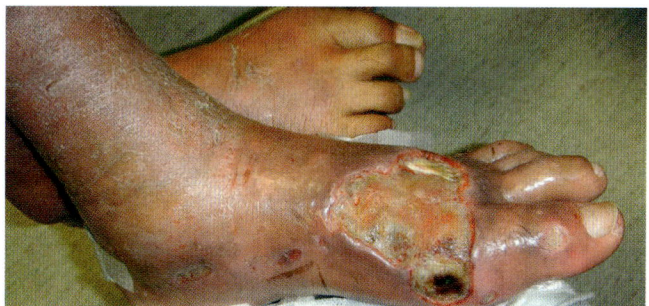

Fig. 16.31 *Mycobacterium haemophilum* cellulitis and ulcer. *Courtesy Dr. Ang Chia Chun.*

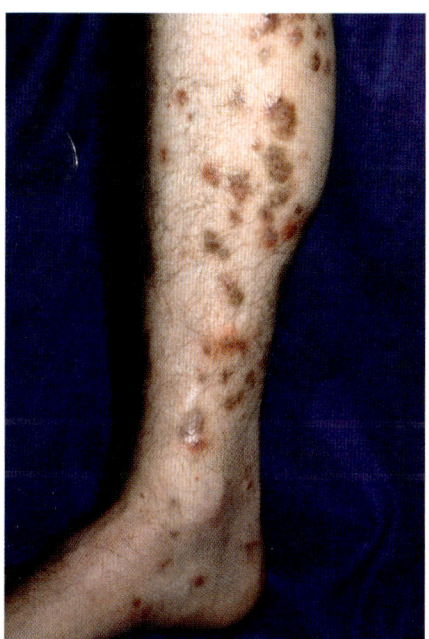

Fig. 16.32 *Mycobacterium fortuitum* infection.

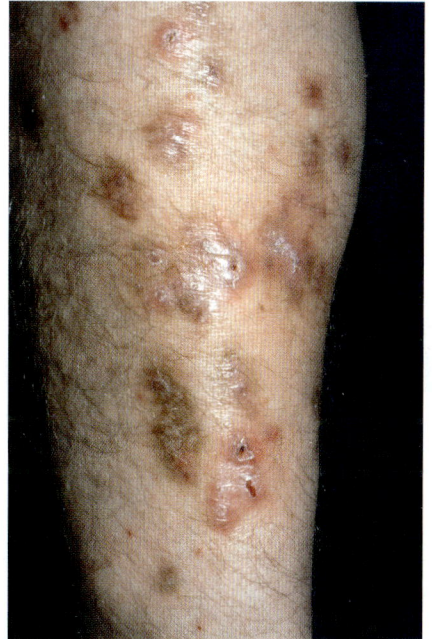

Fig. 16.33 *Mycobacterium fortuitum* infection.

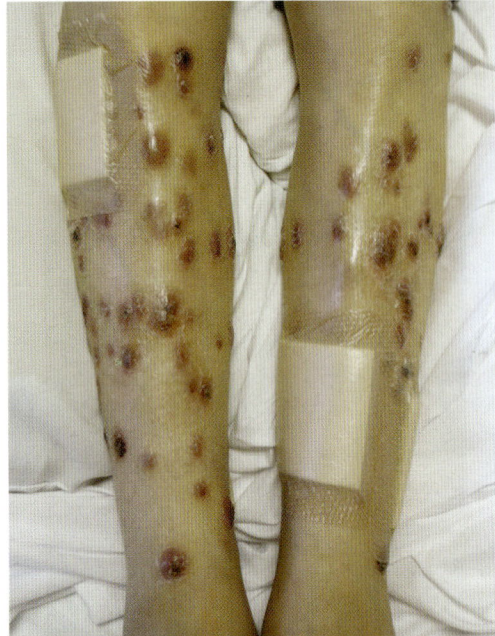

Fig. 16.34 *Mycobacterium* abscessus infection in a lung transplant recipient.

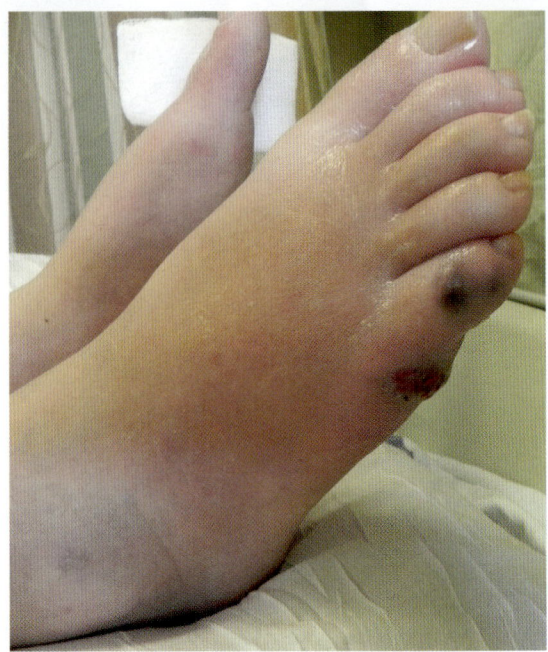

Fig. 16.35 *Mycobacterium chelonae* infection in a lung transplant patient.

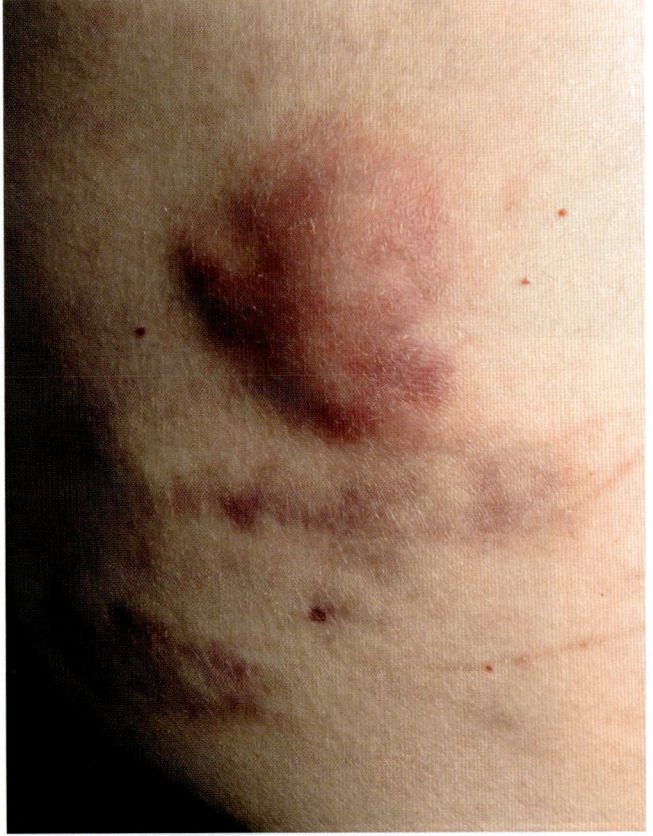

Fig. 16.36 *Mycobacterium abscessus* infection in an otherwise healthy patient.

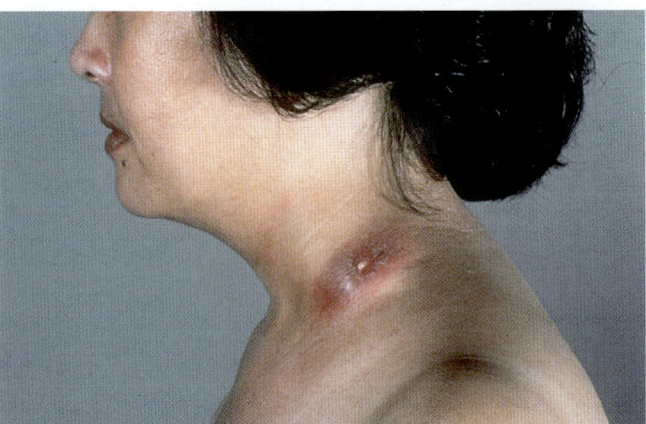

Fig. 16.37 *Mycobacterium chelonae* infection. *Courtesy Edward C. Oldfield III, MD.*

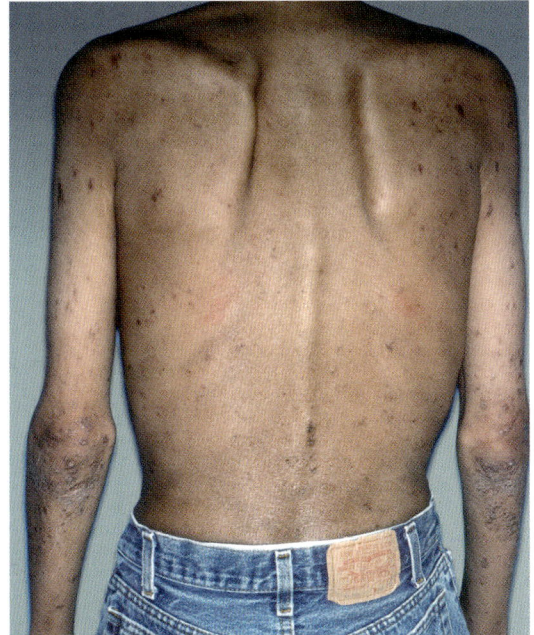

Fig. 16.38 Generalized *Mycobacterium avium-intracellulare* infection in an HIV-infected patient. *Courtesy Curt Samlaska, MD.*

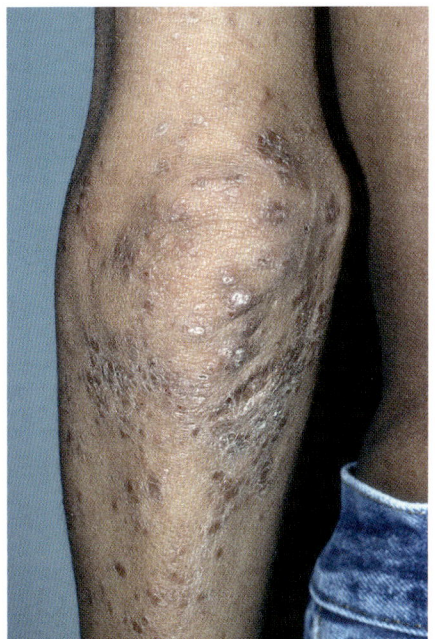

Fig. 16.39 Generalized *Mycobacterium avium-intracellulare* infection in an HIV-infected patient. *Courtesy Curt Samlaska, MD.*

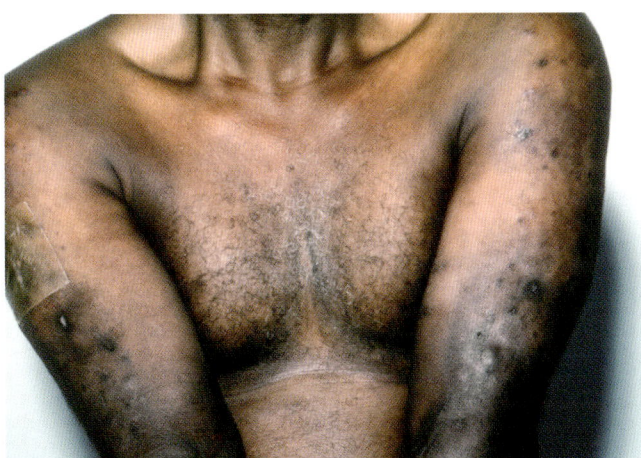

Fig. 16.40 Cutaneous *Mycobacterium avium-intracellulare* infection.

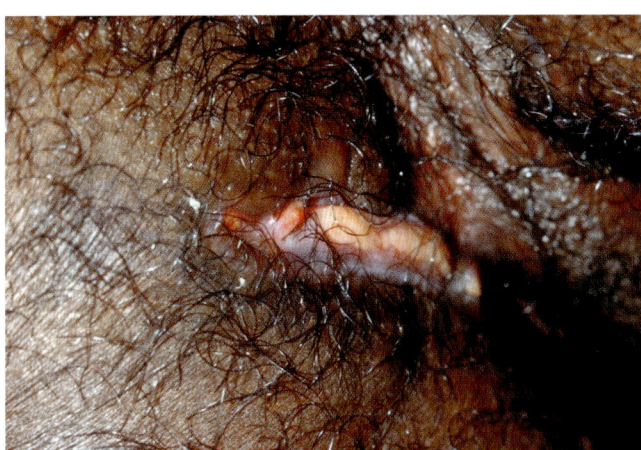

Fig. 16.41 Cutaneous *Mycobacterium kansasii* infection.

Hansen Disease 17

Clinical manifestations of leprosy vary from the subtle hypopigmented patches of indeterminate leprosy to the diffuse facial infiltration and nodules of lepromatous leprosy. The clinical and histologic manifestations of the disease are a reflection of the immune response and bacterial burden. Indeterminate leprosy demonstrates sparse perivascular lymphoid infiltrates and onion skin fibrosis as a manifestation of chronicity. The clinical findings are also subtle with little to no erythema or induration. Tuberculoid leprosy presents as indurated erythematous anesthetic plaques; borderline disease is characterized by annular erythematous indurated lesions, and the lepromatous pole by papules, nodules, and diffuse induration with loss of lateral eyebrows and progression to leonine facies. Diffuse induration correlates with a diffuse dermal histiocytic infiltrate. Globi (clusters of organisms) are easily identified in tissue sections.

Reactional states include reversal reactions characterized by increasing induration, pain, and neurologic manifestations as a reflection of a heightened cell-mediated immune response. In contrast, erythema nodosum leprosum represents a reaction to locally formed immune complexes and is characterized histologically by leukocytoclastic vasculitis in areas of high bacterial burden. Lucio phenomenon demonstrates thrombosis of large and small vessels with variable vasculitis and presents with stellate ulcers and retiform purpura on a background of indurated skin. This portion of the atlas will guide you through the various clinical presentations of Hansen disease.

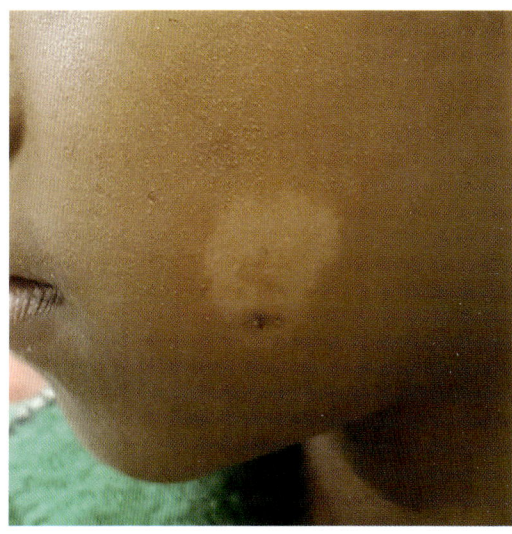

Fig. 17.2 Indeterminate leprosy. *Courtesy Archana Singal, MD.*

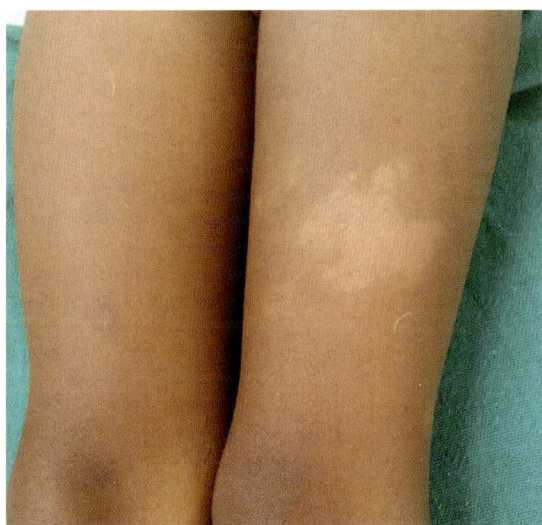

Fig. 17.1 Indeterminate leprosy. *Courtesy Archana Singal, MD.*

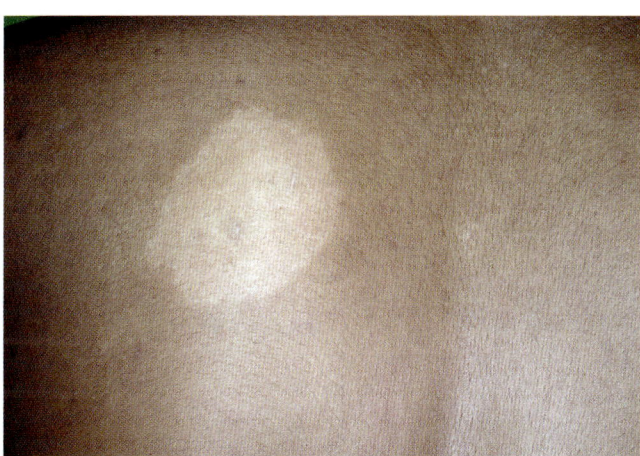

Fig. 17.3 Early tuberculoid leprosy. *Courtesy Shyam Verma, MBBS, DVD.*

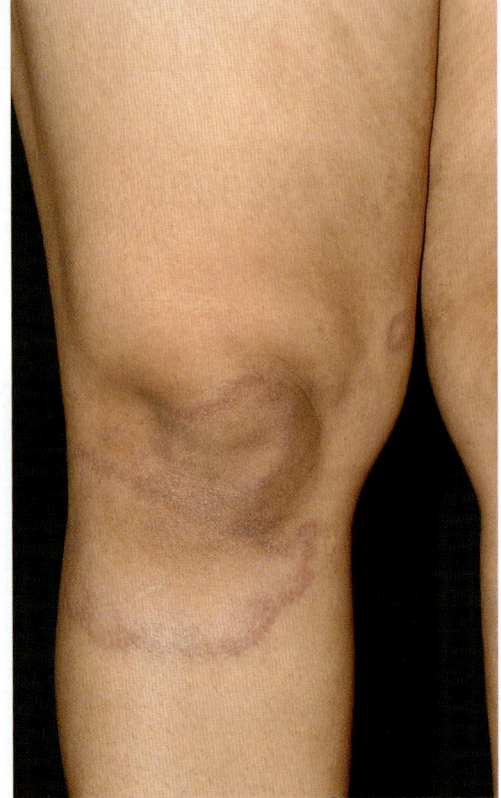

Fig. 17.4 Tuberculoid leprosy. *Courtesy National Cheng Kung University, Taiwan.*

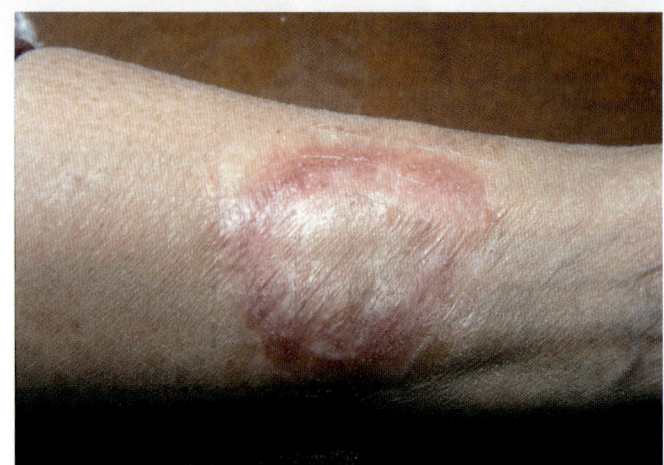

Fig. 17.5 Tuberculoid leprosy. *Courtesy Steven Binnick, MD.*

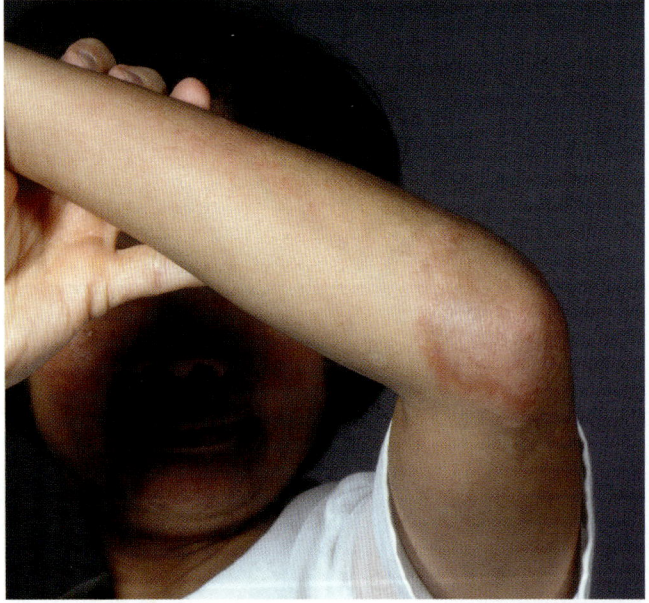

Fig. 17.6 Tuberculoid leprosy.

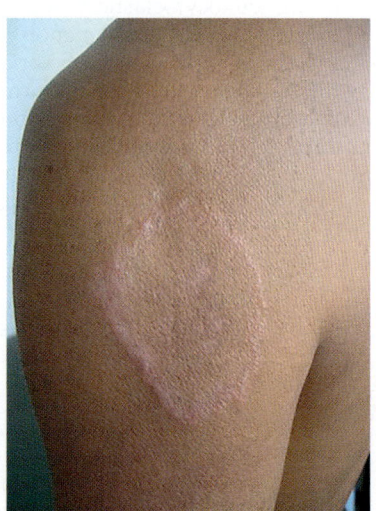

Fig. 17.7 Tuberculoid leprosy. *Courtesy Dermatology Division, University of Campinas, Brazil.*

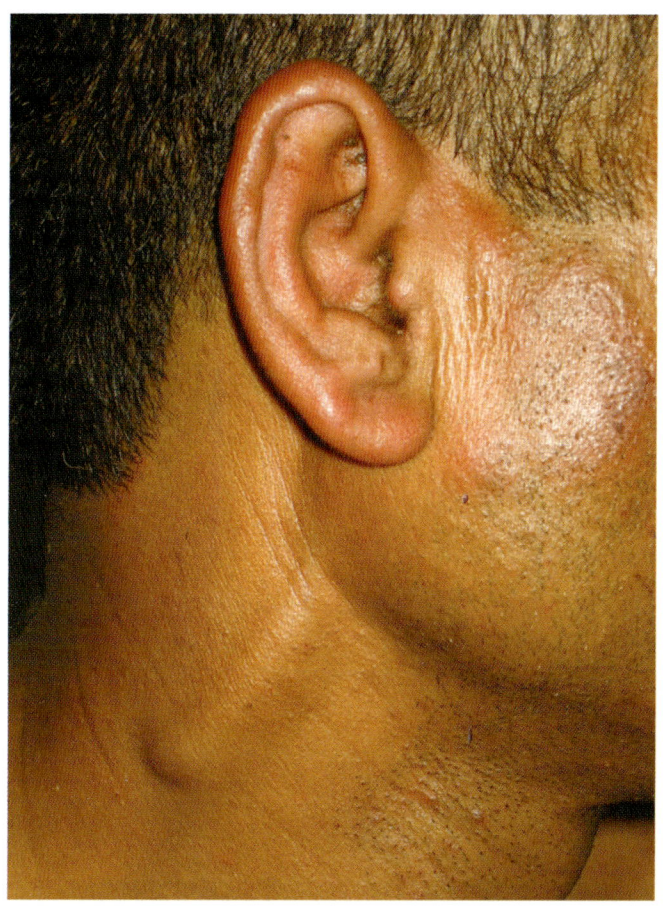

Fig. 17.8 Greater auricular nerve enlargement in leprosy. *Courtesy Archana Singal, MD.*

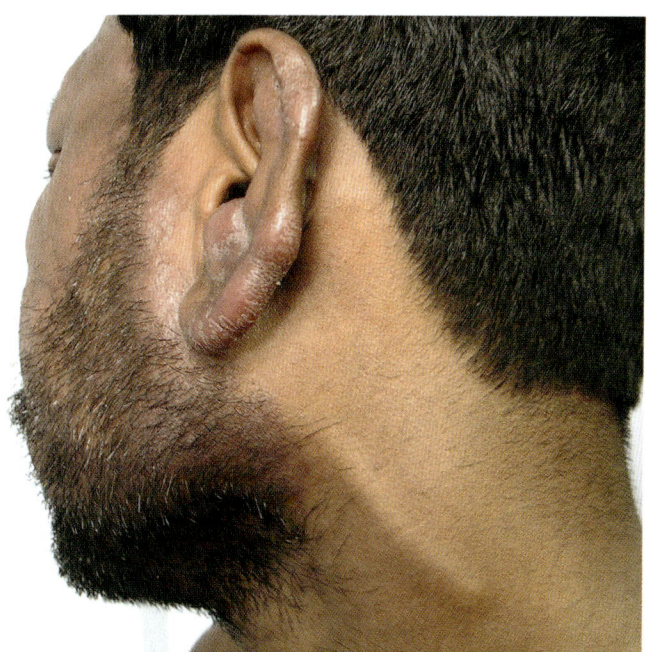

Fig. 17.9 Nerve enlargement in leprosy. *Courtesy Debabrata Bandyopadhyay.*

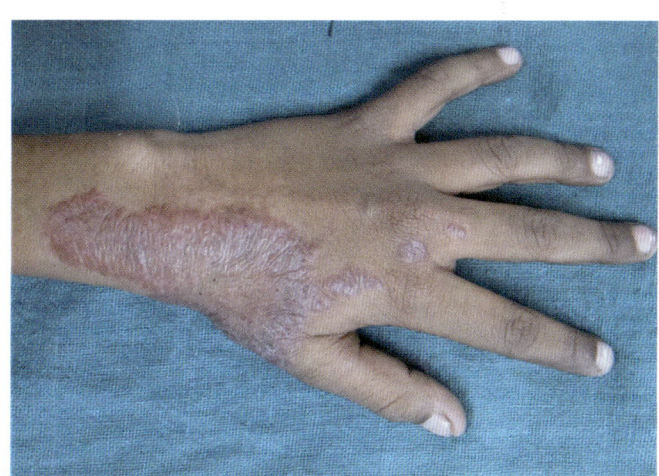

Fig. 17.10 Borderline tuberculoid leprosy. *Courtesy Archana Singal, MD.*

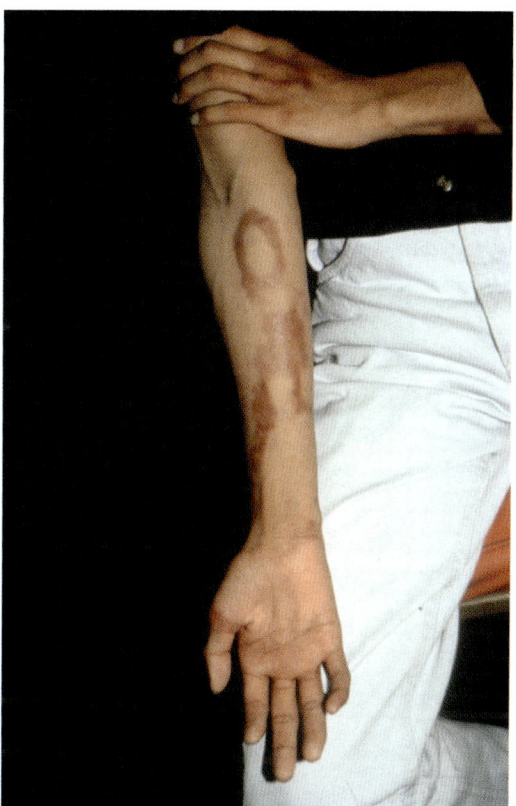

Fig. 17.11 Borderline tuberculoid leprosy.

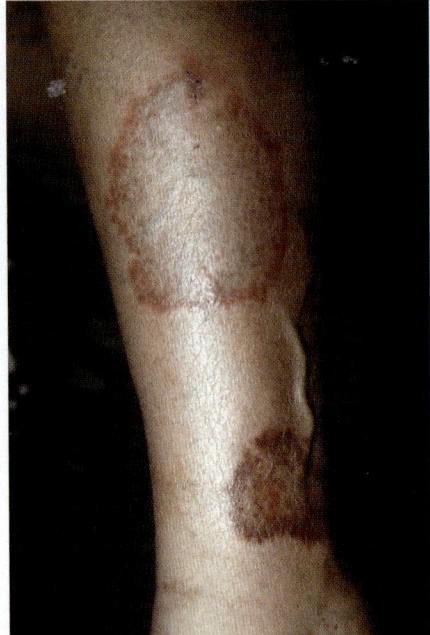

Fig. 17.12 Borderline tuberculoid leprosy.

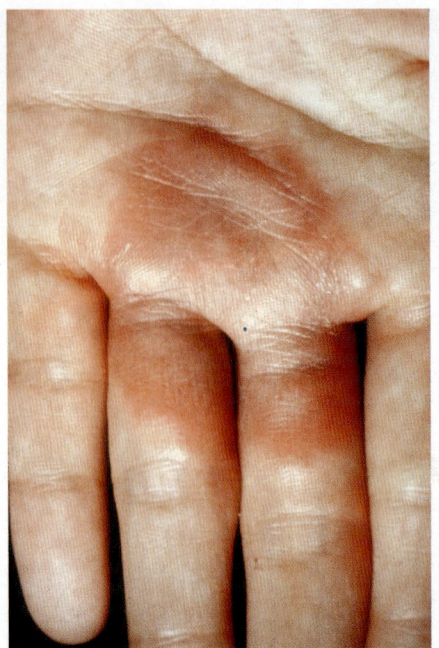

Fig. 17.13 Borderline tuberculoid leprosy.

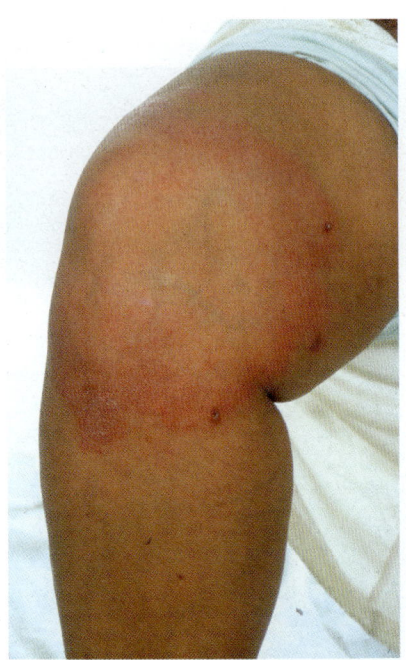

Fig. 17.14 Borderline tuberculoid leprosy.

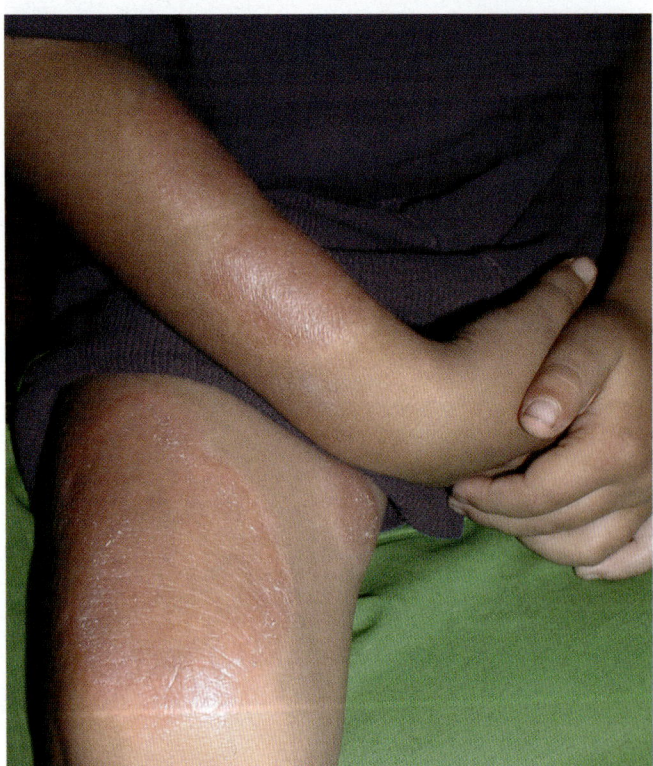

Fig. 17.15 Borderline tuberculoid leprosy. *Courtesy Shyam Verma, MBBS, DVD.*

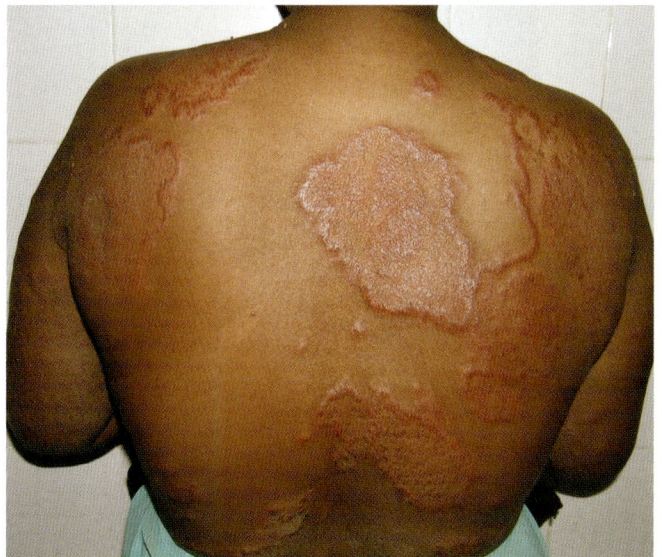

Fig. 17.16 Borderline leprosy. *Courtesy Archana Singal, MD.*

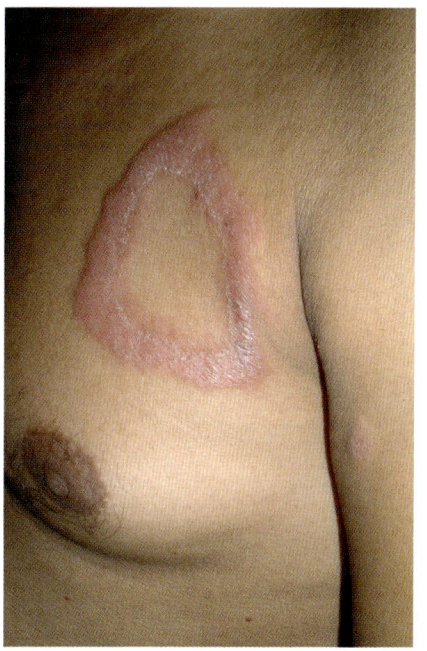

Fig. 17.17 Borderline leprosy. *Courtesy Shyam Verma, MBBS, DVD.*

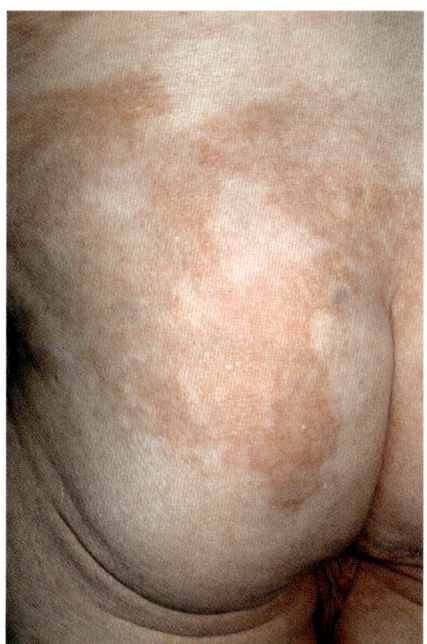

Fig. 17.18 Borderline lepromatous leprosy.

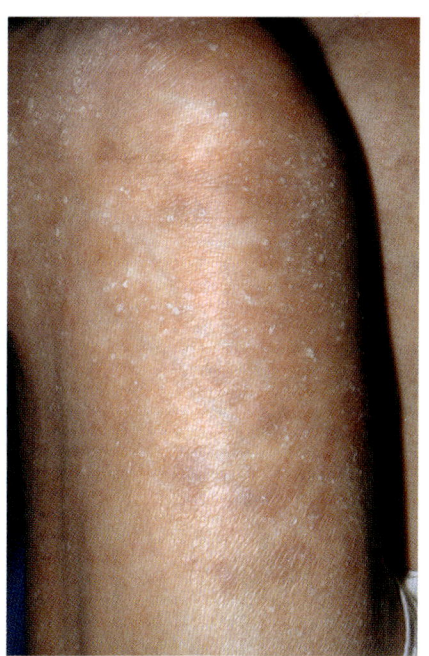

Fig. 17.19 Borderline lepromatous leprosy.

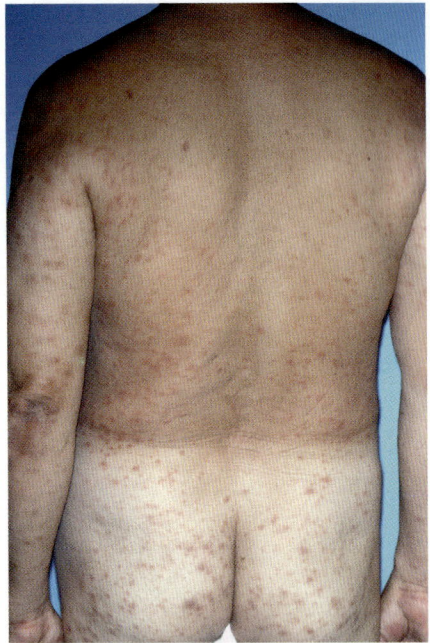

Fig. 17.20 Borderline lepromatous leprosy. *Courtesy Curt Samlaska, MD.*

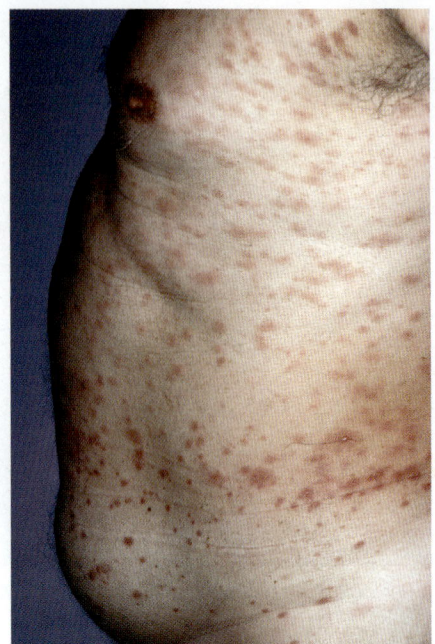

Fig. 17.21 Borderline lepromatous leprosy. *Courtesy Curt Samlaska, MD.*

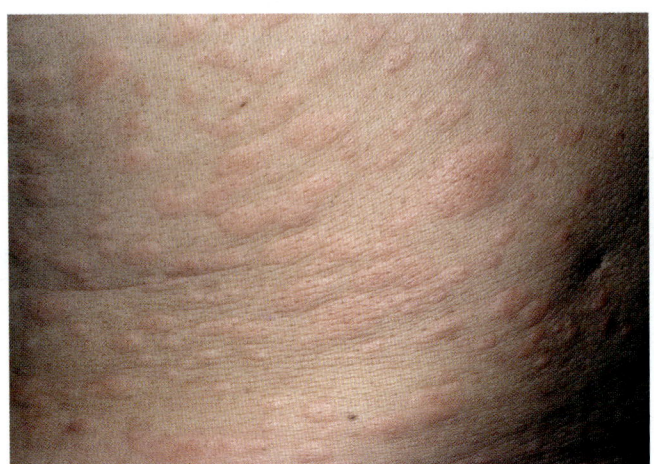

Fig. 17.22 Borderline lepromatous leprosy. *Courtesy Curt Samlaska, MD.*

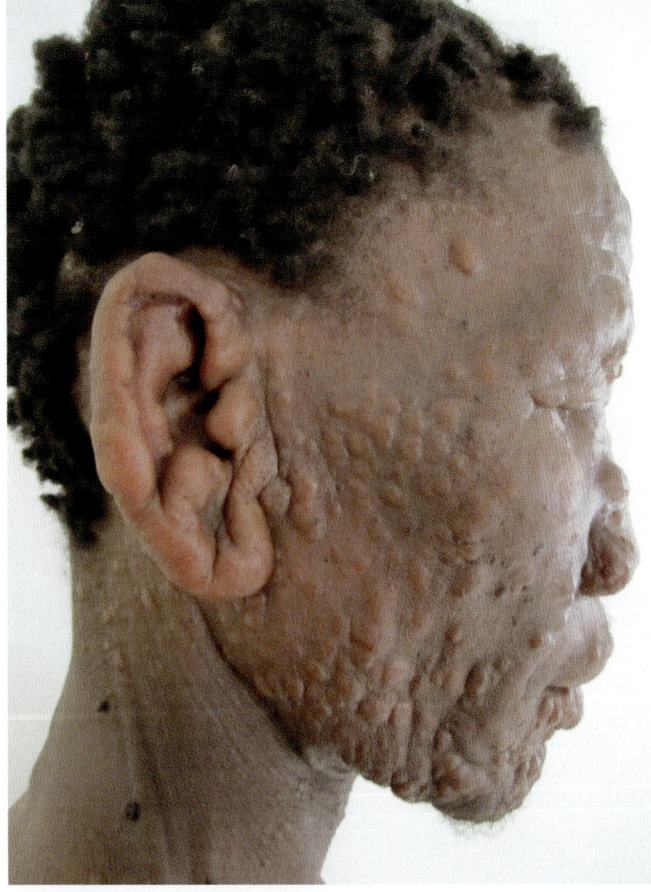

Fig. 17.23 Lepromatous leprosy. *Courtesy Michelle Weir, MD.*

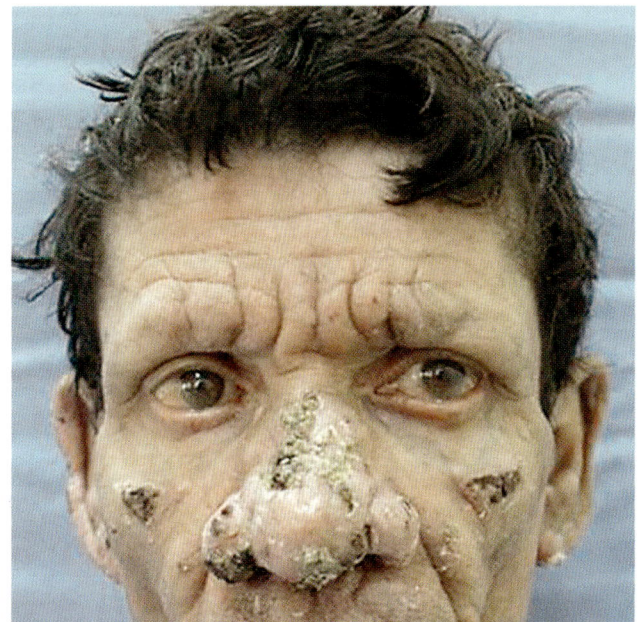

Fig. 17.24 Lepromatous leprosy. *Courtesy Tatiana C. P. Cordeiro de Andrade, MD.*

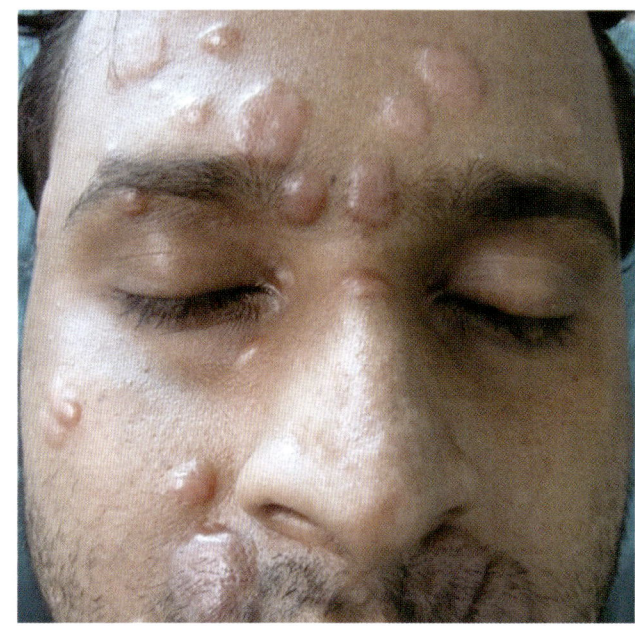

Fig. 17.25 Lepromatous leprosy. *Courtesy Archana Singal, MD.*

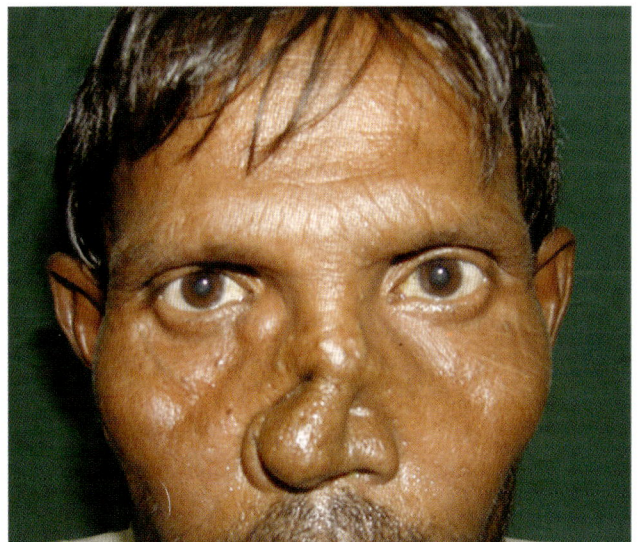

Fig. 17.26 Collapse of the nasal septum from leprosy; destruction of the nose characterizes this and some other infections, including syphilis, leishmaniasis, and tuberculosis. *Courtesy Archana Singal, MD.*

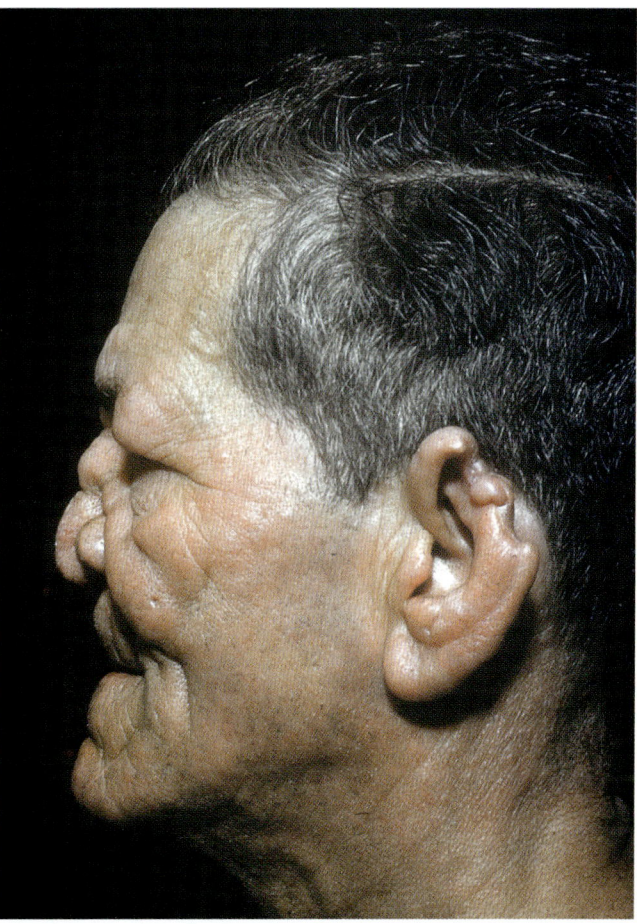

Fig. 17.27 Lepromatous leprosy. *Courtesy Steven Binnick, MD.*

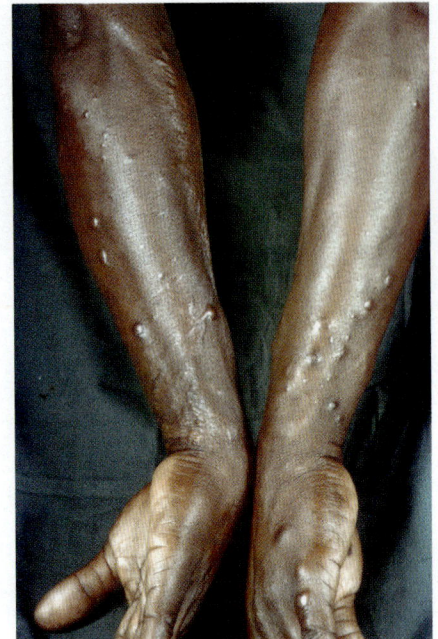

Fig. 17.28 Lepromatous leprosy.

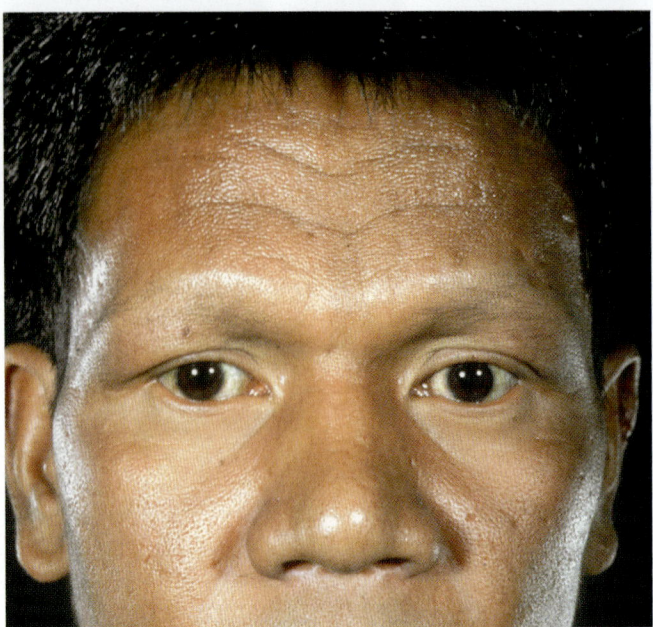

Fig. 17.29 Diffuse leprosy of Lucio. Note loss of eyebrows.

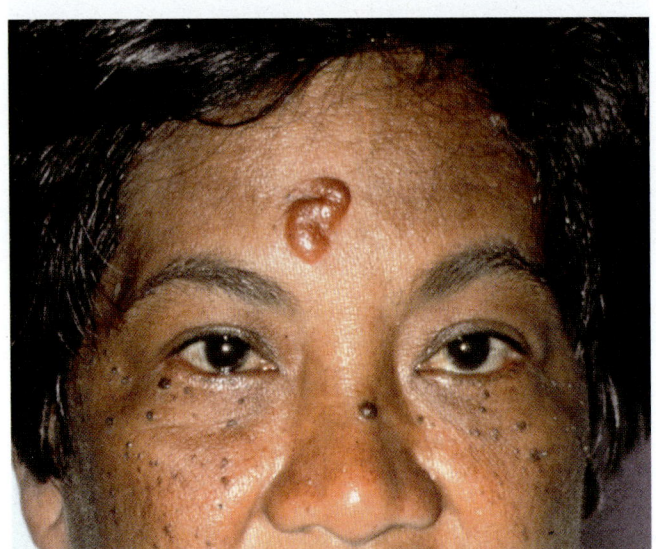

Fig. 17.30 Histiocytoid leprosy.

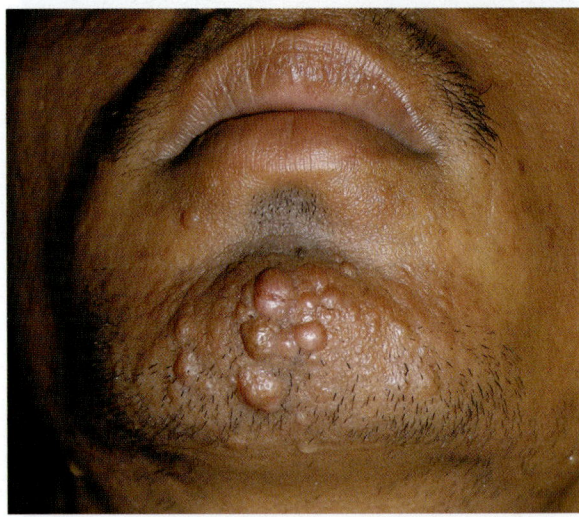

Fig. 17.31 Histiocytoid leprosy. *Courtesy James Steger, MD.*

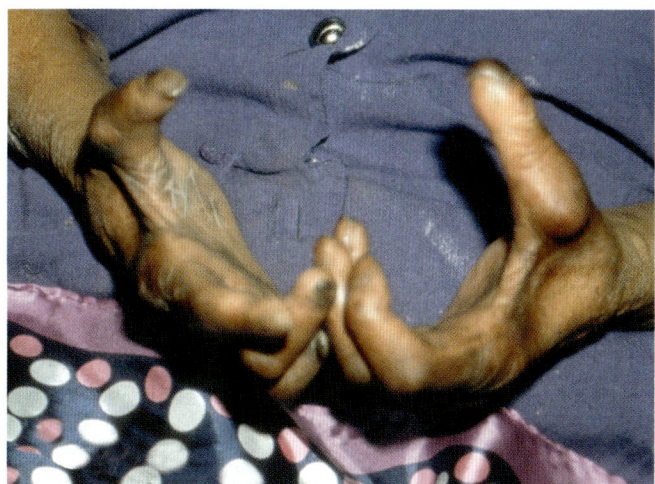

Fig. 17.32 Secondary changes caused by neurologic disease in leprosy.

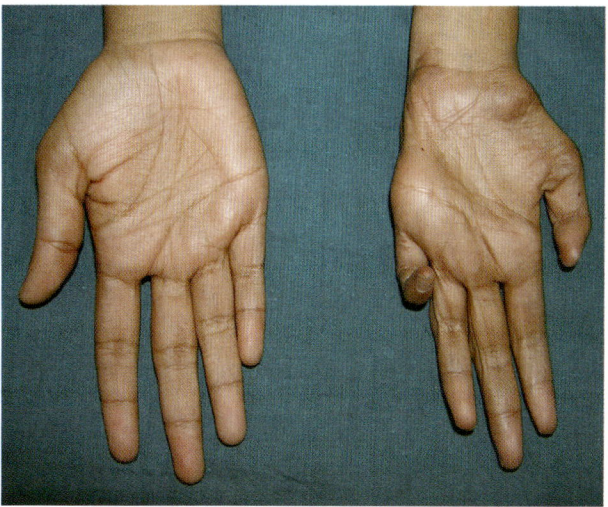

Fig. 17.33 Claw hand (left) complicating neurologic involvement with leprosy. *Courtesy Archana Singal, MD.*

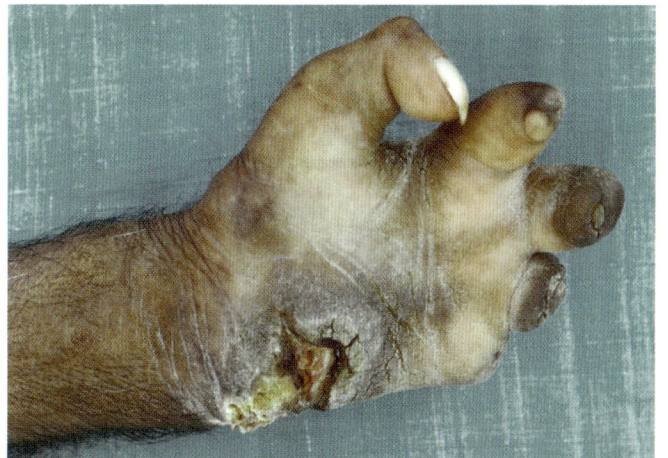

Fig. 17.34 Neuropathic ulcer in leprosy. *Courtesy Shyam Verma, MBBS, DVD.*

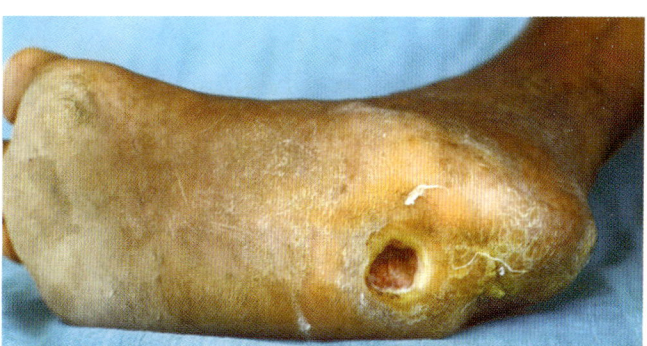

Fig. 17.35 Neuropathic ulcer in leprosy. *Courtesy Shyam Verma, MBBS, DVD.*

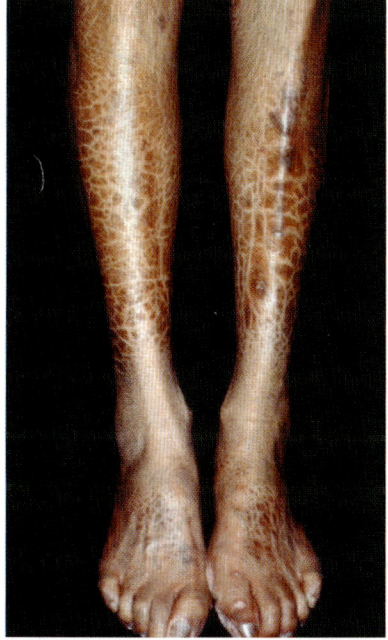

Fig. 17.36 Ichthyosis and pigmentation after clofazimine in leprosy. *Courtesy Scott Norton, MD.*

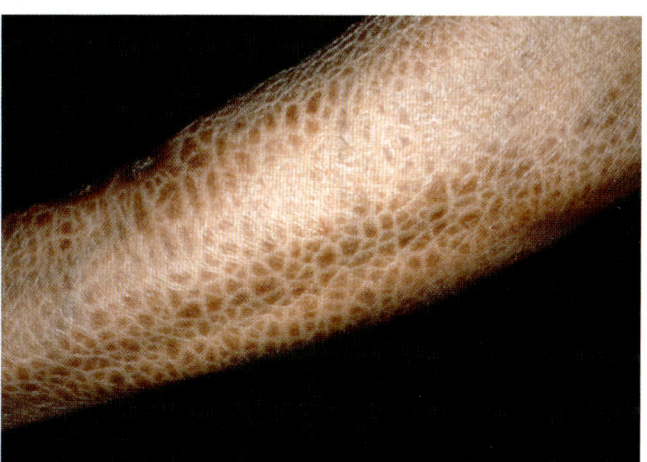

Fig. 17.37 Acquired ichthyosis in leprosy. *Courtesy Scott Norton, MD.*

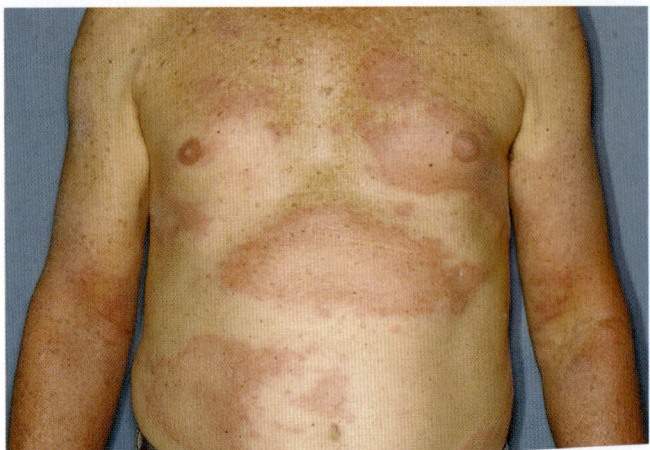

Fig. 17.38 Type 1 reactional leprosy. *Courtesy Lauro de Souza Lima Institute, Brazil.*

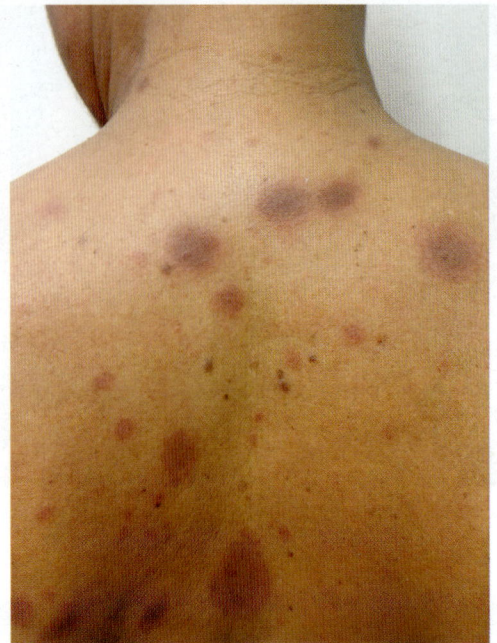

Fig. 17.39 Type 1 reactional leprosy. *Courtesy Lauro de Souza Lima Institute, Brazil.*

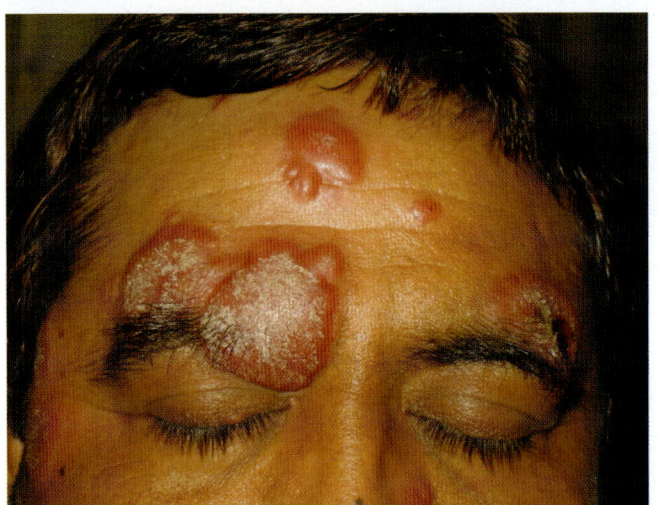

Fig. 17.40 Borderline tuberculoid leprosy with downgrading reaction. *Courtesy Archana Singal, MD.*

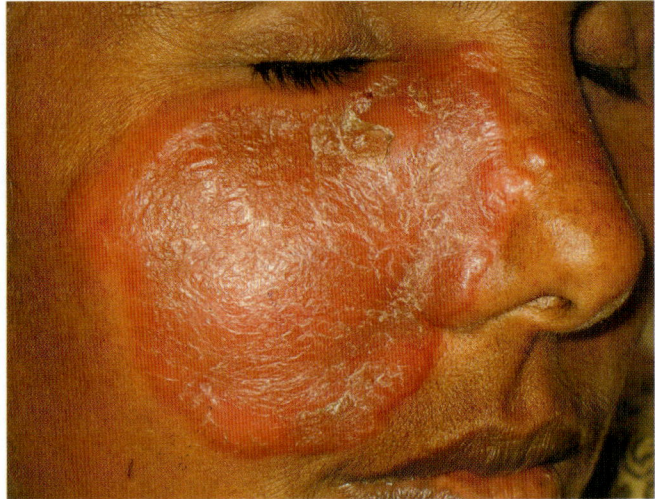

Fig. 17.41 Borderline tuberculoid leprosy with downgrading reaction. *Courtesy Archana Singal, MD.*

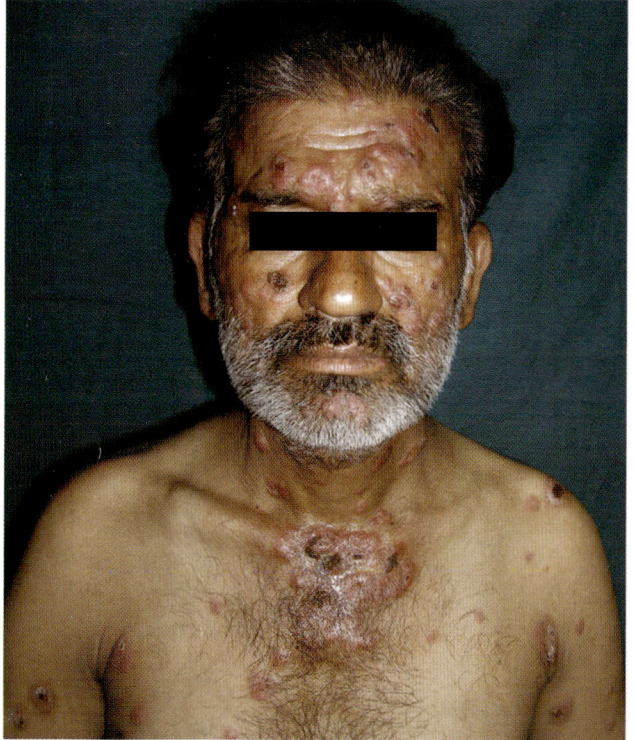

Fig. 17.42 Lepromatous leprosy with erythema nodosum leprosum reaction. *Courtesy Archana Singal, MD.*

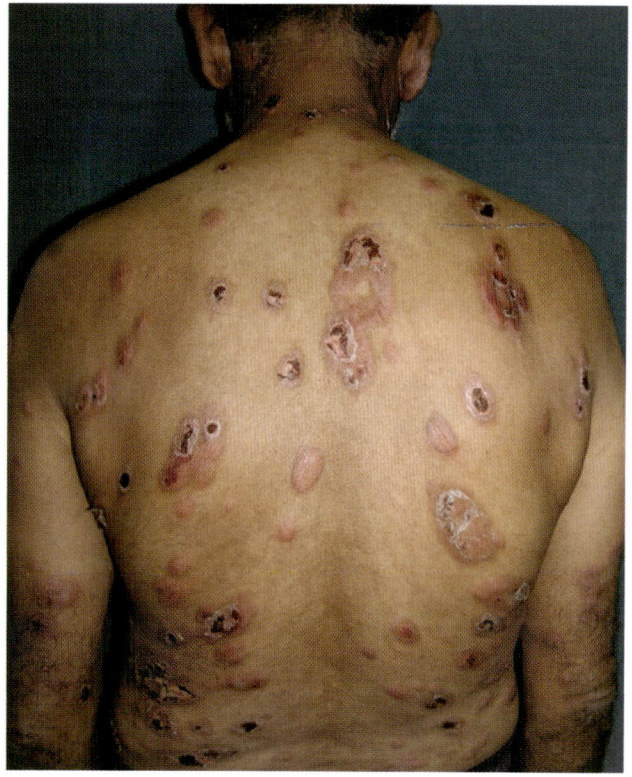

Fig. 17.43 Lepromatous leprosy with erythema nodosum leprosum reaction. *Courtesy Archana Singal, MD.*

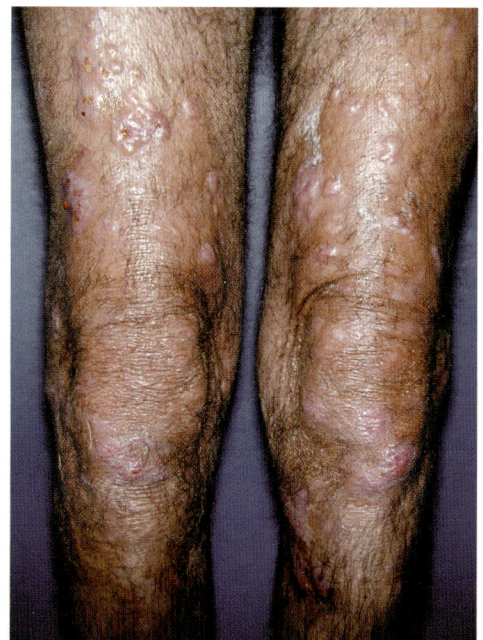

Fig. 17.44 Type 2 reactional leprosy. *Courtesy Lauro de Souza Lima Institute, Brazil.*

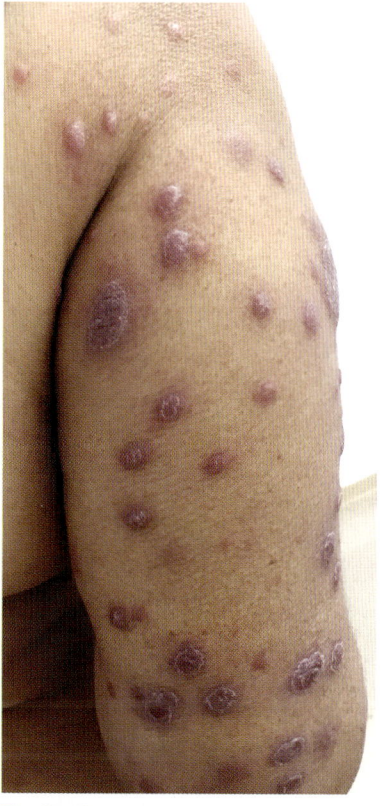

Fig. 17.45 Type 2 reactional leprosy. *Courtesy Aileen Chang, MD.*

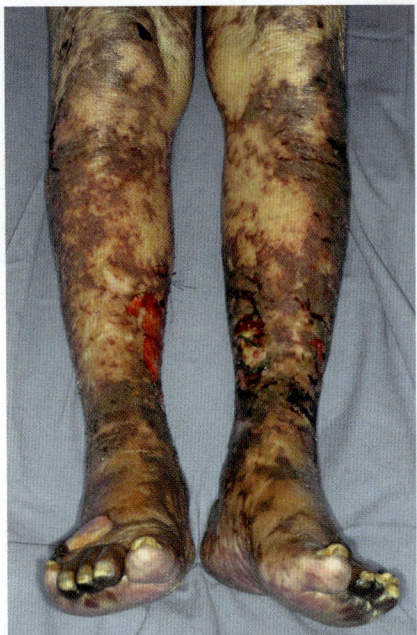

Fig. 17.46 Lucio phenomenon. *Courtesy Lauro de Souza Lima Institute, Brazil.*

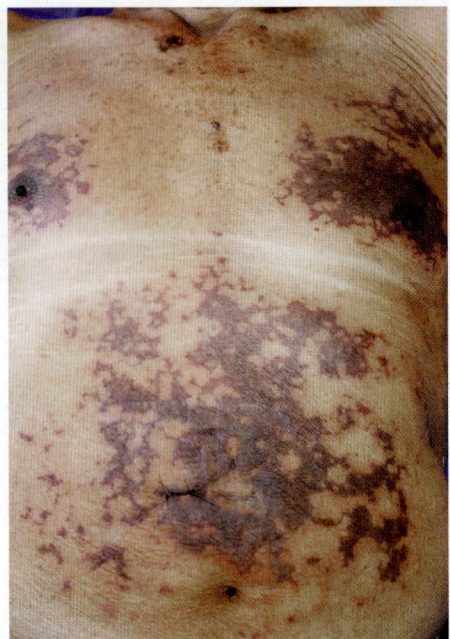

Fig. 17.47 Lucio phenomenon. *Courtesy Lauro de Souza Lima Institute, Brazil.*

Syphilis, Yaws, Bejel, and Pinta 18

Syphilis has been dubbed "the great imitator" for its ability to assume varied morphologies. Primary syphilis is characterized by a chancre—a minimally tender, indurated ulcer—or less commonly by syphilitic balanoposthitis. Secondary syphilis can present with indurated, ham- to copper-colored papulosquamous lesions with peripheral adherent scale, annular and gyrate lesions, patchy alopecia, and gray indurated mucous patches. The palms and soles may be involved. Tertiary syphilis is characterized by destructive granulomatous disease that often involves the central face, causing destruction of the nasal bridge. Congenital syphilis can present with periostitis leading to saber shins and frontal bossing, mucositis, and gray fissured periorificial mucous patches. Vesiculobullous lesions may be seen in congenital syphilis. Pustular and crusted lesions characterize lues maligna and rupioid syphilis, respectively.

A high index of suspicion is required, and serologic testing can be falsely negative (prozone reaction) as a result of very high antibody titers. Recognition of morphologies suggestive of syphilis should prompt appropriate testing to include a skin biopsy.

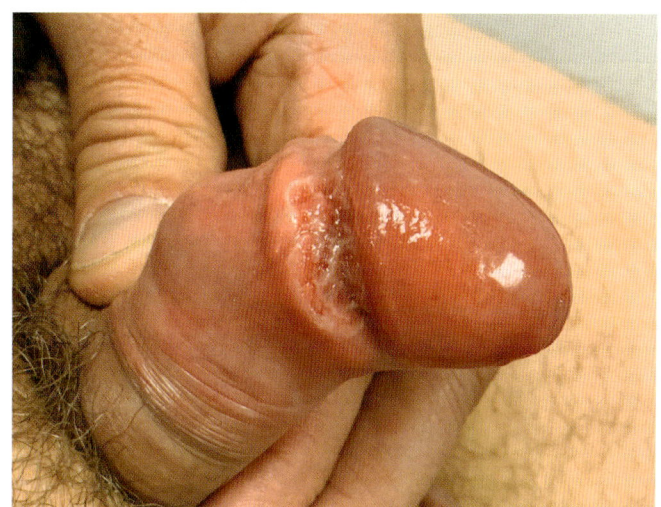

Fig. 18.2 Primary syphilis.

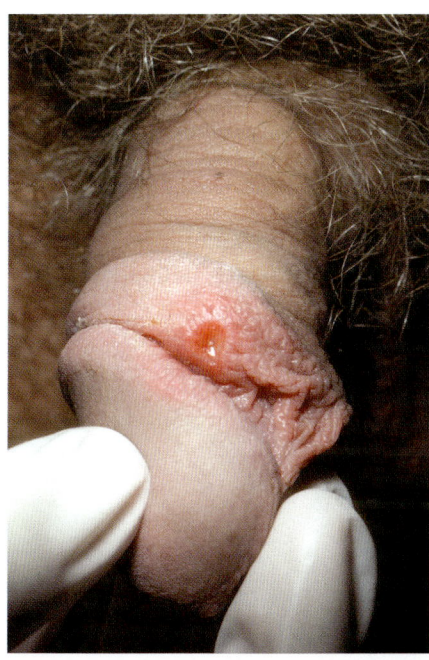

Fig. 18.1 Primary syphilis.

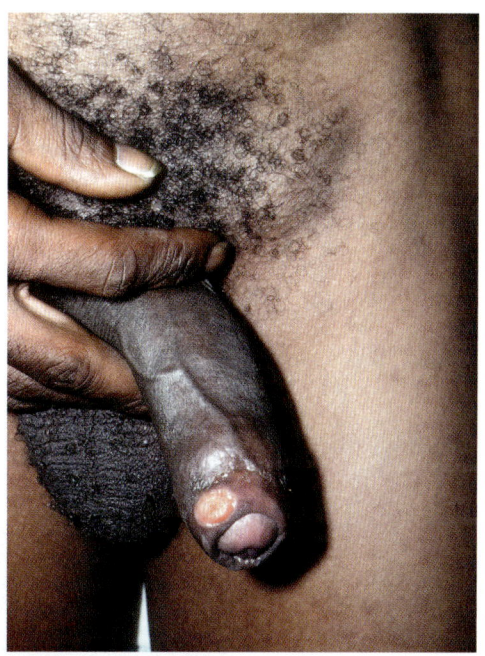

Fig. 18.3 Primary syphilis.

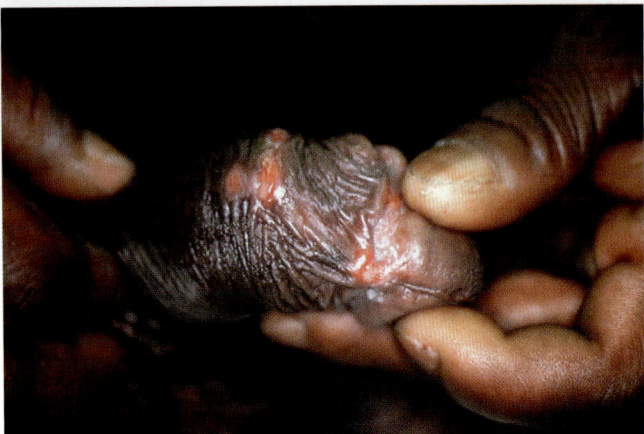

Fig. 18.4 Primary syphilis.

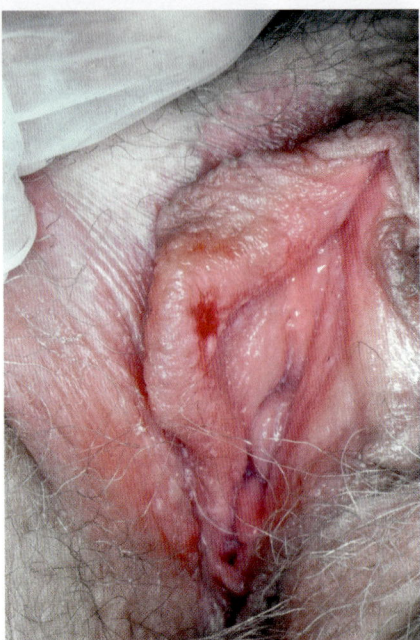

Fig. 18.5 Primary syphilis.

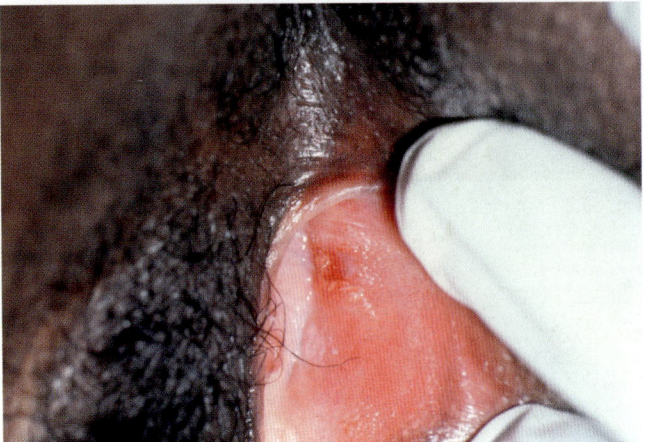

Fig. 18.6 Primary syphilis.

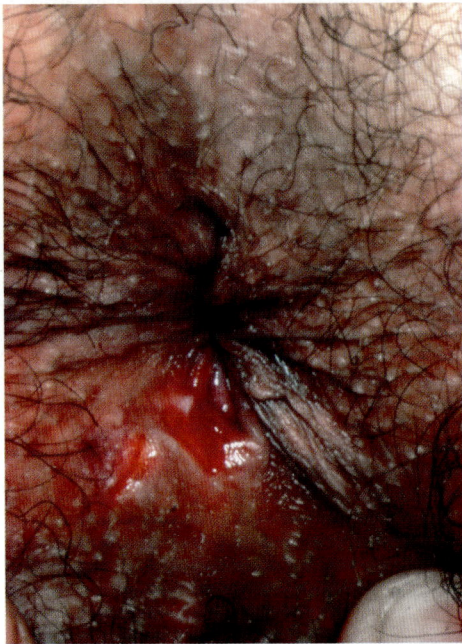

Fig. 18.7 Primary syphilis.

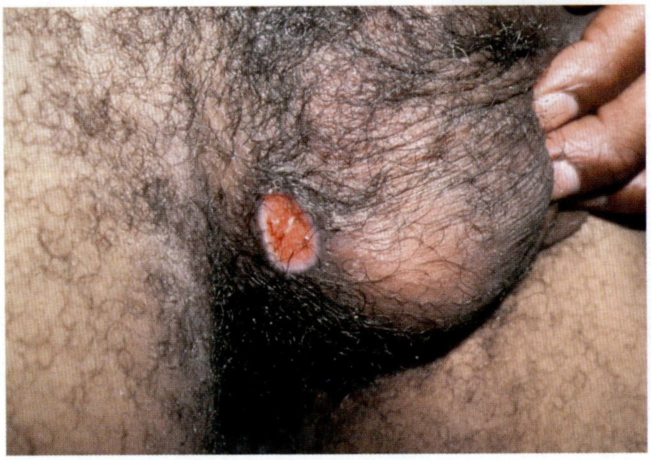

Fig. 18.8 Primary syphilis.

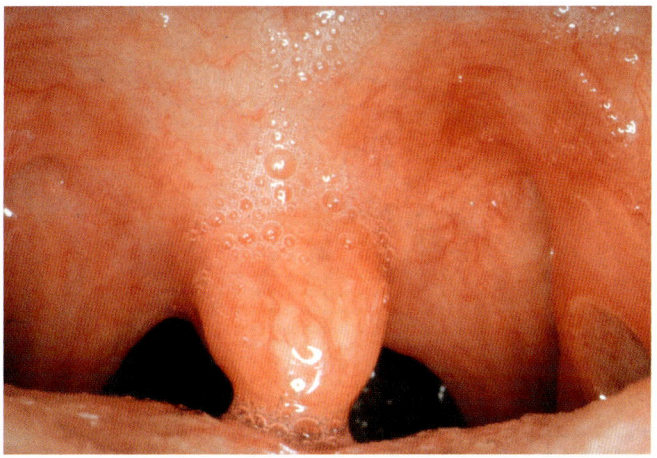

Fig. 18.9 Primary syphilis; chancre is on patient's left palate.

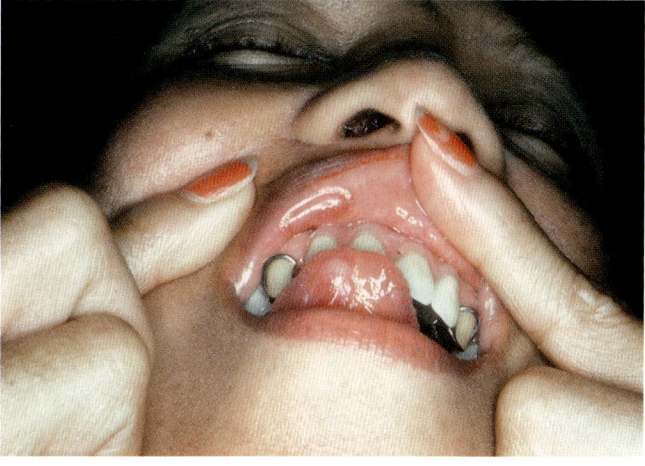

Fig. 18.10 Healing primary syphilis on upper lip; concomitant mucous patch of secondary syphilis on tongue.

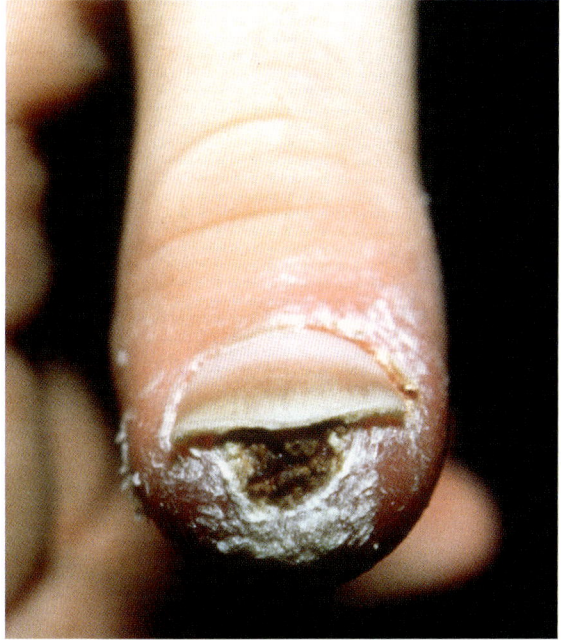

Fig. 18.11 Primary syphilis.

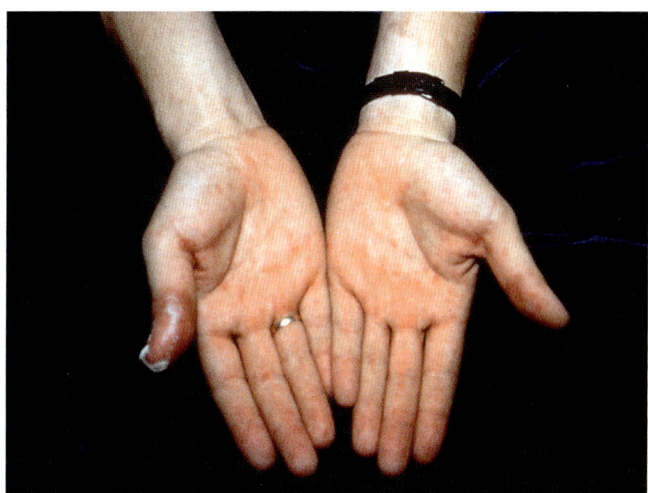

Fig. 18.12 Primary syphilis with secondary lesions on the palms.

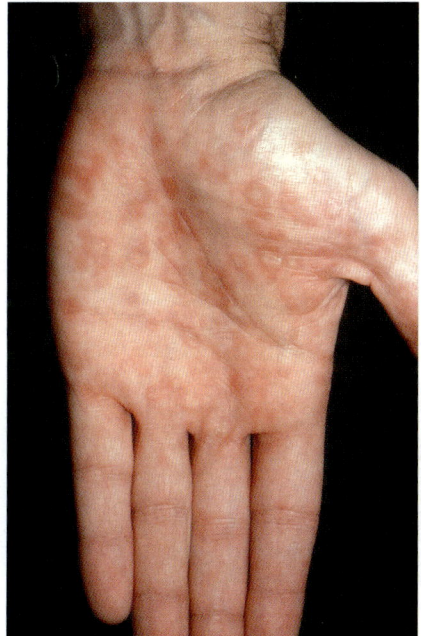

Fig. 18.13 Secondary syphilis.

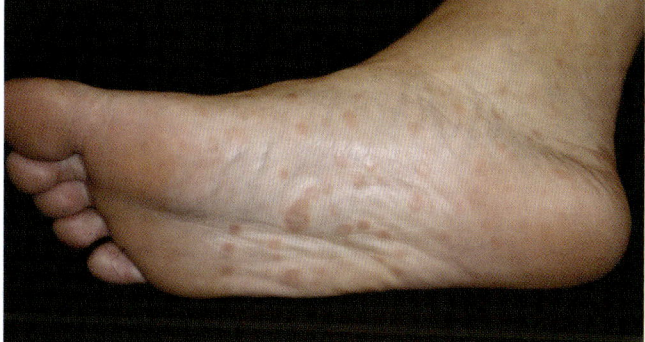

Fig. 18.14 Secondary syphilis. *Courtesy Kaohsiung Chang Gang Memorial Hospital, Taiwan.*

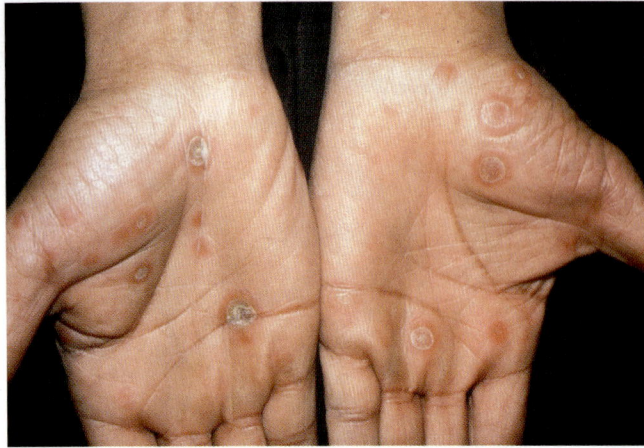

Fig. 18.15 Secondary syphilis.

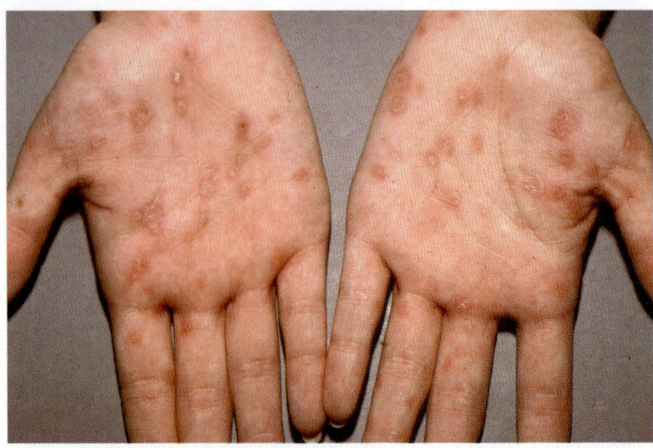

Fig. 18.16 Secondary syphilis. *Courtesy The University of Utah and Oregon Health Sciences University Leonard Swinyer MD image collection.*

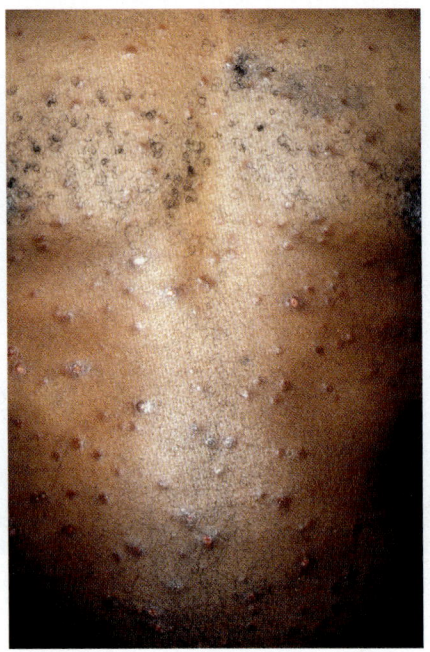

Fig. 18.17 Secondary syphilis.

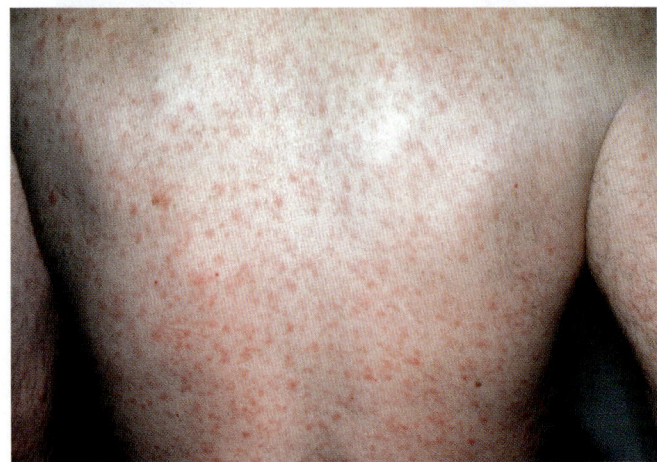

Fig. 18.18 Secondary syphilis.

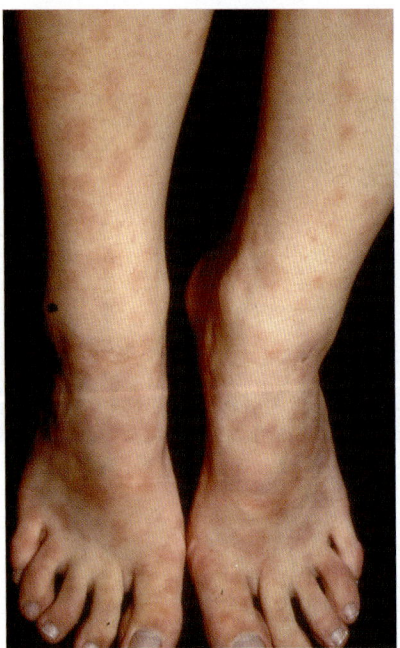

Fig. 18.19 Secondary syphilis. *Courtesy The University of Utah and Oregon Health Sciences University Leonard Swinyer MD image collection.*

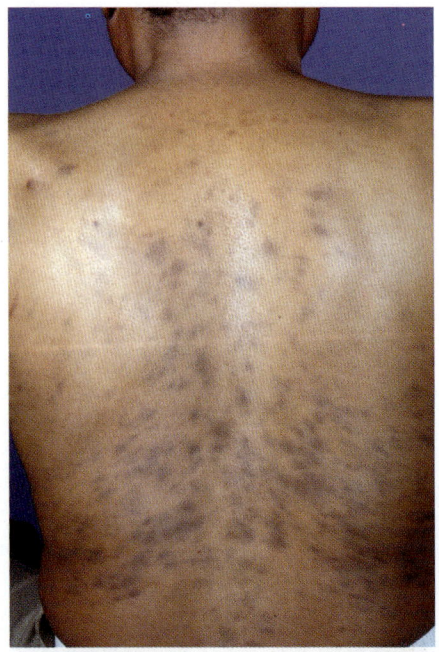

Fig. 18.20 Secondary syphilis.

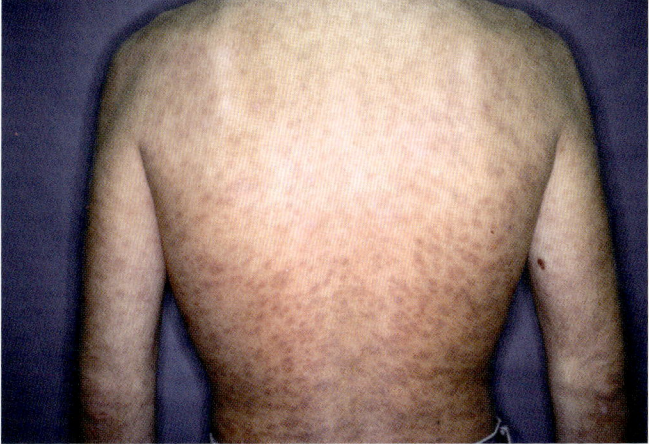

Fig. 18.21 Secondary syphilis and Kaposi sarcoma (on the right arm) of an HIV-infected patient.

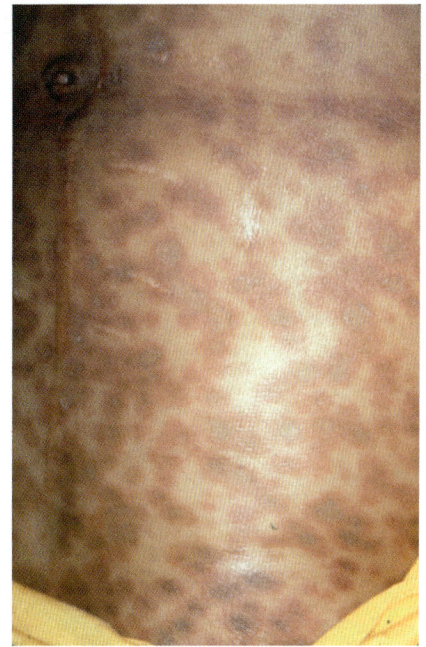

Fig. 18.22 Secondary syphilis in an HIV-infected patient. *Courtesy Scott Norton, MD.*

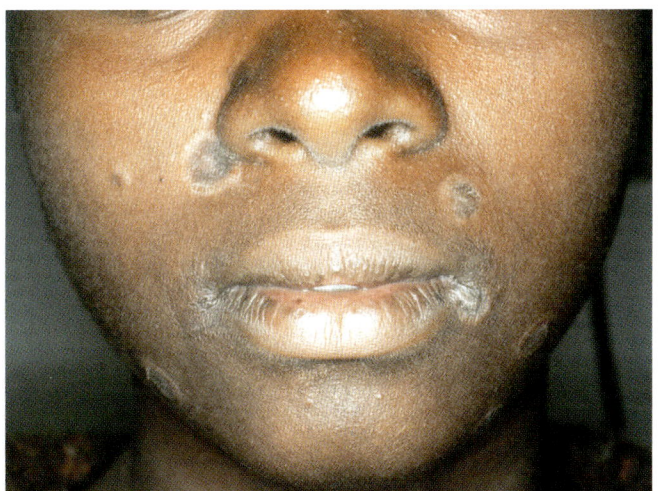

Fig. 18.23 Secondary syphilis.

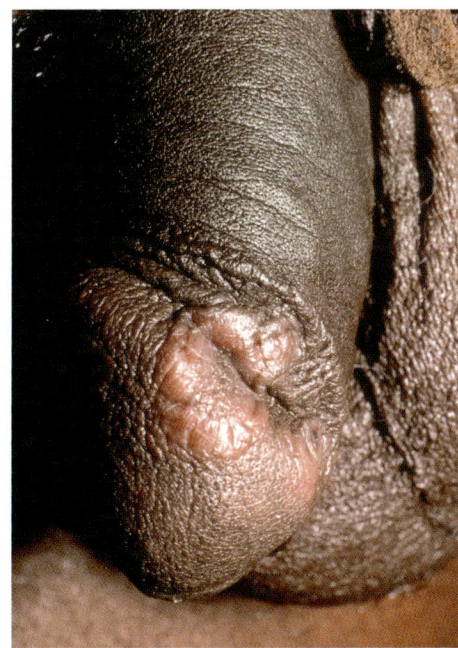

Fig. 18.24 Secondary syphilis.

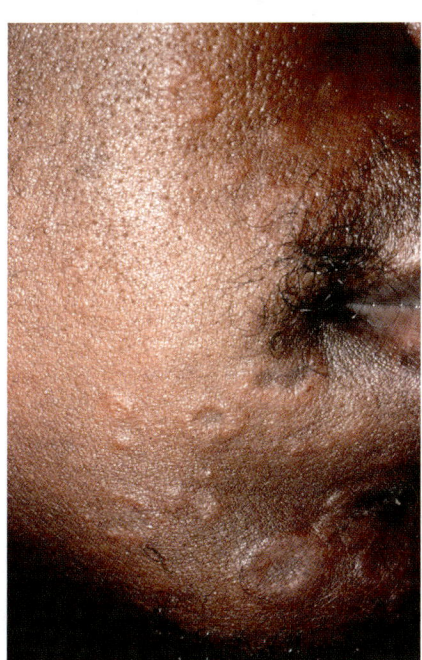

Fig. 18.25 Secondary syphilis.

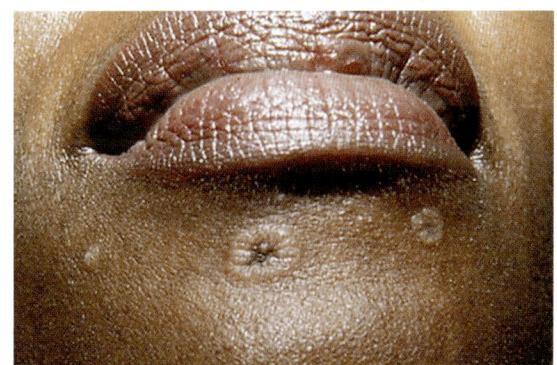

Fig. 18.26 Secondary syphilis.

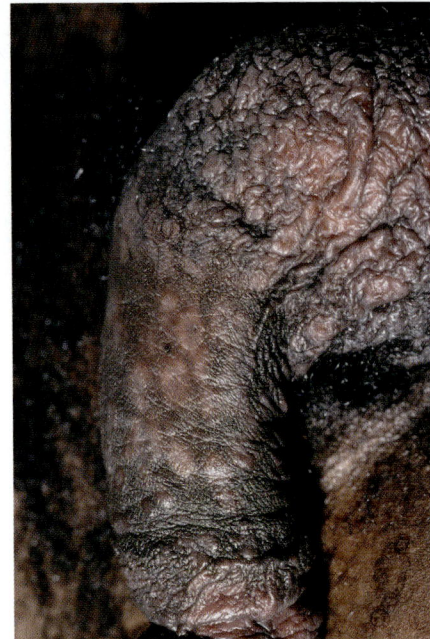

Fig. 18.27 Secondary syphilis.

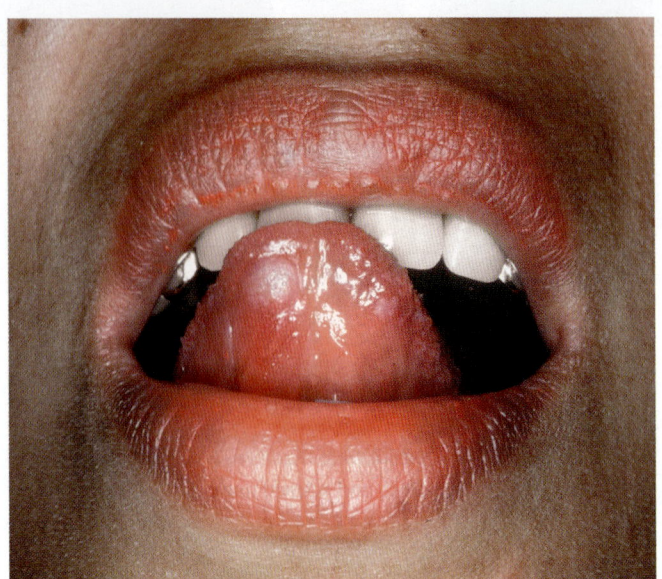

Fig. 18.28 Mucous patch of the tongue in syphilis.

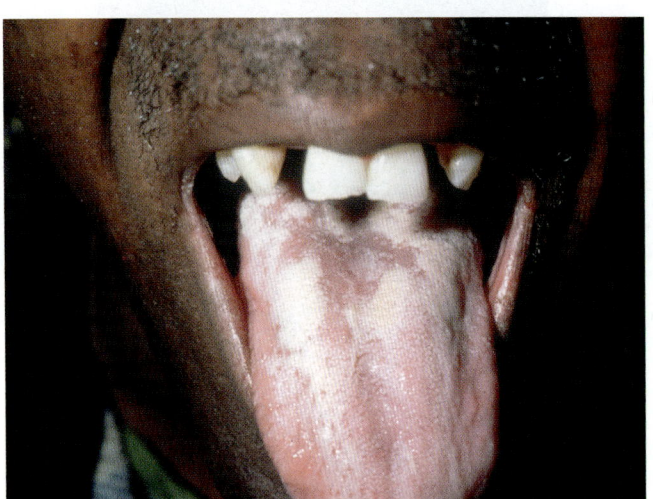

Fig. 18.29 Secondary syphilis, mucous patch. *Courtesy Steven Binnick, MD.*

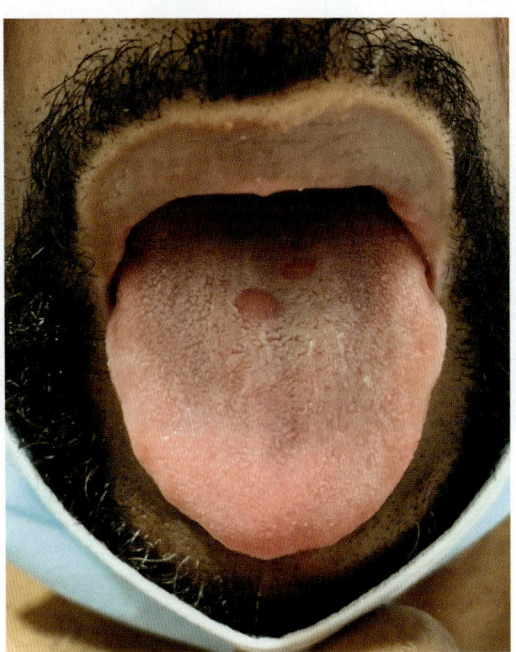

Fig. 18.30 Secondary syphilis, mucous patch.

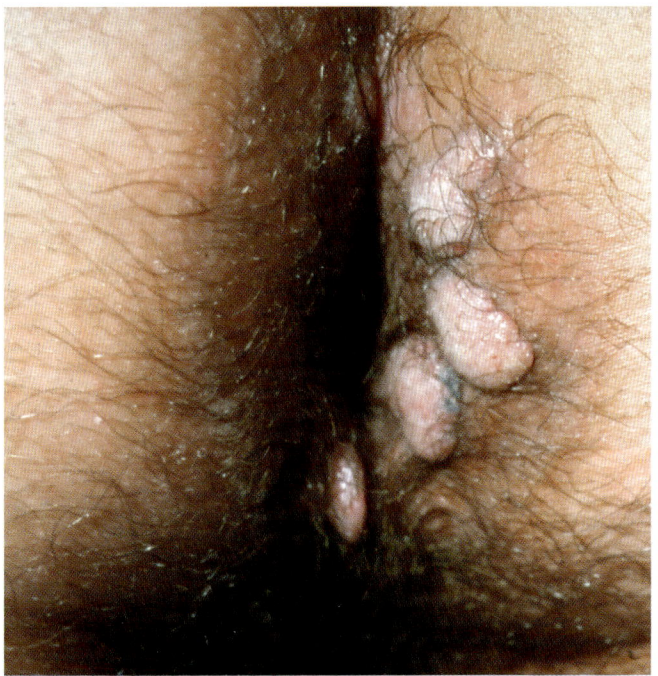

Fig. 18.31 Condyloma lata.

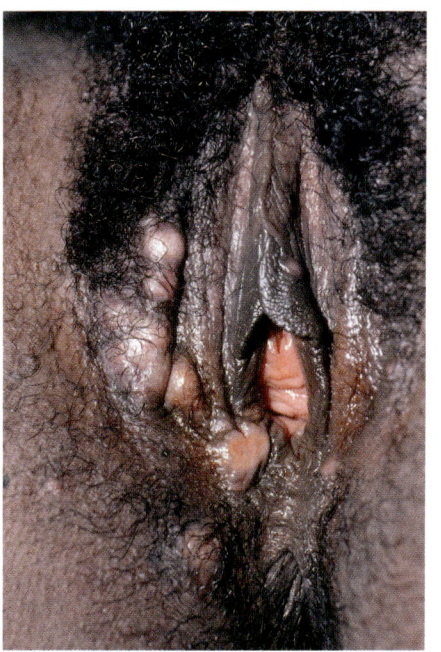

Fig. 18.32 Condyloma lata.

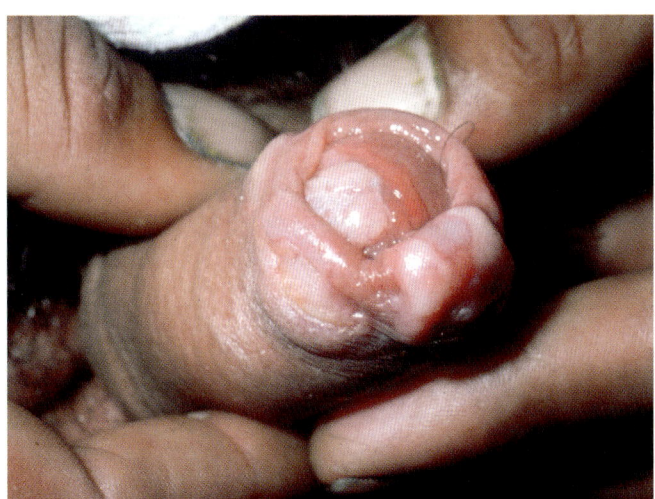

Fig. 18.33 Condyloma lata. *Courtesy Ken Greer, MD.*

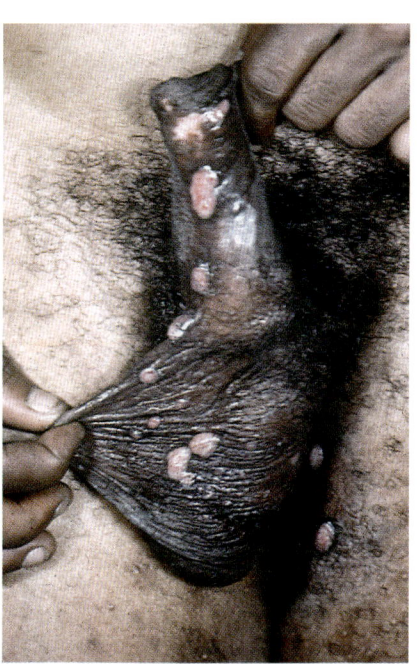

Fig. 18.34 Condyloma lata.

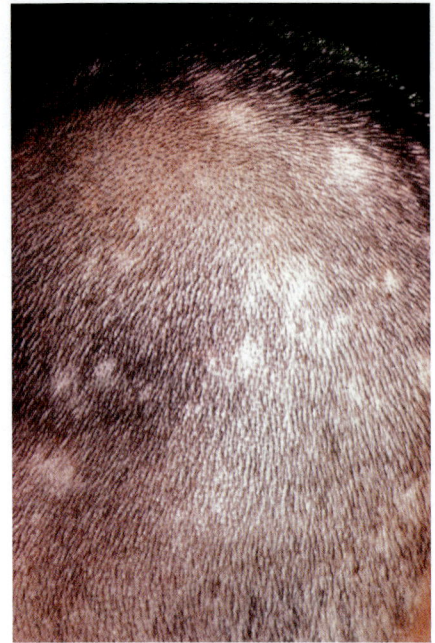

Fig. 18.35 Secondary syphilis alopecia.

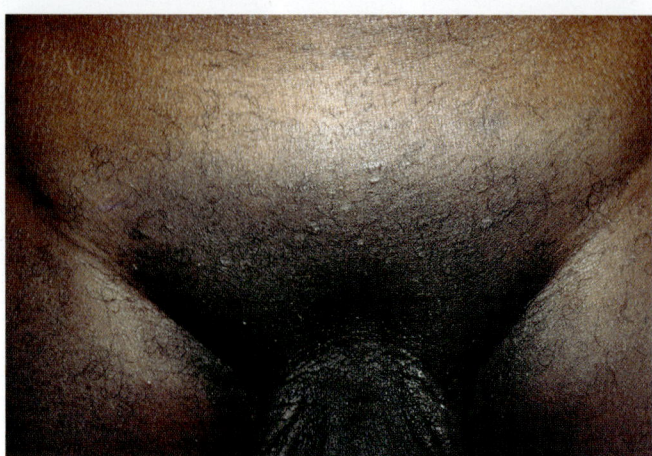

Fig. 18.36 Secondary syphilis alopecia.

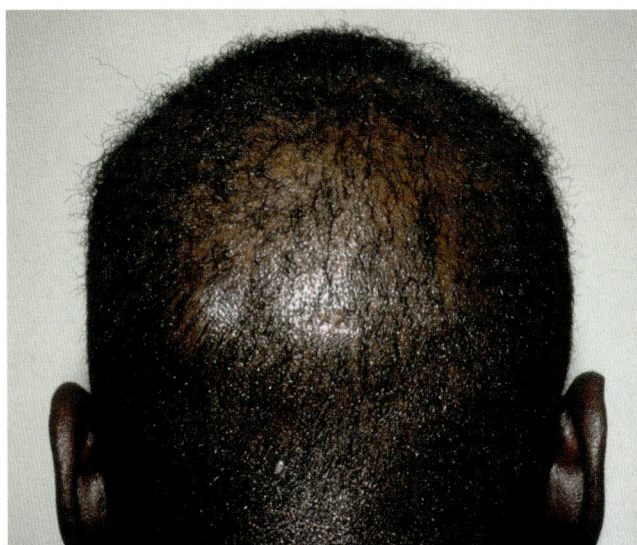

Fig. 18.37 Secondary syphilis alopecia.

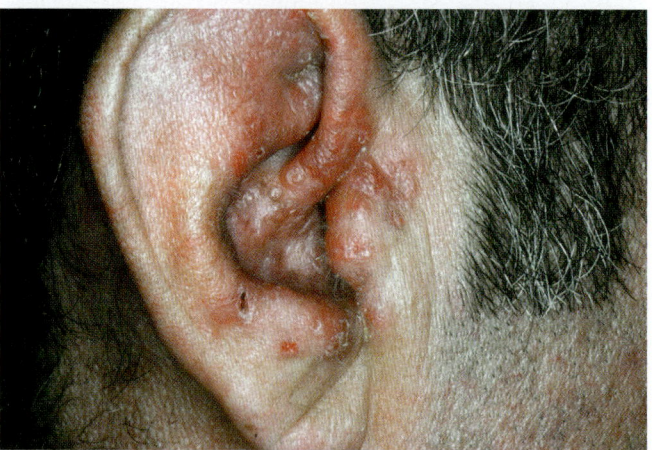

Fig. 18.38 Tertiary syphilis.

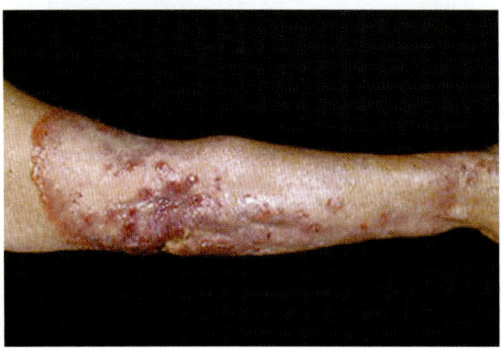

Fig. 18.39 Tertiary syphilis. *Courtesy Lauro de Souza Lima Institute, Brazil.*

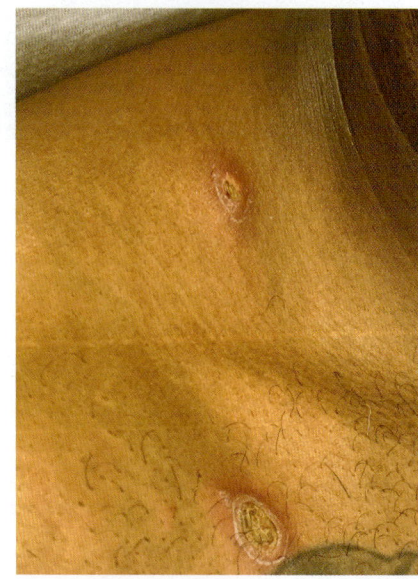

Fig. 18.40 Tertiary syphilis in a patient with advanced HIV who also developed lytic bone lesions.

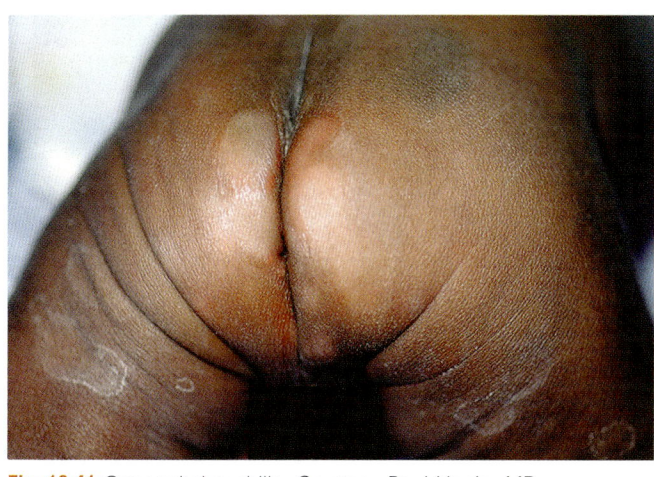

Fig. 18.41 Congenital syphilis. *Courtesy Paul Honig, MD.*

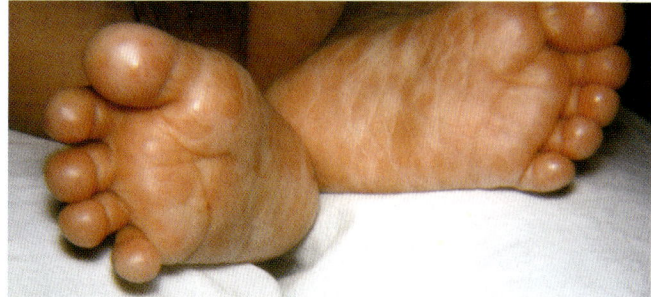

Fig. 18.42 Congenital syphilis. *Courtesy Paul Honig, MD.*

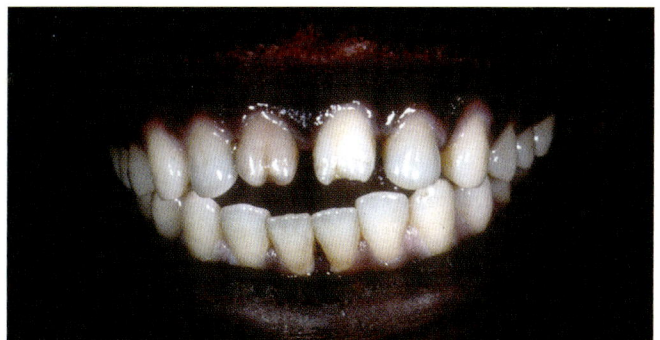

Fig. 18.43 Congenital syphilis with Hutchinson teeth.

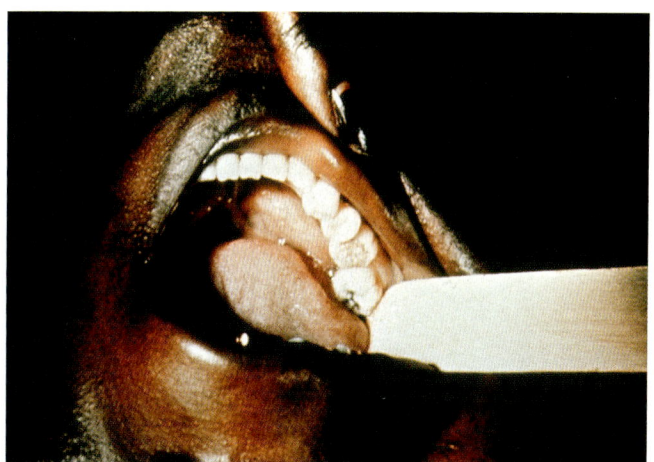

Fig. 18.44 Congenital syphilis with mulberry molar.

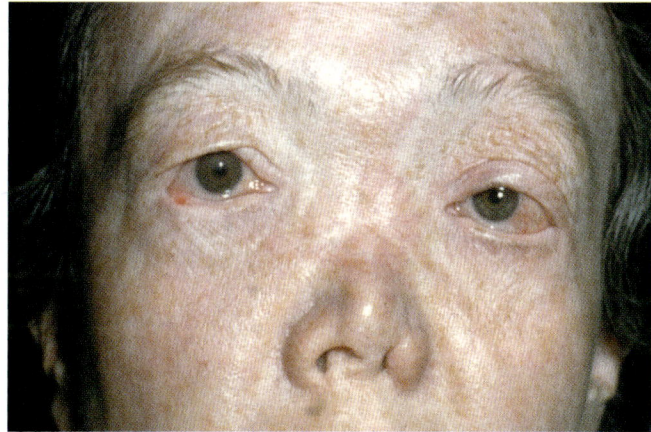

Fig. 18.45 Congenital syphilis.

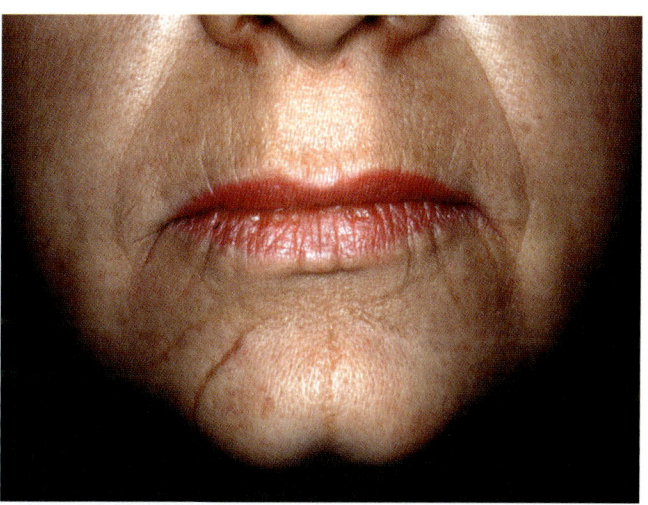

Fig. 18.46 Congenital syphilis; scars from rhagades.

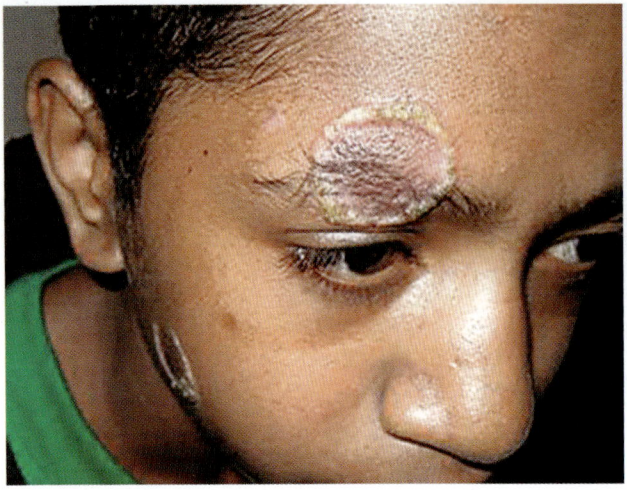

Fig. 18.47 Yaws.

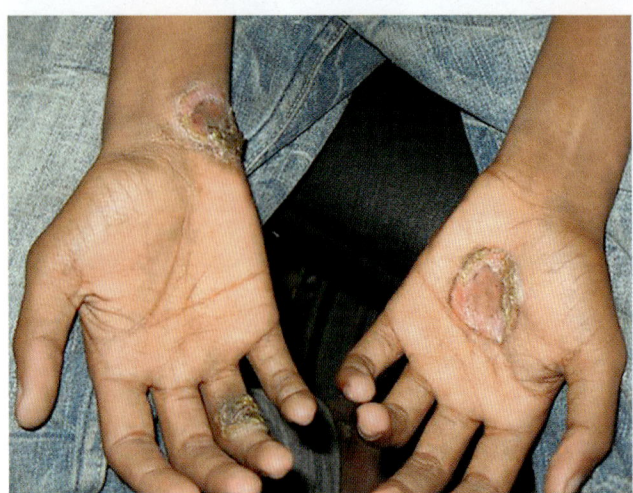

Fig. 18.48 Yaws.

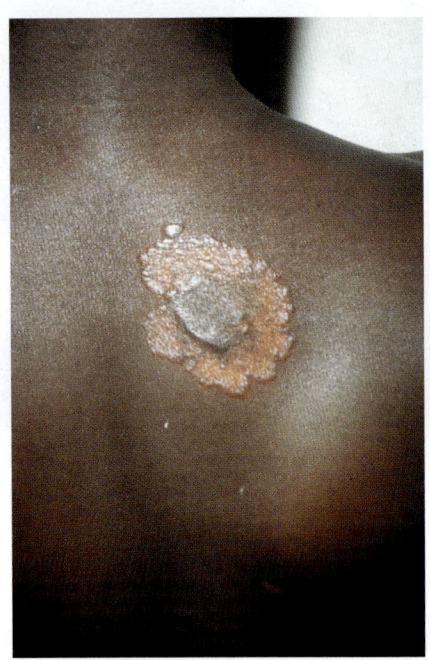

Fig. 18.49 Yaws.

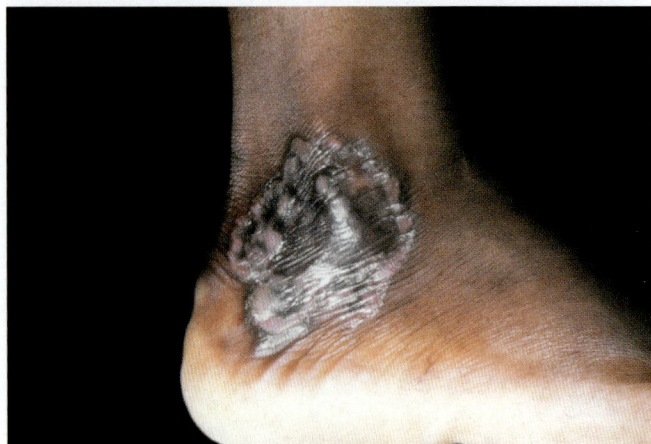

Fig. 18.50 Yaws.

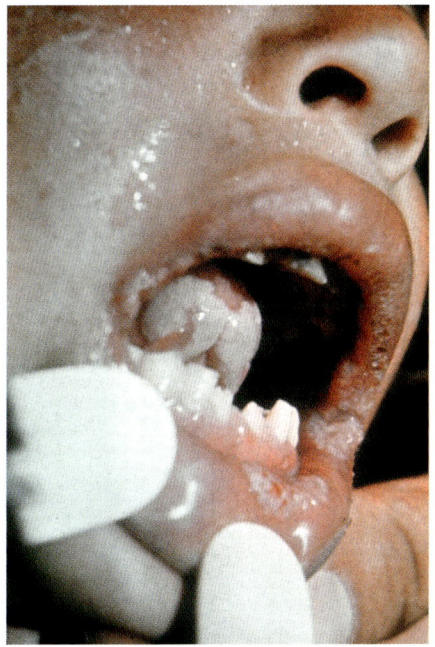

Fig. 18.51 Bejel. *Courtesy Steven Binnick, MD.*

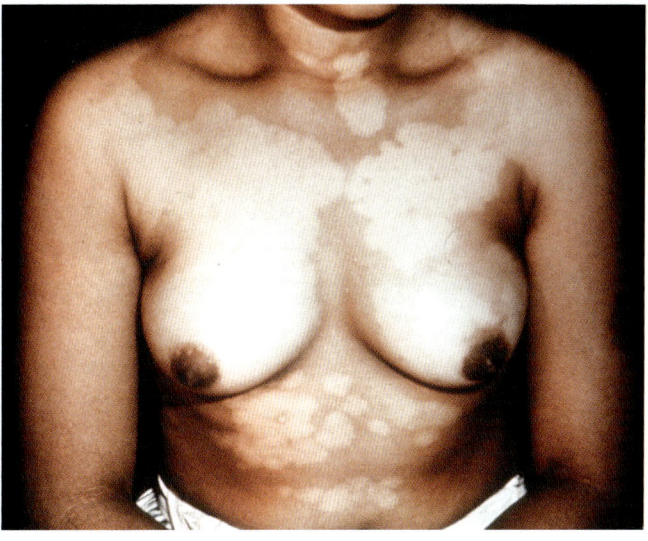

Fig. 18.52 Pinta. *Courtesy Steven Binnick, MD.*

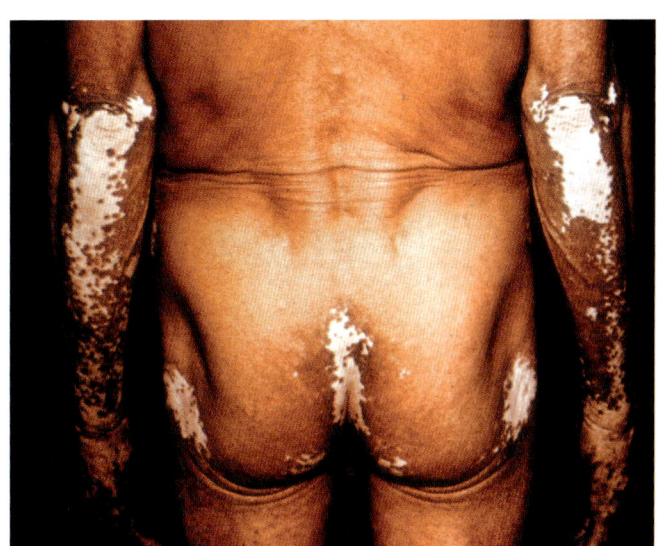

Fig. 18.53 Pinta. *Courtesy Steven Binnick, MD.*

Viral Diseases 19

Viral diseases can manifest as nonspecific exanthems, such as in measles and many other morbilliform eruptions, or more specific patterned eruptions, such as the papules on the cheeks, elbows, knees, and buttocks seen in Gianotti-Crosti syndrome. Primary lesions of viral infections vary from the vesicles seen in many herpetic and enteroviral conditions to the petechiae seen in the papular-purpuric gloves-and-socks syndrome due to parvovirus B19.

Skin lesion distribution is helpful when distinguishing between common vesicular eruptions, including the grouped localized vesicles and erosions seen in herpes simplex virus, compared with the dermatomal vesicular eruptions secondary to herpes zoster virus. As with other infections, the patient's underlying immune status also plays a role in the clinical findings, as evidenced by the verrucous herpetic lesions or severe disseminated herpes zoster seen in immunocompromised patients. Other underlying conditions, such as concurrent eczema, can also contribute to the patterns of involvement as seen in eczema herpeticum and the newly coined *eczema coxsackium* due to Coxsackie virus A6. Obtaining viral cultures and polymerase chain reaction specimens from these lesions is a common way to establish the exact cause of many vesicular viral eruptions.

The age of the patient can particularly affect the cutaneous manifestations of viral illnesses, including the extramedullary hematopoiesis presenting as purple nodules in congenital cytomegalovirus infections ("blueberry muffin baby") or the classic "slapped cheek" appearance due to erythema infectiosum (parvovirus B19) seen most commonly in school-aged children.

Uncommon viral infections are included, such as the zoonotic poxviruses like Orf that cause self-limited papulonodules, as well as even more exotic arthropod-borne viral infections such as Dengue and Chikungunya virus. Common viral conditions are included here as well, such as the dome-shaped, umbilicated, shiny papules of molluscum contagiosum and verruca vulgaris in its many forms secondary to human papillomavirus.

Finally, amid the many viral illnesses included in this portion of the atlas, human immunodeficiency virus deserves particular mention because it can cause a polymorphous primary eruption in the skin and is also associated with many other coinfections such as human herpesvirus 8 in the form of Kaposi sarcoma.

This portion of the atlas highlights the vast range of skin manifestations produced by viral illnesses.

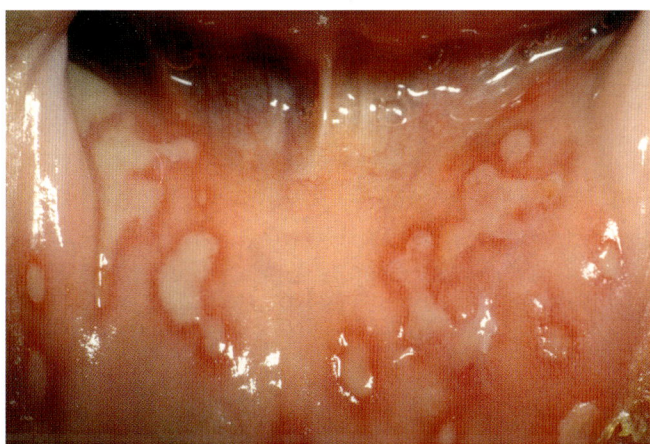

Fig. 19.1 Primary herpes simplex infection.

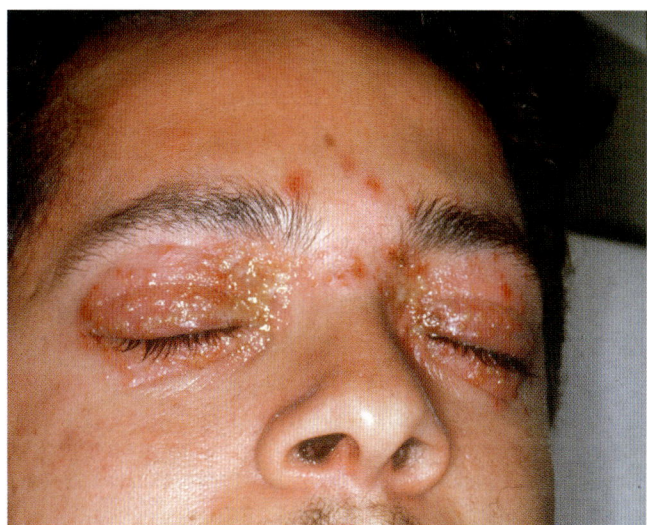

Fig. 19.2 Primary herpes simplex infection.

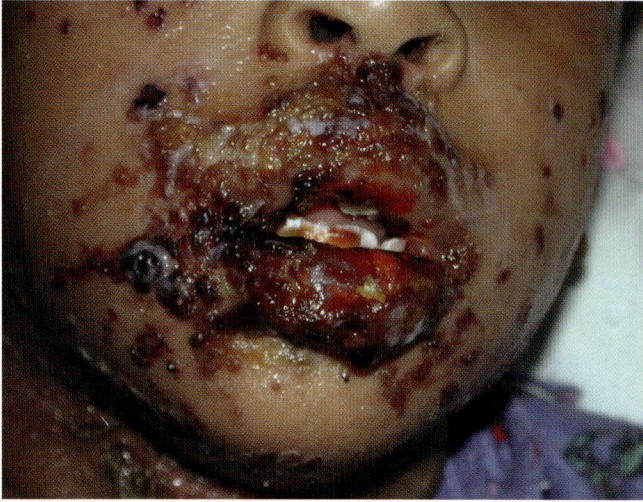

Fig. 19.3 Primary herpes simplex infection.

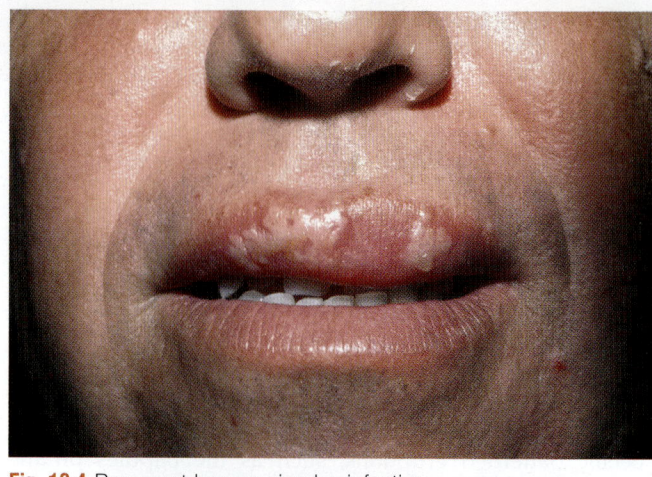

Fig. 19.4 Recurrent herpes simplex infection.

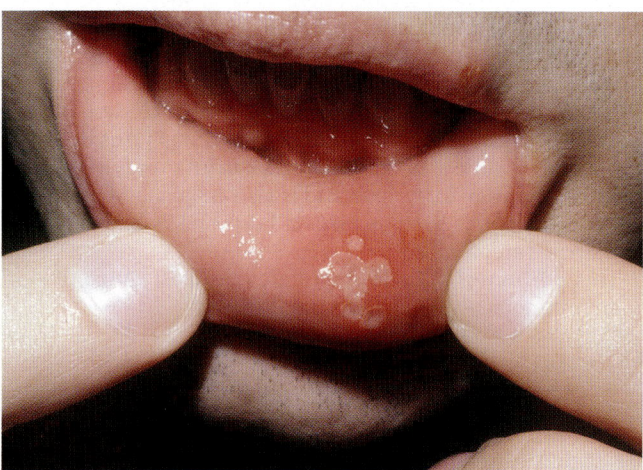

Fig. 19.5 Recurrent herpes simplex infection. *Courtesy Steven Binnick, MD.*

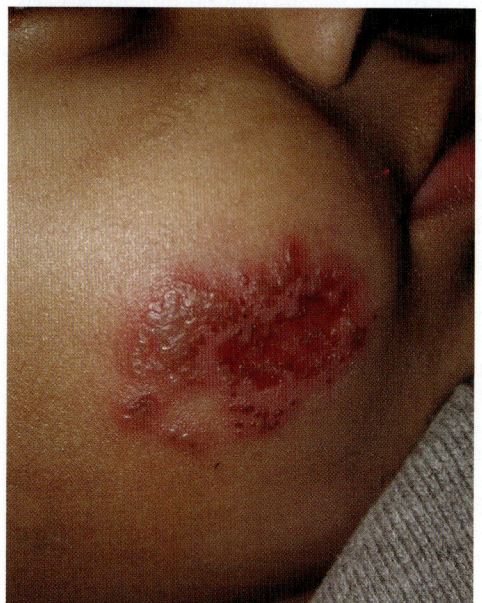

Fig. 19.6 Recurrent herpes simplex infection.

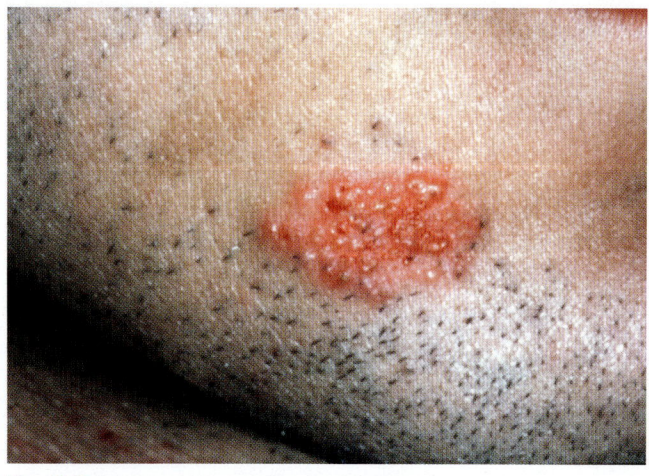

Fig. 19.7 Recurrent herpes simplex infection.

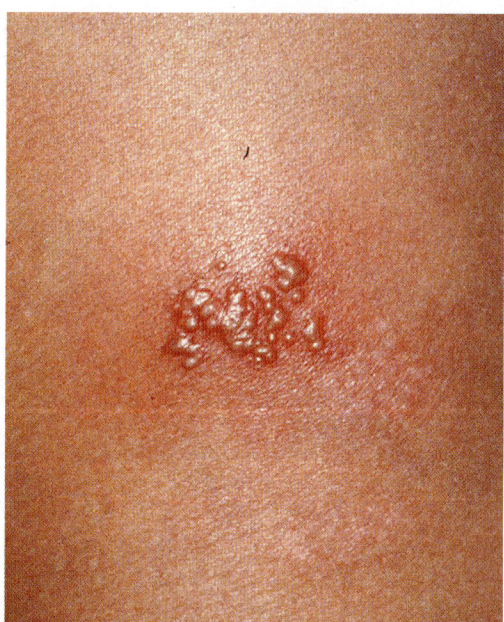

Fig. 19.8 Recurrent herpes simplex on the leg. *Courtesy The University of Utah and Oregon Health Sciences University Leonard Swinyer MD image collection.*

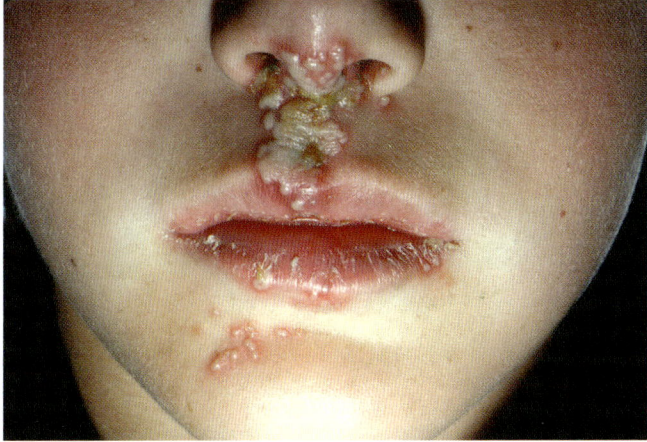

Fig. 19.9 Recurrent herpes simplex infection. *Courtesy The University of Utah and Oregon Health Sciences University Leonard Swinyer MD image collection.*

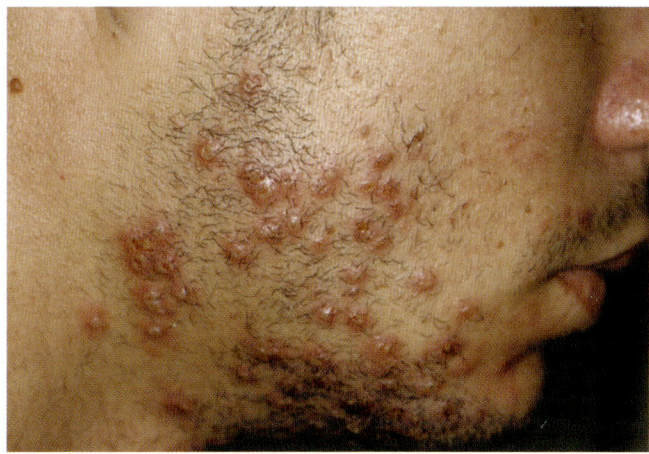

Fig. 19.10 Herpetic sycosis.

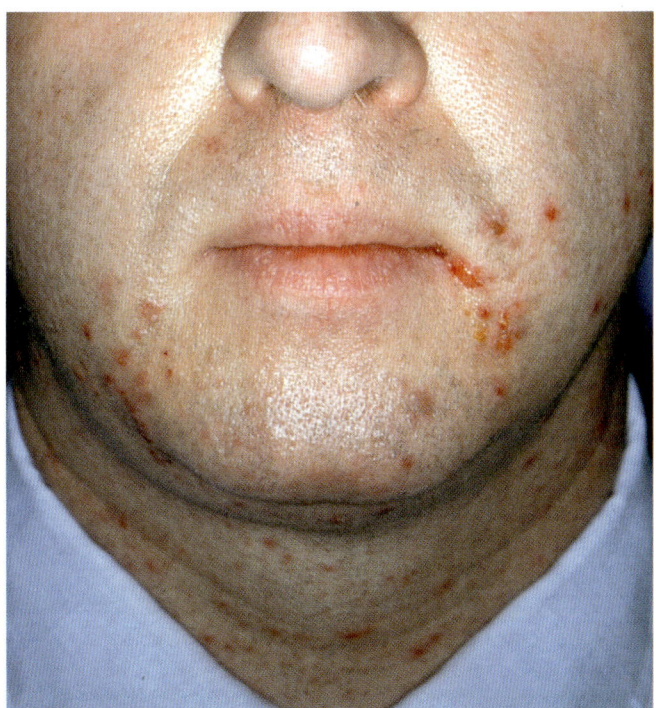

Fig. 19.11 Herpetic sycosis.

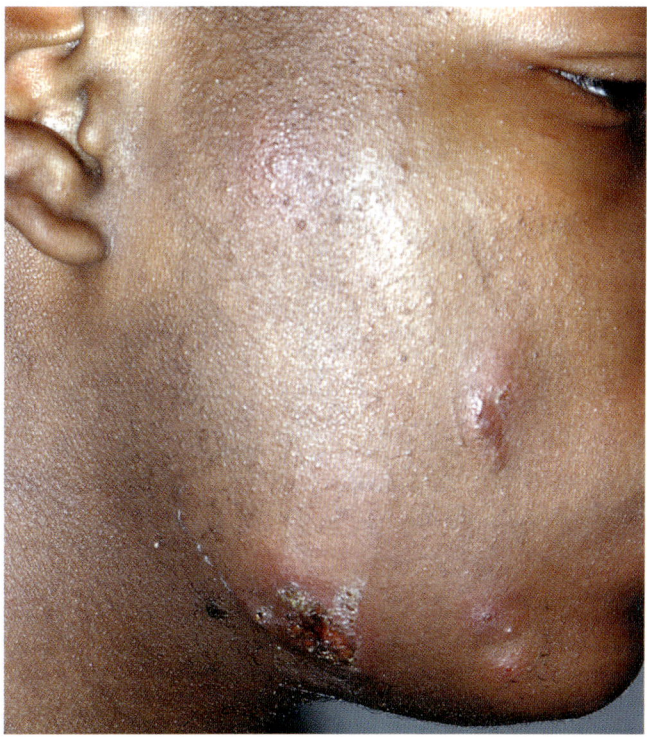

Fig. 19.12 Herpes gladiatorum.

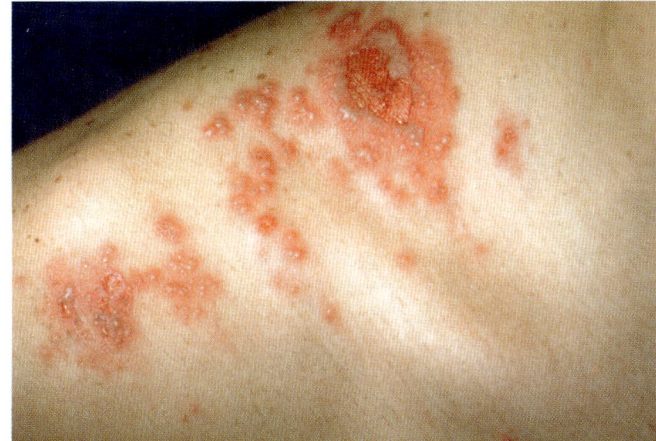

Fig. 19.13 Herpes gladiatorum.

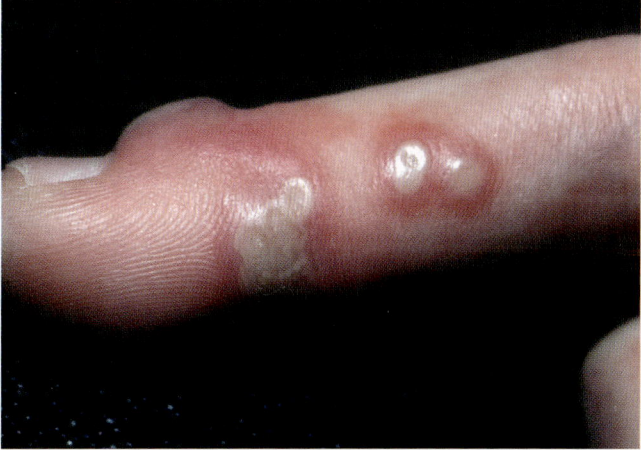

Fig. 19.14 Herpetic whitlow. *Courtesy Steven Binnick, MD.*

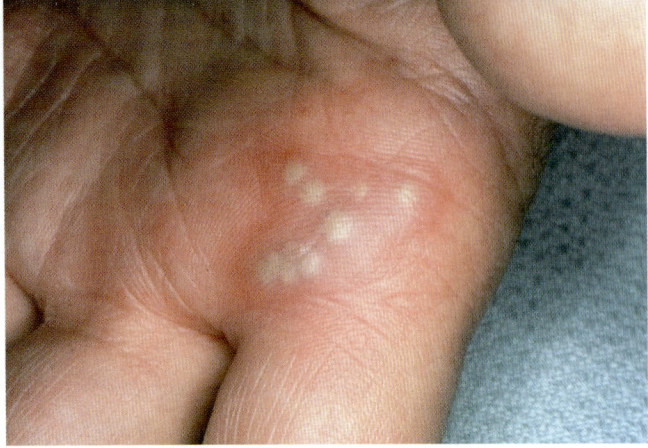

Fig. 19.15 Herpetic infection of the palm.

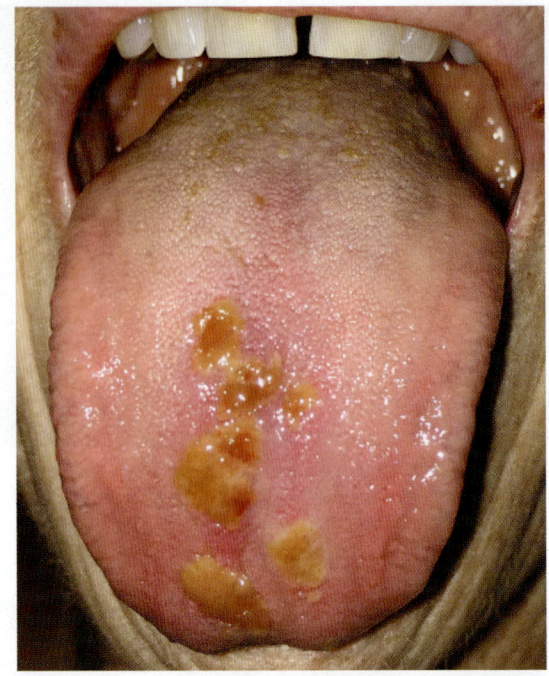

Fig. 19.16 Herpes simplex infection of the tongue.

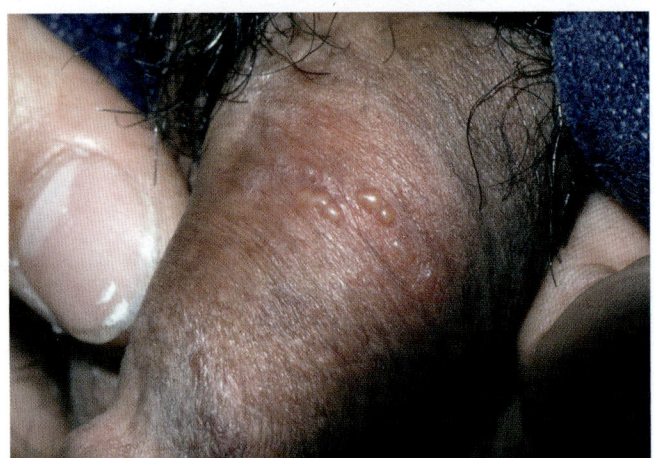

Fig. 19.17 Herpes genitalis. *Courtesy Steven Binnick, MD.*

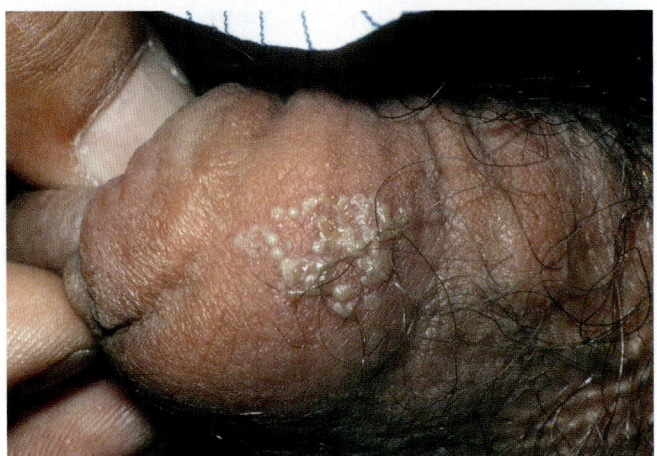

Fig. 19.18 Herpes genitalis. *Courtesy Steven Binnick, MD.*

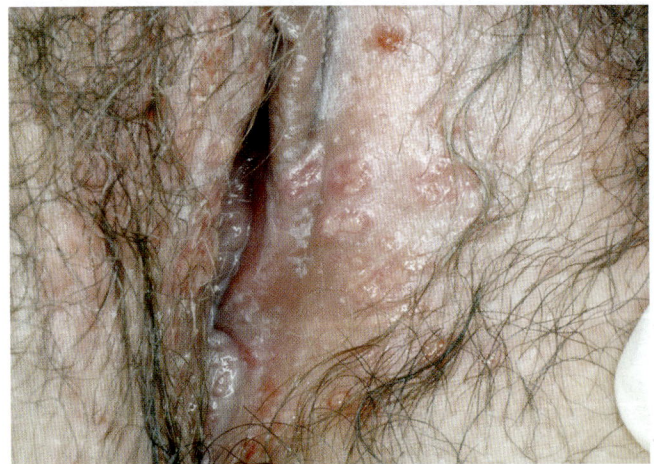

Fig. 19.19 Herpes genitalis. *Courtesy Steven Binnick, MD.*

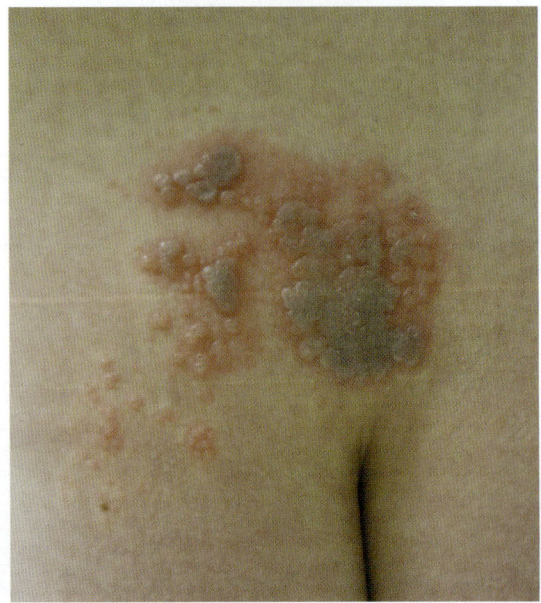

Fig. 19.20 Recurrent herpes simplex, buttock.

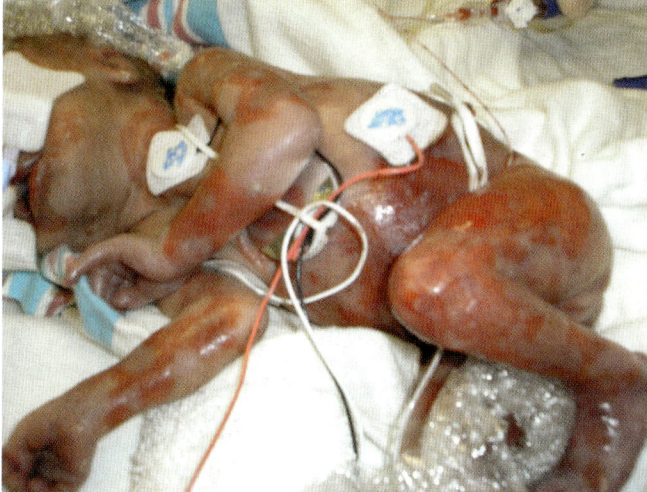
Fig. 19.21 Intrauterine herpes simplex infection.

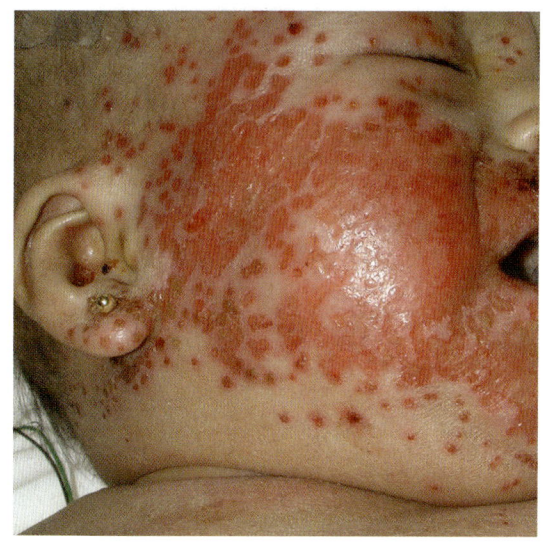
Fig. 19.22 Eczema herpeticum.

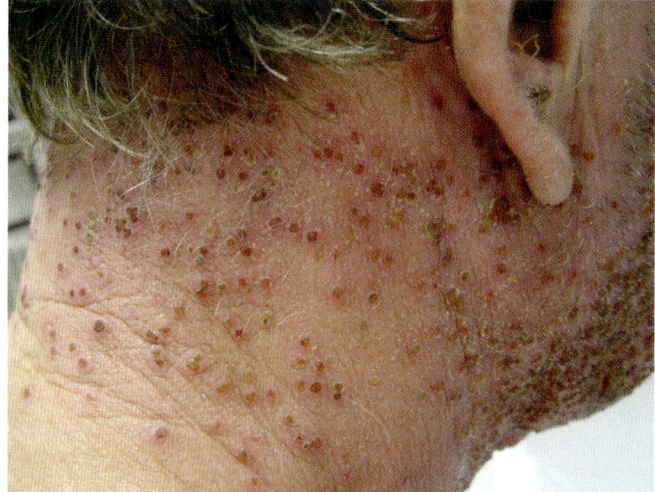
Fig. 19.23 Eczema herpeticum.

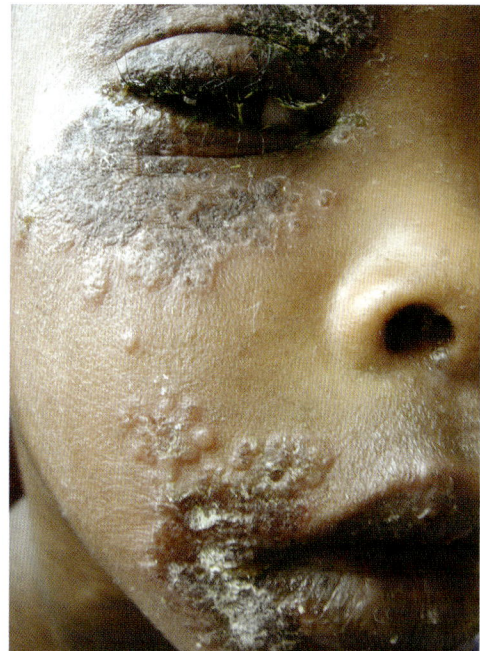
Fig. 19.24 Eczema herpeticum.

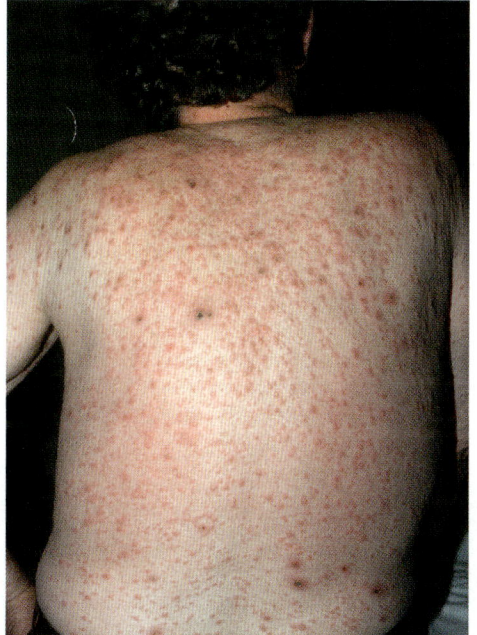
Fig. 19.25 Disseminated herpes simplex infection.

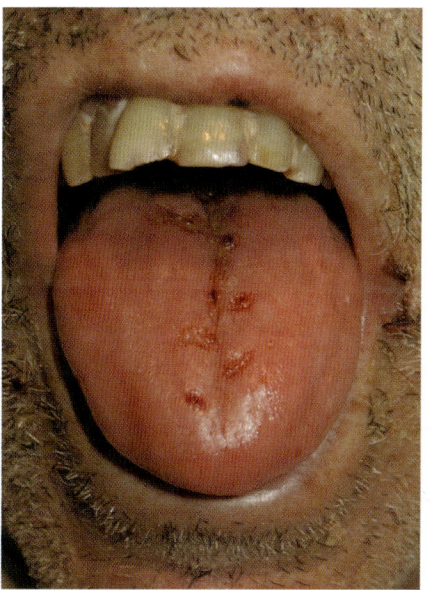
Fig. 19.26 Herpetic geometric glossitis in a neutropenic patient.

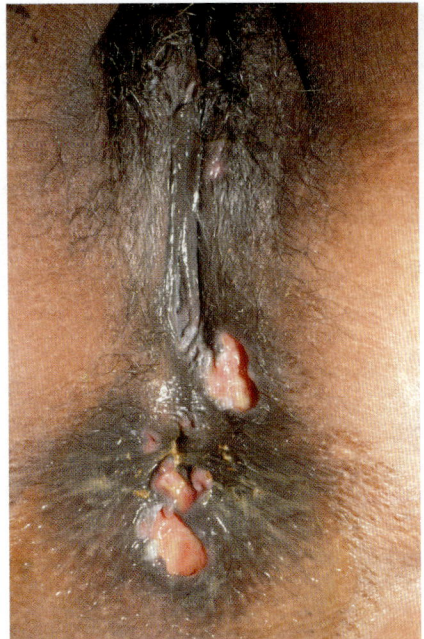

Fig. 19.27 Ulcerative herpes simplex in an HIV-infected patient.

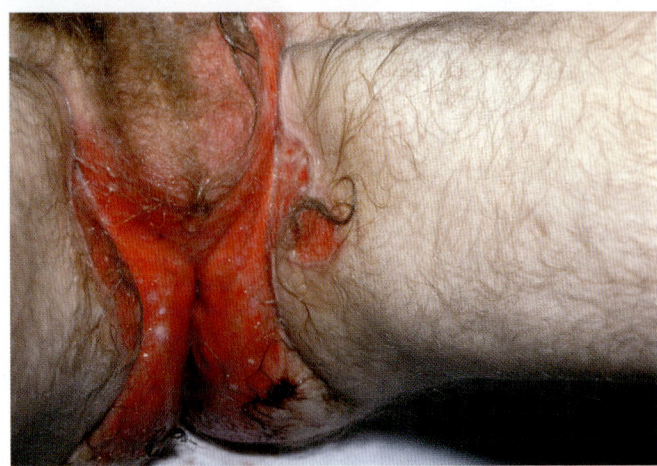

Fig. 19.28 Ulcerative herpes simplex in an HIV-infected patient.

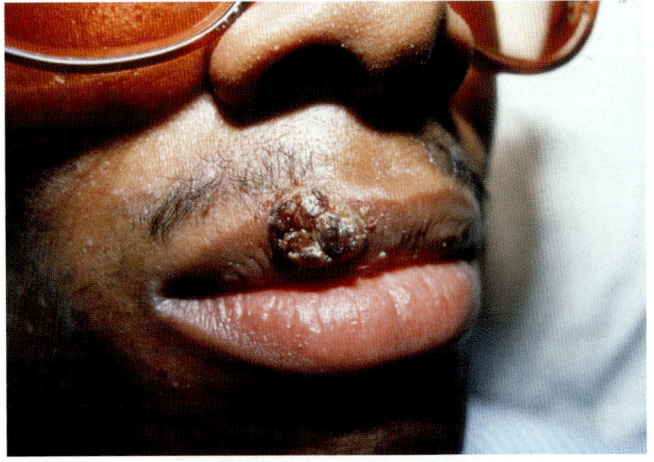

Fig. 19.29 Crusted ulcerative herpes simplex in an HIV-infected patient.

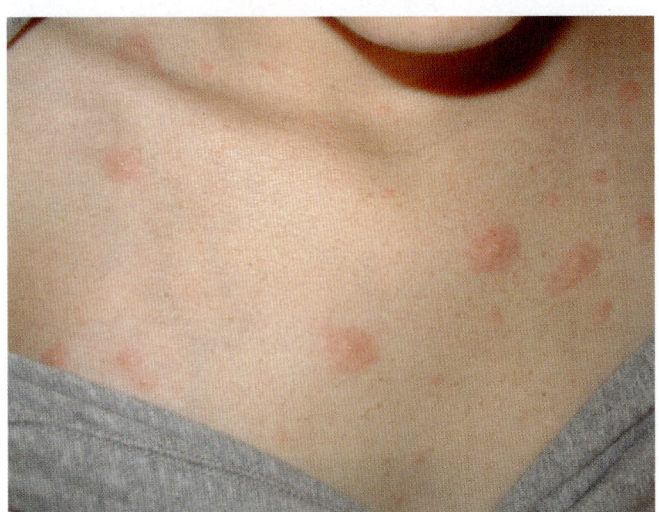

Fig. 19.30 Varicella.

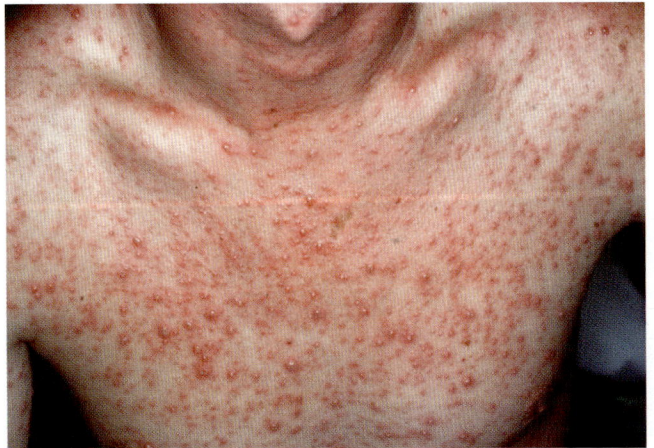

Fig. 19.31 Varicella.

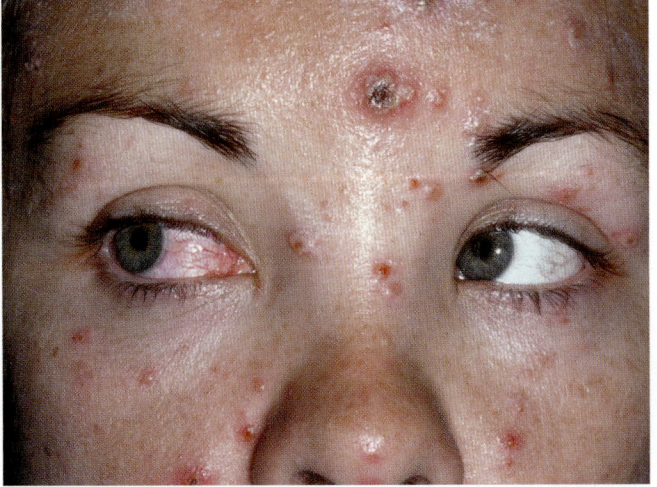

Fig. 19.32 Varicella.

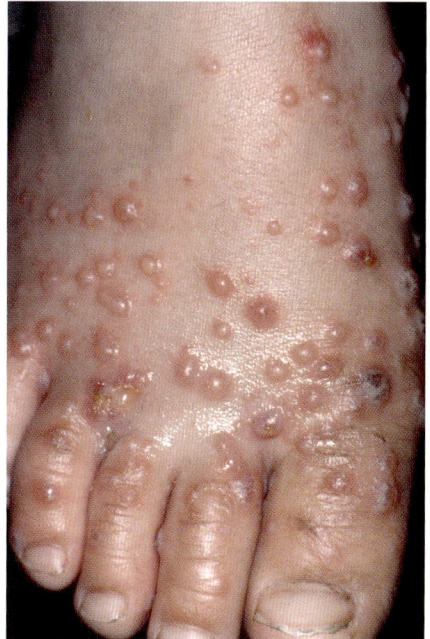

Fig. 19.33 Varicella. *Courtesy Steven Binnick, MD.*

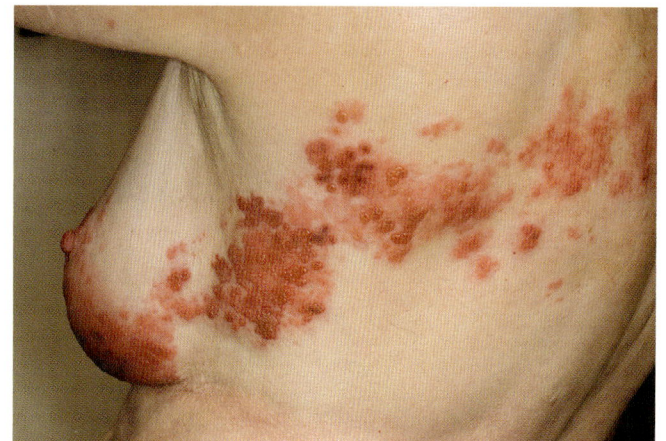

Fig. 19.34 Herpes zoster.

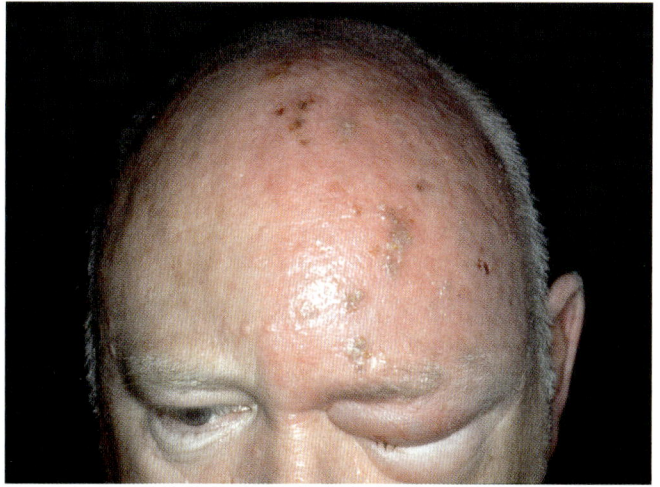

Fig. 19.35 Herpes zoster.

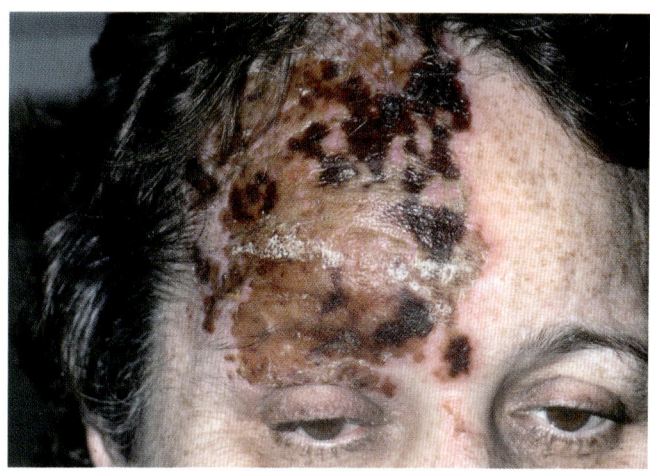

Fig. 19.36 Herpes zoster. *Courtesy Steven Binnick, MD.*

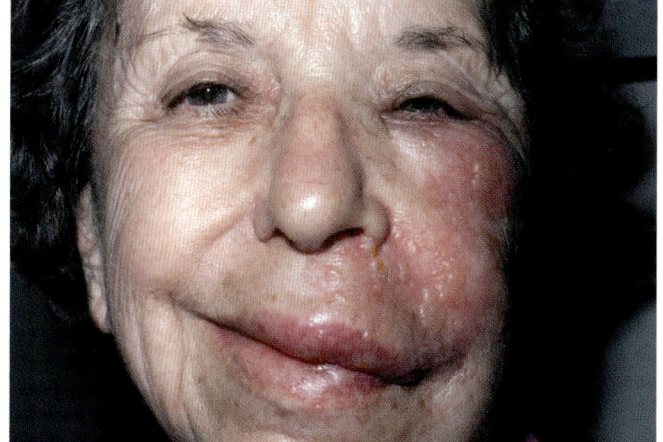

Fig. 19.37 Herpes zoster with Ramsay Hunt syndrome. *Courtesy Steven Binnick, MD.*

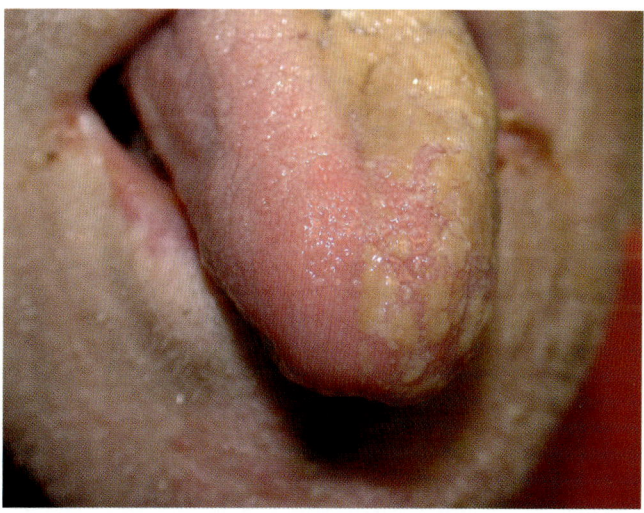

Fig. 19.38 Herpes zoster. *Courtesy Steven Binnick, MD.*

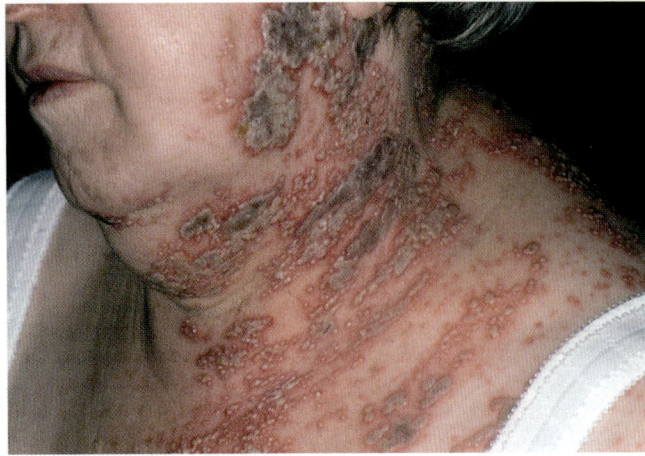

Fig. 19.39 Herpes zoster.

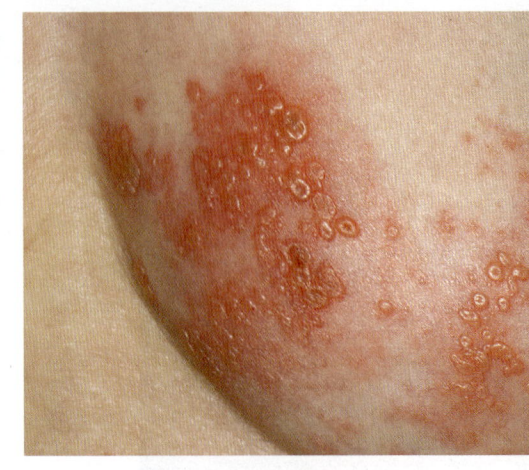

Fig. 19.40 Herpes zoster.

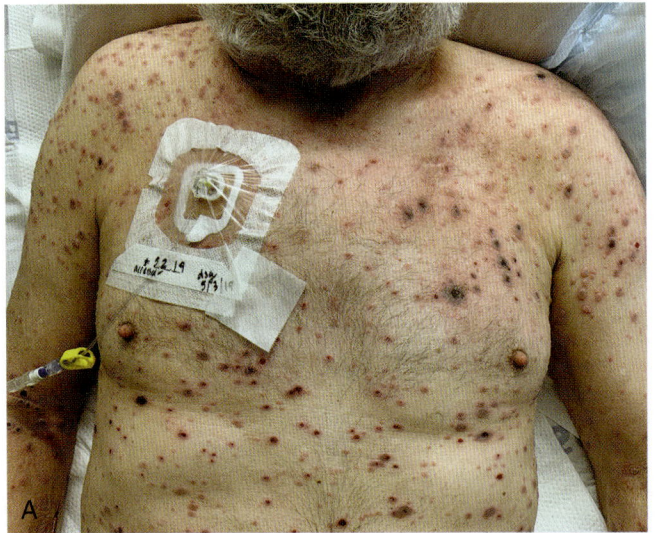

Fig. 19.41 (A) Disseminated varicella in a patient with leukemia. (B) Close-up of the same patient.

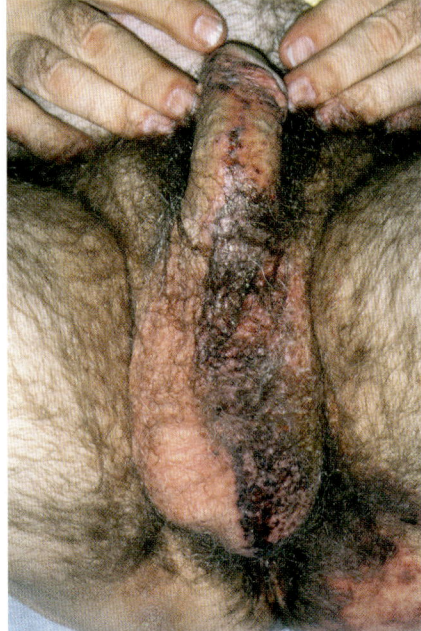

Fig. 19.42 Herpes zoster.

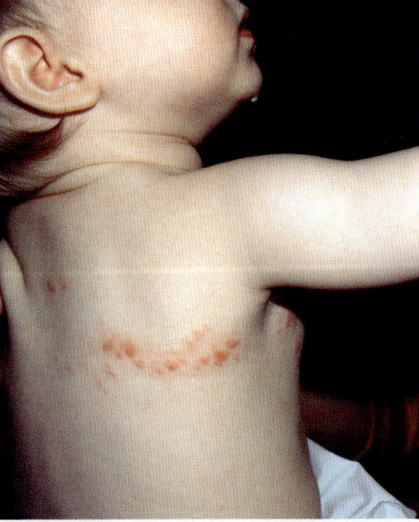

Fig. 19.43 Herpes zoster in an 11-month-old patient.

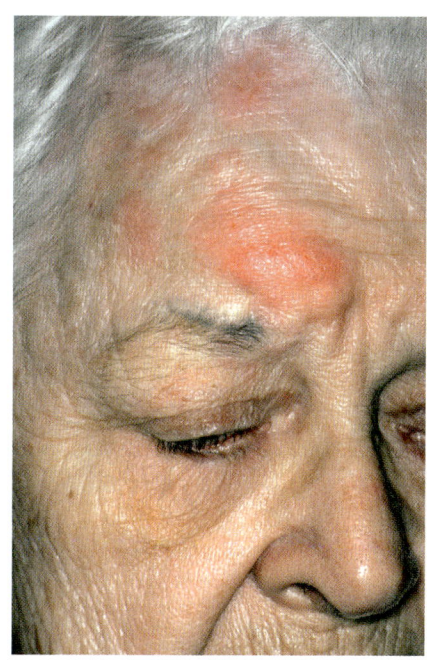

Fig. 19.44 Herpes zoster, prevesicular.

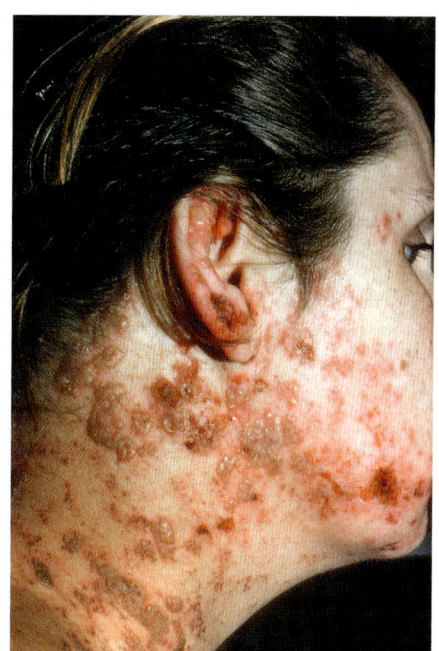

Fig. 19.45 Herpes zoster in a patient with Hodgkin disease.

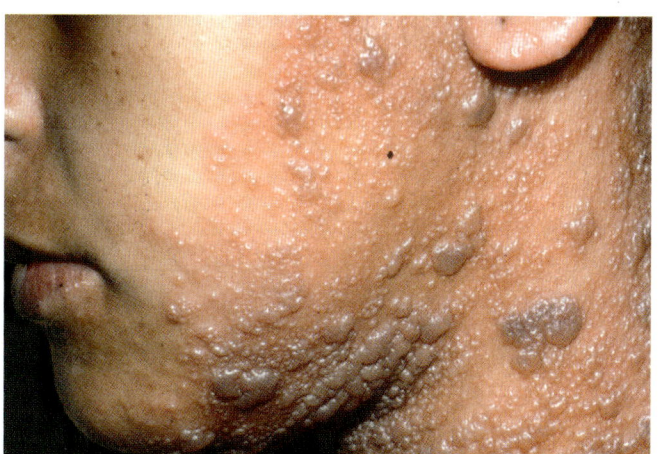

Fig. 19.46 Herpes zoster in an HIV-infected patient.

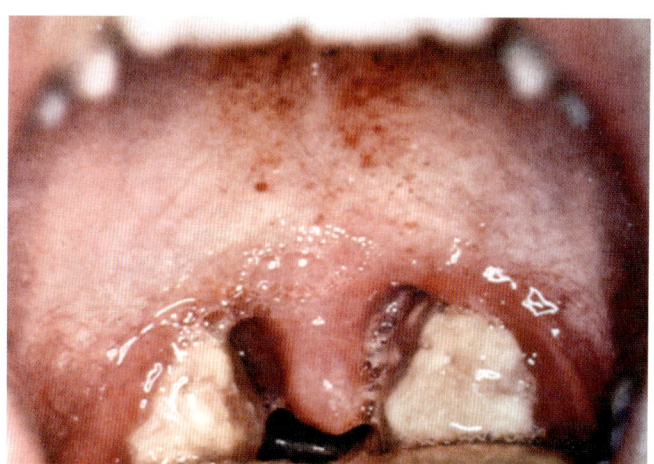

Fig. 19.47 Mononucleosis. *Courtesy Steven Binnick, MD.*

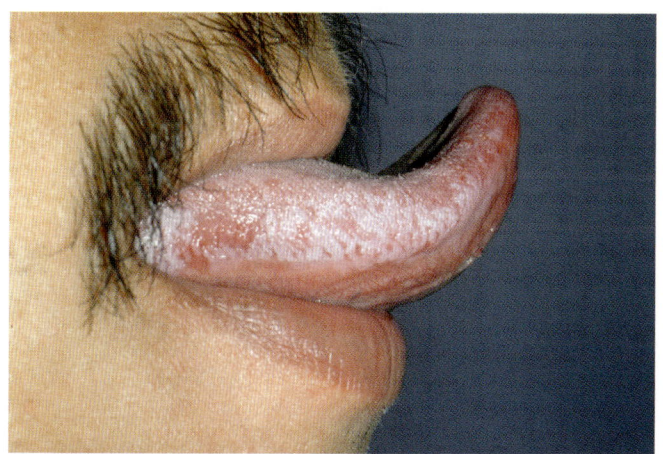

Fig. 19.48 Oral hairy leukoplakia.

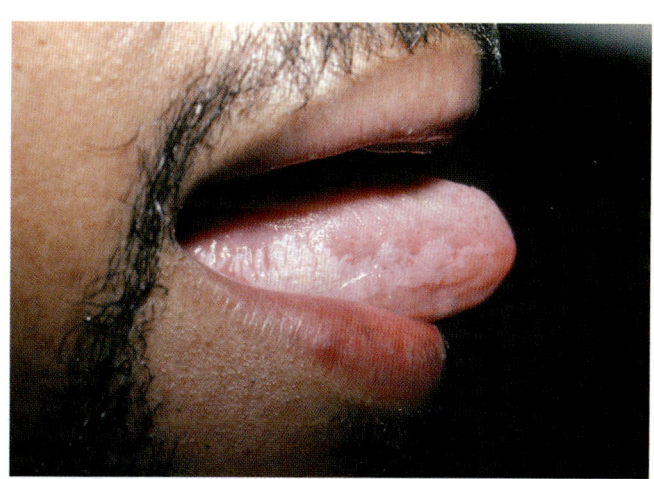

Fig. 19.49 Oral hairy leukoplakia.

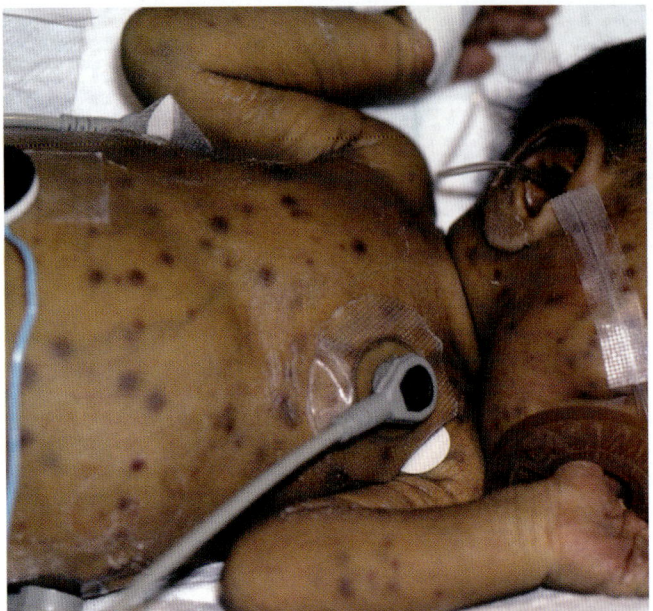

Fig. 19.50 Cytomegaloviral infection in a newborn. *Courtesy Paul Honig, MD.*

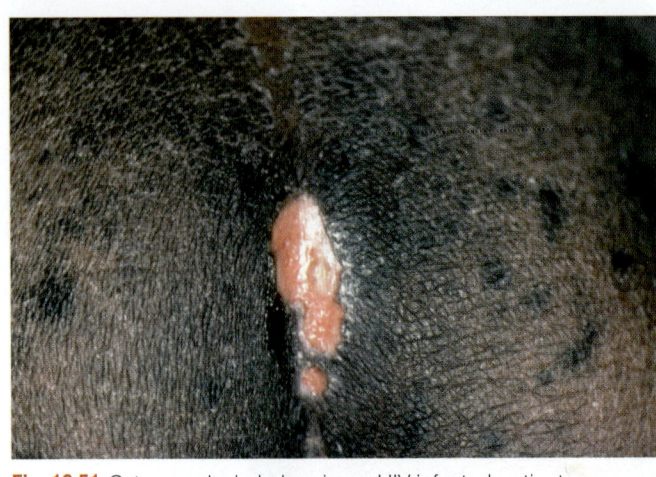

Fig. 19.51 Cytomegaloviral ulcer in an HIV-infected patient.

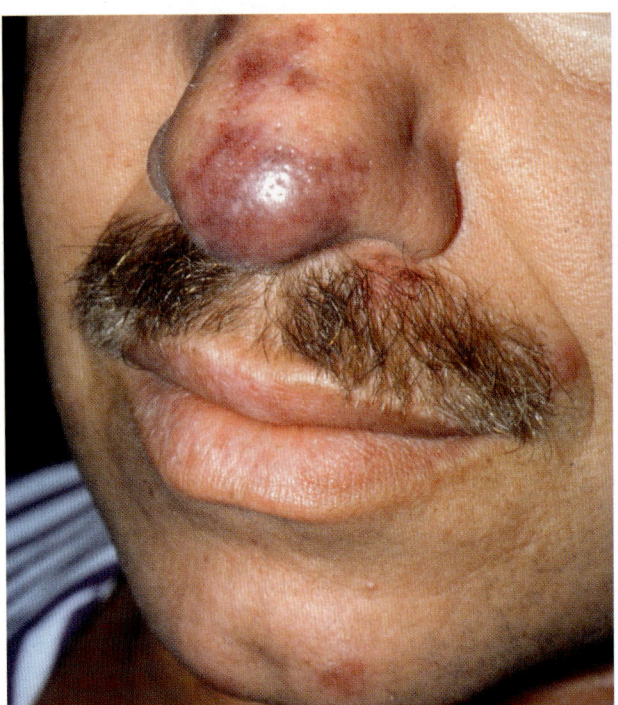

Fig. 19.52 Kaposi sarcoma in an HIV-infected patient.

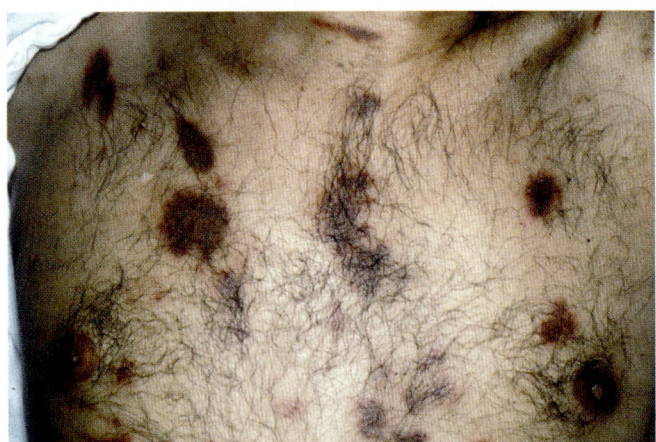

Fig. 19.53 Kaposi sarcoma in an HIV-infected patient.

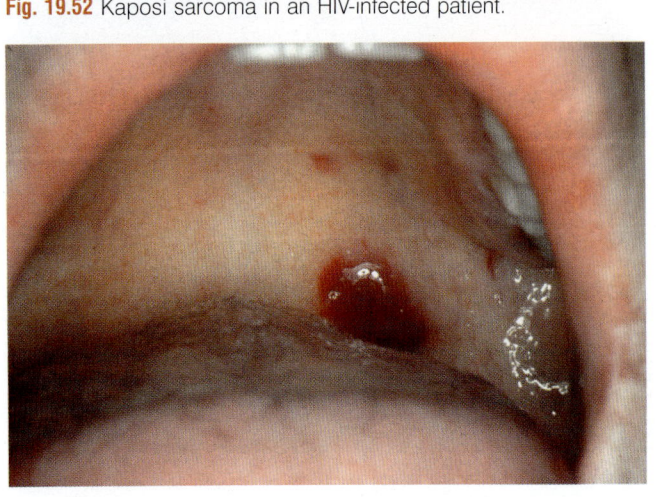

Fig. 19.54 Kaposi sarcoma in an HIV-infected patient.

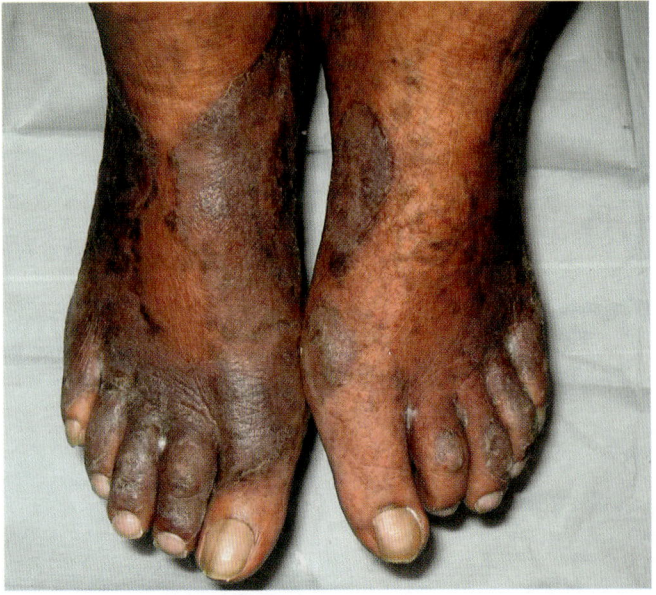

Fig. 19.55 Necrolytic acral erythema. *Courtesy Carrie Kovarik, MD.*

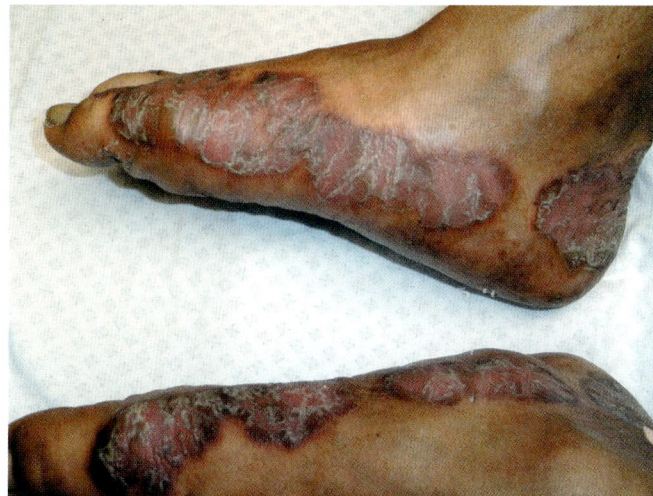

Fig. 19.56 Necrolytic acral erythema. *Courtesy Scott Norton, MD.*

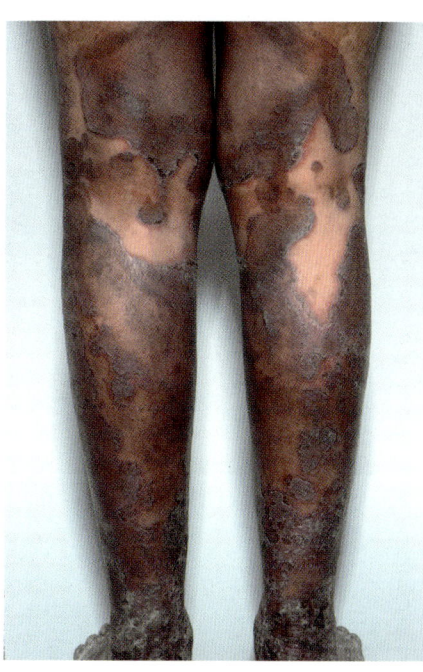

Fig. 19.57 Necrolytic acral erythema. (First published in Hivnor CM, Yan AC, Junkins-Hopkins JM, Honig PJ: Necrolytic acral erythema. *J Am Acad Dermatol* 2004;50(suppl) S121–124.)

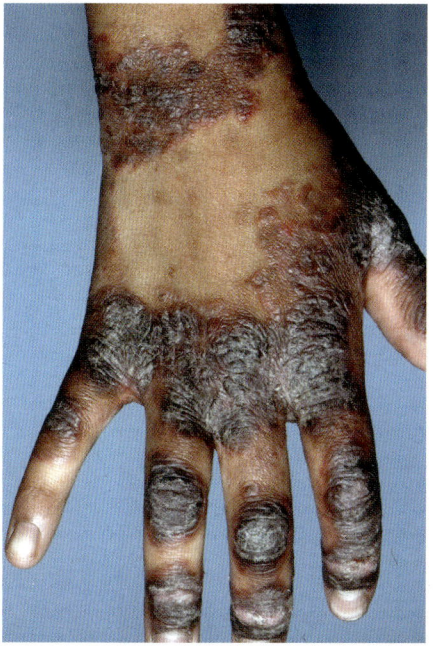

Fig. 19.58 Necrolytic acral erythema. (First published in Hivnor CM, Yan AC, Junkins-Hopkins JM, Honig PJ: Necrolytic acral erythema. *J Am Acad Dermatol* 2004;50(suppl) S121–124.)

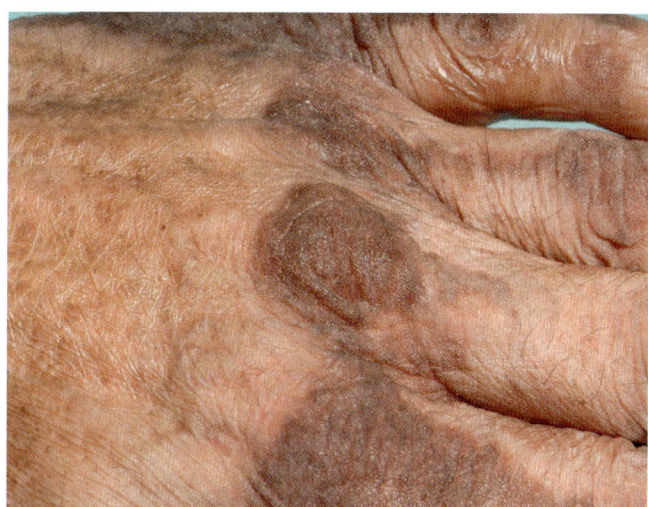

Fig. 19.59 Necrolytic acral erythema.

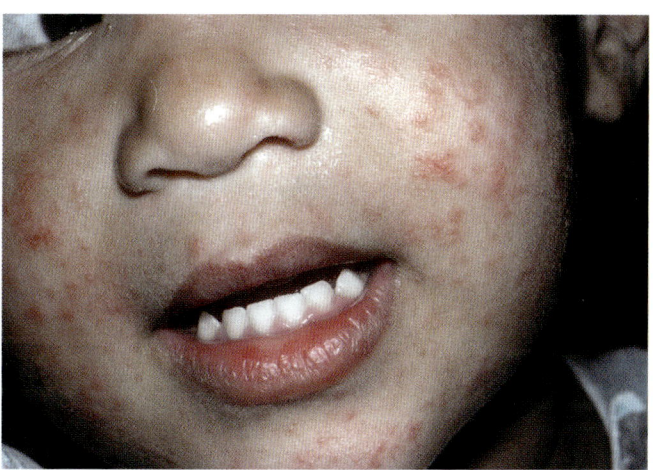

Fig. 19.60 Gianotti-Crosti syndrome. *Courtesy Curt Samlaska, MD.*

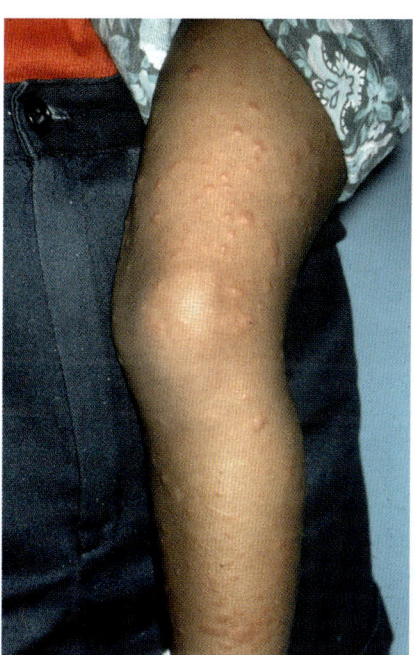

Fig. 19.61 Gianotti-Crosti syndrome.

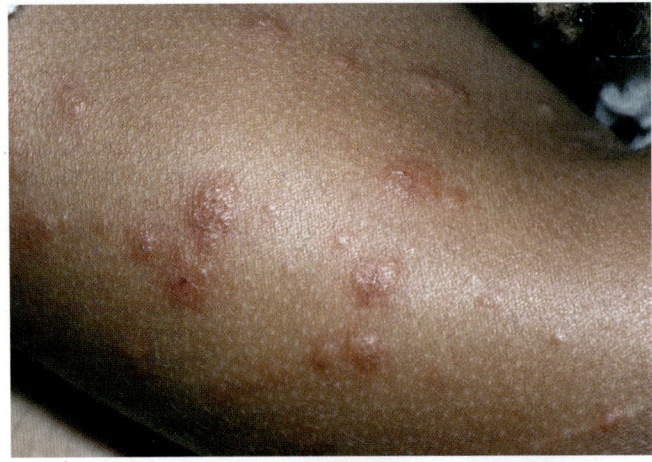

Fig. 19.62 Gianotti-Crosti syndrome. *Courtesy Curt Samlaska, MD.*

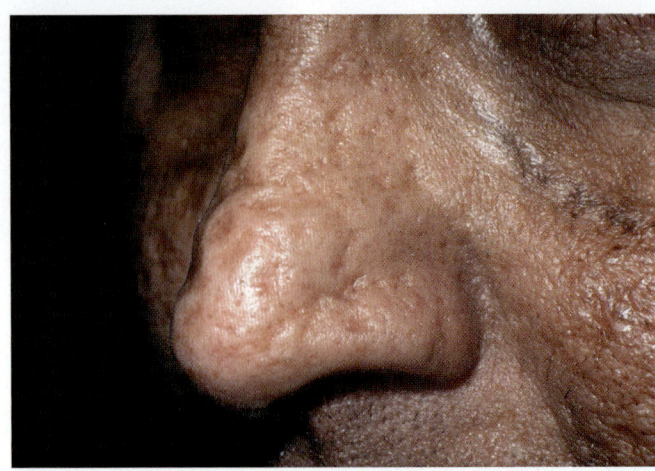

Fig. 19.63 Smallpox scarring. *Courtesy Steven Binnick, MD.*

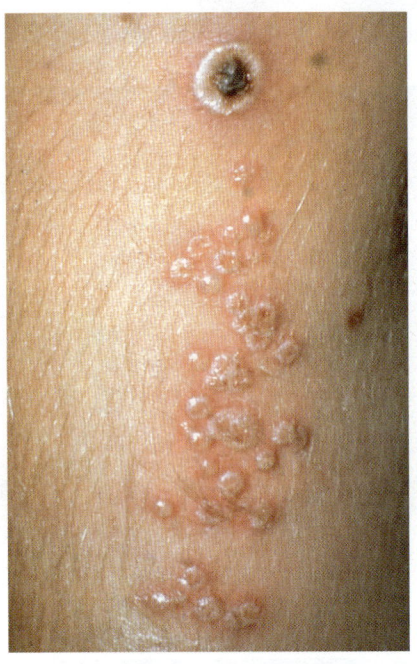

Fig. 19.64 Vaccinia vaccination with autoinoculation.

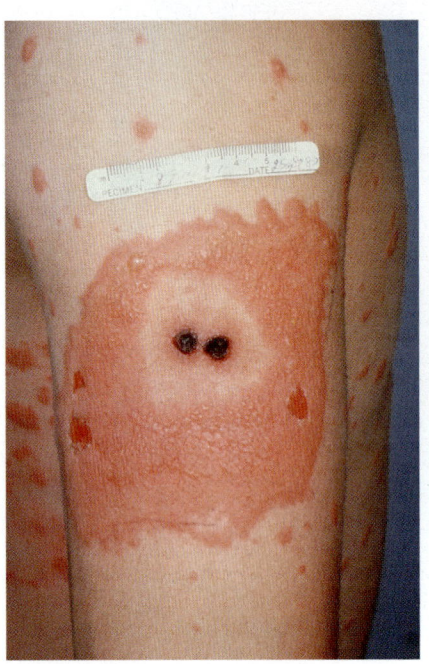

Fig. 19.65 Vaccinia vaccination site with reactive erythema.

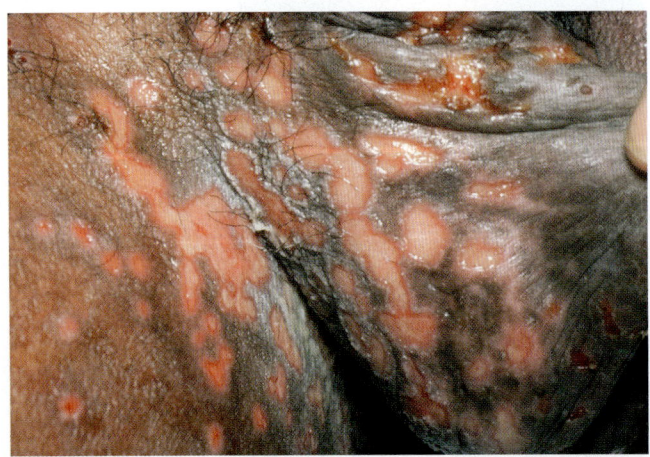

Fig. 19.66 Disseminated vaccinia.

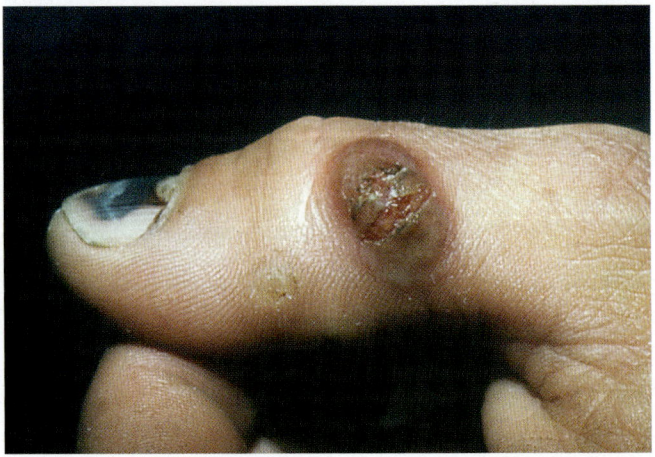

Fig. 19.67 Orf.

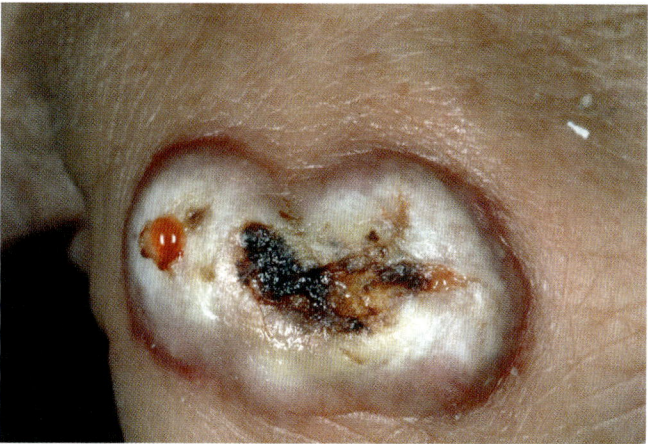

Fig. 19.68 Milker nodule.

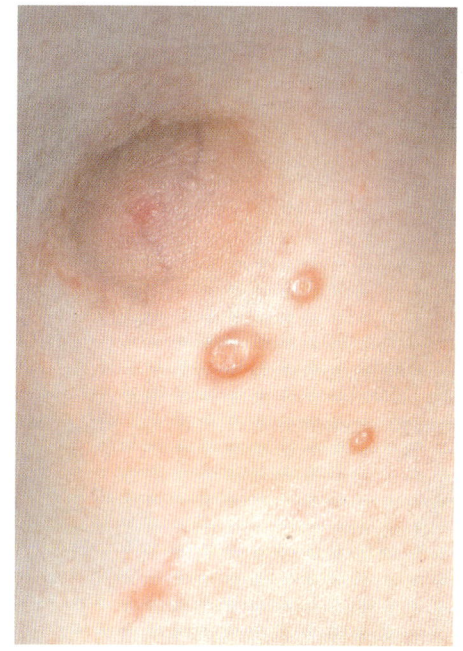

Fig. 19.69 Molluscum contagiosum. *Courtesy Steven Binnick, MD.*

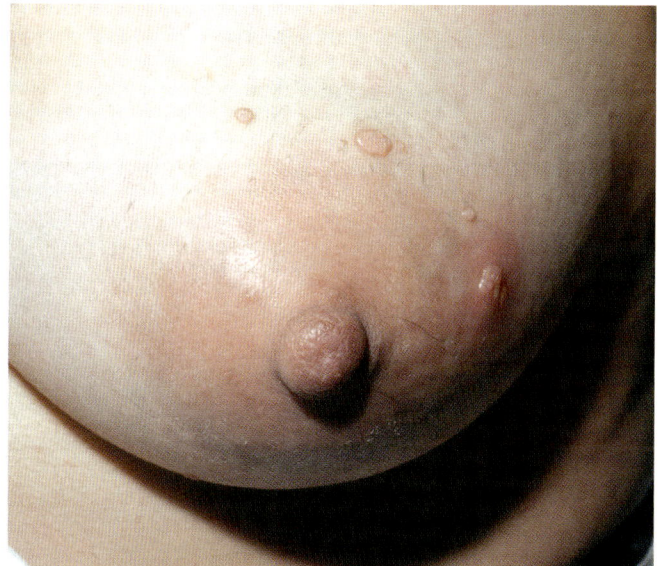

Fig. 19.70 Molluscum contagiosum. *Courtesy Steven Binnick, MD.*

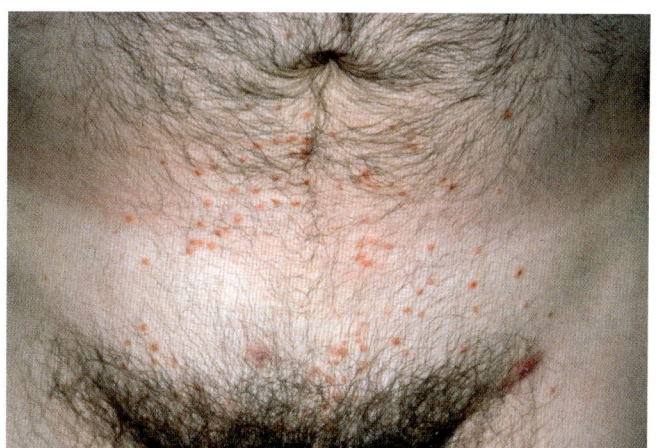

Fig. 19.71 Molluscum contagiosum.

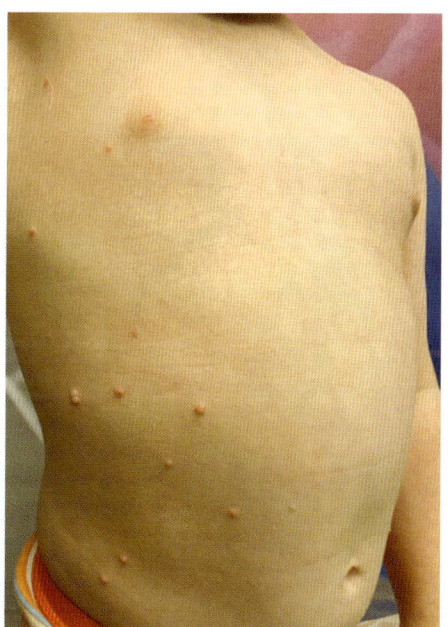

Fig. 19.72 Molluscum contagiosum.

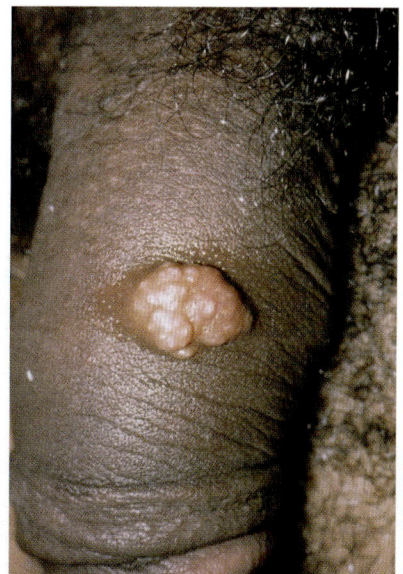

Fig. 19.73 Giant molluscum contagiosum.

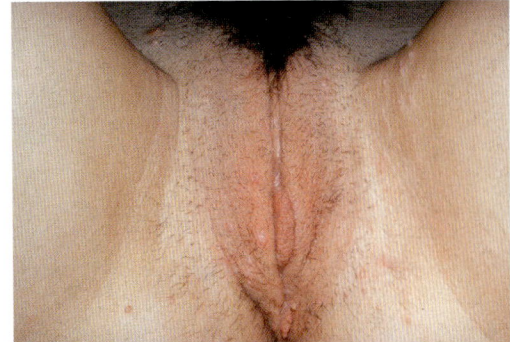

Fig. 19.74 Molluscum contagiosum.

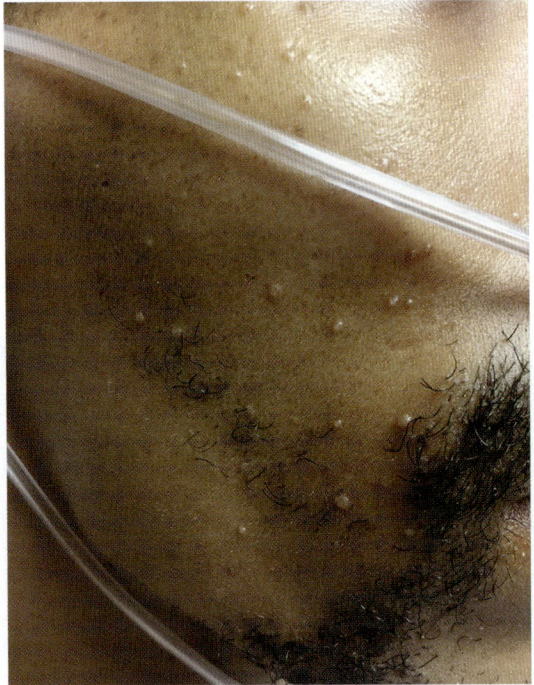

Fig. 19.76 Molluscum contagiosum in an HIV-infected patient.

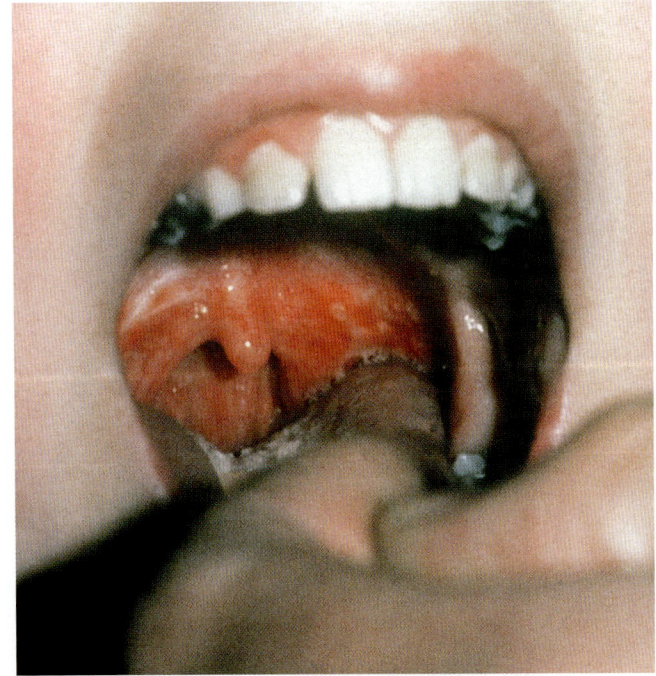

Fig. 19.78 Herpangina.

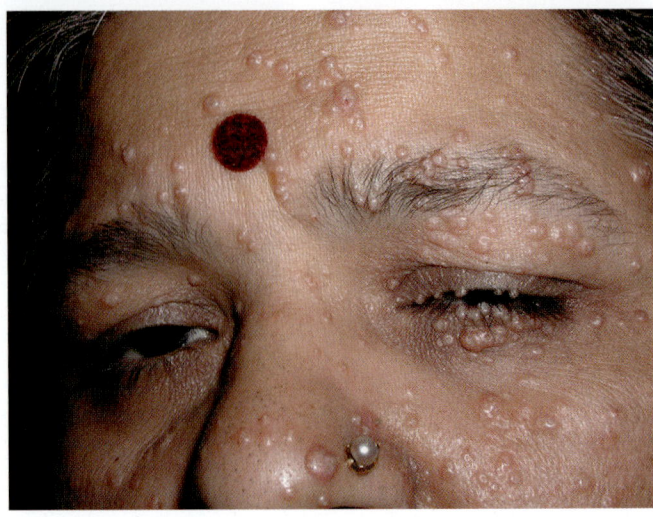

Fig. 19.75 Giant molluscum contagiosum. *Courtesy Shyam Verma, MBBS, DVD.*

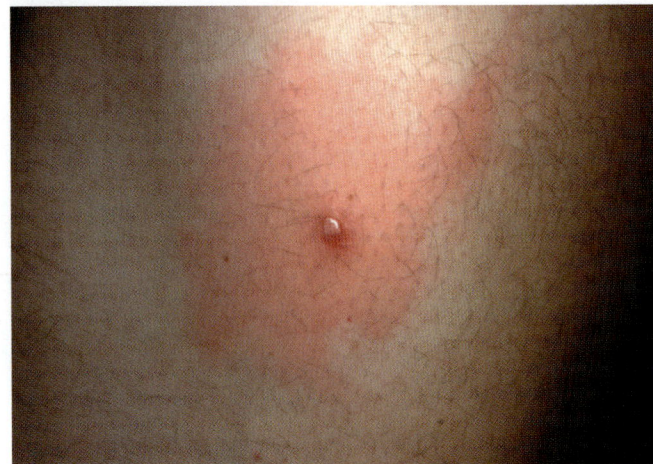

Fig. 19.77 Molluscum dermatitis.

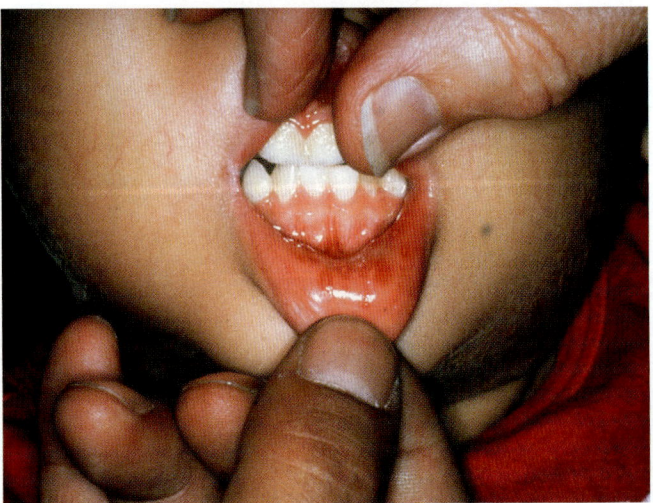

Fig. 19.79 Hand, foot, and mouth disease.

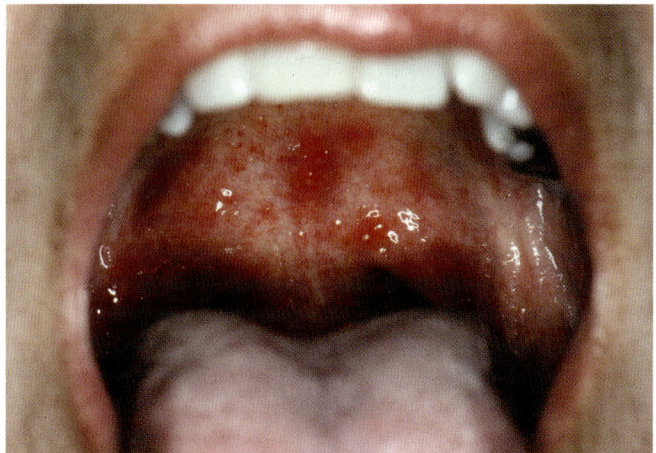

Fig. 19.80 Hand, foot, and mouth disease.

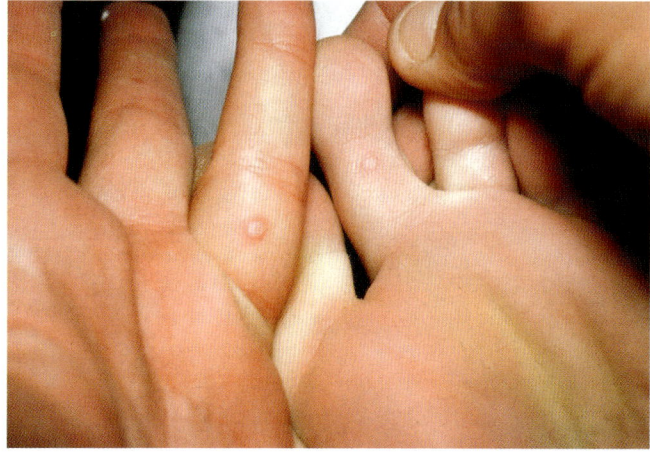

Fig. 19.81 Hand, foot, and mouth disease. *Courtesy Steven Binnick, MD.*

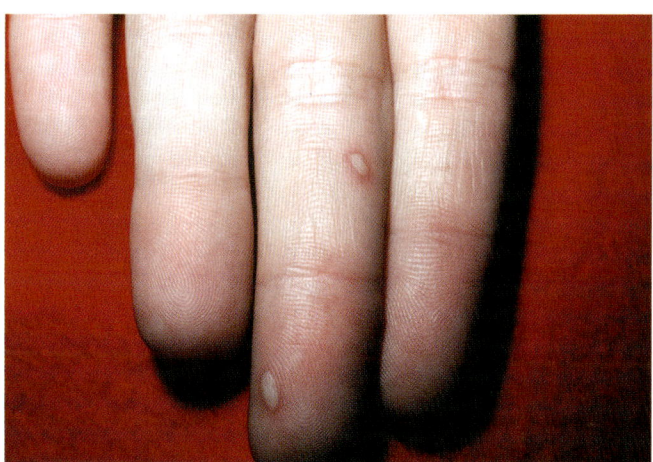

Fig. 19.82 Hand, foot, and mouth disease. *Courtesy Steven Binnick, MD.*

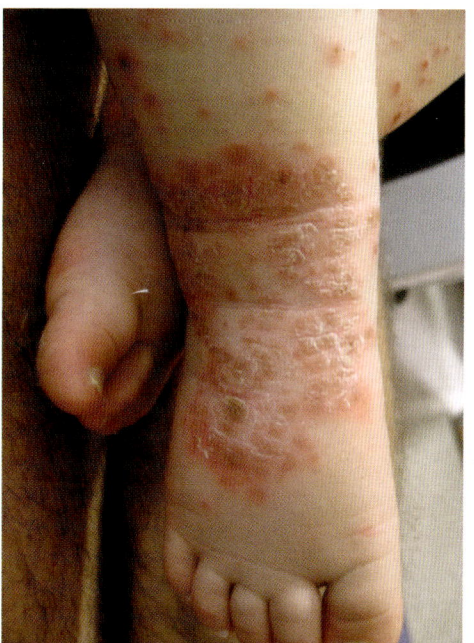

Fig. 19.83 Coxsackie A6 hand, foot, and mouth disease.

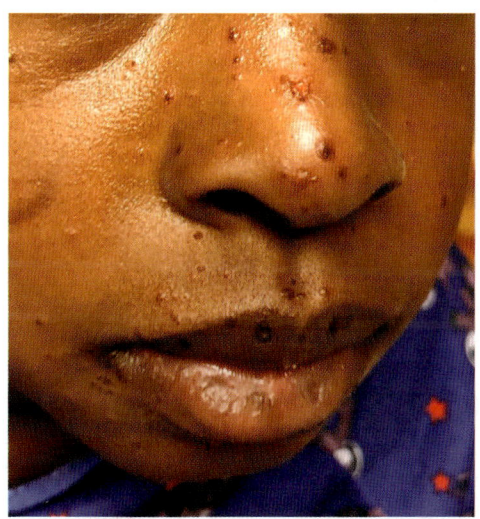

Fig. 19.84 Enterovirus hand, foot, and mouth disease.

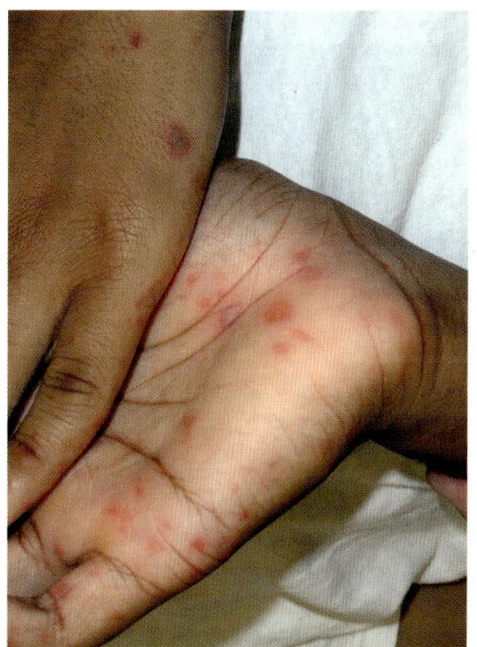

Fig. 19.85 Coxsackie A6 hand, foot, and mouth disease. *Courtesy Scott Norton, MD.*

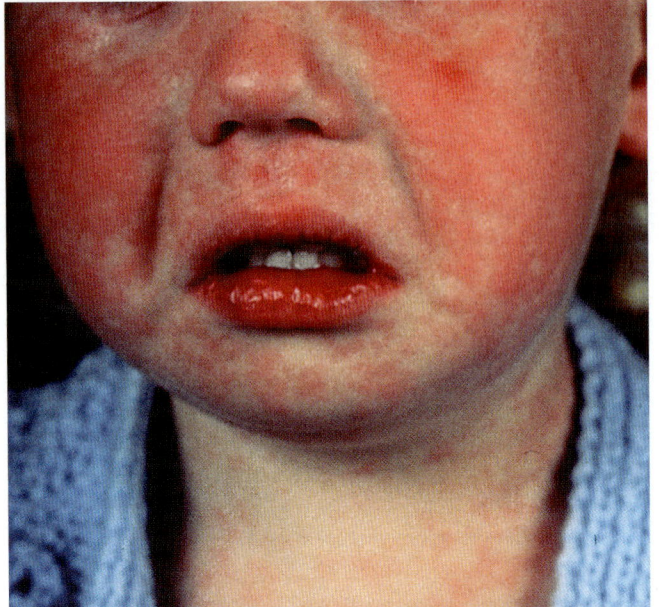

Fig. 19.86 Rubeola (measles).

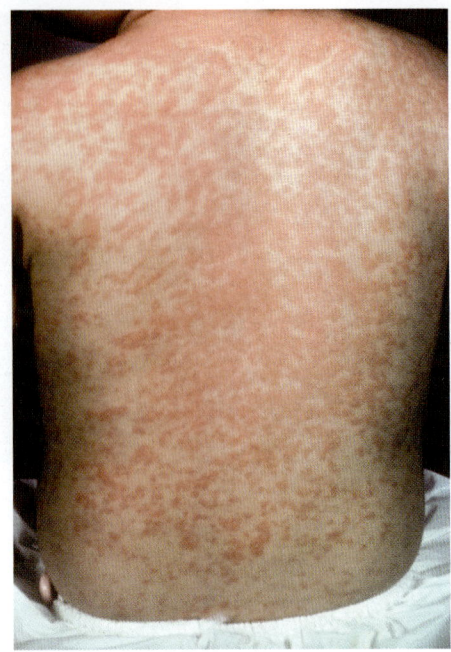

Fig. 19.87 Rubeola (measles).

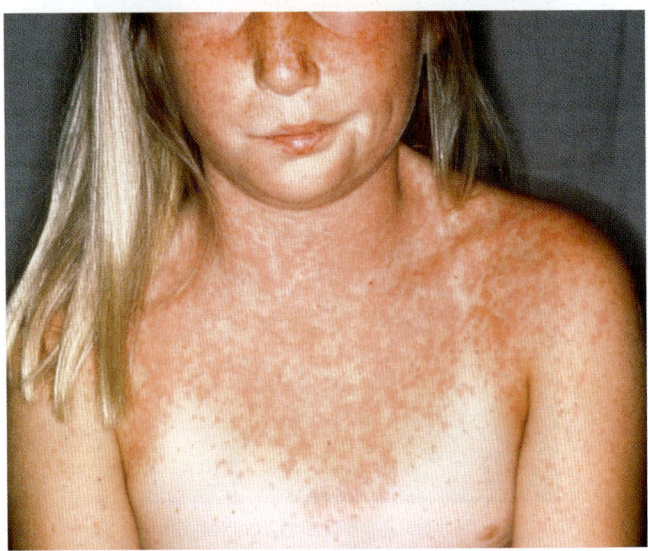

Fig. 19.88 Rubeola (measles) in a photodistribution.

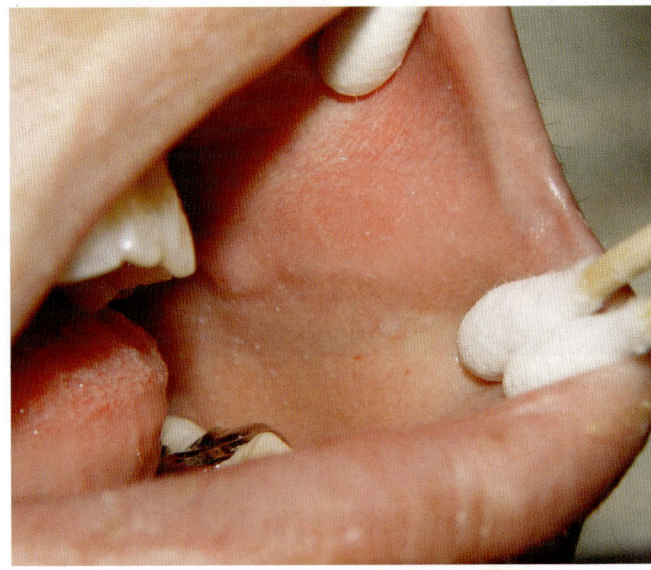

Fig. 19.89 Koplik spots (measles). *Courtesy National Cheng Kung University, Taiwan.*

Fig. 19.90 Rubella.

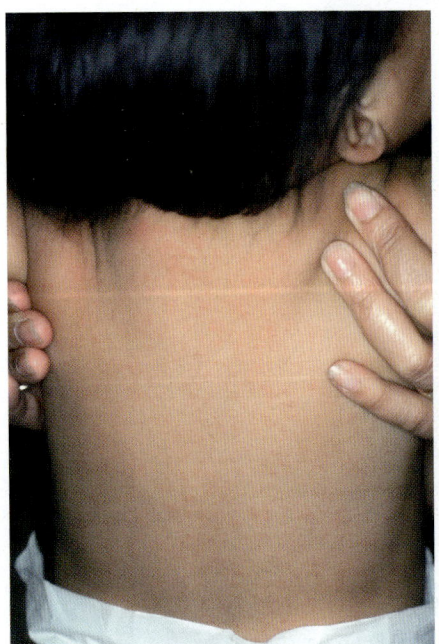

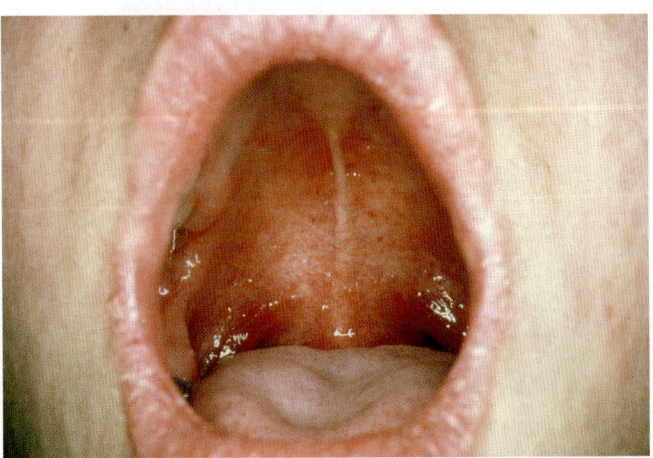

Fig. 19.91 Forchheimer spots in rubella.

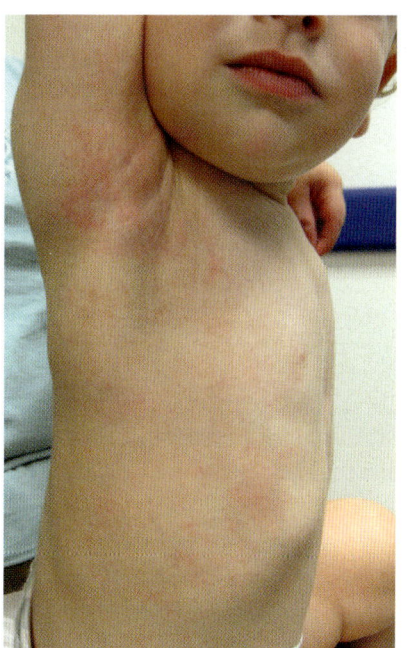

Fig. 19.92 Asymmetric periflexural exanthem of childhood.

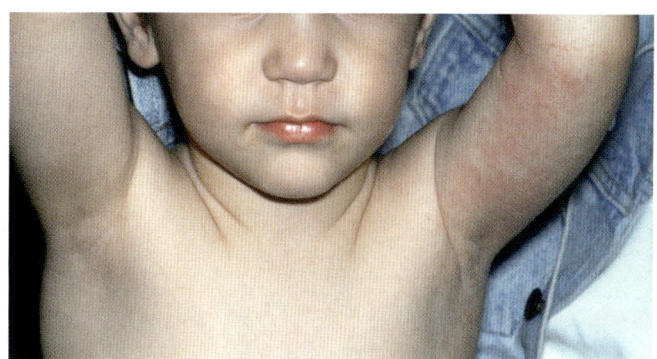

Fig. 19.93 Asymmetric periflexural exanthem of childhood. *Courtesy Steven Binnick, MD.*

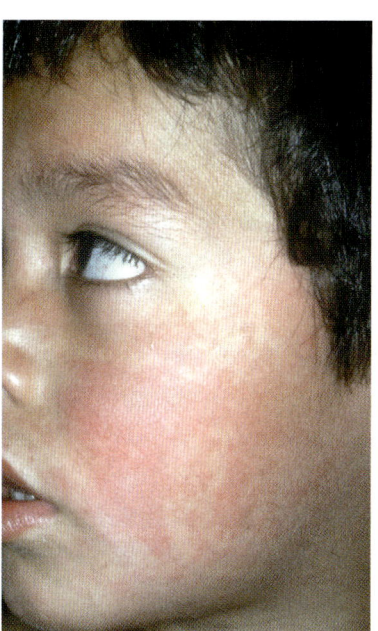

Fig. 19.94 Erythema infectiosum.

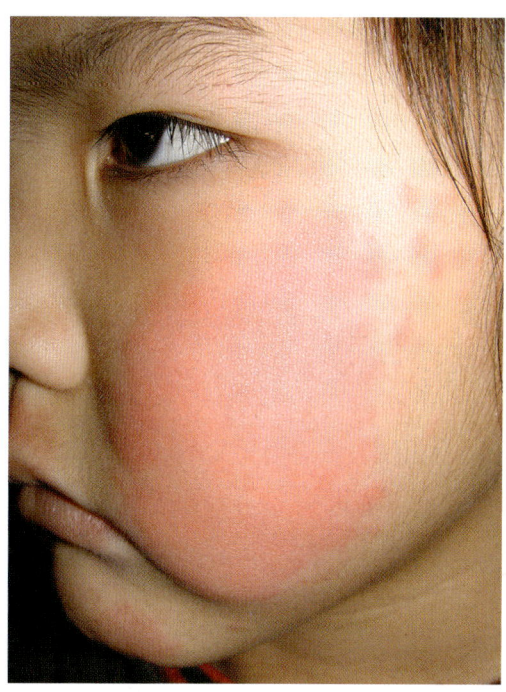

Fig. 19.95 Erythema infectiosum. *Courtesy Chia-Yu Chu, MD, PhD.*

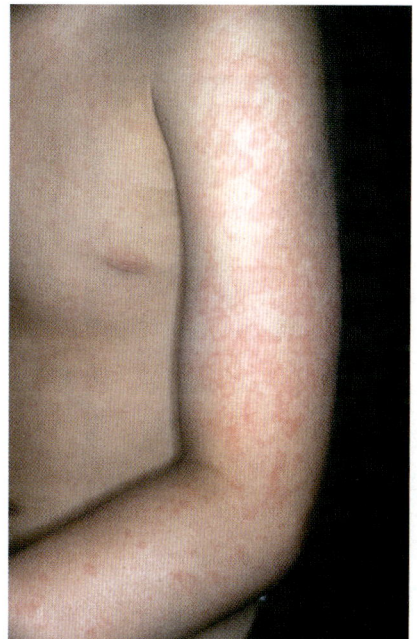

Fig. 19.97 Erythema infectiosum.

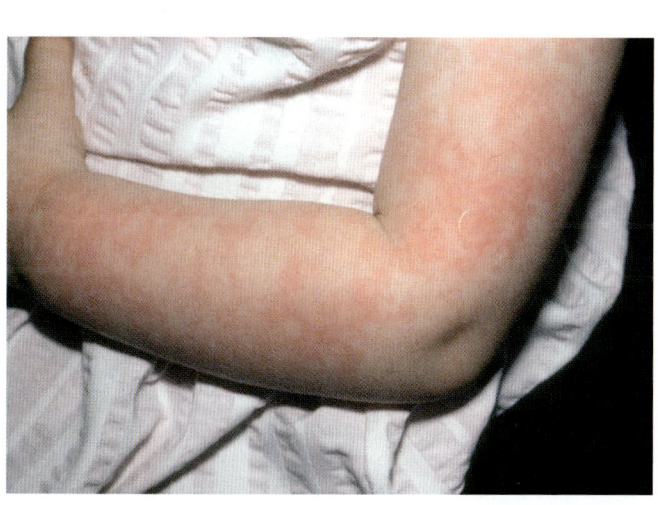

Fig. 19.96 Erythema infectiosum. *Courtesy Steven Binnick, MD.*

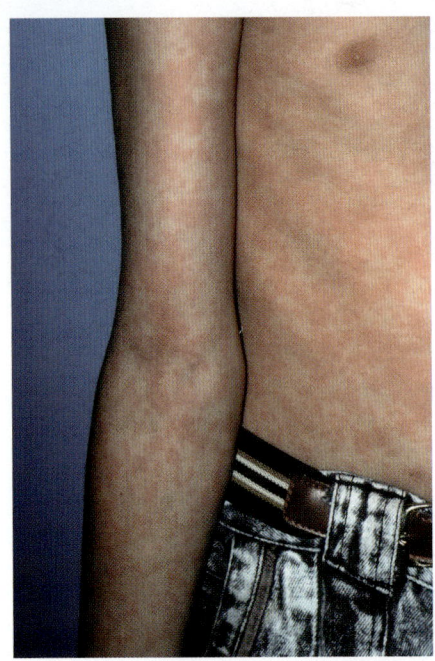

Fig. 19.98 Erythema infectiosum. *Courtesy Curt Samlaska, MD.*

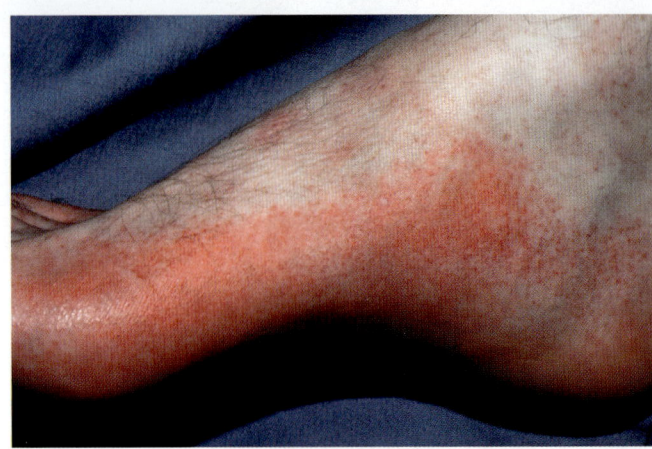

Fig. 19.99 Purpuric gloves and socks syndrome.

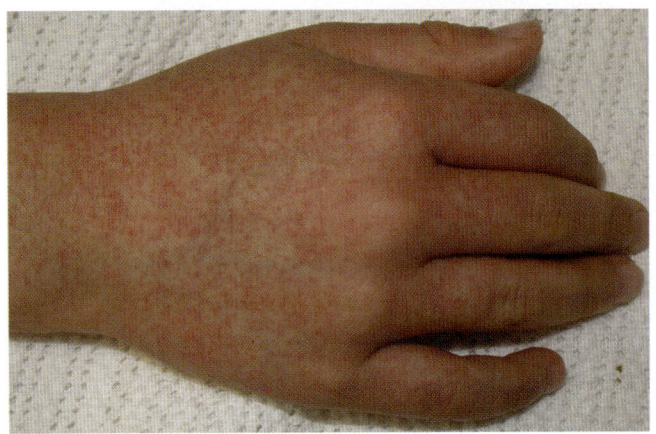

Fig. 19.100 Parvovirus B19 gloves and socks syndrome.

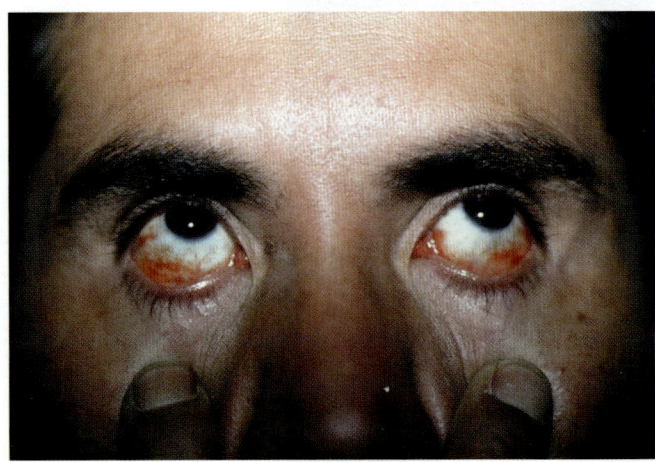

Fig. 19.101 Dengue fever.

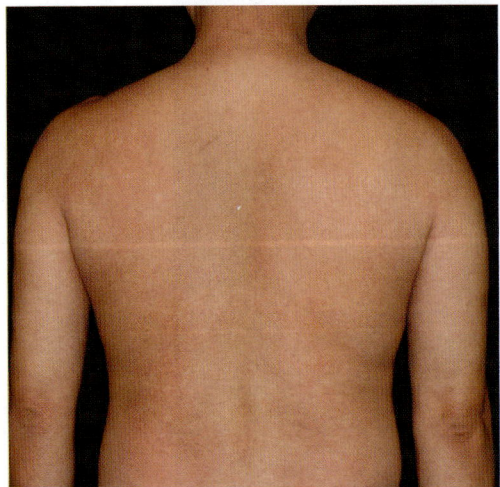

Fig. 19.102 Dengue fever (note islands of sparing). *Courtesy Kaohsiung Chang Gang Memorial Hospital, Taiwan.*

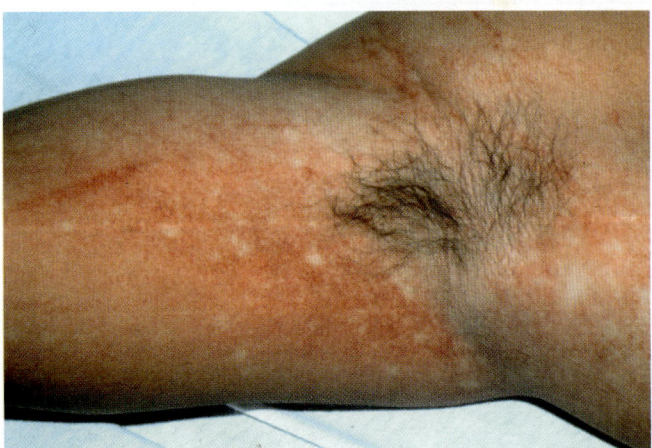

Fig. 19.103 Dengue fever (note islands of sparing and linear petechiae).

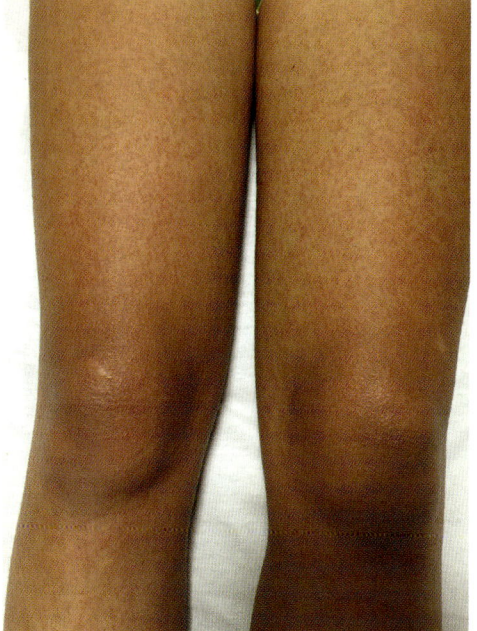

Fig. 19.104 Chikungunya fever. *Courtesy Warren R. Heymann, MD.*

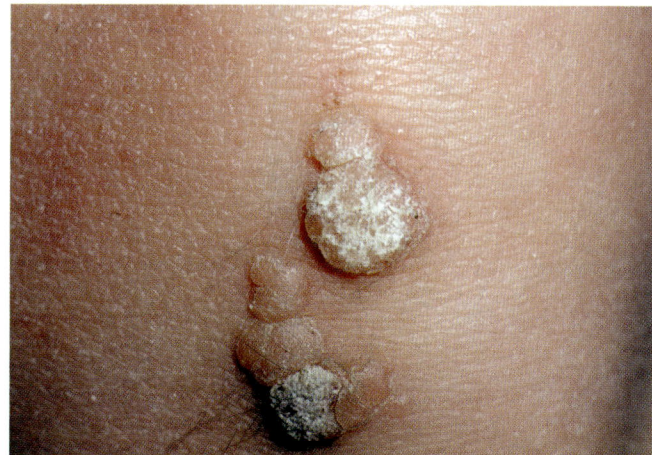

Fig. 19.105 Warts. *Courtesy Steven Binnick, MD.*

Fig. 19.106 Warts.

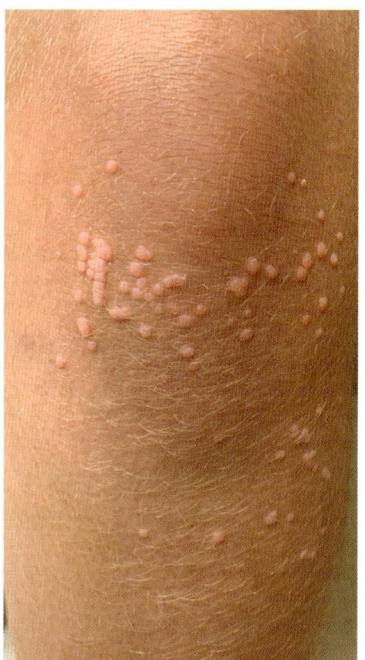

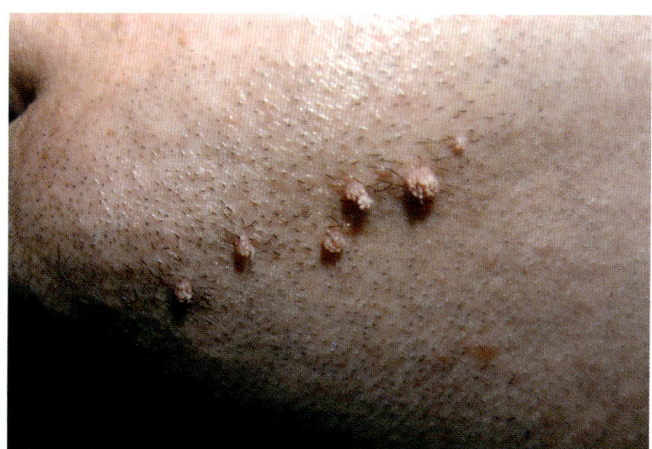

Fig. 19.107 Warts.

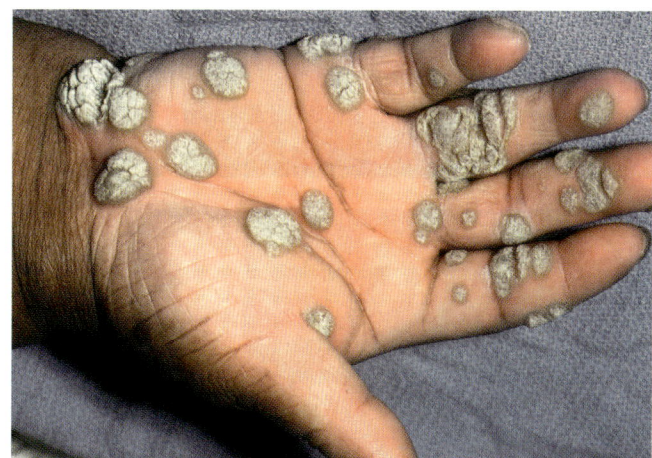

Fig. 19.109 Warts.

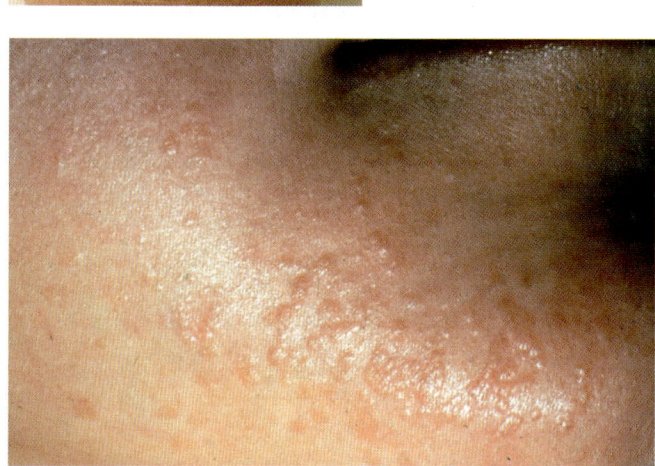

Fig. 19.108 Flat warts.

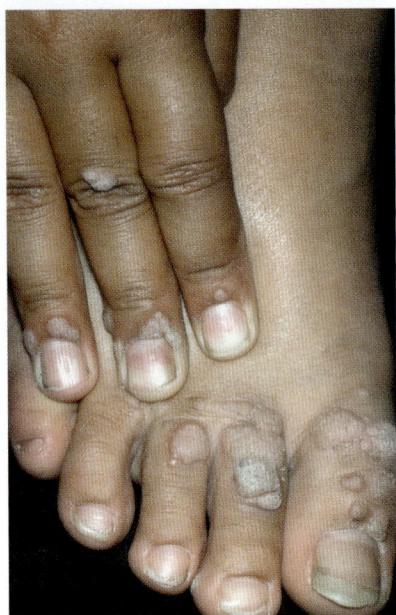

Fig. 19.110 Warts. *Courtesy Scott Norton, MD.*

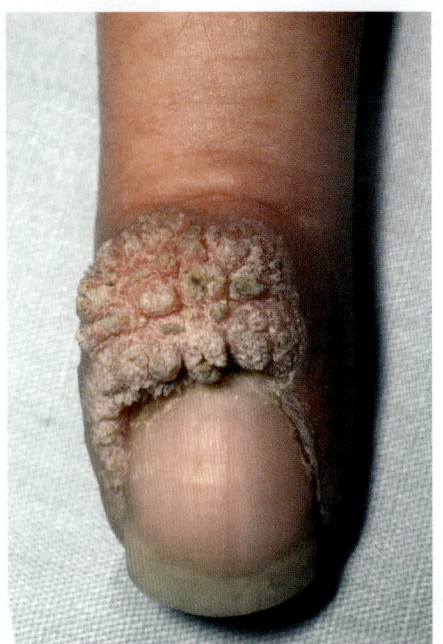

Fig. 19.111 Periungual warts. *Courtesy Steven Binnick, MD.*

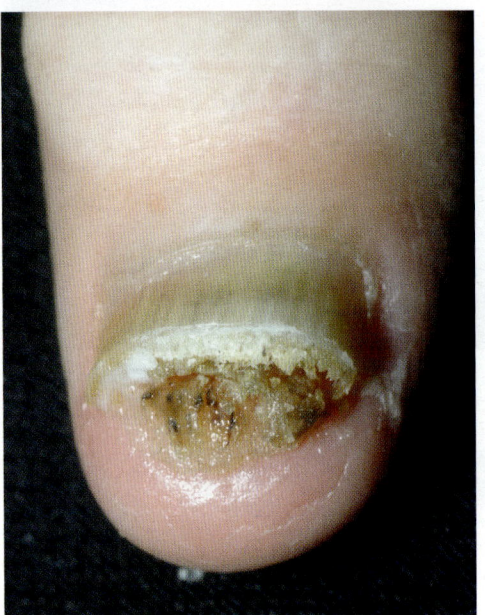

Fig. 19.112 Subungual wart. *Courtesy Curt Samlaska, MD.*

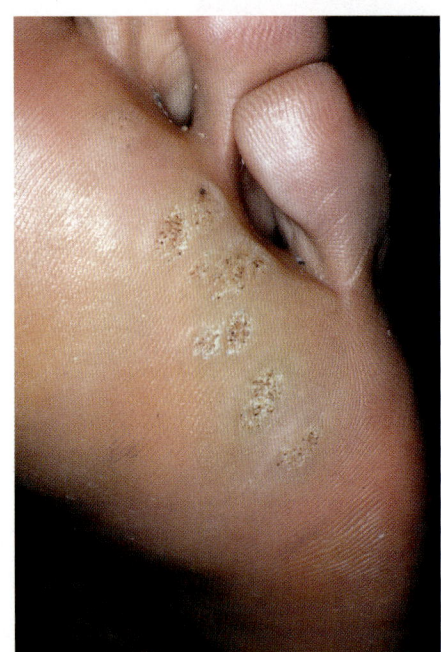

Fig. 19.113 Plantar warts.

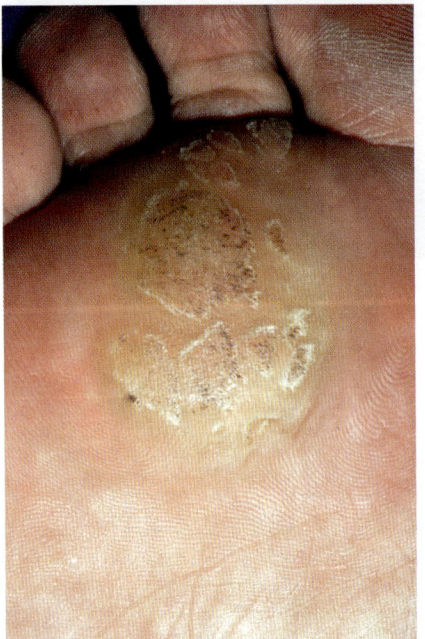

Fig. 19.114 Plantar warts.

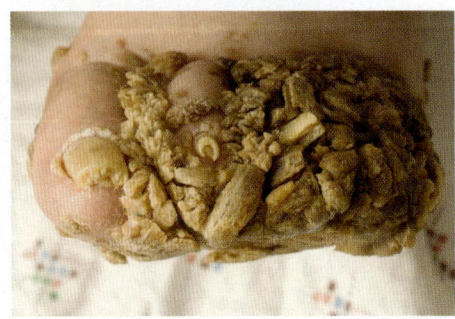

Fig. 19.115 Extensive warts in a patient with gastrointestinal lymphangiomatosis.

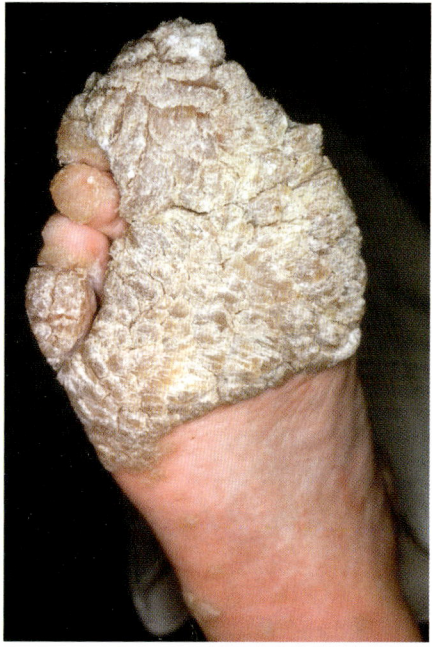

Fig. 19.116 Extensive warts as seen in immunodeficiencies such as WHIM and DOCK8 deficiency syndromes.

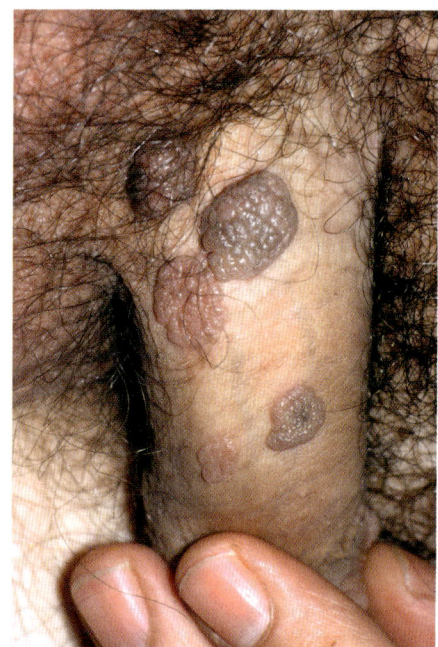

Fig. 19.117 Condylomata acuminata. *Courtesy Steven Binnick, MD.*

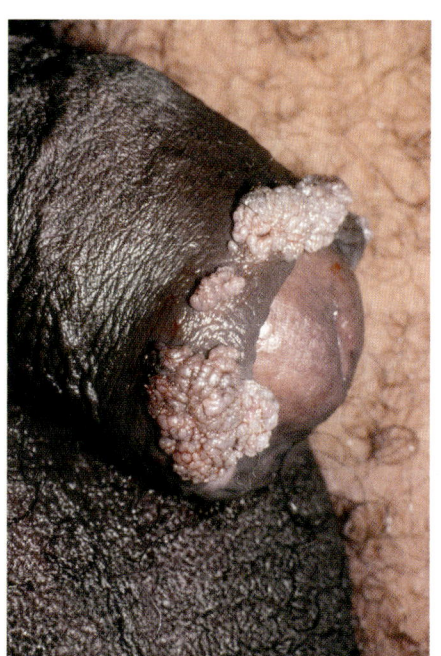

Fig. 19.118 Condylomata acuminata. *Courtesy Steven Binnick, MD.*

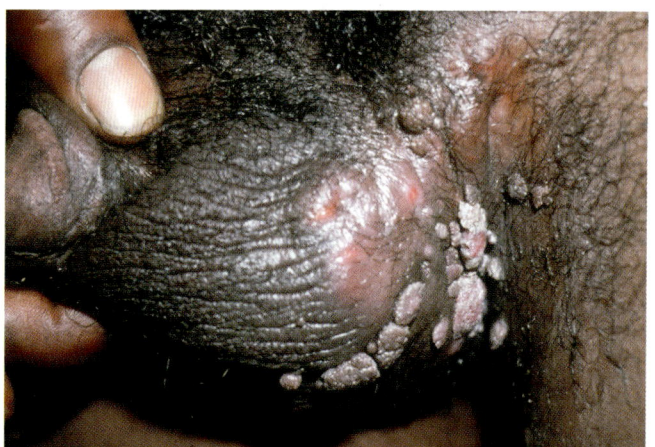

Fig. 19.119 Condylomata acuminata. *Courtesy Steven Binnick, MD.*

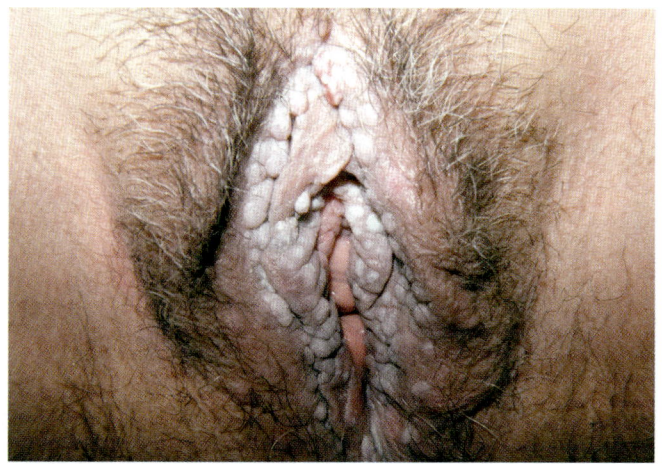

Fig. 19.120 Condylomata acuminata. *Courtesy Steven Binnick, MD.*

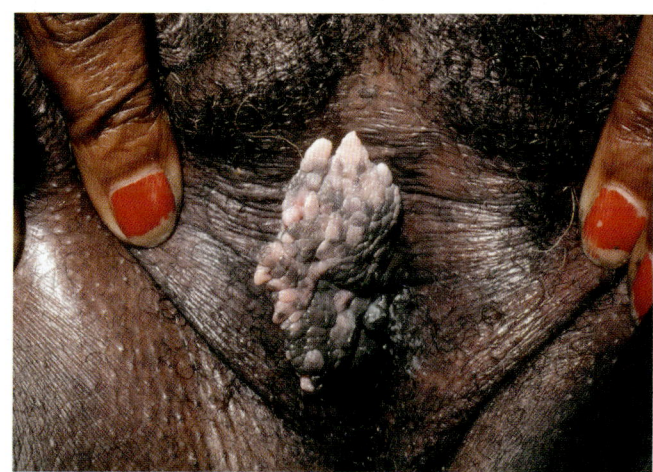

Fig. 19.121 Condylomata acuminata.

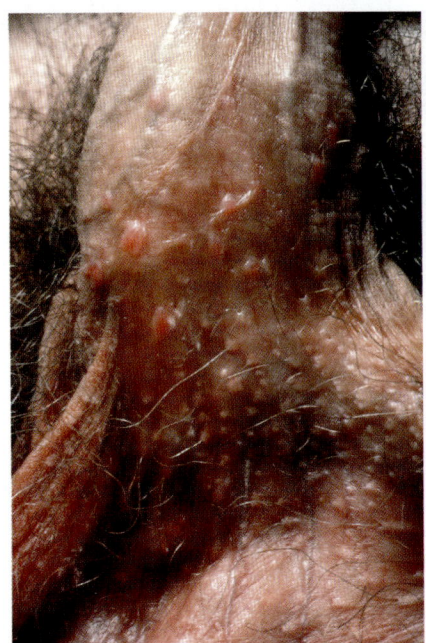

Fig. 19.122 Bowenoid papulosis.

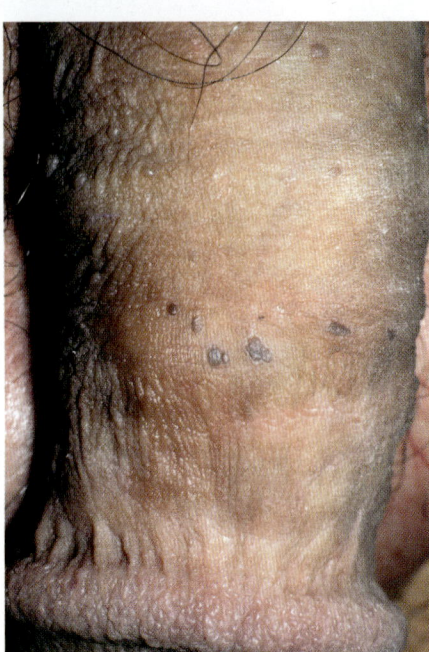

Fig. 19.123 Bowenoid papulosis. *Courtesy Steven Binnick, MD.*

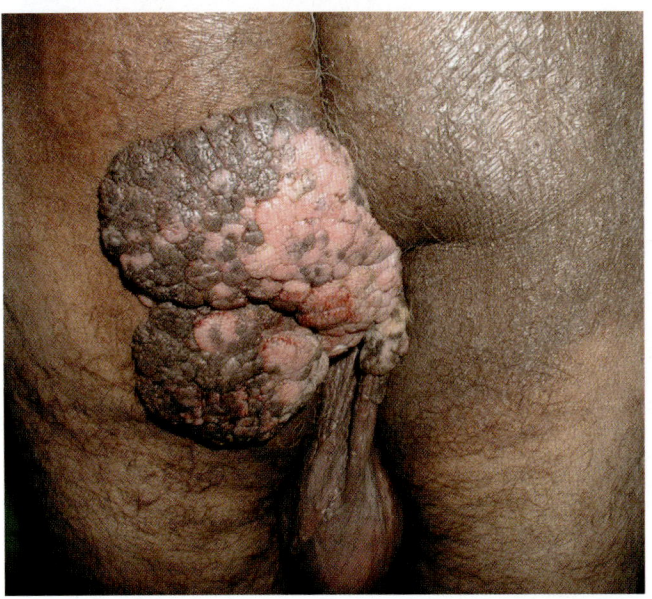

Fig. 19.124 Buschke-Lowenstein tumor. *Courtesy Shyam Verma, MBBS, DVD.*

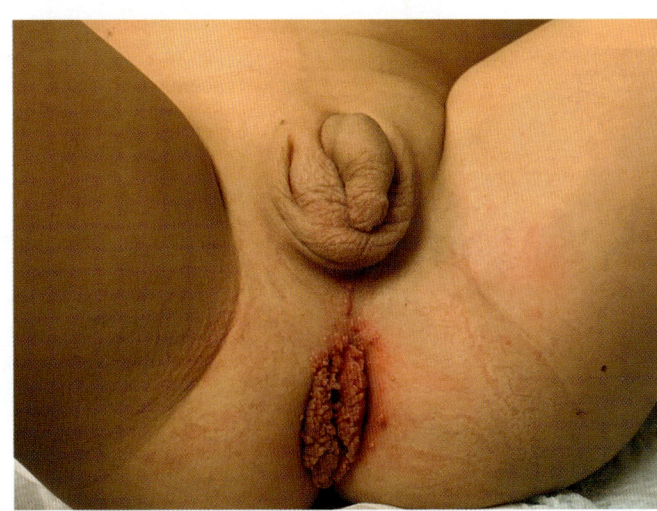

Fig. 19.125 Perianal condylomata acuminata in a young child.

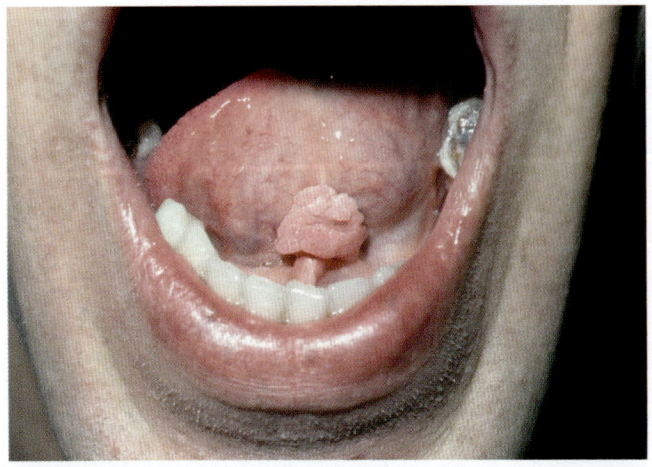

Fig. 19.126 Oral wart.

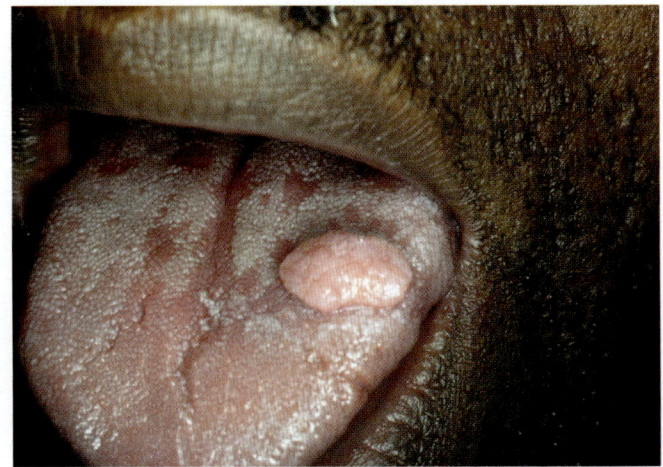

Fig. 19.127 Oral wart.

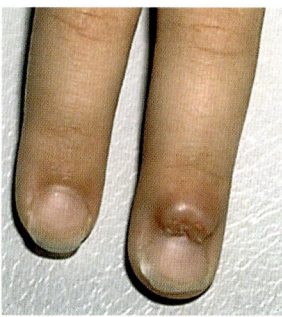

Fig. 19.128 Myrmecia.

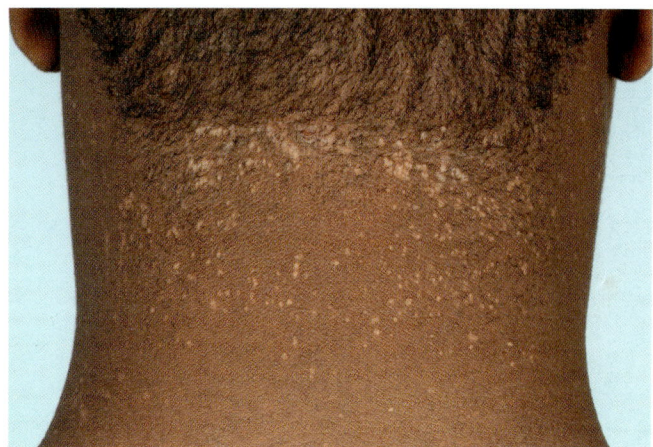

Fig. 19.129 Epidermodysplasia verruciformis in an HIV-infected patient.

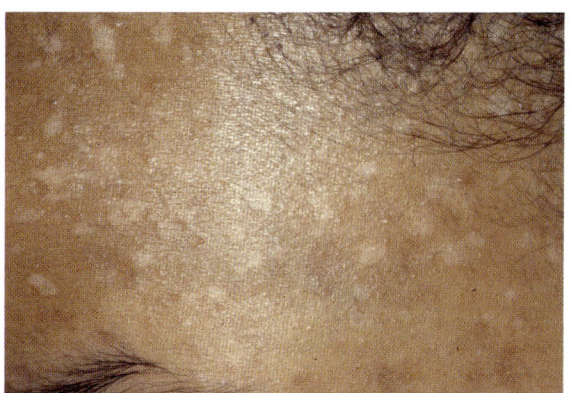

Fig. 19.130 Epidermodysplasia verruciformis in an HIV-infected patient.

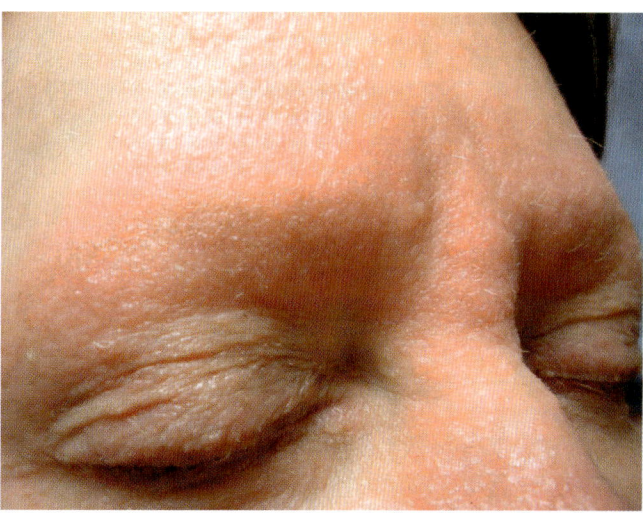

Fig. 19.131 Trichodysplasia spinulosa. *Courtesy Kari Wanat, MD.*

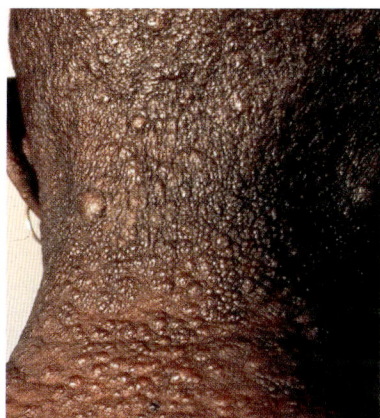

Fig. 19.132 Human T-lymphotropic virus 1 dermatosis. *Courtesy Alain Rook, MD.*

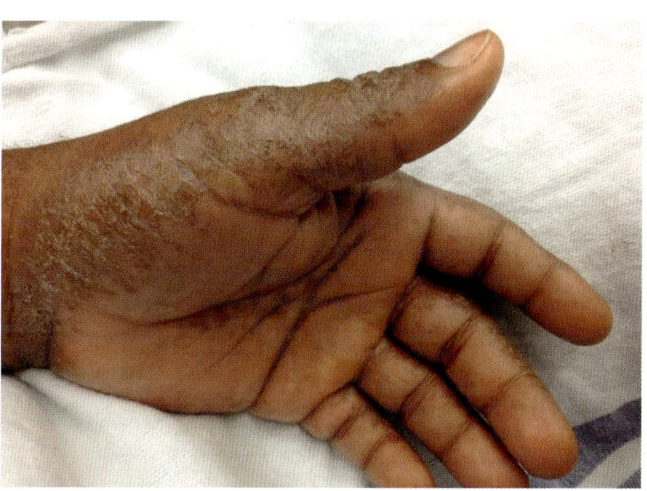

Fig. 19.133 Human T-lymphotropic virus 1 dermatosis.

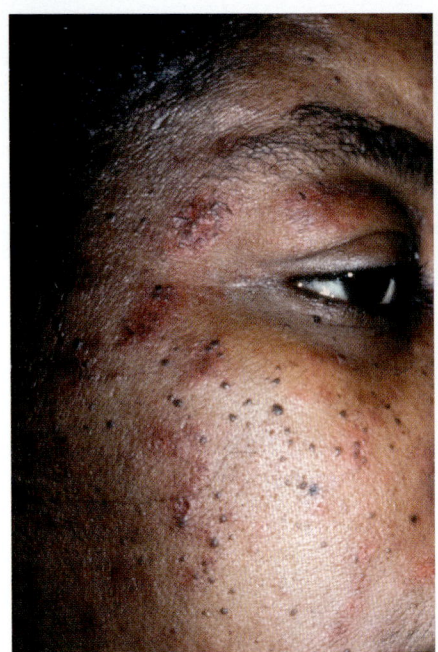

Fig. 19.134 Primary HIV infection.

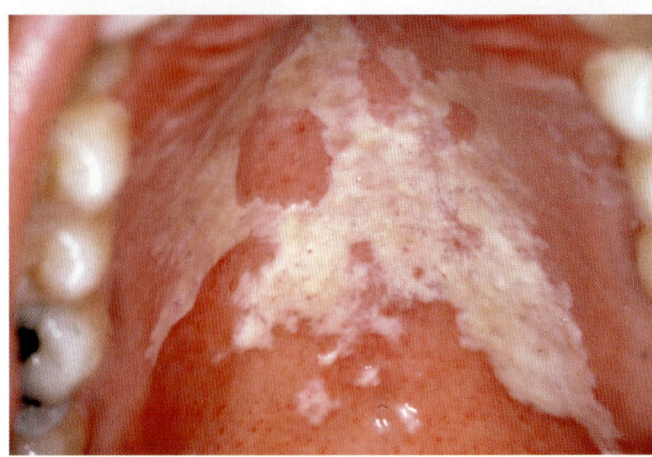

Fig. 19.135 Thrush in an HIV-infected patient. *Courtesy Steven Binnick, MD.*

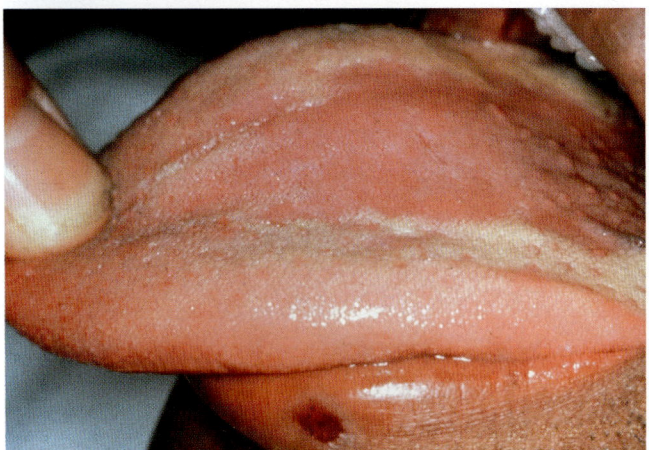

Fig. 19.136 Thrush and resolving chancre in an HIV-infected patient.

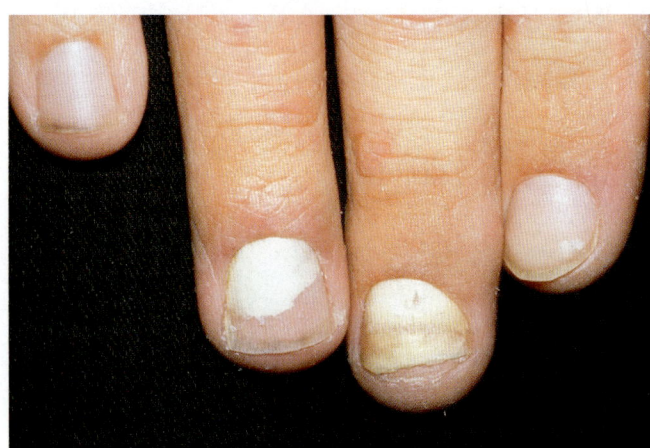

Fig. 19.137 Proximal white onychomycosis in an HIV-infected patient.

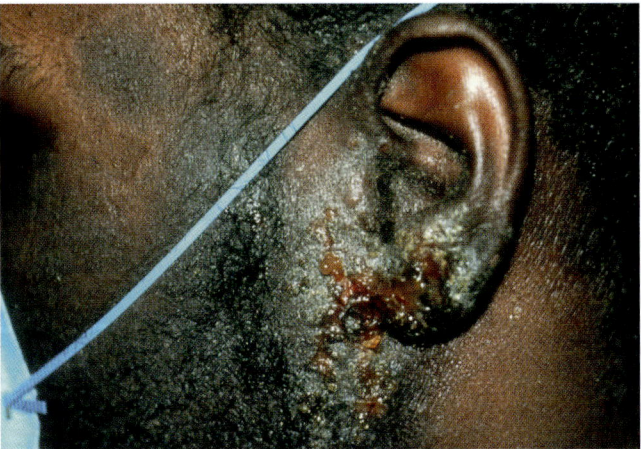

Fig. 19.138 Herpes simplex and seborrheic dermatitis in an HIV-infected patient.

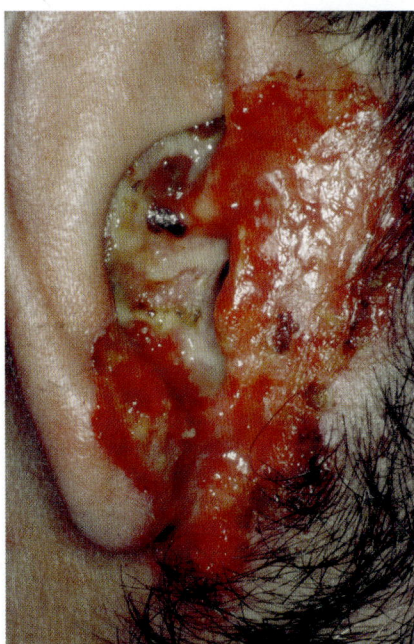

Fig. 19.139 Chronic herpes simplex in an HIV-infected patient.

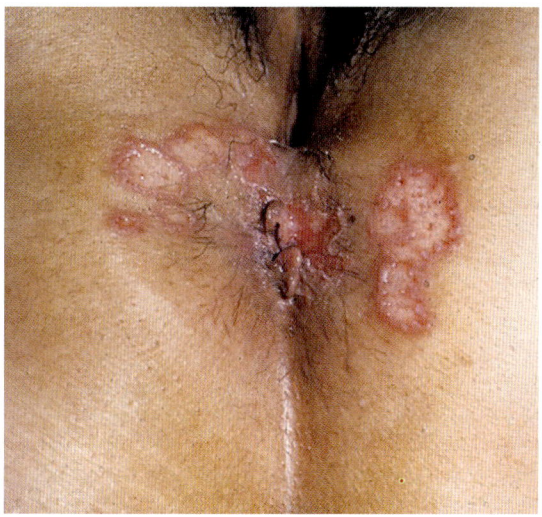

Fig. 19.140 Chronic ulcerative herpes simplex in an HIV-infected patient.

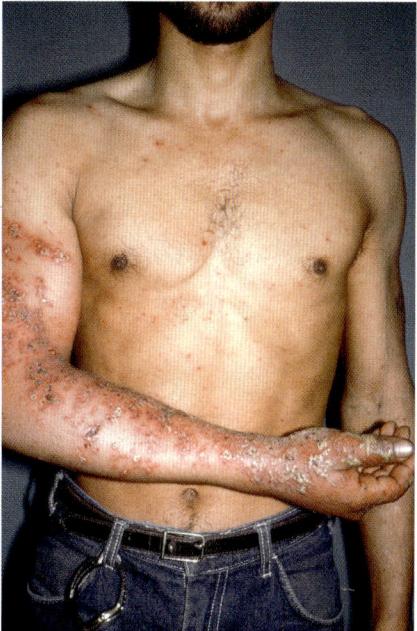

Fig. 19.141 Herpes zoster in an HIV-infected patient.

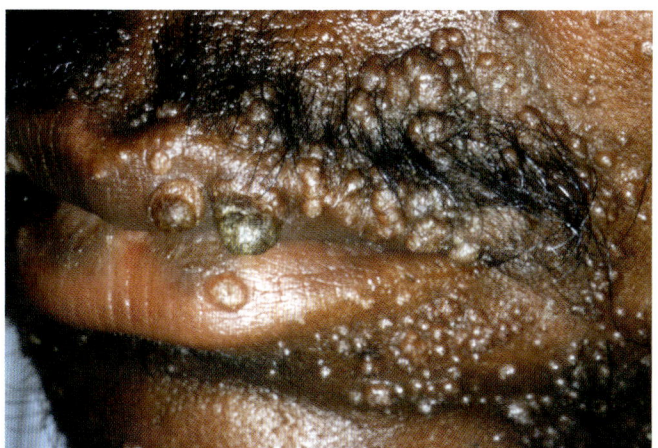

Fig. 19.142 Molluscum contagiosum in an HIV-infected patient.

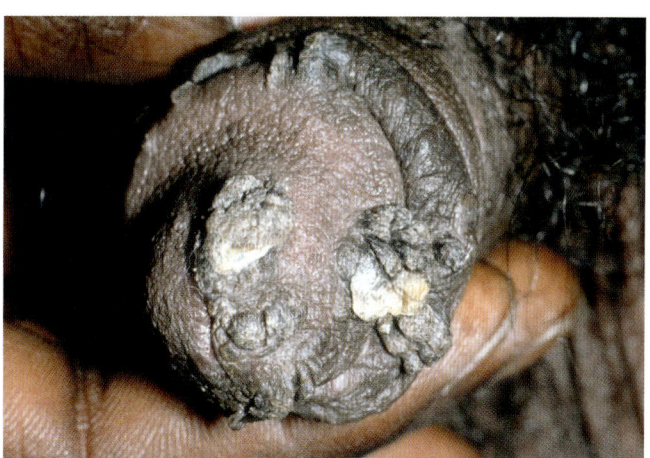

Fig. 19.143 Condylomata acuminata in an HIV-infected patient.

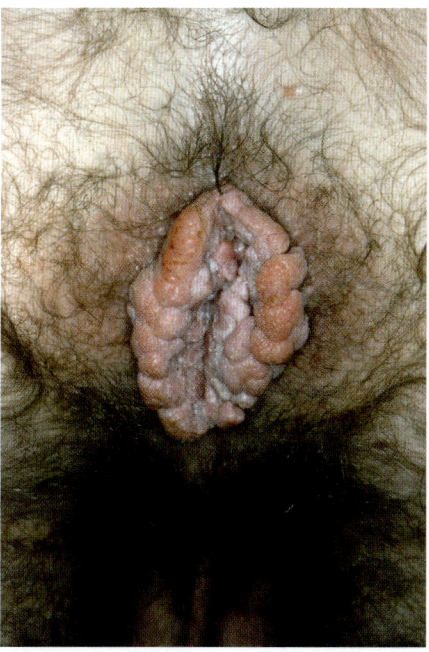

Fig. 19.144 Condylomata acuminata in an HIV-infected patient.

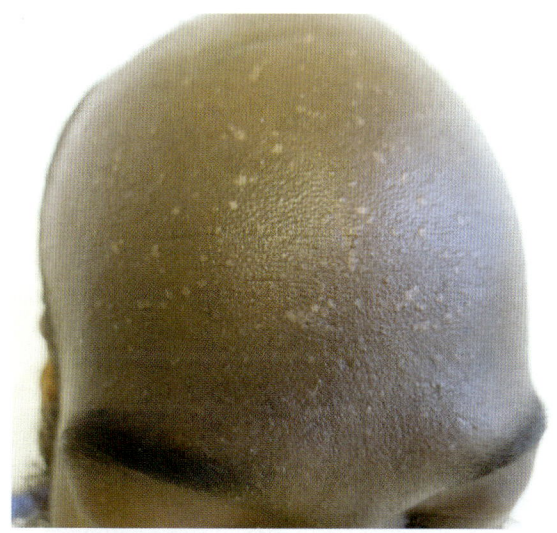

Fig. 19.145 Epidermodysplasia verruciformis–like flat warts in a patient with HIV.

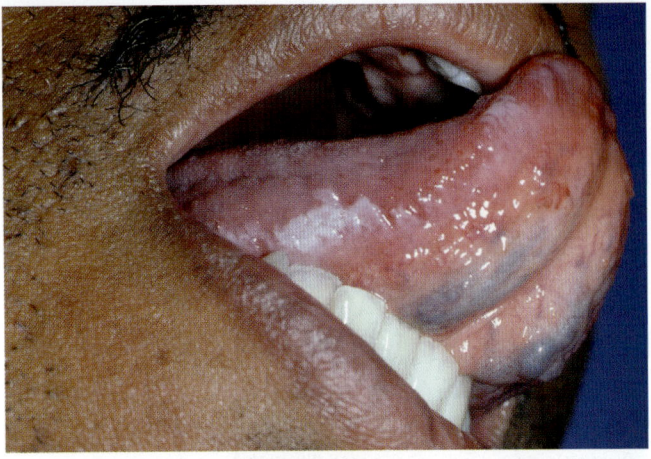

Fig. 19.146 Oral hairy leukoplakia in an HIV-infected patient.

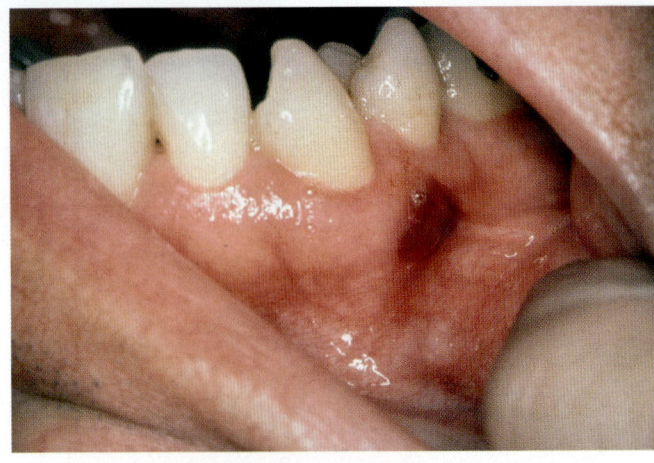

Fig. 19.147 Oral Kaposi sarcoma in an HIV-infected patient.

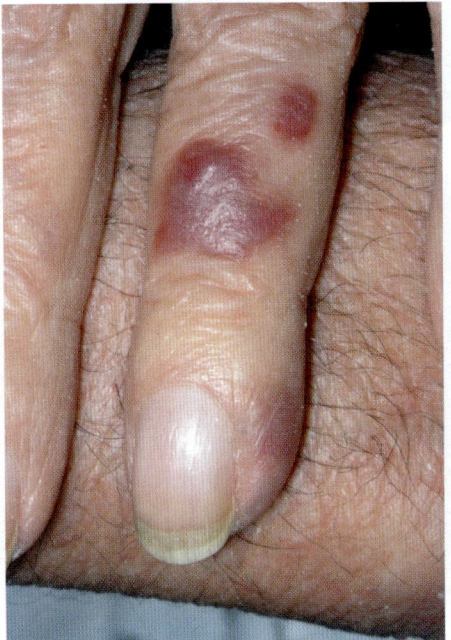

Fig. 19.148 Kaposi sarcoma in an HIV-infected patient.

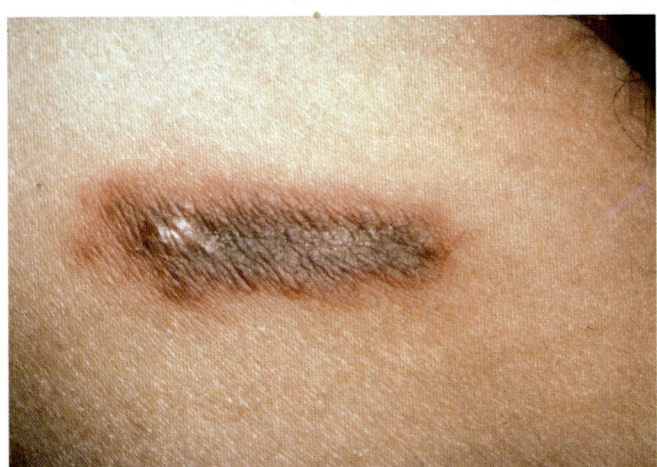

Fig. 19.149 Kaposi sarcoma in an HIV-infected patient.

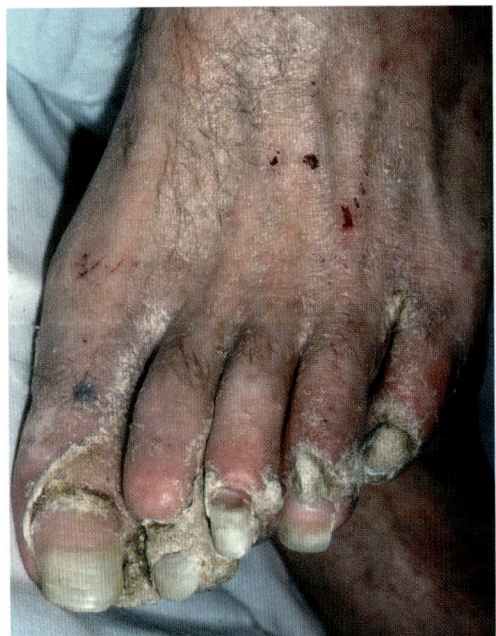

Fig. 19.150 Crusted scabies in an HIV-infected patient.

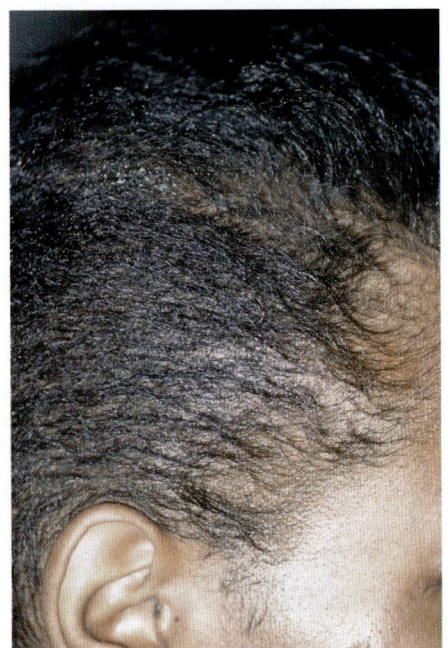

Fig. 19.151 Hair straightening in an HIV-infected patient.

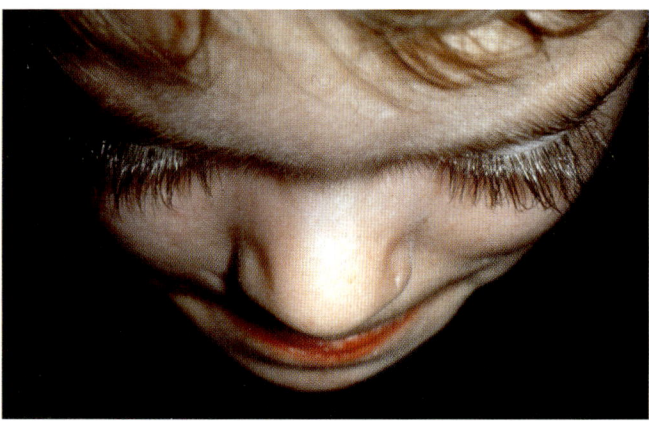

Fig. 19.152 Long eyelashes in an HIV-infected patient.

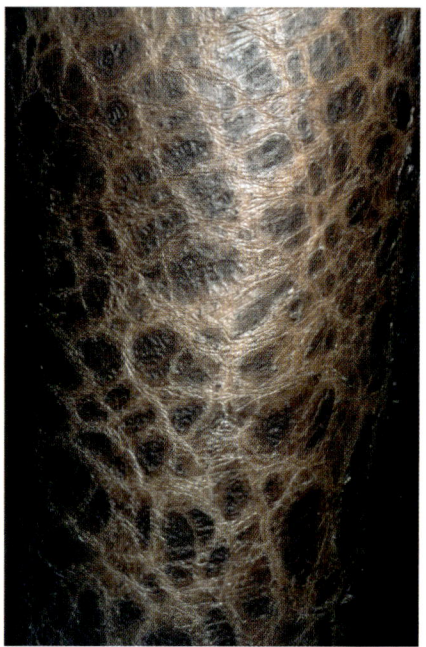

Fig. 19.153 Acquired ichthyosis in an HIV-infected patient.

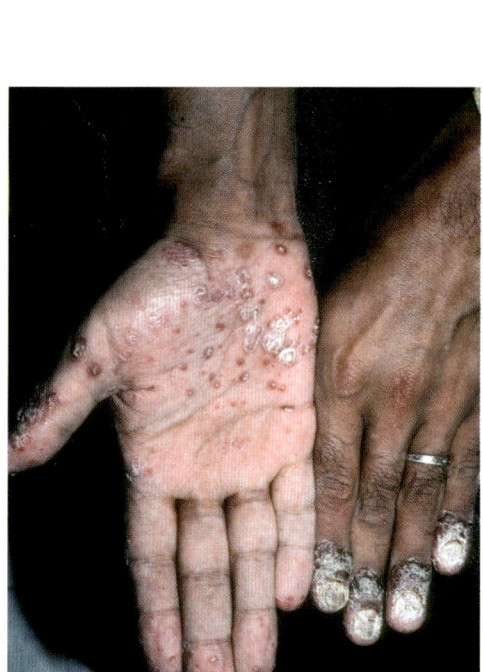

Fig. 19.154 Reactive arthritis in an HIV-infected patient.

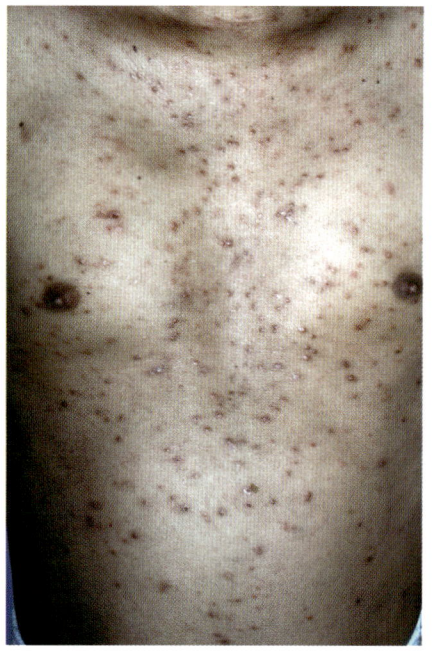

Fig. 19.155 Eosinophilic folliculitis in an HIV-infected patient.

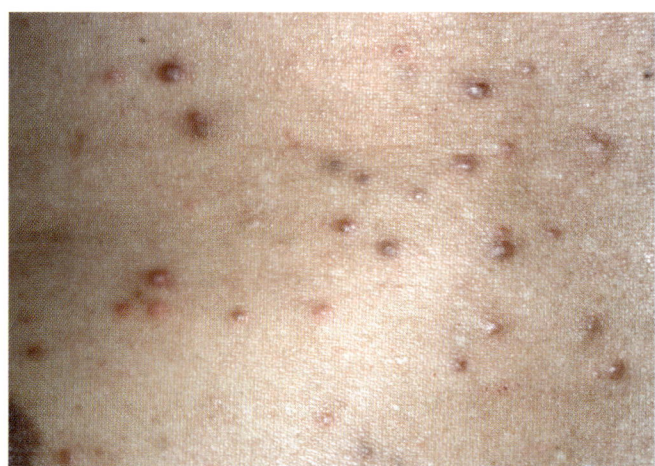

Fig. 19.156 Eosinophilic folliculitis in an HIV-infected patient.

Fig. 19.157 Eosinophilic folliculitis in an HIV-infected patient. *Courtesy Vasanop Vachiramon, MD.*

Parasitic Infestations, Stings, and Bites 20

Bites and infestations present with wide-ranging manifestations, including papules, vesicles, excoriations, and urticarial lesions. Bedbug bites often involve the arms and develop clinical features of prurigo nodularis. A biopsy will demonstrate a wedge-shaped perivascular lymphoid infiltrate with endothelial swelling and eosinophils, suggesting the correct diagnosis.

Cutaneous larva migrans demonstrates an erythematous serpiginous lesion. The worm is located ahead of the advancing border of the lesion, as the cutaneous reaction is a manifestation of a delayed-type immune response to the organism.

Recognition of arthropods of medical importance is critical to allow assessment of the risk of vector-borne disease and guide management. The skin is often affected by ectoparasites as well as endoparasites, and this section of the atlas will provide a guide to identification of the most important organisms.

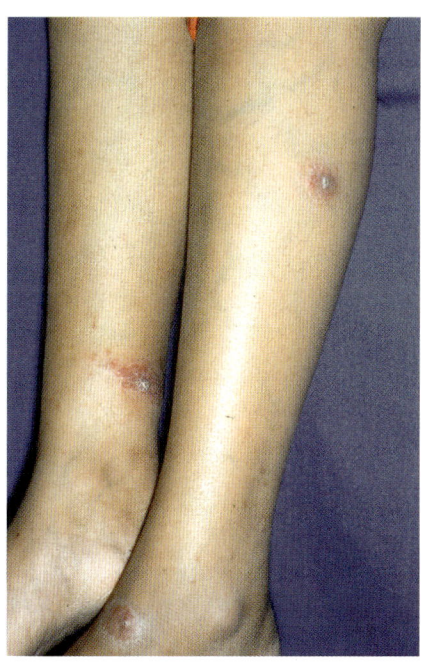

Fig. 20.1 Old World leishmaniasis.

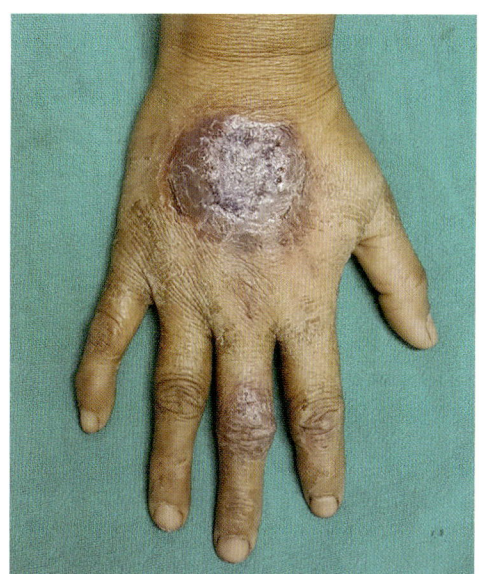

Fig. 20.2 Old World leishmaniasis. *Courtesy Archana Singal, MD.*

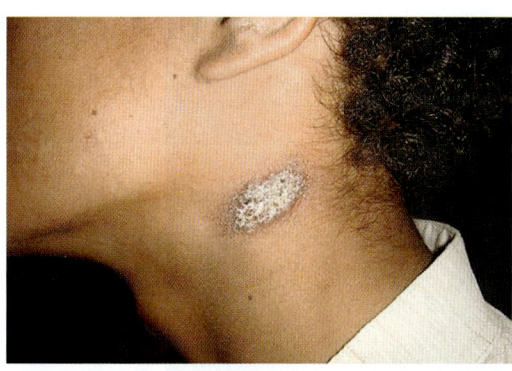

Fig. 20.3 Old World leishmaniasis.

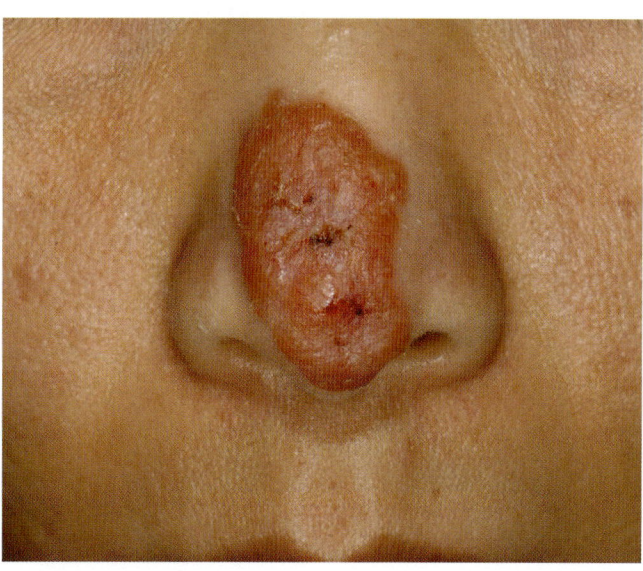

Fig. 20.4 New World leishmaniasis. *Courtesy Kaohsiung Chang Gang Memorial Hospital, Taiwan.*

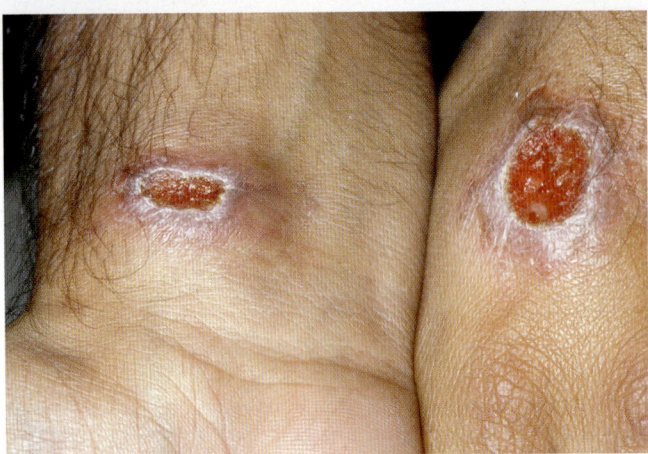

Fig. 20.5 New World leishmaniasis.

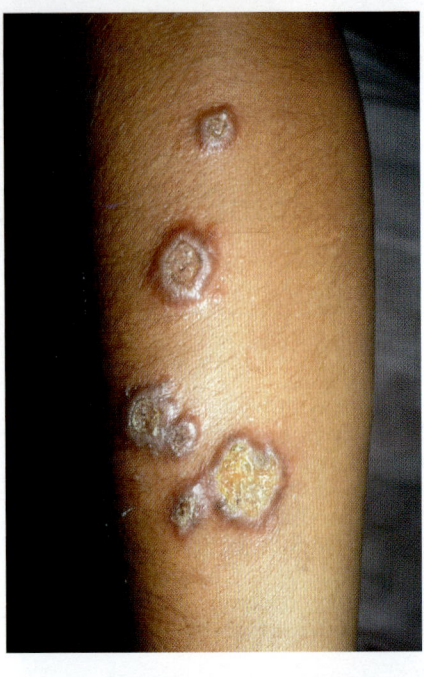

Fig. 20.6 New World leishmaniasis.

Fig. 20.7 New World leishmaniasis.

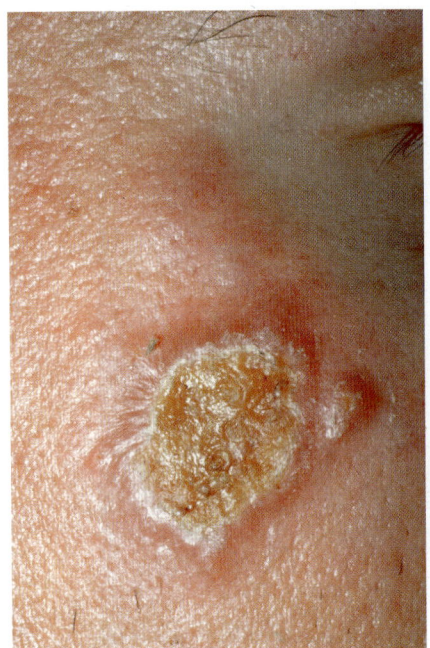

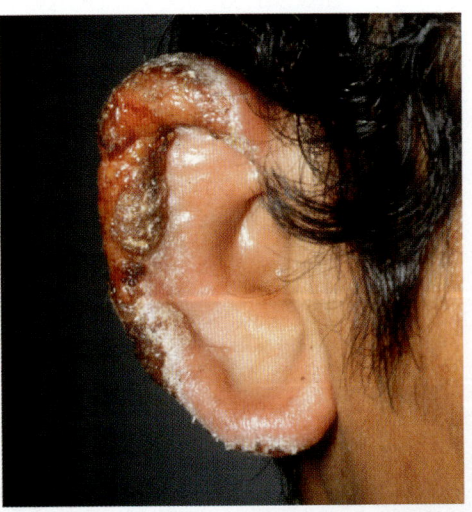

Fig. 20.8 New World leishmaniasis. *Courtesy Scott Norton, MD.*

Fig. 20.9 New World leishmaniasis.

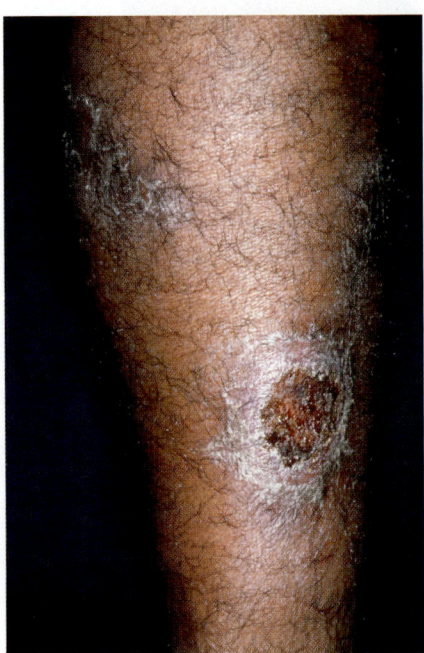

Fig. 20.10 New World leishmaniasis.

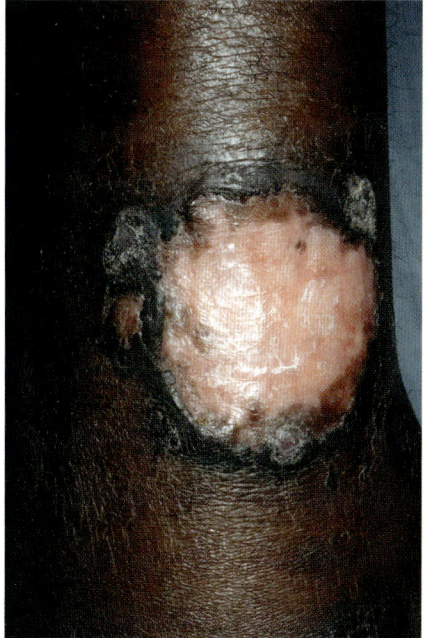

Fig. 20.11 New World leishmaniasis.

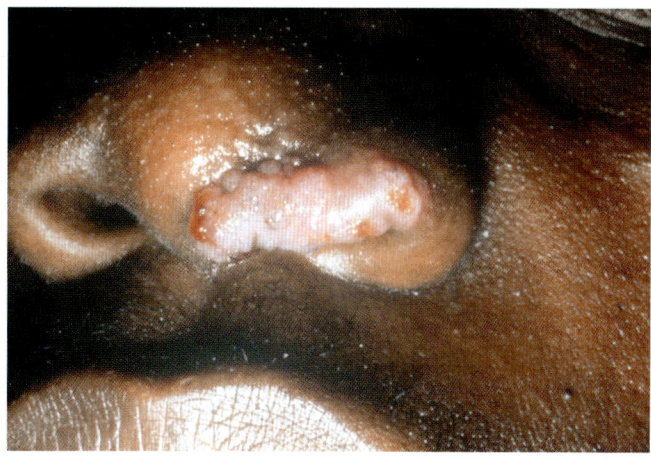

Fig. 20.12 Mucocutaneous leishmaniasis in the same patient as Fig. 20.11.

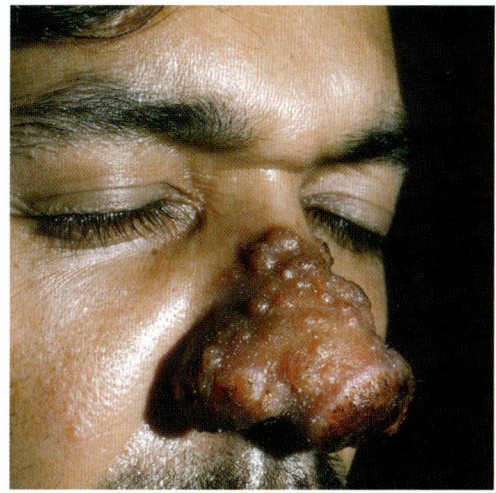

Fig. 20.13 Mucocutaneous leishmaniasis.

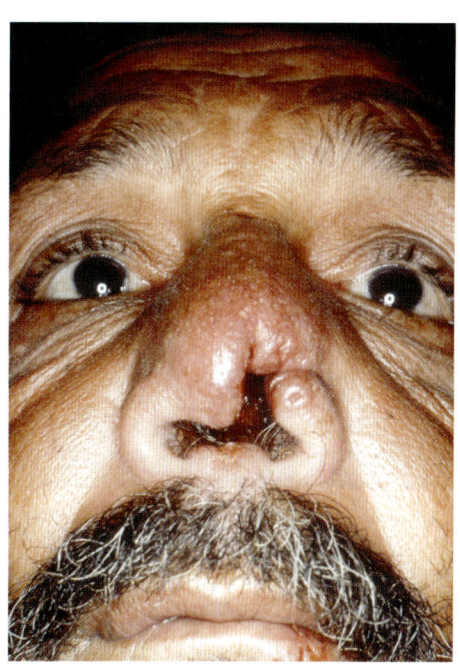

Fig. 20.14 Mucocutaneous leishmaniasis.

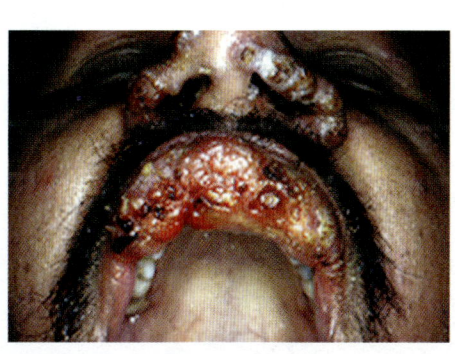

Fig. 20.15 Mucocutaneous leishmaniasis.
Courtesy Lauro de Souza Lima Institute, Brazil.

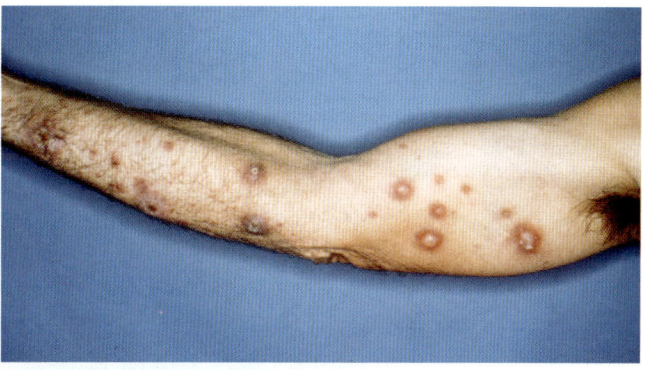

Fig. 20.16 Anergic leishmaniasis.

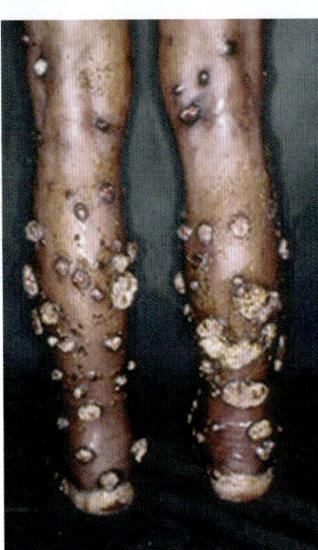

Fig. 20.17 Anergic leishmaniasis. *Courtesy Lauro de Souza Lima Institute, Brazil.*

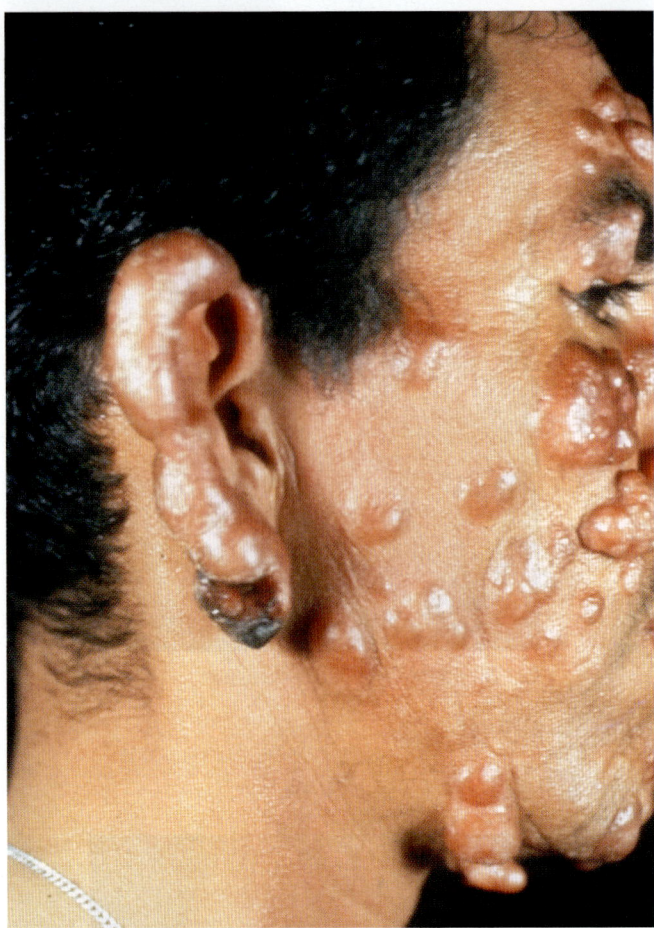

Fig. 20.18 Anergic leishmaniasis.

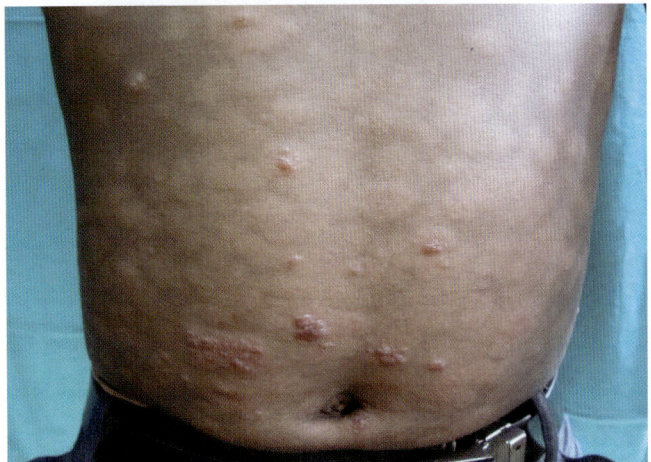

Fig. 20.19 Post-kala-azar dermal leishmaniasis. *Courtesy Archana Singal, MD.*

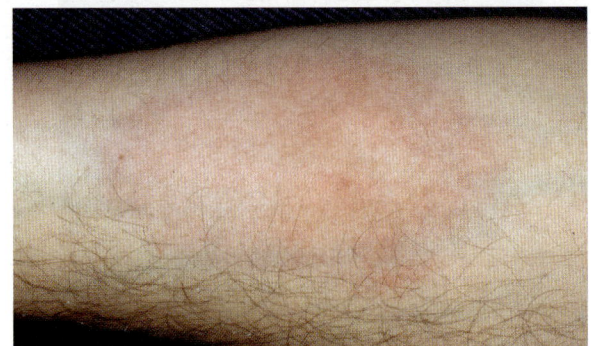

Fig. 20.20 Triatome bite.

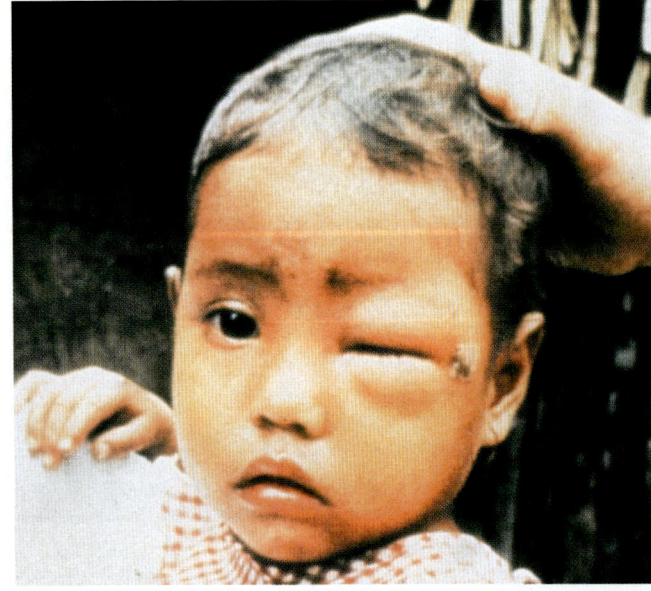

Fig. 20.21 Romana sign, Chagas disease.

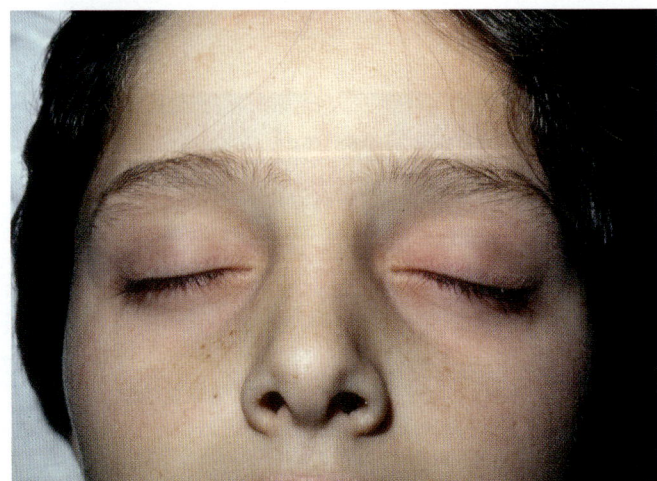

Fig. 20.22 Toxoplasmosis. Note erythema of eyelids. *Courtesy Steven Binnick, MD.*

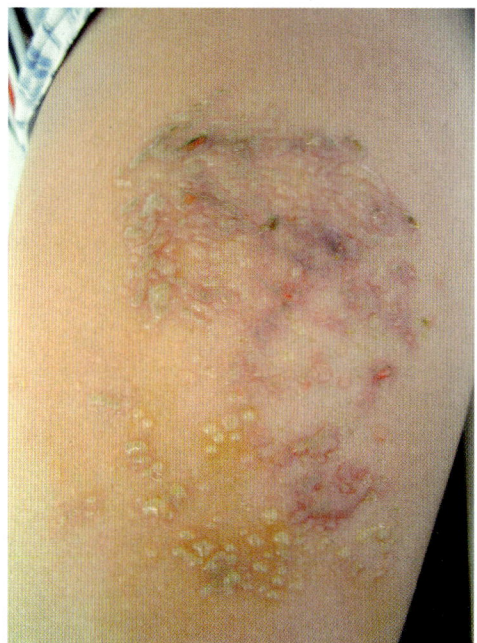

Fig. 20.23 Portuguese man of war dermatitis. *Courtesy Rui Tavares Bello, MD.*

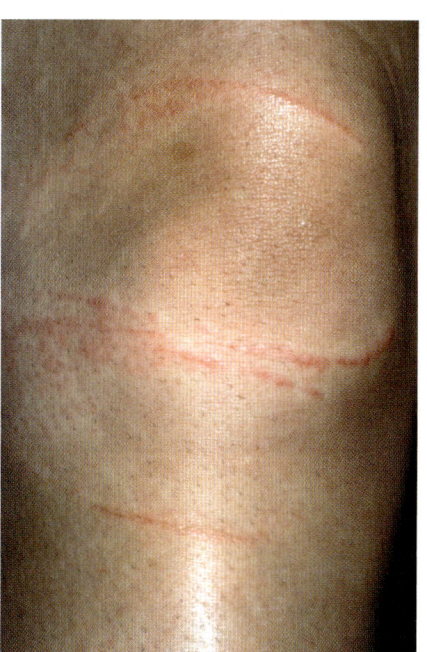

Fig. 20.24 Jellyfish dermatitis. *Courtesy Steven Binnick, MD.*

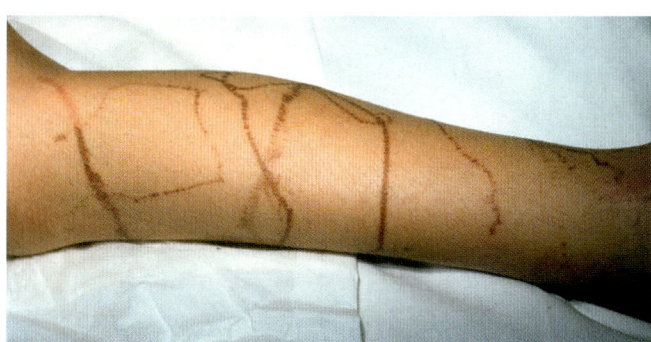

Fig. 20.25 Sea wasp dermatitis. *Courtesy Curt Samlaska, MD.*

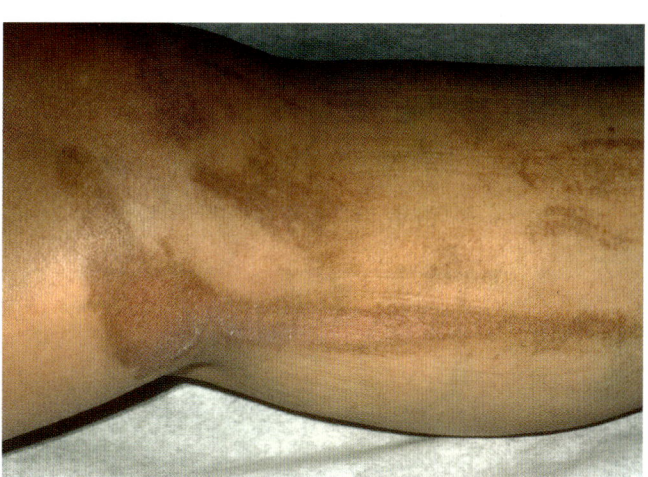

Fig. 20.26 Healed jellyfish dermatitis. *Courtesy Steven Binnick, MD.*

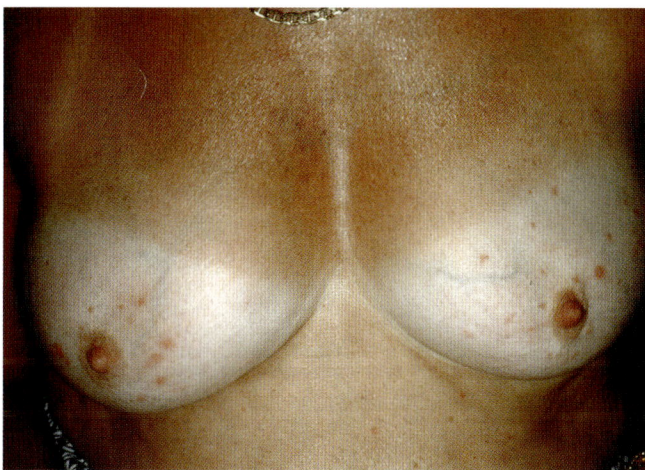

Fig. 20.27 Seabather eruption. *Courtesy Scott Norton, MD.*

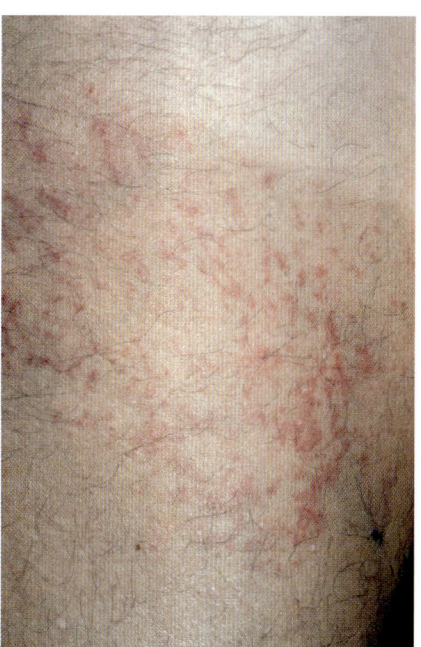

Fig. 20.28 Fire coral dermatitis. *Courtesy Steven Binnick, MD.*

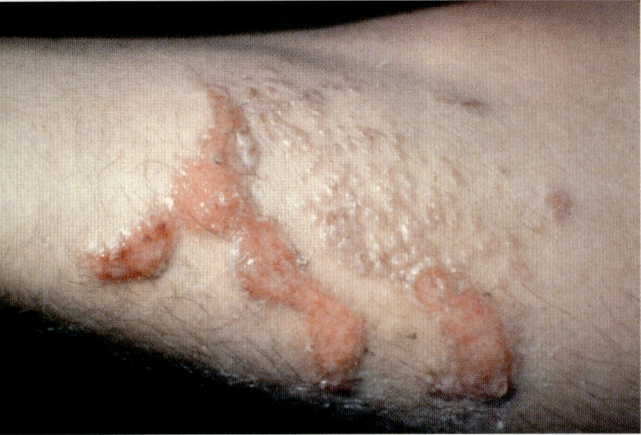

Fig. 20.29 Coral granuloma.

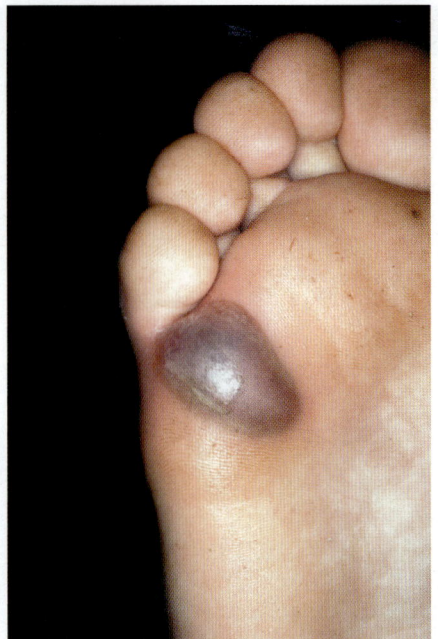

Fig. 20.30 Sea urchin injury. *Courtesy Scott Norton, MD.*

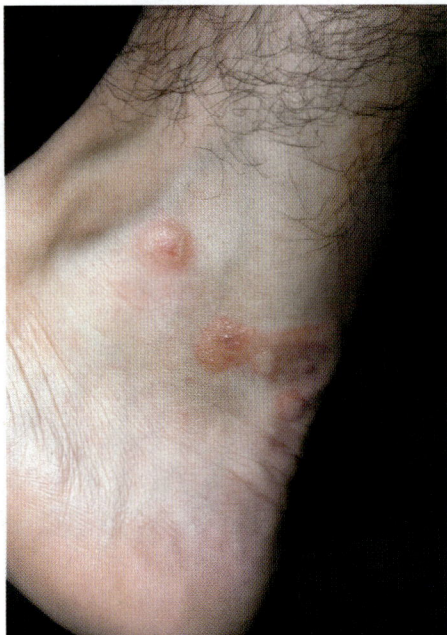

Fig. 20.31 Sea urchin granuloma. *Courtesy Steven Binnick, MD.*

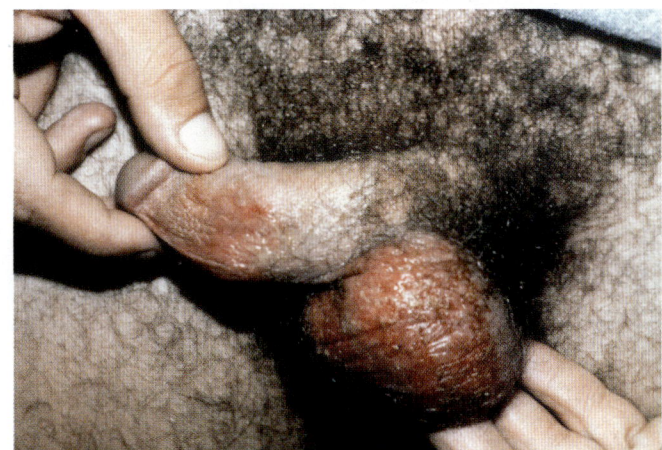

Fig. 20.32 Seaweed dermatitis. *Courtesy Curt Samlaska, MD.*

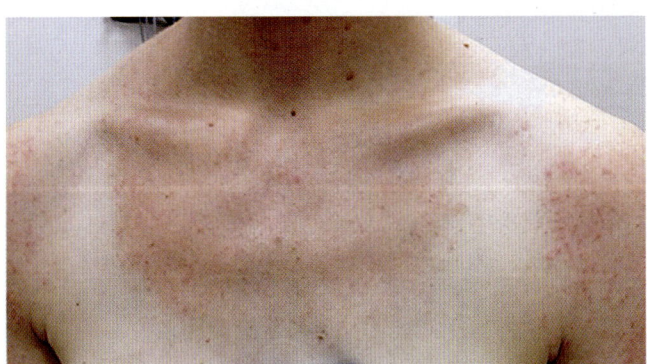

Fig. 20.33 Swimmer itch. *Courtesy Camille Introcaso, MD.*

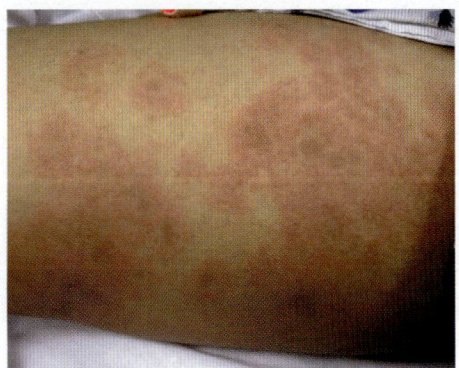

Fig. 20.34 Katayama fever–associated dermatitis. *Courtesy Scott Norton, MD.*

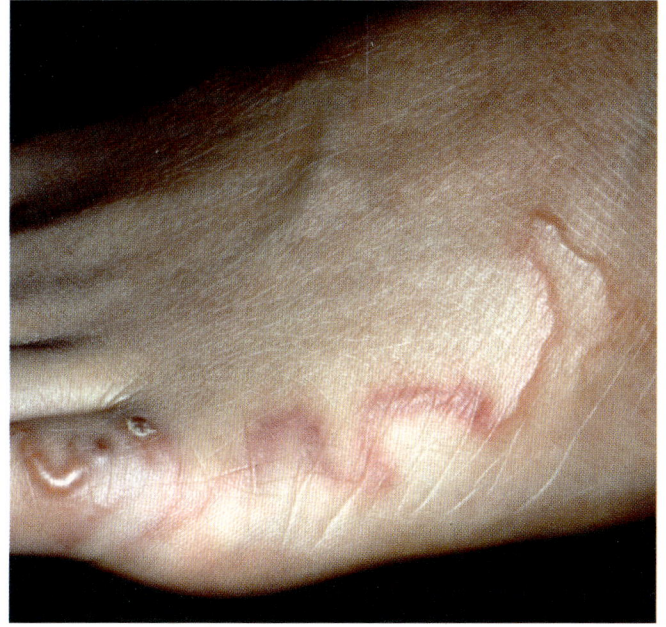

Fig. 20.35 Cutaneous larva migrans.

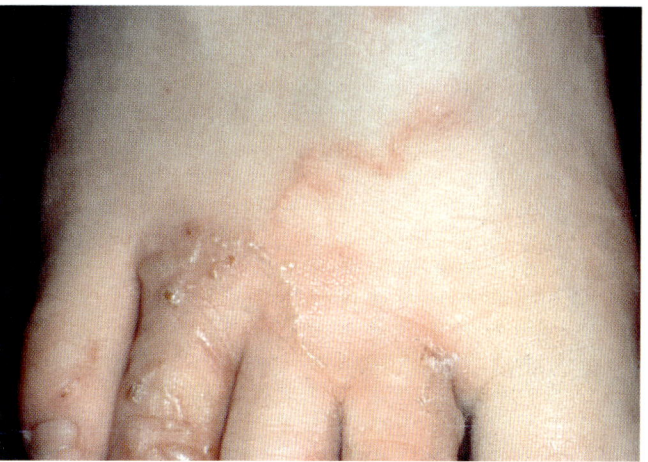

Fig. 20.36 Cutaneous larva migrans.

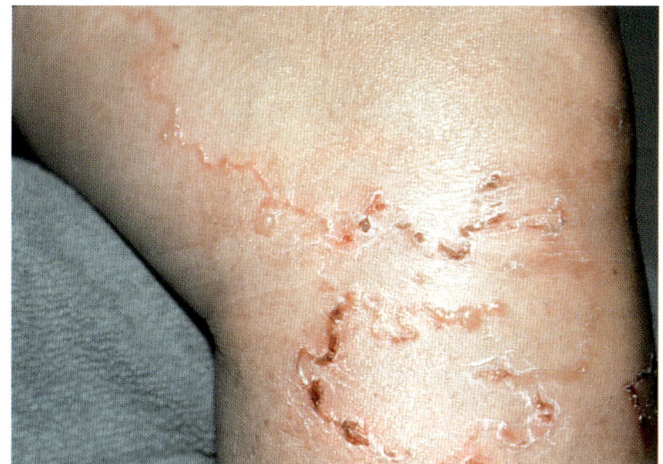

Fig. 20.37 Cutaneous larva migrans.

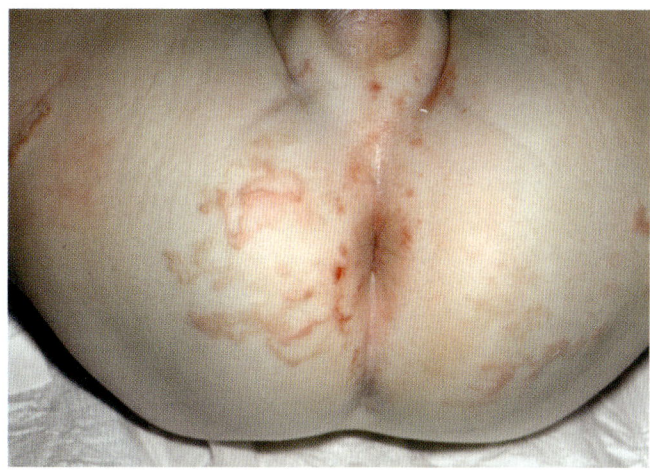

Fig. 20.38 Cutaneous larva migrans. *Courtesy Steven Binnick, MD.*

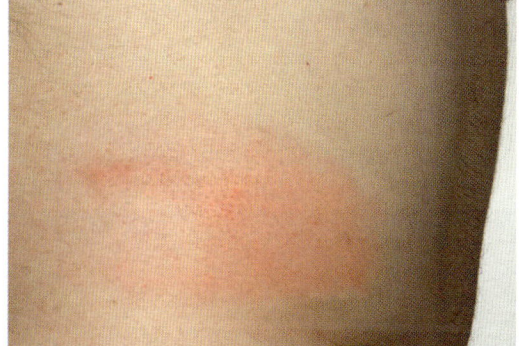

Fig. 20.39 Gnathostomiasis. *Courtesy Scott Norton, MD.*

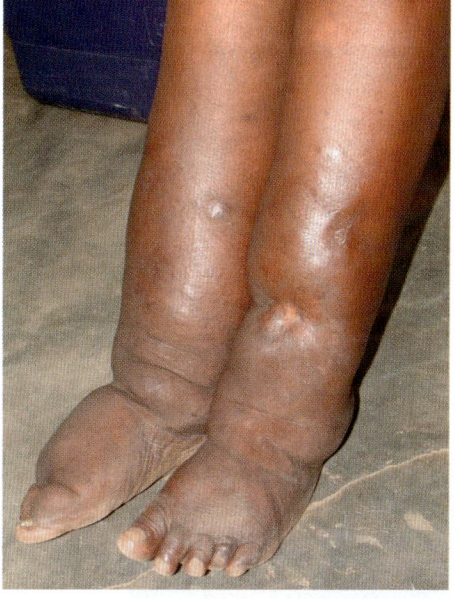

Fig. 20.40 Filariasis. *Courtesy Scott Norton, MD.*

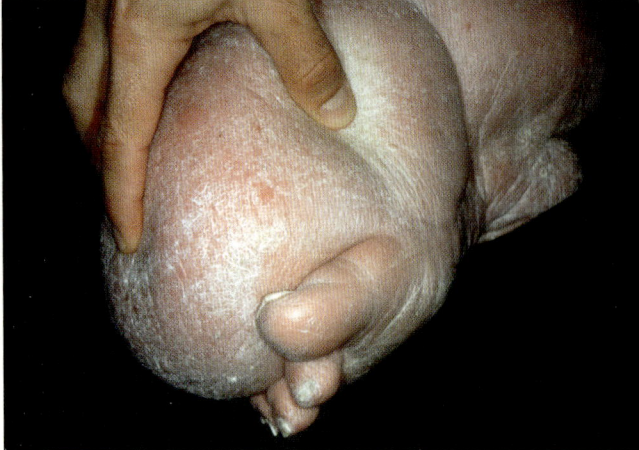

Fig. 20.41 Filariasis.

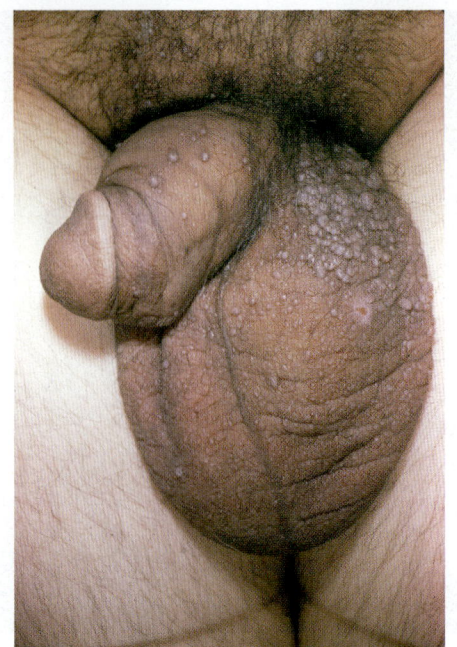

Fig. 20.42 Filariasis.

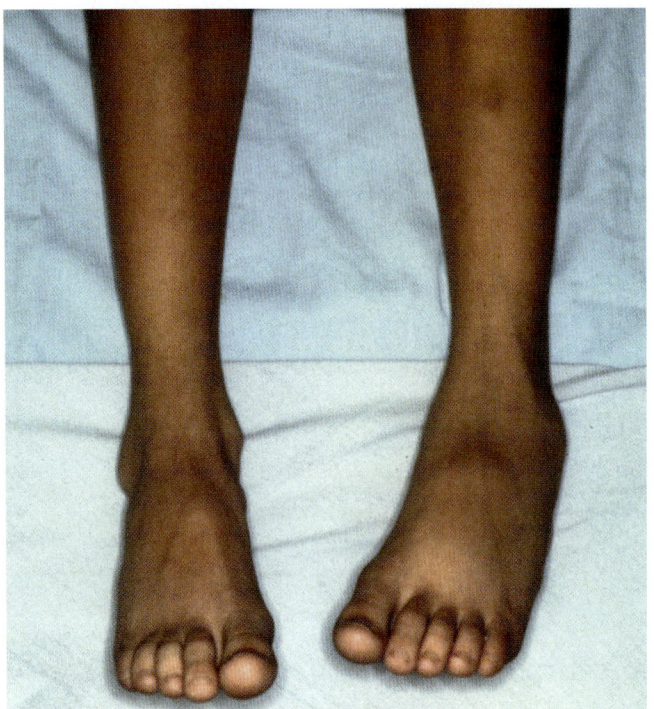

Fig. 20.43 Calabar swelling. *Courtesy Curt Samlaska, MD.*

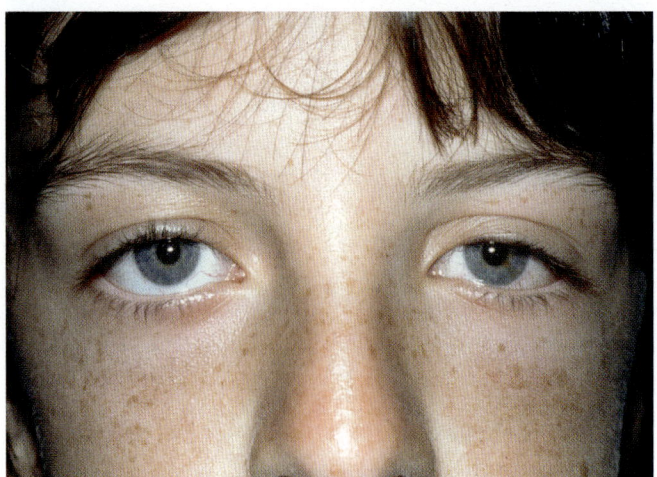

Fig. 20.44 Loiasis; worm is in patient's left upper eyelid. *Courtesy Curt Samlaska, MD.*

Fig. 20.45 Onchocerciasis with acute papular eruption.

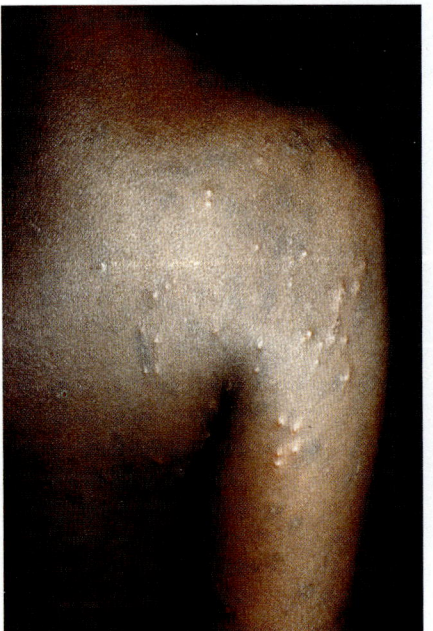

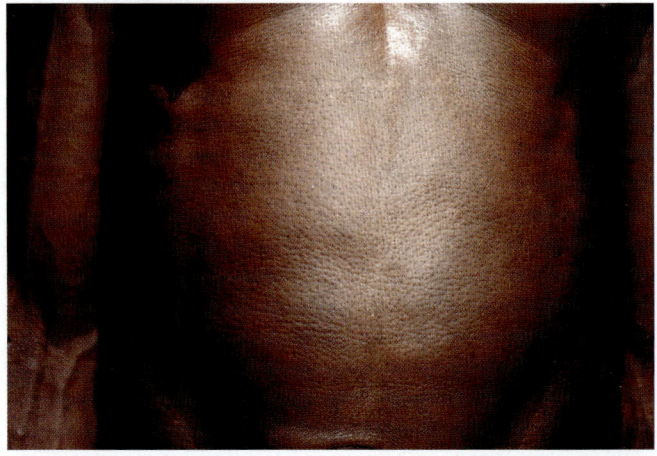

Fig. 20.46 Onchocerciasis with peau d'orange edema.

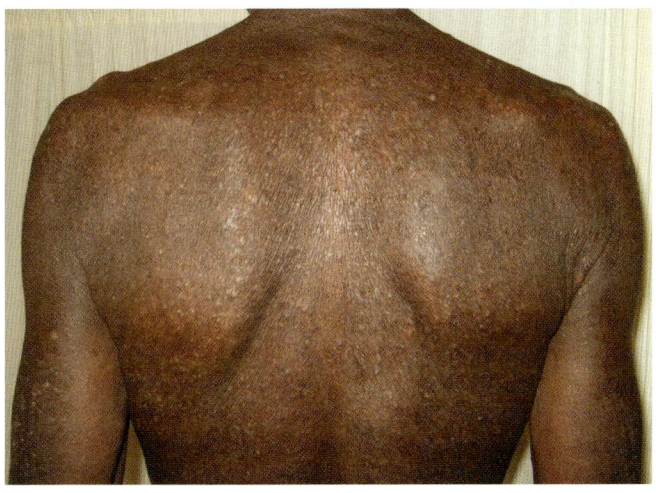

Fig. 20.47 Onchocerciasis with papules and dyspigmentation. *Courtesy Scott Norton, MD.*

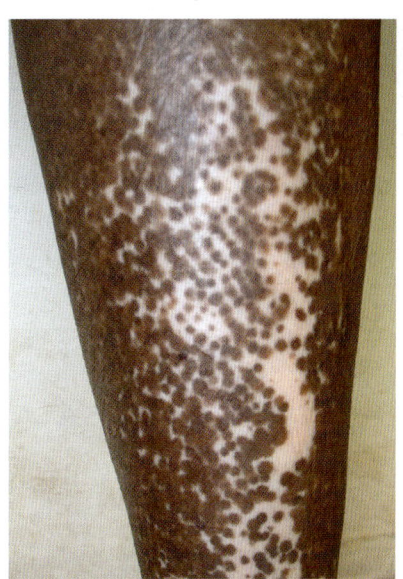

Fig. 20.48 Onchocerciasis with dyspigmentation. *Courtesy Scott Norton, MD.*

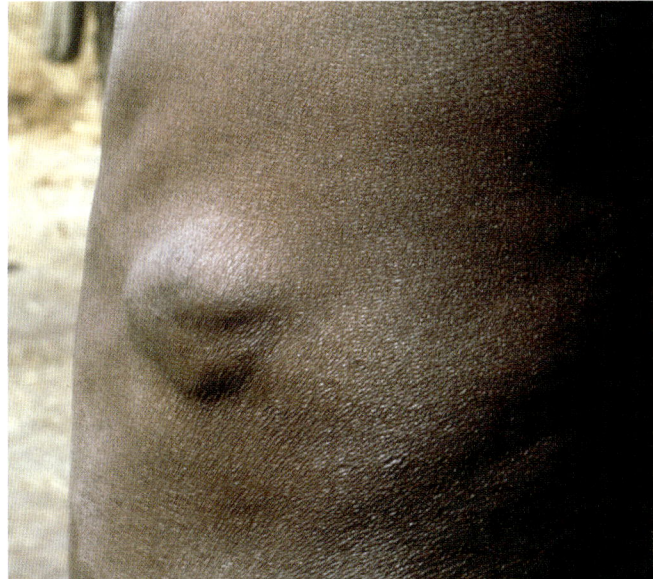

Fig. 20.49 Onchocercoma.

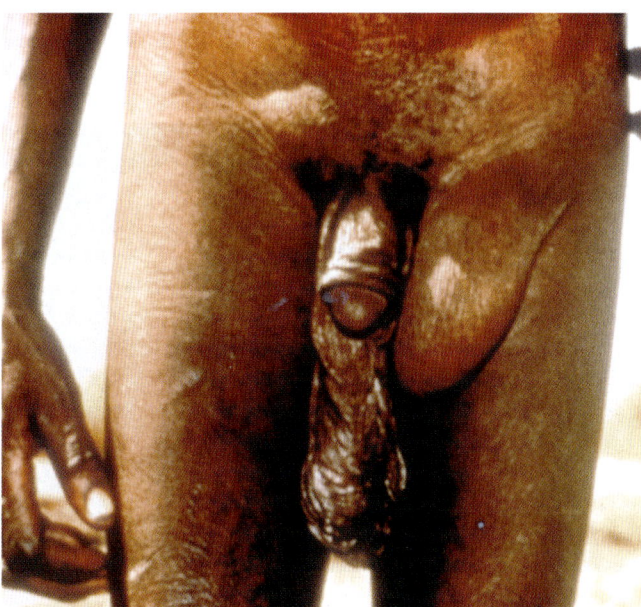

Fig. 20.50 Onchocerciasis with hanging groin.

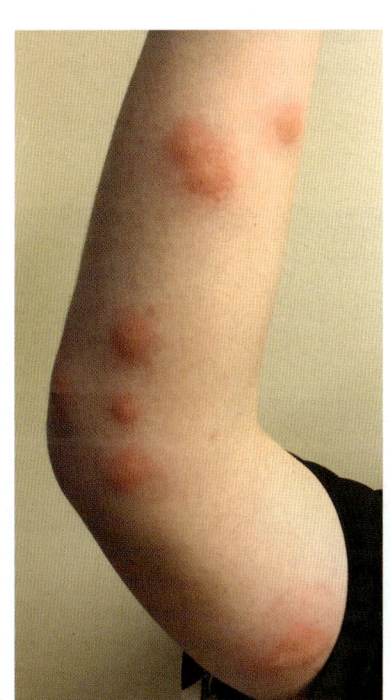

Fig. 20.51 Insect bite reaction.

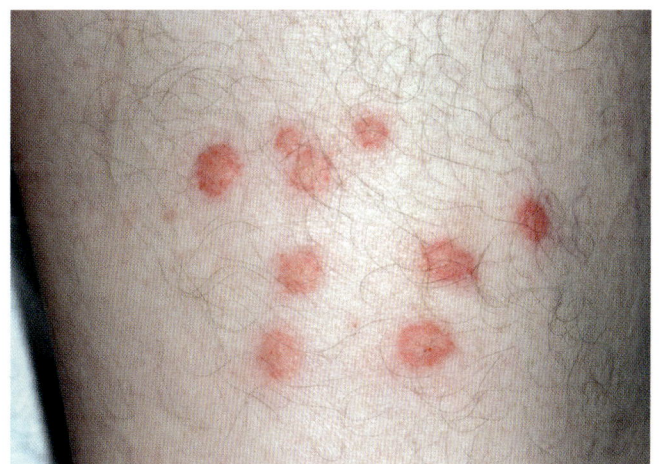

Fig. 20.52 Insect bites.

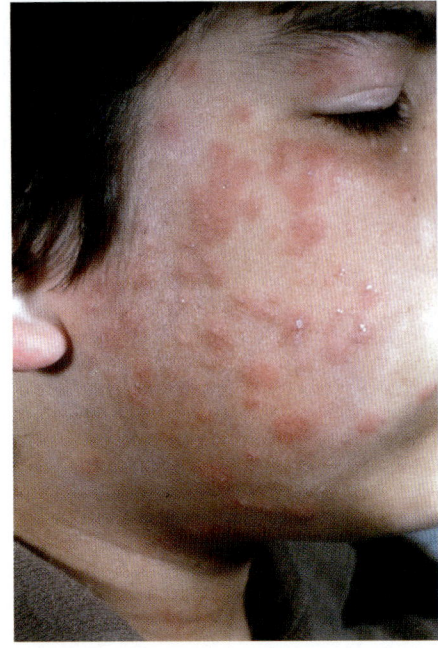

Fig. 20.53 Bedbug bites.

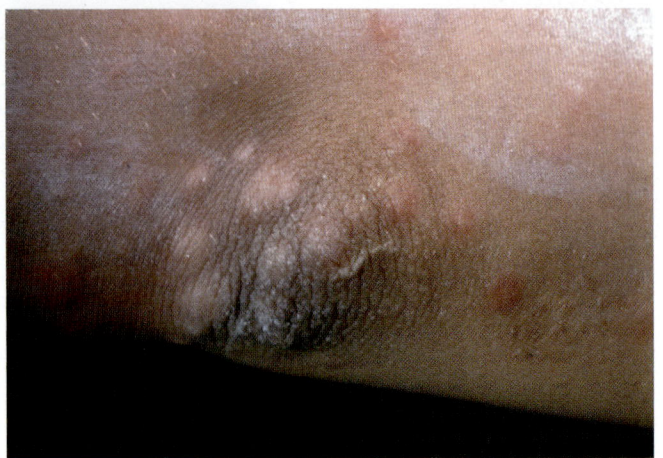

Fig. 20.54 Bedbug bites.

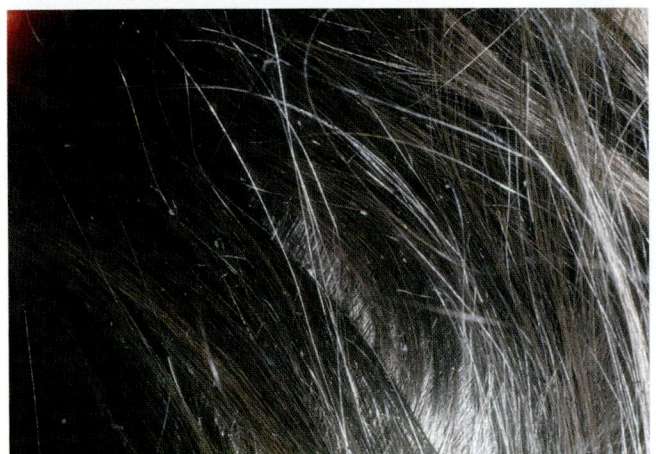

Fig. 20.55 Pediculosis capitis.

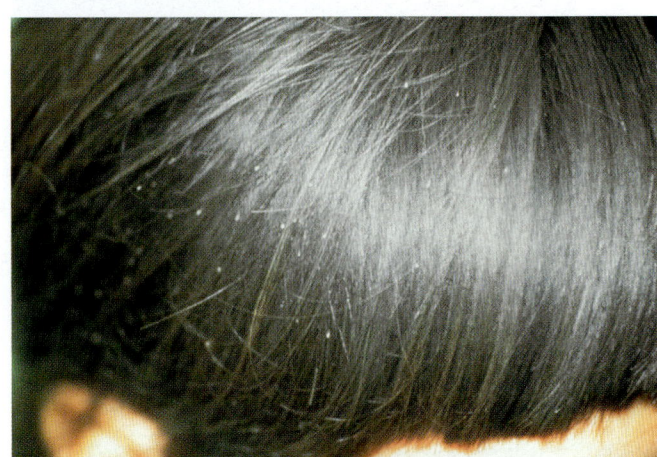

Fig. 20.56 Pediculosis capitis.

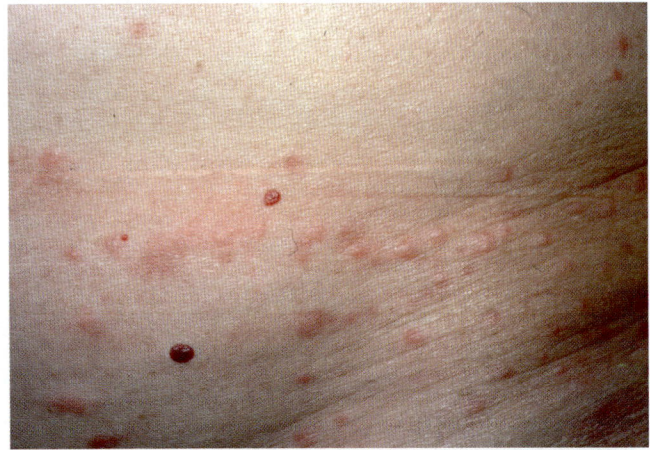

Fig. 20.57 Pediculosis corporis.

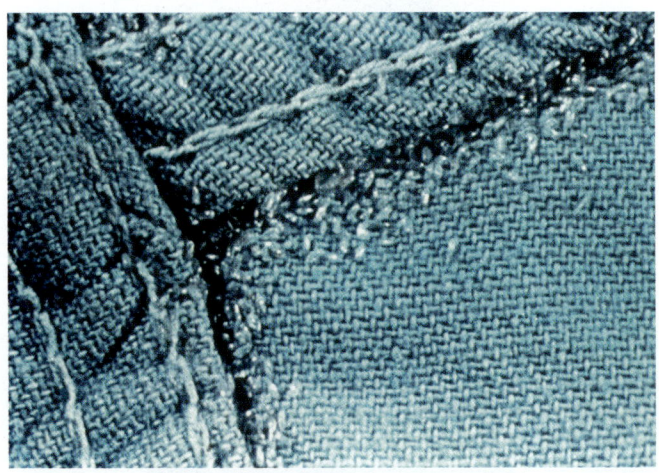

Fig. 20.58 Pediculosis; nits in clothing.

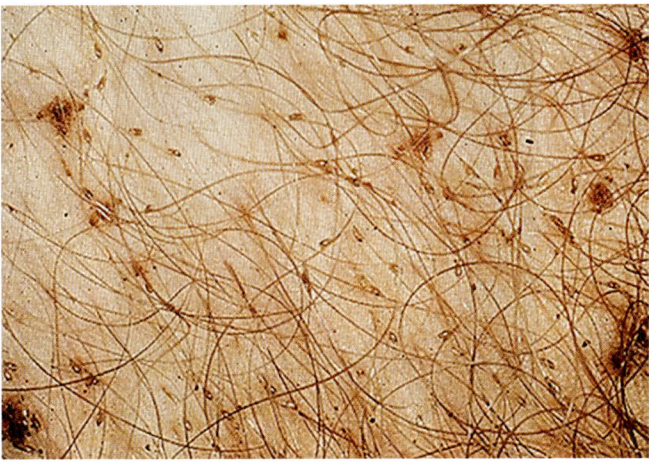

Fig. 20.59 Pediculosis pubis.

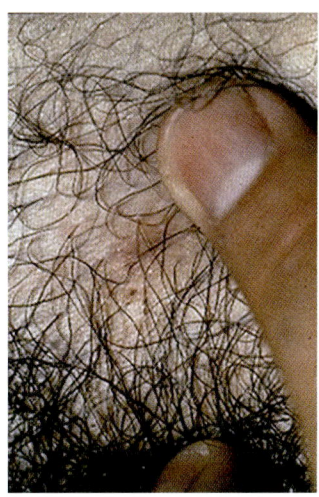

Fig. 20.60 Maculae ceruleae.

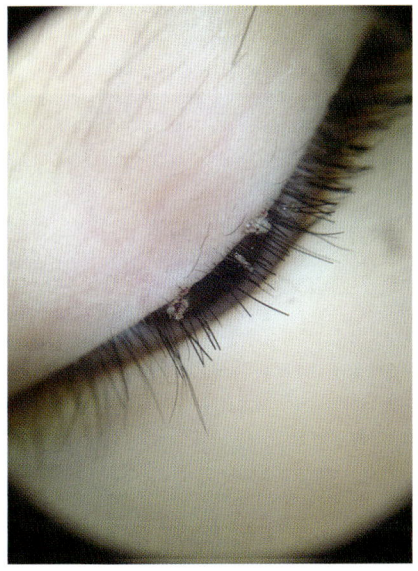

Fig. 20.61 Pubic lice on the eyelashes. *Courtesy Dr. Yi-Shuan Sheen.*

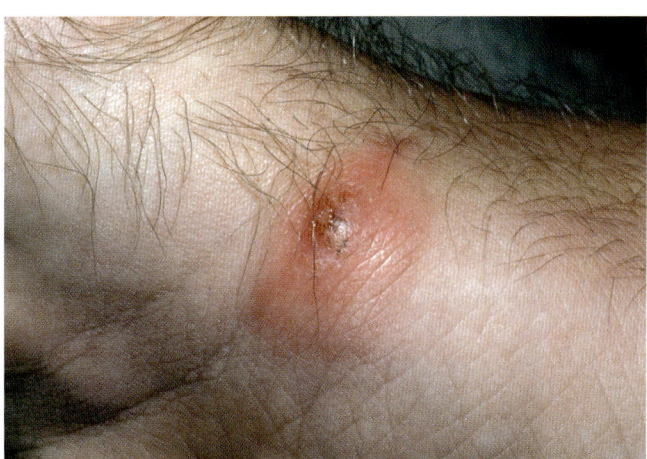

Fig. 20.62 Myiasis. *Courtesy Steven Binnick, MD.*

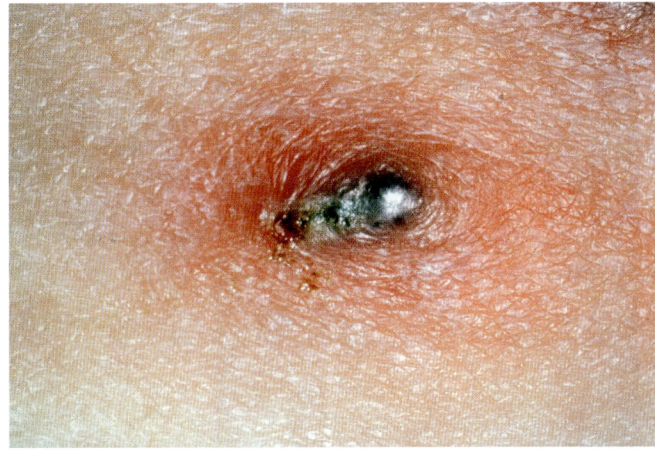

Fig. 20.63 Myiasis.

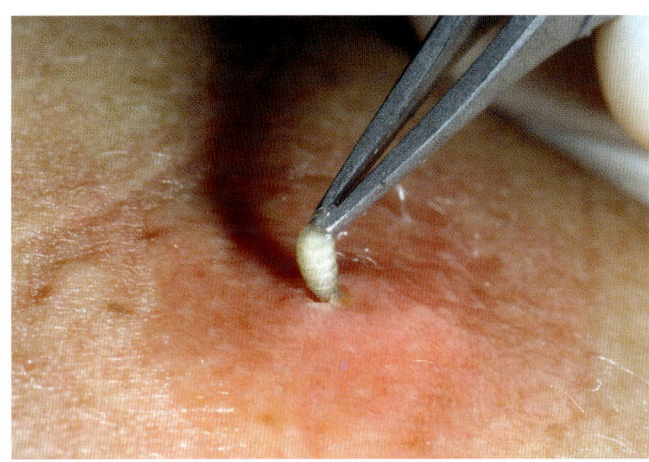

Fig. 20.64 Extraction of larva after treating with petrolatum.

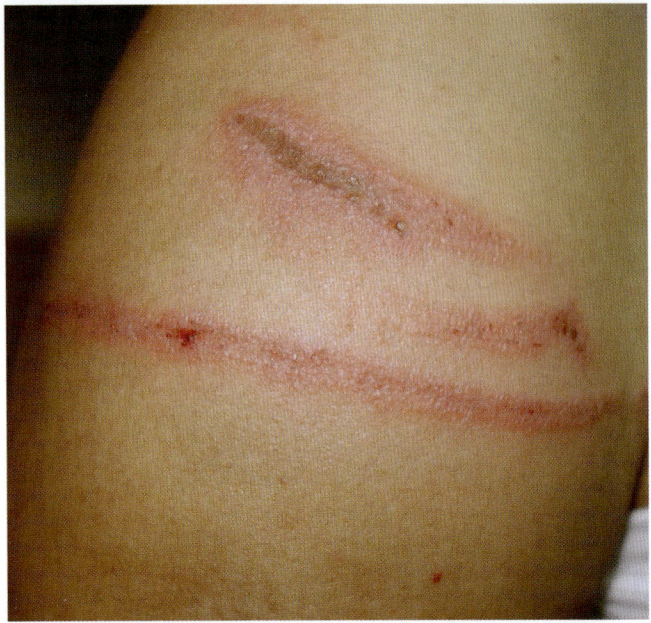

Fig. 20.65 Paederus (beetle) dermatitis. *Courtesy Shyam Verma, MBBS, DVD.*

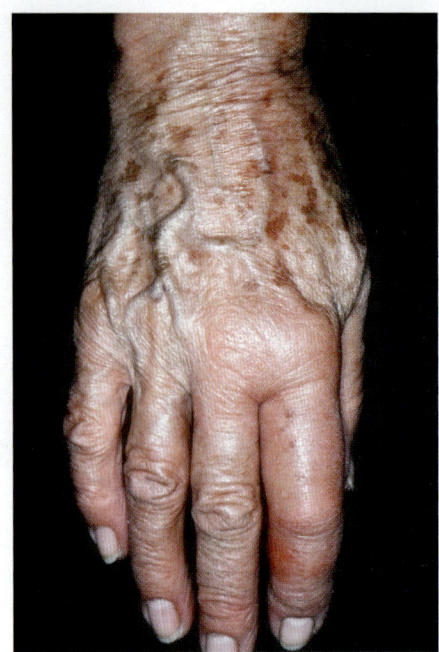

Fig. 20.66 Wasp sting.

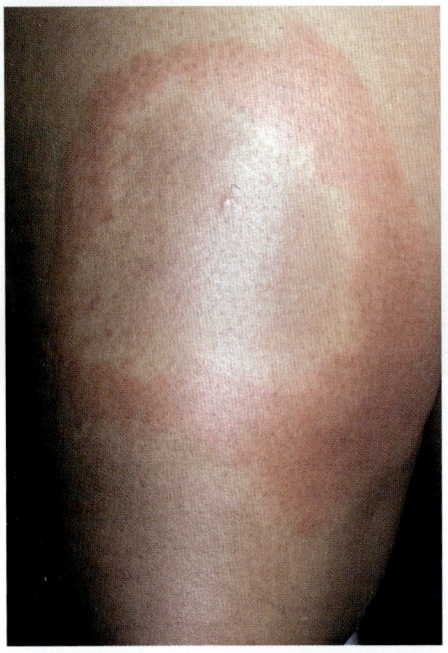

Fig. 20.67 Bee sting. *Courtesy Steven Binnick, MD.*

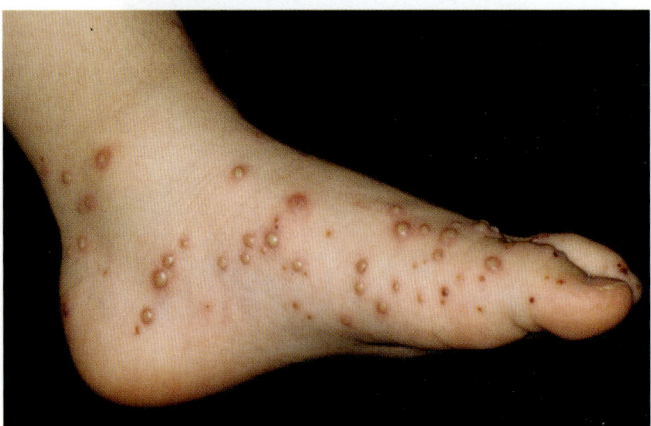

Fig. 20.68 Fire ant stings.

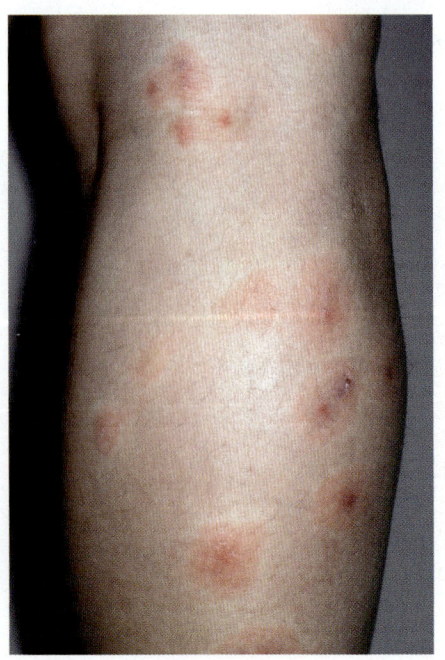

Fig. 20.69 Flea bites. *Courtesy Curt Samlaska, MD.*

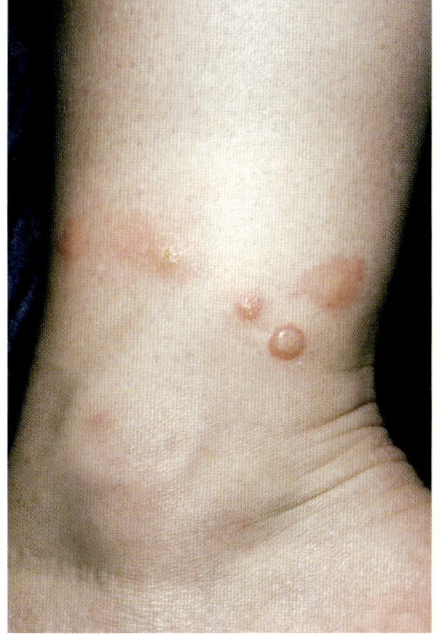

Fig. 20.70 Flea bites.

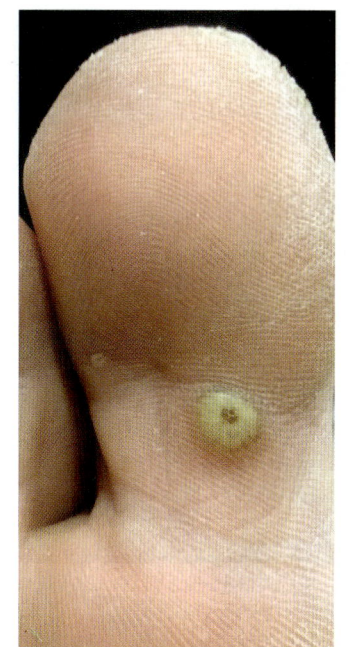

Fig. 20.71 Tungiasis. *Courtesy Catherine Quirk, MD.*

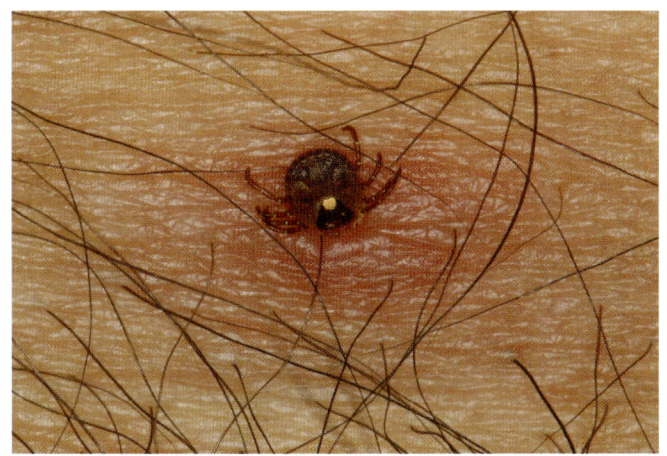

Fig. 20.72 *Amblyomma americanum*.

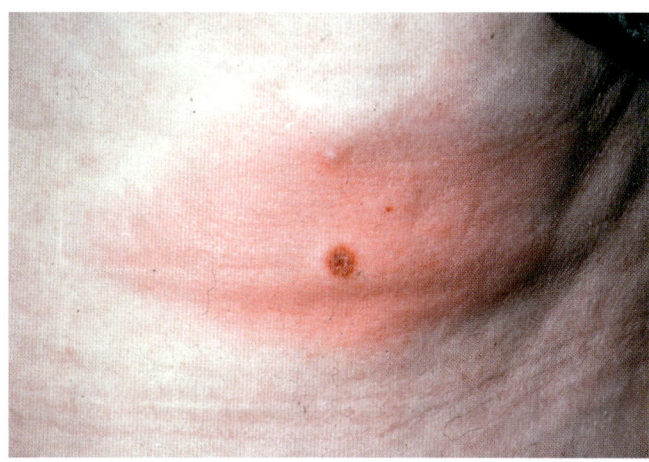

Fig. 20.73 Tick bite site.

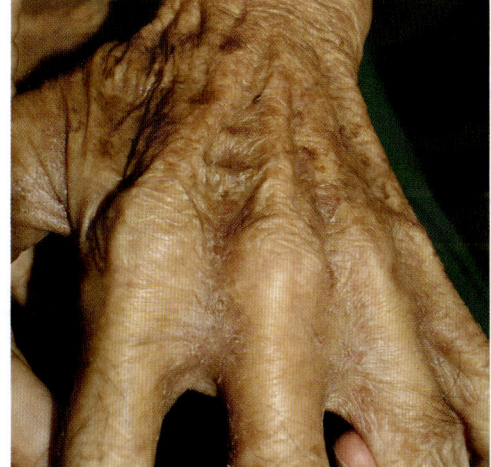

Fig. 20.74 Scabies. *Courtesy National Cheng Kung University, Taiwan.*

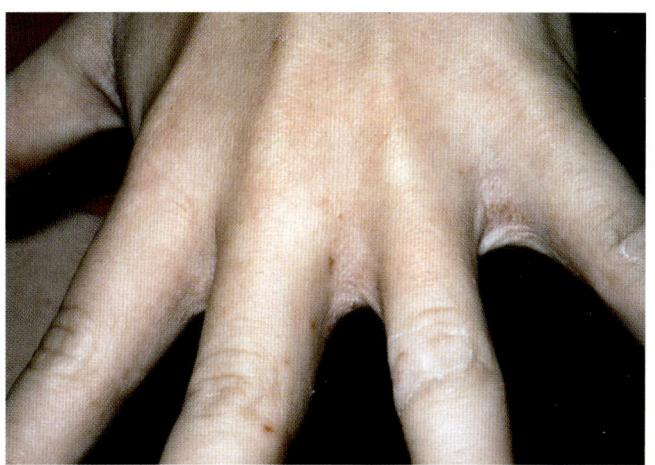

Fig. 20.75 Scabies.

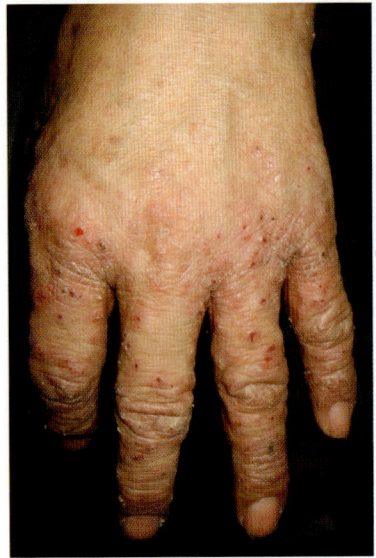

Fig. 20.76 Scabies. *Courtesy National Cheng Kung University, Taiwan.*

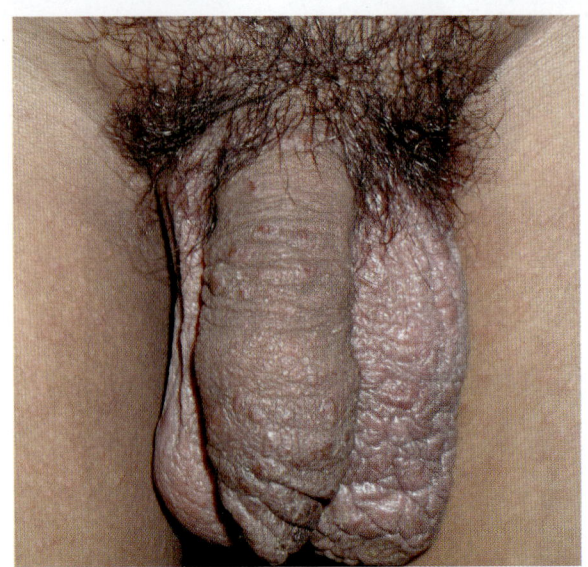

Fig. 20.77 Scabies. *Courtesy Shyam Verma, MBBS, DVD.*

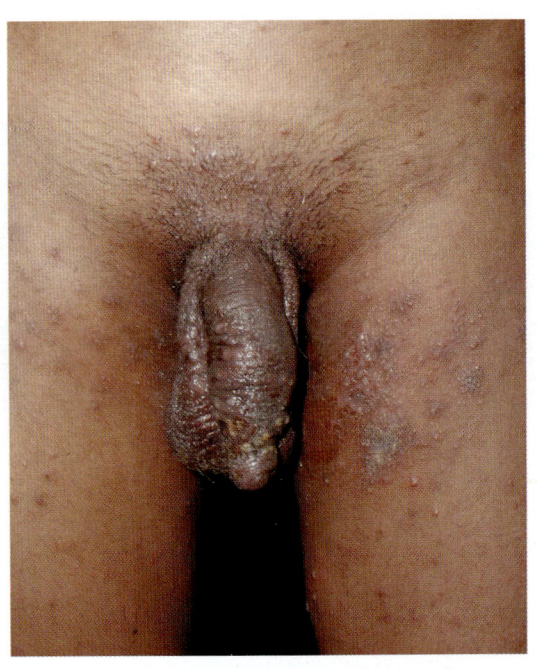

Fig. 20.78 Scabies. *Courtesy Shyam Verma, MBBS, DVD.*

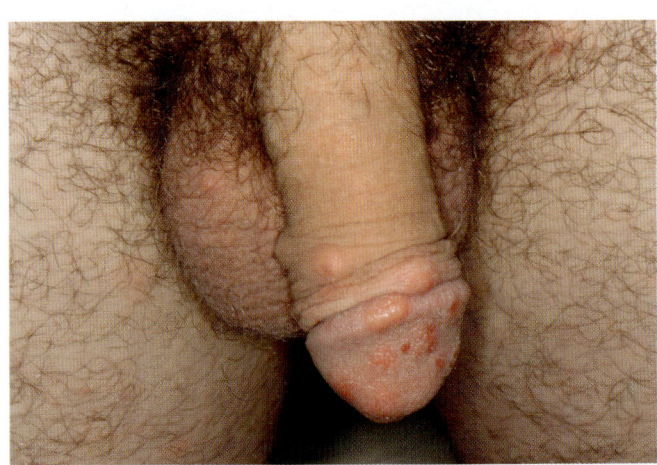

Fig. 20.79 Nodular scabies.

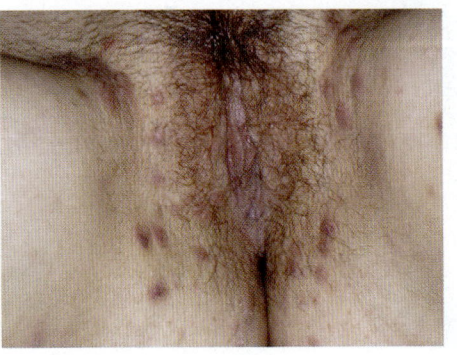

Fig. 20.80 Nodular scabies.

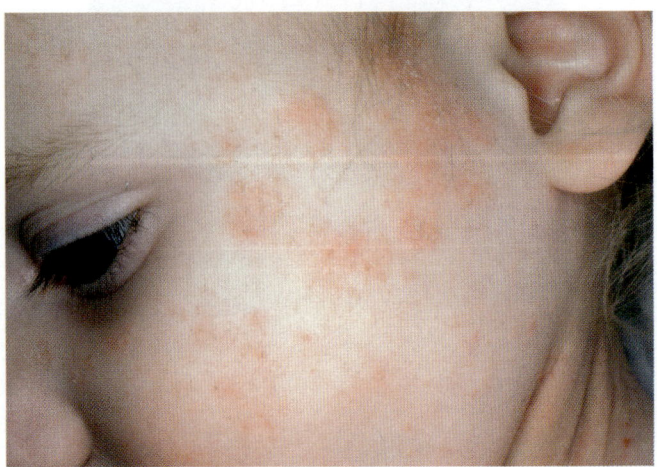

Fig. 20.81 Scabies.

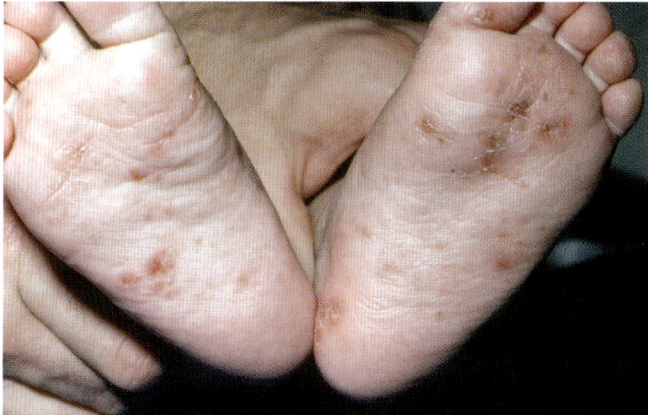

Fig. 20.82 Scabies.

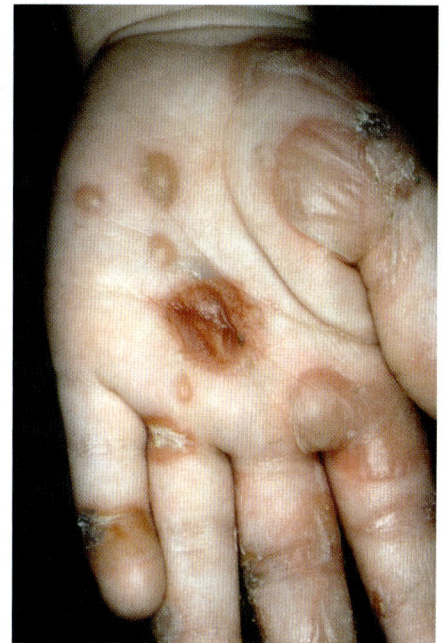

Fig. 20.83 Scabies.

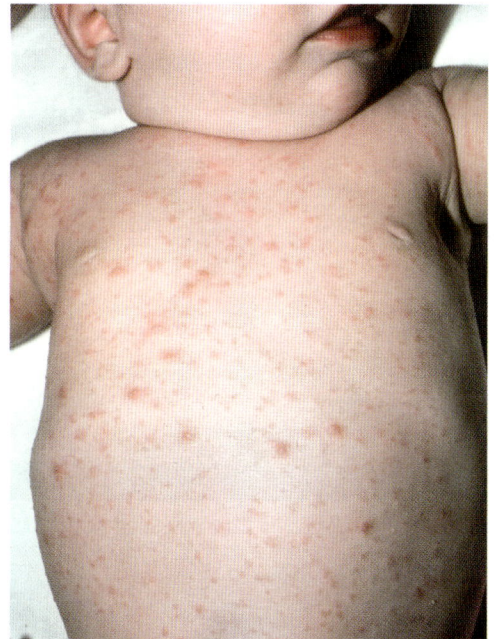

Fig. 20.84 Scabies.

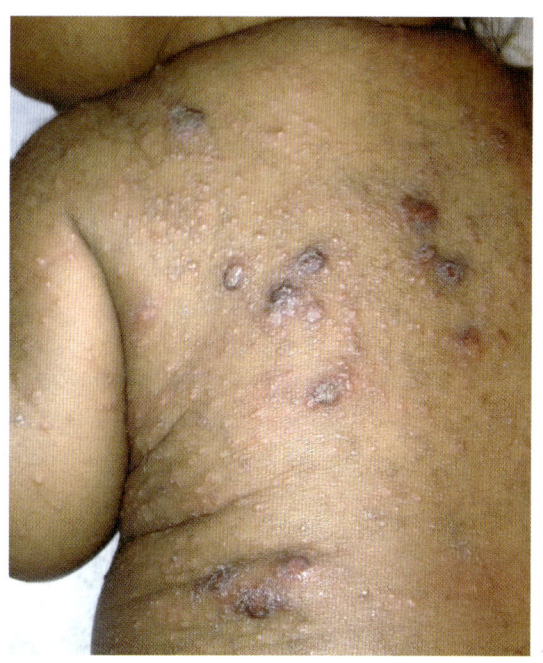

Fig. 20.85 Scabies.

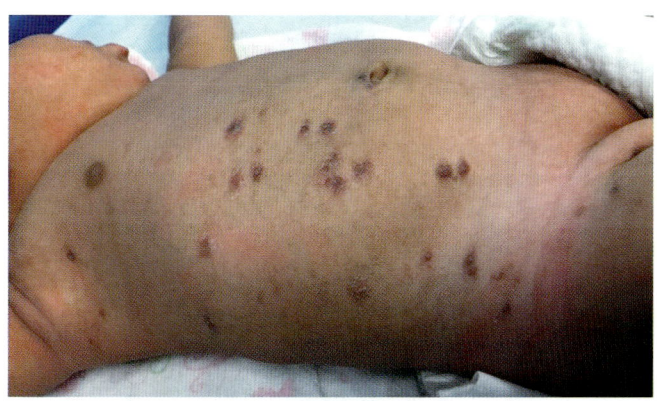

Fig. 20.86 Scabies.

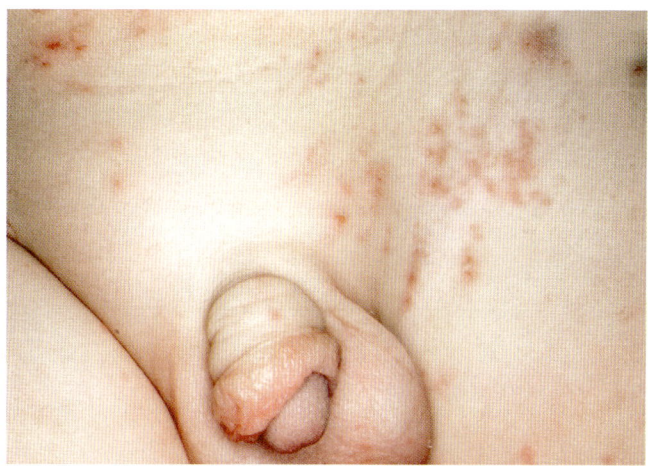

Fig. 20.87 Scabies.

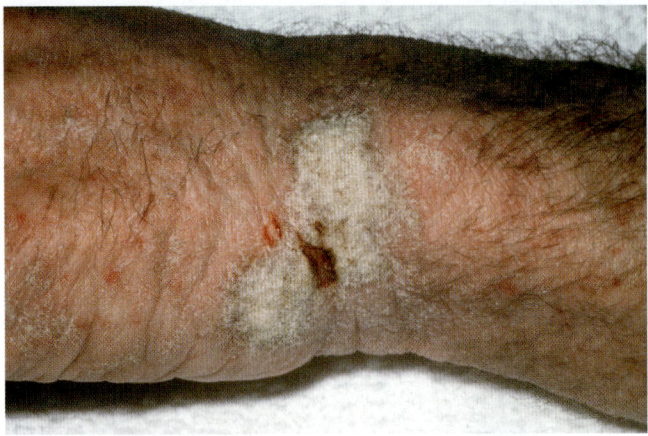

Fig. 20.88 Crusted scabies in an HIV-infected patient.

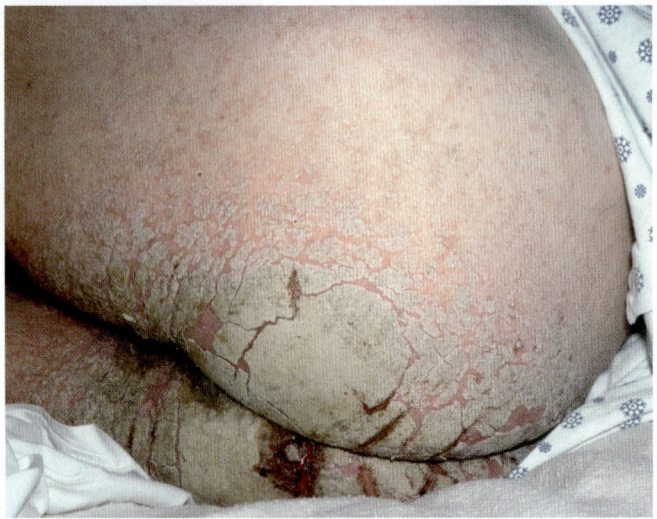

Fig. 20.89 Crusted scabies in an HIV-infected patient. *Courtesy Curt Samlaska, MD.*

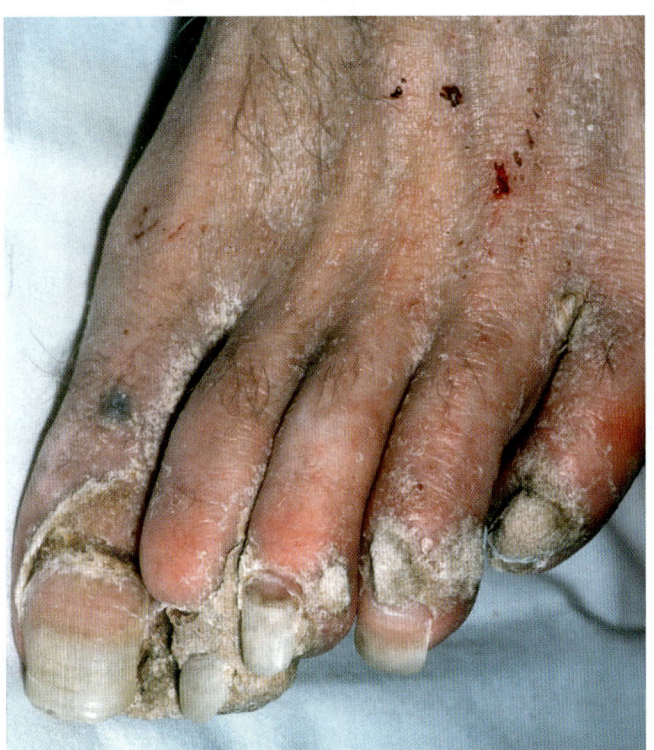

Fig. 20.90 Crusted scabies in an HIV-infected patient.

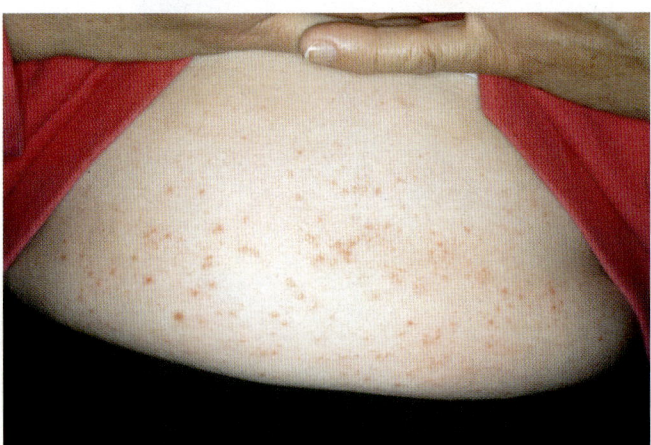

Fig. 20.91 Cheyletiella mite bites. *Courtesy Scott Norton, MD.*

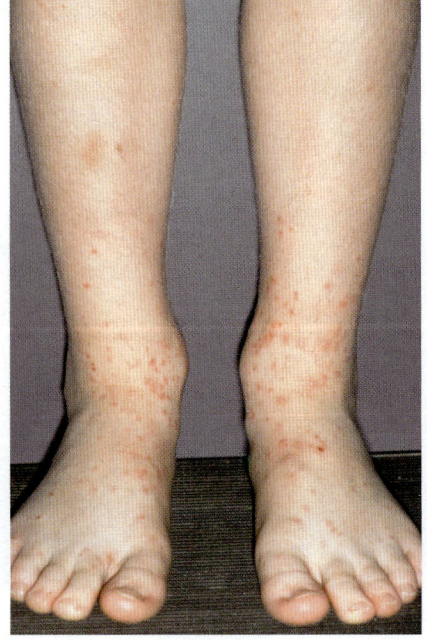

Fig. 20.92 Chigger bites.

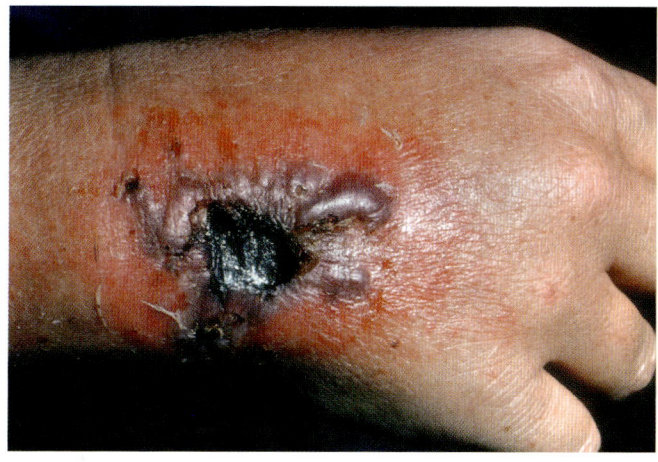

Fig. 20.93 Brown recluse spider bite. *Courtesy Steven Binnick, MD.*

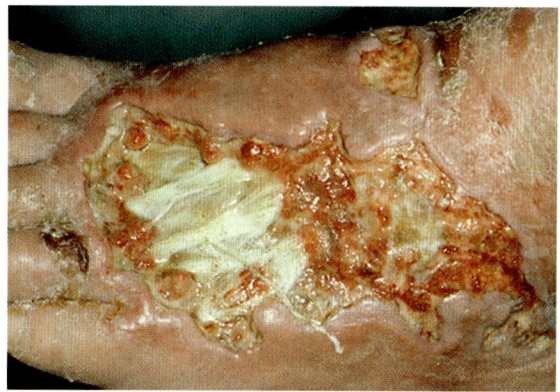

Fig. 20.94 Brown recluse spider bite.

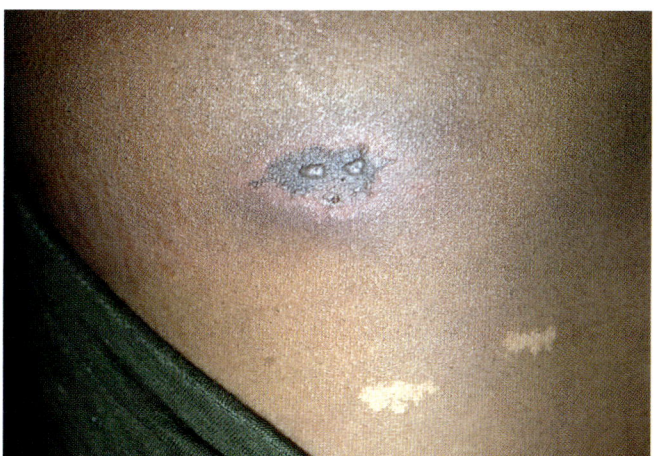

Fig. 20.95 Spider bite.

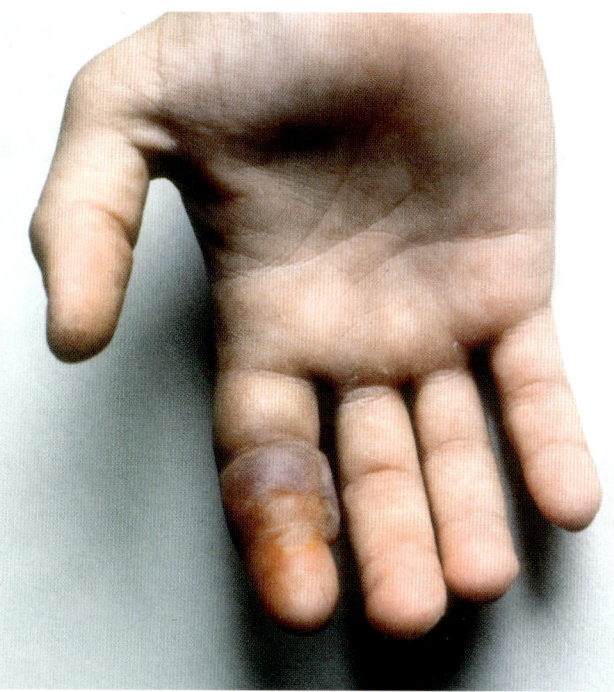

Fig. 20.96 Snake bite.

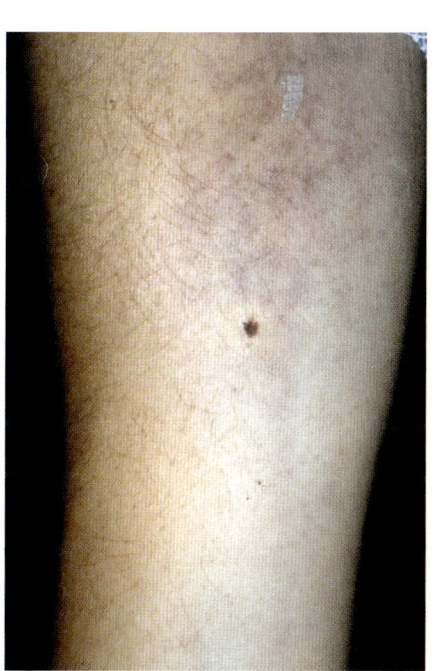

Fig. 20.97 Russell pit viper bite. *Courtesy Scott Norton, MD.*

Chronic Blistering Dermatoses 21

Immunobullous dermatoses may present with urticarial lesions, blisters, erosions, or pustules. IgA-mediated disease is characterized by annular lesions with a "string of pearls" morphology—bullous in the case of linear IgA bullous dermatosis and pustular or erosive in the case of IgA pemphigus. Pemphigoid typically presents with tense blisters forming on erythematous patches or urticarial plaques. Pemphigus vulgaris often initially appears with oral erosions, but can progress to widely denuded areas of skin. In contrast, pemphigus foliaceus presents with superficial erosions and adherent crusts that resemble macerated cornflakes allowed to dry at the bottom of the bowl. Pemphigus vegetans is characterized by localized, moist, heaped-up crusts, sometimes studded with pustules. Dermatitis herpetiformis presents with intense itching with excoriation and erosions clustered on the posterior scalp, extensor surfaces, and buttocks. Itching is intense, so it is rare to identify intact blisters. This portion of the atlas will guide you through the various clinical presentations of bullous disorders of the skin.

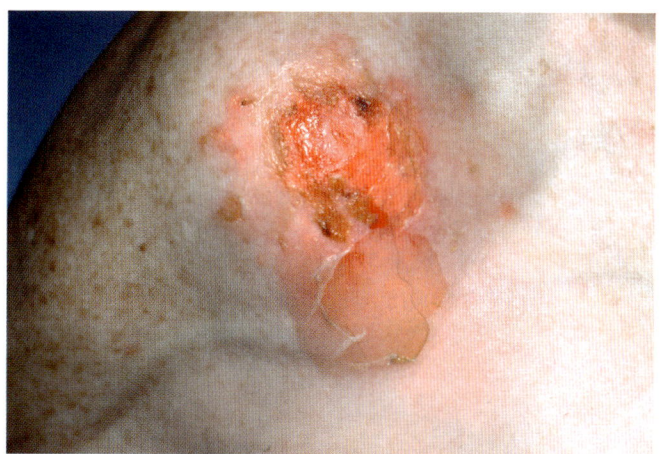

Fig. 21.1 Pemphigus vulgaris. *Courtesy Curt Samlaska, MD.*

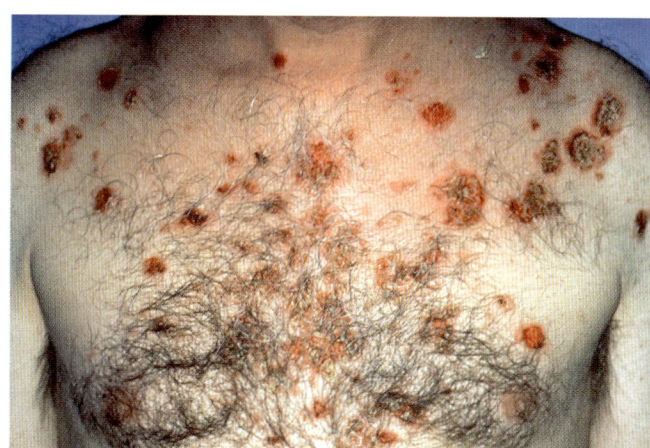

Fig. 21.2 Pemphigus vulgaris.

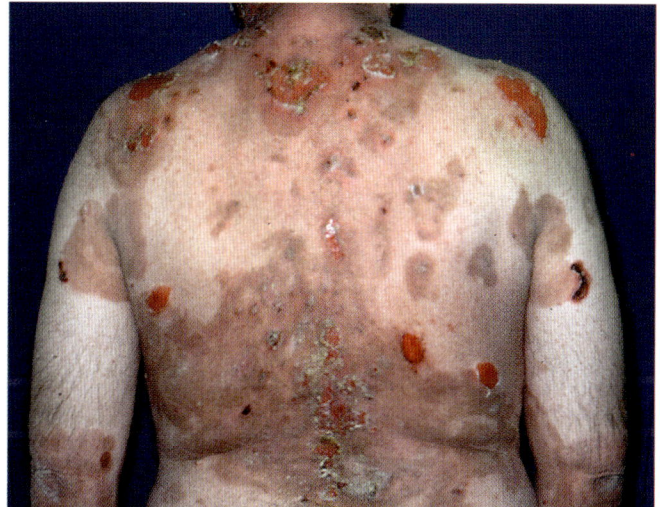

Fig. 21.3 Pemphigus vulgaris with hyperpigmentation.

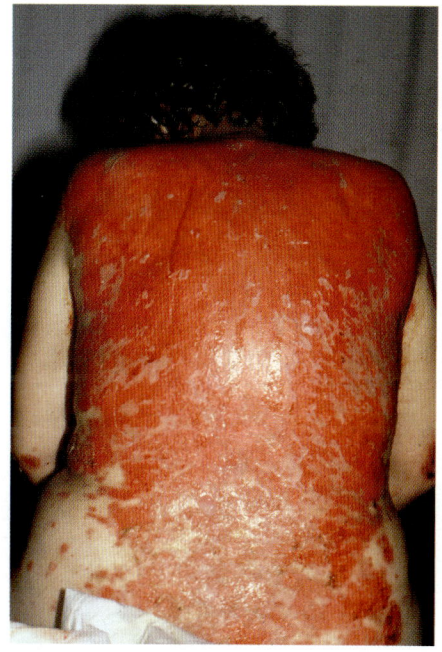

Fig. 21.4 Pemphigus vulgaris.

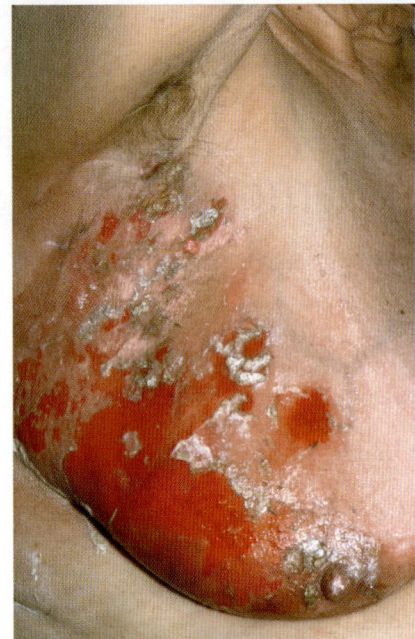

Fig. 21.5 Pemphigus vulgaris after radiation therapy.

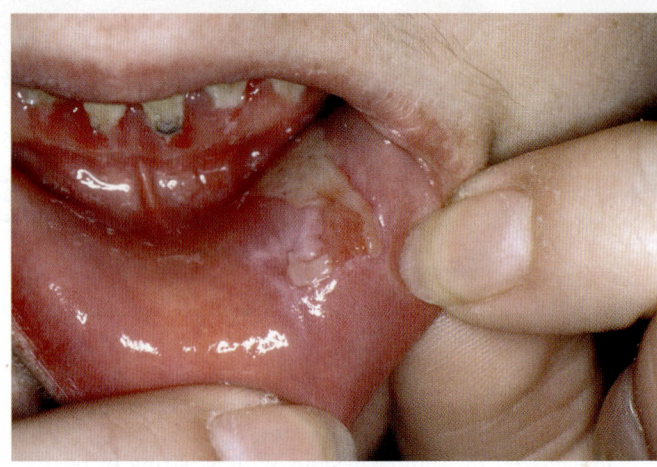

Fig. 21.6 Oral pemphigus vulgaris. *Courtesy Steven Binnick, MD.*

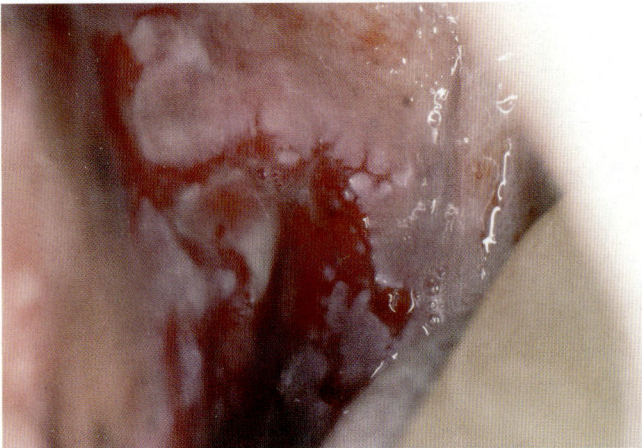

Fig. 21.7 Oral pemphigus vulgaris. *Courtesy Curt Samlaska, MD.*

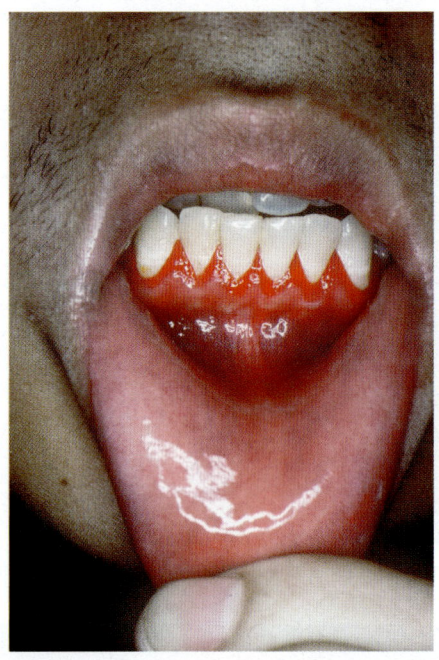

Fig. 21.8 Oral pemphigus vulgaris.

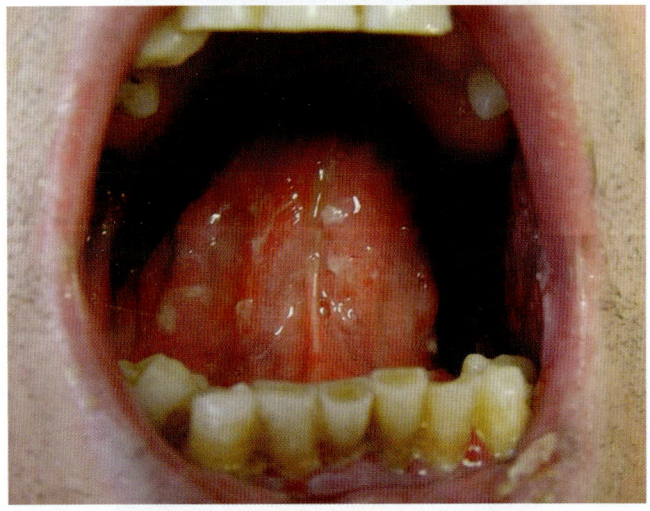

Fig. 21.9 Oral pemphigus vulgaris. *Courtesy Dr. Rui Carlos Taveres Bello.*

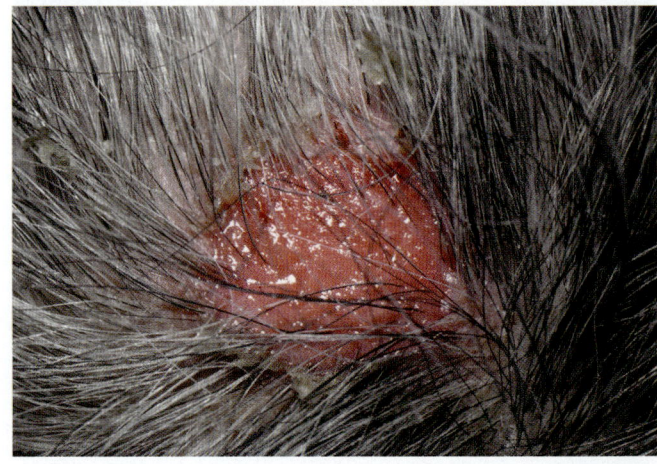

Fig. 21.10 Scalp pemphigus vulgaris. *Courtesy Curt Samlaska, MD.*

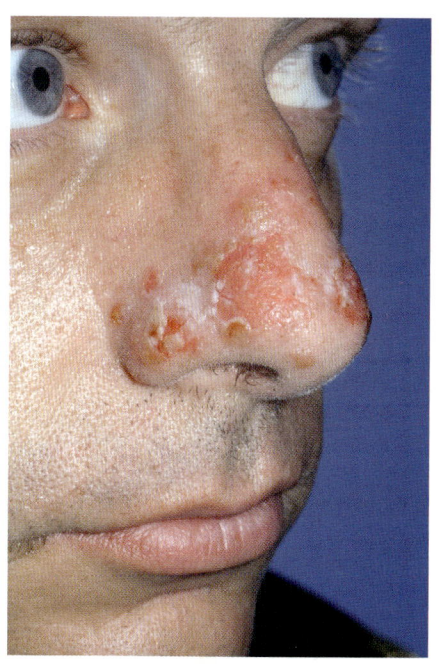

Fig. 21.11 Pemphigus vulgaris. *Courtesy Curt Samlaska, MD.*

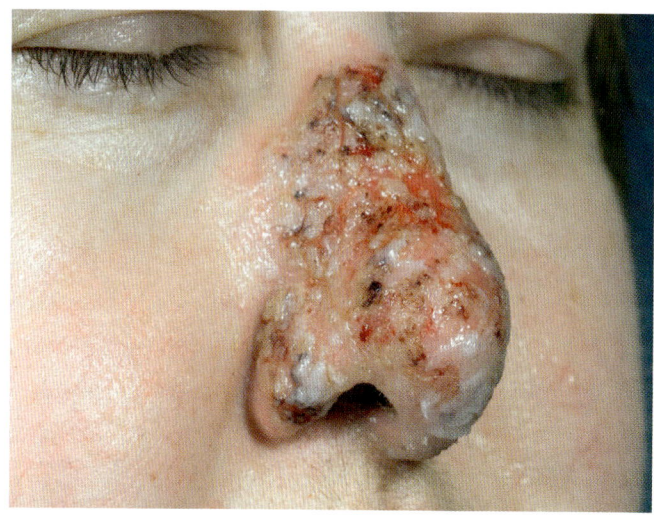

Fig. 21.12 Pemphigus vulgaris.

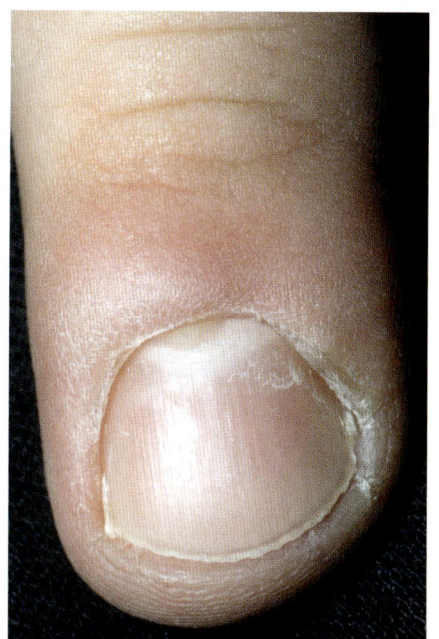

Fig. 21.13 Nail pemphigus vulgaris, paronychia type.

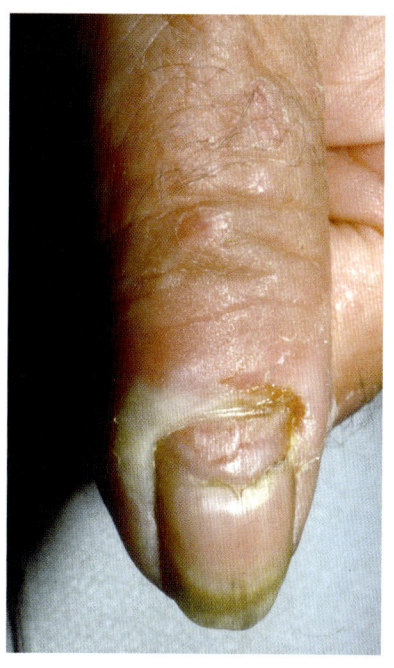

Fig. 21.14 Nail pemphigus vulgaris, onychomadesis type.

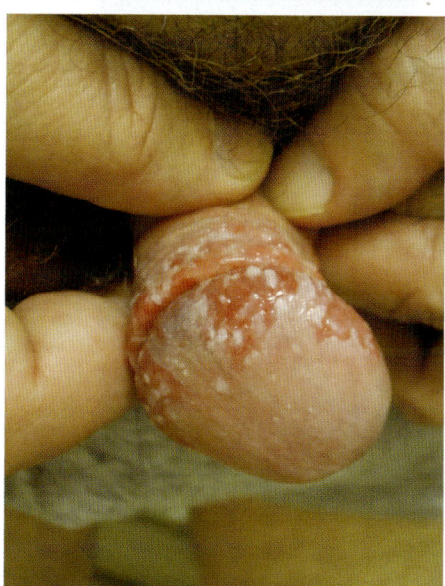

Fig. 21.15 Pemphigus vulgaris.

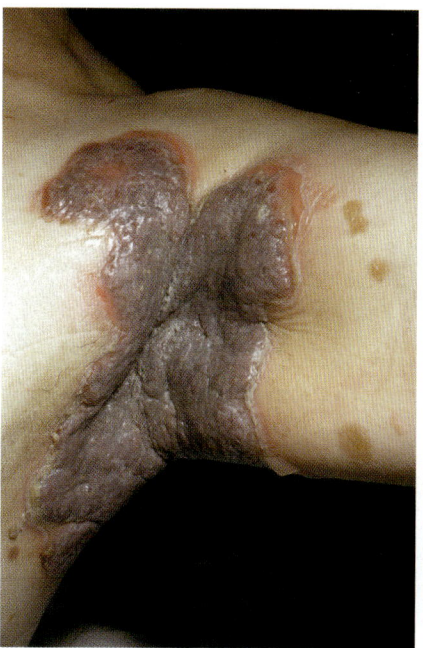

Fig. 21.16 Pemphigus vegetans. *Courtesy Steven Binnick, MD.*

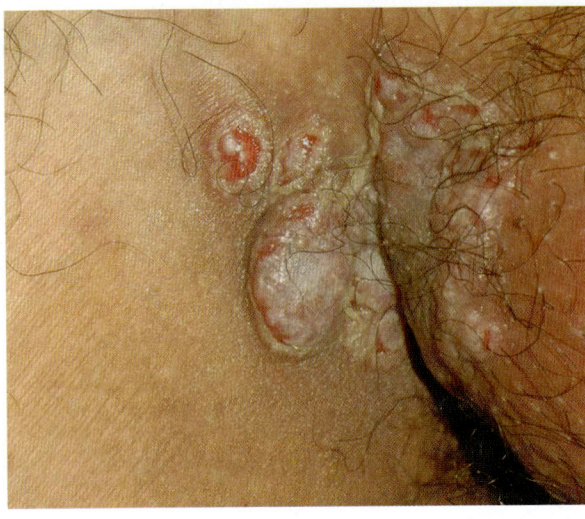

Fig. 21.17 Pemphigus vegetans. *Courtesy Yung-Tsu Cho, MD.*

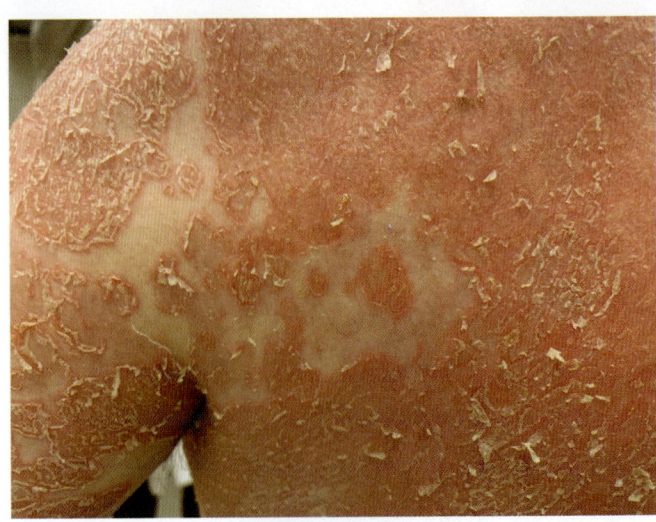

Fig. 21.18 Pemphigus foliaceus.

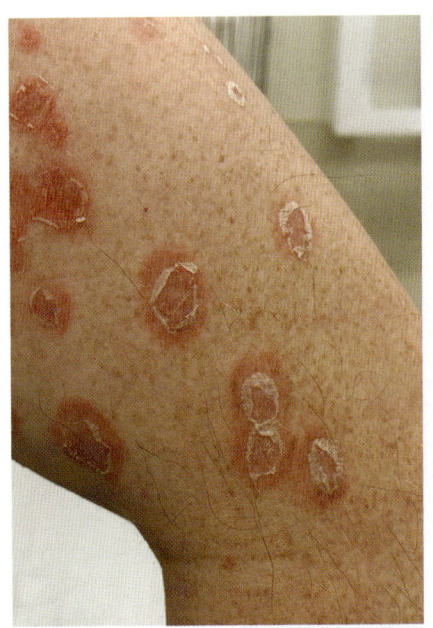

Fig. 21.19 Pemphigus foliaceus.

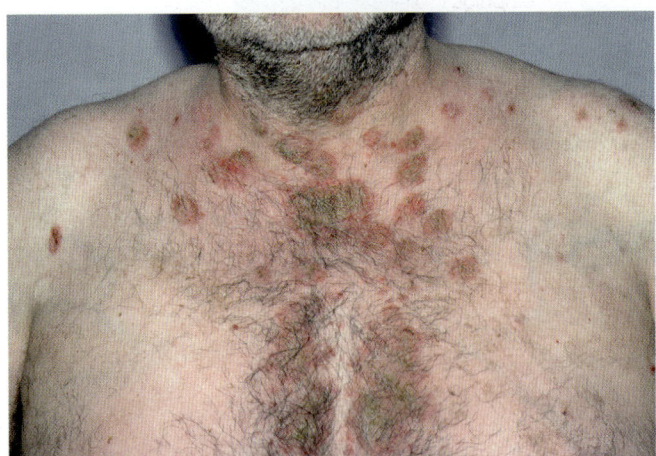

Fig. 21.20 Pemphigus foliaceus.

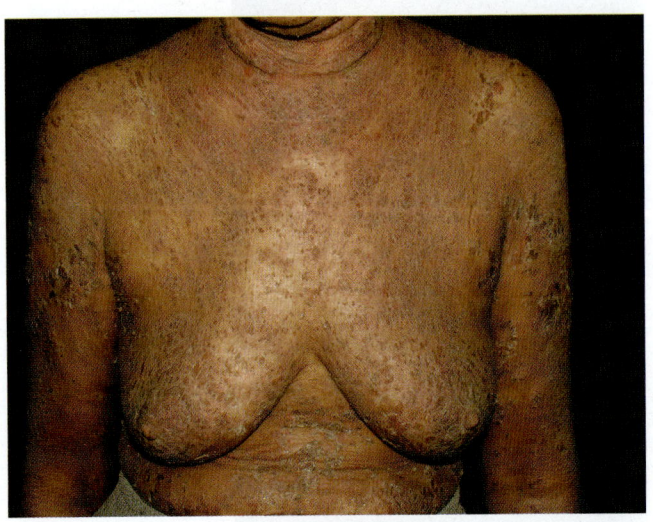

Fig. 21.21 Pemphigus foliaceus. *Courtesy Vasanop Vachiramon, MD.*

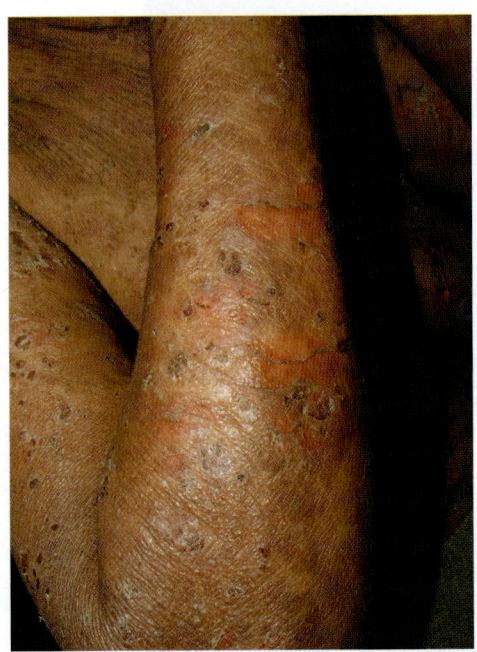

Fig. 21.22 Pemphigus foliaceus. *Courtesy Vasanop Vachiramon, MD.*

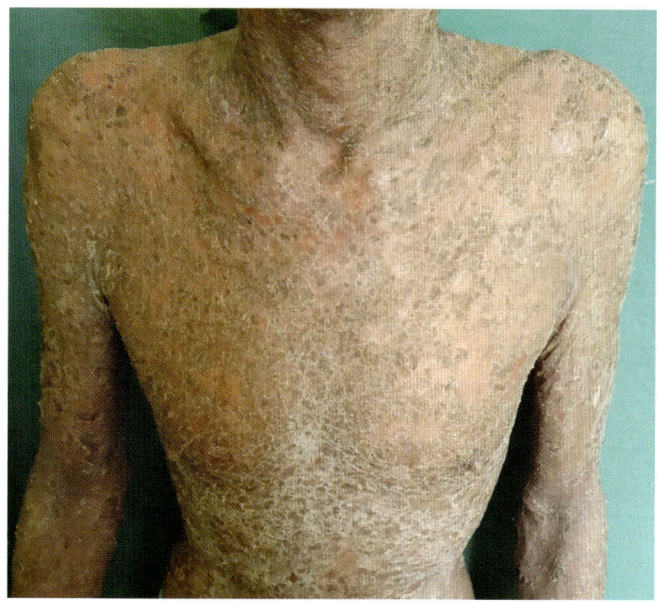

Fig. 21.23 Pemphigus foliaceus. *Courtesy Debabrata Bandyopadhyay.*

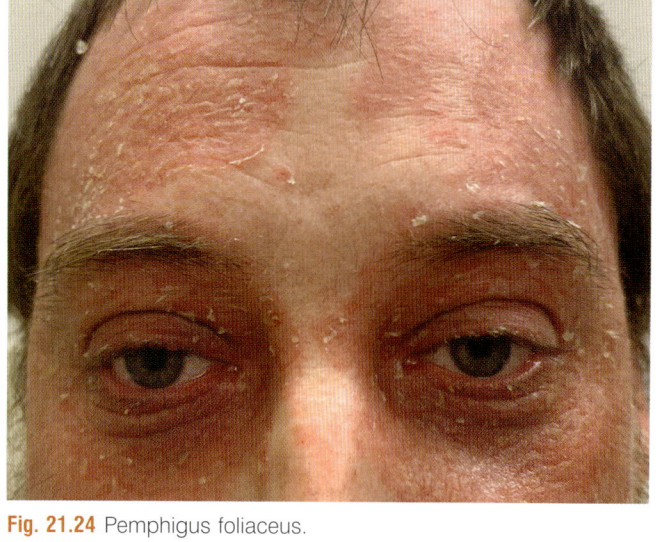

Fig. 21.24 Pemphigus foliaceus.

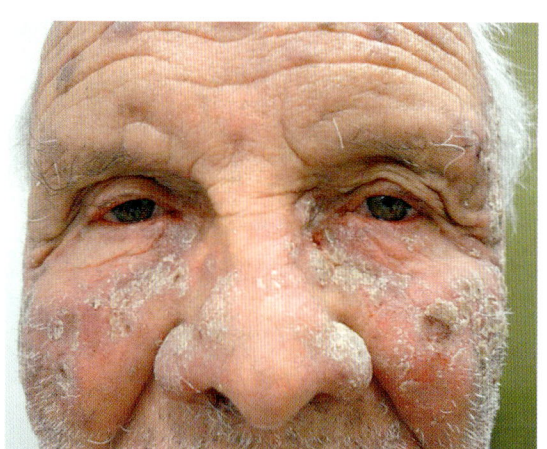

Fig. 21.25 Fogo selvagem. *Courtesy Dermatology Division, University of Campinas, Brazil.*

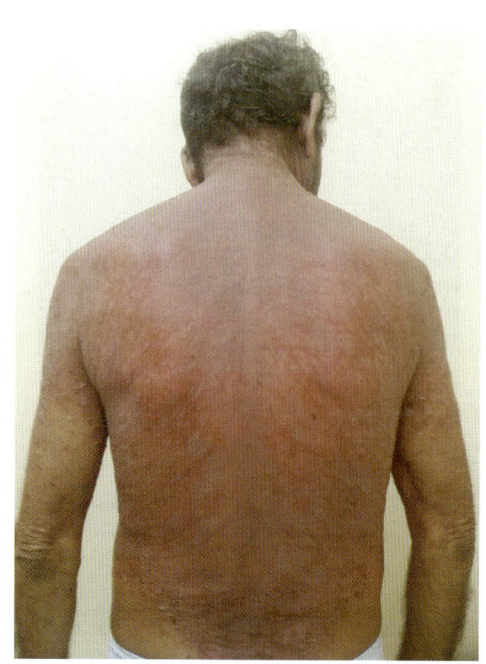

Fig. 21.26 Fogo selvagem.

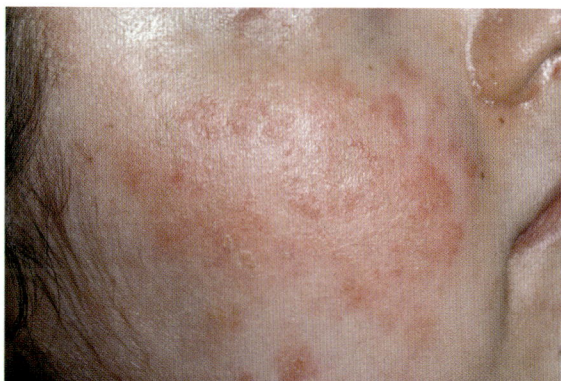

Fig. 21.27 Pemphigus erythematosus–like pemphigus foliaceus. *Courtesy John Stanley, MD.*

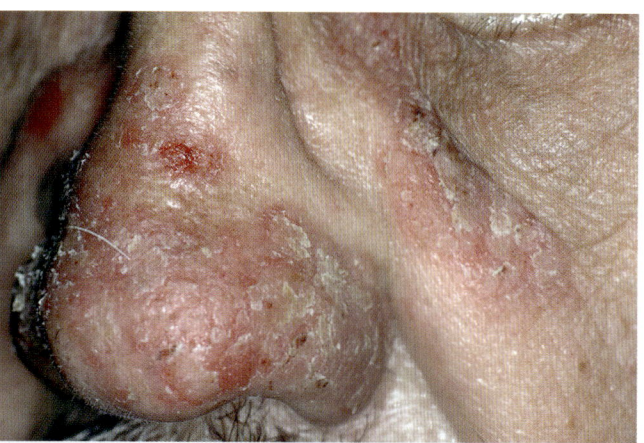

Fig. 21.28 Pemphigus erythematosus. *Courtesy Steven Binnick, MD.*

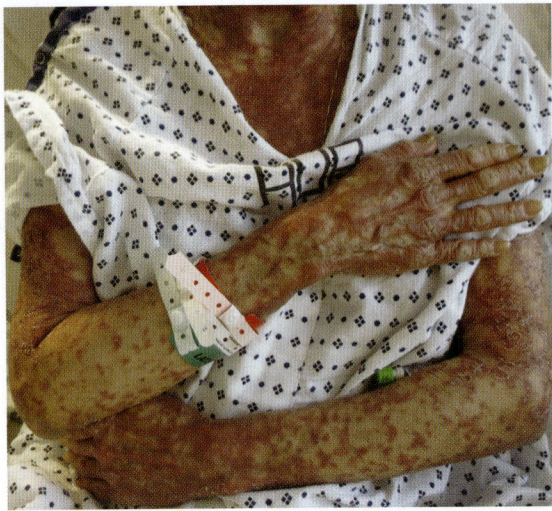

Fig. 21.29 Paraneoplastic pemphigus, lichenoid variant.

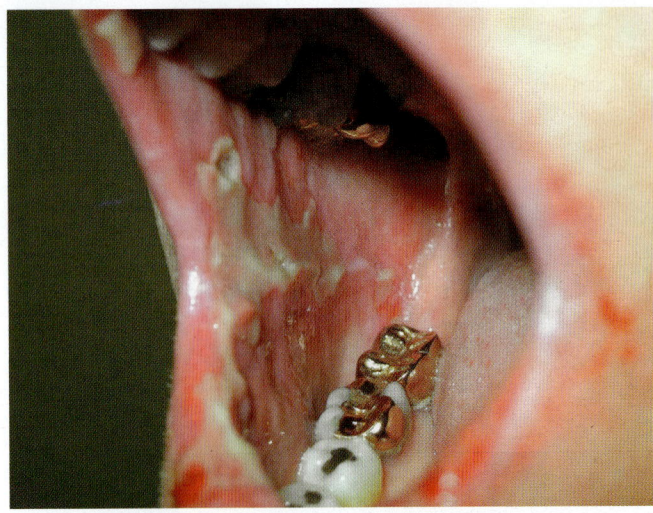

Fig. 21.30 Paraneoplastic pemphigus.

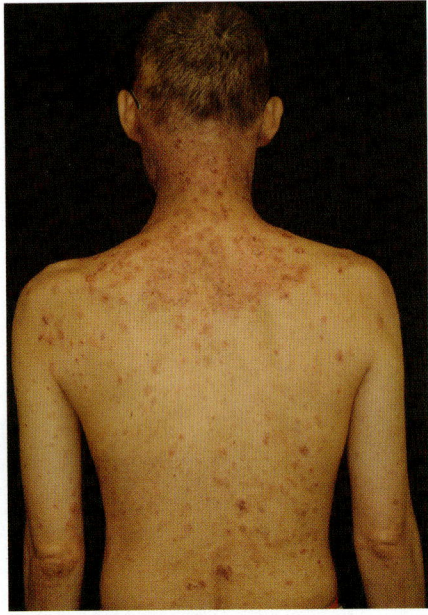

Fig. 21.31 Paraneoplastic pemphigus. *Courtesy Kaohsiung Chang Gang Memorial Hospital, Taiwan.*

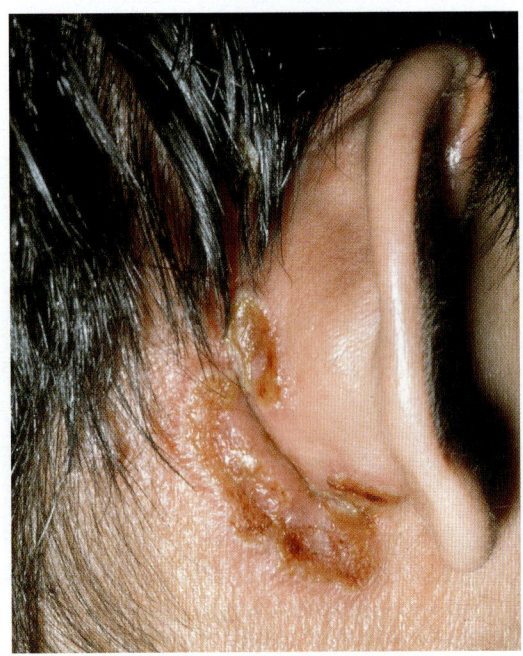

Fig. 21.33 Intraepidermal neutrophilic IgA dermatosis. *Courtesy John Stanley, MD.*

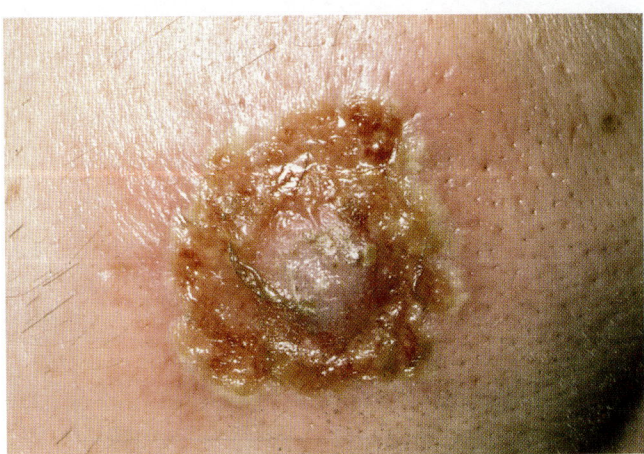

Fig. 21.32 Intraepidermal neutrophilic IgA dermatosis. *Courtesy John Stanley, MD.*

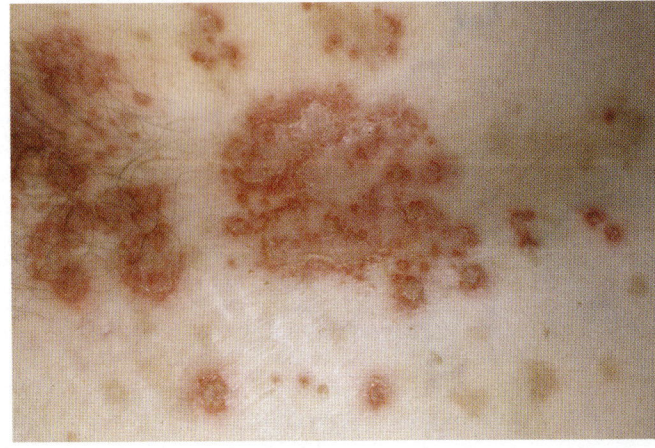

Fig. 21.34 Intraepidermal neutrophilic IgA dermatosis.

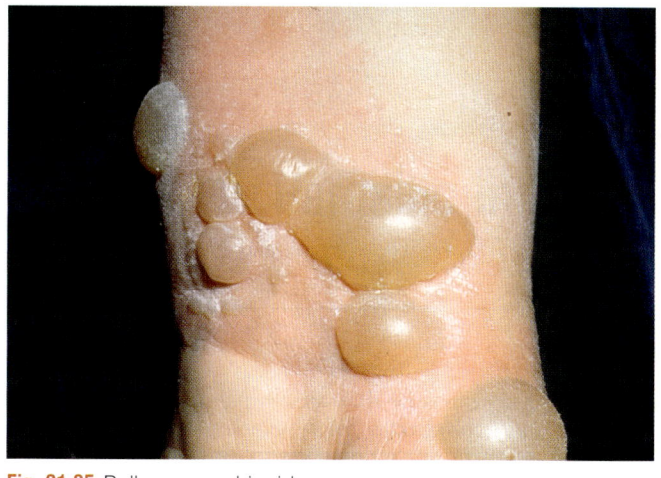

Fig. 21.35 Bullous pemphigoid.

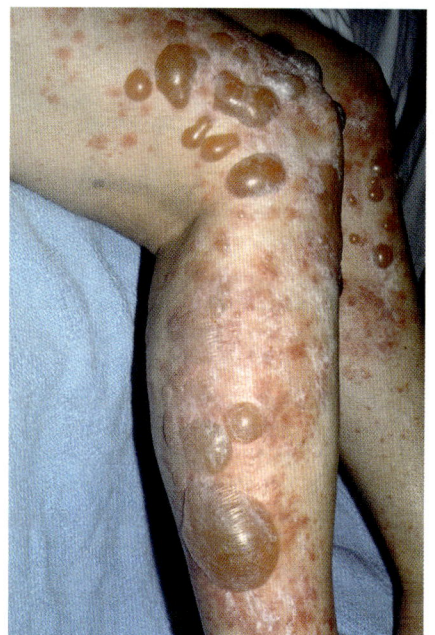

Fig. 21.36 Bullous pemphigoid.

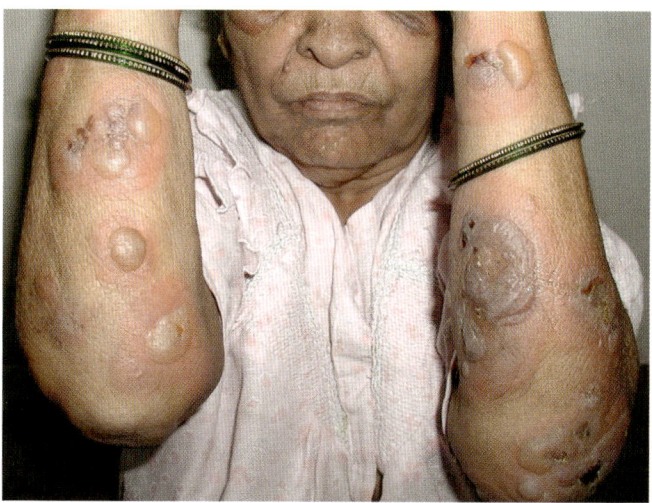

Fig. 21.37 Bullous pemphigoid. *Courtesy Shyam Verma, MBBS, DVD.*

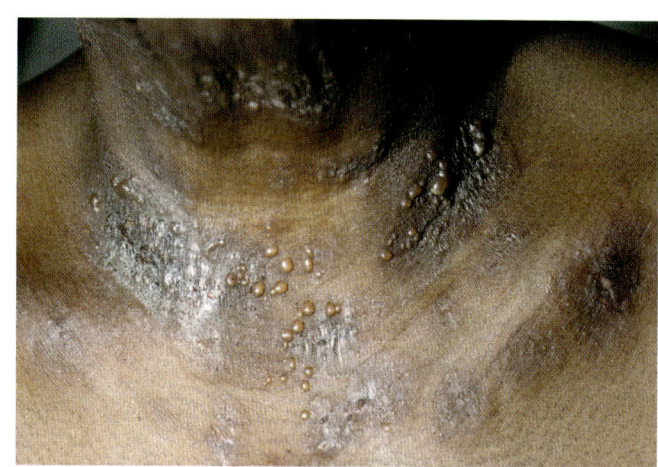

Fig. 21.38 Bullous pemphigoid.

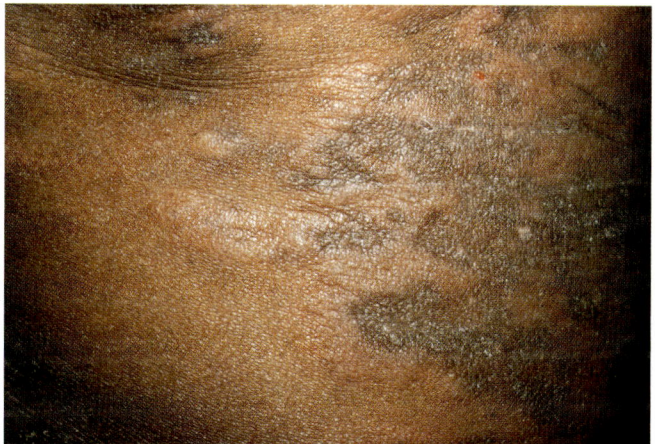

Fig. 21.39 Urticarial bullous pemphigoid.

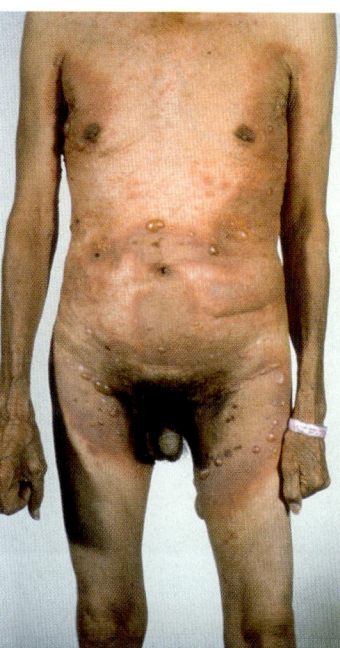

Fig. 21.40 Urticarial bullous pemphigoid with bullae.

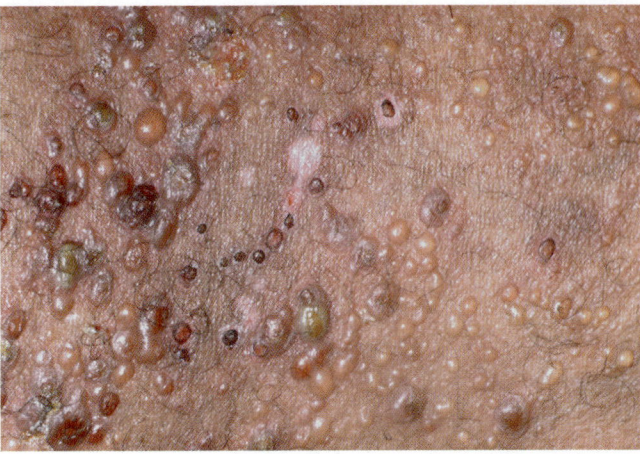

Fig. 21.41 Vesicular bullous pemphigoid. *Courtesy Steven Binnick, MD.*

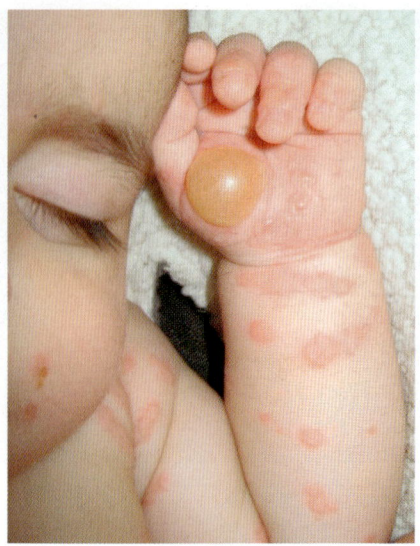

Fig. 21.42 Infantile bullous pemphigoid.

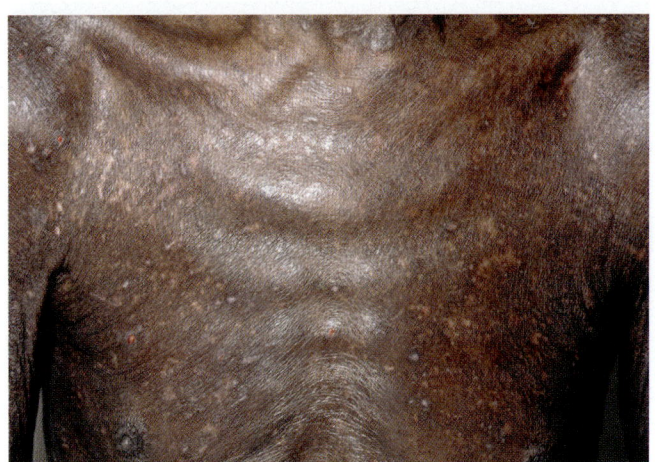

Fig. 21.43 Erythrodermic bullous pemphigoid.

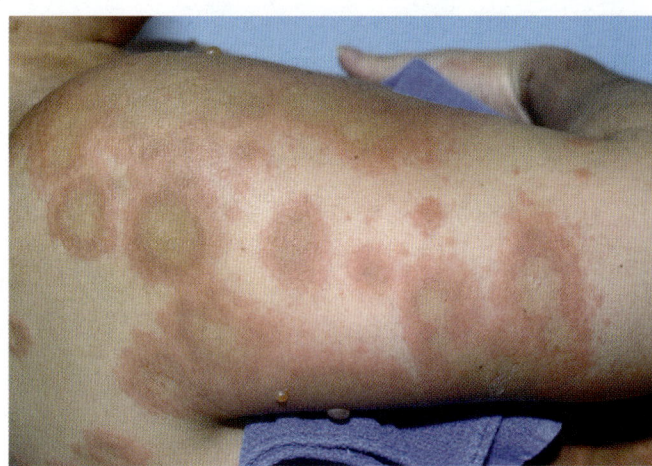

Fig. 21.44 Pemphigoid gestationis.

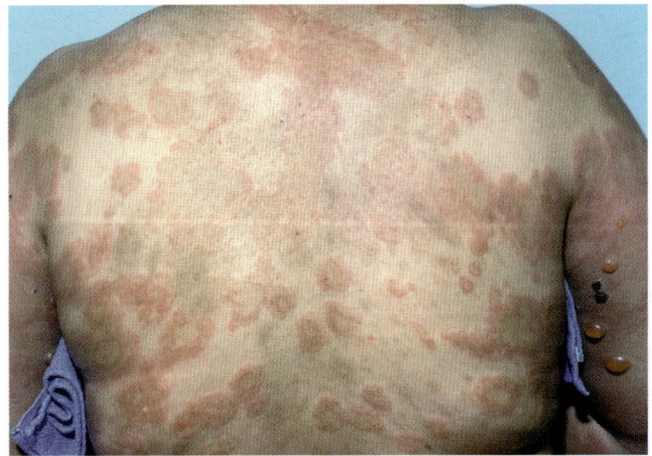

Fig. 21.45 Pemphigoid gestationis.

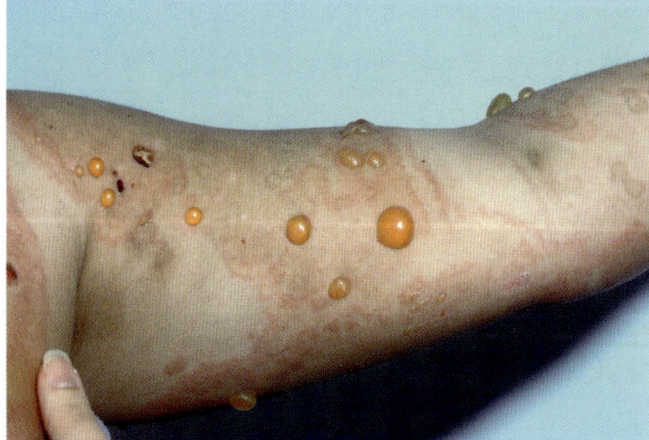

Fig. 21.46 Pemphigoid gestationis.

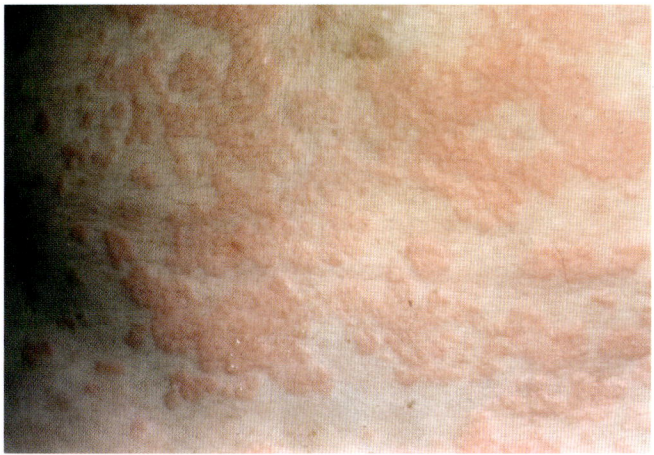
Fig. 21.47 Pemphigoid gestationis. *Courtesy Ken Greer, MD.*

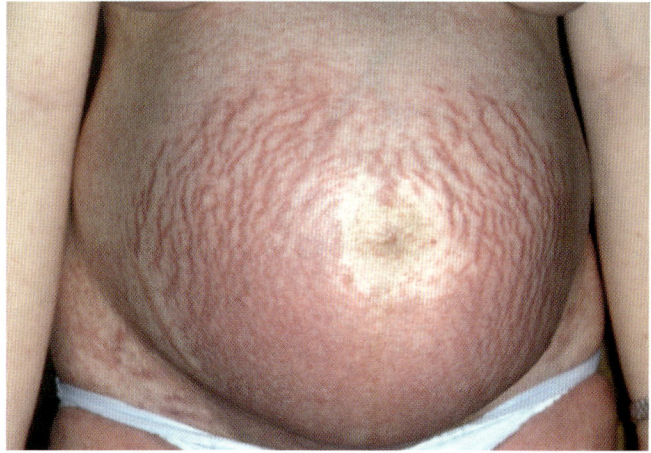
Fig. 21.48 Pruritic urticarial papules and plaques of pregnancy.

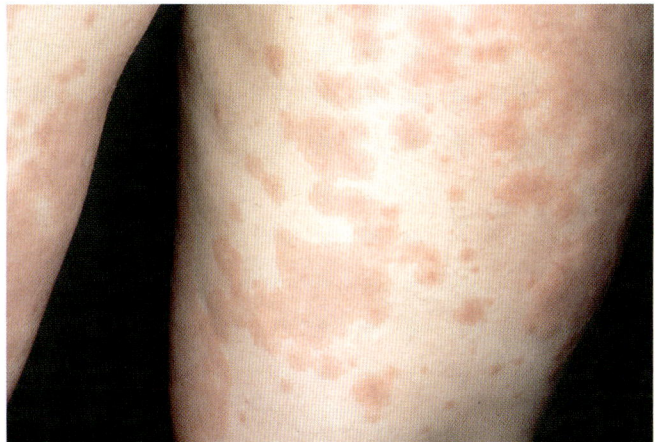
Fig. 21.49 Pruritic urticarial papules and plaques of pregnancy.

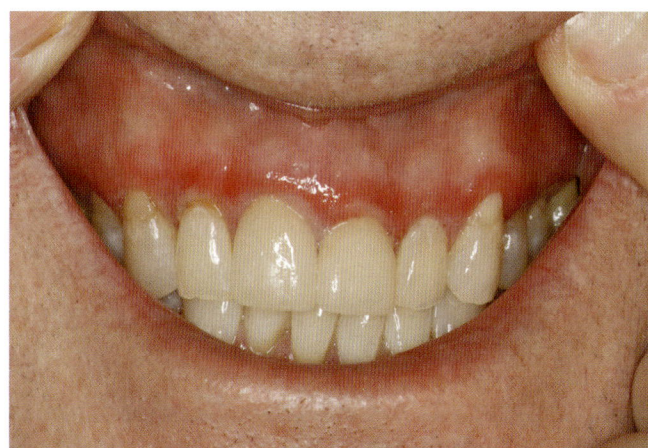
Fig. 21.50 Cicatricial pemphigoid.

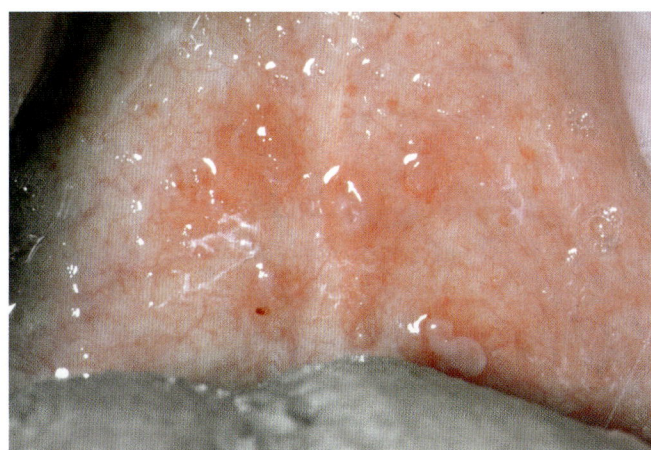
Fig. 21.51 Cicatricial pemphigoid.

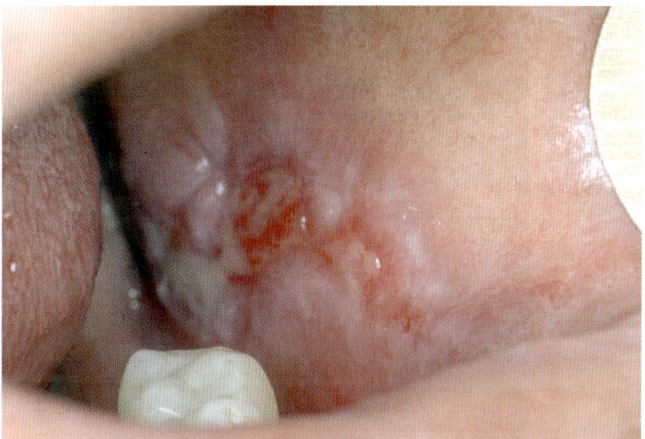
Fig. 21.52 Cicatricial pemphigoid. *Courtesy Curt Samlaska, MD.*

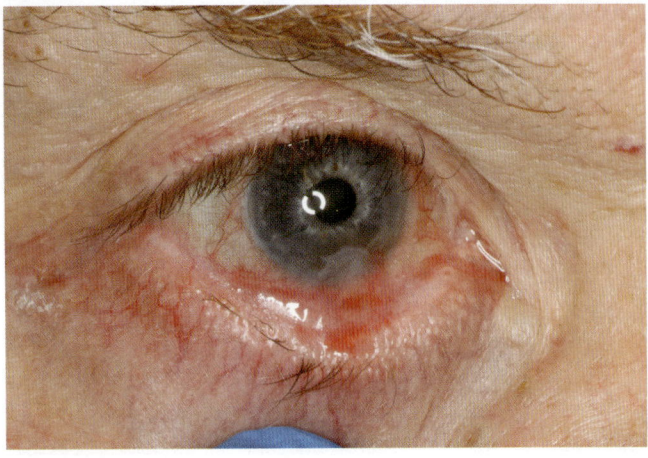

Fig. 21.53 Cicatricial pemphigoid.

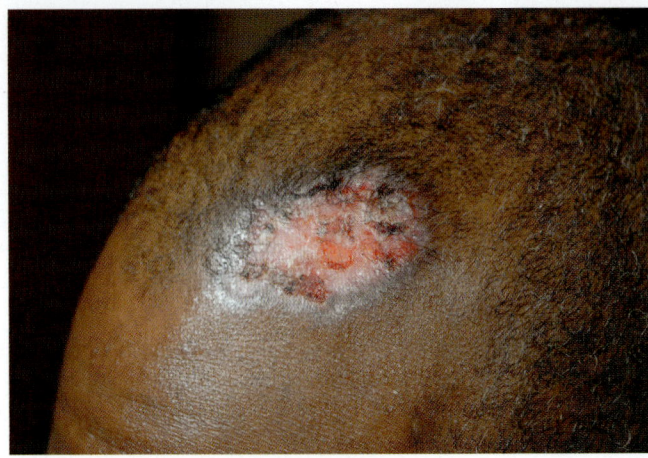

Fig. 21.54 Brunsting-Perry pemphigoid.

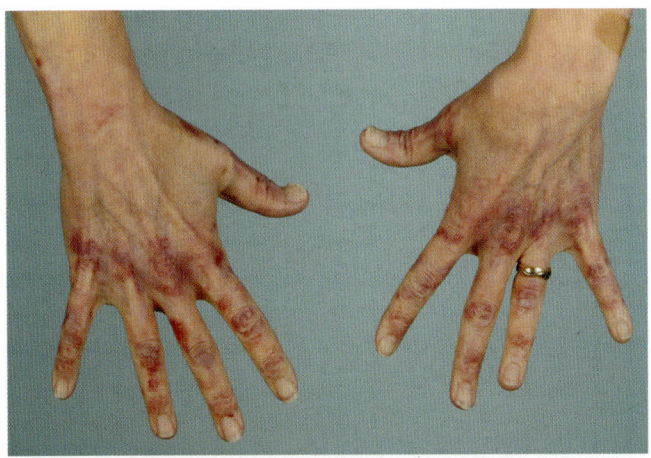

Fig. 21.55 Epidermolysis bullosa acquisita.

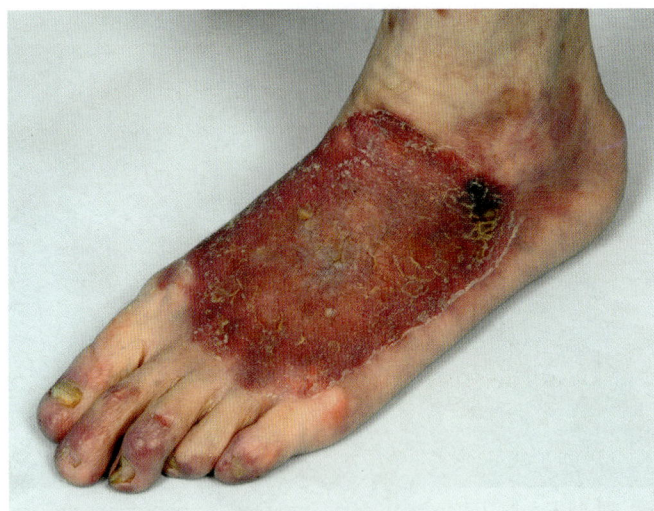

Fig. 21.56 Epidermolysis bullosa acquisita.

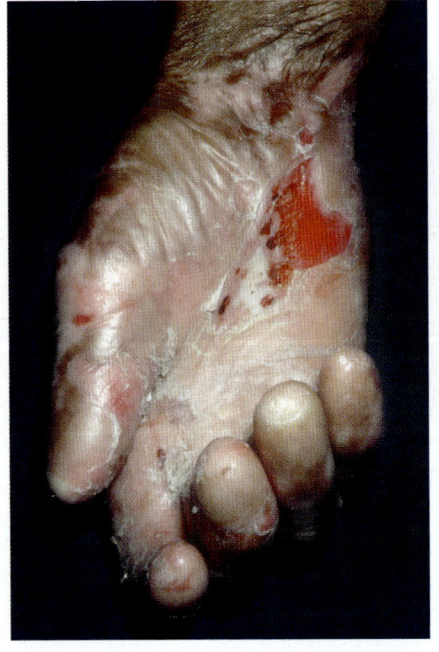

Fig. 21.57 Epidermolysis bullosa acquisita.

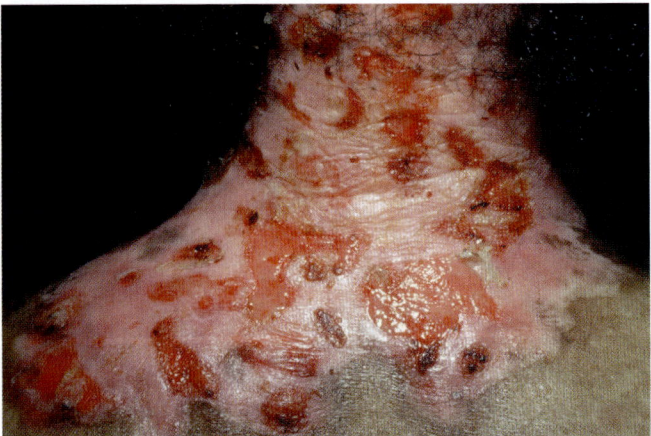

Fig. 21.58 Epidermolysis bullosa acquisita.

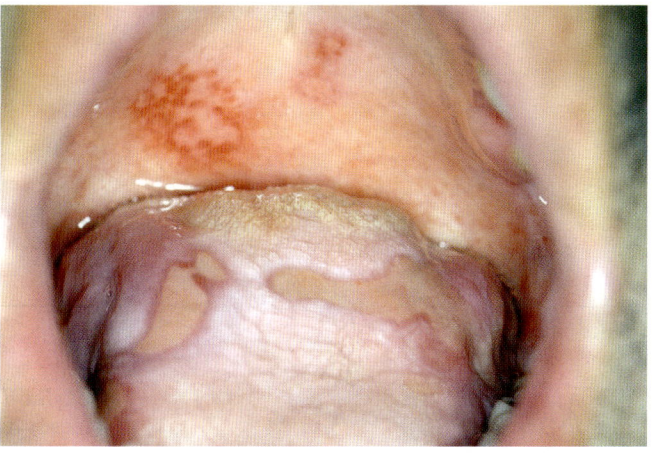

Fig. 21.59 Epidermolysis bullosa acquisita.

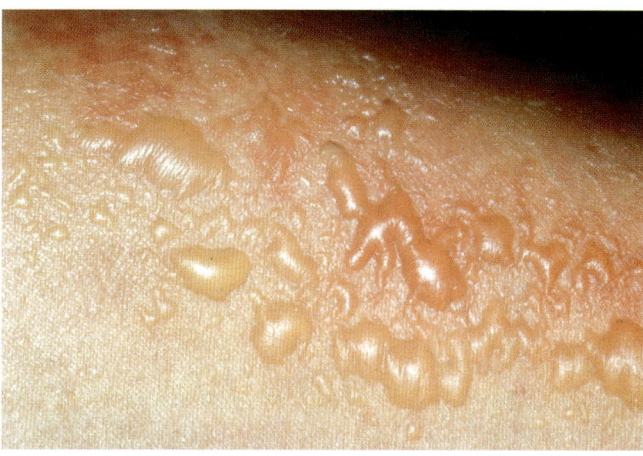

Fig. 21.60 Inflammatory epidermolysis bullosa acquisita.

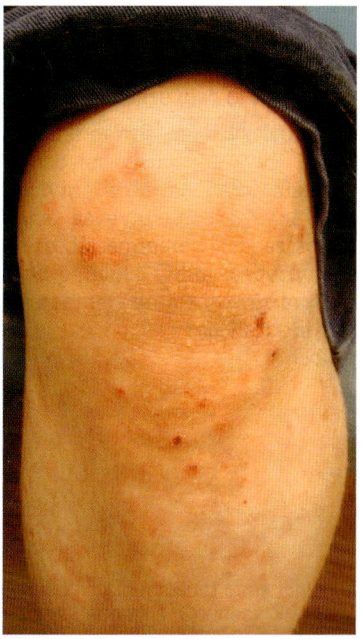

Fig. 21.61 Dermatitis herpetiformis.

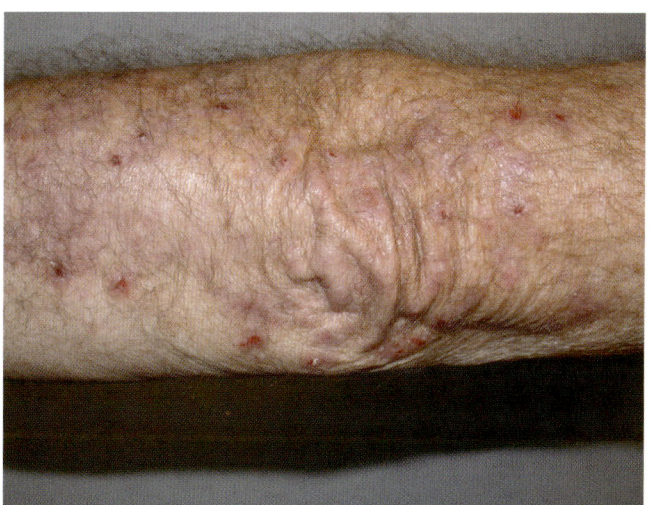

Fig. 21.62 Dermatitis herpetiformis.

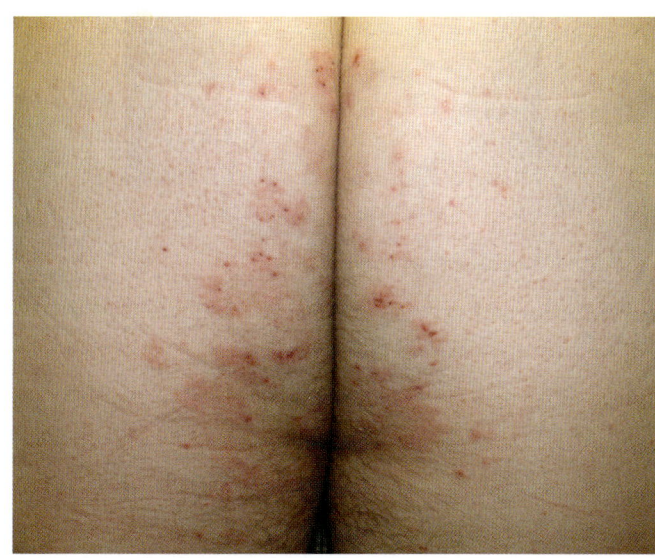

Fig. 21.63 Dermatitis herpetiformis.

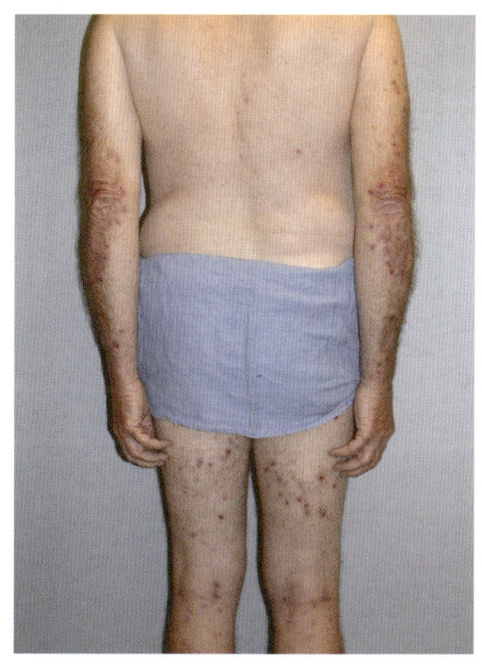

Fig. 21.64 Dermatitis herpetiformis.

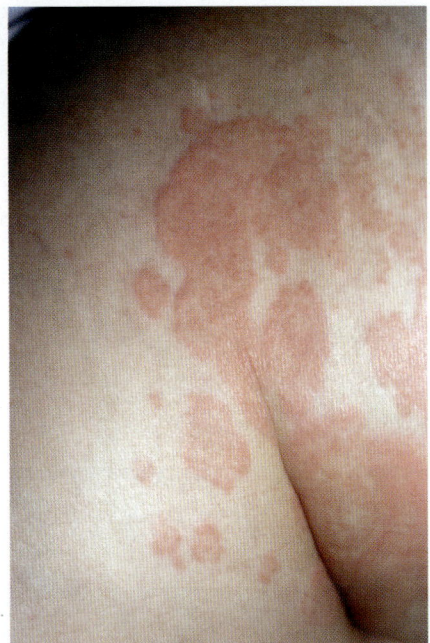

Fig. 21.65 Urticarial lesions of dermatitis herpetiformis.

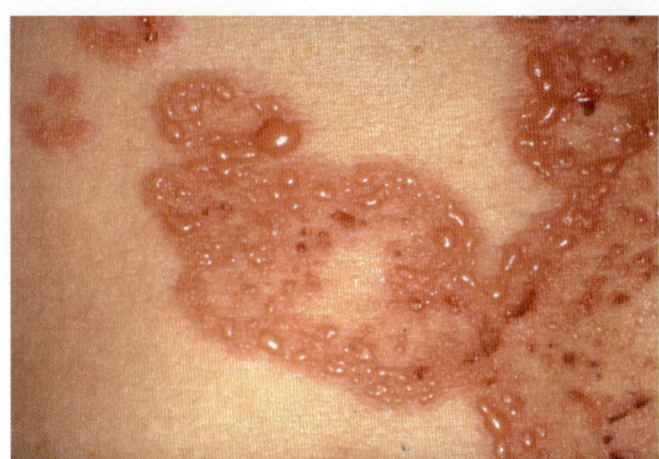

Fig. 21.66 Unusual configuration in dermatitis herpetiformis.

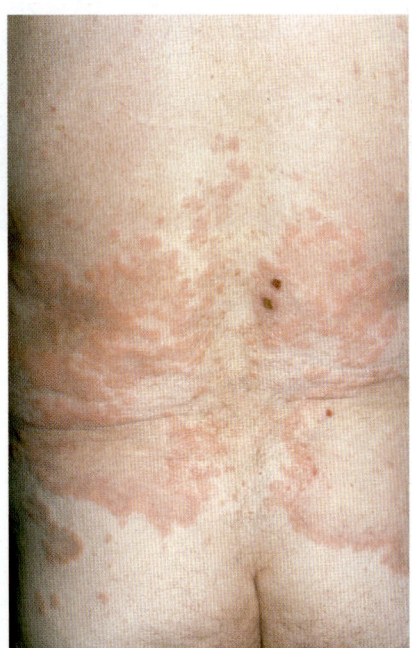

Fig. 21.67 Adult linear IgA disease, urticarial type.

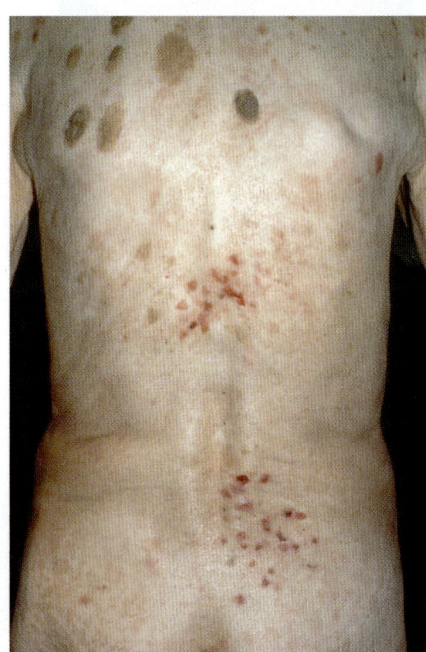

Fig. 21.68 Adult linear IgA disease, which is indistinguishable from dermatitis herpetiformis.

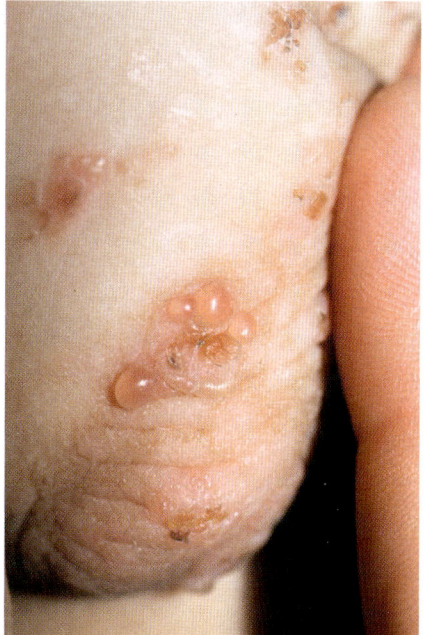

Fig. 21.69 Childhood linear IgA disease.

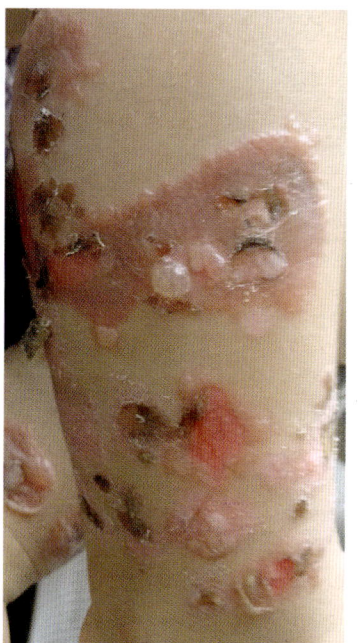

Fig. 21.70 Childhood linear IgA disease.

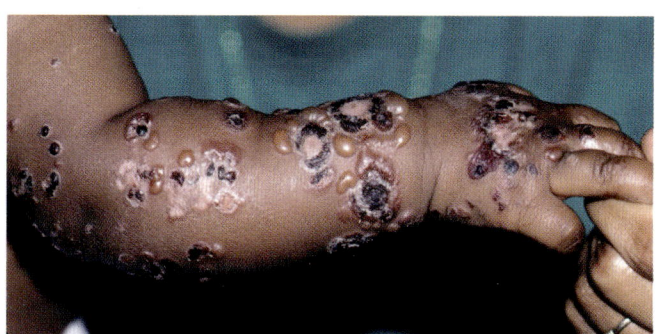

Fig. 21.71 Childhood linear IgA disease. *Courtesy Paul Honig, MD.*

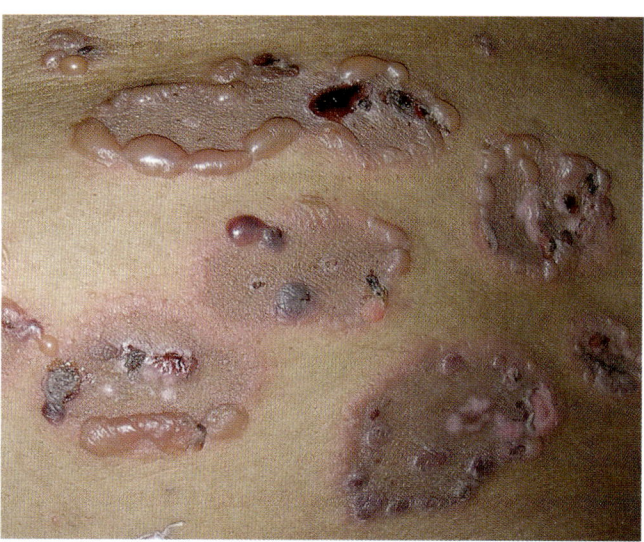

Fig. 21.72 Childhood linear IgA disease. *Courtesy Debabrata Bandyopadhyay, MD.*

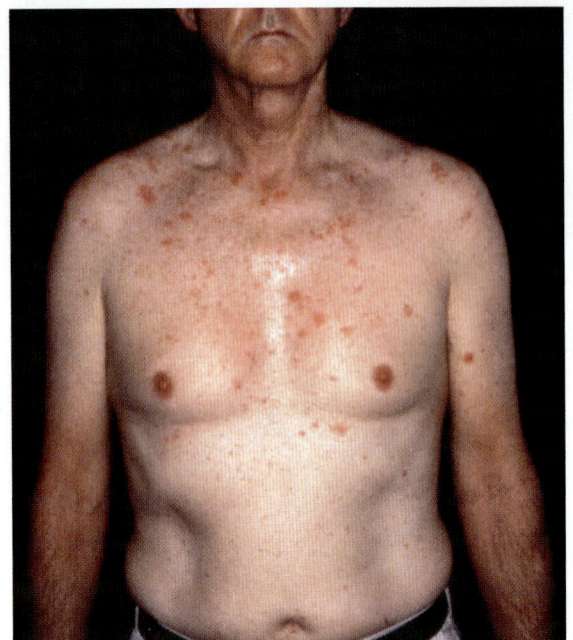

Fig. 21.73 Transient acantholytic dermatosis.

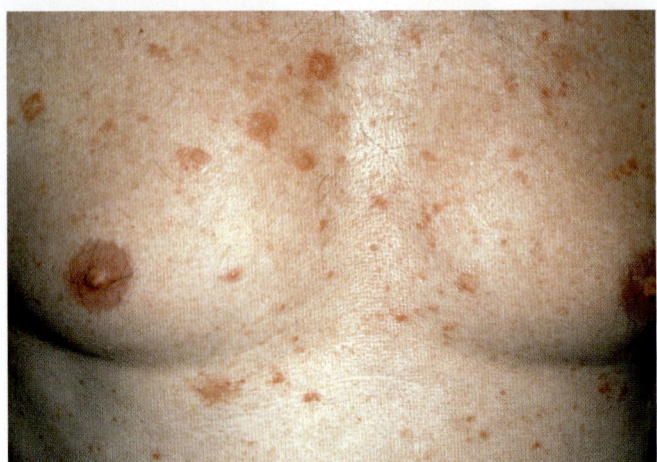

Fig. 21.74 Transient acantholytic dermatosis.

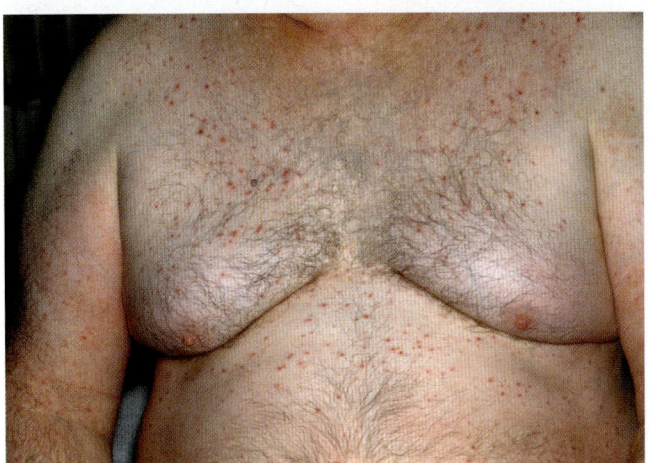

Fig. 21.75 Transient acantholytic dermatosis. *Courtesy Steven Binnick, MD.*

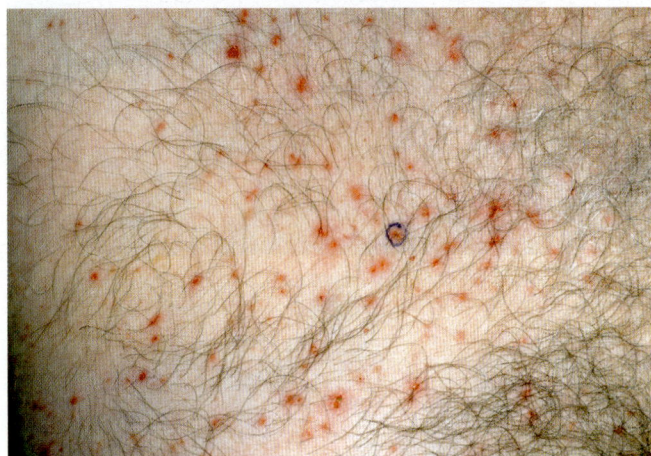

Fig. 21.76 Transient acantholytic dermatosis. *Courtesy Steven Binnick, MD.*

Nutritional Diseases 22

A deficiency or excess of certain required vitamins or minerals can cause specific findings in the skin, hair, nails, and mucosae. This chapter provides images of many of these findings, both common and rare.

Deficiencies in some essential nutrients cause a particular constellation of mucocutaneous and systemic signs and symptoms worth outlining. These include the bleeding gums, corkscrew hairs, easy bruising, and perifollicular hemorrhages seen in the setting of vitamin C deficiency, or scurvy. In pellagra, or vitamin B_3 (niacin) deficiency, a combination of a photodistributed eruption appearing sunburn-like, scaly, hyperpigmented, or atrophic can be seen along with protracted diarrhea, weakness, dementia, paresthesias, and depression. Kwashiorkor, or protein-energy malnutrition, may present with general lightening of the skin and hair, a scaly eruption with superficial peeling of skin resembling flaking paint, and a dermatitis with cracked skin resembling "crazy pavement" in the setting of a patient with signs of edema and poor growth. These nutritional deficiencies can occur due to general malnutrition where food is scarce, but can also occur in individuals with restricted diets or eating disorders (e.g. anorexia nervosa). Lastly, malabsorption states as found in inflammatory bowel diseases can lead to nutritional deficiencies.

Another relatively common deficiency that presents most commonly during infancy is zinc deficiency leading to acrodermatitis enteropathica. In this condition, scaly and erosive patches tend to be well demarcated with heaped-up, sometimes crusted, borders that consistently affect the perioral region, distal extremities, and groin. Affected infants with acrodermatitis enteropathica are notably irritable.

Acrodermatitis enteropathica-like conditions can be seen in some inherited metabolic conditions, including those leading to biotin deficiency.

This portion of the atlas highlights these and other nutrition-related diseases that affect the skin, hair, nails, and mucosal surfaces.

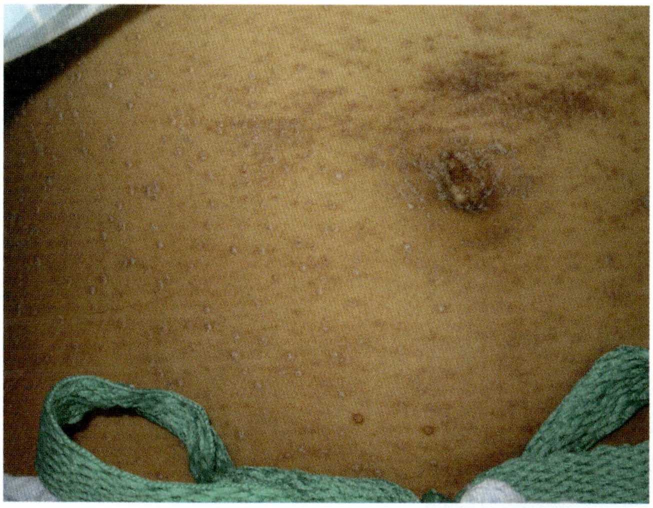

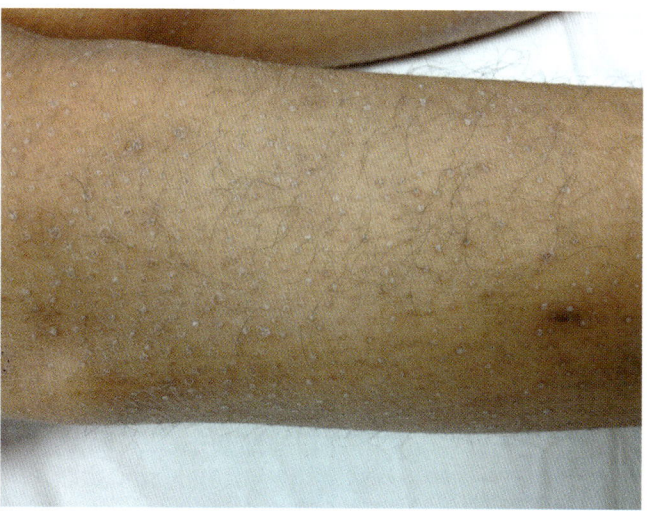

Fig. 22.2 Phrynoderma in a patient with inflammatory bowel disease.

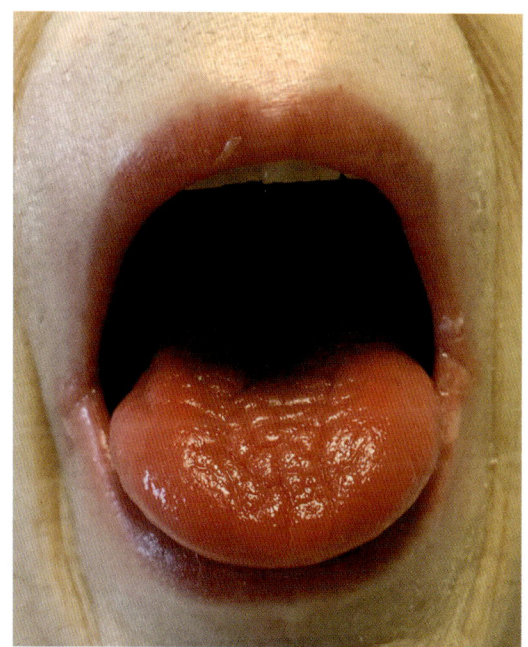

Fig. 22.1 Phrynoderma in a patient with inflammatory bowel disease.

Fig. 22.3 Atrophic glossitis as seen in vitamin B deficiencies.

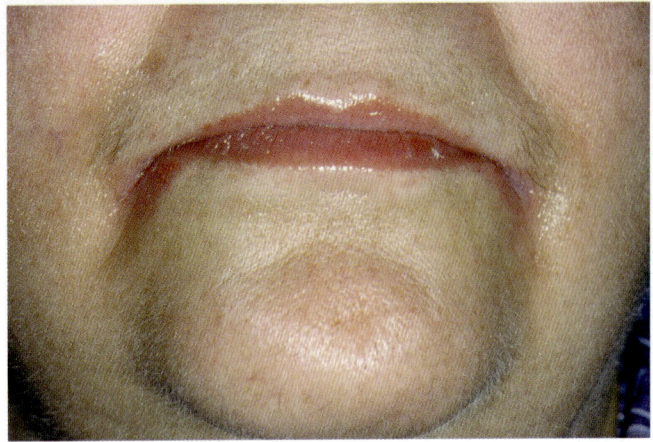

Fig. 22.4 Perlèche as seen in vitamin B deficiencies.

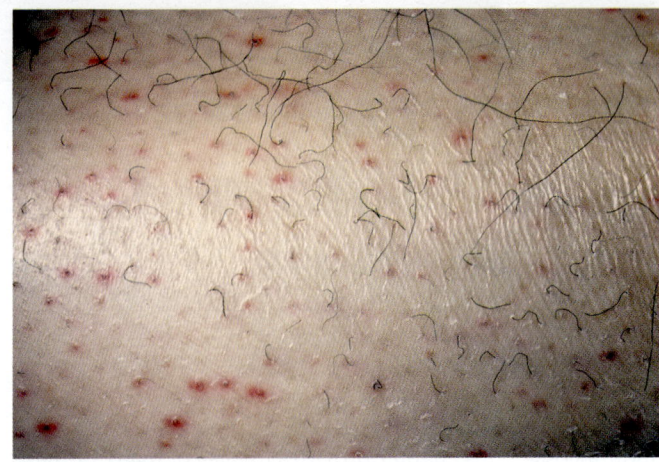

Fig. 22.5 Scurvy.

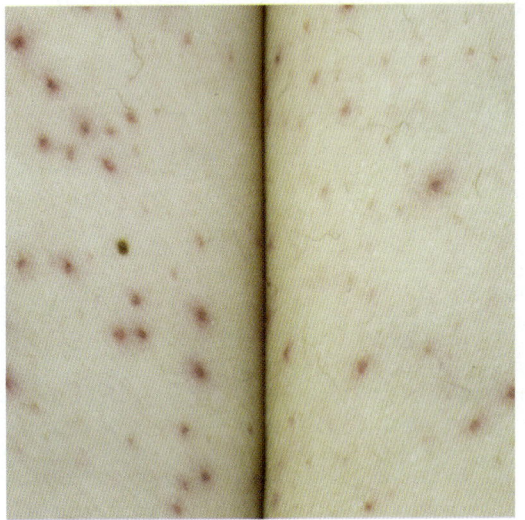

Fig. 22.6 Scurvy.

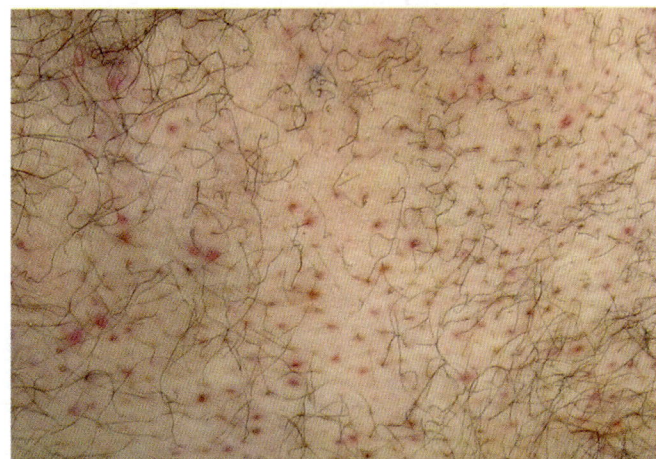

Fig. 22.7 Scurvy.

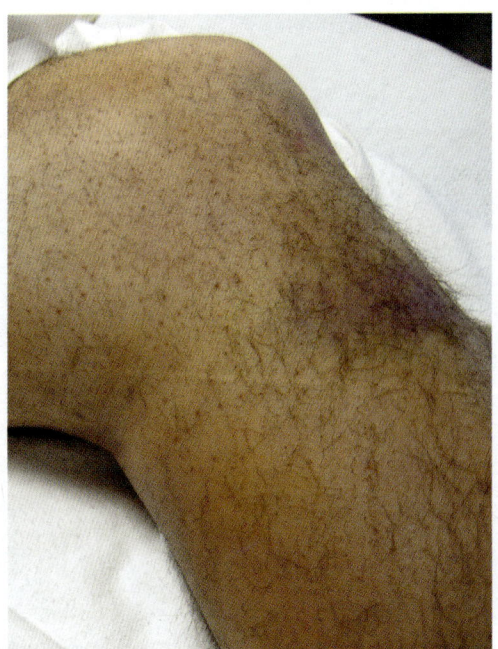

Fig. 22.8 Scurvy.

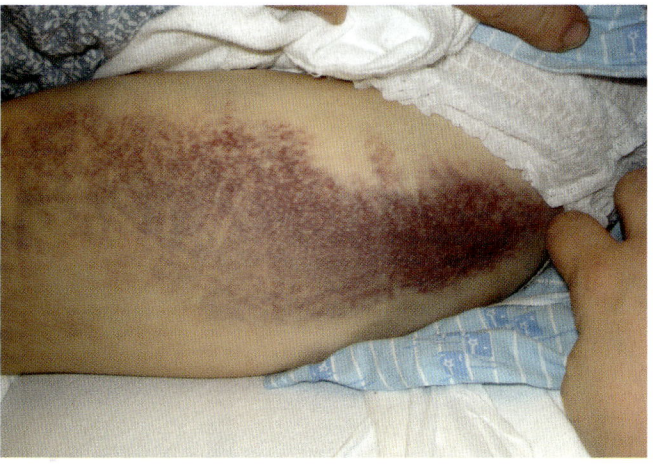

Fig. 22.10 Scurvy.

Fig. 22.9 Scurvy.

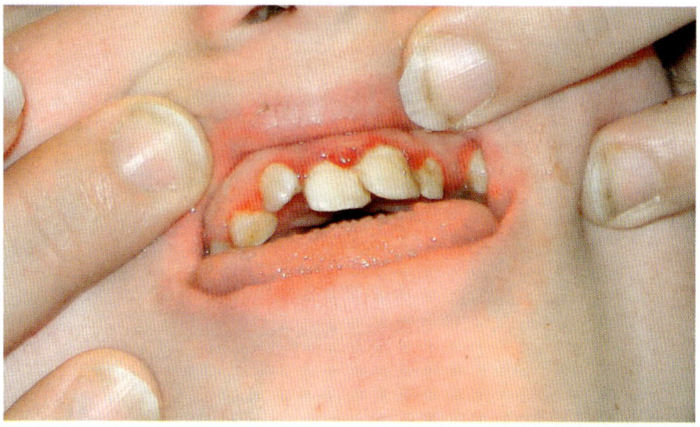

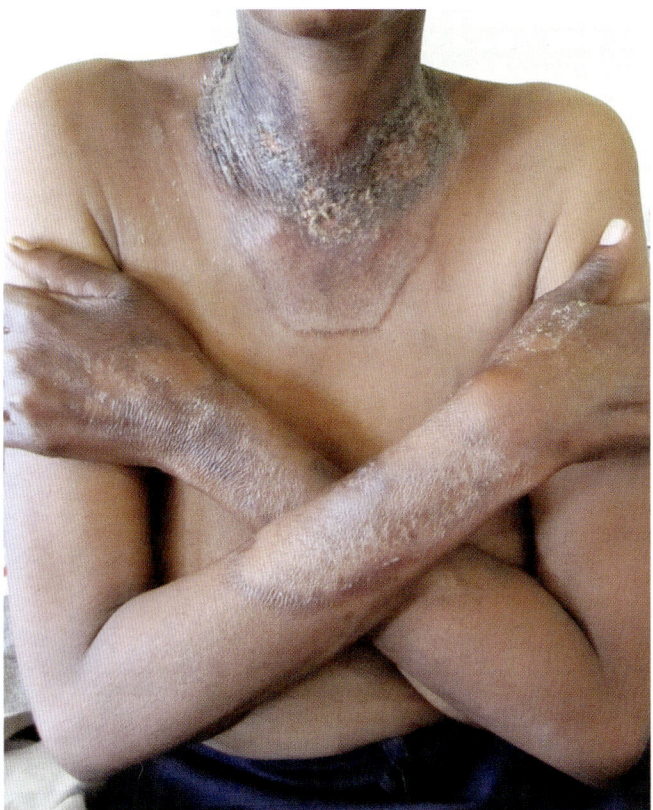

Fig. 22.11 Pellagra. *Courtesy Michelle Weir, MD.*

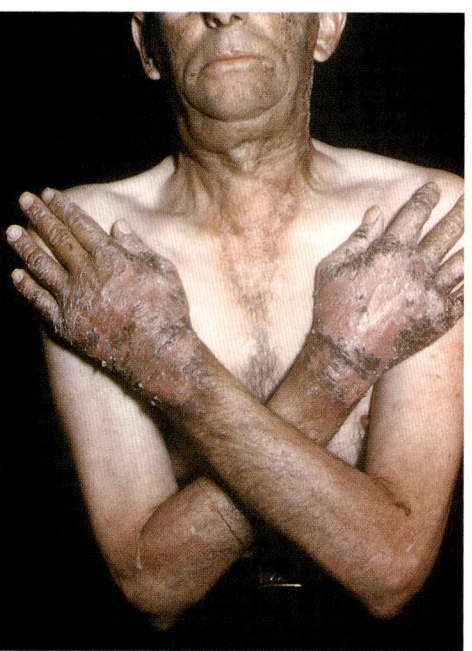

Fig. 22.12 Pellagra. *Courtesy Steven Binnick, MD.*

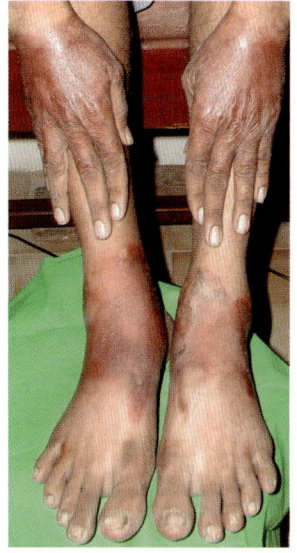

Fig. 22.13 Pellagra. *Courtesy Shyam Verma, MBBS, DVD.*

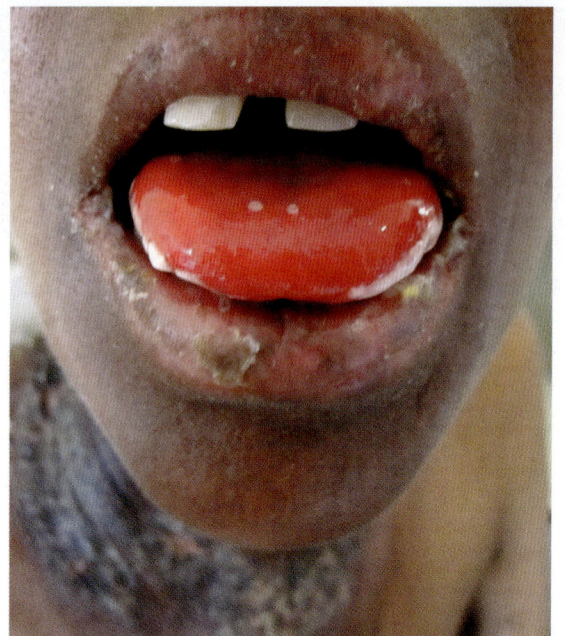

Fig. 22.14 Pellagra. *Courtesy Michelle Weir, MD.*

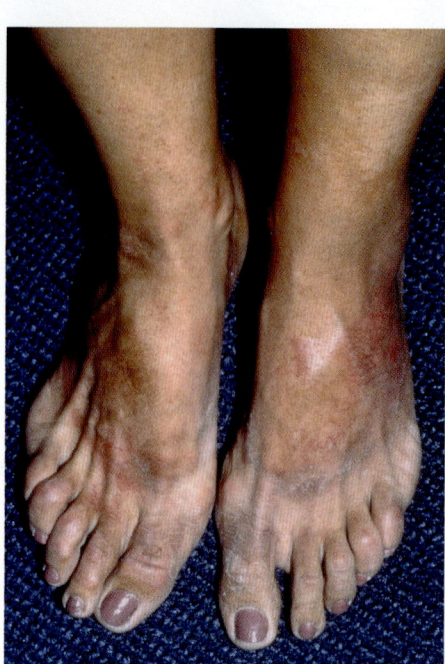

Fig. 22.15 Isoniazid-induced pellagra-like reaction.

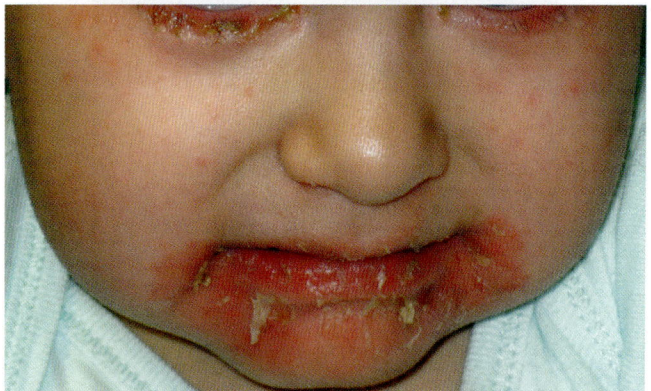

Fig. 22.16 Multiple carboxylase deficiency.

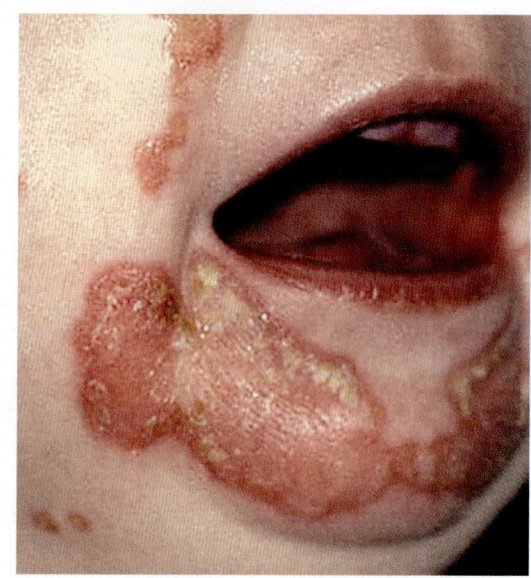

Fig. 22.17 Acrodermatitis enteropathica. *Courtesy Paul Honig, MD.*

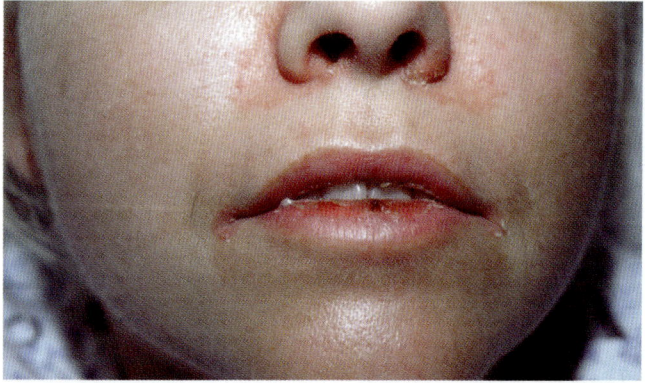

Fig. 22.18 Acrodermatitis enteropathica.

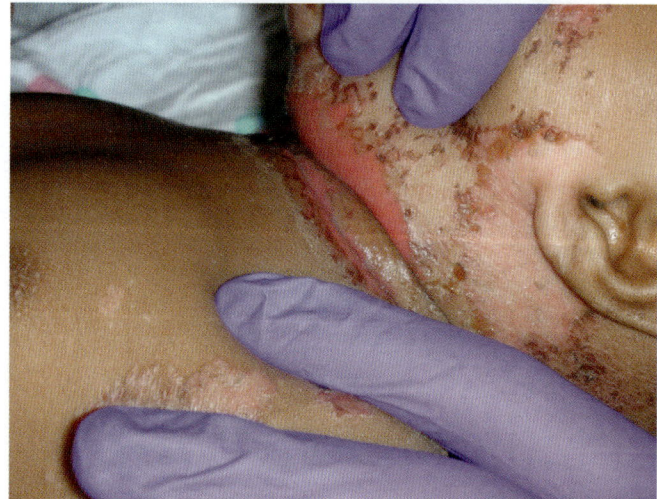

Fig. 22.19 Acrodermatitis enteropathica.

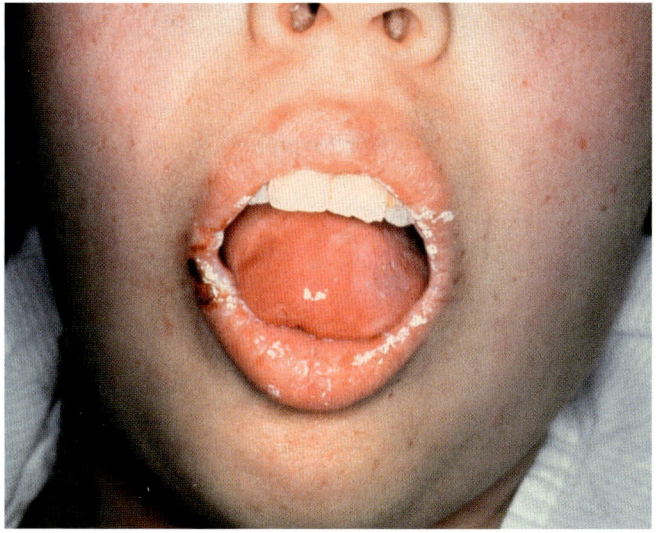

Fig. 22.20 Acrodermatitis enteropathica.

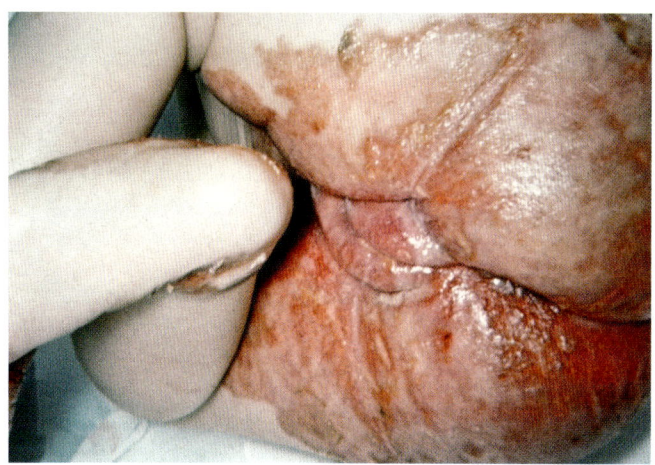

Fig. 22.21 Acrodermatitis enteropathica.

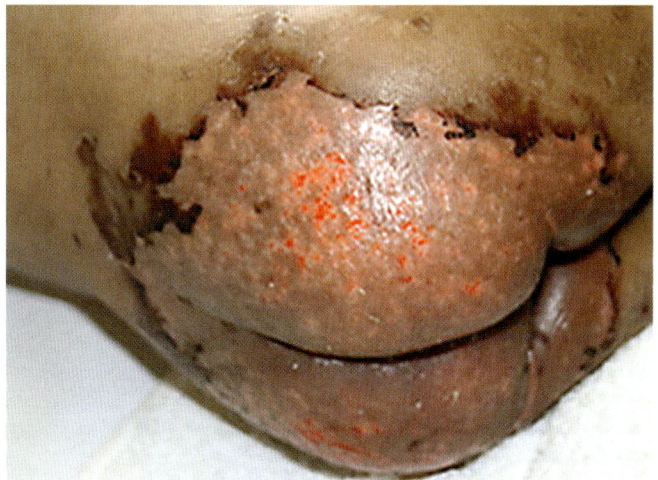

Fig. 22.22 Acrodermatitis enteropathica. *Courtesy Carrie Kovarik, MD.*

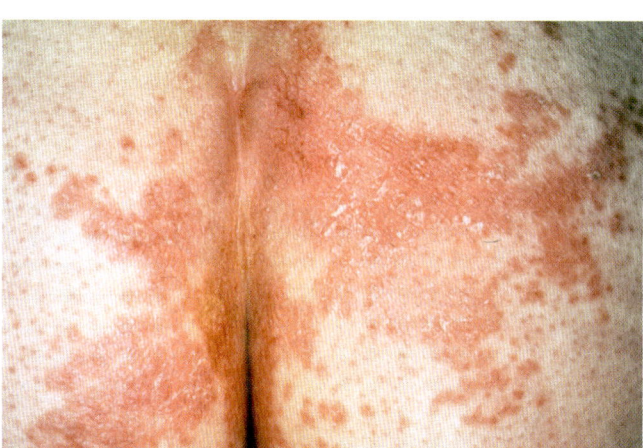

Fig. 22.23 Acrodermatitis enteropathica.

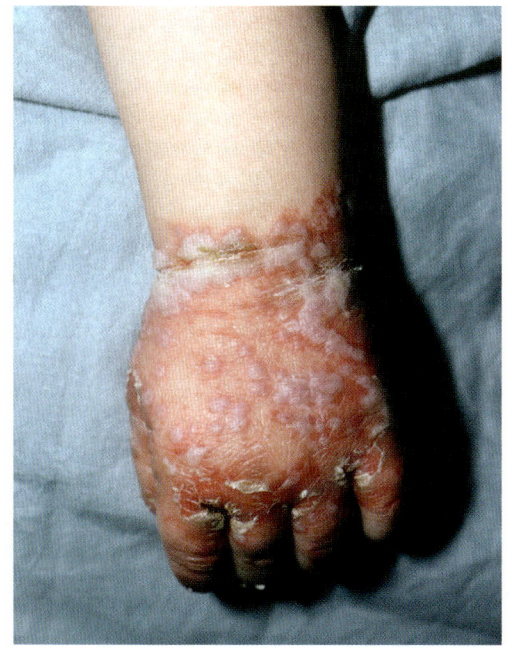

Fig. 22.24 Acrodermatitis enteropathica.

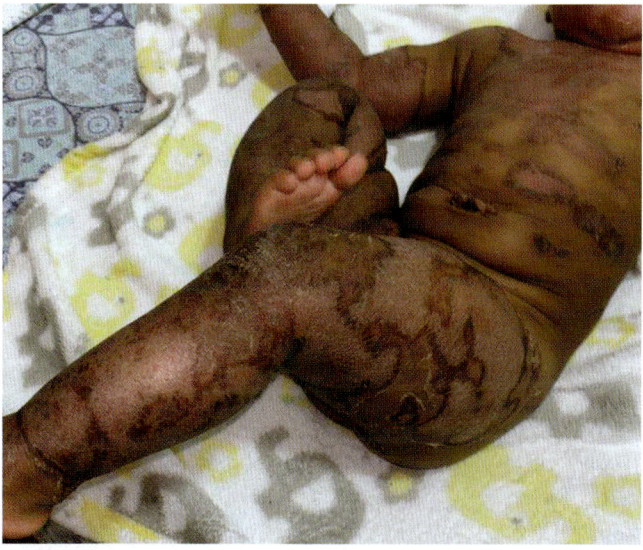

Fig. 22.25 Acrodermatitis enteropathica.

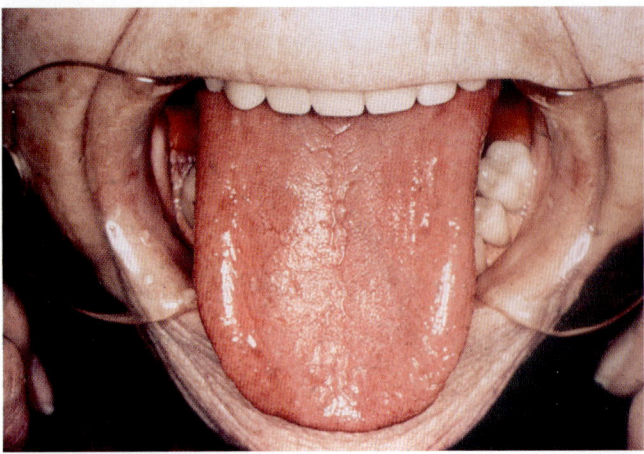

Fig. 22.26 Smooth tongue in anemia.

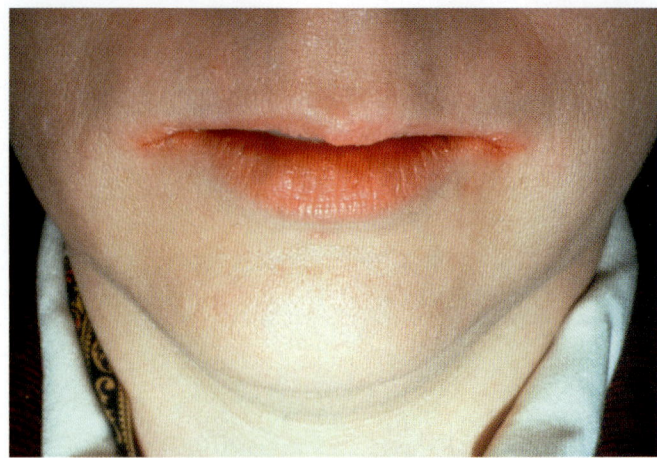

Fig. 22.27 Angular cheilitis as seen in iron deficiency.

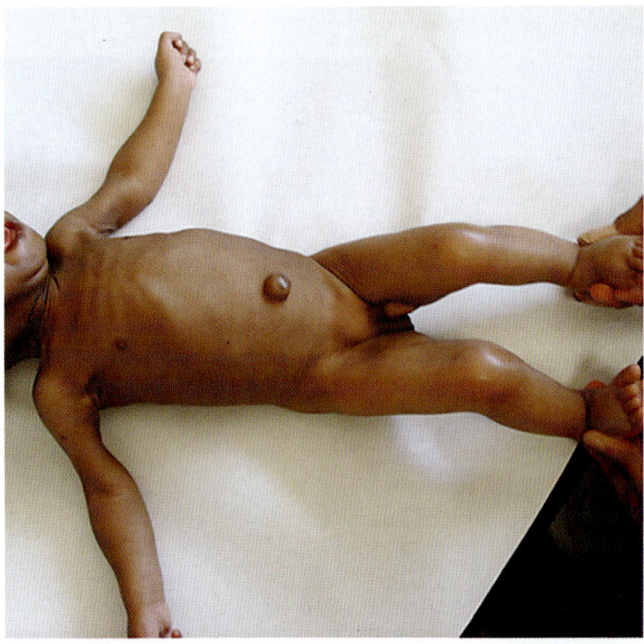

Fig. 22.28 Marasmus.

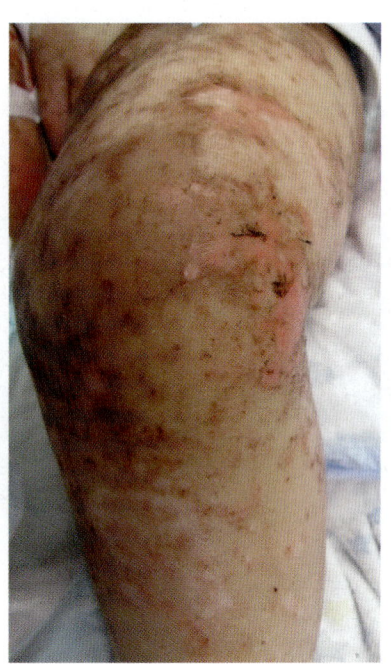

Fig. 22.29 Kwashiorkor. *Courtesy Campbell Stewart, MD.*

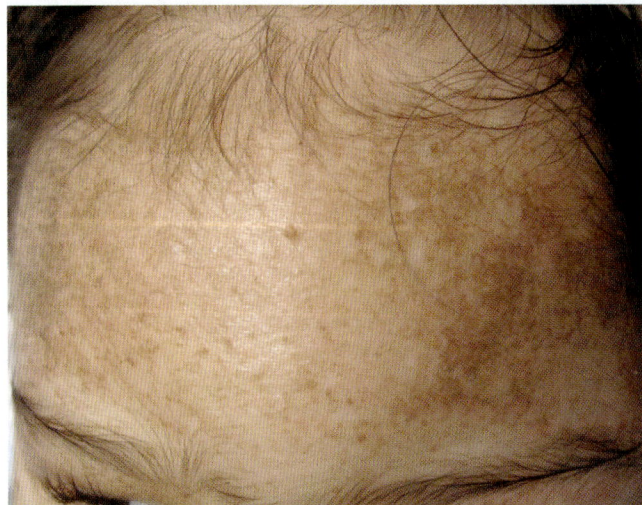

Fig. 22.30 Kwashiorkor. *Courtesy Campbell Stewart, MD.*

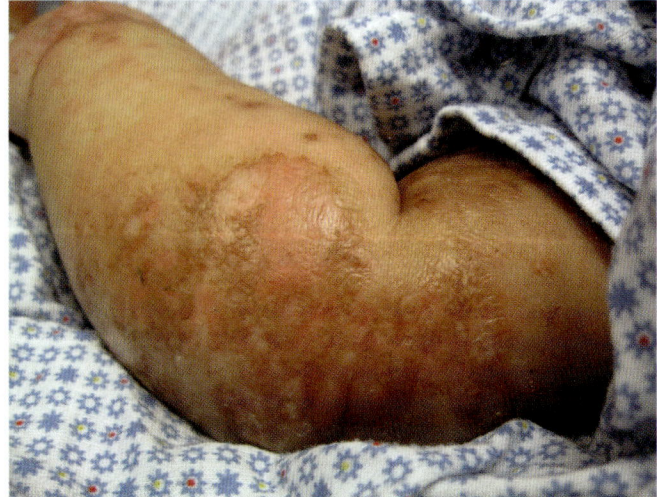

Fig. 22.31 Kwashiorkor. *Courtesy Campbell Stewart, MD.*

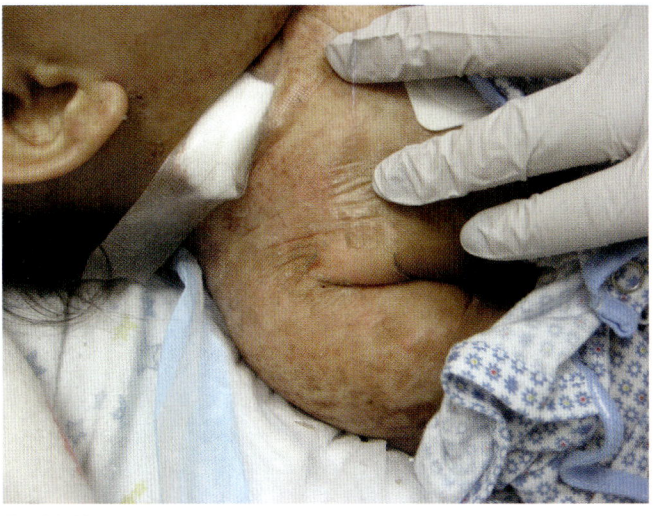

Fig. 22.32 Kwashiorkor.

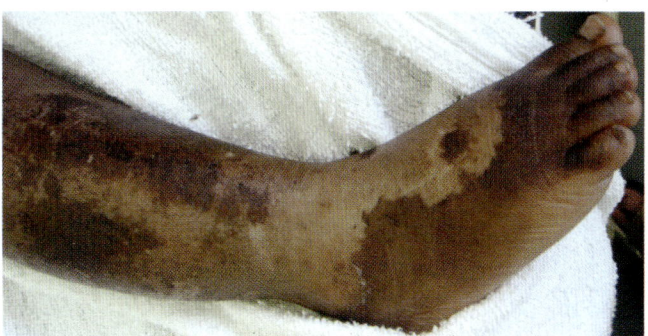

Fig. 22.33 Kwashiorkor. *Courtesy Carrie Kovarik, MD.*

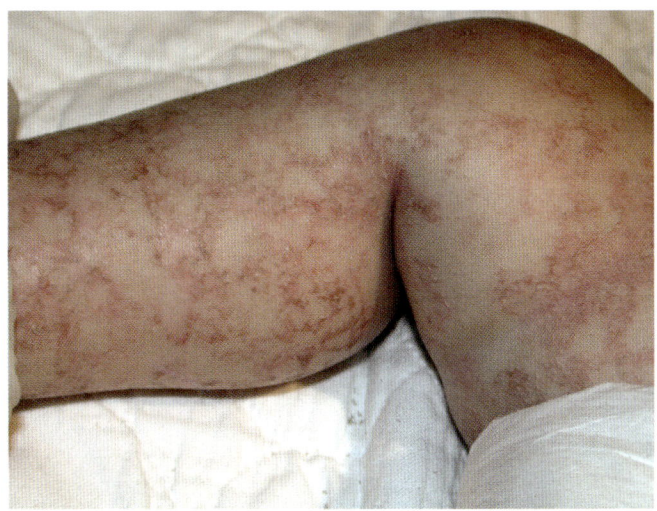

Fig. 22.34 Kwashiorkor.

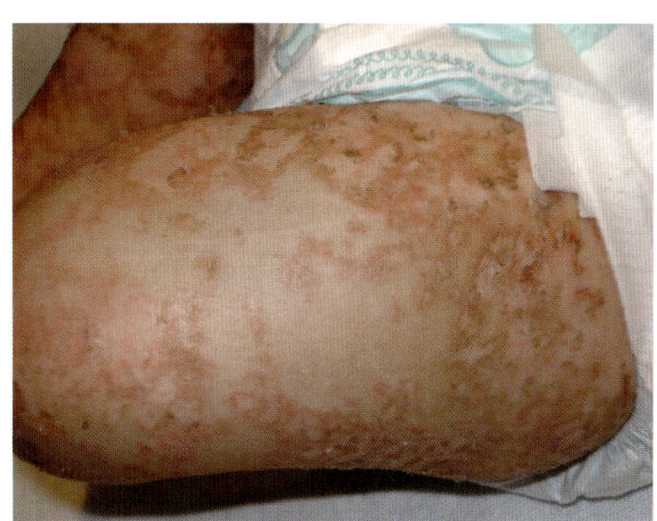

Fig. 22.35 Kwashiorkor.

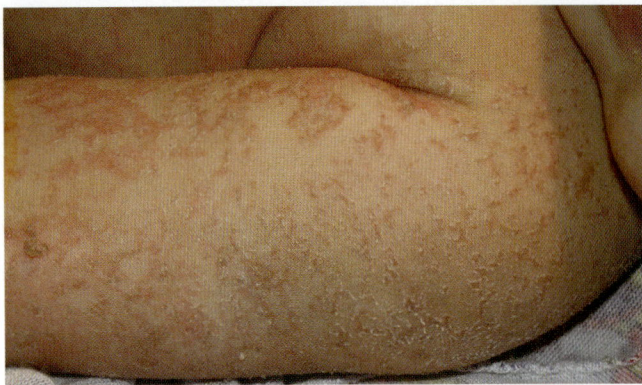

Fig. 22.36 Kwashiorkor.

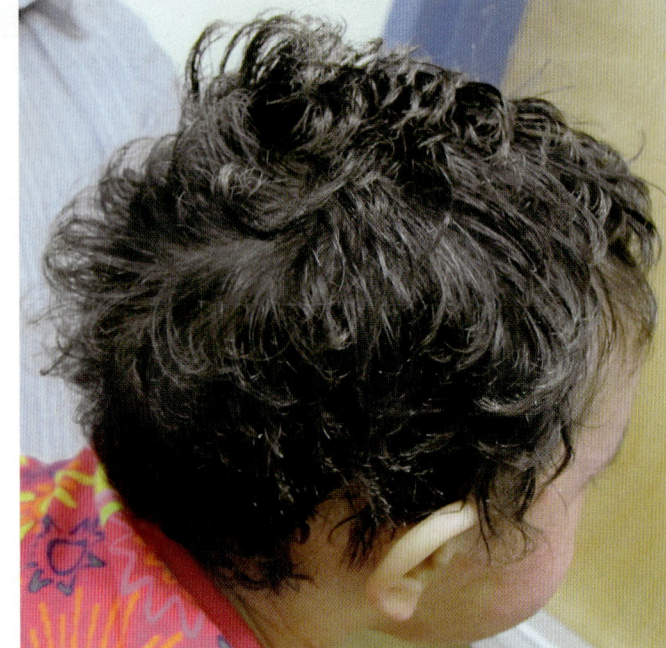

Fig. 22.37 Kwashiorkor flag sign.

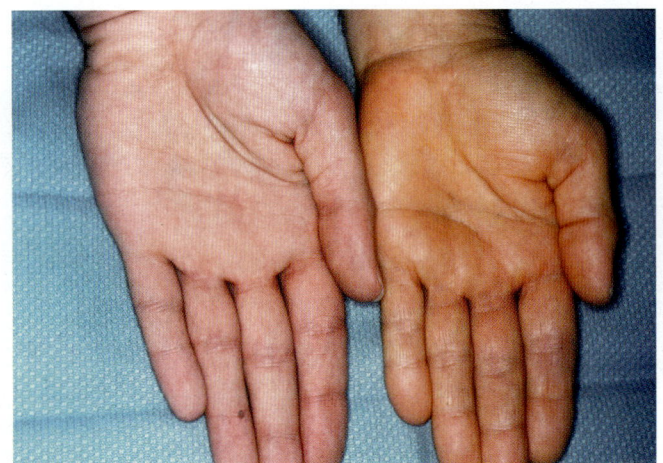

Fig. 22.38 Carotenemia.

Diseases of Subcutaneous Fat 23

Panniculitis presents with deep erythematous nodules, induration, and tenderness. Clinical lesions of erythema nodosum can appear as deep-seated, erythematous, tender nodules or can resemble bruises, giving rise to the term *erythema contusiforme*. The lesions tend to be bilateral except in erythema nodosum migrans, which is generally unilateral and slowly expands to form an annular plaque.

Erythema induratum favors the calves, and ulceration is frequent. Oily fluid often drains from the ulcers. Pancreatic panniculitis presents as indurated plaques, most commonly on the lower legs. The subcutaneous fat elsewhere may also be affected, and multiple areas may be affected. Tenderness of the ankles is commonly reported. Another form of panniculitis is subcutaneous fat necrosis of the newborn, which also presents as hard, indurated areas and demonstrates characteristic intracellular crystalline rosettes histologically.

Lipodermatosclerosis represents ischemic fat necrosis associated with venous stasis. Early lesions present as tender nodules of the lower leg. Over time, the skin becomes erythematous and indurated, with constriction of the lower leg giving the appearance of an inverted champagne bottle. Factitial and infectious panniculitis range in appearance from erythematous nodules to draining indurated plaques, whereas lipodystrophies present with loss of subcutaneous fat, giving a gaunt and muscular appearance. This section of the atlas will focus on the range of cutaneous findings that accompany diseases of the fat.

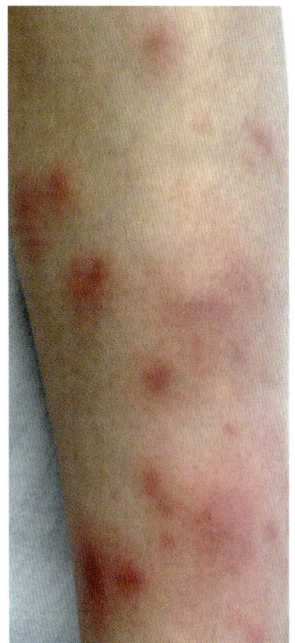

Fig. 23.2 Erythema nodosum.

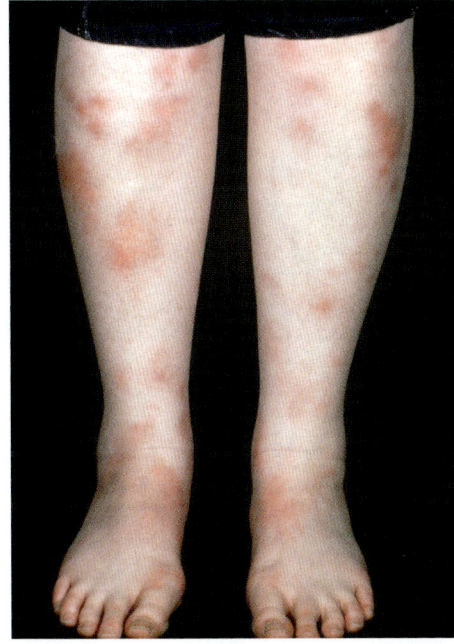

Fig. 23.1 Erythema nodosum. *Courtesy Scott Norton, MD.*

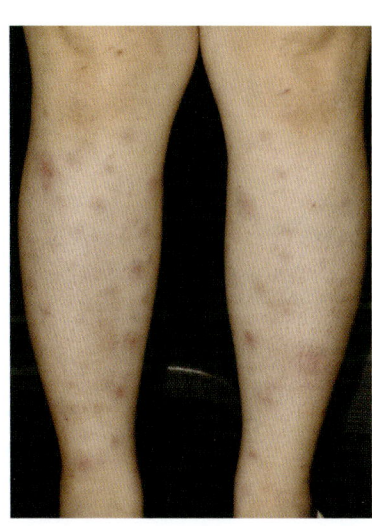

Fig. 23.3 Erythema nodosum. *Courtesy National Cheng Kung University, Taiwan.*

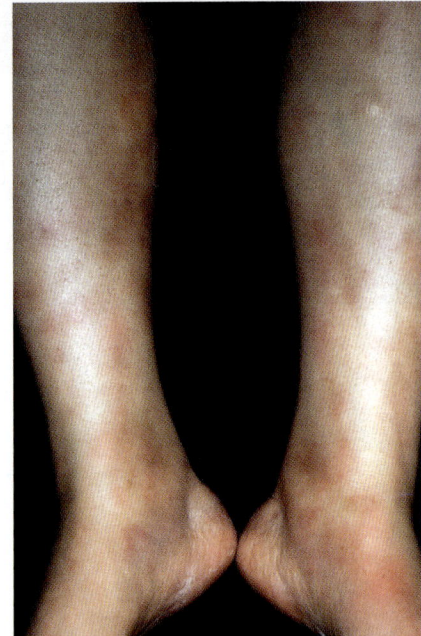

Fig. 23.4 Erythema nodosum.

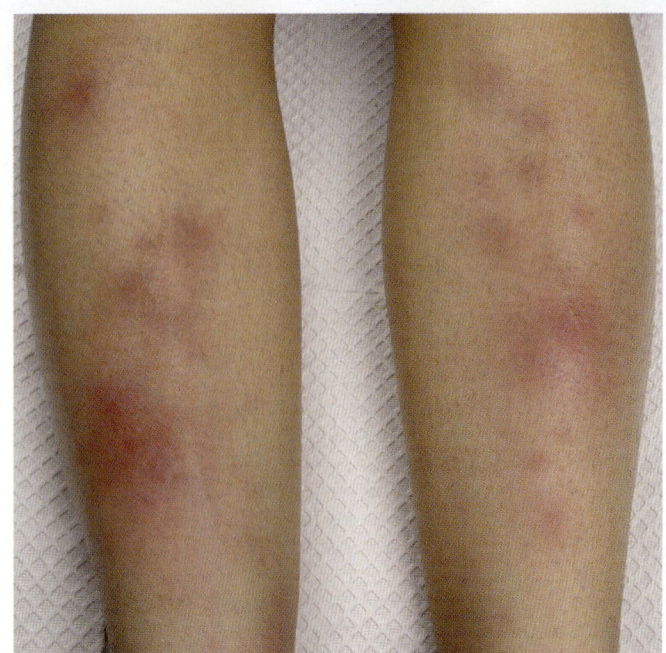

Fig. 23.5 Erythema nodosum.

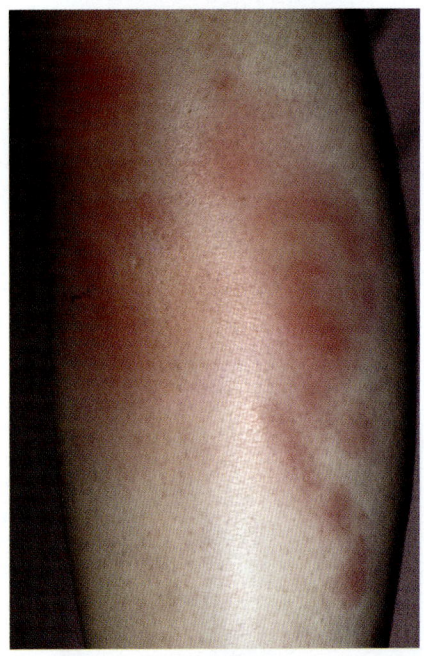

Fig. 23.6 Erythema nodosum. *Courtesy Steven Binnick, MD.*

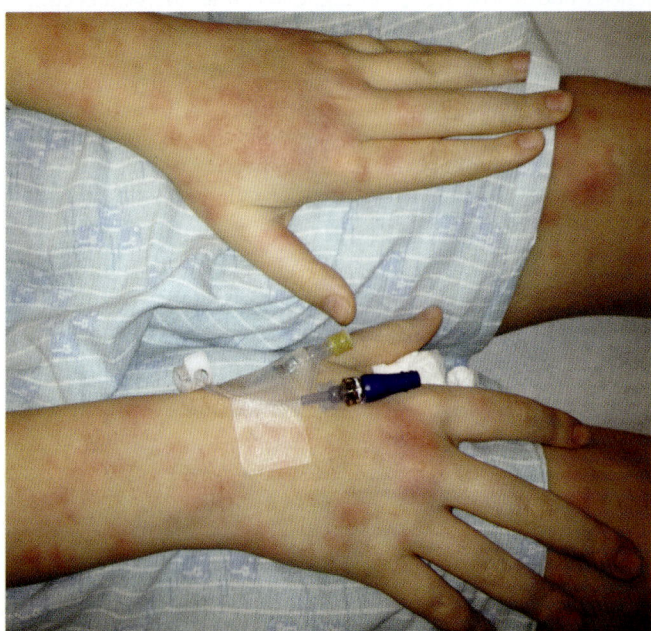

Fig. 23.7 Erythema nodosum.

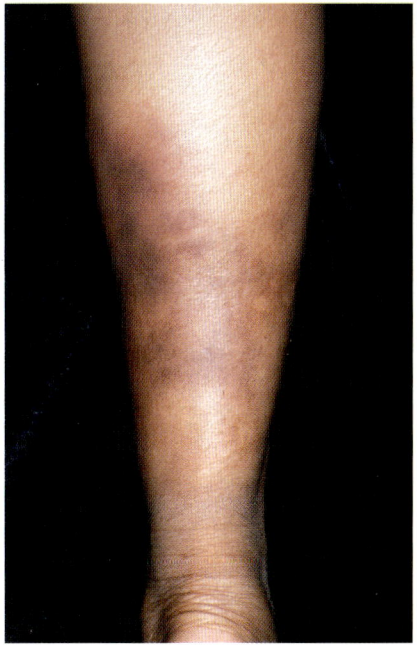

Fig. 23.8 Chronic erythema nodosum.

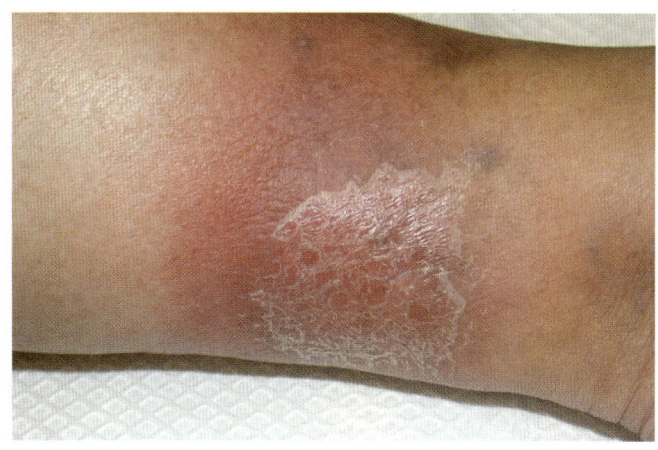

Fig. 23.9 Erythema induratum.

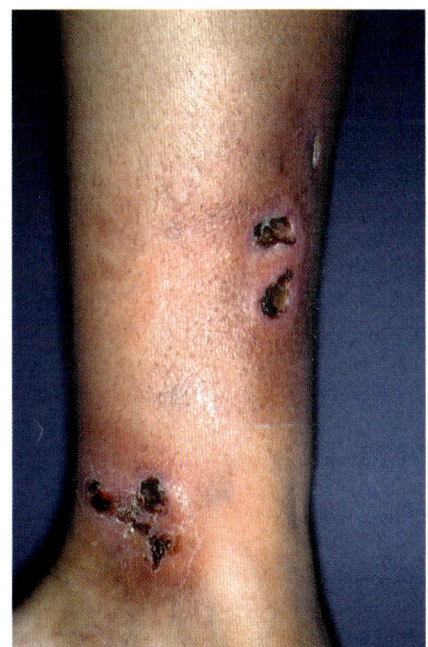

Fig. 23.10 Erythema induratum.

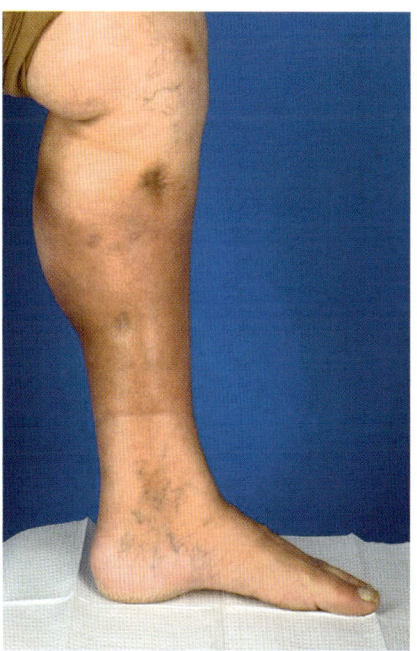

Fig. 23.11 Lipodermatosclerosis. *Courtesy Douglas Pugliese, MD.*

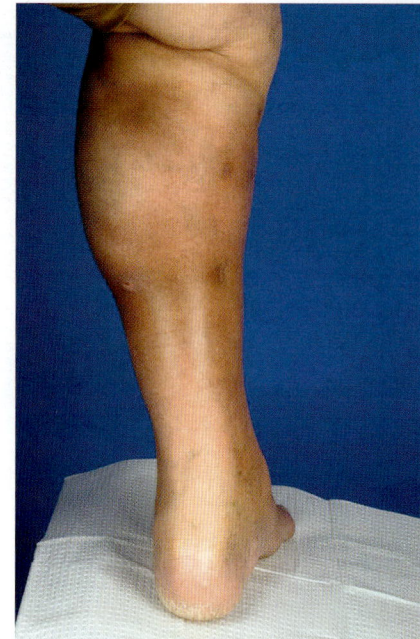

Fig. 23.12 Lipodermatosclerosis. *Courtesy Douglas Pugliese, MD.*

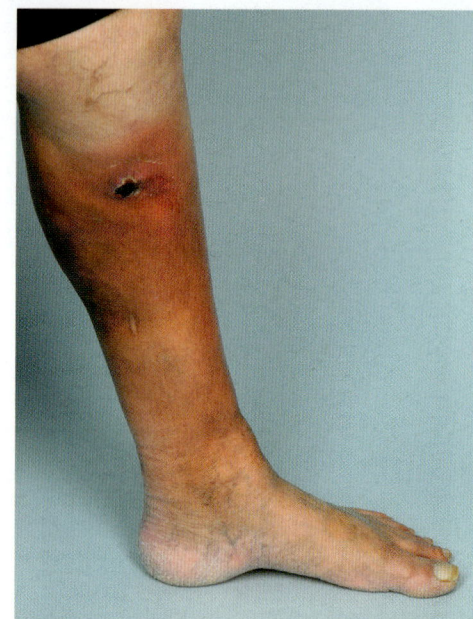

Fig. 23.13 Lipodermatosclerosis. *Courtesy Douglas Pugliese, MD.*

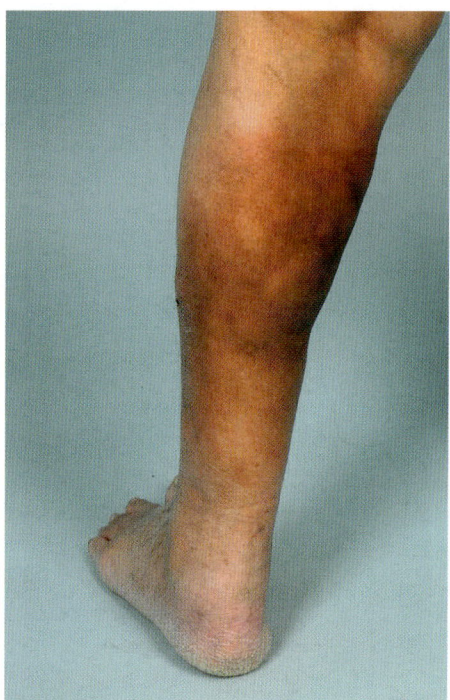

Fig. 23.14 Lipodermatosclerosis. *Courtesy Douglas Pugliese, MD.*

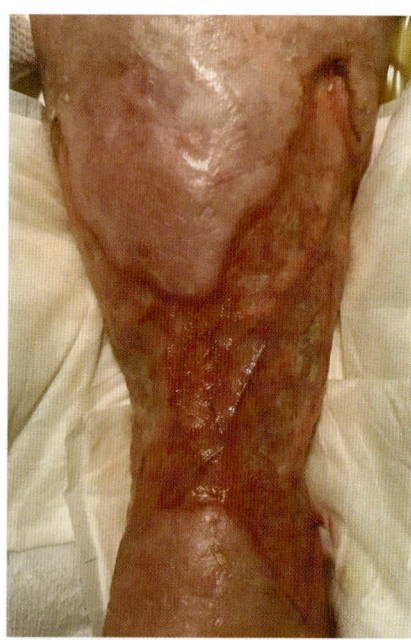

Fig. 23.15 Lipodermatosclerosis with circumferential ulceration.

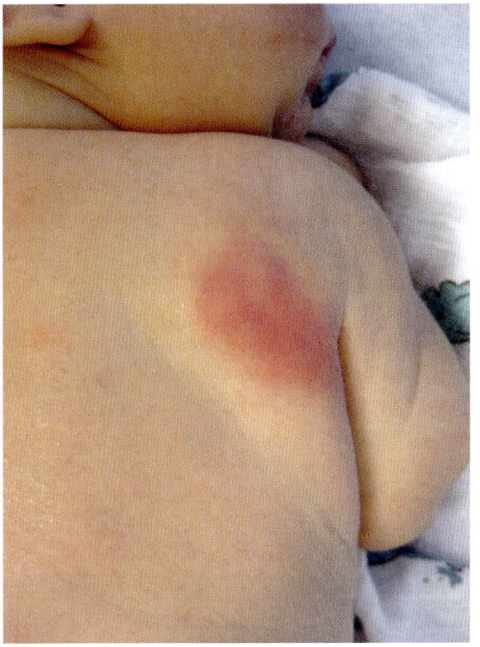

Fig. 23.16 Subcutaneous fat necrosis of the newborn.

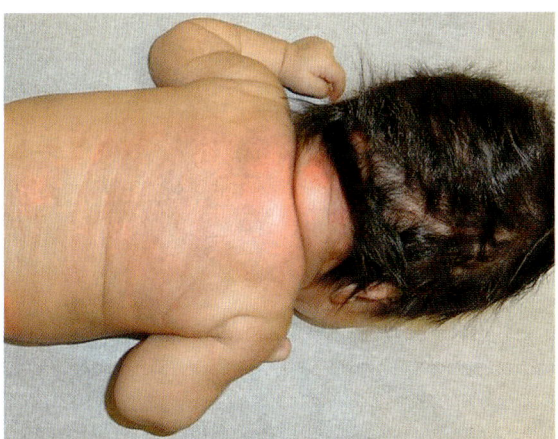

Fig. 23.18 Subcutaneous fat necrosis of the newborn. *Courtesy Scott Norton, MD.*

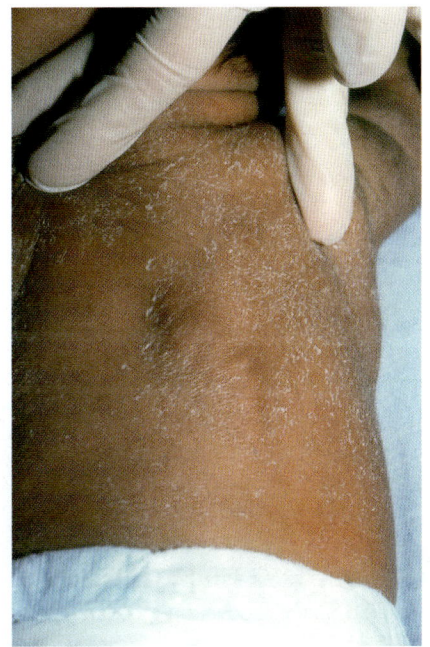

Fig. 23.20 Subcutaneous fat necrosis of the newborn.

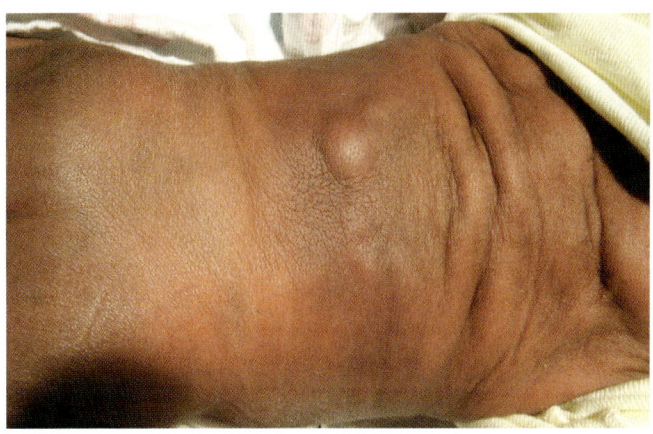

Fig. 23.17 Subcutaneous fat necrosis of the newborn.

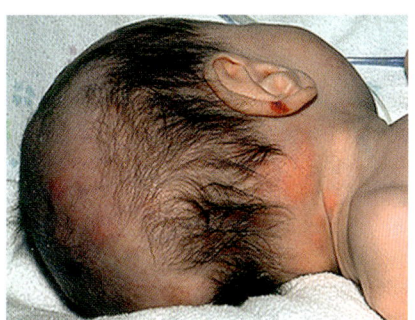

Fig. 23.19 Subcutaneous fat necrosis of the newborn. *Courtesy Paul Honig, MD.*

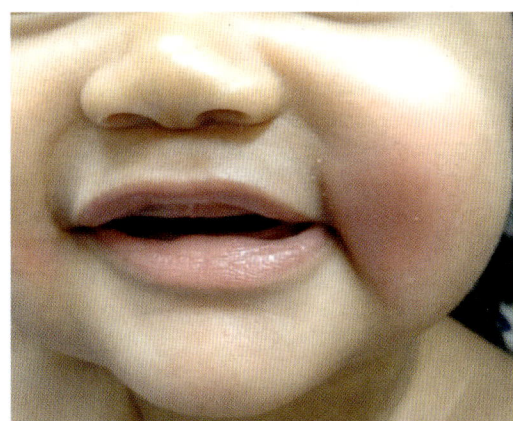

Fig. 23.21 Cold panniculitis.

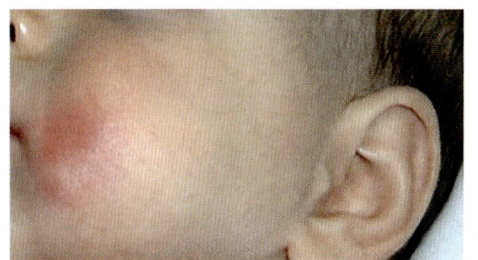

Fig. 23.22 Cold panniculitis.

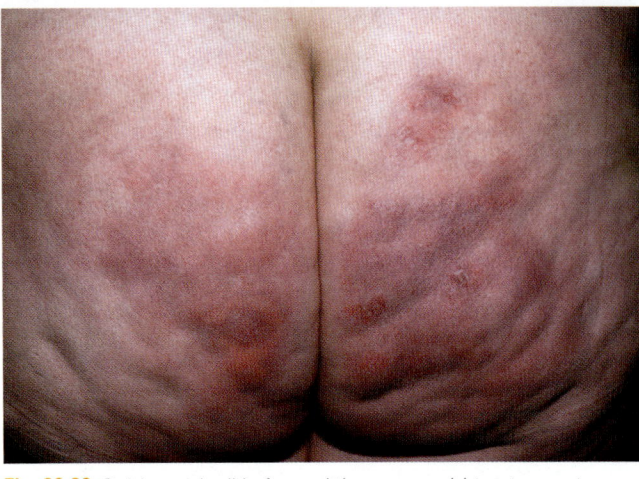

Fig. 23.23 Cold panniculitis from sitting on a cold tractor seat.

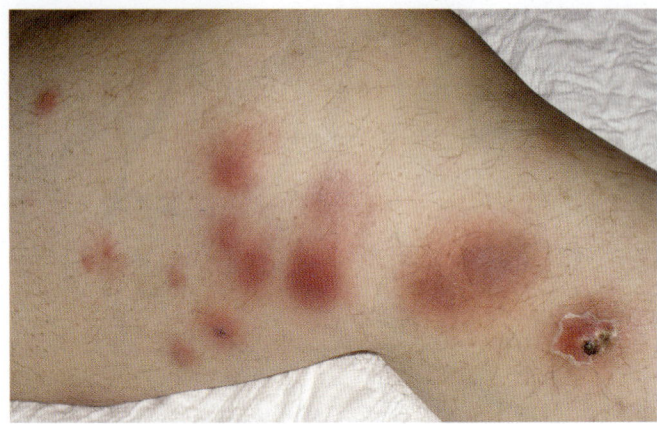

Fig. 23.24 Pancreatic panniculitis. *Courtesy Misha Rosenbach, MD.*

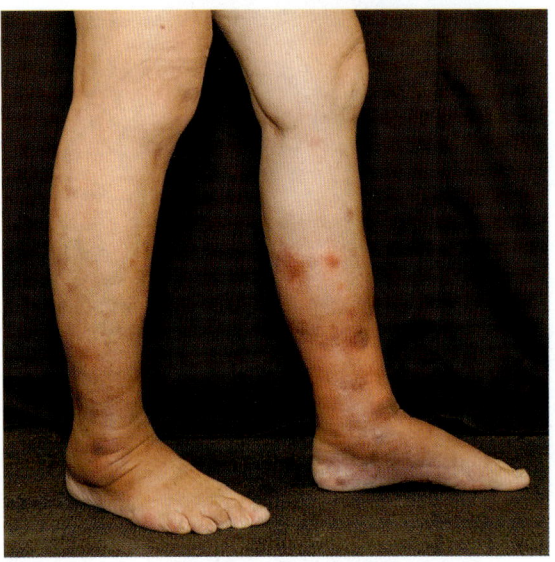

Fig. 23.25 Pancreatic panniculitis. *Courtesy Kaohsiung Chang Gang Memorial Hospital, Taiwan.*

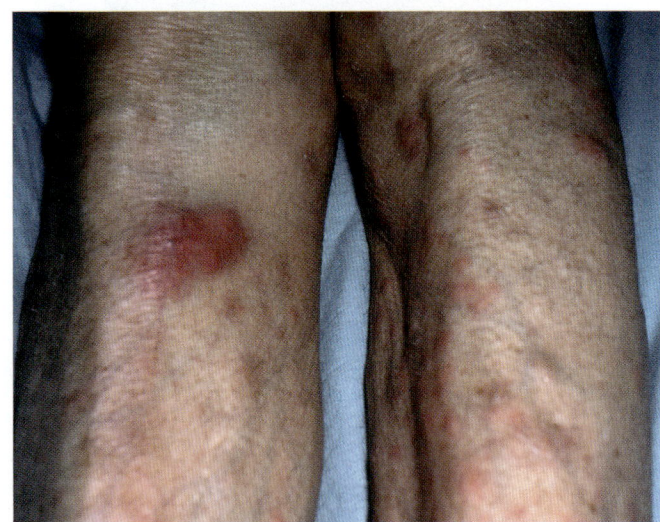

Fig. 23.26 Pancreatic panniculitis. *Courtesy Ken Greer, MD.*

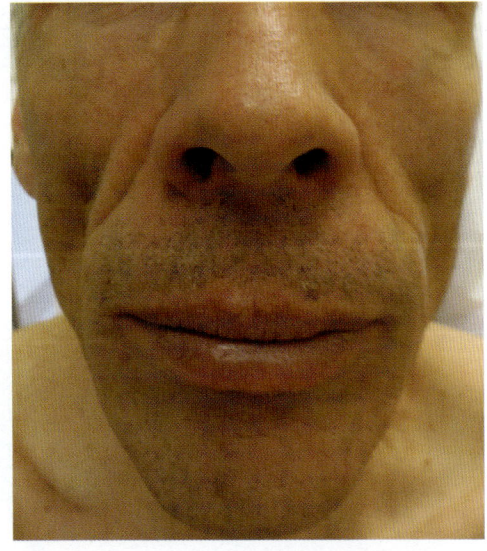

Fig. 23.27 Acquired partial lipodystrophy.

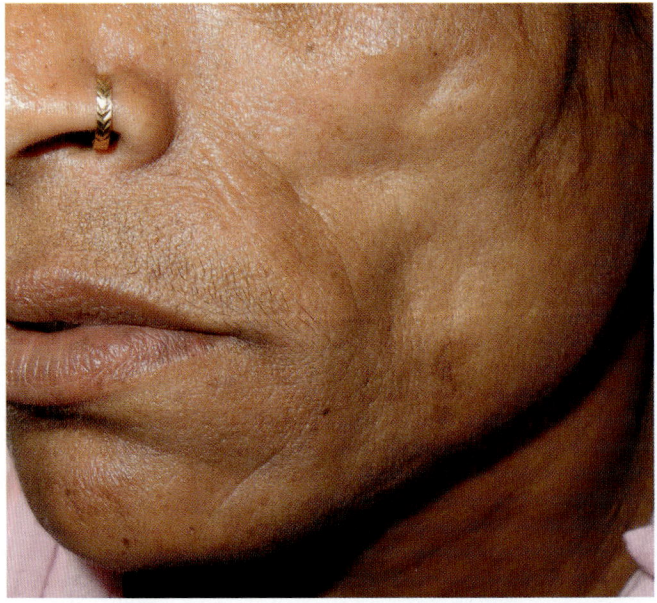

Fig. 23.28 Acquired partial lipodystrophy. *Courtesy Debabrata Bandyopadhyay.*

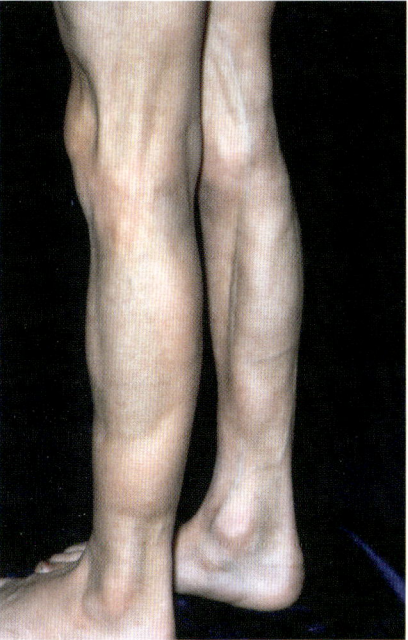

Fig. 23.29 Acquired partial lipodystrophy.

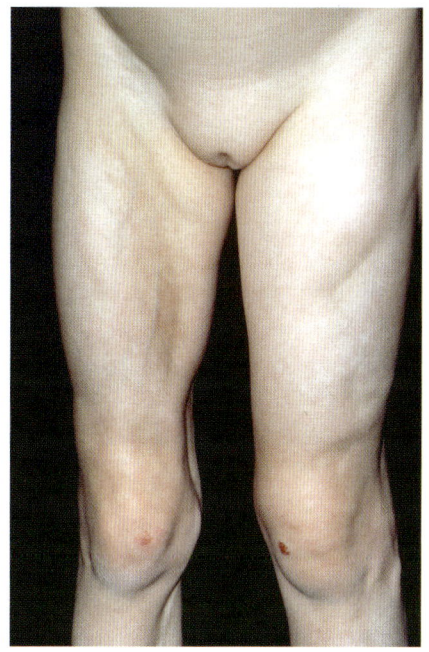

Fig. 23.30 Acquired partial lipodystrophy.

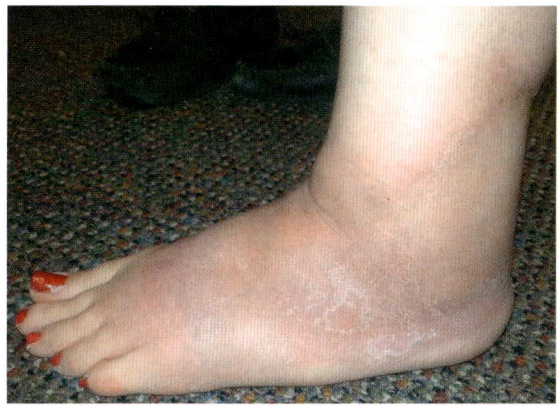

Fig. 23.31 Annular atrophic panniculitis, inflammatory phase. *Courtesy Marie Wagener, DO, and Elise Grgurich, DO.*

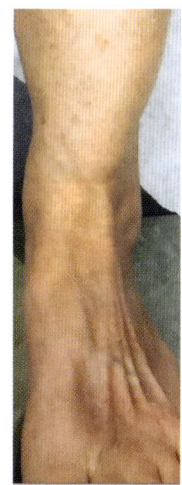

Fig. 23.32 Annular atrophic panniculitis, lipoatrophic phase. *Courtesy Marie Wagener, DO, and Elise Grgurich, DO.*

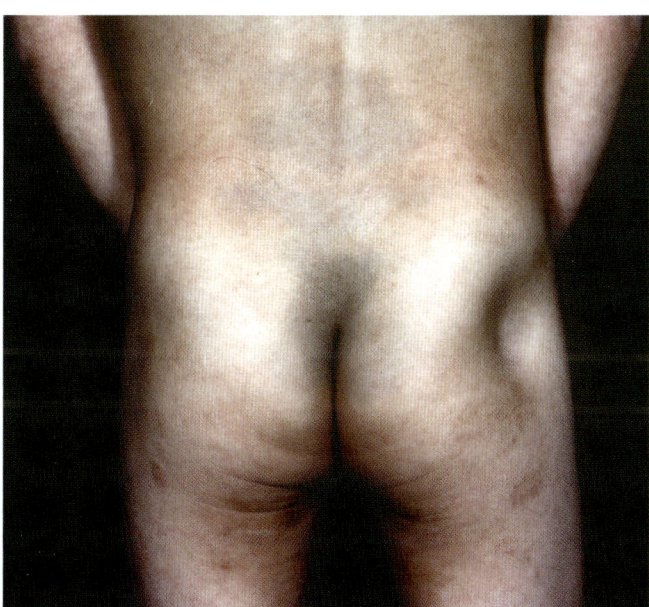

Fig. 23.33 Post–steroid injection atrophy.

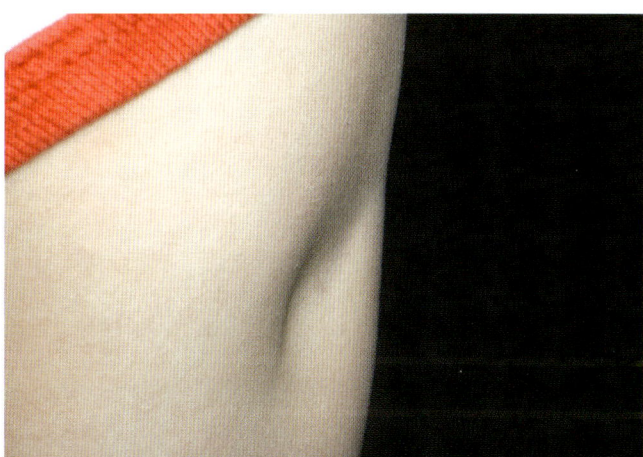

Fig. 23.34 Post–steroid injection atrophy. *Courtesy Steven Binnick, MD.*

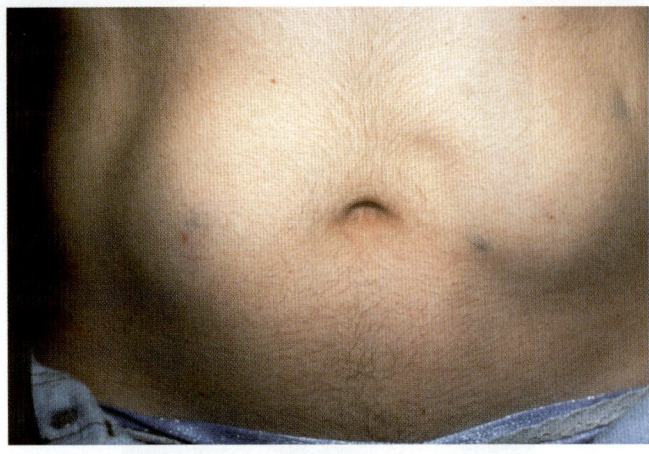
Fig. 23.35 Insulin lipohypertrophy.

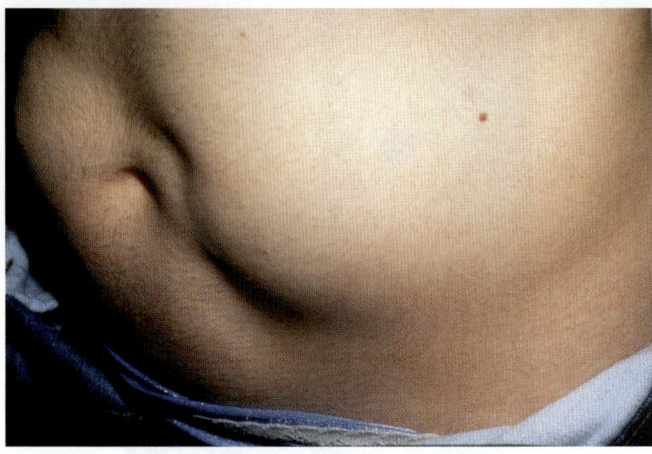
Fig. 23.36 Insulin lipohypertrophy.

Endocrine Diseases 24

Endocrine disorders present with a range of findings that may affect any layer of the skin. The associated skin changes can lead the astute physician to suspect the underlying disorder and order appropriate confirmatory tests.

Excess growth hormone before closure of the epiphyses leads to gigantism, whereas in adults it leads to acromegaly with hypertrophy of the chin, nose, and supraorbital ridges and thickening and wrinkling of the forehead, sometimes accompanied by cutis verticis gyrata. The distal digits are expanded. Addison disease leads to generalized hyperpigmentation as well as orolabial pigmented macules and nail streaks, whereas Cushing disease results in moon facies, fat redistribution giving rise to a buffalo hump, and hirsutism. An appreciation of the range of clinical findings in these conditions can lead to the early diagnosis of systemic disease.

Thyroid disease can present with subtle edema, most prominent around the eyes, in the case of hypothyroid myxedema, or with pebbly thickening of the skin of the shins and dorsal foot in Graves disease–associated pretibial myxedema. Necrobiosis lipoidica presents as atrophic, orange-to-yellow plaques with prominent vascularity and occasional ulceration. The plaques often involve the shins. Diabetes can cause acanthosis nigricans, a velvety thickening and darkening of the skin, noted most prominently over the flexures.

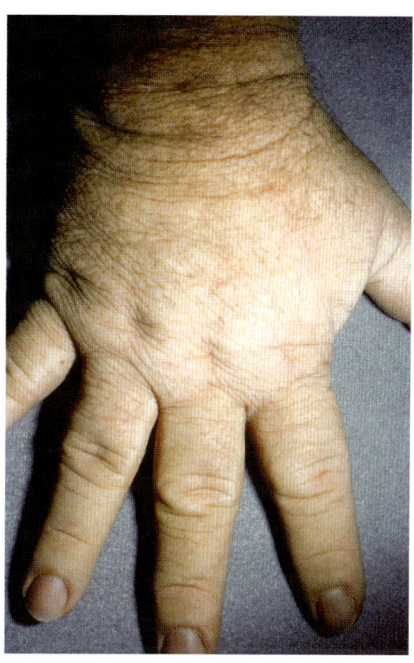

Fig. 24.2 Acromegaly.

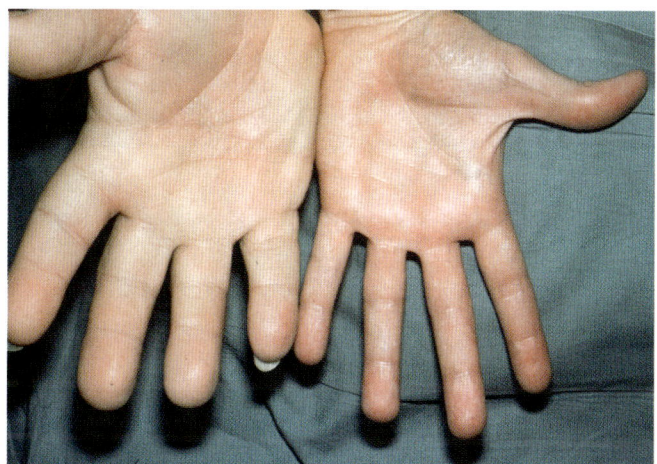

Fig. 24.1 Acromegalic hand compared with normal.

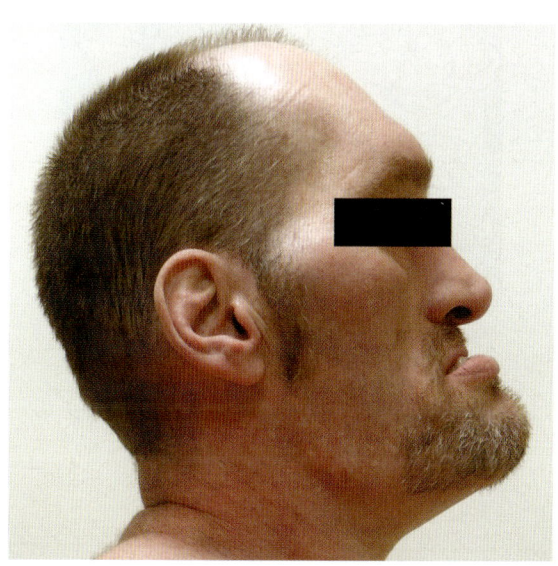

Fig. 24.3 Acromegaly.

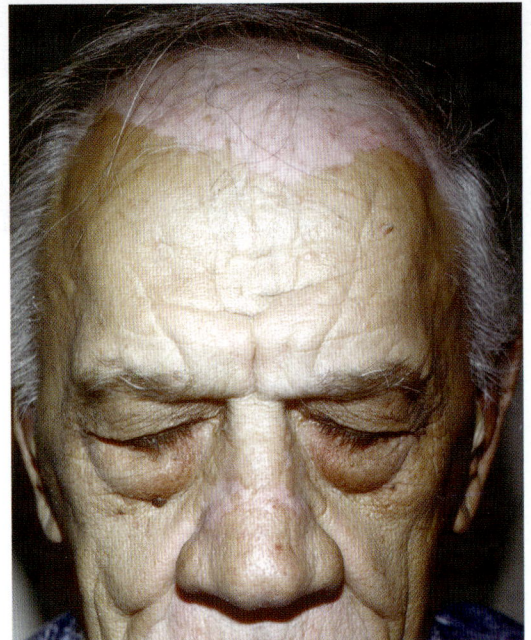

Fig. 24.4 Patient with acromegaly with vitiligo.
Courtesy Steven Binnick, MD.

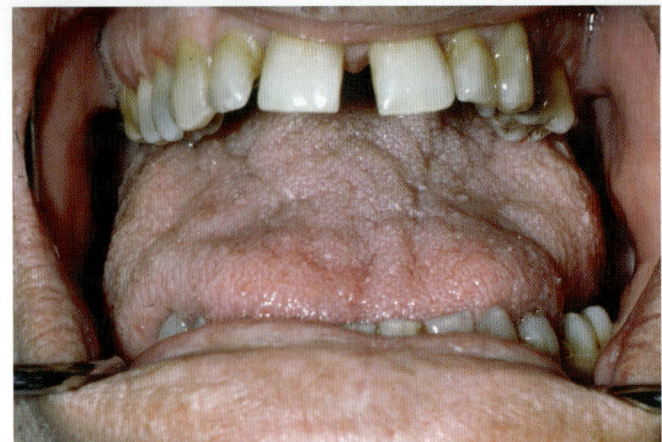

Fig. 24.5 Enlarged tongue in acromegaly.

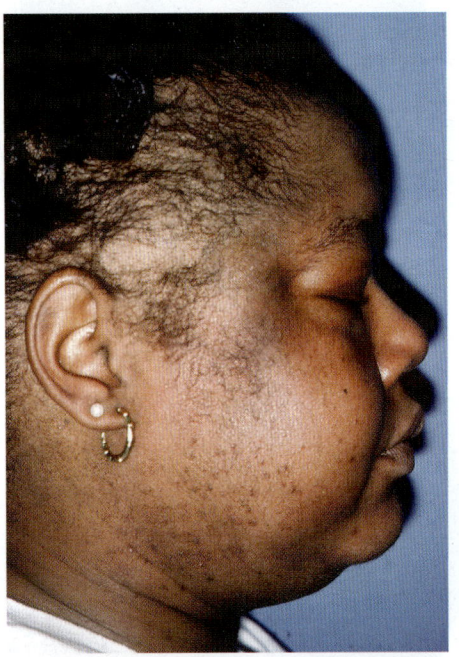

Fig. 24.6 Patient with Cushing disease with round face, thin hair, hypertrichosis, and acne.

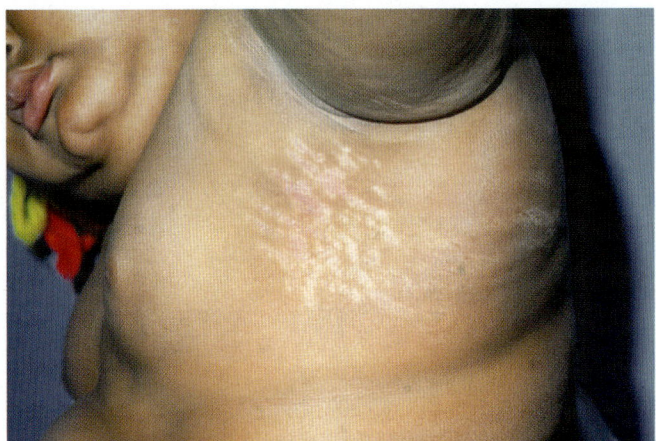

Fig. 24.7 Cushing disease with striae.

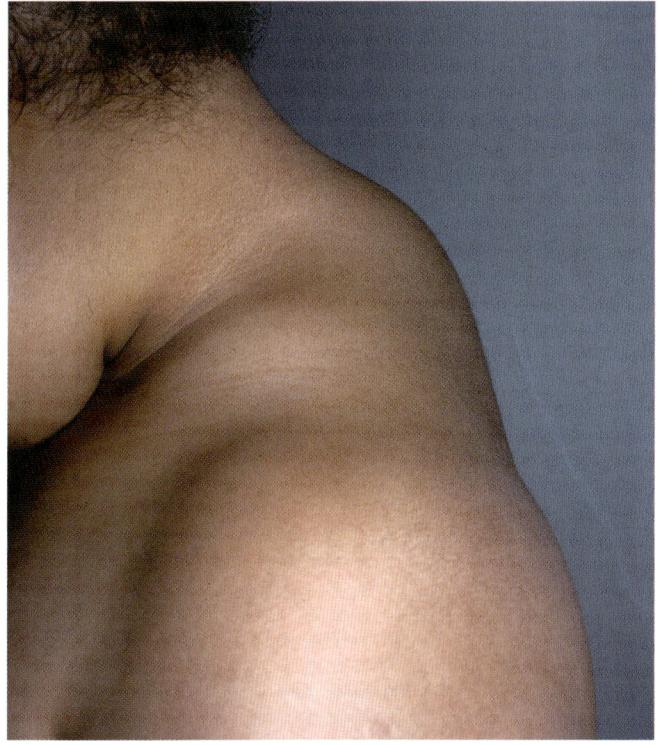

Fig. 24.8 Buffalo hump secondary to increased glucocorticoids.

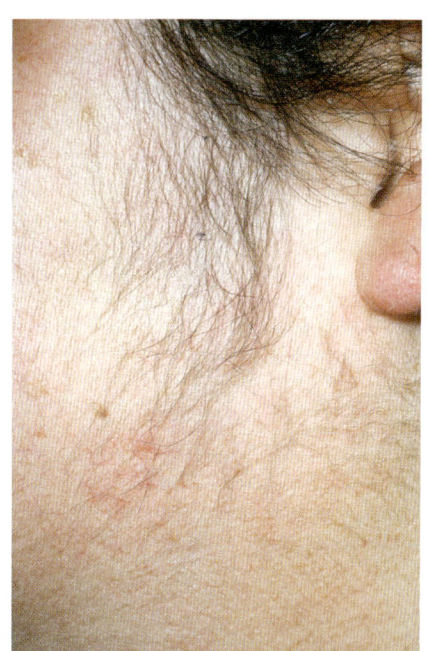

Fig. 24.9 Hypertrichosis in Cushing disease.

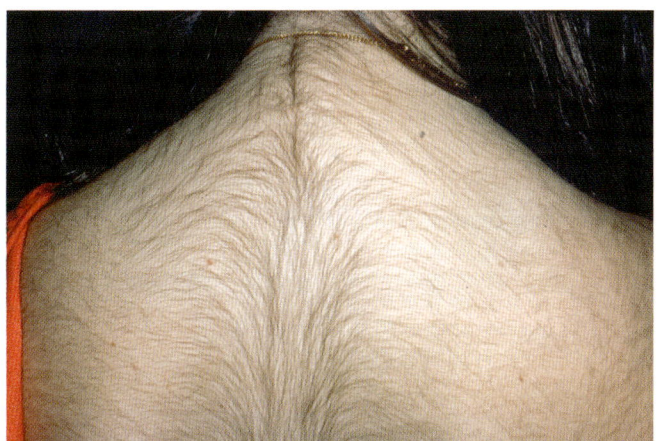

Fig. 24.10 Hypertrichosis in Cushing disease.

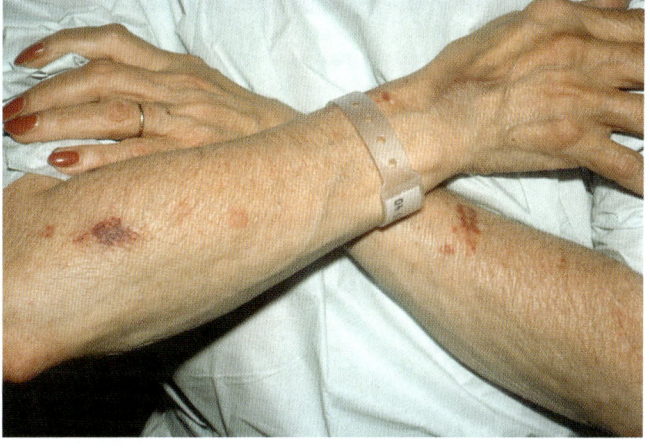

Fig. 24.11 Skin thinning and ecchymoses in Cushing disease.

Fig. 24.12 Striae in glucocorticoid excess.

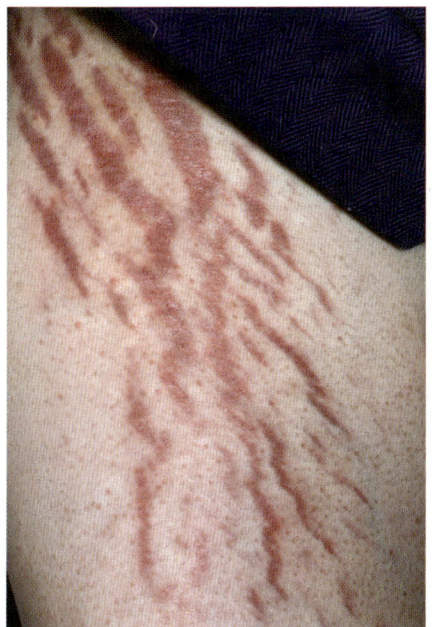

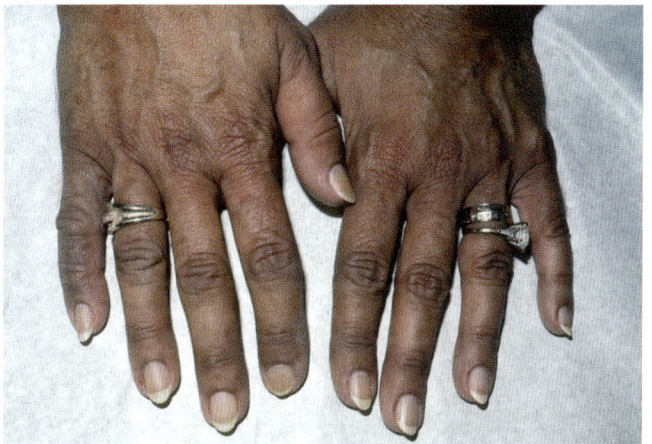

Fig. 24.13 Hyperpigmentation in Addison disease. *Courtesy Steven Binnick, MD.*

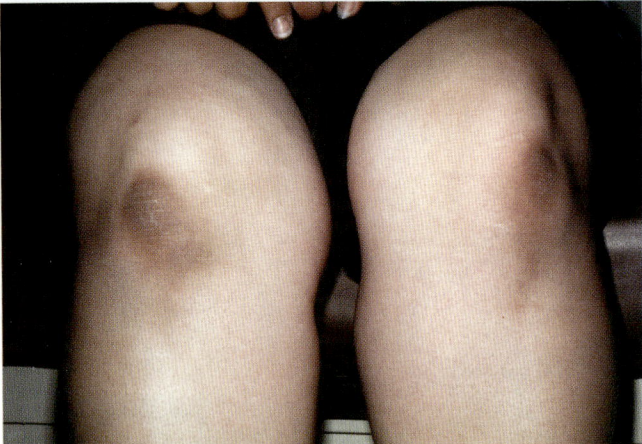

Fig. 24.14 Hyperpigmentation of chronic traumatic sites in Addison disease. *Courtesy Steven Binnick, MD.*

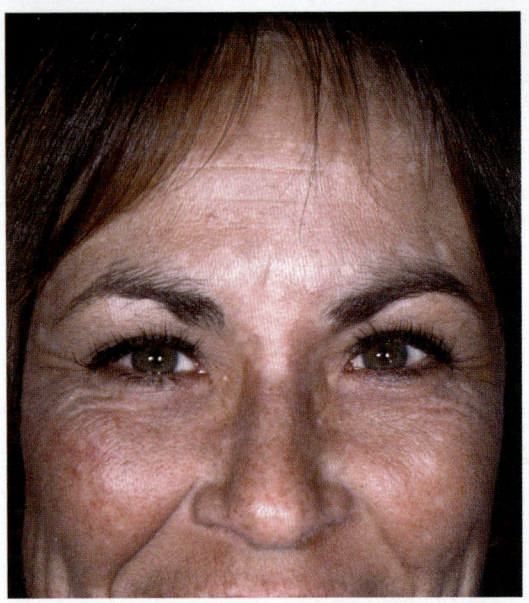

Fig. 24.15 Hyperpigmentation secondary to Addison disease. *Courtesy The University of Utah and Oregon Health Sciences University Leonard Swinyer MD image collection.*

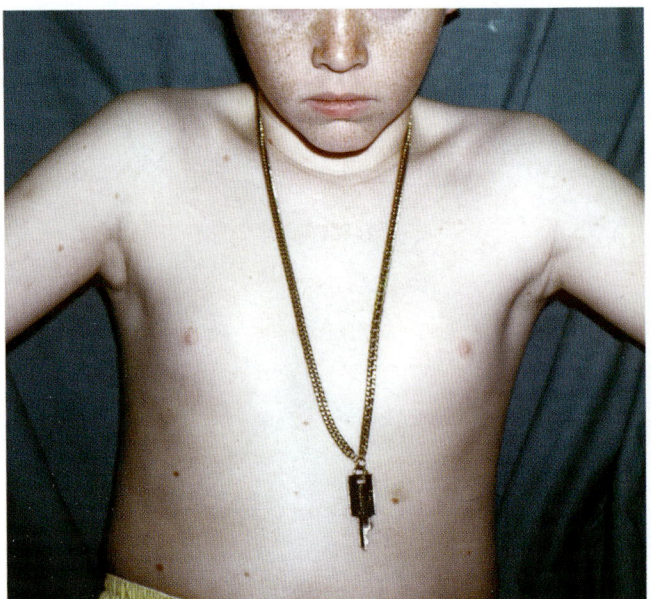

Fig. 24.16 Panhypopituitarism with pale, thin skin.

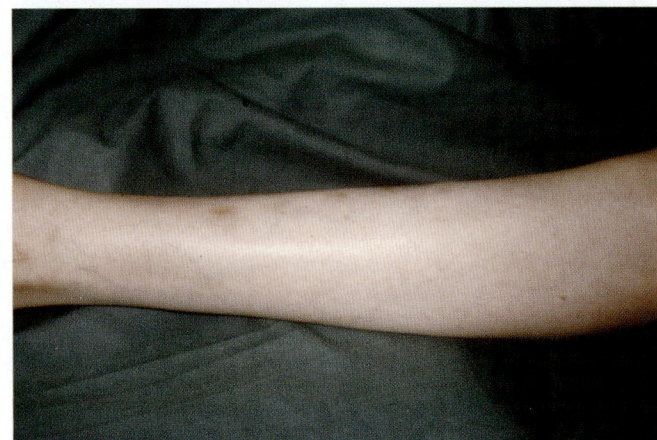

Fig. 24.17 Panhypopituitarism with pale, thin skin.

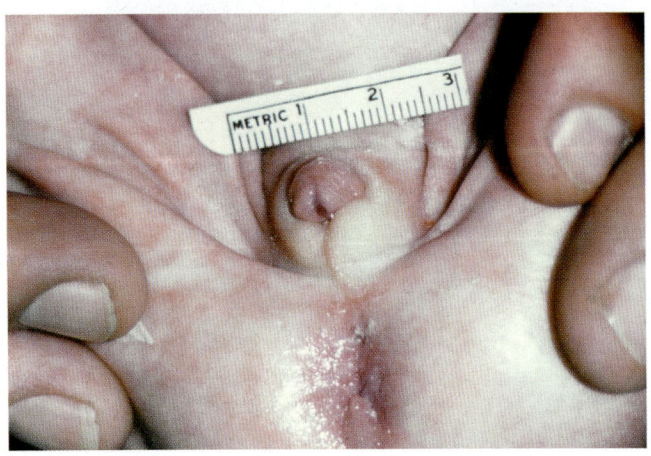

Fig. 24.18 Adrenogenital syndrome. *Courtesy Ken Greer, MD.*

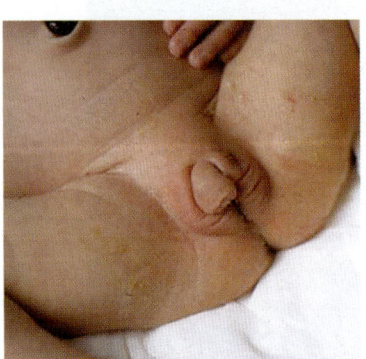

Fig. 24.19 Adrenogenital syndrome with ambiguous genitalia. *Courtesy Paul Honig, MD.*

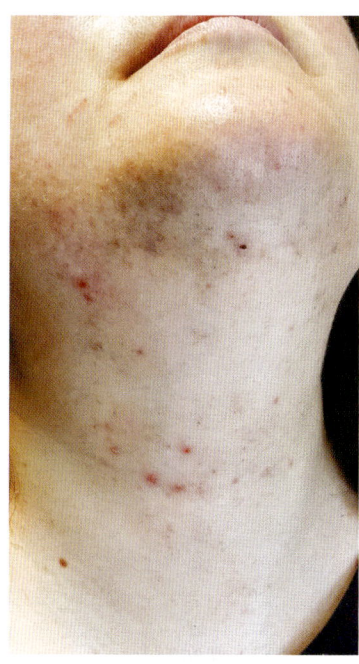

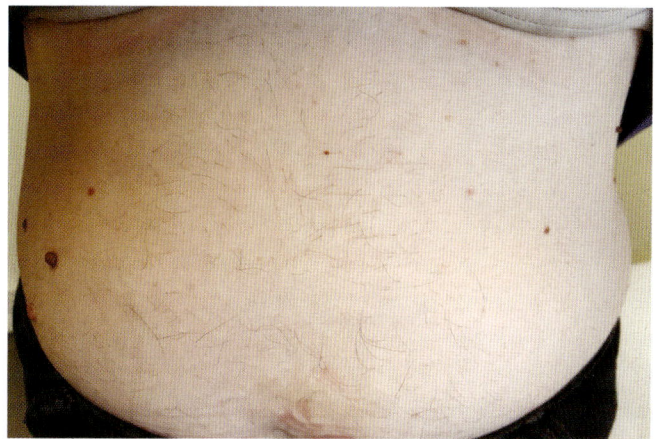

Fig. 24.20 Adrenogenital syndrome. *Courtesy Rui Tavares Bello, MD.*

Fig. 24.21 Adrenogenital syndrome. *Courtesy Rui Tavares Bello, MD.*

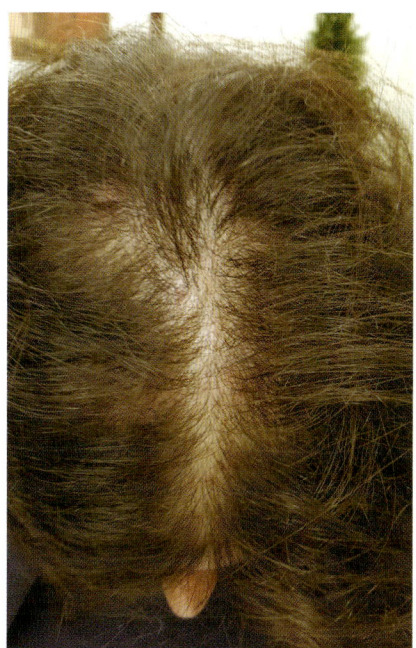

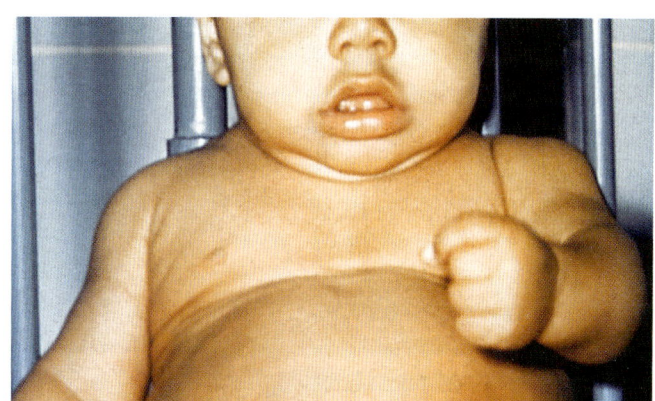

Fig. 24.22 Adrenogenital syndrome. *Courtesy Rui Tavares Bello, MD.*

Fig. 24.23 Congenital hypothyroidism.

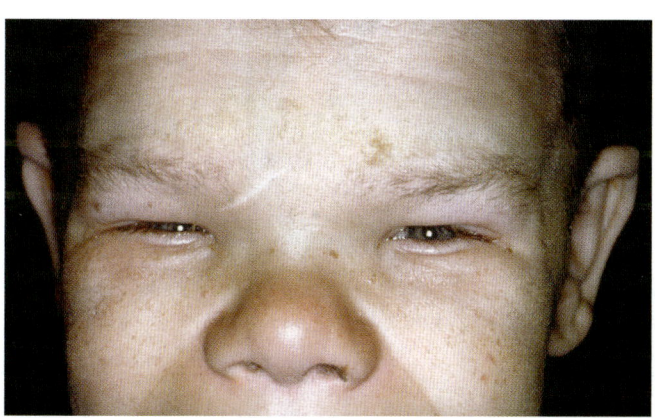

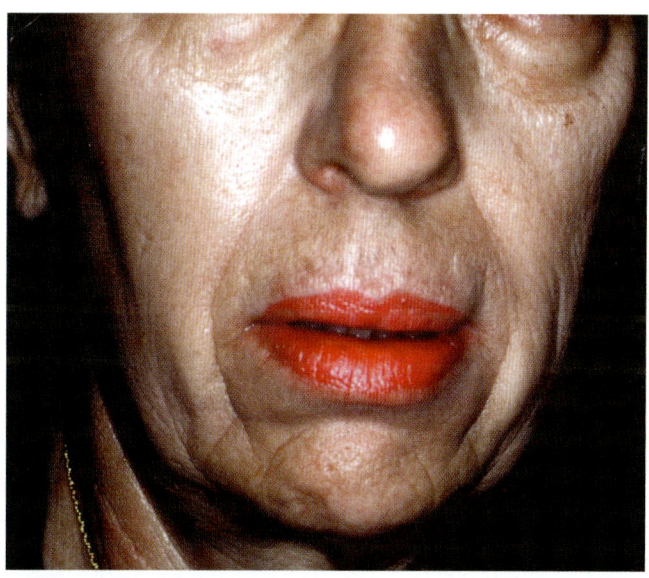

Fig. 24.24 Congenital hypothyroidism.

Fig. 24.25 Myxedema.

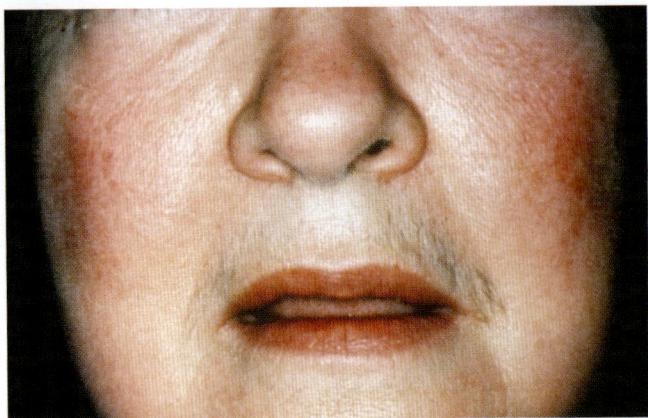

Fig. 24.26 Myxedema.

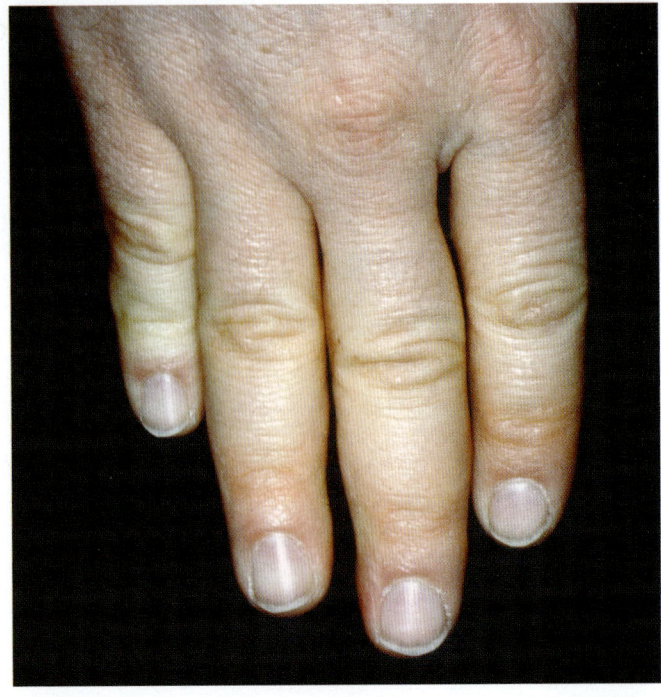

Fig. 24.27 Puffy, yellow hands in myxedema.

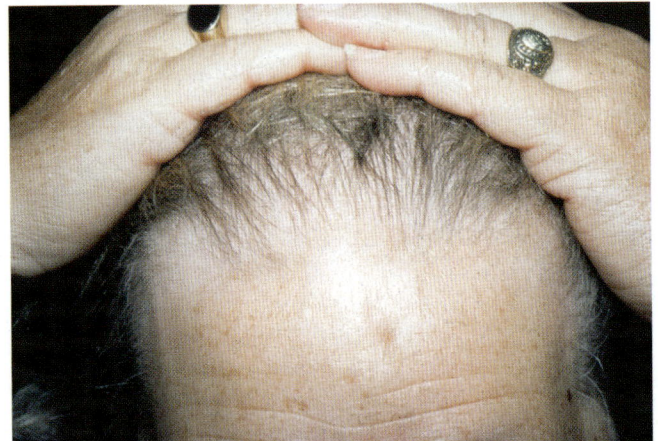

Fig. 24.28 Hair thinning in hypothyroidism.

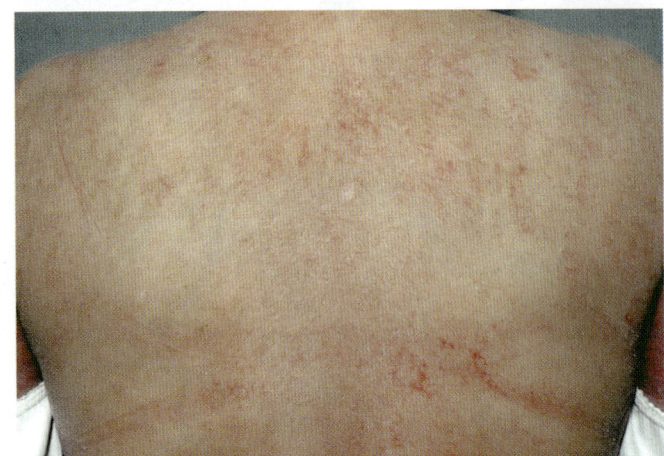

Fig. 24.29 Dry skin in hypothyroidism.

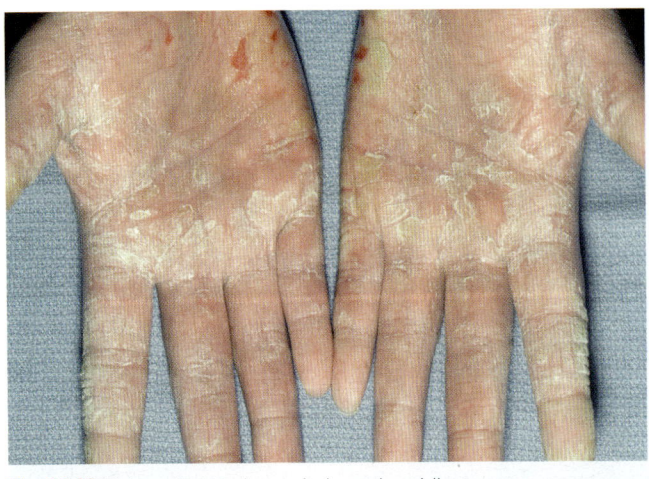

Fig. 24.30 Palmar keratoderma in hypothyroidism.

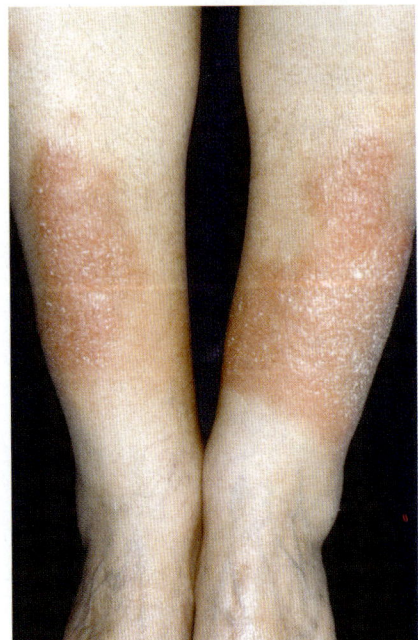

Fig. 24.31 Pretibial myxedema.

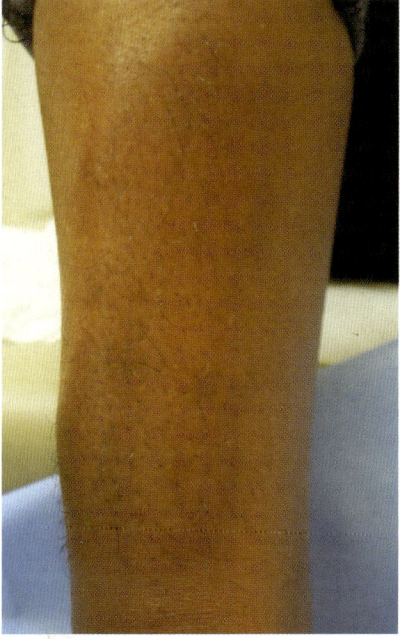

Fig. 24.32 Pretibial myxedema.

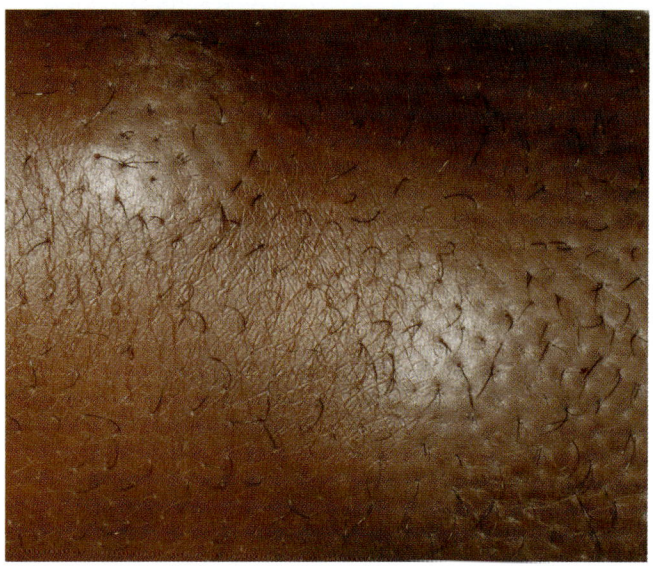

Fig. 24.33 Pretibial myxedema.

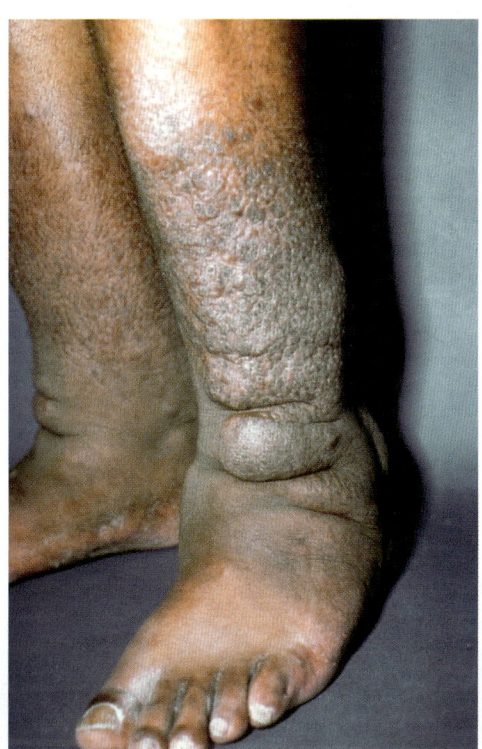

Fig. 24.34 Pretibial myxedema.

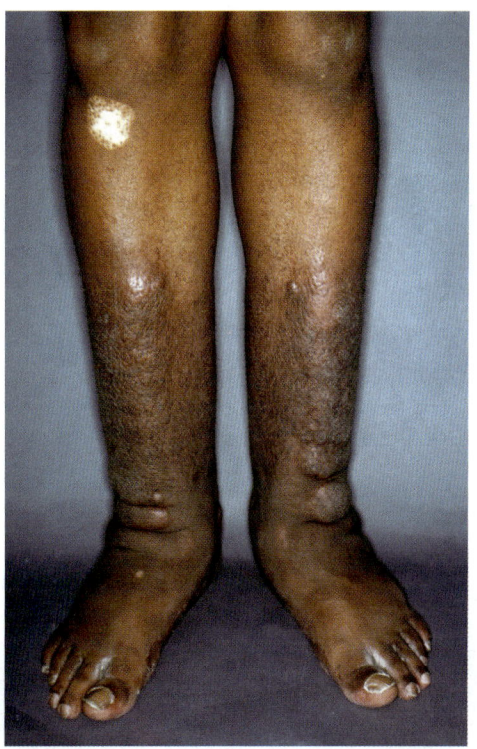

Fig. 24.35 Pretibial myxedema.

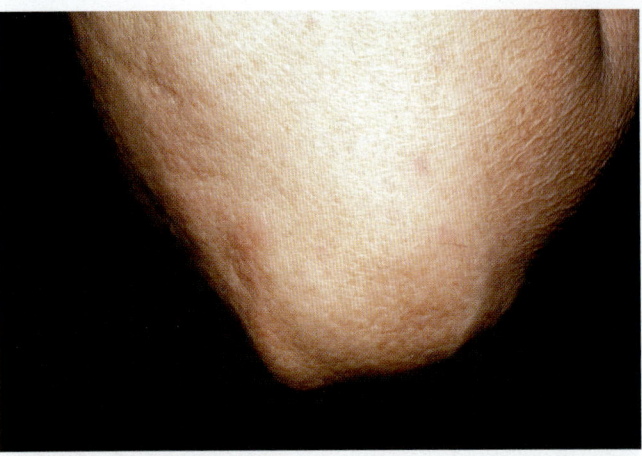

Fig. 24.36 Preradial myxedema.

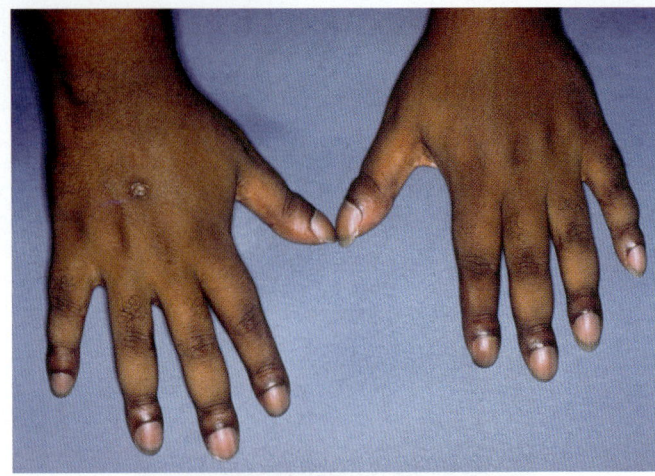

Fig. 24.37 Thyroid acropachy.

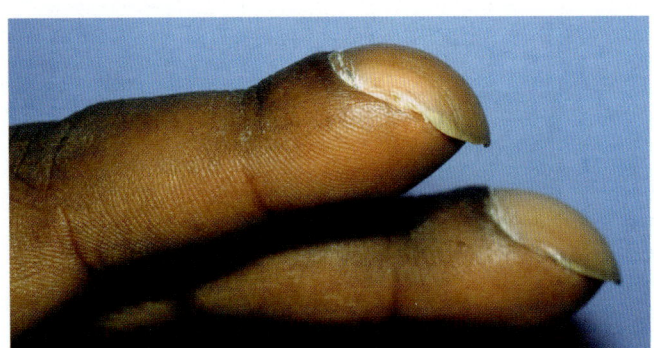

Fig. 24.38 Thyroid acropachy.

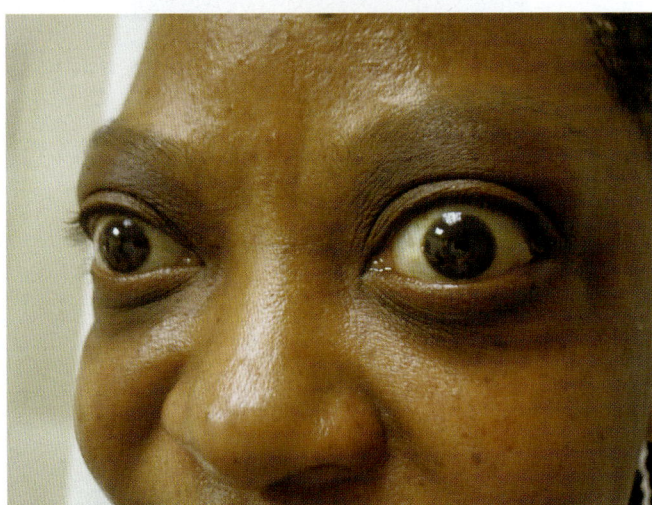

Fig. 24.39 Graves ophthalmopathy.

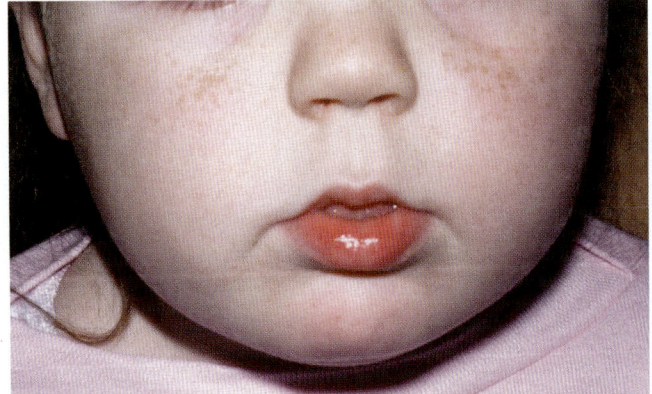

Fig. 24.40 Pseudohypoparathyroidism with typical facies. *Courtesy Steven Binnick, MD.*

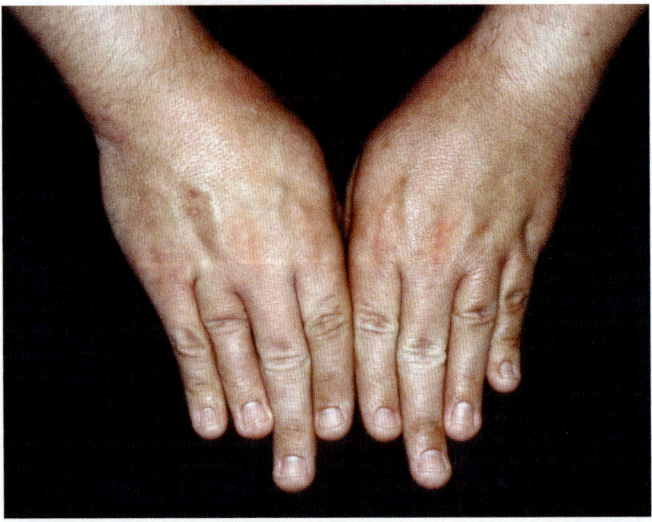

Fig. 24.41 Pseudohypoparathyroidism.

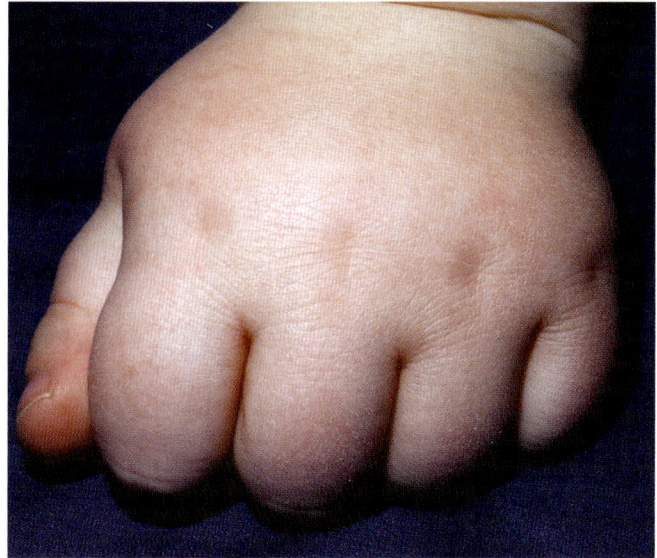

Fig. 24.42 Pseudohypoparathyroidism.

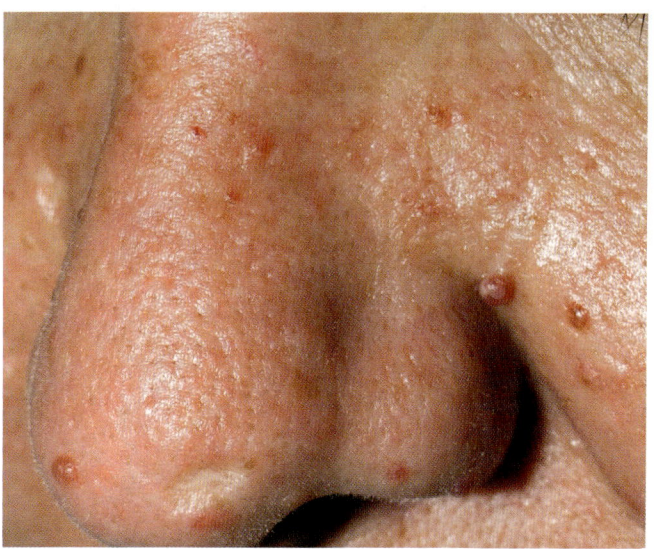

Fig. 24.43 Multiple endocrine neoplasia type 1 angiofibromas. *Courtesy Thomas Darling, MD, PhD.*

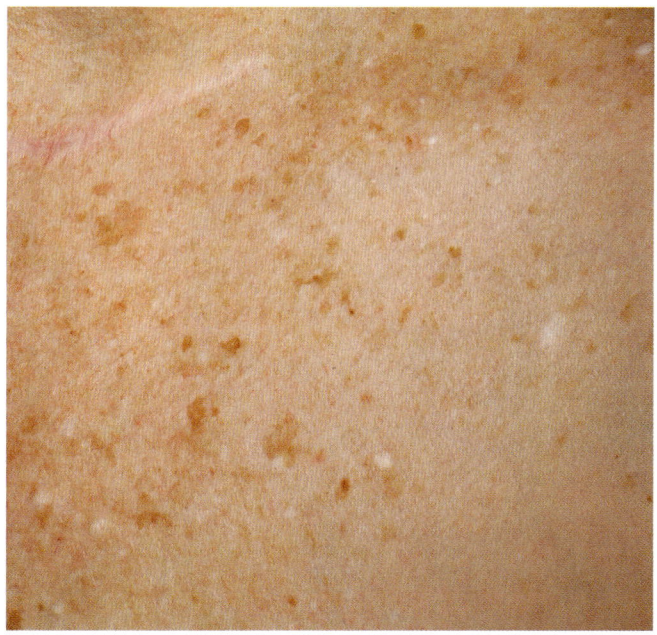

Fig. 24.44 Multiple endocrine neoplasia type 1, collagenomas. *Courtesy Thomas Darling, MD, PhD.*

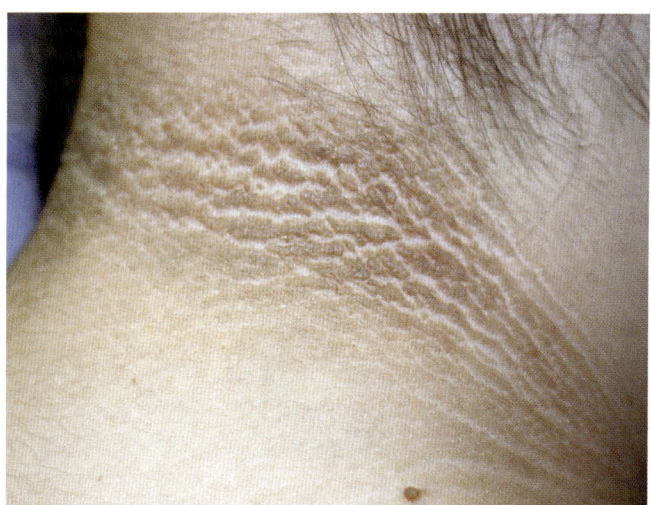

Fig. 24.45 Acanthosis nigricans.

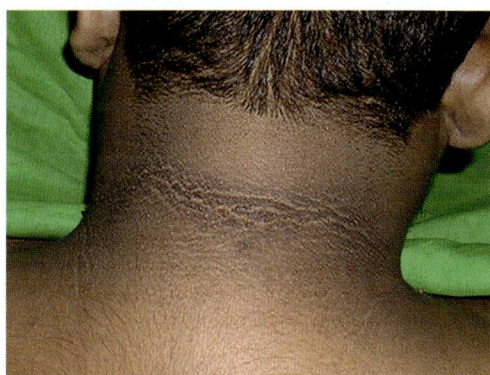

Fig. 24.46 Acanthosis nigricans. *Courtesy Shyam Verma, MBBS, DVD.*

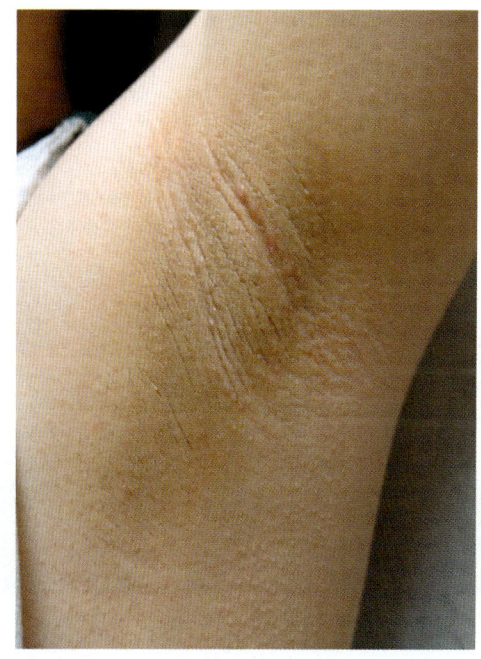

Fig. 24.47 Acanthosis nigricans.

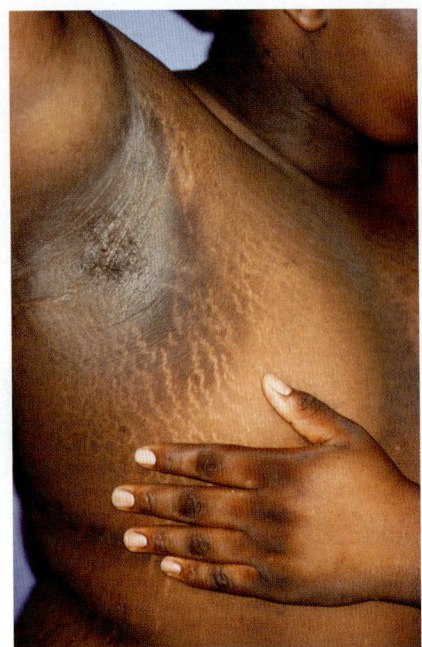
Fig. 24.48 Acanthosis nigricans.

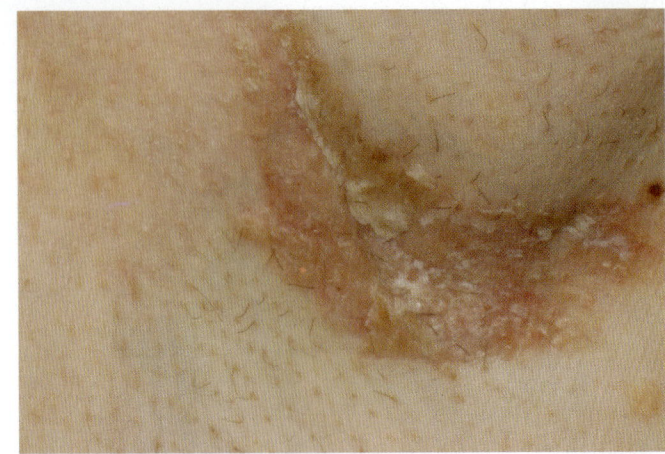
Fig. 24.49 Axillary granular parakeratosis.

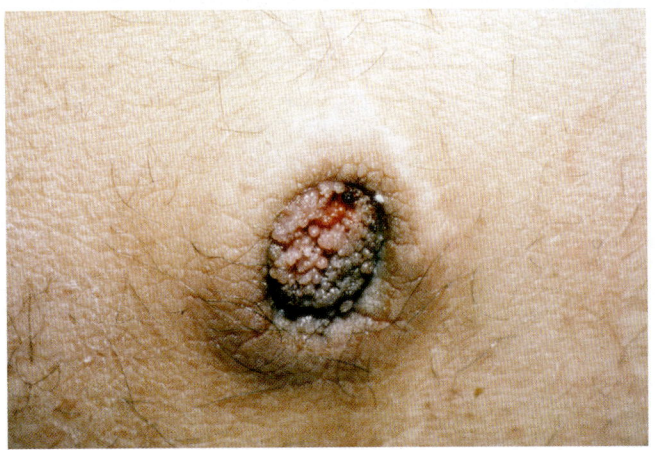
Fig. 24.50 Acanthosis nigricans with malignancy.

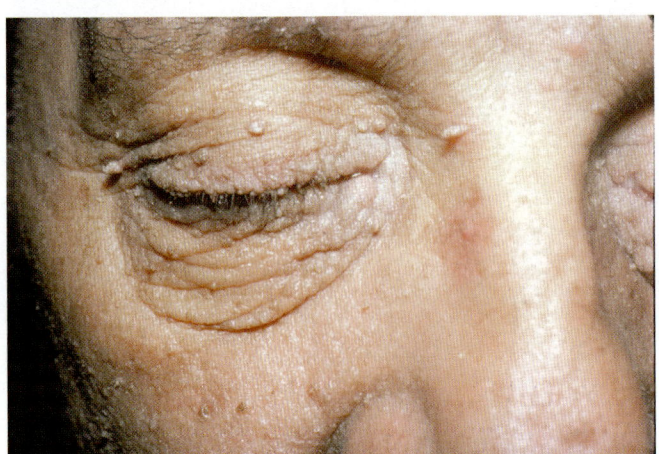
Fig. 24.51 Acanthosis nigricans with malignancy.

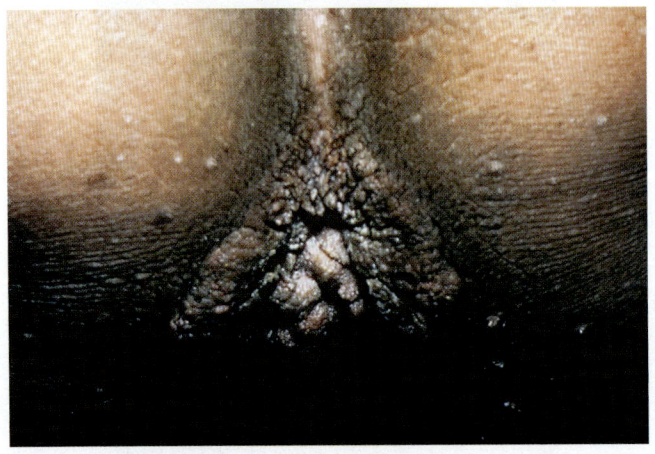
Fig. 24.52 Acanthosis nigricans with malignancy.

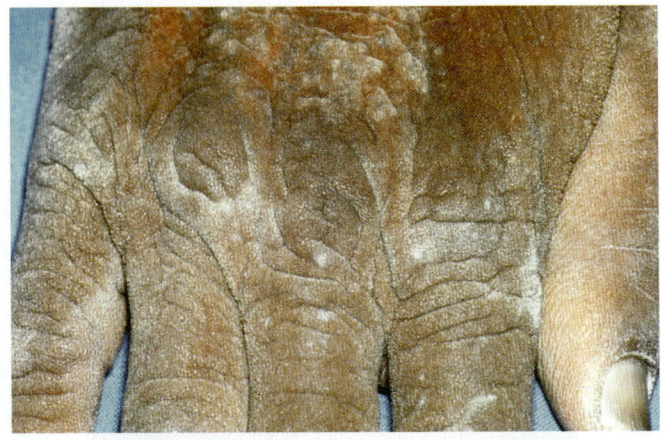
Fig. 24.53 Type B syndrome.

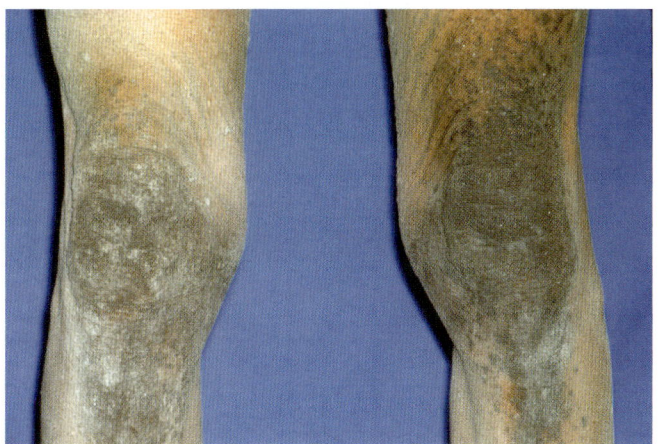

Fig. 24.54 Type B syndrome.

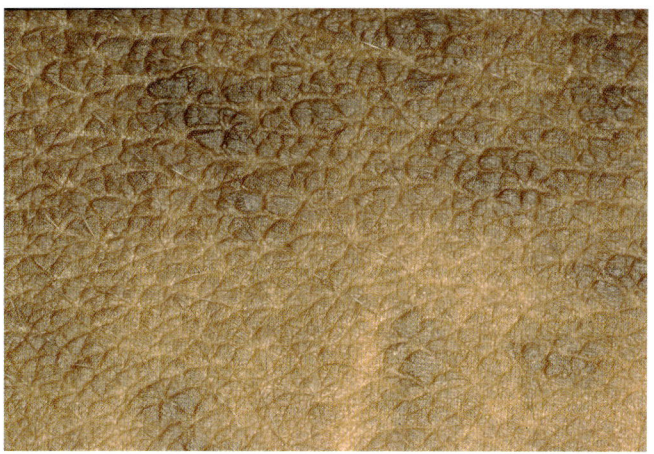

Fig. 24.55 Type B syndrome (close-up of acanthosis nigricans on the back).

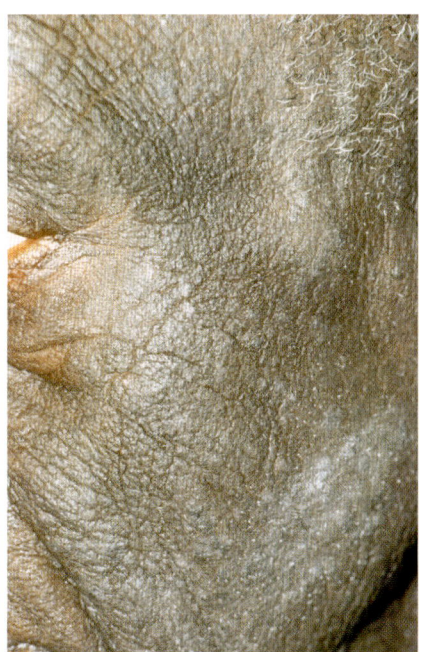

Fig. 24.56 Type B syndrome.

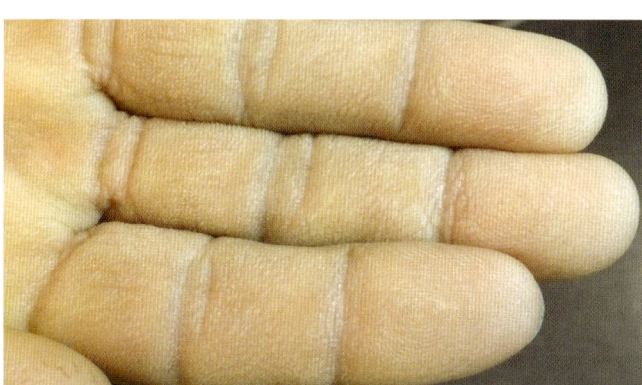

Fig. 24.57 Tripe palms in a patient with gastric adenocarcinoma. *Courtesy Dr. Rui Carlos Taveres Bello.*

Abnormalities of Dermal Fibrous and Elastic Tissue 25

This chapter includes a variety of conditions, all resulting from either inherited or acquired changes in the collagen or elastic tissue of the skin.

Some inherited syndromes with particularly unique skin findings include forms of Ehlers-Danlos syndrome (EDS). Affected individuals are noted to have doughy skin that is hyperextensible. Skin is prone to wide "fish-mouth" wounds, molluscoid pseudotumors, and atrophic scars. In contrast, those patients with inherited forms of cutis laxa produce widespread drooping, redundant skin with pendulous folds. Pseudoxanthoma elasticum (PXE) can present with yellowish papules predominantly on the lateral neck said to resemble "plucked chicken skin," as well as lax skin akin to that seen in some forms of cutis laxa. Marfan syndrome is included here due to its underlying genetic mutation in fibrillin-1 that affects connective tissues. In Marfan syndrome characteristic physical findings include tall stature, high-arched palate, and arachnodactyly. Knowledge of the skin findings of these genetic conditions is important to aid in an early diagnosis, especially given that they all have the potential to involve internal organs such as the cardiovascular system and lungs.

More localized skin conditions are also represented here, including the serpiginous keratotic papules seen in elastosis perforans serpiginosa. This rare condition is more common in those with trisomy 21 (Down syndrome), but can also be seen in patients with some of the aforementioned connective tissue conditions such as EDS and Marfan syndrome.

Skin biopsy with subsequent staining for connective tissue fibers can be necessary and diagnostic for some of these conditions such as PXE. However, those patients with a suspected inherited condition with known gene mutation should be offered confirmatory genetic testing from the blood.

This portion of the atlas features these connective tissue diseases, among others, that affect the dermal fibrous and elastic tissues.

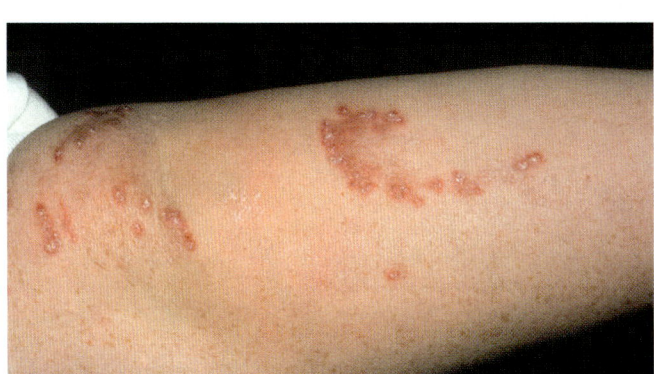

Fig. 25.1 Elastosis perforans serpiginosa.

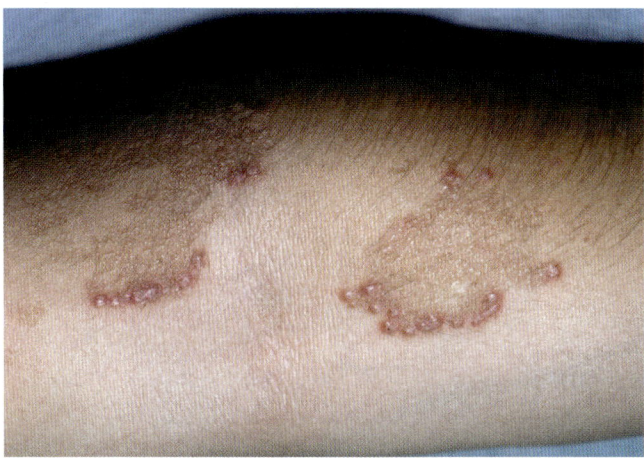

Fig. 25.2 Elastosis perforans serpiginosa. *Courtesy Ken Greer, MD.*

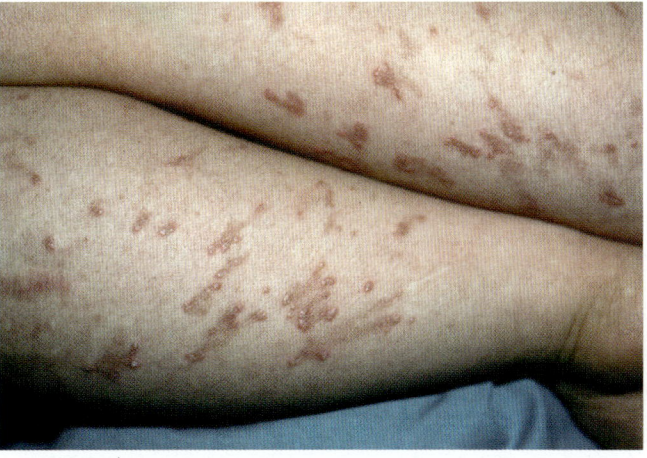

Fig. 25.3 Elastosis perforans serpiginosa. *Courtesy Ken Greer, MD.*

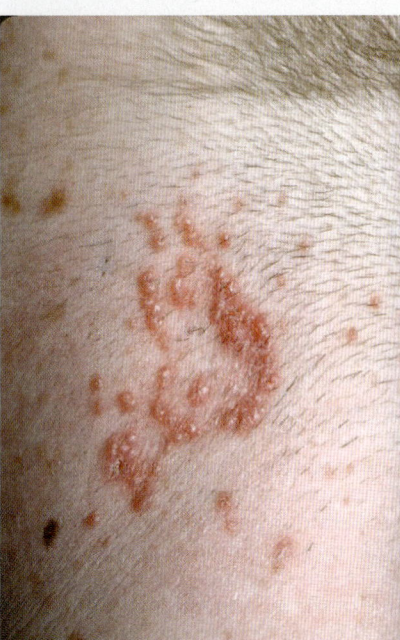

Fig. 25.4 Elastosis perforans serpiginosa. *Courtesy The University of Utah and Oregon Health Sciences University Leonard Swinyer MD image collection.*

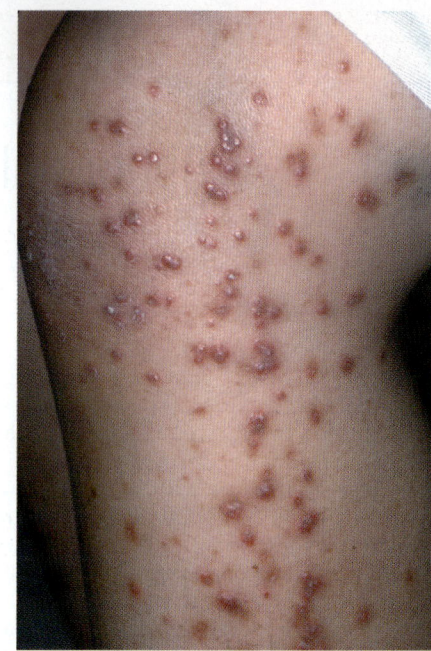

Fig. 25.5 Reactive perforating collagenosis. *Courtesy Steven Binnick, MD.*

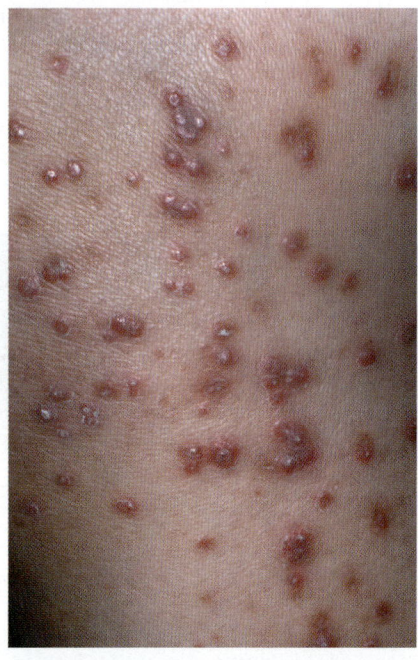

Fig. 25.6 Reactive perforating collagenosis. *Courtesy Steven Binnick, MD.*

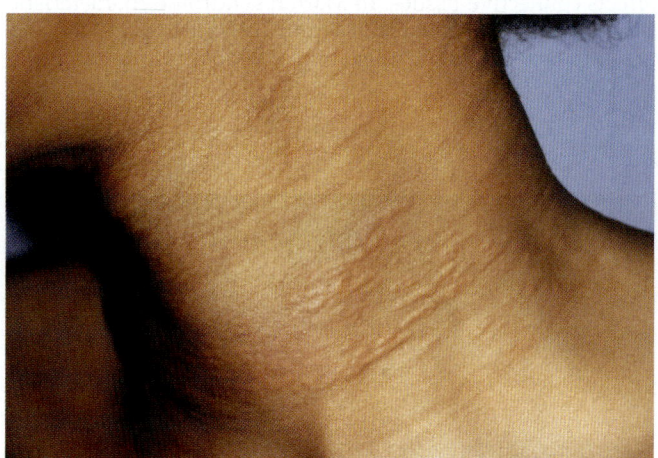

Fig. 25.7 Pseudoxanthoma elasticum.

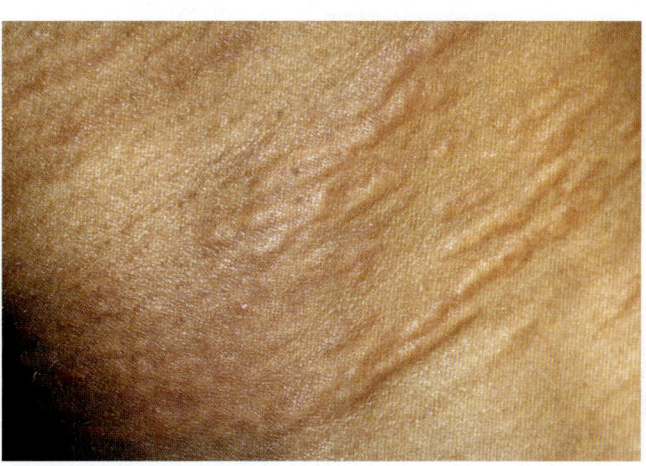

Fig. 25.8 Pseudoxanthoma elasticum.

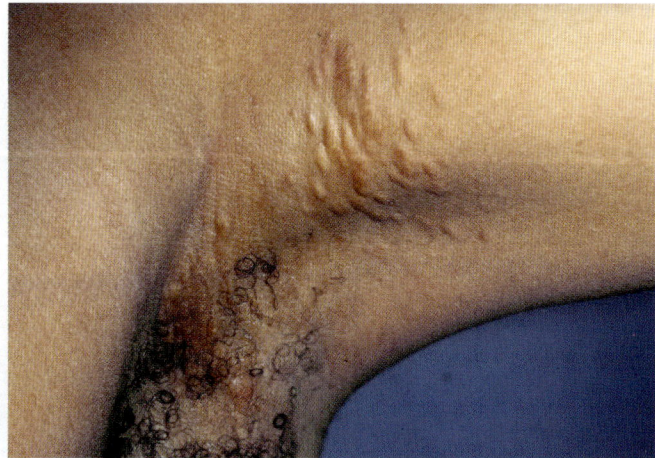

Fig. 25.9 Pseudoxanthoma elasticum.

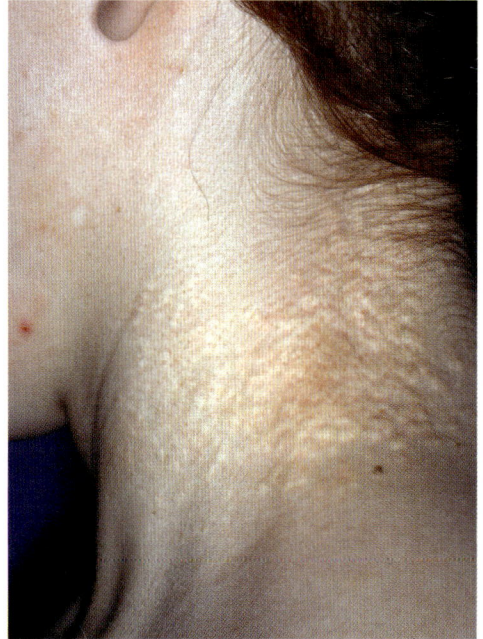

Fig. 25.10 Pseudoxanthoma elasticum.

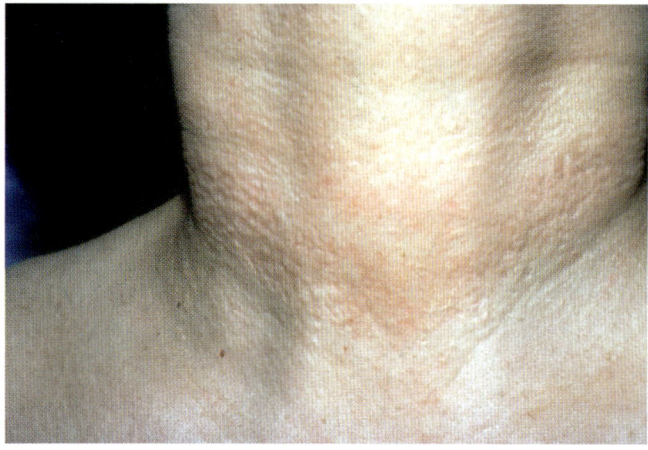

Fig. 25.11 Pseudoxanthoma elasticum.

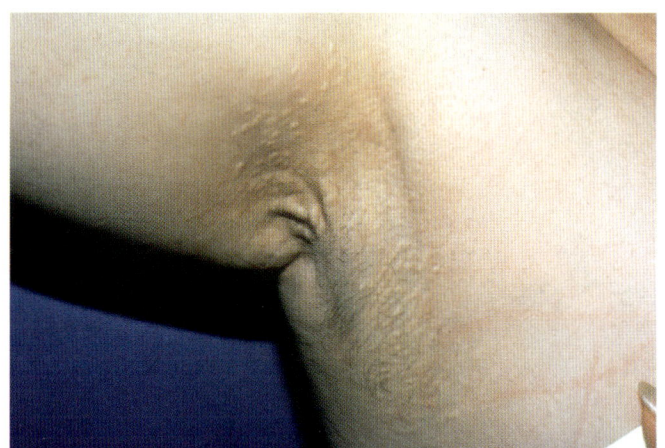

Fig. 25.12 Pseudoxanthoma elasticum.

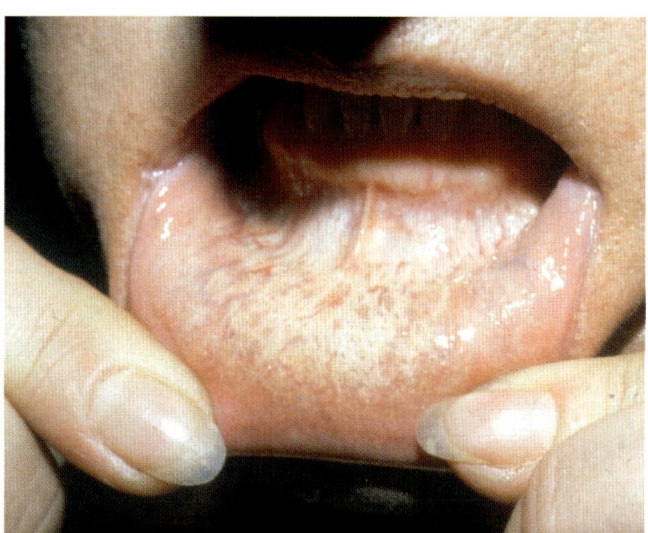

Fig. 25.13 Pseudoxanthoma elasticum.

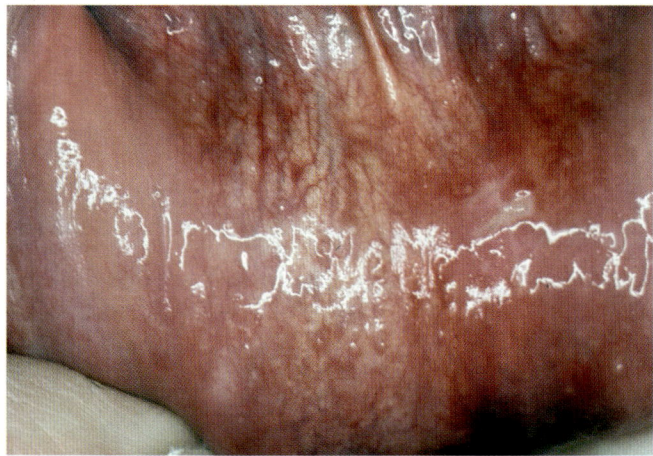

Fig. 25.14 Pseudoxanthoma elasticum.

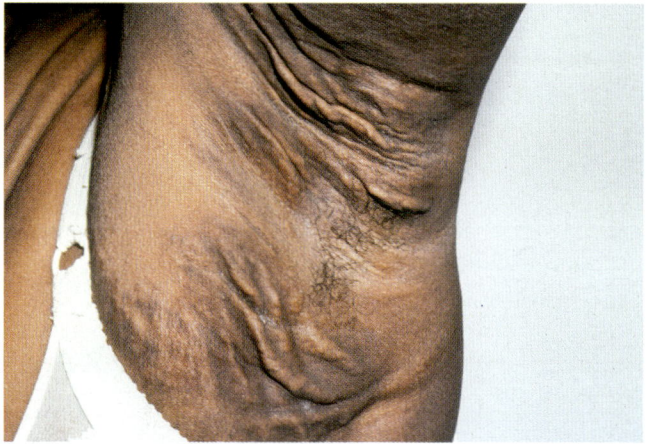

Fig. 25.15 Pseudoxanthoma elasticum.

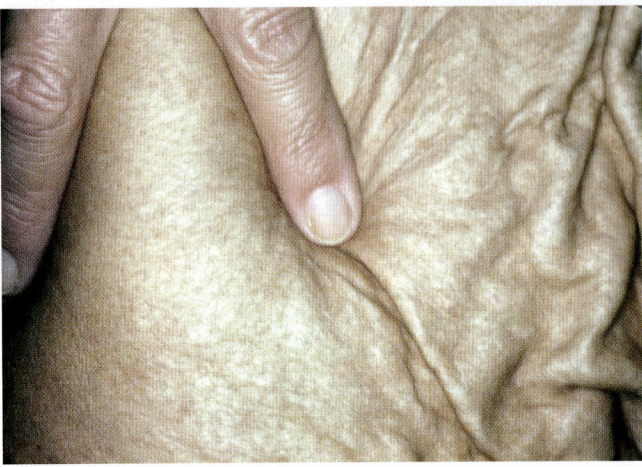

Fig. 25.16 Pseudoxanthoma elasticum.

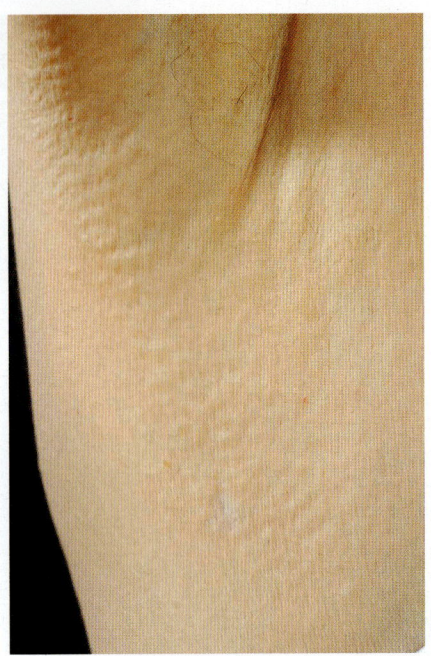

Fig. 25.17 Pseudoxanthoma elasticum–like papillary dermal elastolysis.

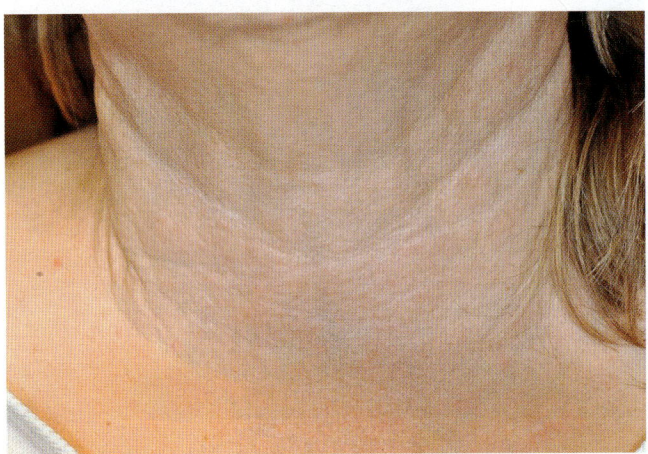

Fig. 25.18 Penicillamine elastopathy.

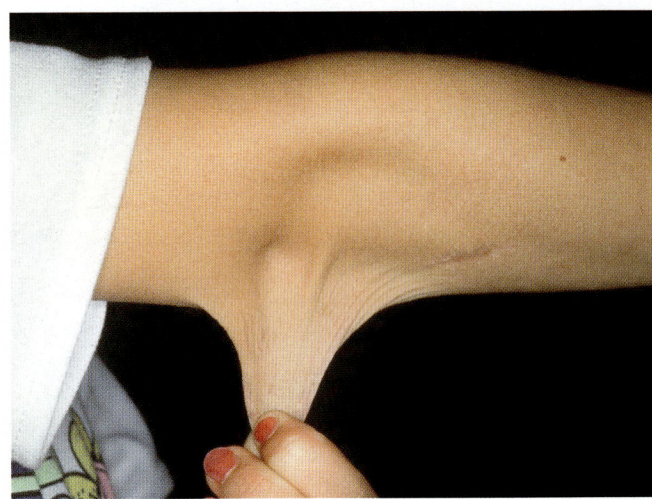

Fig. 25.19 Ehlers-Danlos syndrome.

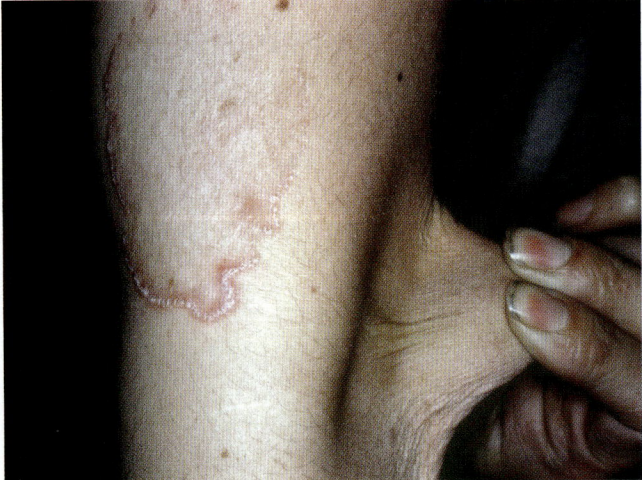

Fig. 25.20 Ehlers-Danlos syndrome and elastosis perforans serpiginosa.

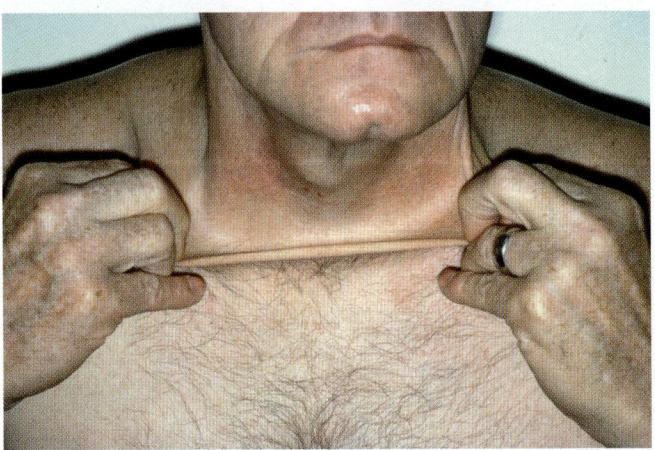

Fig. 25.21 Ehlers-Danlos syndrome.

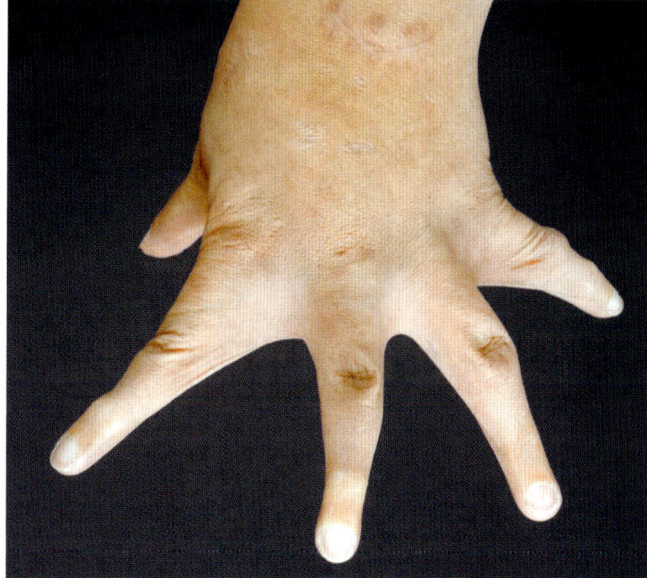

Fig. 25.22 Ehlers-Danlos syndrome.

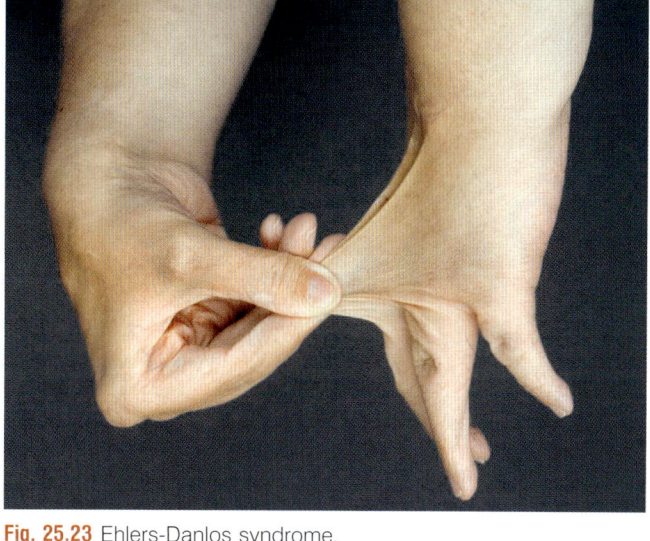

Fig. 25.23 Ehlers-Danlos syndrome.

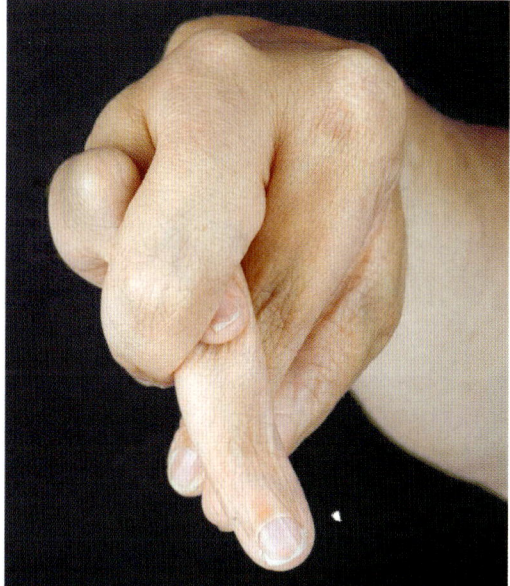

Fig. 25.24 Ehlers-Danlos syndrome.

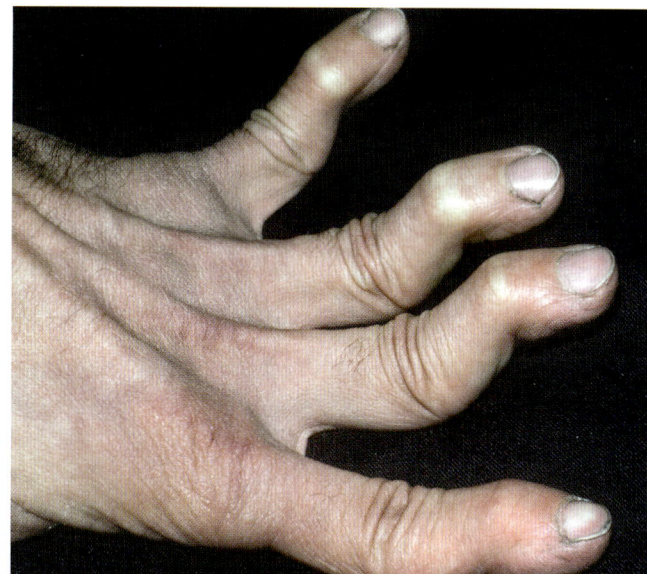

Fig. 25.25 Ehlers-Danlos syndrome. *Courtesy Steven Binnick, MD.*

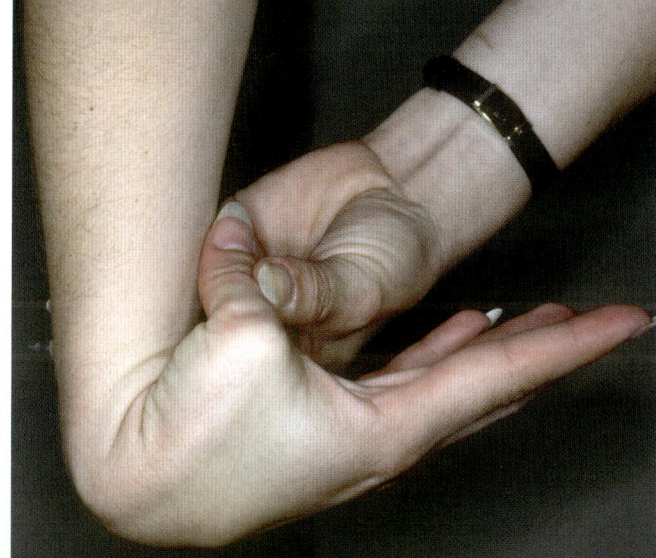

Fig. 25.26 Ehlers-Danlos syndrome.

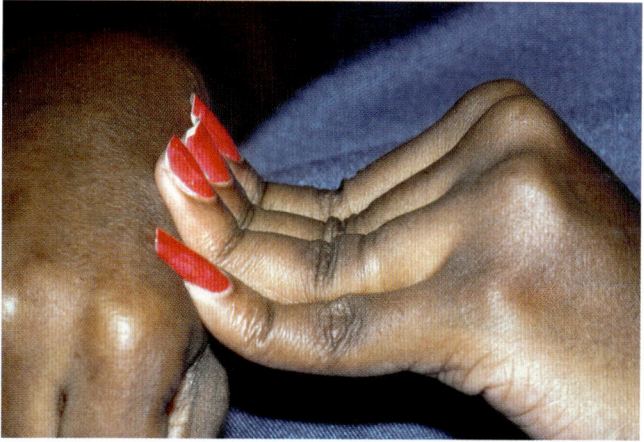

Fig. 25.27 Ehlers-Danlos syndrome.

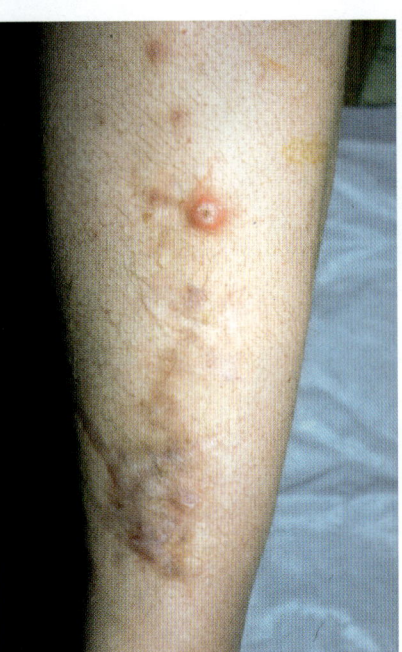

Fig. 25.28 Ehlers-Danlos syndrome with scarring and molluscoid pseudotumor.

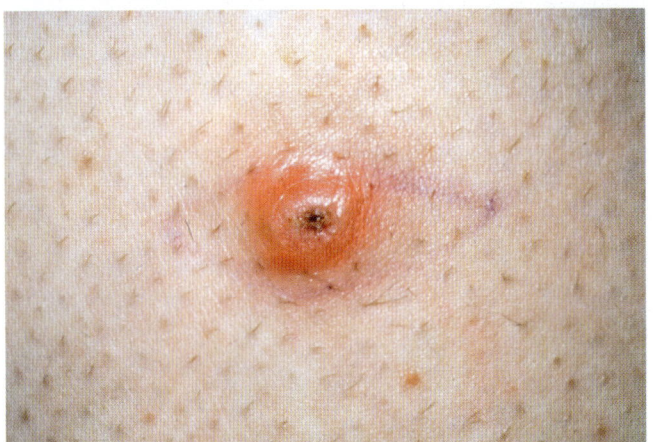

Fig. 25.29 Molluscoid pseudotumor.

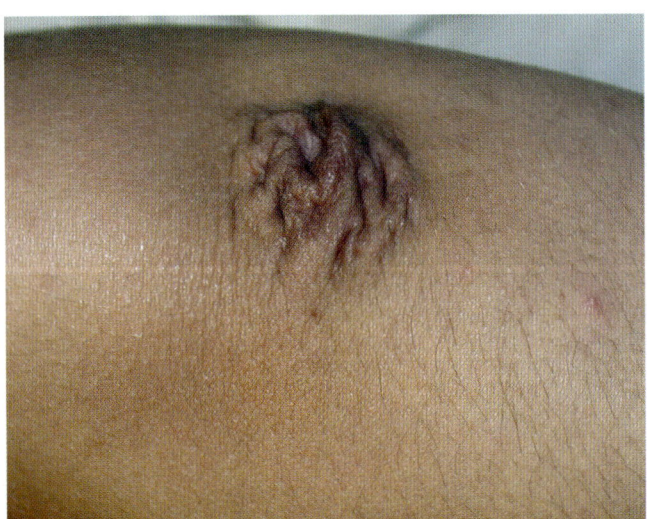

Fig. 25.31 Ehlers Danlos syndrome with atrophic scar.

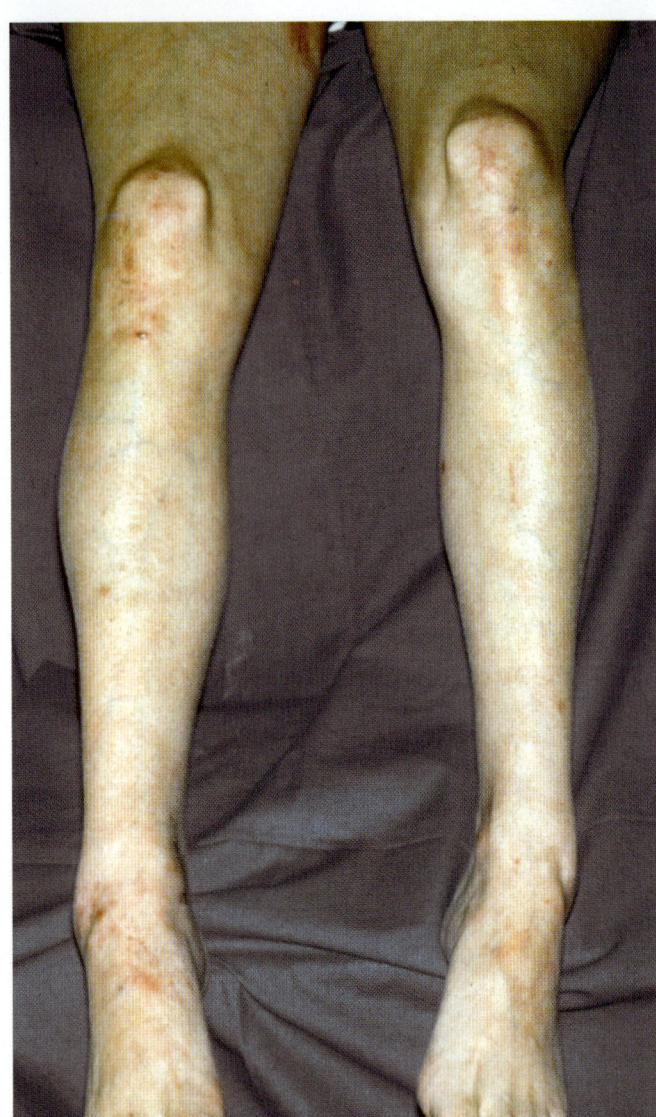

Fig. 25.30 Ehlers-Danlos syndrome type IV with translucent skin.

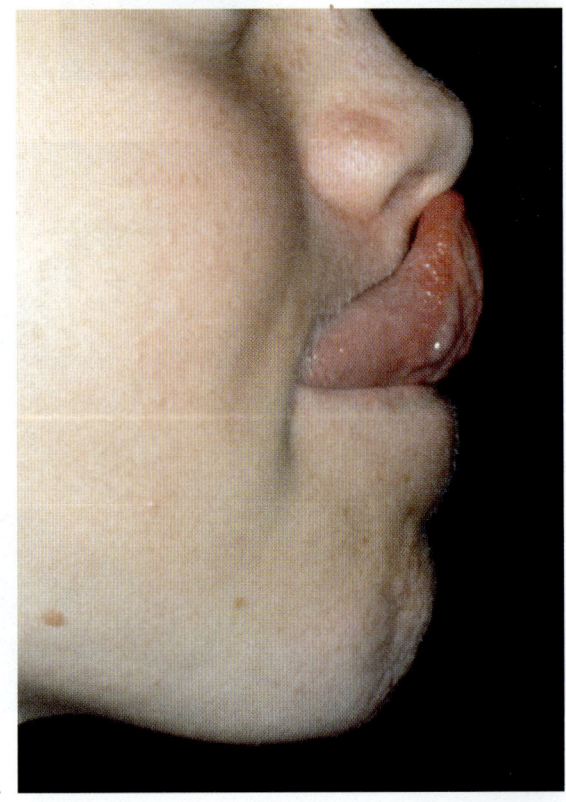

Fig. 25.32 Ehlers-Danlos syndrome.

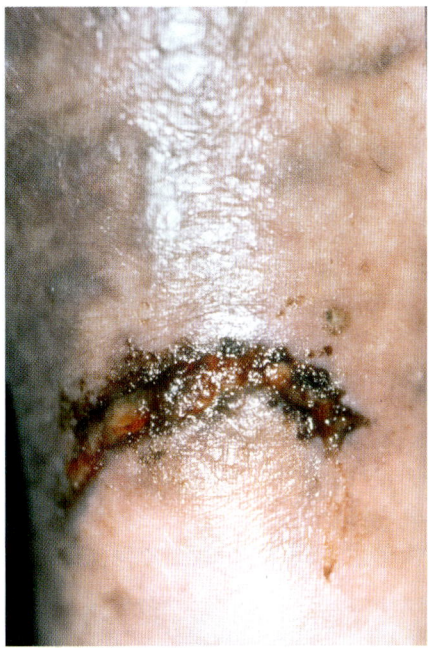

Fig. 25.33 Shin of a patient with Ehlers-Danlos type VIII.

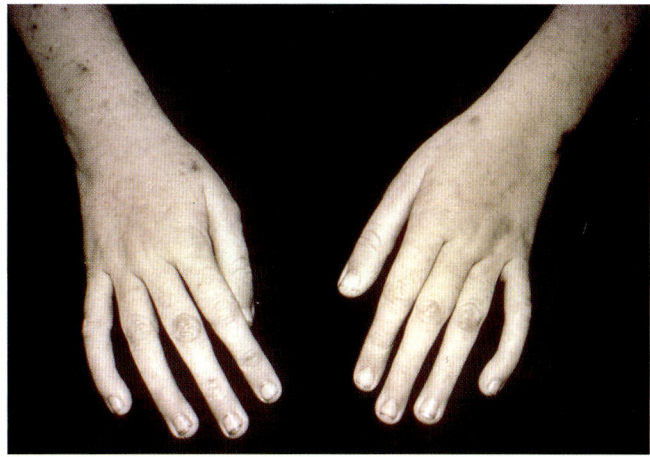

Fig. 25.34 Marfan syndrome.

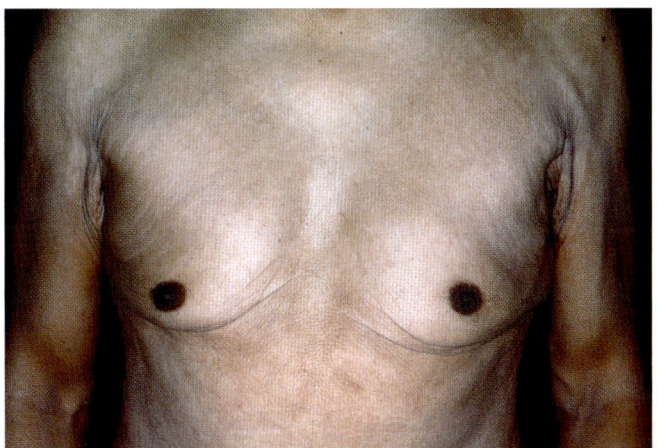

Fig. 25.35 Cutis laxa.

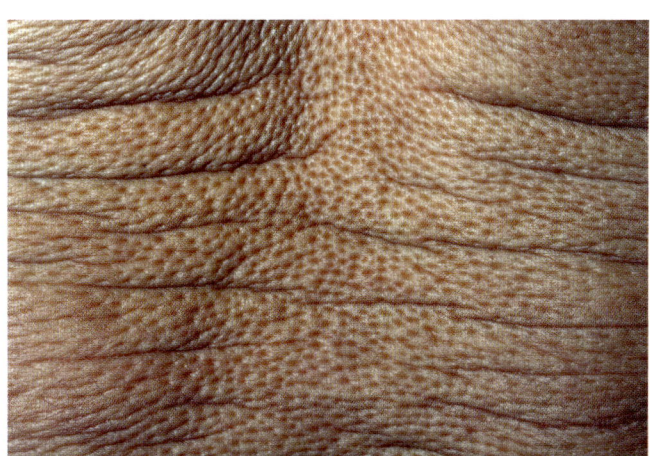

Fig. 25.36 Cutis laxa.

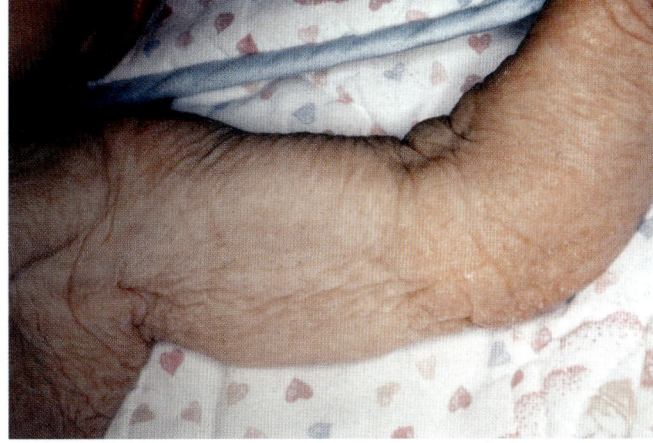

Fig. 25.37 Neonatal cutis laxa.

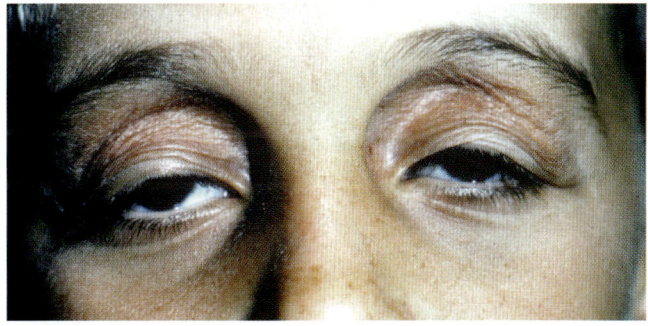

Fig. 25.38 Blepharochalasis in Ascher syndrome. *Courtesy Ken Greer, MD.*

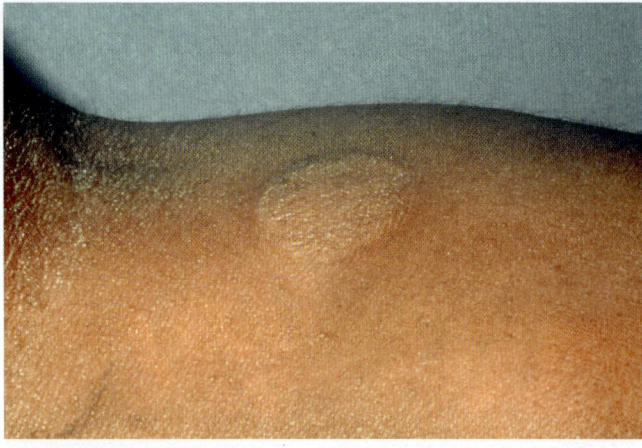

Fig. 25.39 Anetoderma.

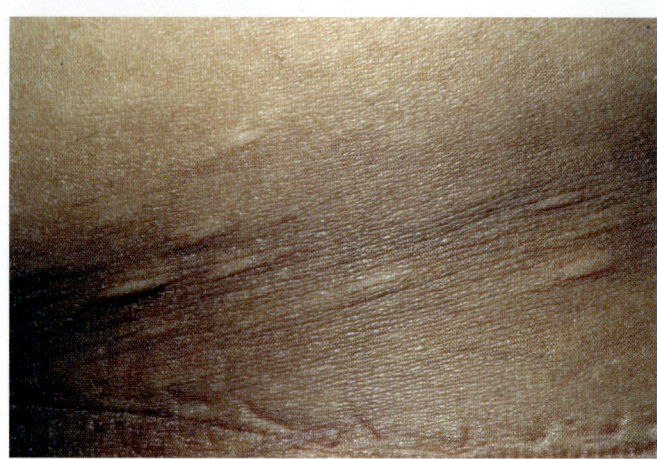

Fig. 25.40 Anetoderma.

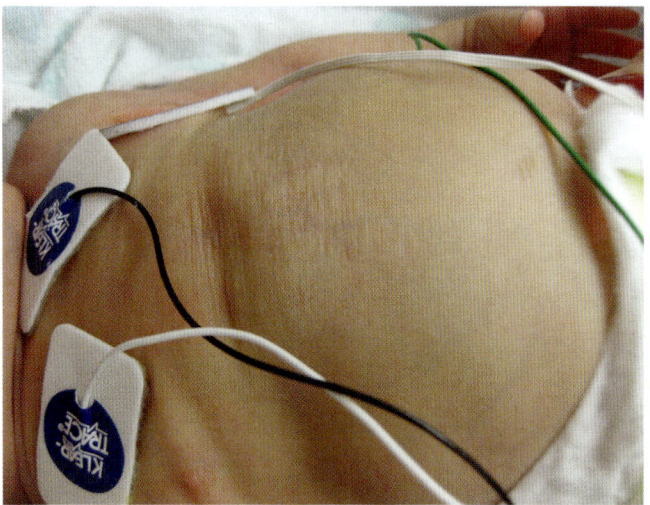

Fig. 25.41 Anetoderma of prematurity.

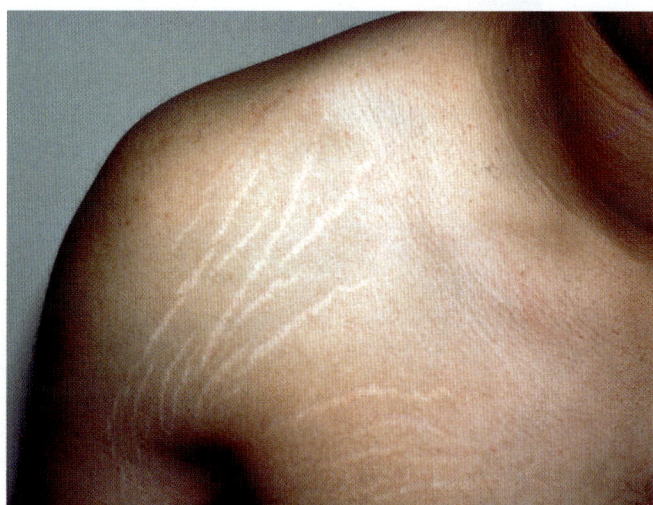

Fig. 25.42 Striae distensae.

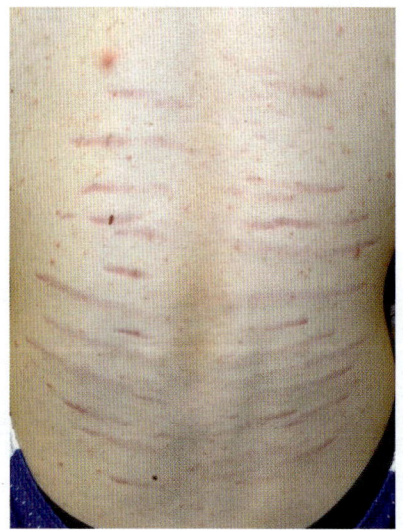

Fig. 25.43 Striae distensae. *Courtesy Scott Norton, MD.*

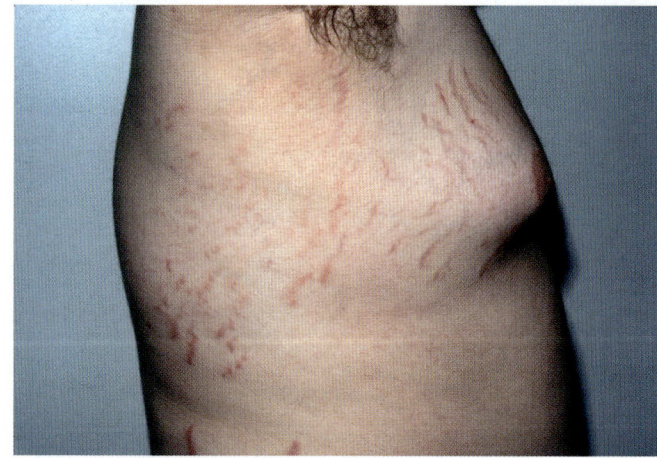

Fig. 25.44 Striae distensae.

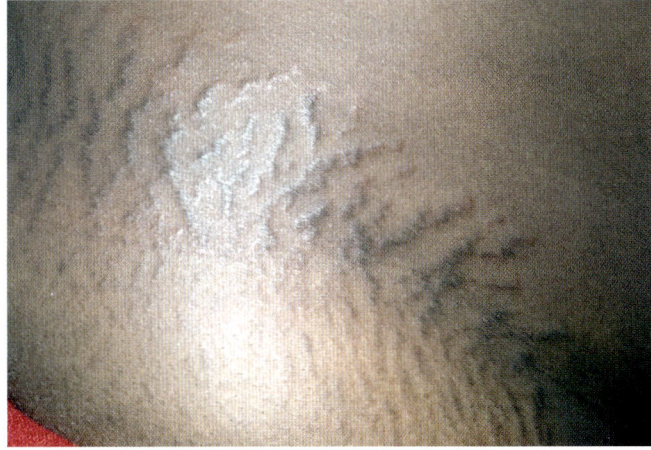

Fig. 25.45 Striae distensae.

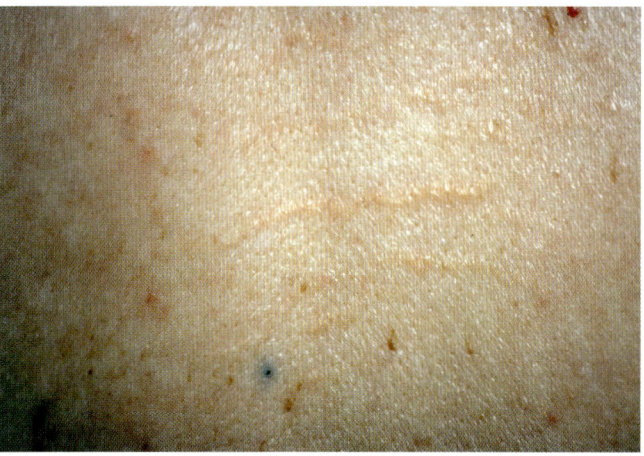

Fig. 25.46 Elastotic striae.

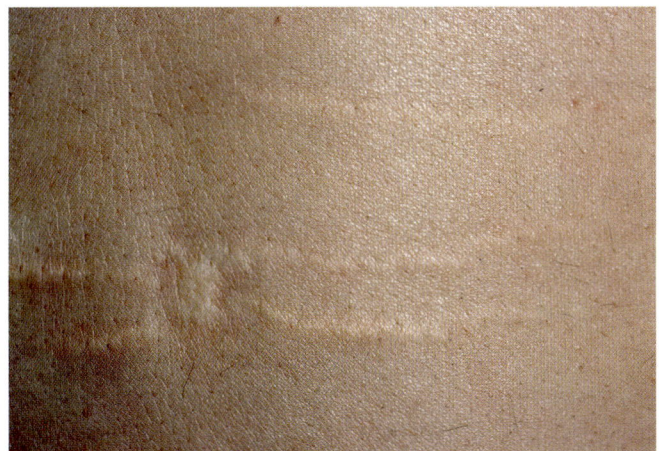

Fig. 25.47 Elastotic striae.

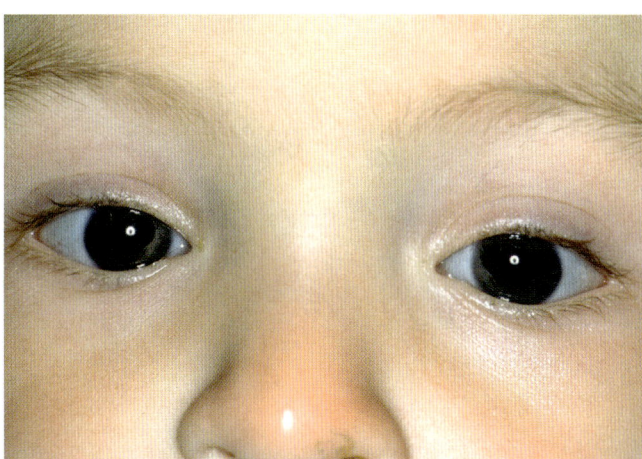

Fig. 25.48 Osteogenesis imperfecta with blue sclerae. *Courtesy Scott Norton, MD.*

Errors in Metabolism — 26

This chapter provides images of a collection of conditions that result from errors in metabolism. Many of these diseases manifest in the skin secondary to the deposition of material such as amyloid, porphyrin, calcium, lipid, and urate crystals.

Amyloidosis includes systemic and localized cutaneous forms. Systemic amyloidosis is characterized clinically by scattered shiny, firm papules, plaques, and nodules; macroglossia; and, most commonly, easy bruising with the typical "pinched purpura." Cutaneous amyloidosis includes the keratinocyte-derived amyloid deposited in macular and lichenoid patterns, as well as the nodular, plasma cell-derived form.

Porphyrins are required to build heme, but when specific enzyme defects cause them to accumulate, they can cause tissue damage after being activated by visible light (400-410 nm). This interaction with light explains why porphyrias are conditions that demonstrate photosensitivity with vesicles, bullae, and erosions in the typical photodistributed pattern on the face, upper chest, and dorsal hands and forearms. Other clinical findings of note in porphyrias include hyperpigmentation, skin fragility, and hypertrichosis.

Calcinosis cutis has been categorized into dystrophic, metastatic, and iatrogenic, depending on the cause. All forms present with rock-hard papules, nodules, or plaques that can extrude whitish chalky material. Patient history, full physical examination, and laboratory investigations will help distinguish between these forms of calcinosis. Idiopathic calcinosis cutis also occurs in specific locations, such as the scrotum, where it often does not require further clinical workup.

Deposition of lipid in the skin leads to yellow- or orange-colored papules, plaques, or masses that are categorized clinically based on their anatomic location and morphology. These include tuberous and tendinous xanthomas that often occur over joints requiring differentiation from gout. Eruptive xanthomas present with widespread papules, whereas plane xanthomas are characterized by larger yellowish patches. Other more localized xanthomas include palmar xanthomas on the hands and xanthelasma palpebrarum on the eyelids. Although xanthelasmas can be found in the setting of normal lipid levels, all patients with xanthomas require a workup to confirm the diagnosis and screen for a wide range of hyperlipidemias.

This portion of the atlas includes the previously mentioned deposition-related conditions, the cutaneous manifestations of diabetes mellitus, and rarer syndromes, including lipoid proteinosis and Fabry disease (angiokeratoma corporis diffusum).

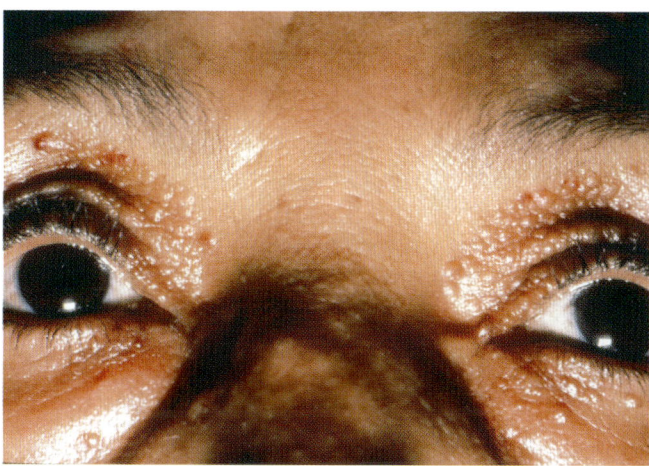

Fig. 26.1 Amyloidosis.

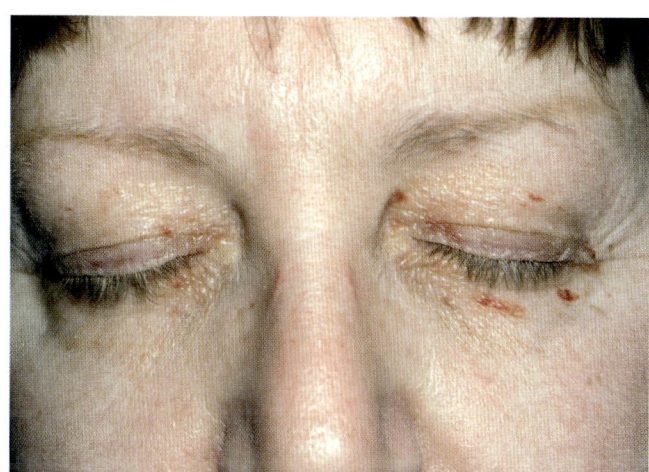

Fig. 26.2 Amyloidosis.

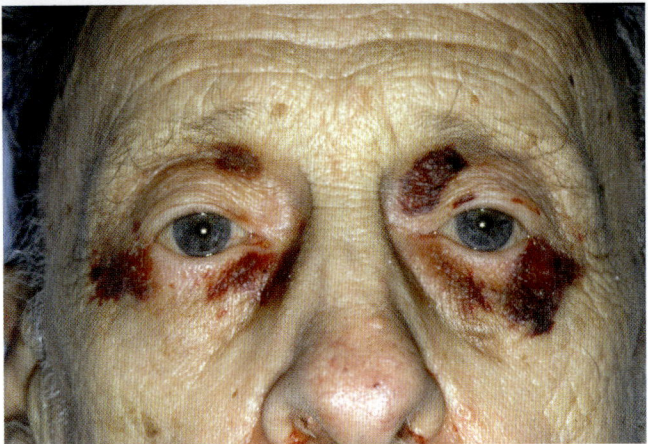

Fig. 26.3 Amyloidosis.

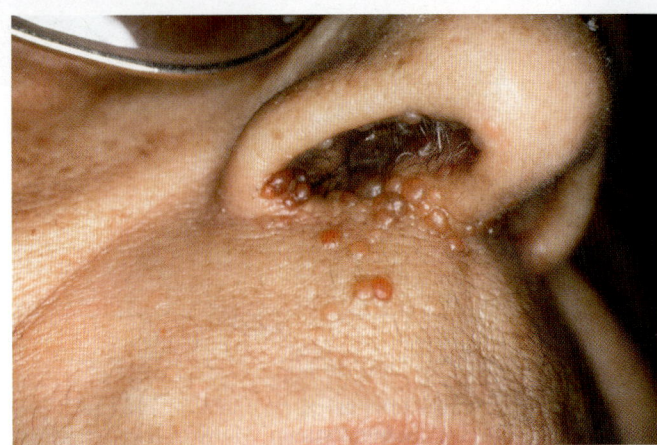

Fig. 26.4 Amyloidosis.

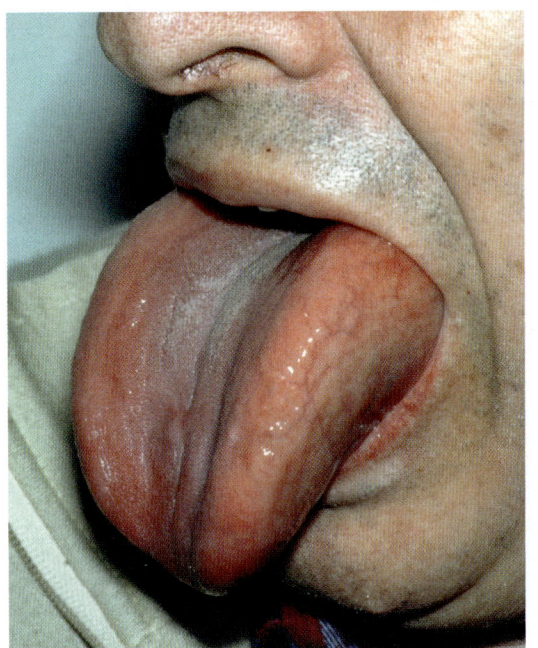

Fig. 26.5 Macroglossia in amyloidosis.

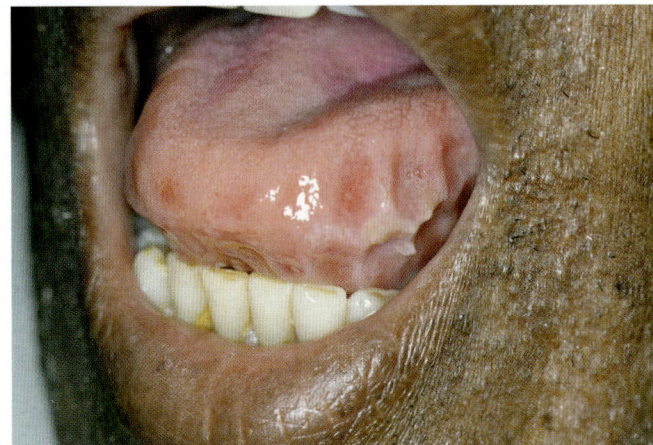

Fig. 26.6 Macroglossia in amyloidosis.

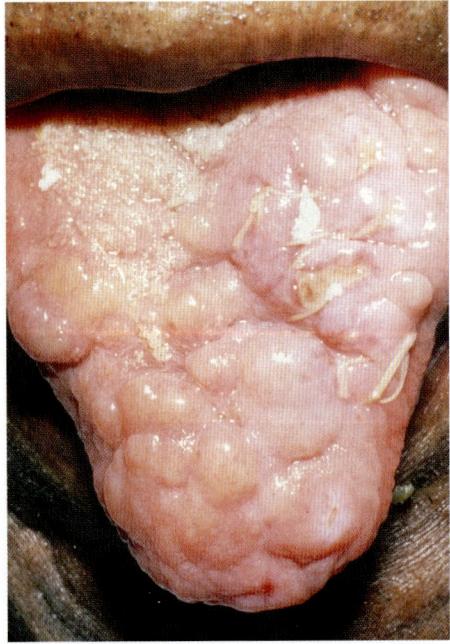

Fig. 26.7 Amyloidosis of the tongue.

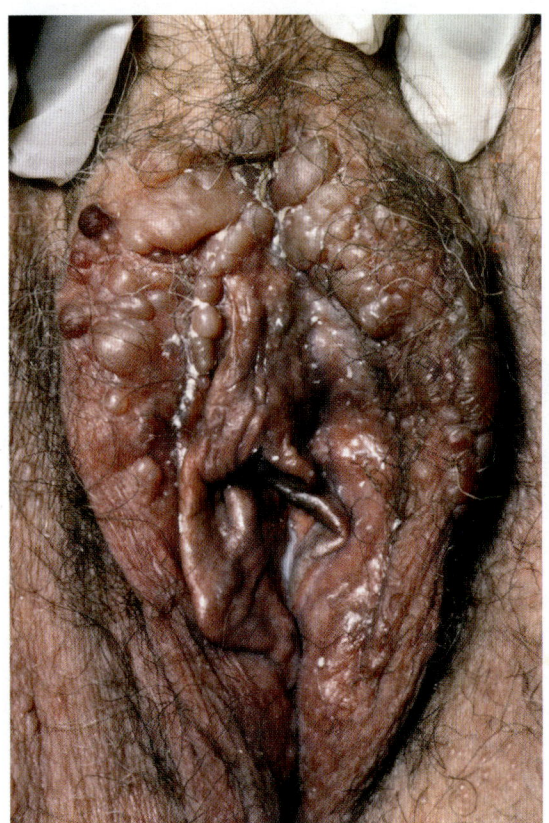

Fig. 26.8 Amyloidosis.

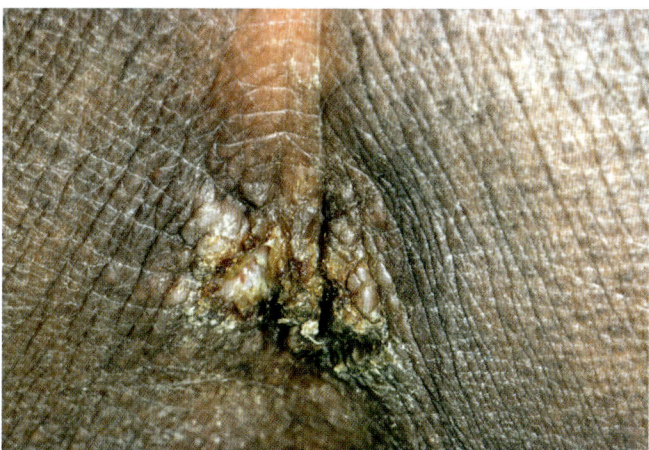
Fig. 26.9 Amyloidosis.

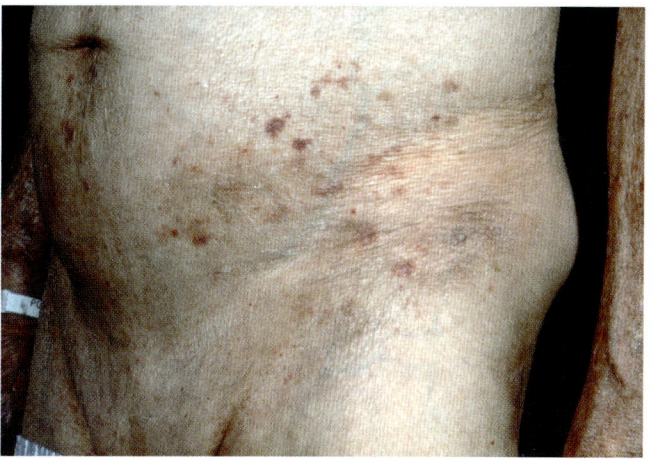
Fig. 26.10 Amyloidosis.

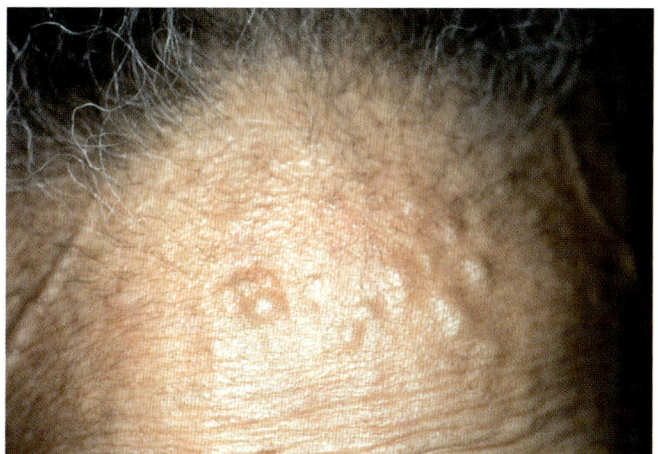
Fig. 26.11 Amyloidosis.

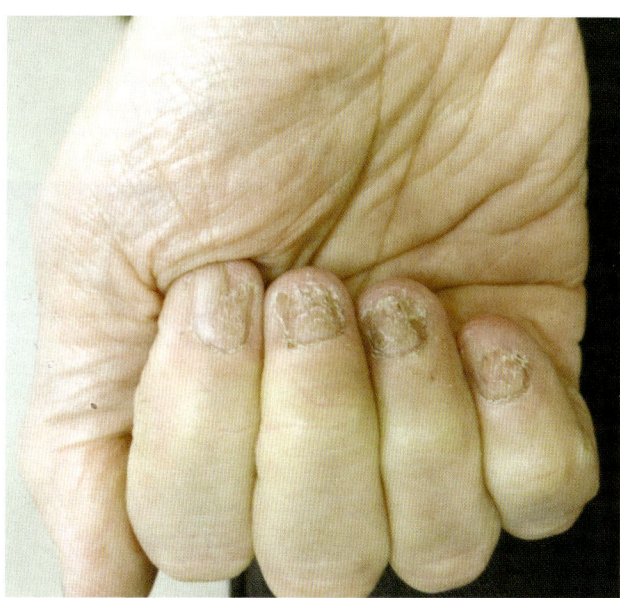
Fig. 26.12 Amyloidosis with involvement of the nail matrix with resultant dystrophy.

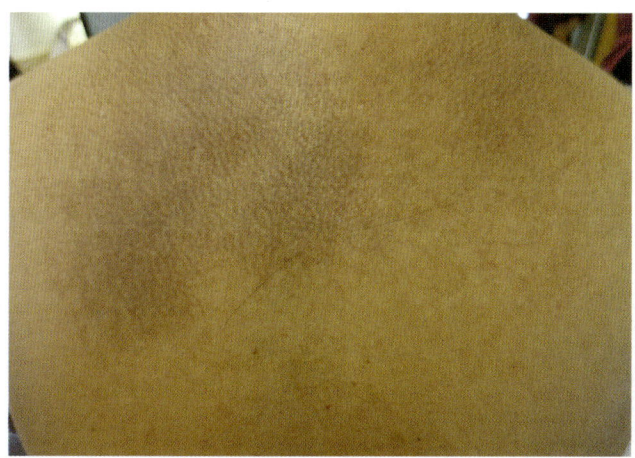
Fig. 26.13 Macular amyloidosis.

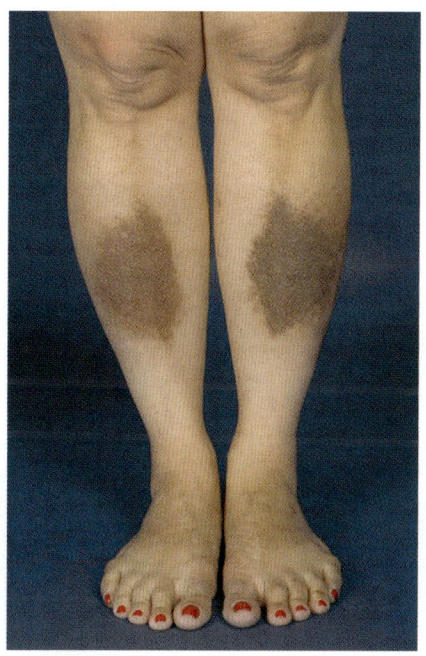
Fig. 26.14 Lichen amyloidosis.

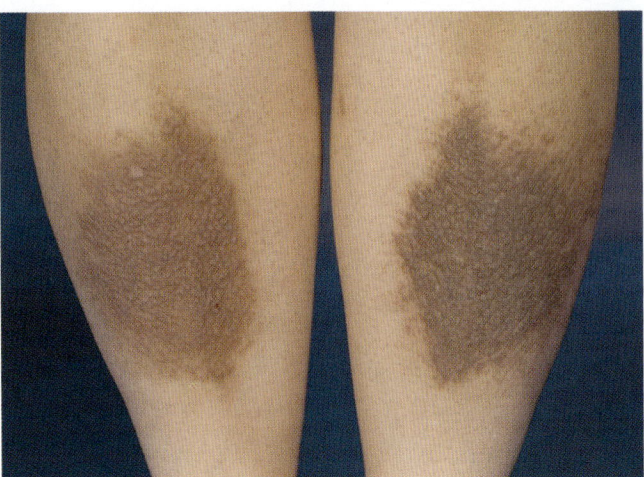

Fig. 26.15 Lichen amyloidosis.

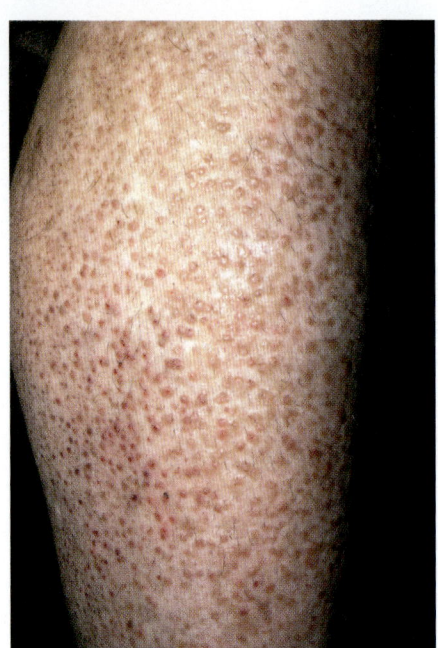

Fig. 26.16 Lichen amyloidosis.

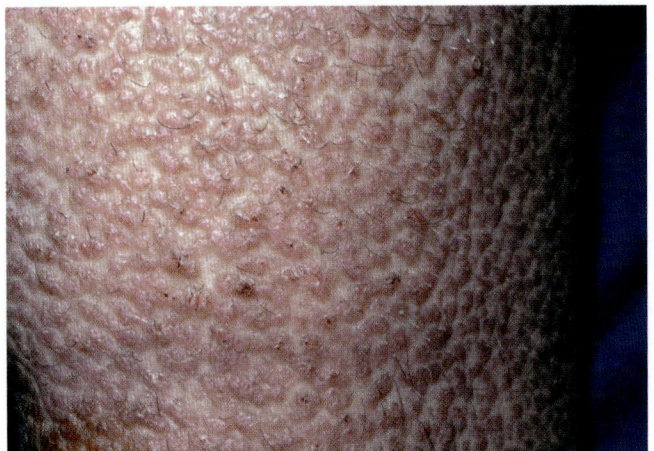

Fig. 26.17 Lichen amyloidosis. *Courtesy Steven Binnick, MD.*

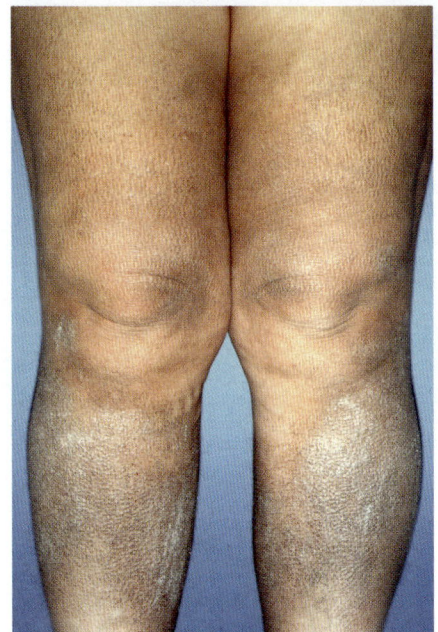

Fig. 26.18 Lichen amyloidosis.

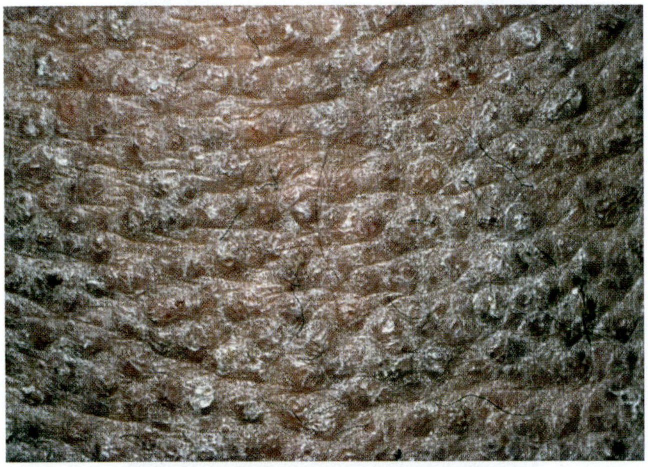

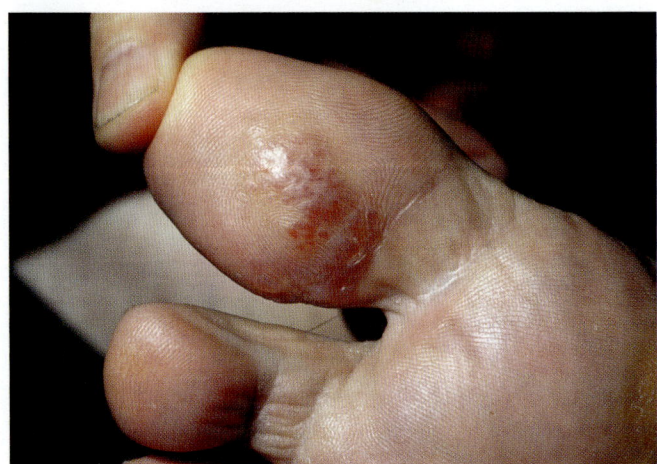

Fig. 26.19 Lichen amyloidosis.

Fig. 26.20 Nodular amyloidosis.

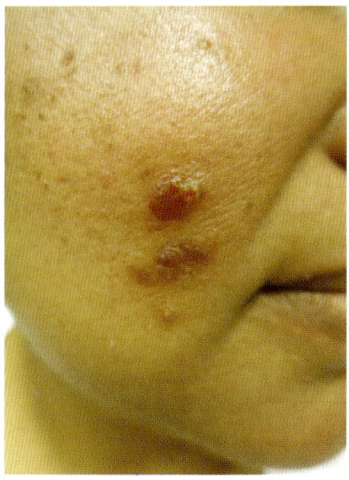

Fig. 26.21 Nodular amyloidosis.

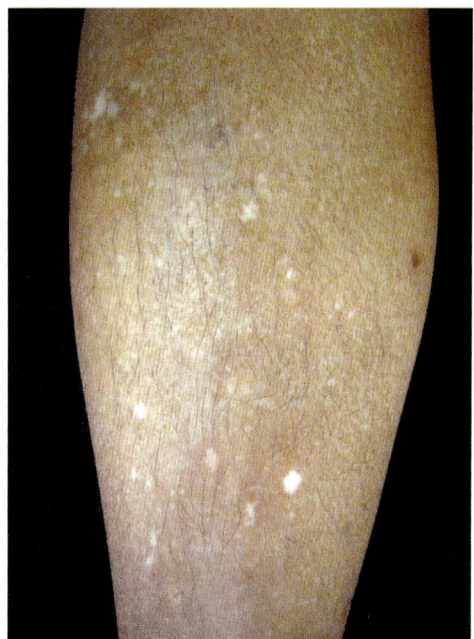

Fig. 26.22 Dyschromic amyloidosis. *Courtesy Vasanop Vachiramon, MD.*

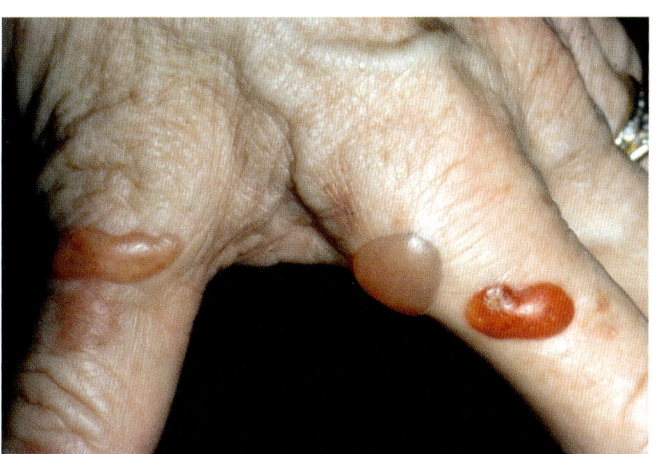

Fig. 26.23 Porphyria cutanea tarda.

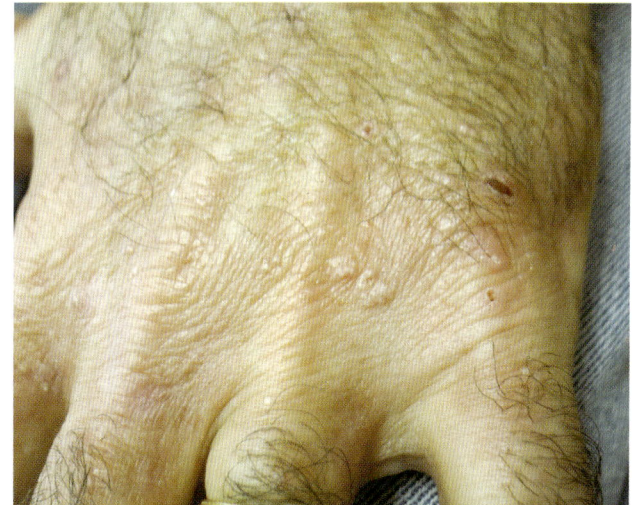

Fig. 26.24 Milia and scarring in porphyria cutanea tarda.

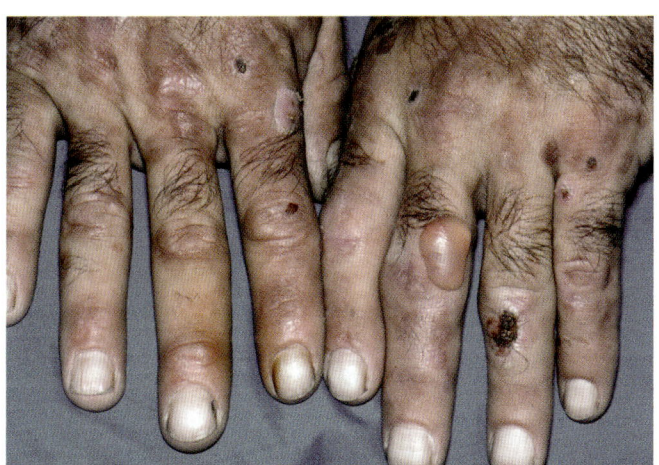

Fig. 26.25 Porphyria cutanea tarda. *Courtesy Steven Binnick, MD.*

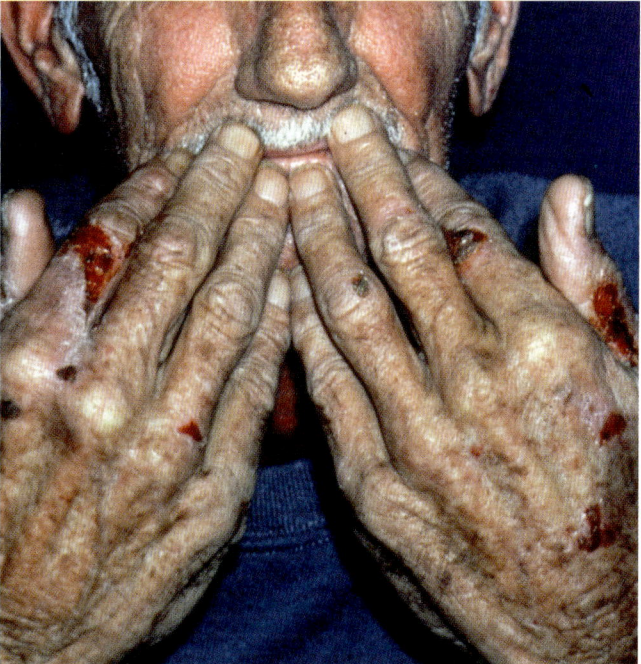

Fig. 26.26 Porphyria cutanea tarda in a patient with hepatoma.

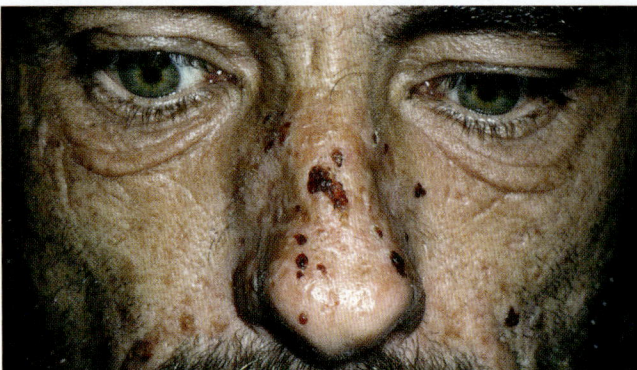

Fig. 26.27 Porphyria cutanea tarda in a patient with hepatoma. *Courtesy Steven Binnick, MD.*

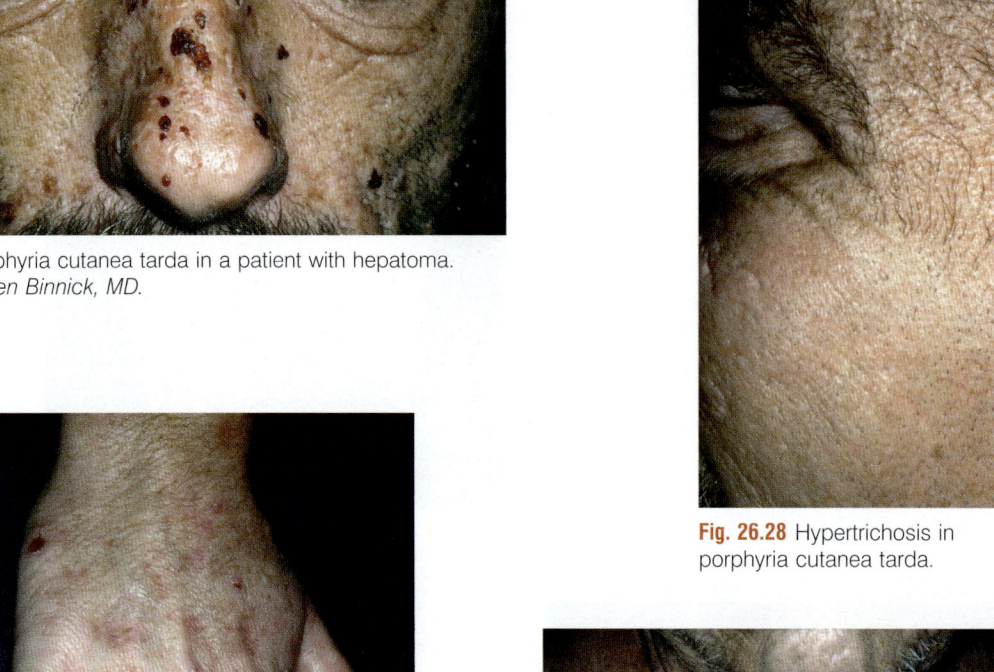

Fig. 26.28 Hypertrichosis in porphyria cutanea tarda.

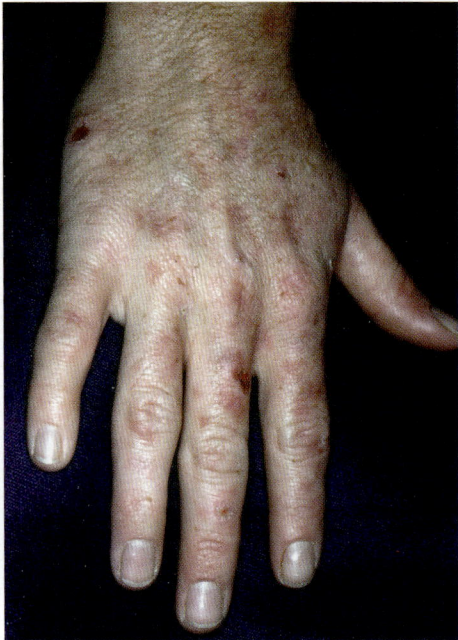

Fig. 26.29 Pseudo–porphyria cutanea tarda in a 16-year-old young woman who was taking tetracycline for acne.

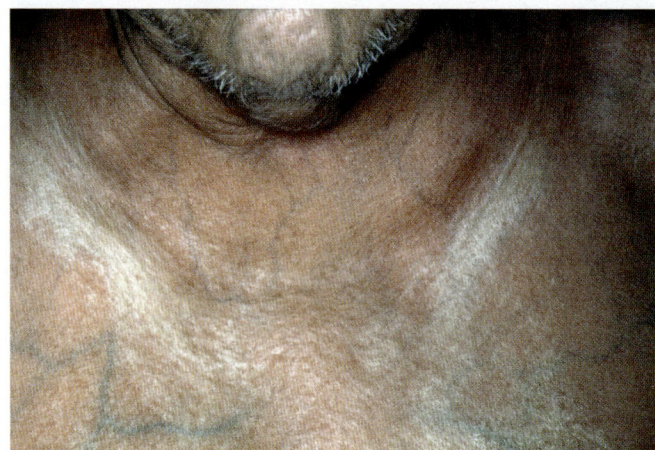

Fig. 26.30 Sclerodermoid lesions in a patient with porphyria cutanea tarda.

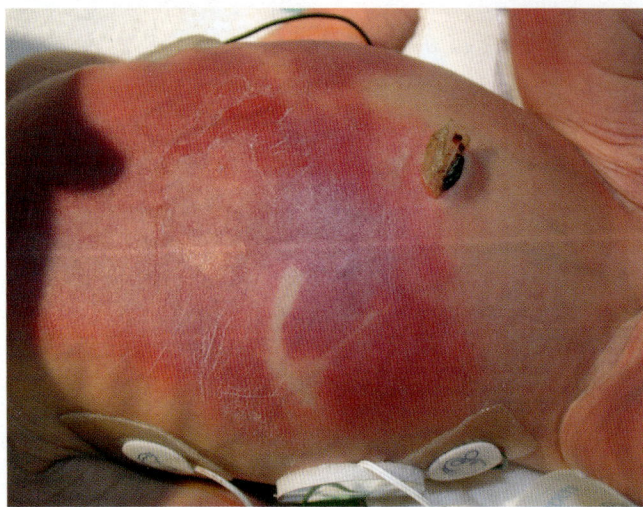

Fig. 26.31 Erythropoietic protoporphyria in a neonate after bili-light exposure.

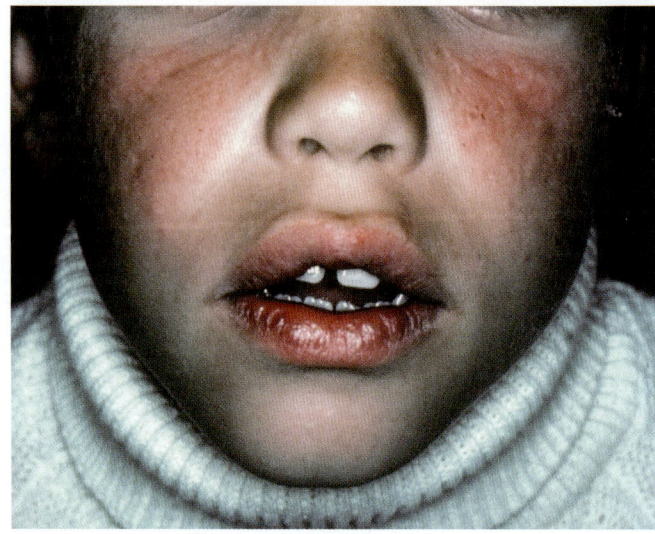

Fig. 26.32 Erythropoietic protoporphyria with scarring.

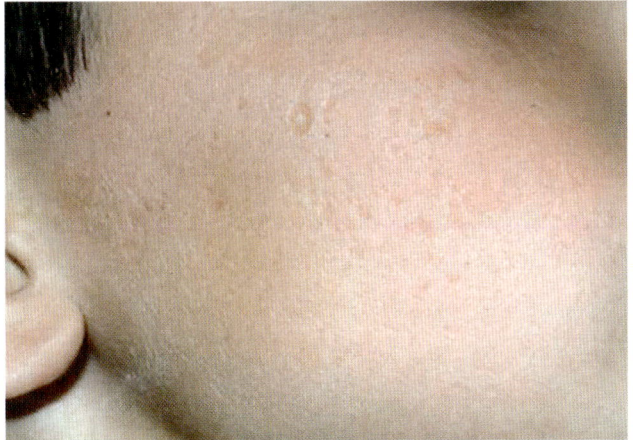

Fig. 26.33 Erythropoietic protoporphyria with scarring.

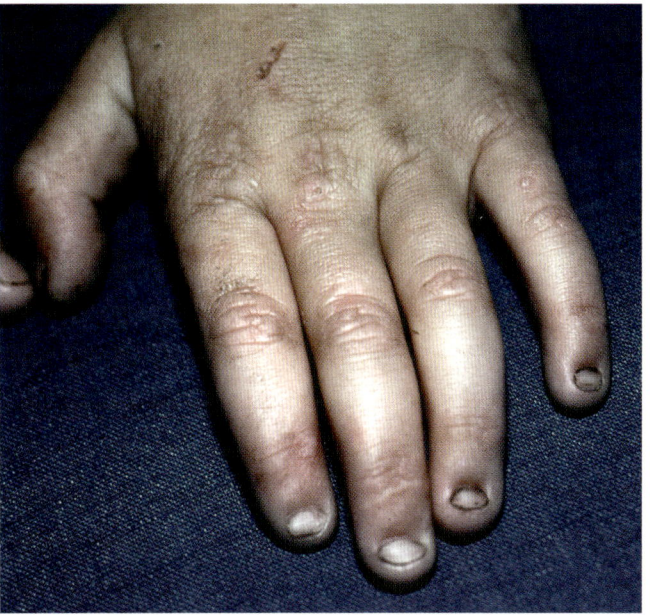

Fig. 26.34 Erythropoietic protoporphyria with scarring.

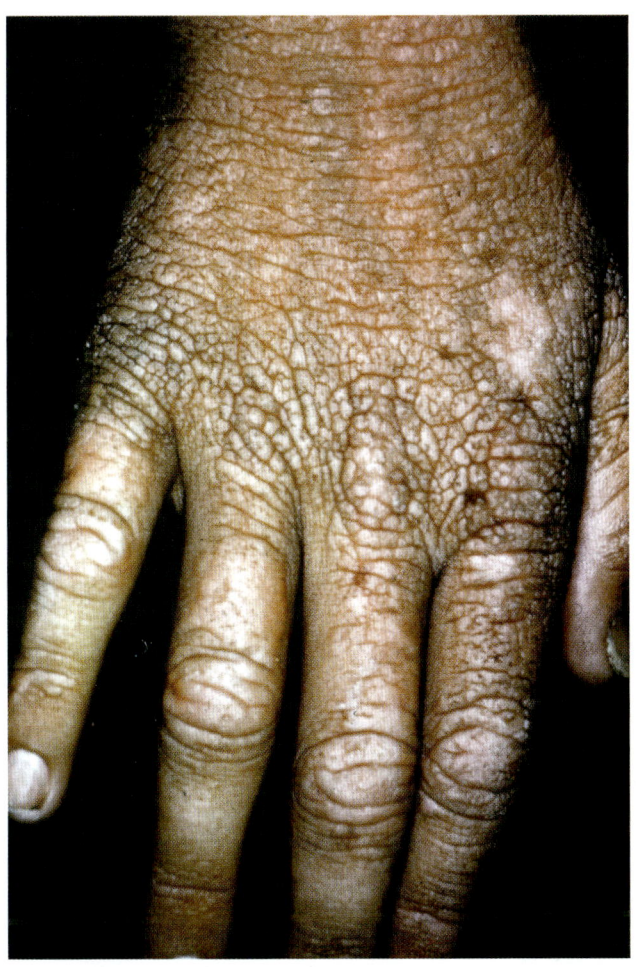

Fig. 26.35 Erythropoietic protoporphyria with scarring, thickening, and pebbling of the skin.

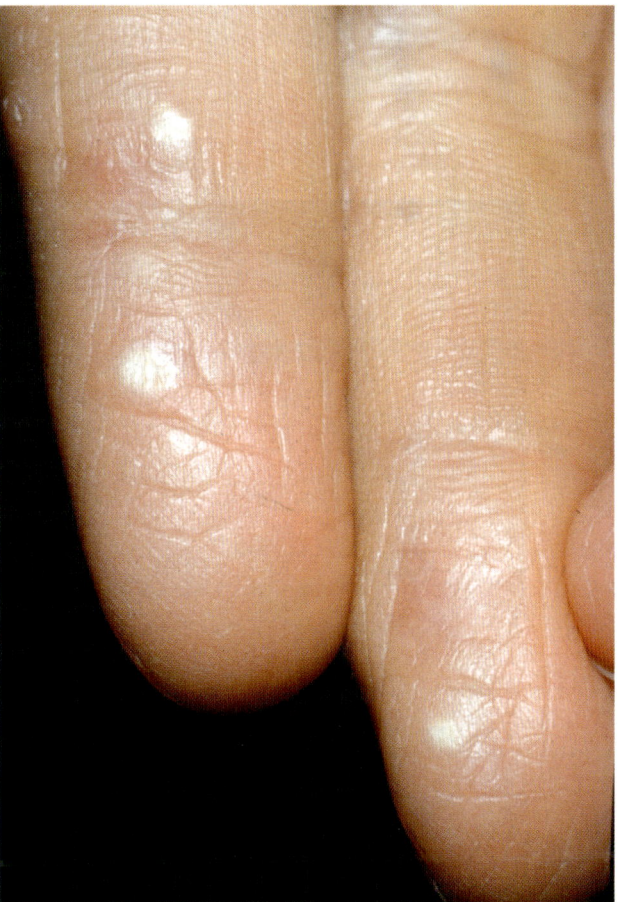

Fig. 26.36 Dystrophic calcinosis cutis.

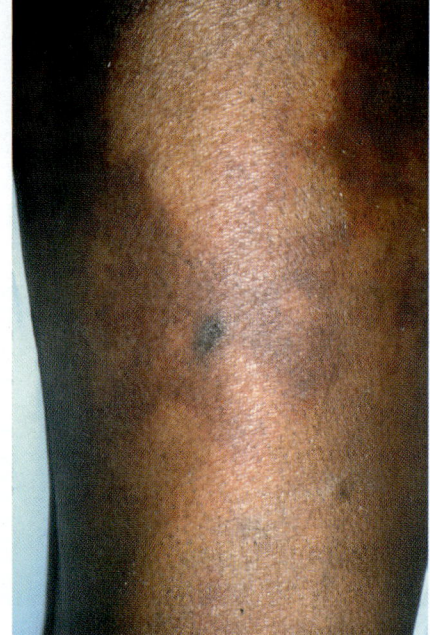

Fig. 26.37 Calciphylaxis.

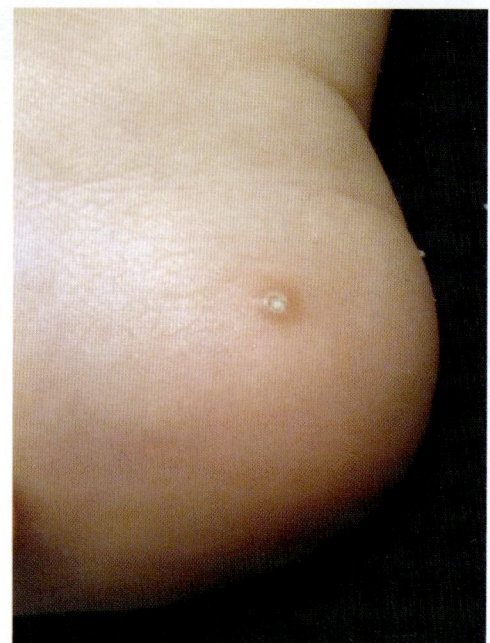

Fig. 26.38 Heel stick calcinosis.

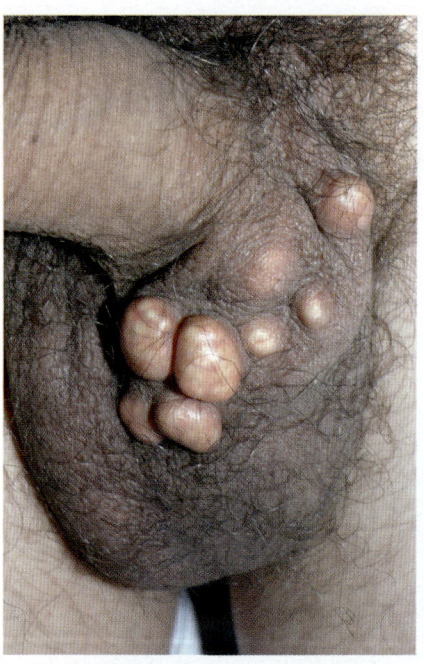

Fig. 26.39 Scrotal calcinosis. *Courtesy Steven Binnick, MD.*

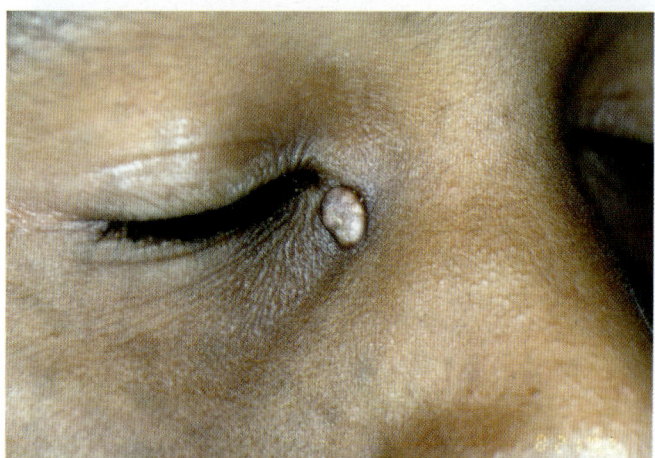

Fig. 26.40 Subepidermal calcified nodule.

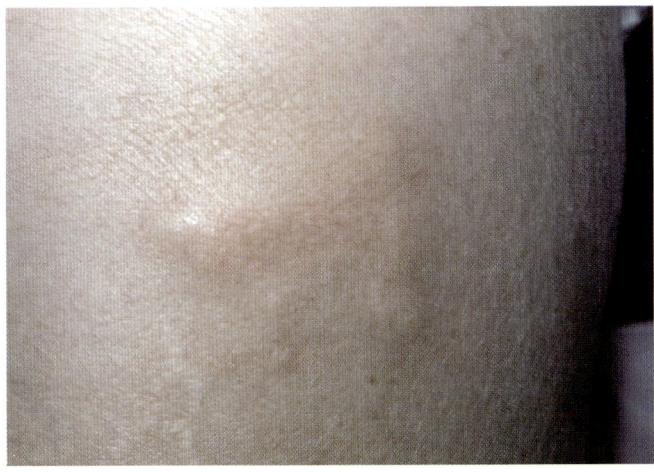

Fig. 26.41 Calcinosis cutis.

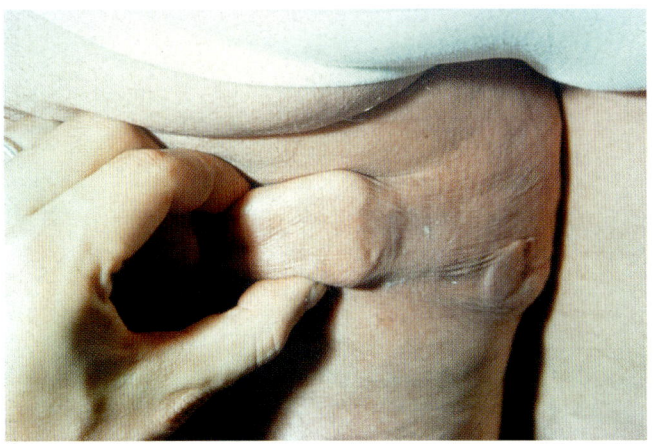

Fig. 26.42 Tumoral calcinosis cutis.

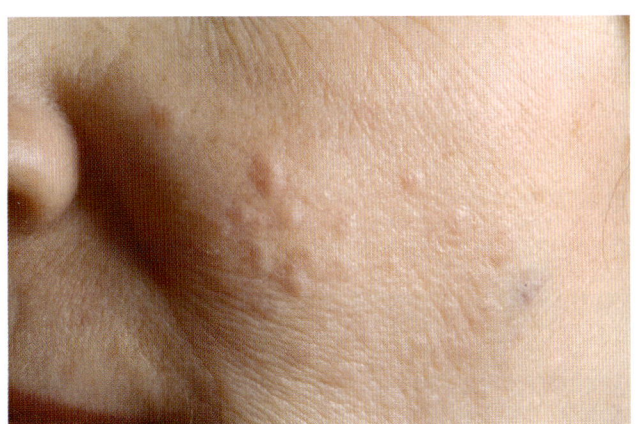

Fig. 26.43 Osteoma cutis.

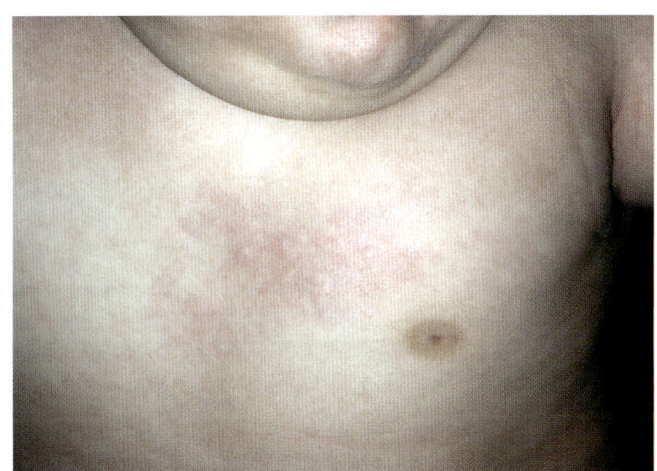

Fig. 26.44 Osteoma cutis.

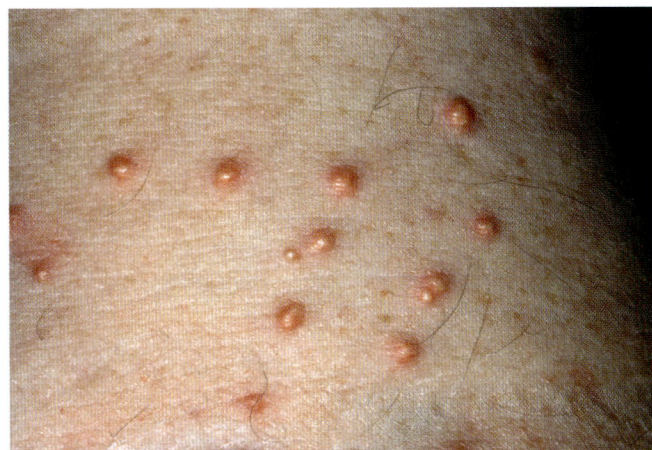

Fig. 26.45 Eruptive xanthomas.

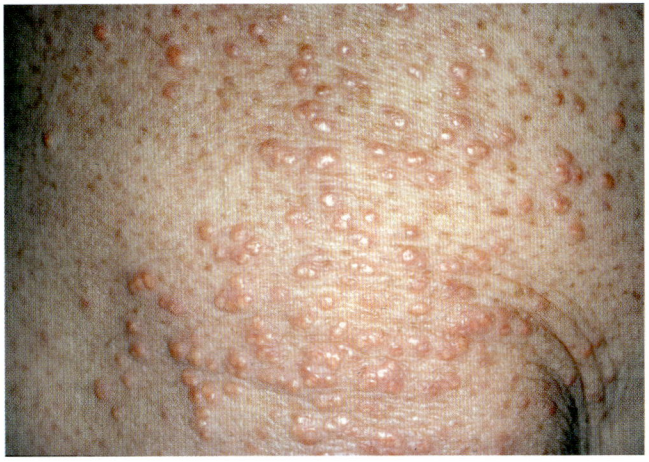

Fig. 26.46 Eruptive xanthomas.

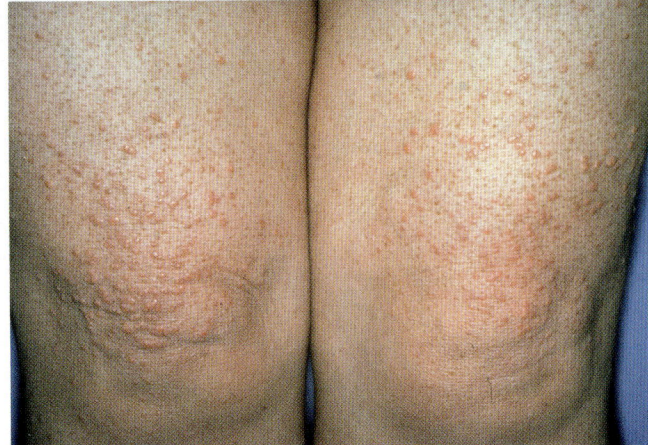

Fig. 26.47 Eruptive xanthomas.

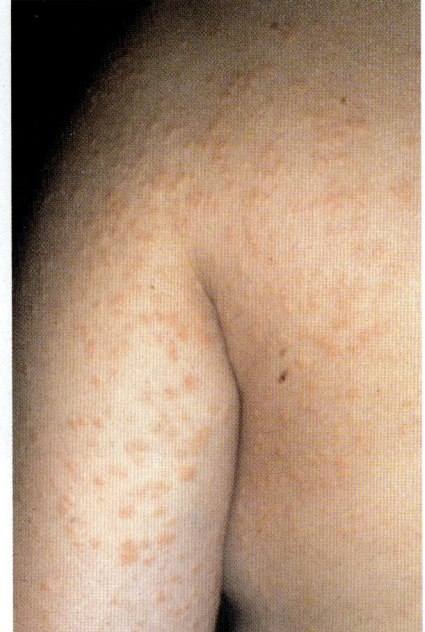

Fig. 26.48 Type I hyperlipidemic eruptive xanthomas.

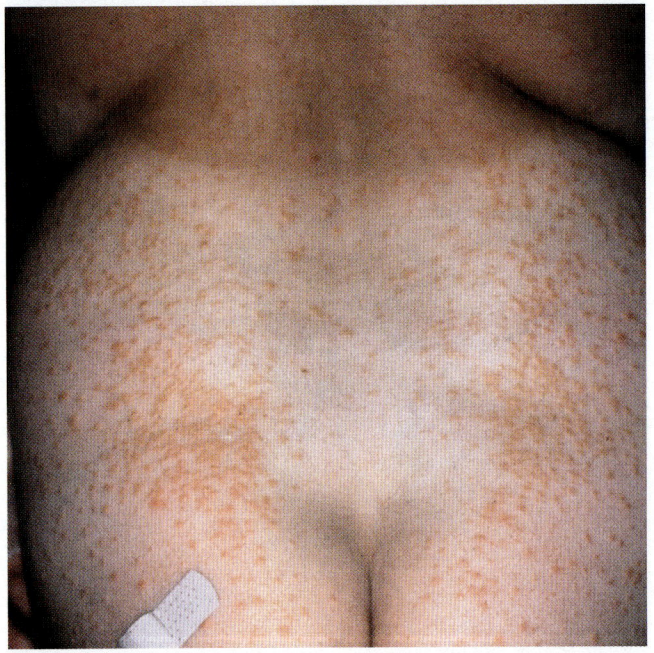

Fig. 26.49 Type I hyperlipidemic eruptive xanthomas.

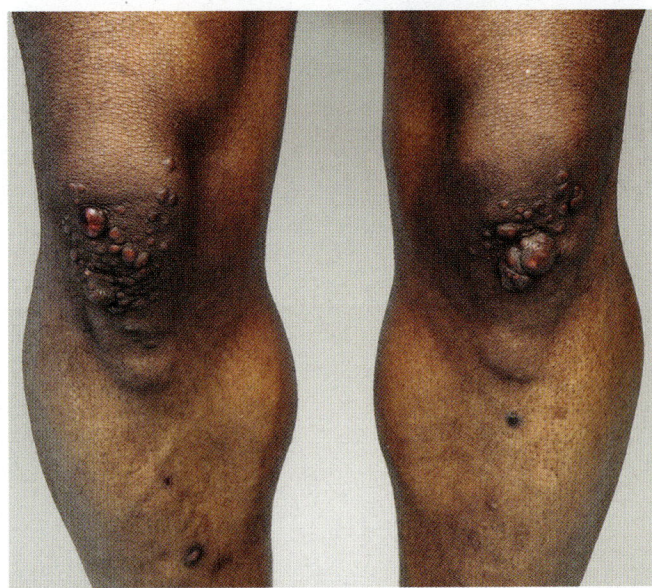

Fig. 26.50 Tuberous xanthomas.

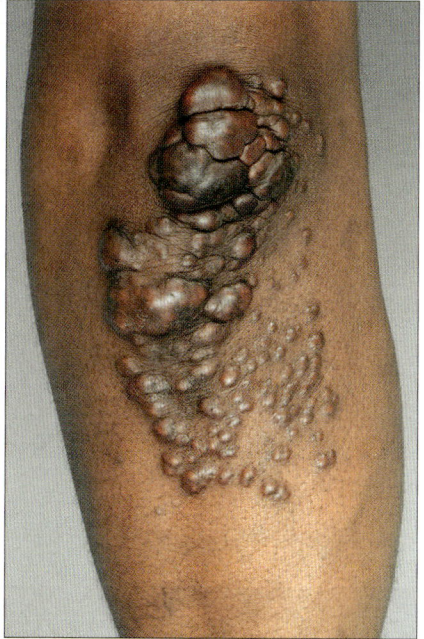

Fig. 26.51 Tuberous xanthomas.

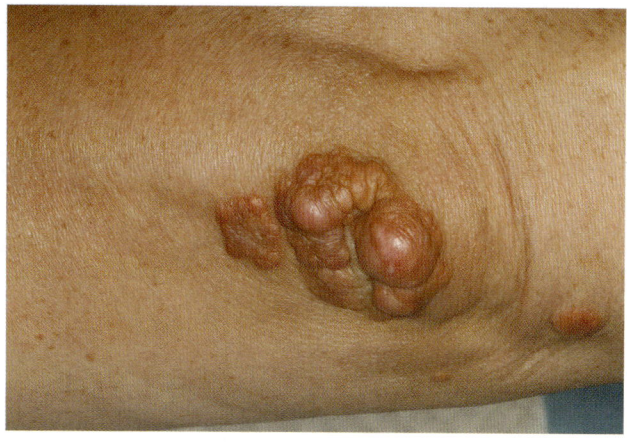

Fig. 26.52 Tuberous xanthomas.

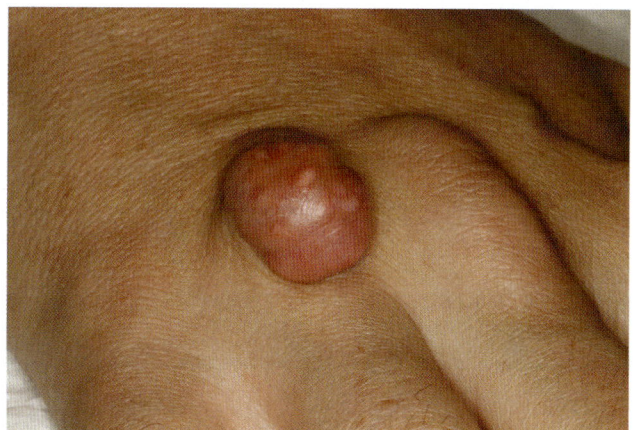

Fig. 26.53 Tuberous xanthoma.

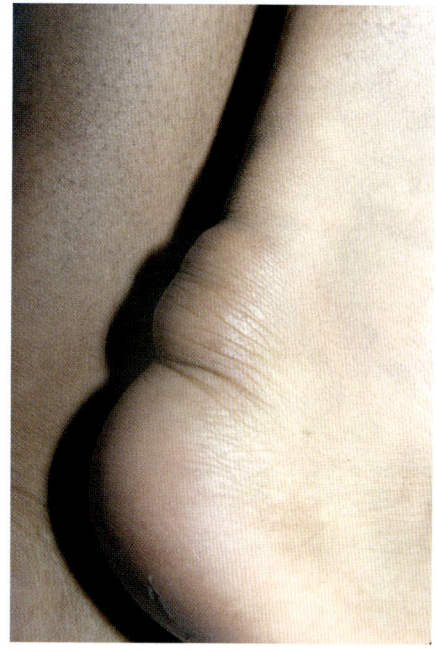

Fig. 26.54 Tendinous xanthoma.

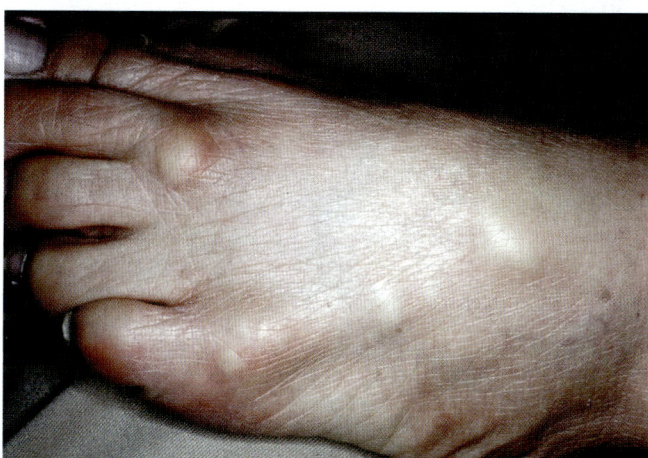

Fig. 26.55 Tendinous xanthomas.

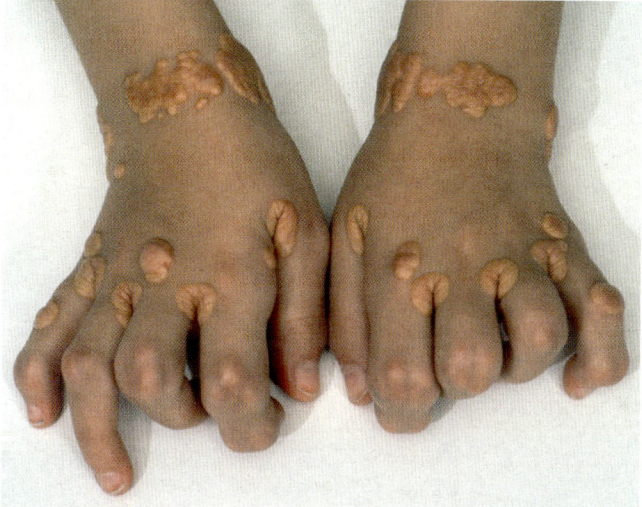

Fig. 26.56 Homozygous hypercholesterolemia with intertriginous xanthomas.

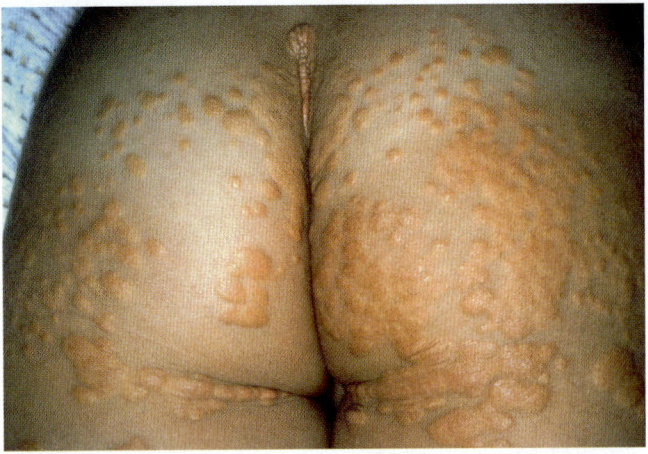

Fig. 26.57 Homozygous hypercholesterolemia with intertriginous xanthomas.

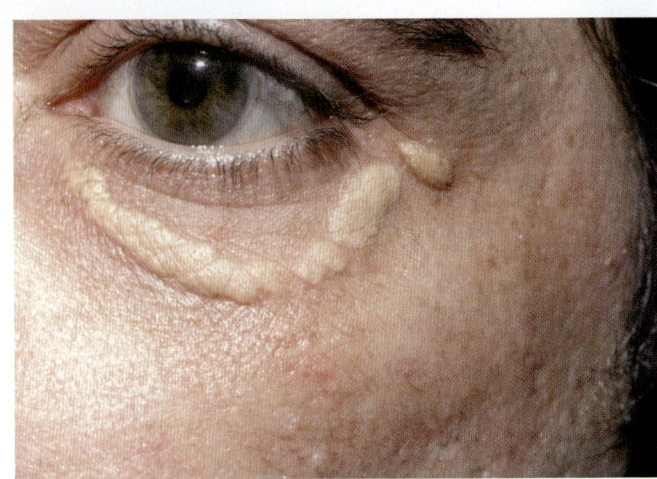

Fig. 26.58 Xanthelasma.

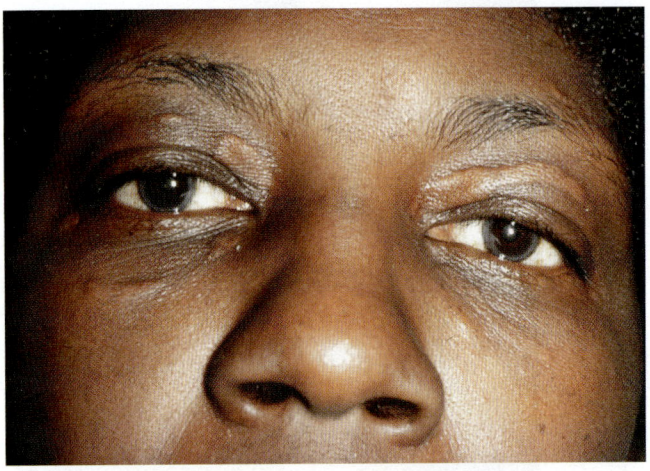

Fig. 26.59 Xanthelasma.

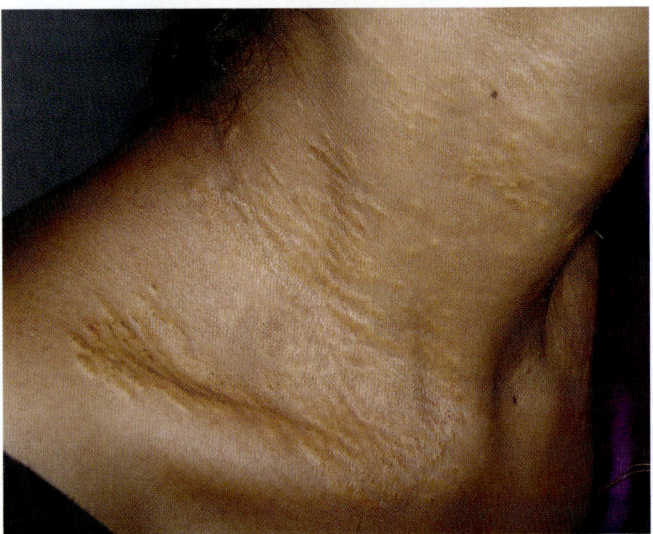

Fig. 26.60 Plane xanthoma.

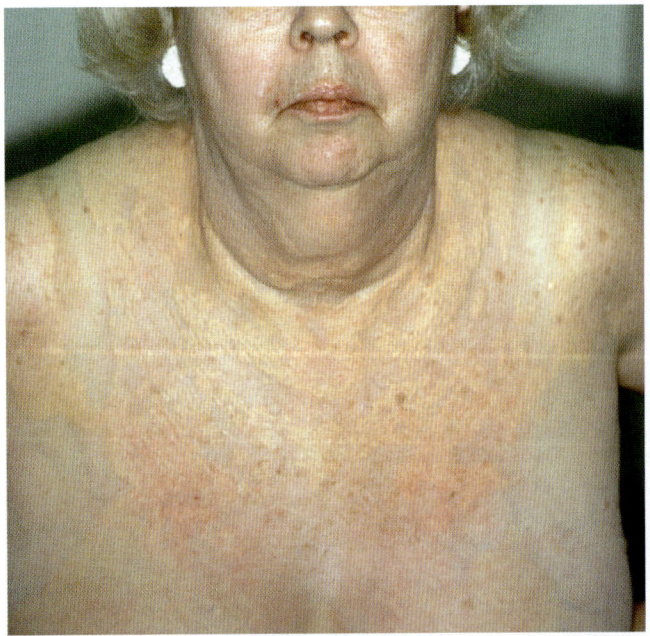

Fig. 26.61 Plane xanthoma.

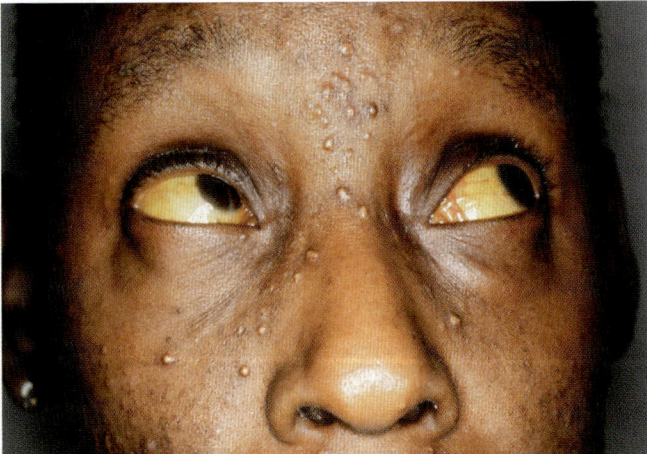

Fig. 26.62 Primary biliary cirrhosis and tuberoeruptive xanthomas. *Courtesy Scott Norton, MD.*

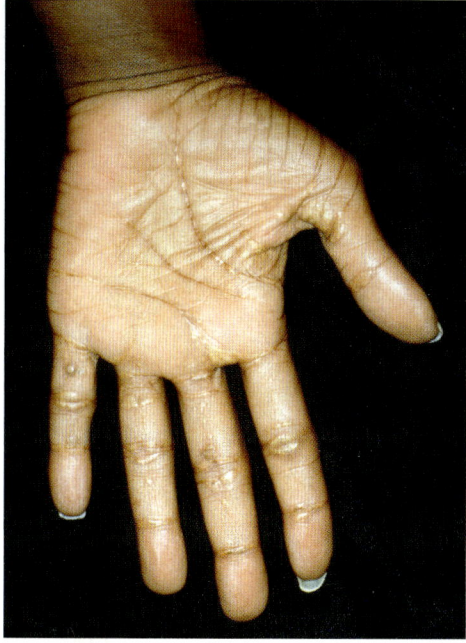

Fig. 26.63 Palmar xanthomas in biliary cirrhosis.

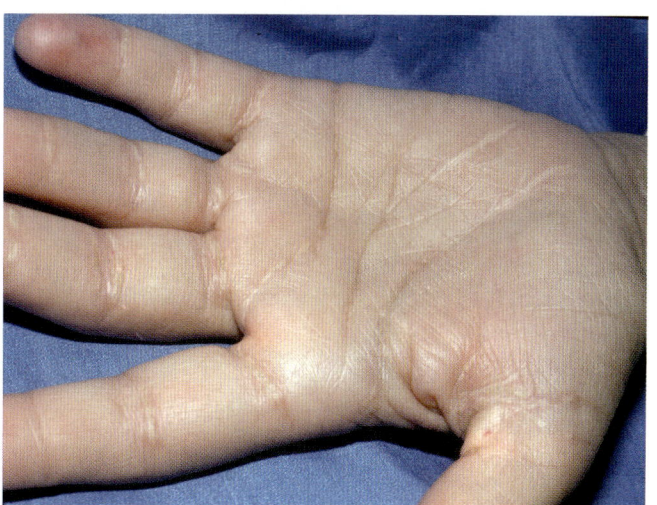

Fig. 26.64 Palmar xanthomas in biliary cirrhosis. *Courtesy Steven Binnick, MD.*

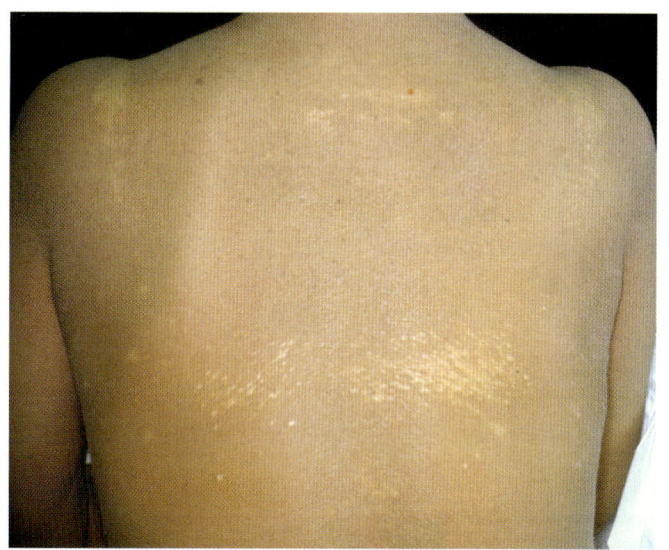

Fig. 26.65 Plane xanthoma in biliary cirrhosis. *Courtesy Steven Binnick, MD.*

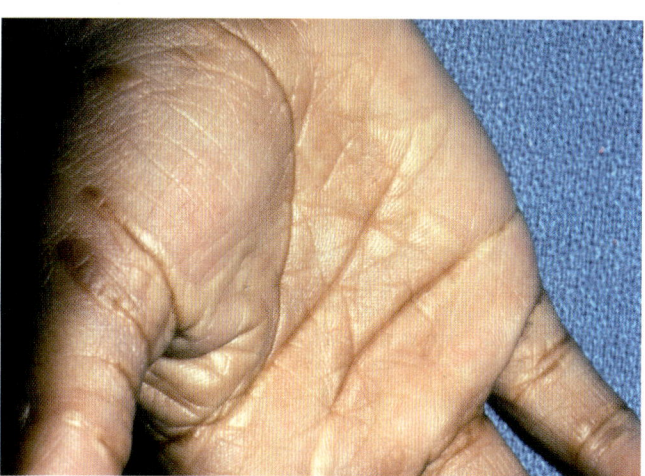

Fig. 26.66 Palmar xanthomas in Alagille syndrome. *Courtesy Steven Binnick, MD.*

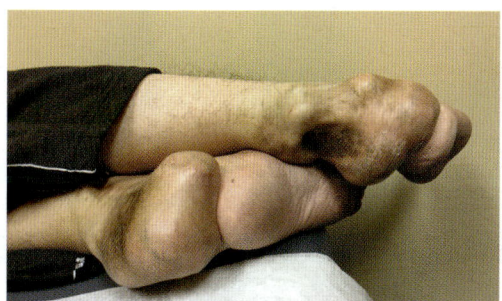

Fig. 26.67 Cerebrotendinous xanthomas. *Courtesy Vikash Oza, MD.*

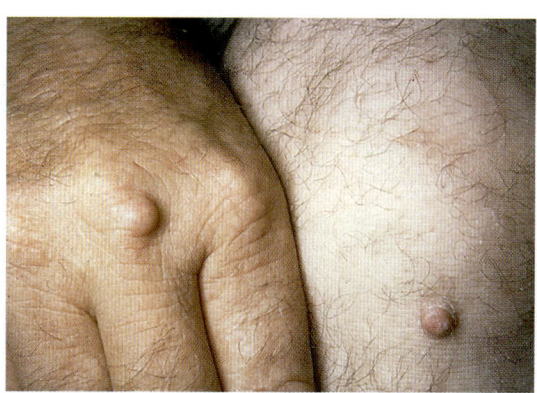

Fig. 26.68 Sitosterolemia.

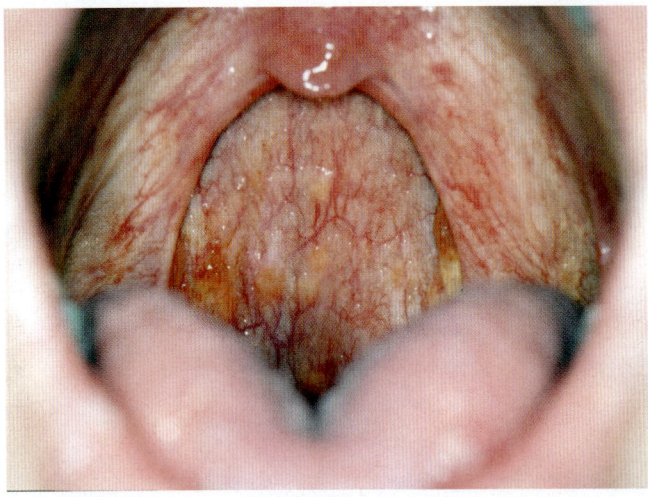

Fig. 26.69 Tangier disease with residual yellow tonsils.

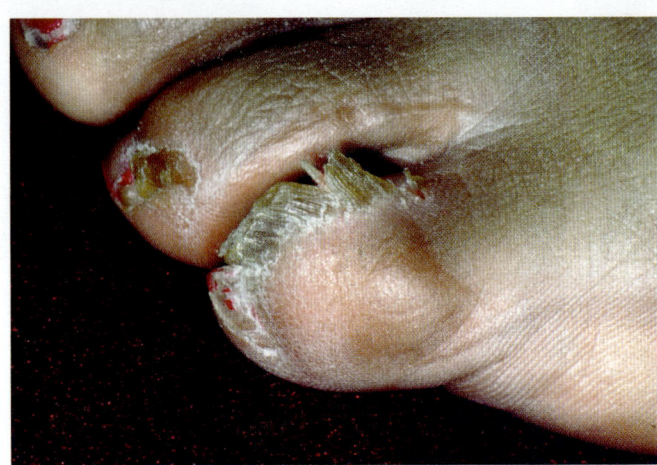

Fig. 26.70 Verruciform xanthoma.

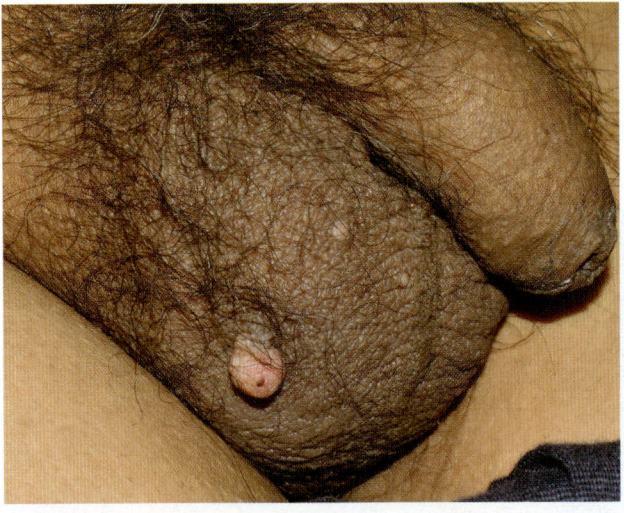

Fig. 26.71 Verruciform xanthoma. *Courtesy National Taiwan University Hospital.*

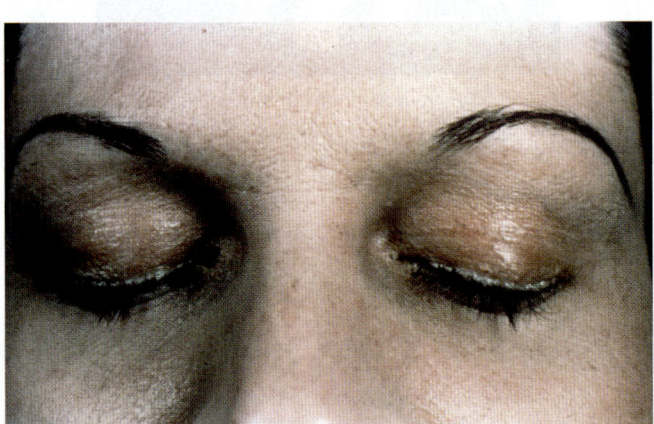

Fig. 26.72 Lipoid proteinosis.

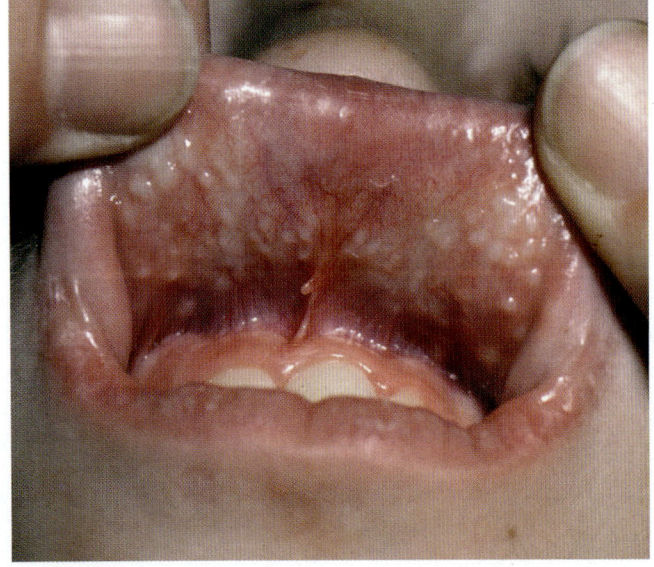

Fig. 26.73 Lipoid proteinosis.

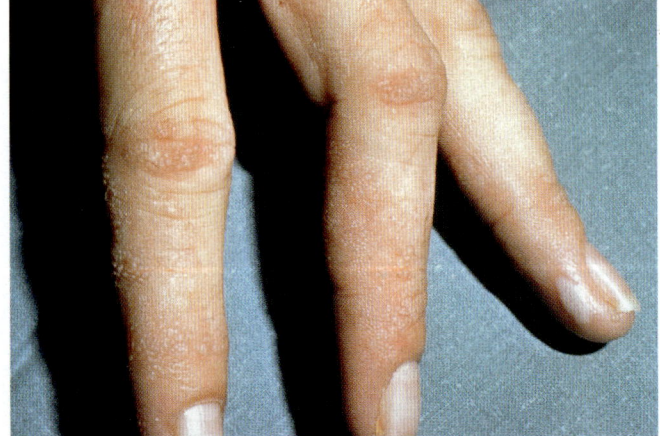

Fig. 26.74 Lipoid proteinosis.

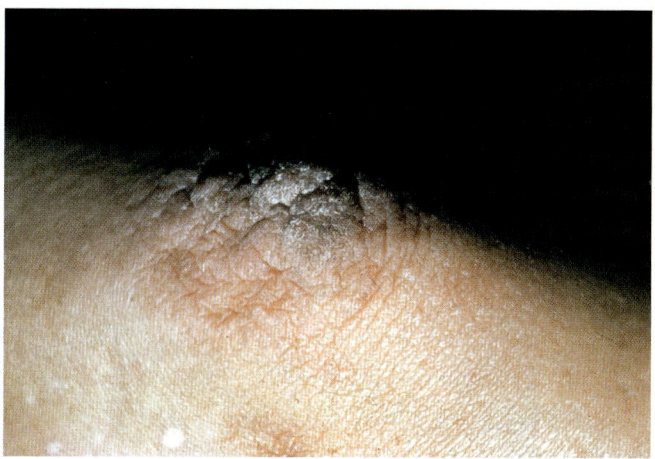
Fig. 26.75 Lipoid proteinosis.

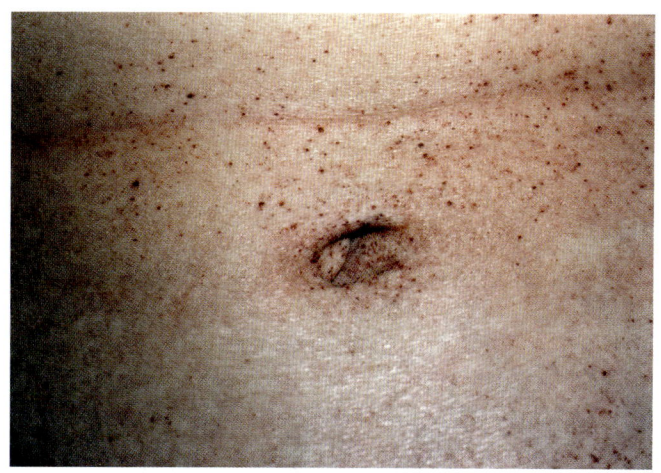
Fig. 26.76 Fabry disease. *Courtesy Ken Greer, MD.*

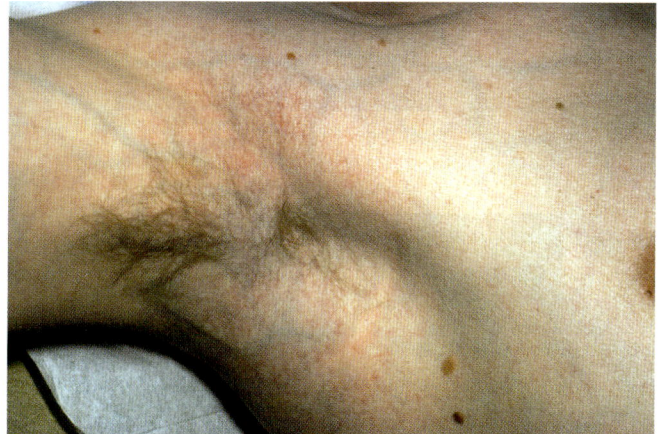
Fig. 26.77 Fabry disease.

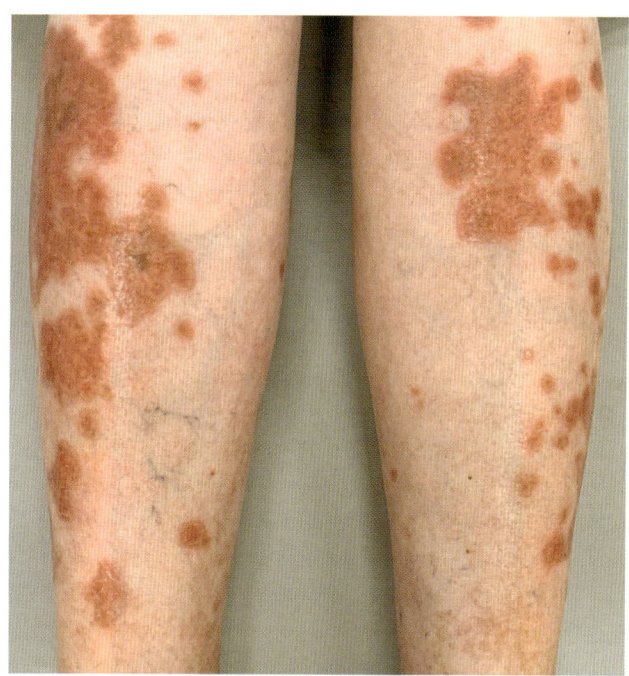
Fig. 26.78 Necrobiosis lipoidica.

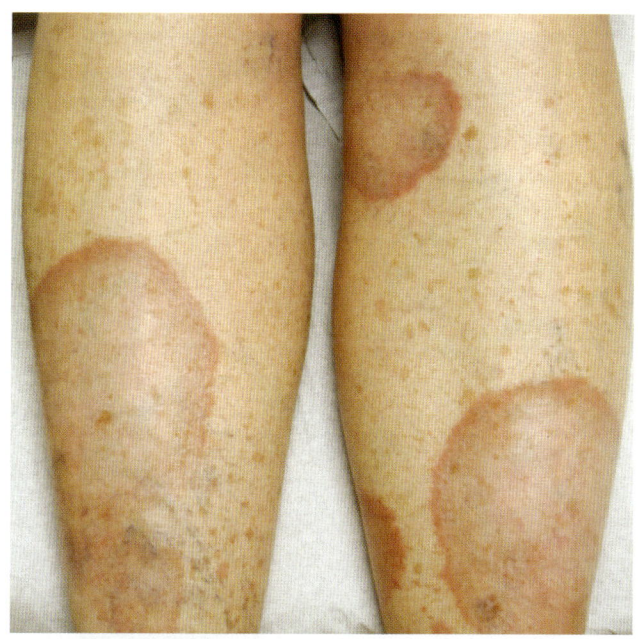
Fig. 26.79 Necrobiosis lipoidica.

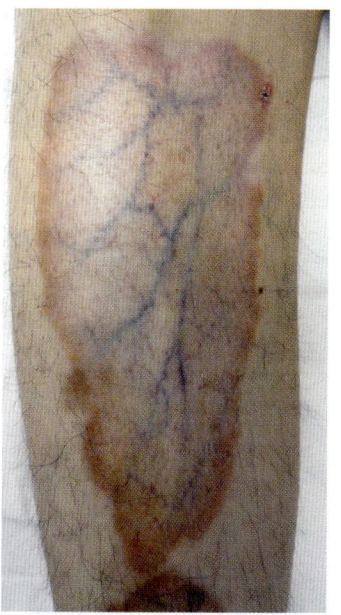
Fig. 26.80 Necrobiosis lipoidica. *Courtesy Scott Norton, MD.*

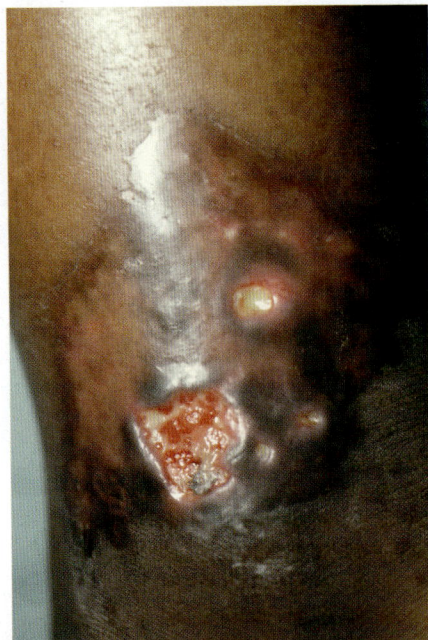

Fig. 26.81 Necrobiosis lipoidica.

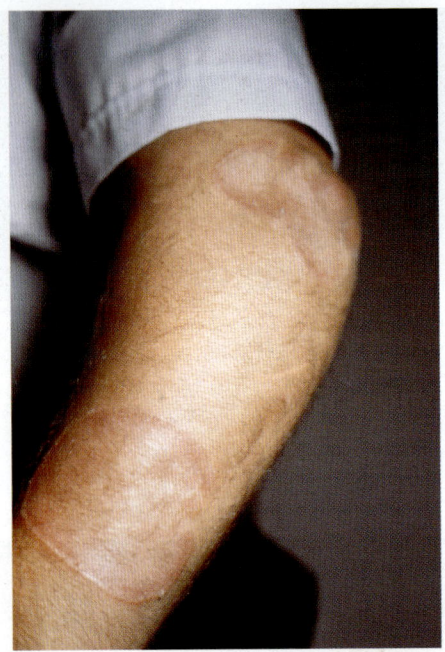

Fig. 26.82 Necrobiosis lipoidica.

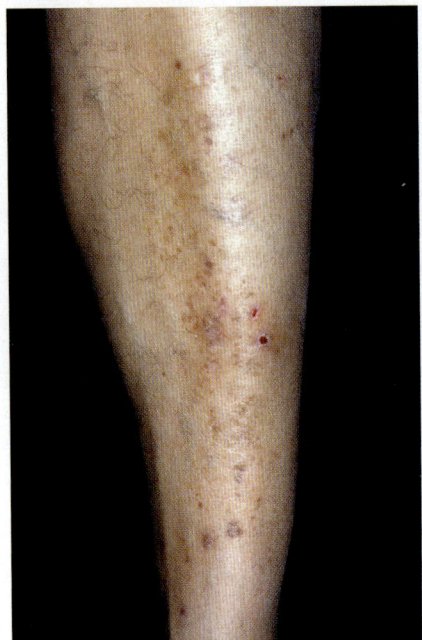

Fig. 26.83 Diabetic dermopathy.

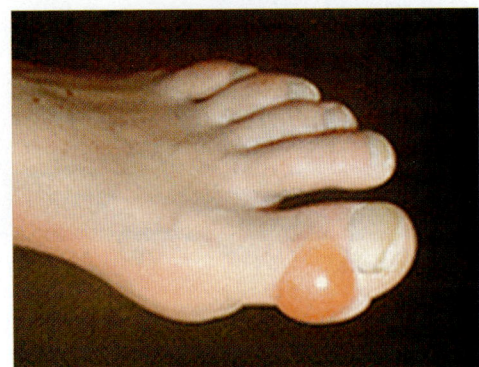

Fig. 26.84 Bullous diabetic dermatosis.

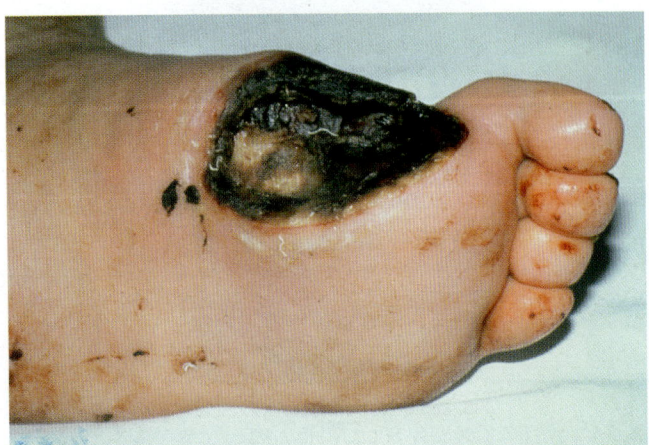

Fig. 26.85 Diabetic gangrene.

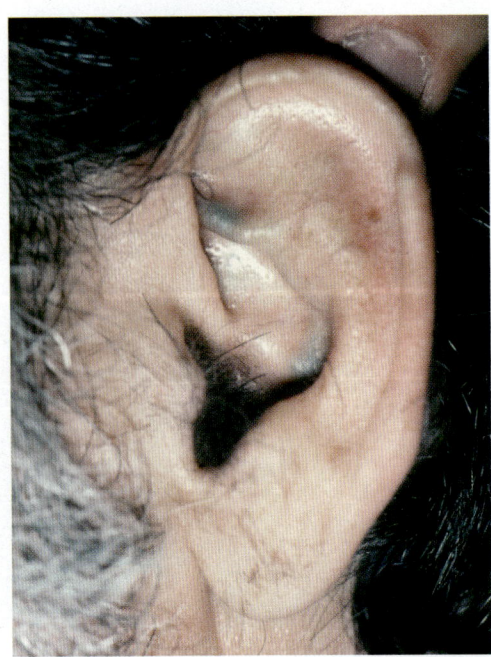

Fig. 26.86 Alkaptonuria.

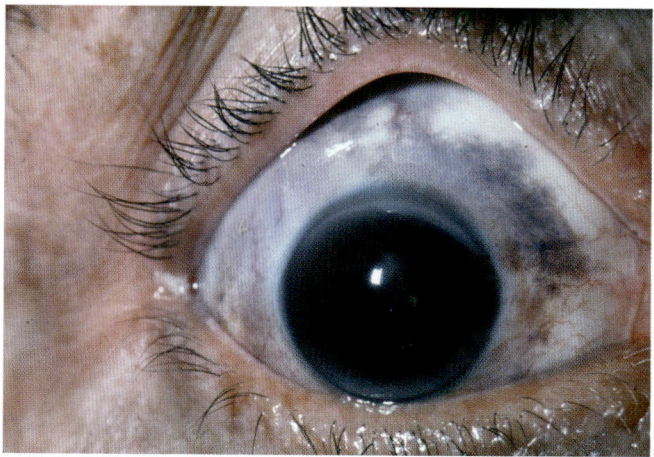
Fig. 26.87 Alkaptonuria.

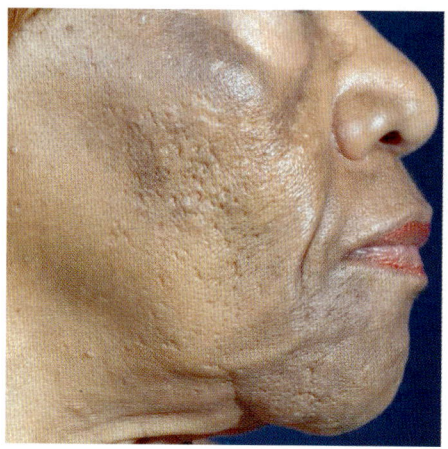
Fig. 26.88 Exogenous ochronosis.

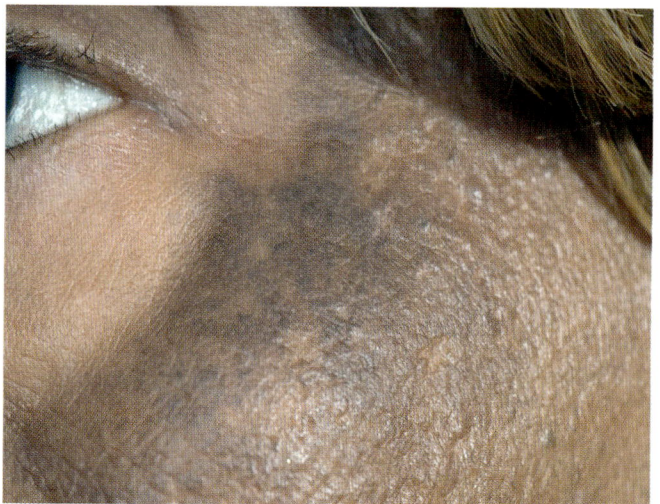
Fig. 26.89 Exogenous ochronosis.

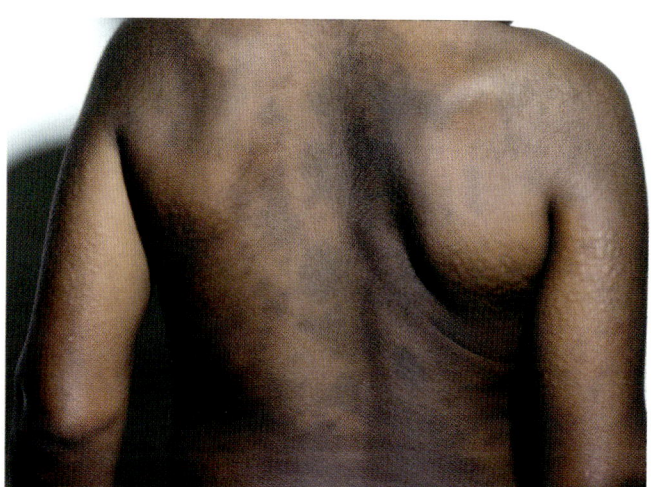
Fig. 26.90 Hunter syndrome. *Courtesy Paul Honig, MD.*

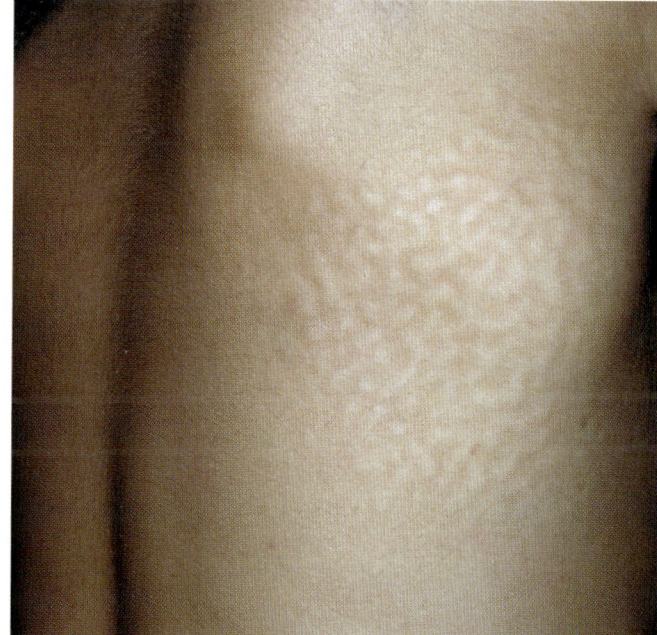
Fig. 26.91 Hunter syndrome.

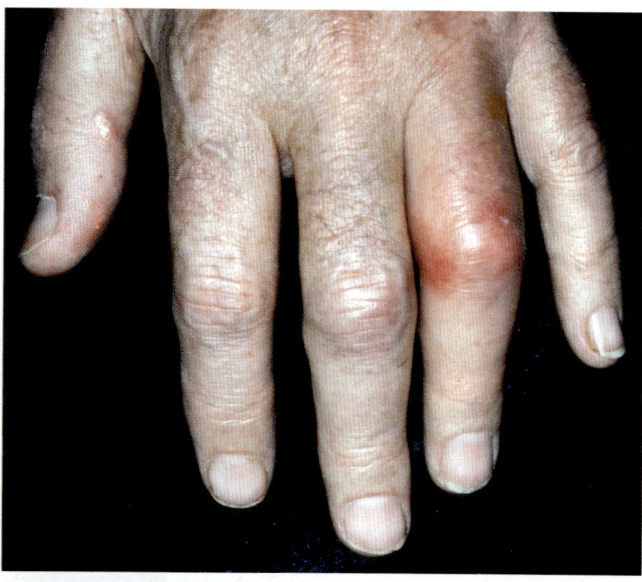
Fig. 26.92 Gout.

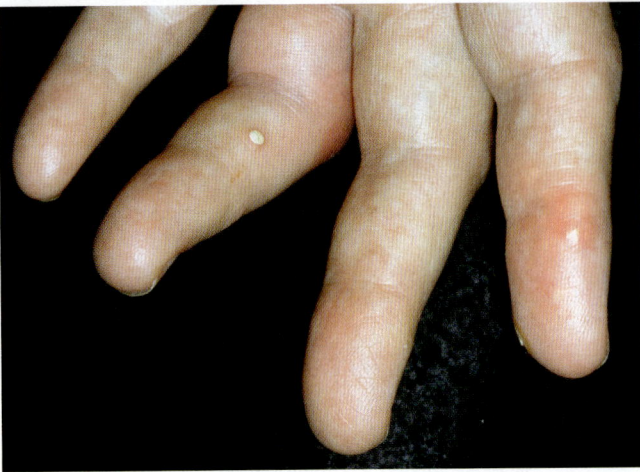

Fig. 26.93 Gout.

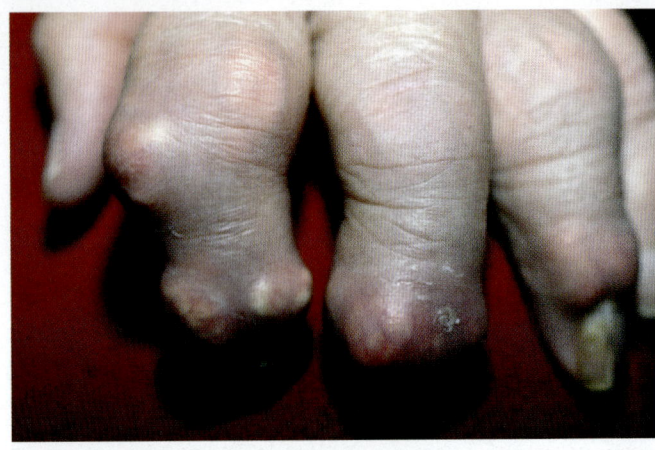

Fig. 26.94 Gout.

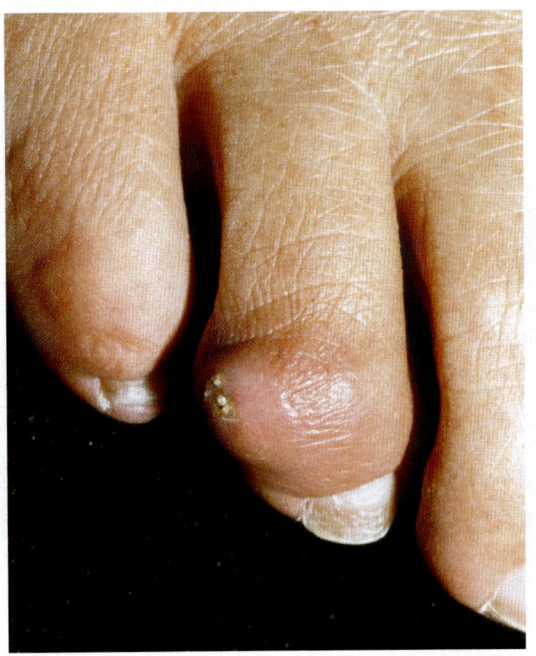

Fig. 26.95 Gout.

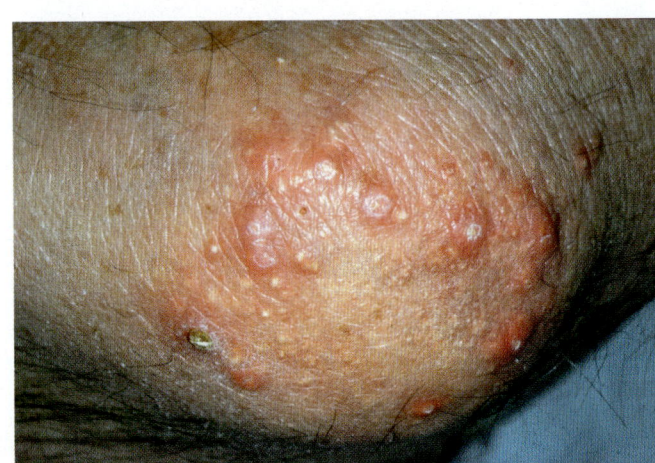

Fig. 26.96 Gout.

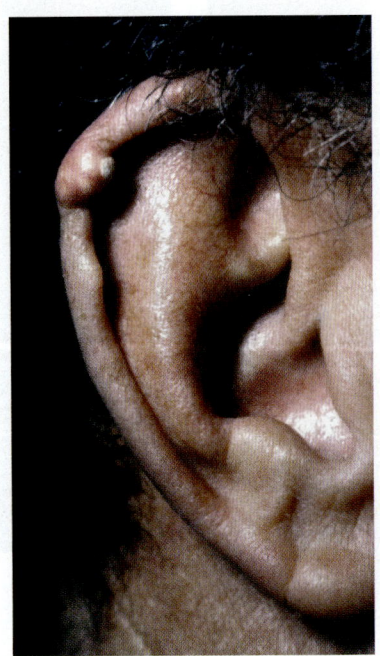

Fig. 26.97 Gout.

Genodermatoses and Congenital Anomalies   27

Genodermatoses include a variety of skin conditions due to underlying genetic mutations with and without associated systemic findings. New gene mutations are being discovered rapidly and allow for more definitive diagnoses in many of these conditions; however, recognizing the salient features on physical examination allows for more directed genetic testing.

Some genodermatoses will present at birth, such as epidermolysis bullosa with skin fragility or congenital ichthyoses with the presence of a collodion membrane. Other conditions manifest distinctive clinical findings in the neonatal period, as seen in the Blaschko linear vesicular and verrucous eruptions indicative of incontentia pigmenti. Childhood onset is more common for conditions like tuberous sclerosis (TS) or neurofibromatosis when patients begin to demonstrate more noticeable clinical stigmata such as angiofibromas or neurofibromas, respectively. Still other genodermatoses can present later during adolescence or early adulthood, including Darier disease with keratotic and crusted papules and plaques and Hailey-Hailey disease (familial benign chronic pemphigus) with reticulated, eroded flexural plaques.

Photosensitivity can be seen in several genodermatoses, including the telangiectatic patches of Bloom syndrome; the poikiloderma of Rothmund-Thomson syndrome; and the lentigines, sun damage, and early skin cancers seen in xeroderma pigmentosa.

A thorough evaluation of these conditions should include examination of the hair, nails, mucosa, and teeth. Screening for associated symptoms is important, such as lack of sweating present in several forms of ectodermal dysplasia or developmental delays and seizures that can be present in several genodermatoses such as epidermal nevus syndrome or TS. Finally, family history can be useful in determining the inheritance pattern and to narrow genetic testing.

This portion of the atlas includes a wide variety of genodermatoses and congenital anomalies to aid the clinician in identifying the clinical clues that help differentiate these diseases and often guide genetic testing when appropriate.

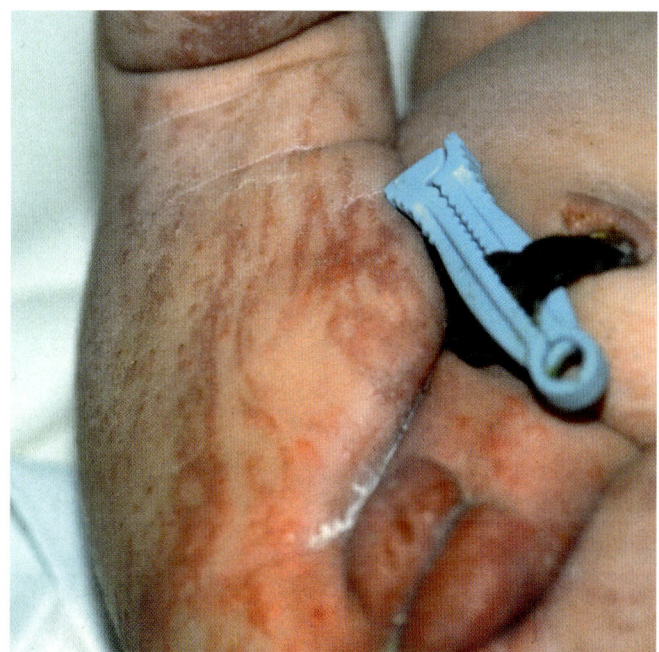

Fig. 27.1 Incontinentia pigmenti, early inflammatory phase.

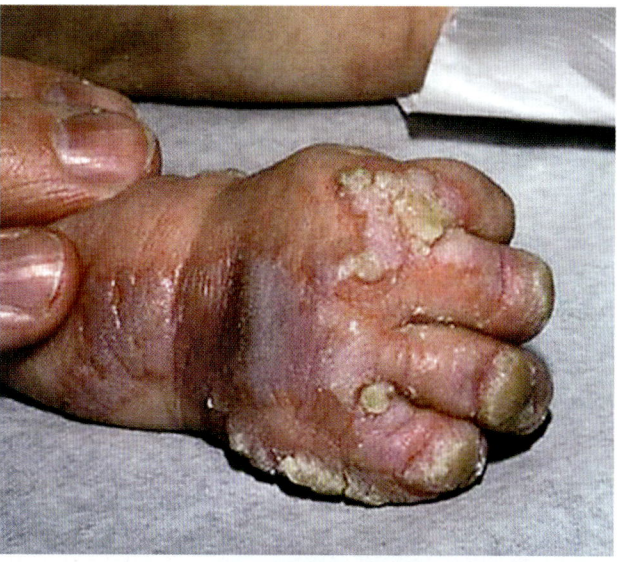

Fig. 27.2 Incontinentia pigmenti with verrucous lesions. *Courtesy Paul Honig, MD.*

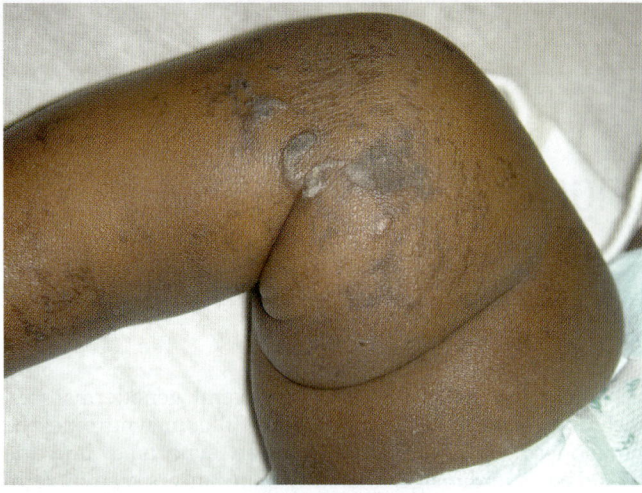

Fig. 27.3 Incontinentia pigmenti with verrucous lesions.

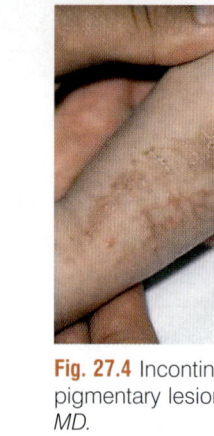

Fig. 27.4 Incontinentia pigmenti with pigmentary lesions. *Courtesy Paul Honig, MD.*

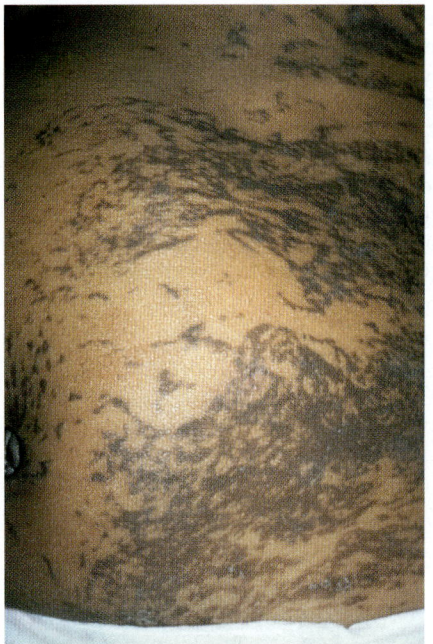

Fig. 27.5 Incontinentia pigmenti with pigmentary lesions.

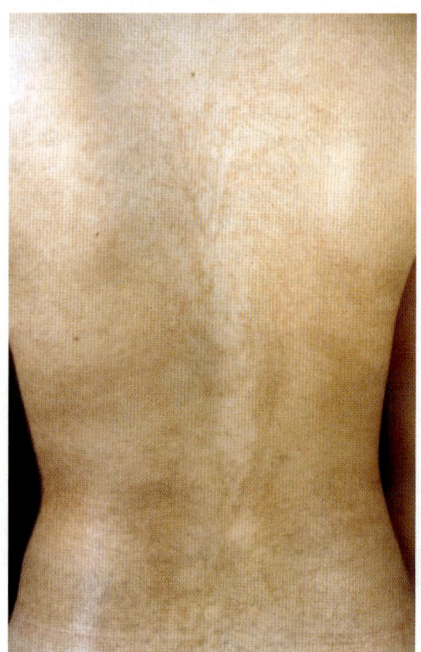

Fig. 27.6 Pigmentary mosaicism (previously hypomelanosis of Ito). *Courtesy Department of Dermatology, Keio University School of Medicine, Tokyo, Japan.*

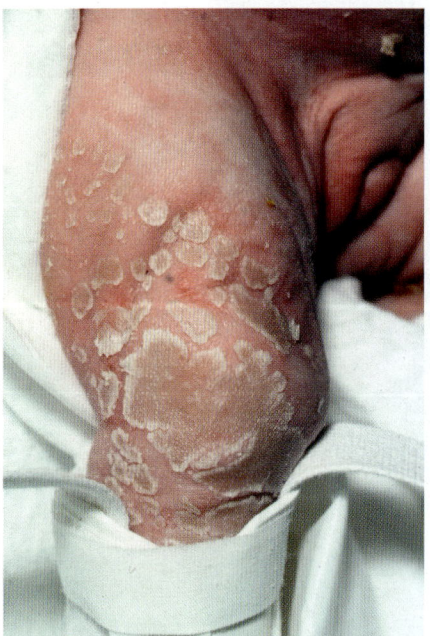

Fig. 27.7 Conradi-Hunermann syndrome.

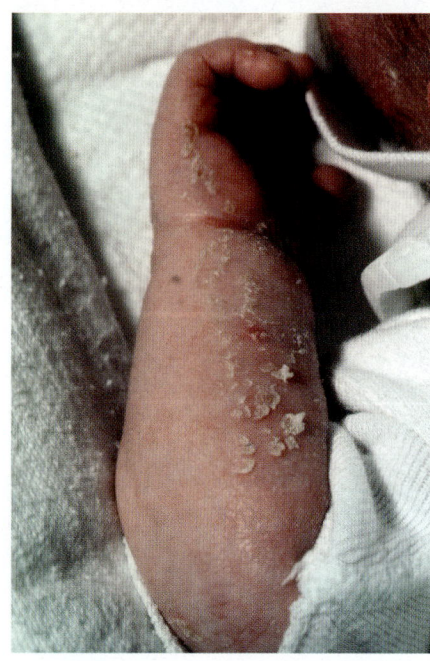

Fig. 27.8 Conradi-Hunermann syndrome.

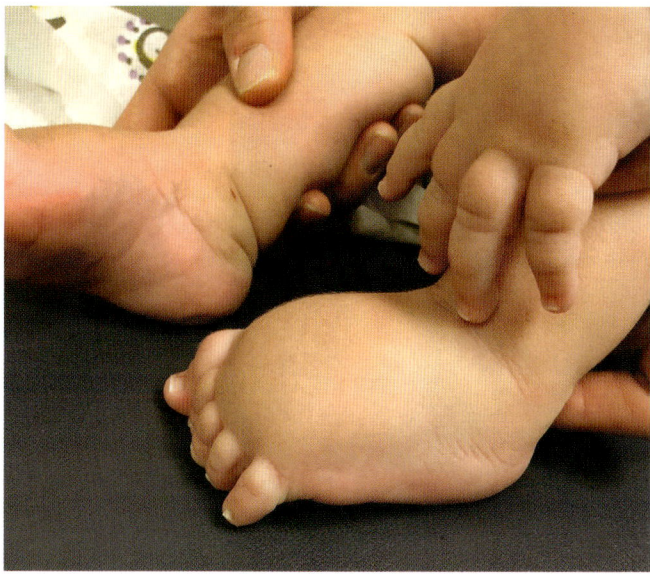

Fig. 27.9 Lymphedema associated with Turner syndrome.

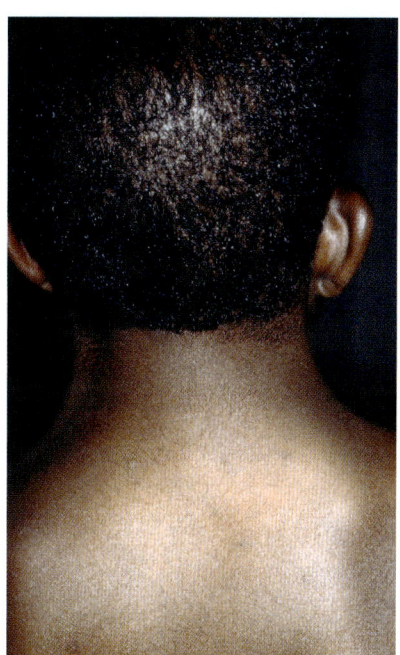

Fig. 27.10 Noonan syndrome.

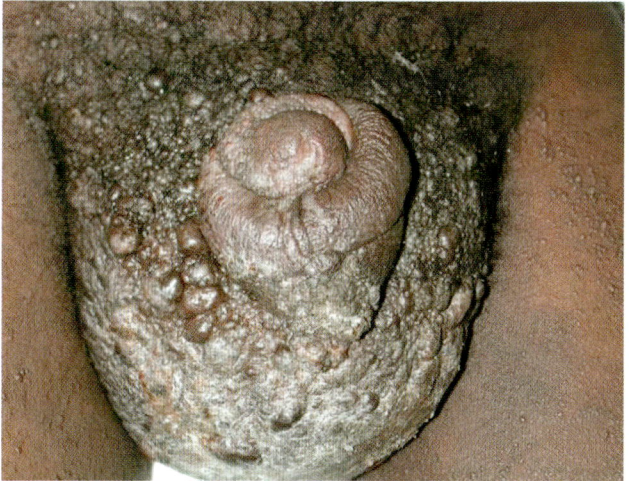

Fig. 27.11 Noonan syndrome with lymphedema and chylous discharge.

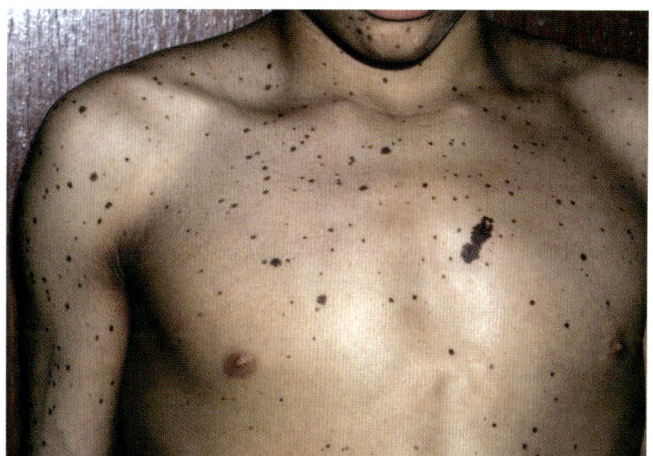

Fig. 27.12 Noonan syndrome with multiple lentigines (previously LEOPARD syndrome). *Courtesy Paul Honig, MD.*

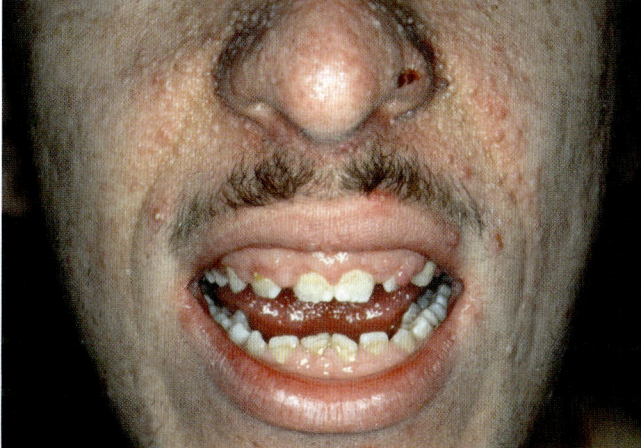

Fig. 27.13 Tuberous sclerosis (TS) with angiofibromas and gingivival hypertrophy from taking phenytoin for his TS-related seizure disorder. *Courtesy Scott Norton, MD.*

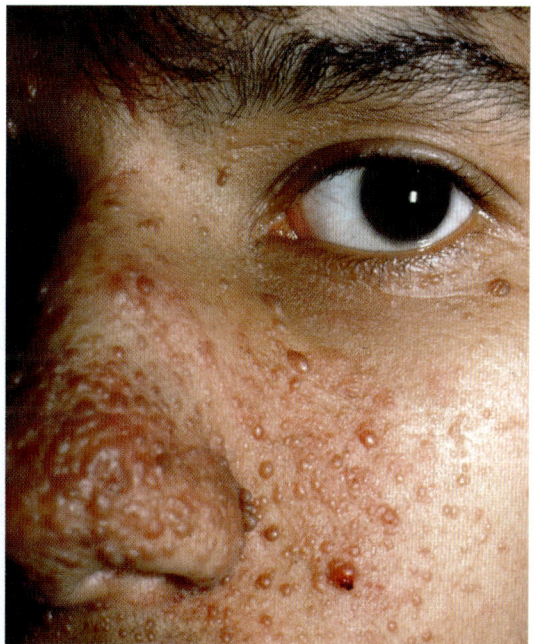

Fig. 27.14 Tuberous sclerosis with angiofibromas.

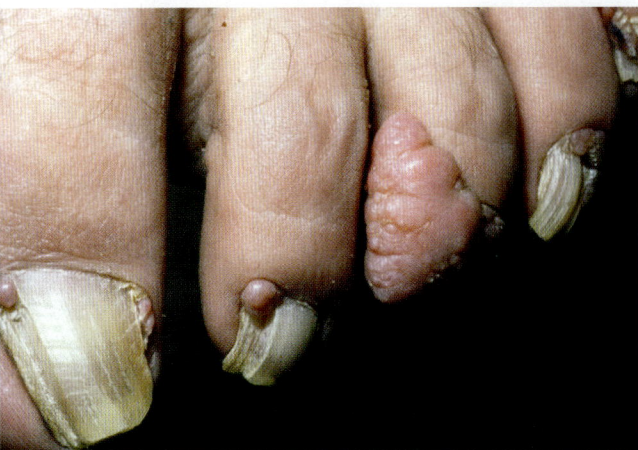

Fig. 27.15 Tuberous sclerosis with periungual fibromas.

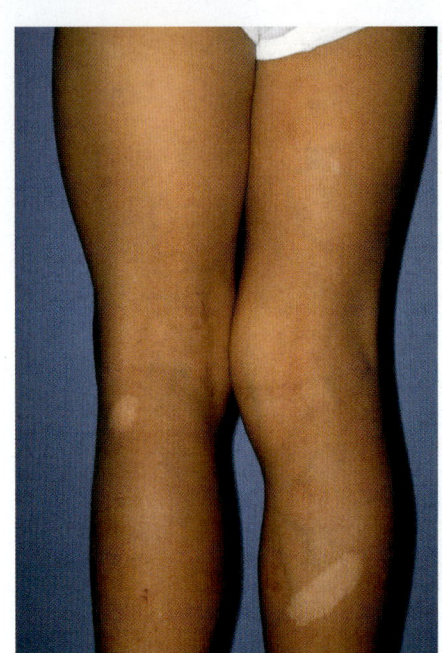

Fig. 27.16 Tuberous sclerosis with ash leaf macule.

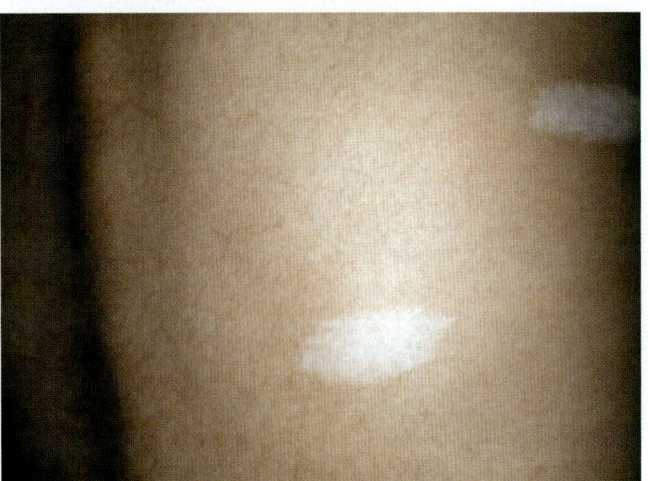

Fig. 27.17 Tuberous sclerosis with ash leaf macule. *Courtesy Steven Binnick, MD.*

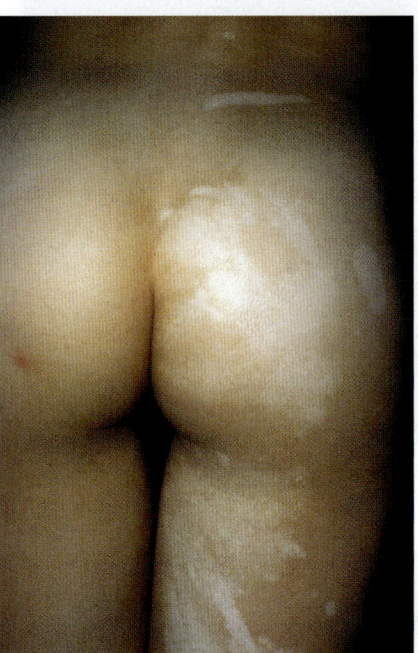

Fig. 27.18 Tuberous sclerosis with paintbrush-type white streaks.

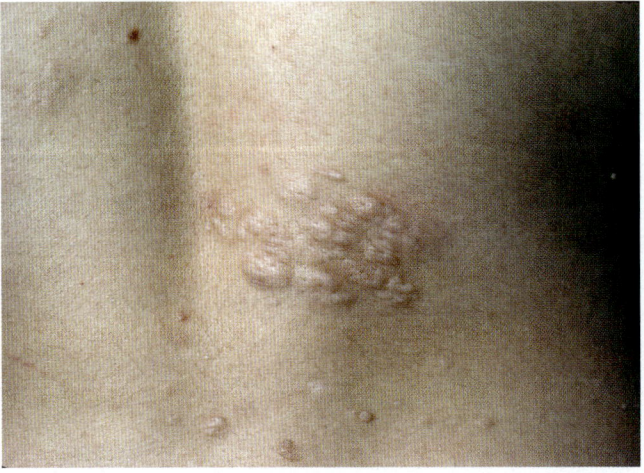

Fig. 27.19 Tuberous sclerosis with shagreen plaque.

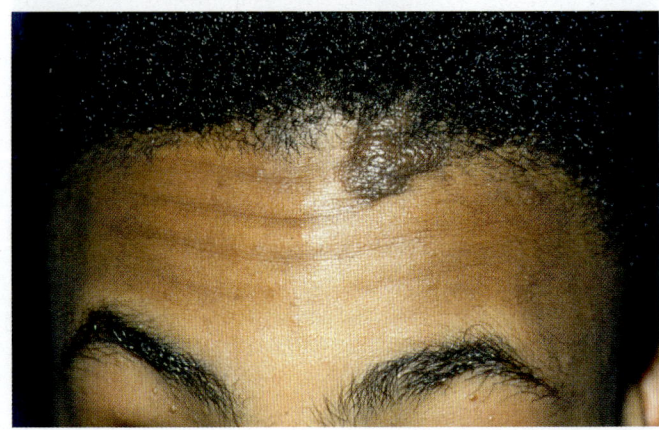

Fig. 27.20 Tuberous sclerosis with fibrous forehead plaque.

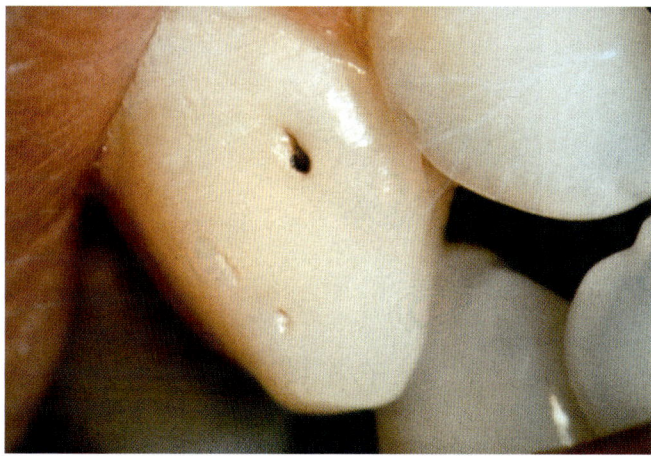

Fig. 27.21 Tuberous sclerosis with dental enamel pit.

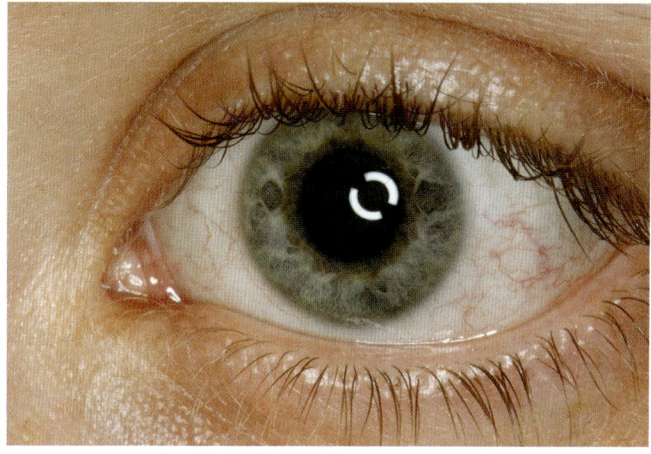

Fig. 27.22 Lisch nodule, neurofibromatosis.

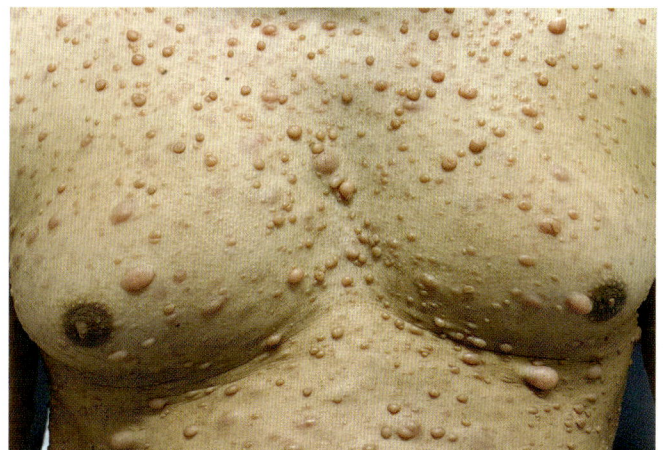

Fig. 27.23 Neurofibromatosis.

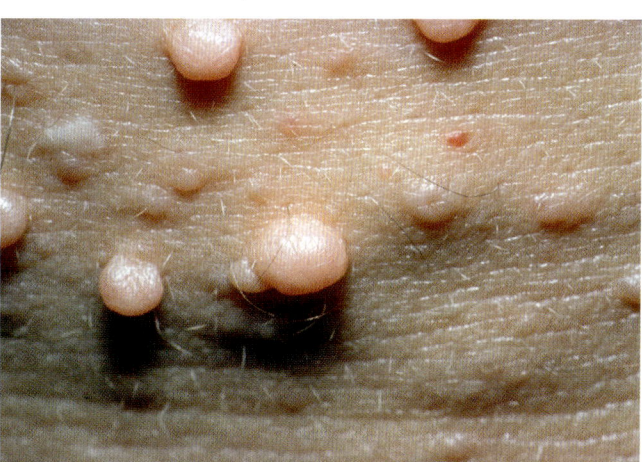

Fig. 27.24 Neurofibromatosis.

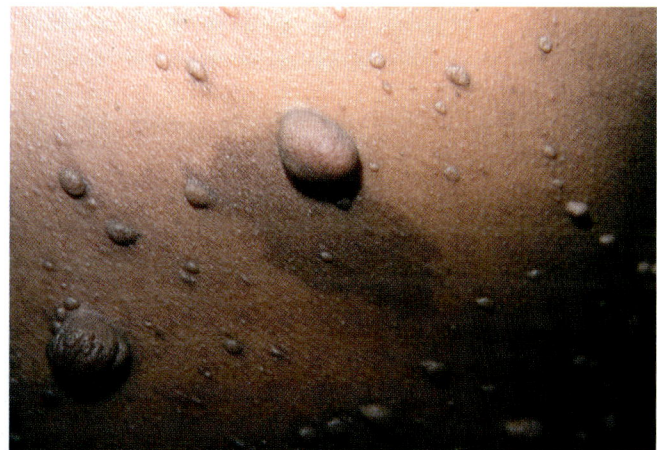

Fig. 27.25 Neurofibromatosis. *Courtesy Steven Binnick, MD.*

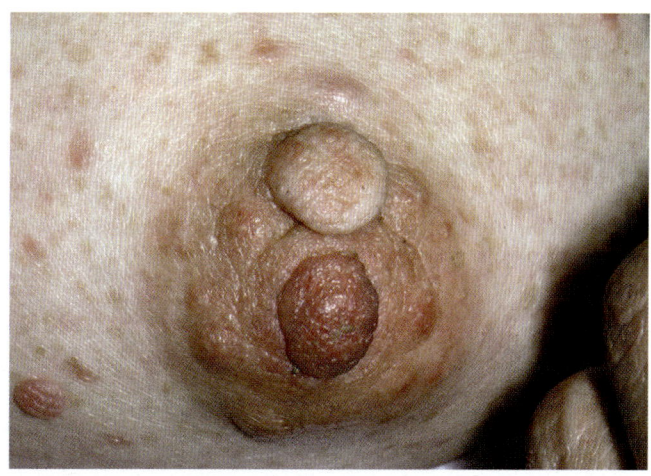

Fig. 27.26 Neurofibromatosis; the areolas are characteristically involved.

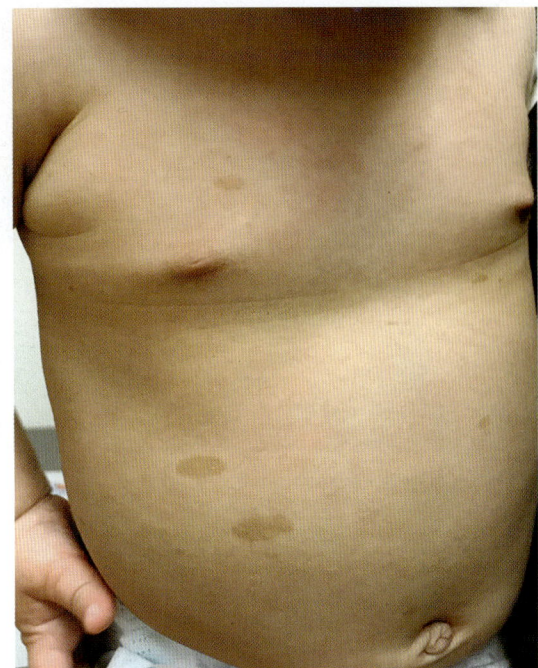

Fig. 27.27 Neurofibromatosis with café-au-lait macule.

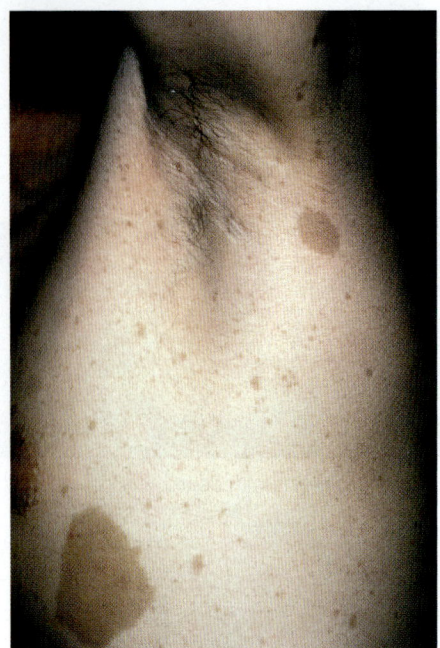

Fig. 27.28 Neurofibromatosis with axillary freckling.

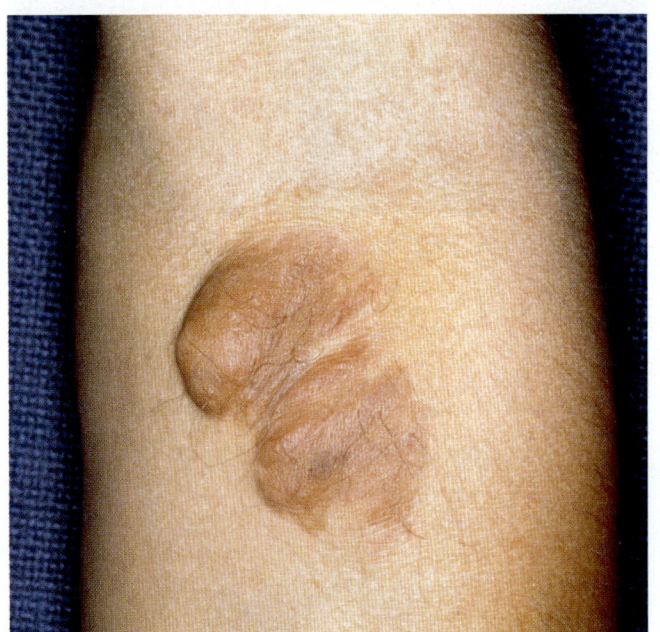

Fig. 27.29 Neurofibromatosis with plexiform neurofibroma.

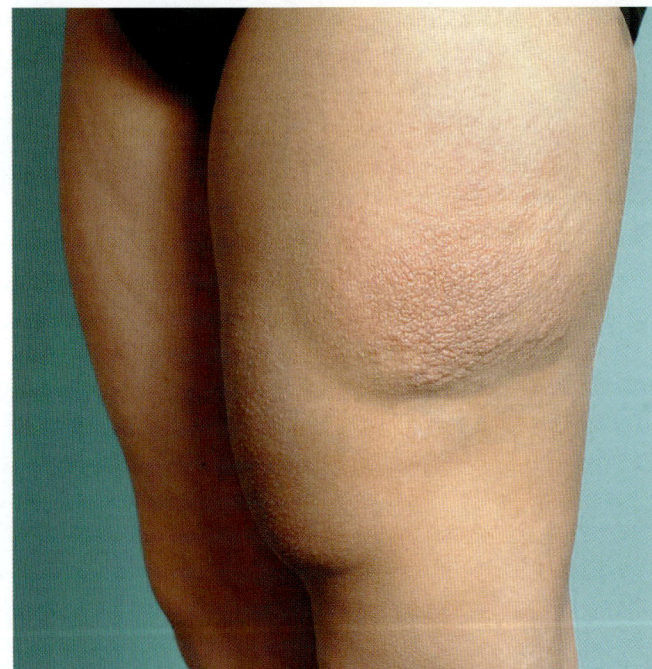

Fig. 27.30 Neurofibromatosis with plexiform neurofibroma.

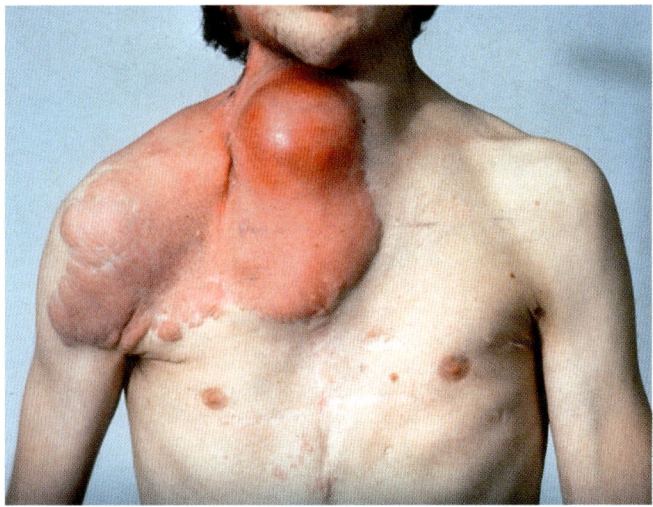

Fig. 27.31 Neurofibromatosis with a malignant peripheral nerve sheath tumor.

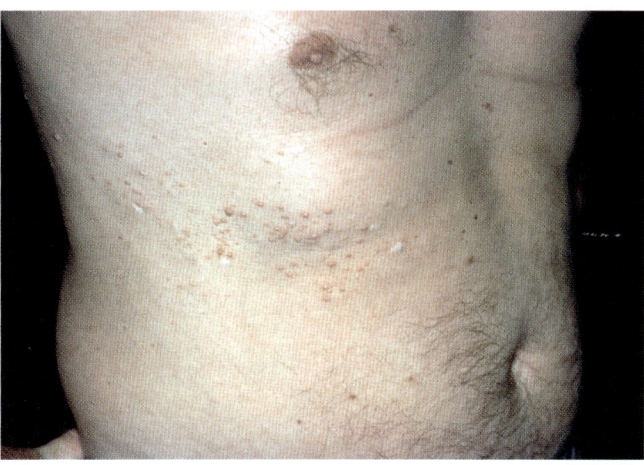

Fig. 27.32 Segmental neurofibromatosis.

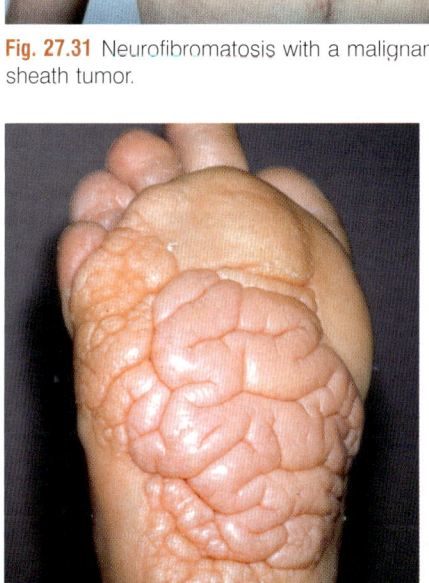

Fig. 27.33 Proteus syndrome with connective tissue nevus.

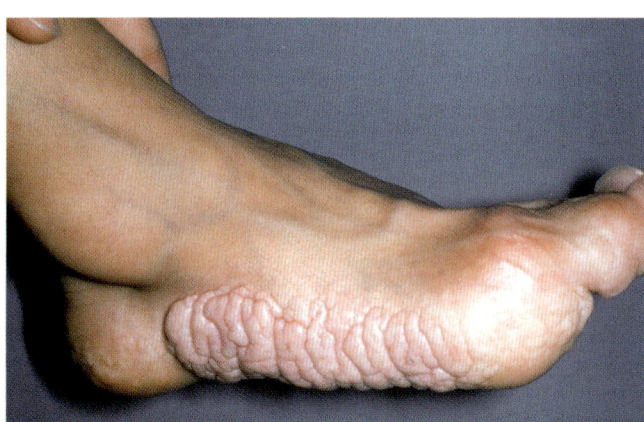

Fig. 27.34 Proteus syndrome with connective tissue nevus.

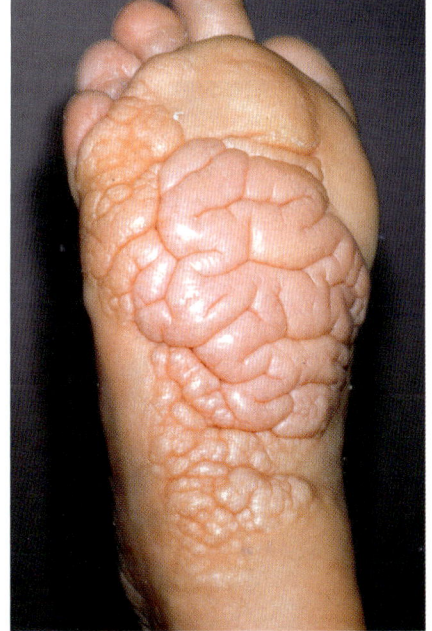

Fig. 27.35 Proteus syndrome with epidermal nevus.

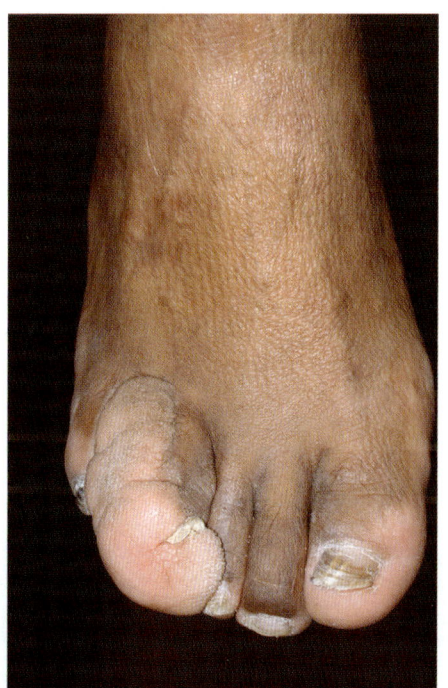

Fig. 27.36 Proteus syndrome. *Courtesy Curt Samlaska, MD.*

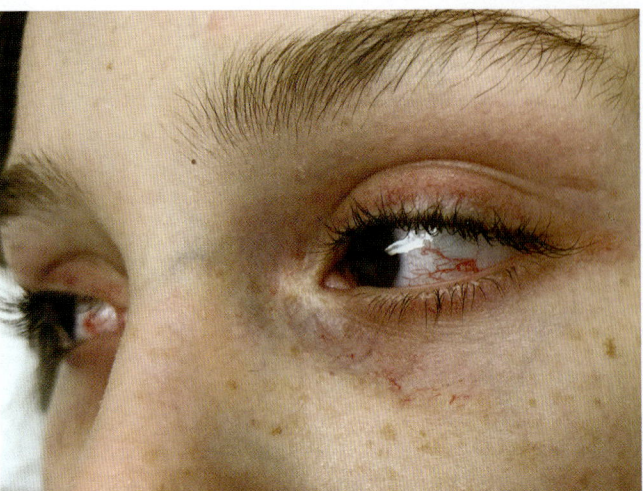

Fig. 27.37 Ataxia telangiectasia.

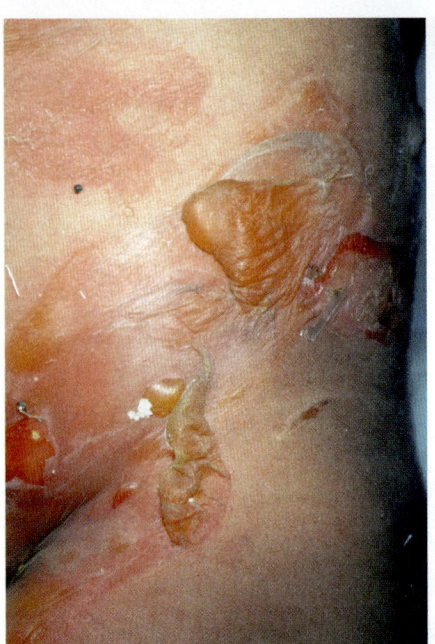

Fig. 27.38 Epidermolysis bullosa simplex, generalized.

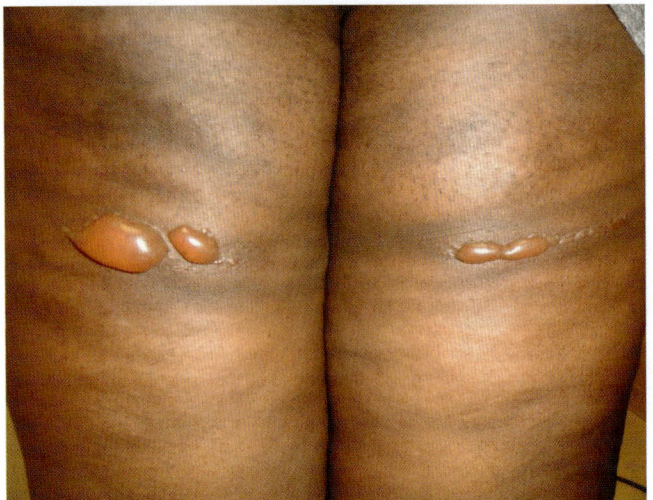

Fig. 27.39 Epidermolysis bullosa simplex, generalized. *Courtesy Scott Norton, MD.*

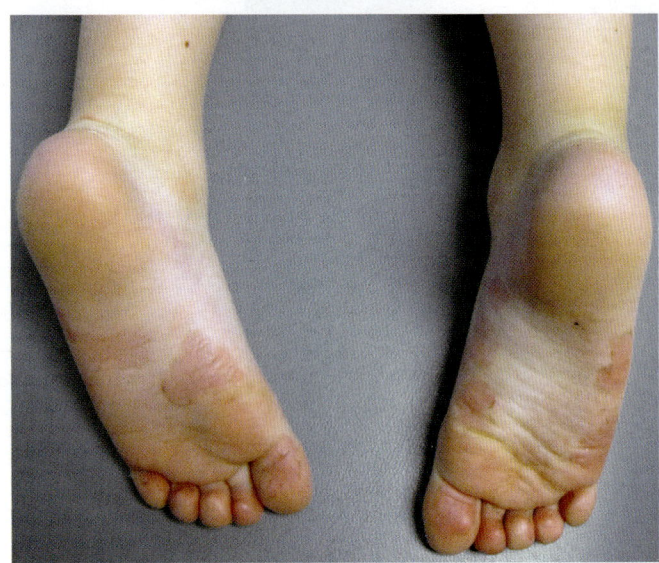

Fig. 27.40 Epidermolysis bullosa simplex, localized.

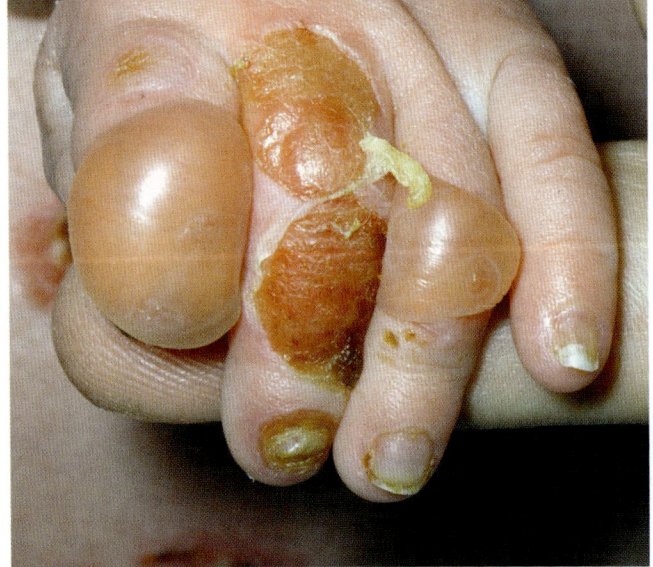

Fig. 27.41 Junctional epidermolysis bullosa.

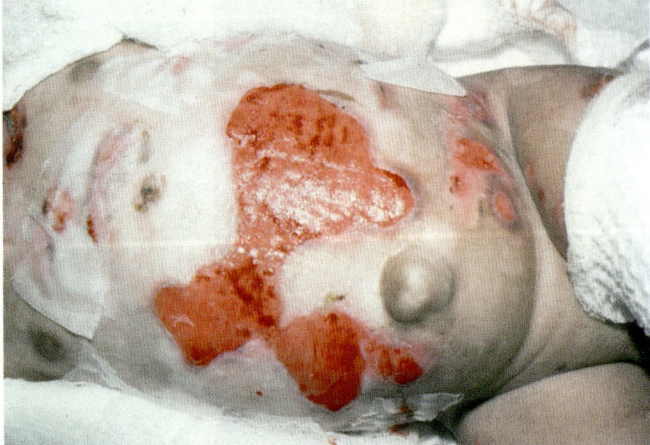

Fig. 27.42 Junctional epidermolysis bullosa.

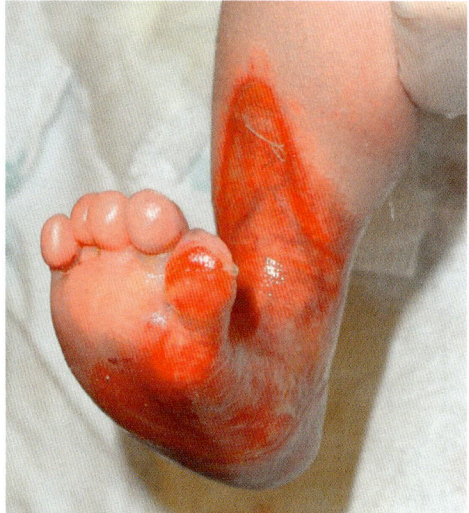

Fig. 27.43 Bart syndrome.

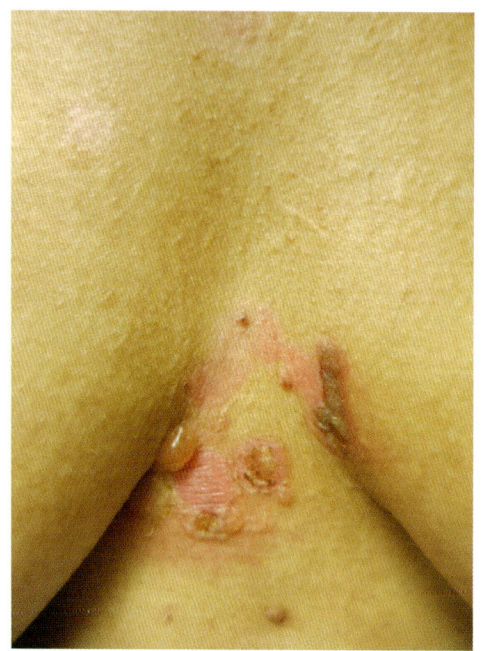

Fig. 27.44 Dominant dystrophic epidermolysis bullosa.

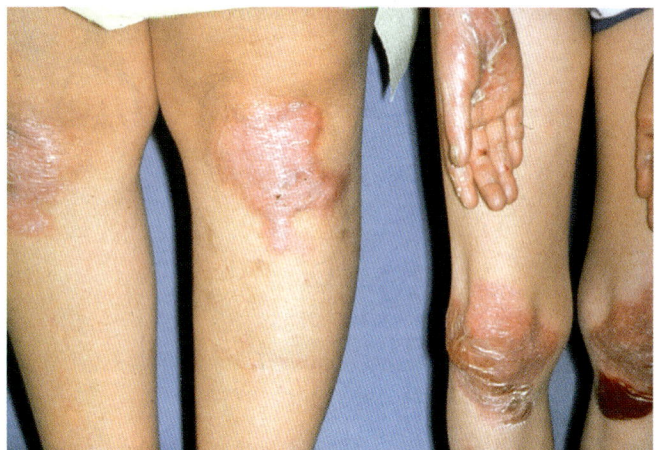

Fig. 27.45 Dominant dystrophic epidermolysis bullosa.

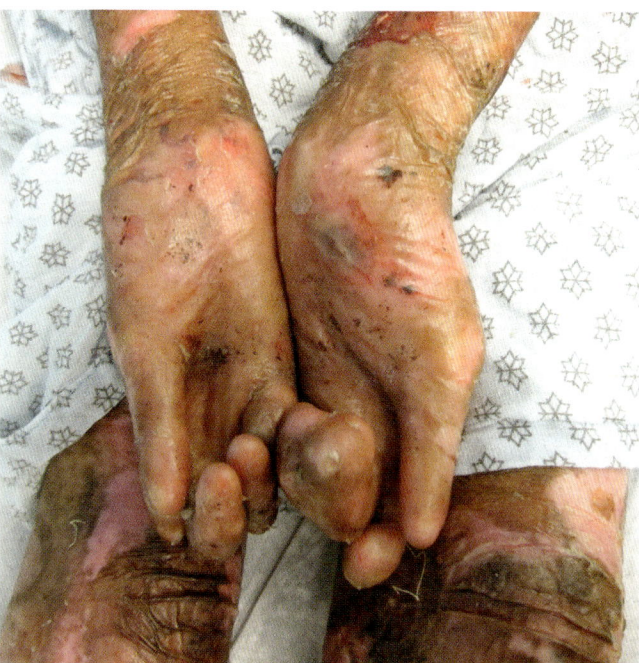

Fig. 27.46 Recessive dystrophic epidermolysis bullosa.

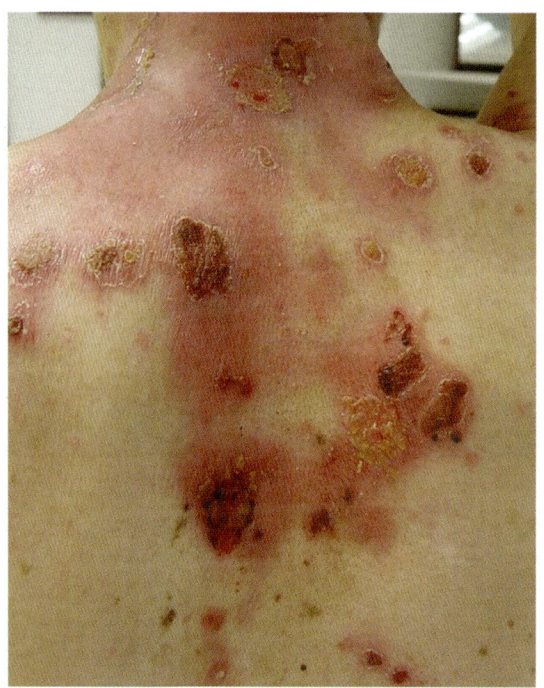

Fig. 27.47 Recessive dystrophic epidermolysis bullosa. *Courtesy Dr. Rui Carlos Taveres Bello.*

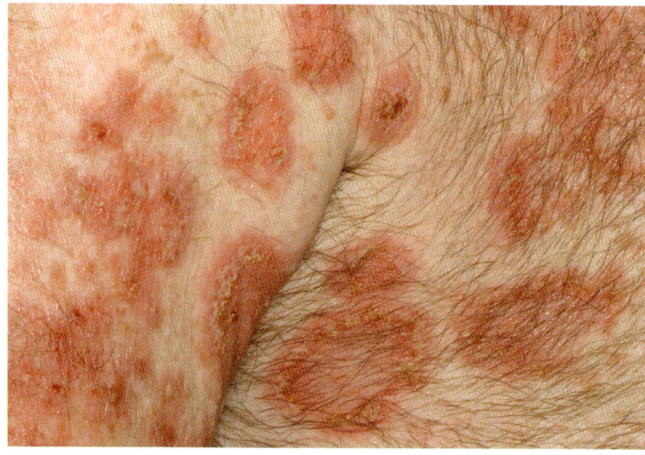

Fig. 27.48 Hailey-Hailey disease.

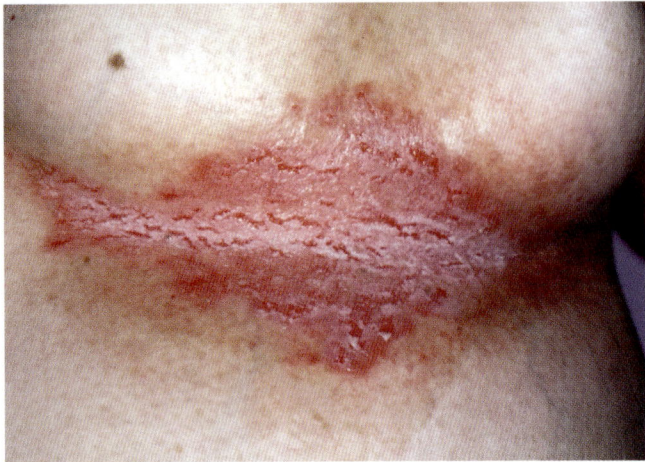

Fig. 27.49 Hailey-Hailey disease.

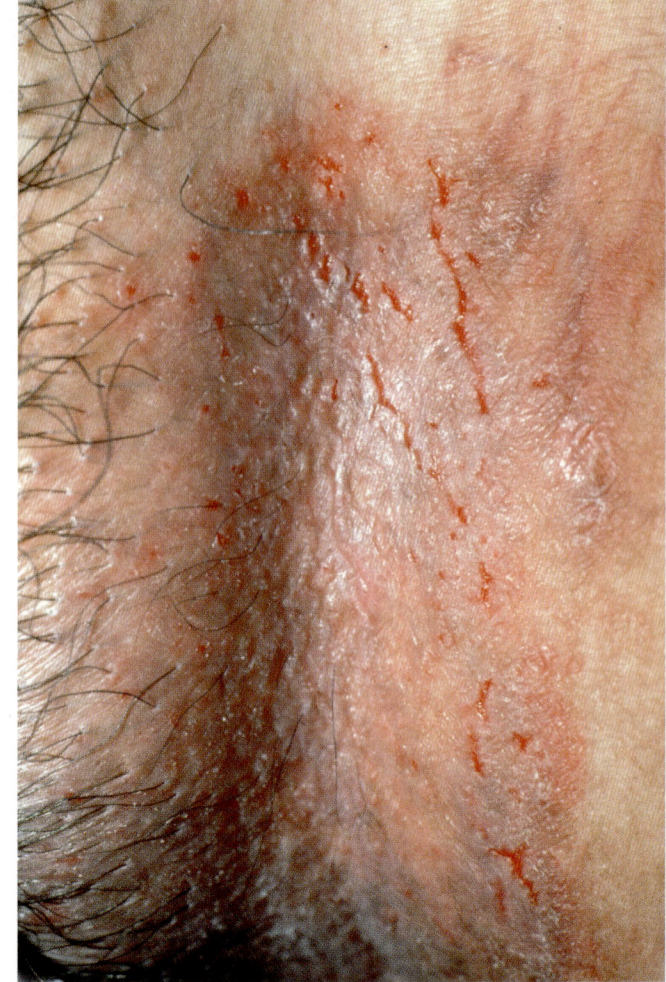

Fig. 27.50 Hailey-Hailey disease.

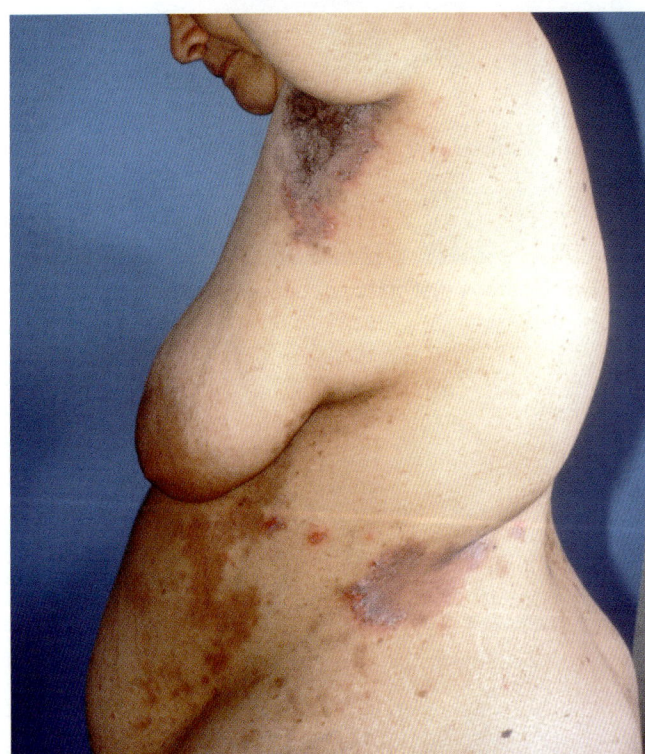

Fig. 27.51 Hailey-Hailey disease.

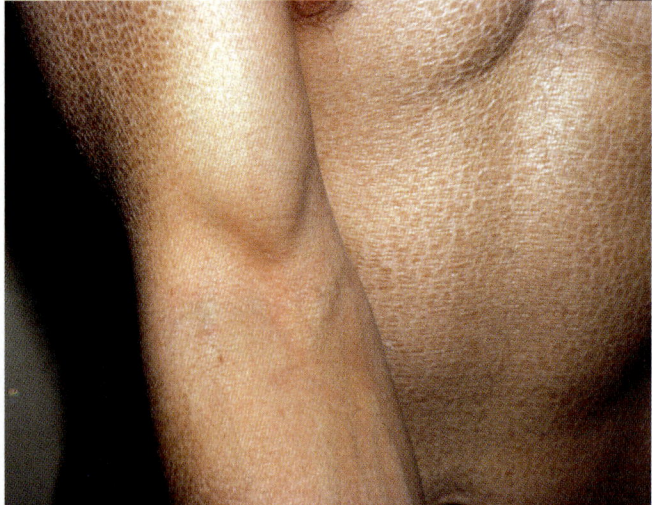

Fig. 27.52 Ichthyosis vulgaris.

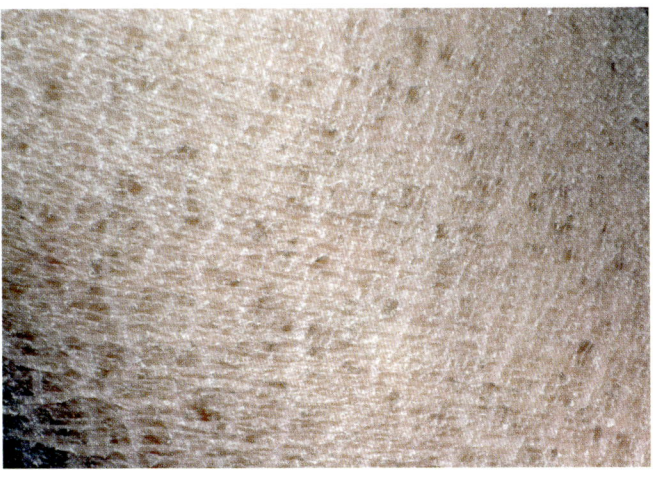

Fig. 27.53 Ichthyosis vulgaris. *Courtesy Steven Binnick, MD.*

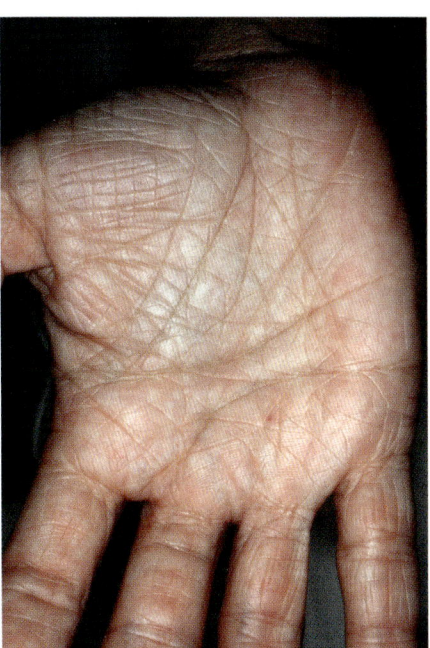

Fig. 27.54 Ichthyosis vulgaris with hyperlinear palms.

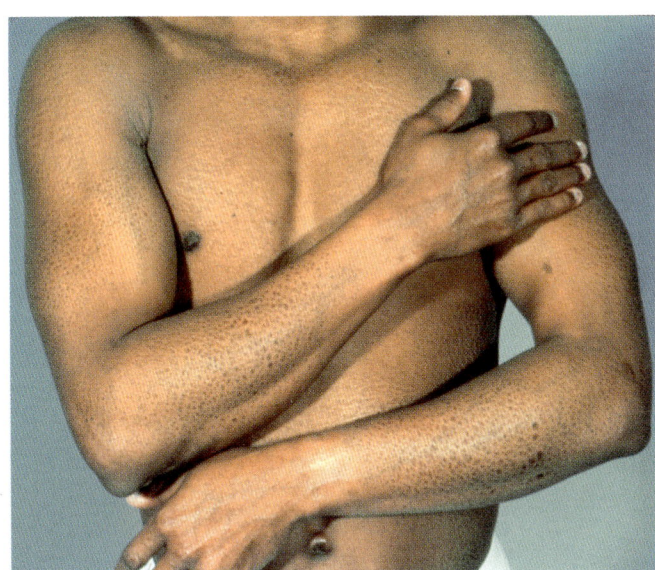

Fig. 27.55 X-linked ichthyosis.

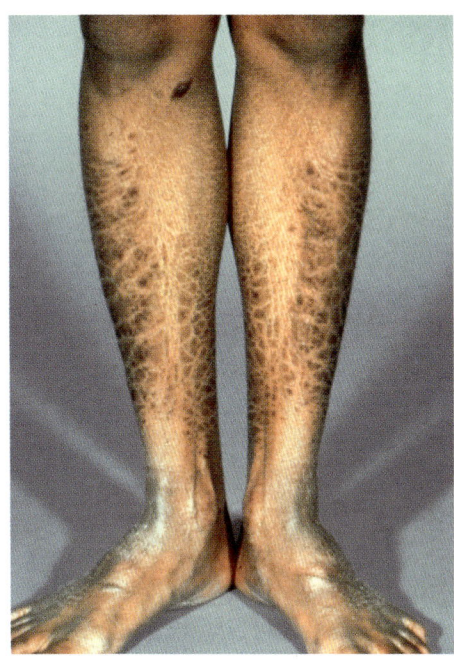

Fig. 27.56 X-linked ichthyosis.

Fig. 27.57 X-linked ichthyosis.

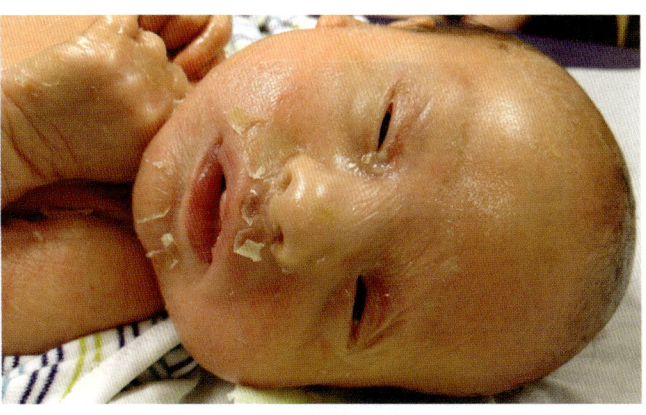

Fig. 27.58 Collodion membrane in congenital ichthyosis.

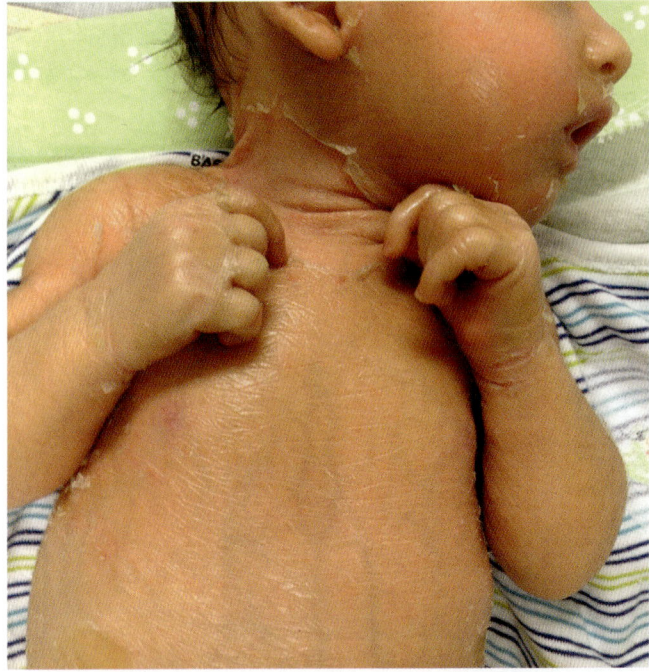

Fig. 27.59 Autosomal-recessive congenital ichthyosis with collodion membrane caused by transglutaminase gene mutation.

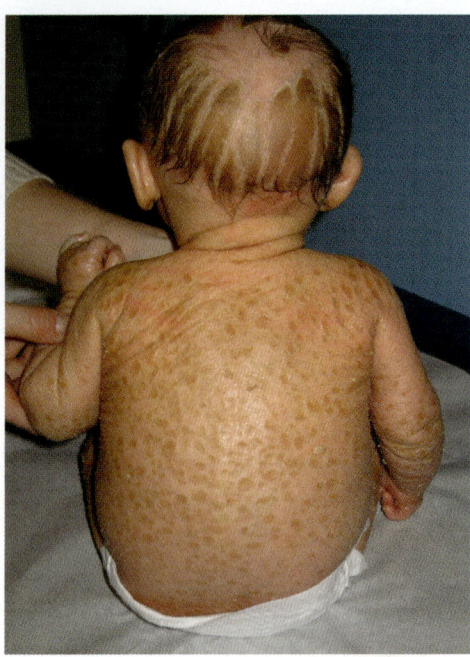

Fig. 27.60 Autosomal-recessive congenital ichthyosis lamellar phenotype caused by transglutaminase gene mutation.

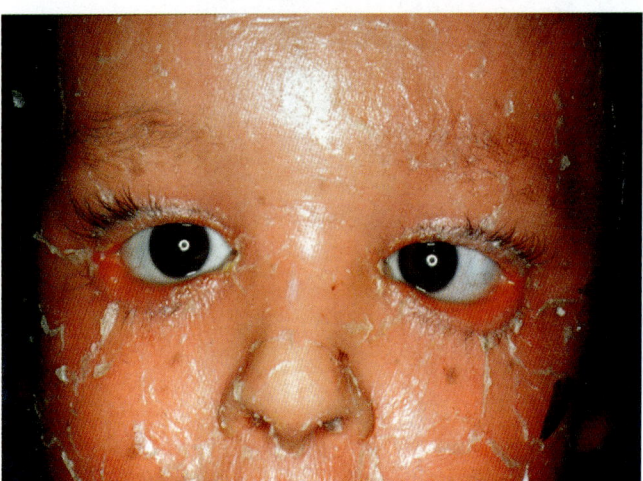

Fig. 27.61 Congenital ichthyosiform erythroderma. *Courtesy Scott Norton, MD.*

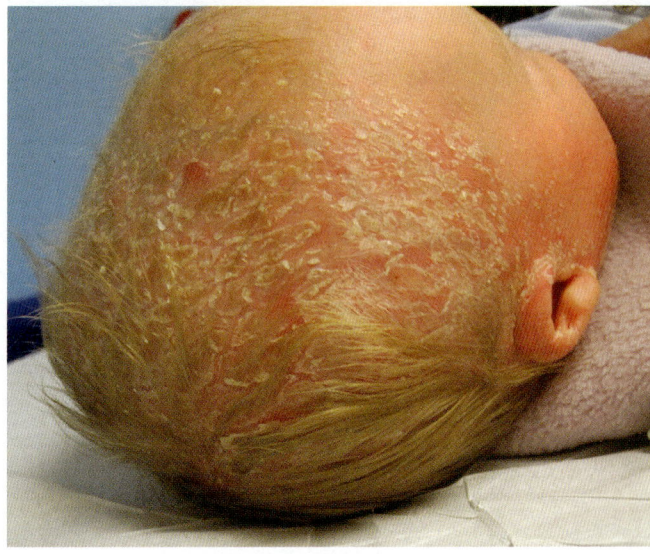

Fig. 27.62 ALOXE3 congenital ichthyosiform erythroderma.

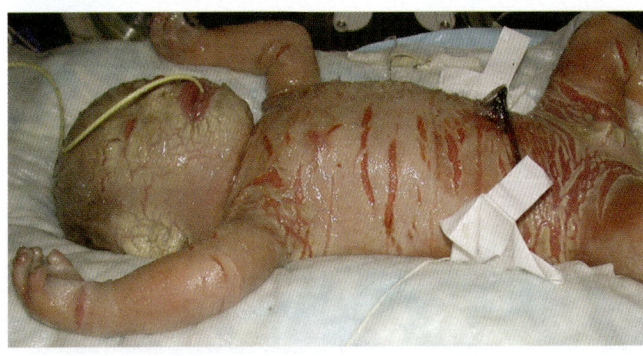

Fig. 27.63 Harlequin ichthyosis.

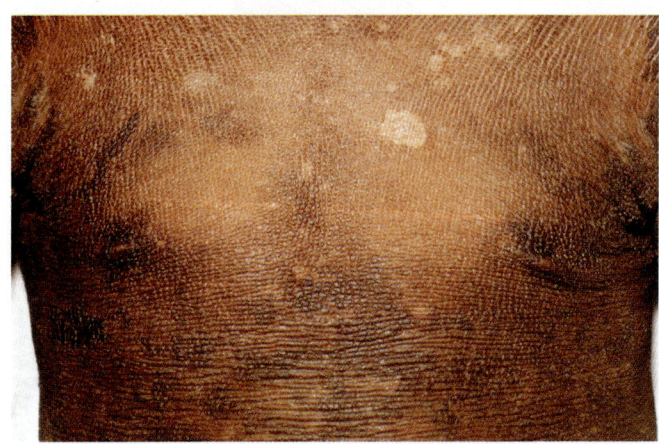

Fig. 27.64 Epidermolytic ichthyosis.

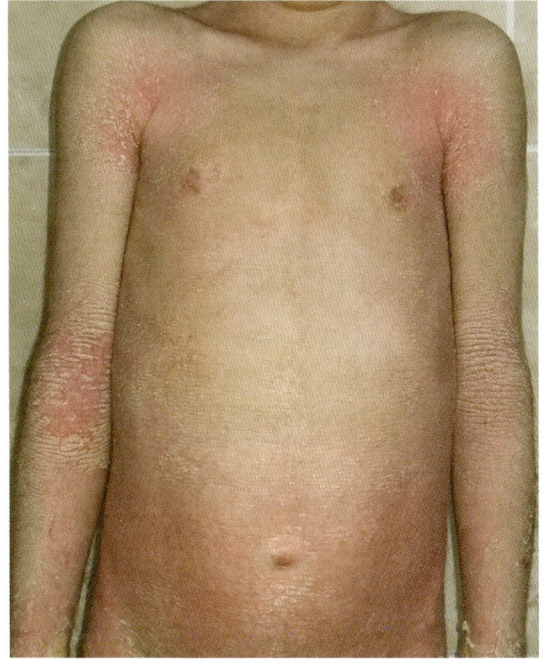

Fig. 27.65 Epidermolytic ichthyosis.

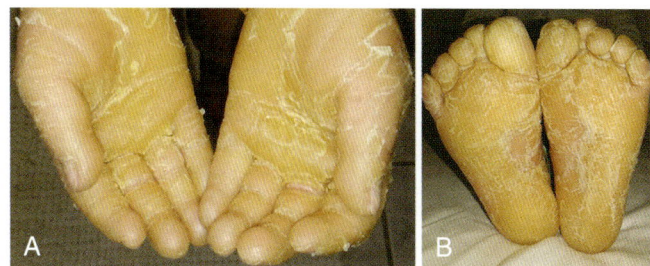

Fig. 27.66 (A) Epidermolytic ichthyosis, palms. (B) Epidermolytic ichthyosis, soles.

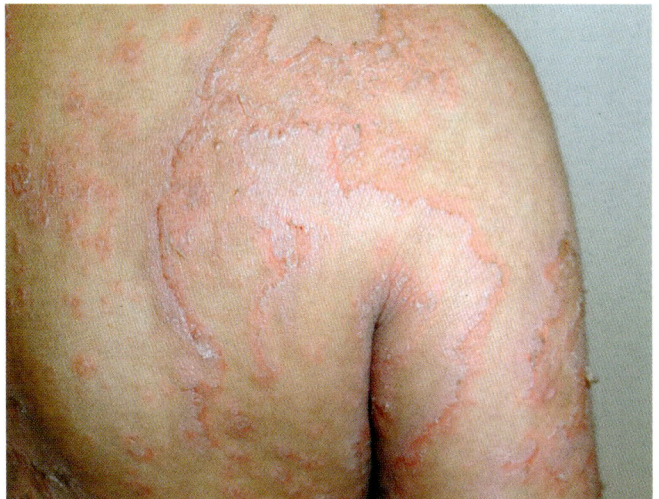

Fig. 27.67 Netherton syndrome. *Courtesy Scott Norton, MD.*

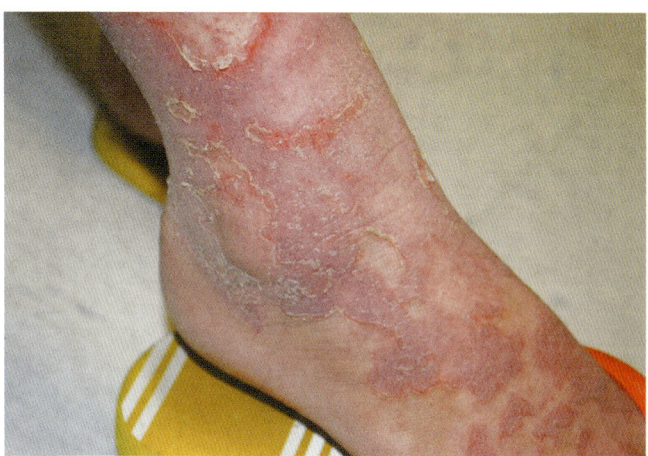

Fig. 27.68 Netherton syndrome.

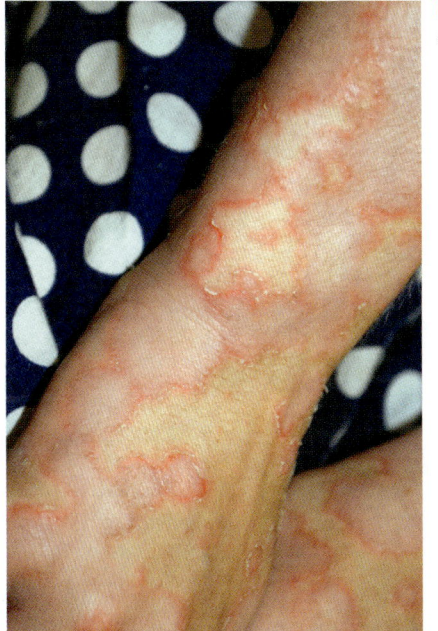

Fig. 27.69 Netherton syndrome.

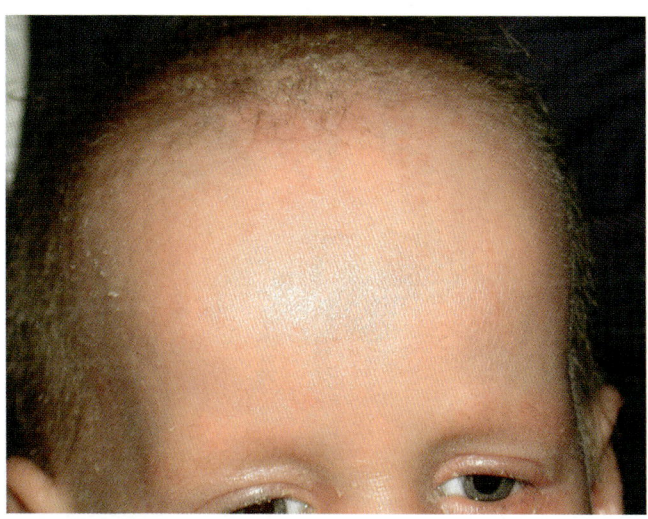

Fig. 27.70 Netherton syndrome.

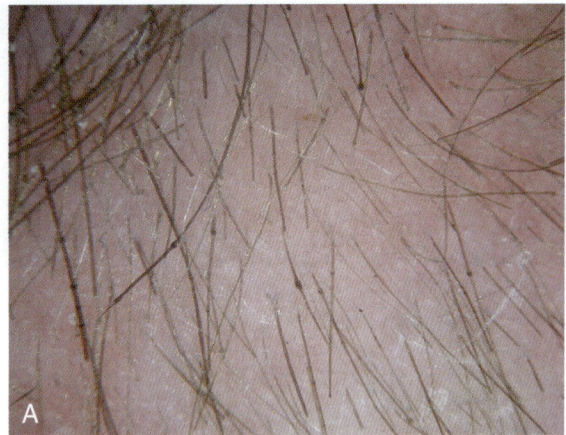
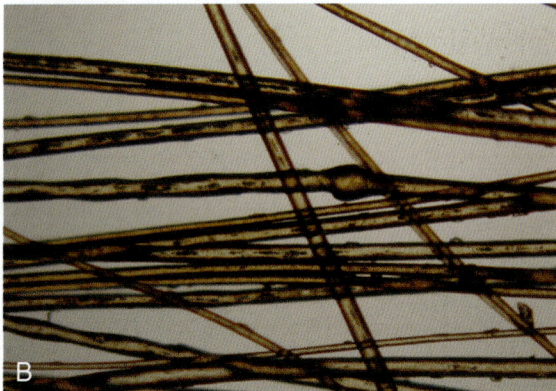

Fig. 27.71 (A) and (B) Trichorrhexis invaginata in Netherton syndrome.

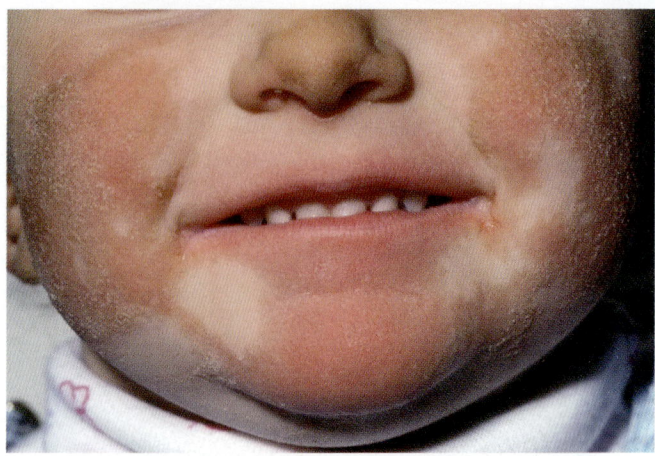

Fig. 27.72 Keratitis ichthyosis deafness syndrome. *Courtesy Paul Honig, MD.*

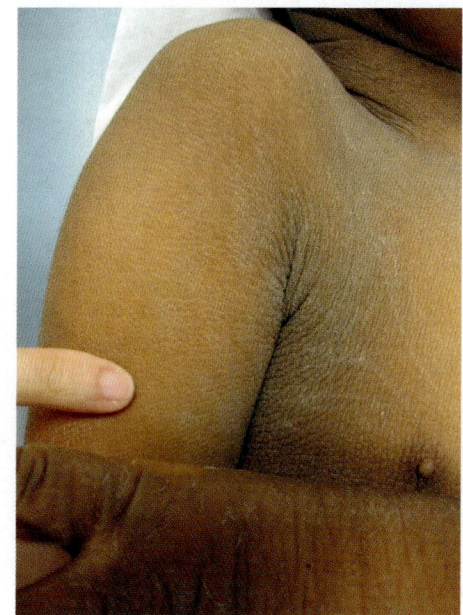

Fig. 27.74 Sjögren-Larsson syndrome.

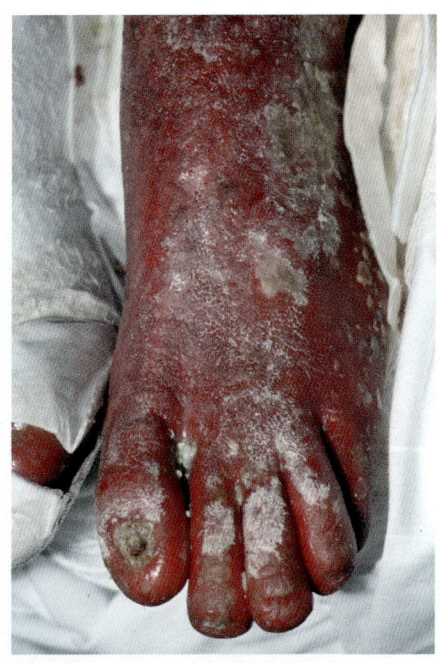

Fig. 27.73 Keratitis ichthyosis deafness syndrome.

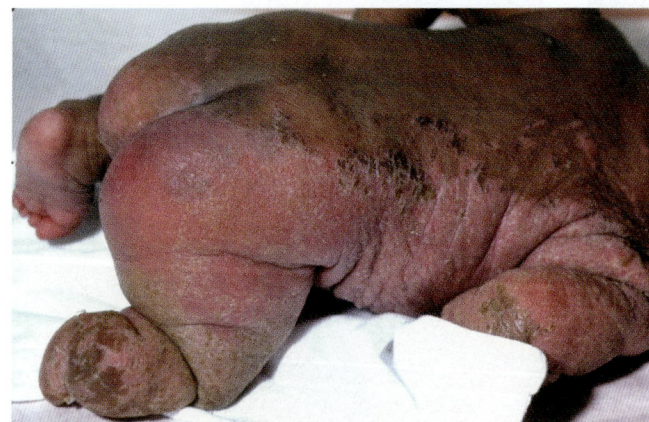

Fig. 27.75 Congenital hemidysplasia with ichthyosiform erythroderma and limb defects (CHILD) syndrome. *Courtesy Paul Honig, MD.*

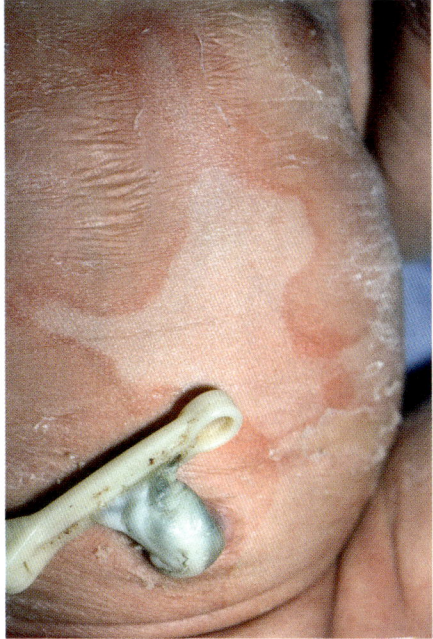

Fig. 27.76 Erythrokeratoderma variabilis. *Courtesy Ken Greer, MD.*

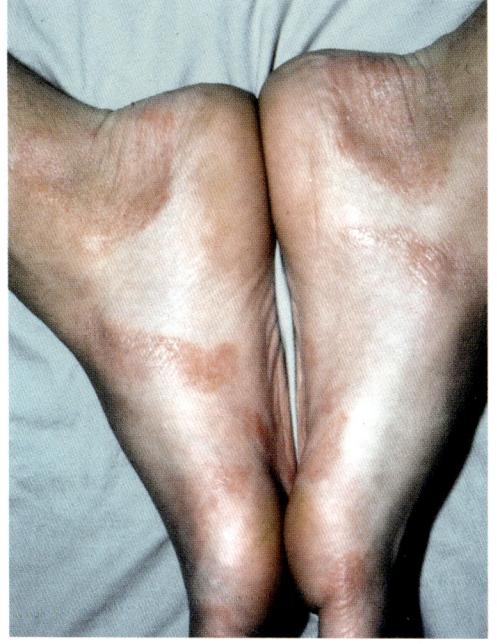

Fig. 27.77 Progressive symmetric erythrokeratoderma. *Courtesy Ken Greer, MD.*

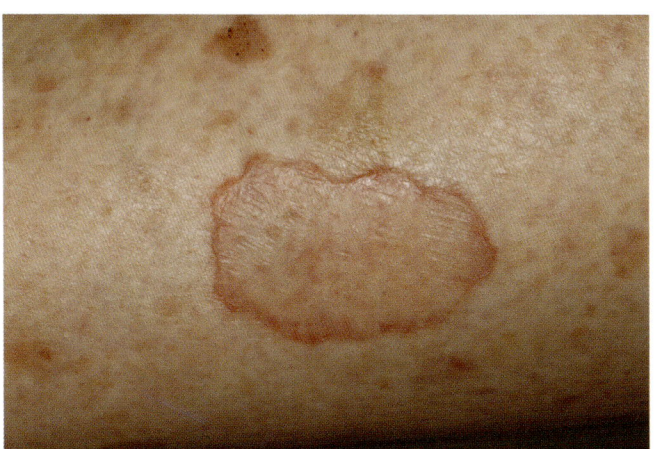

Fig. 27.78 Porokeratosis.

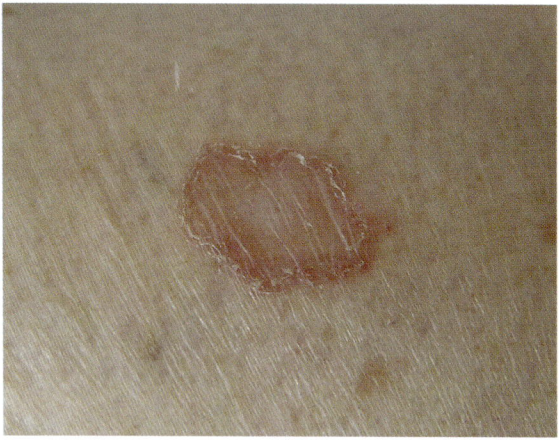

Fig. 27.79 Porokeratosis. *Courtesy Dr. Rui Carlos Taveres Bello.*

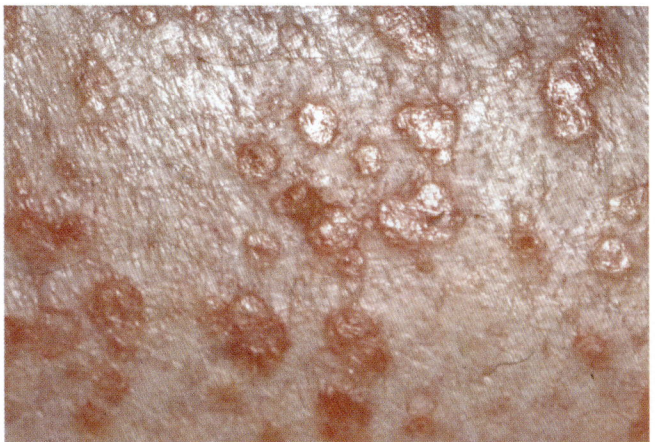

Fig. 27.80 Disseminated superficial actinic porokeratosis.

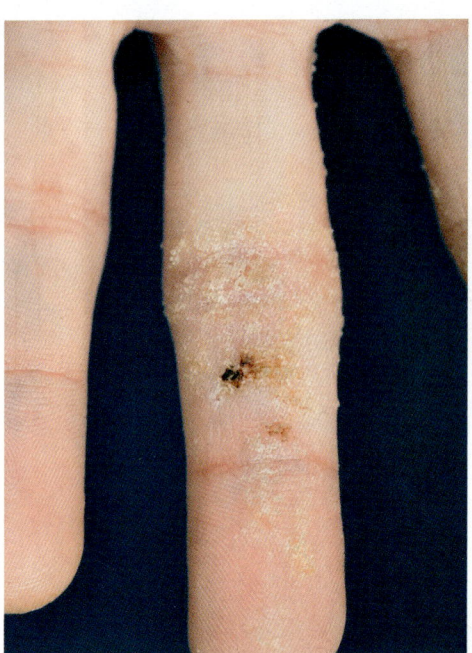

Fig. 27.81 Porokeratotic eccrine and osteal duct nevus.

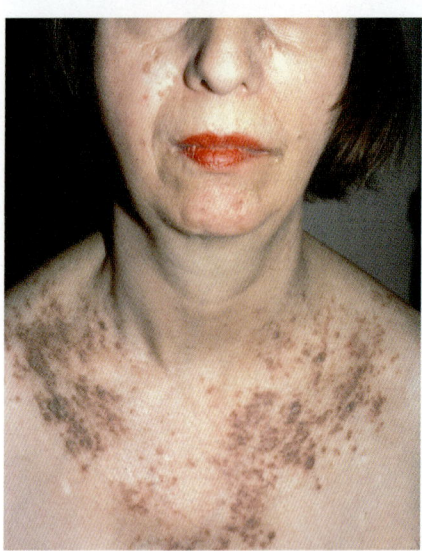

Fig. 27.82 Darier disease.

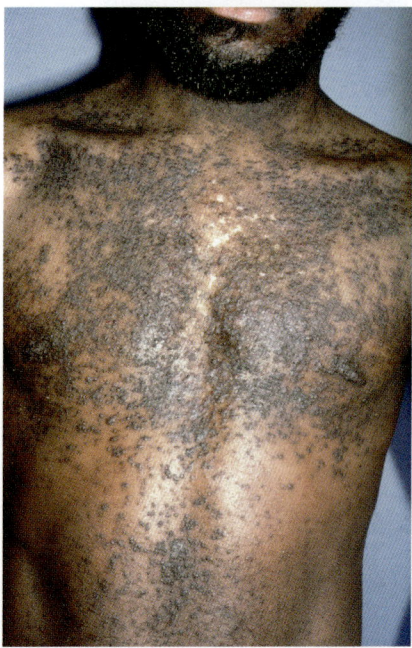

Fig. 27.84 Darier disease.

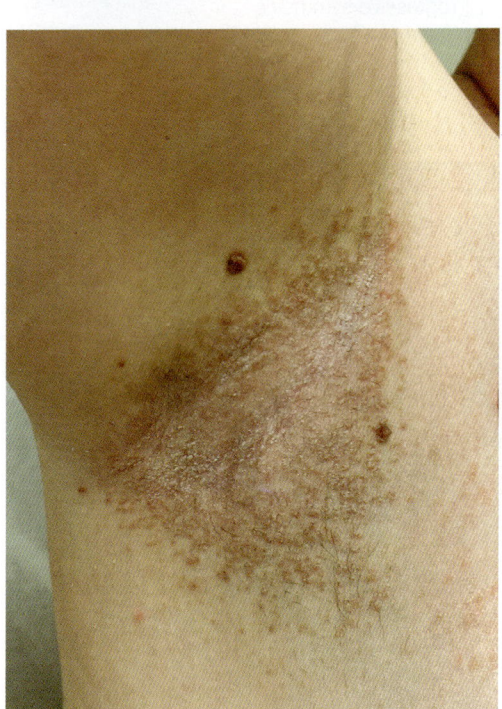

Fig. 27.83 Darier disease.

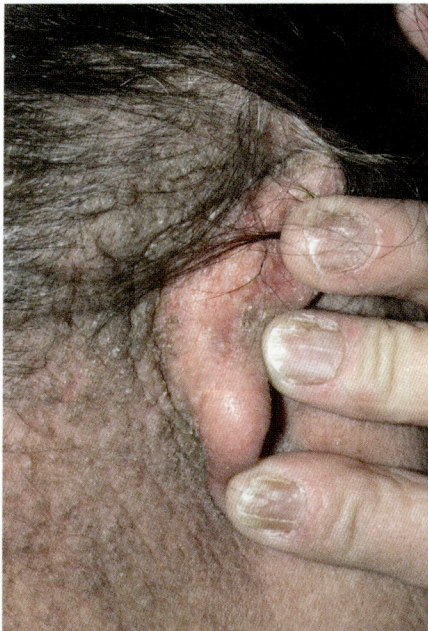

Fig. 27.86 Darier disease. *Courtesy Curt Samlaska, MD.*

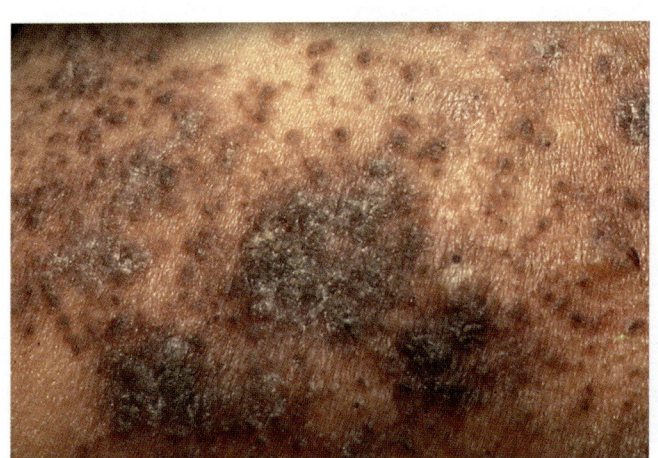

Fig. 27.85 Darier disease.

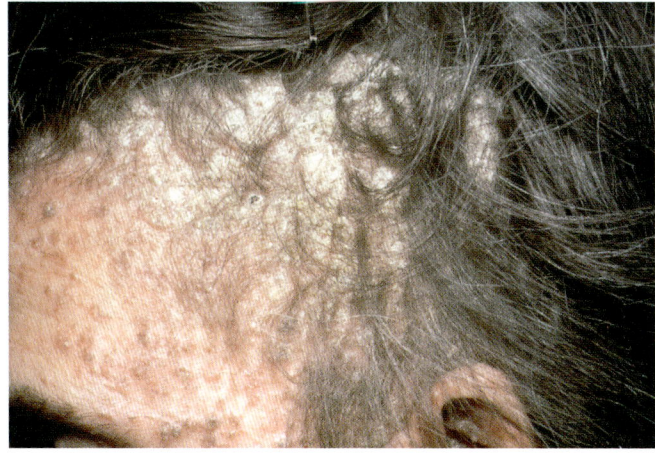

Fig. 27.87 Darier disease.

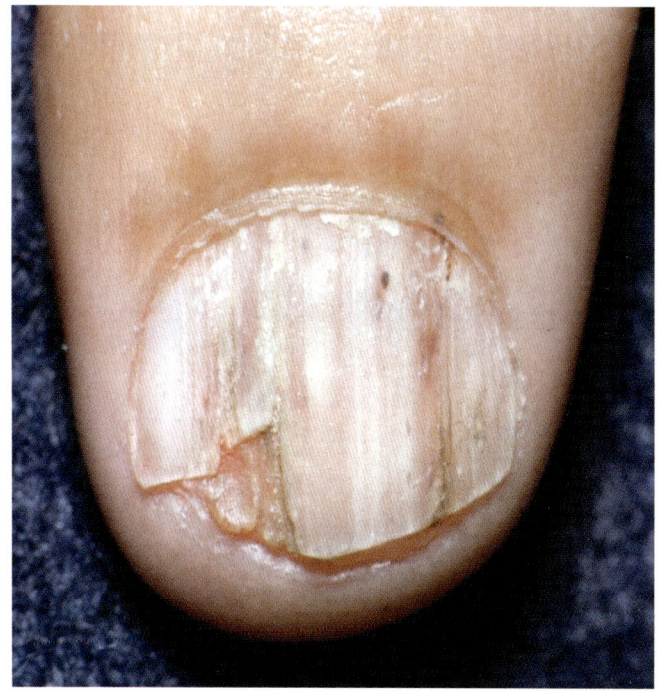

Fig. 27.88 Darier disease.

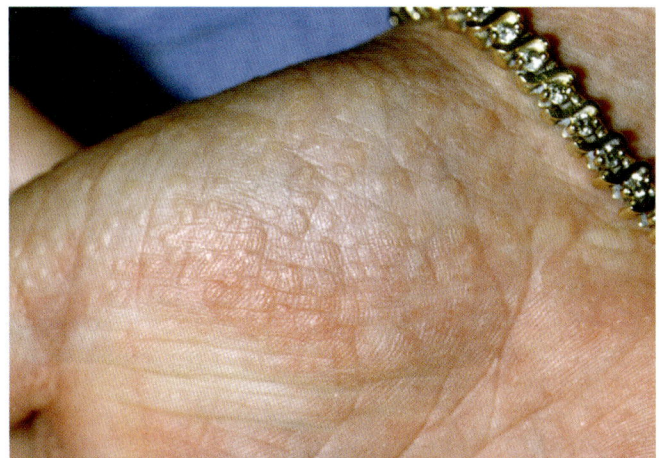

Fig. 27.89 Darier disease.

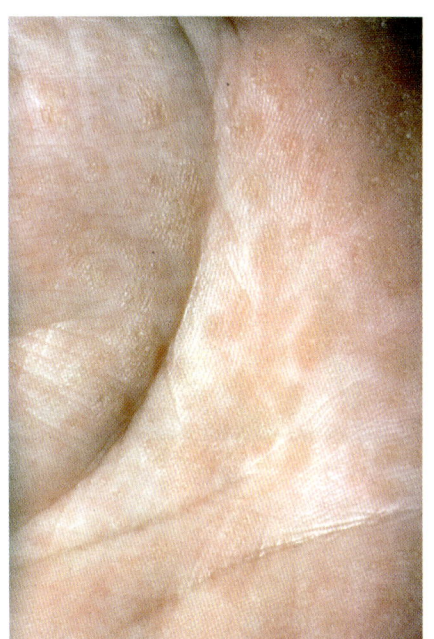

Fig. 27.90 Darier disease.

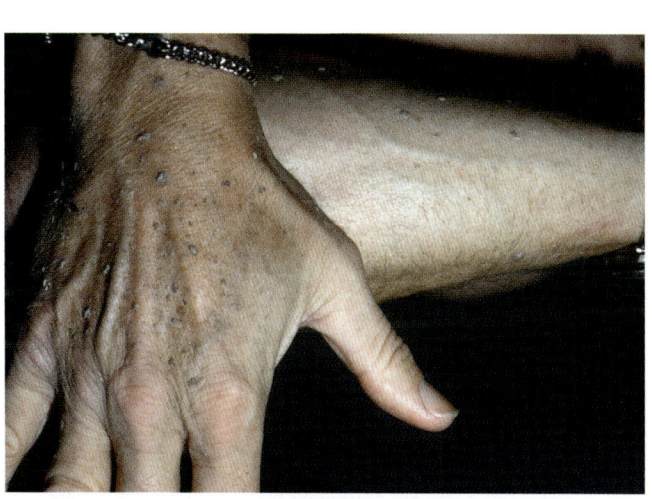

Fig. 27.91 Darier disease.

Fig. 27.92 Acrokeratosis verruciformis of Hopf.

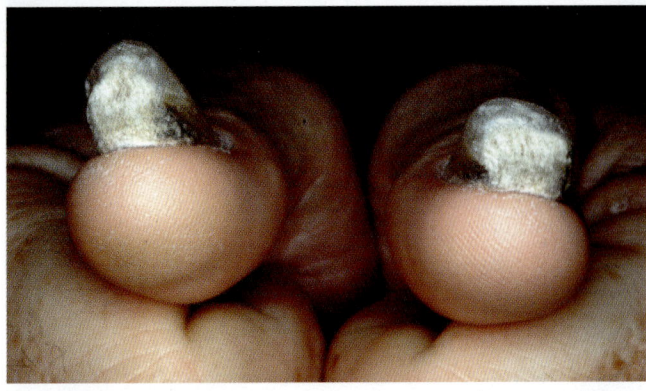

Fig. 27.93 Pachyonychia congenita.

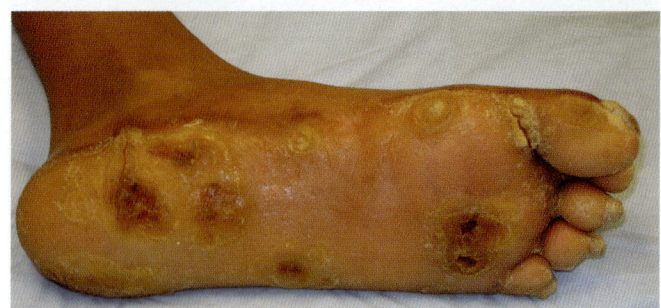

Fig. 27.94 Plantar keratoderma in pachyonychia congenita in a patient with a K16 mutation.

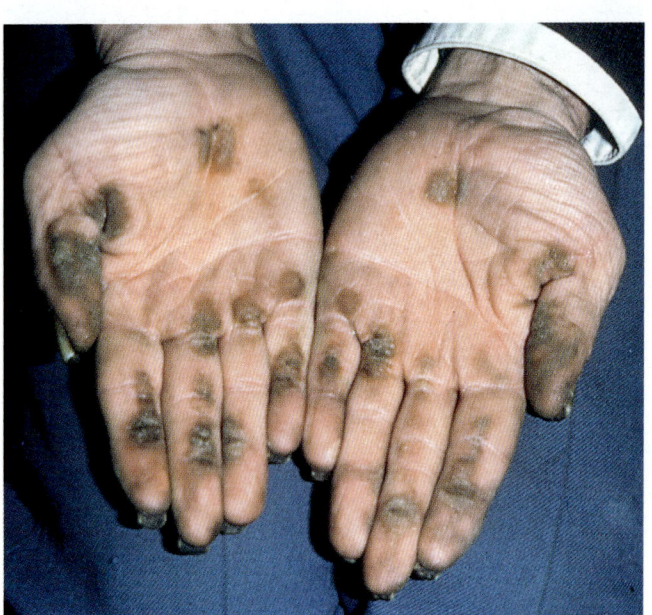

Fig. 27.95 Pachyonychia congenita.

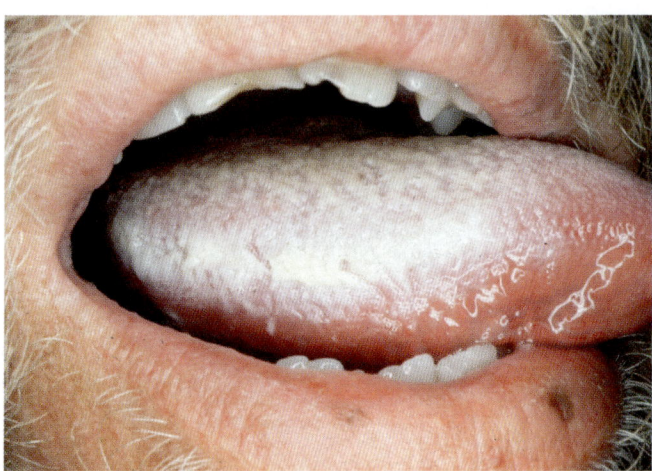

Fig. 27.96 Pachyonychia congenita.

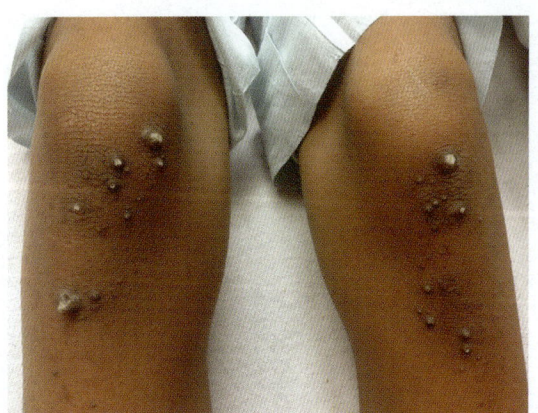

Fig. 27.97 Follicular keratotic papules in pachyonychia congenita with a K16 mutation.

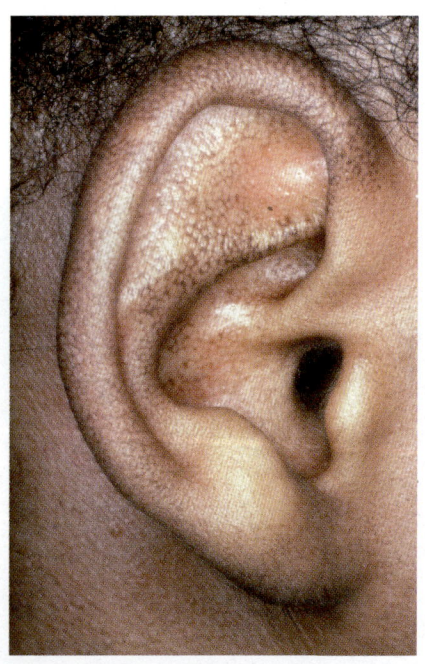

Fig. 27.98 Dyskeratosis congenita.

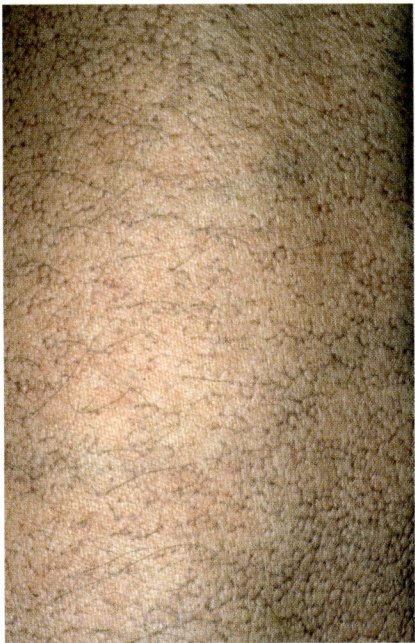

Fig. 27.99 Dyskeratosis congenita.

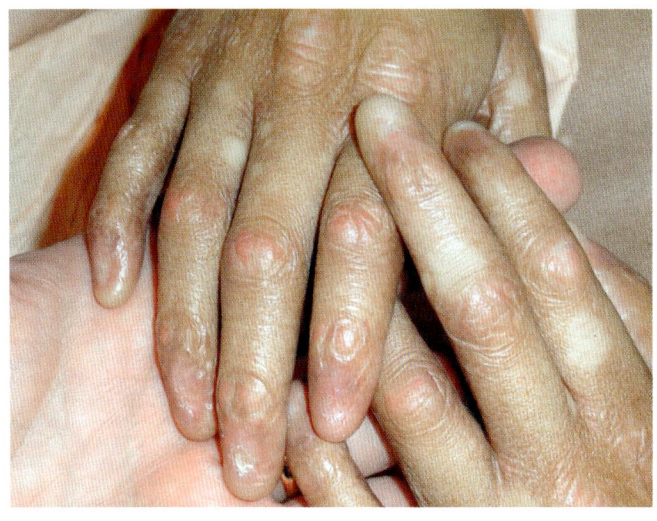

Fig. 27.100 Dyskeratosis congenita.

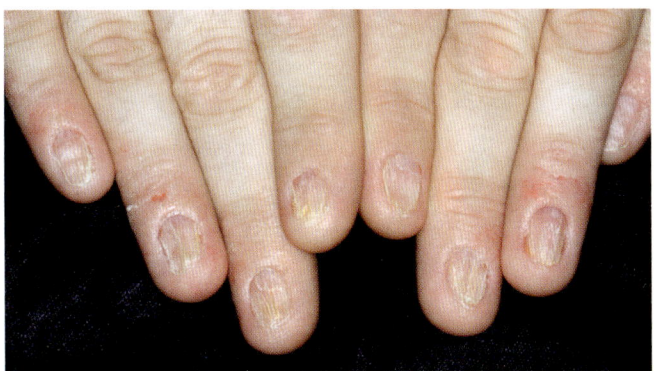

Fig. 27.101 Dyskeratosis congenita.

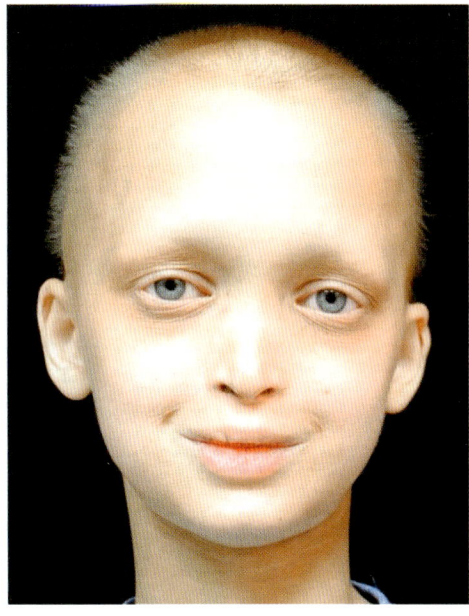

Fig. 27.102 Hypohidrotic X-linked ectodermal dysplasia. *Courtesy Scott Bartlett, MD.*

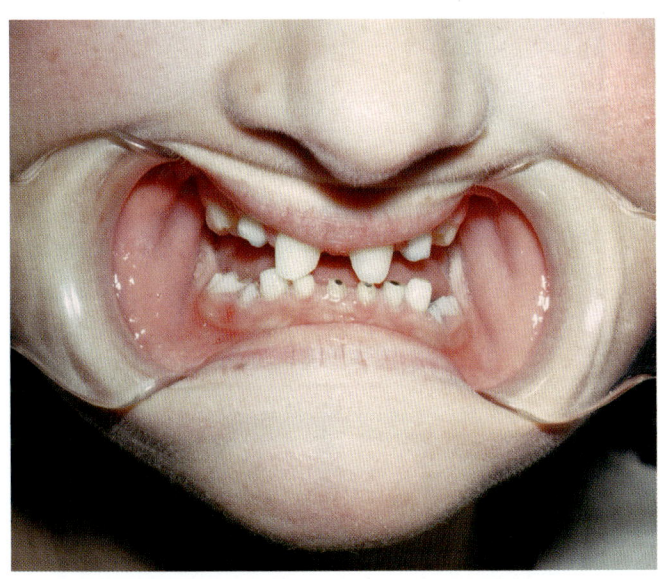

Fig. 27.103 Hypohidrotic X-linked ectodermal dysplasia.

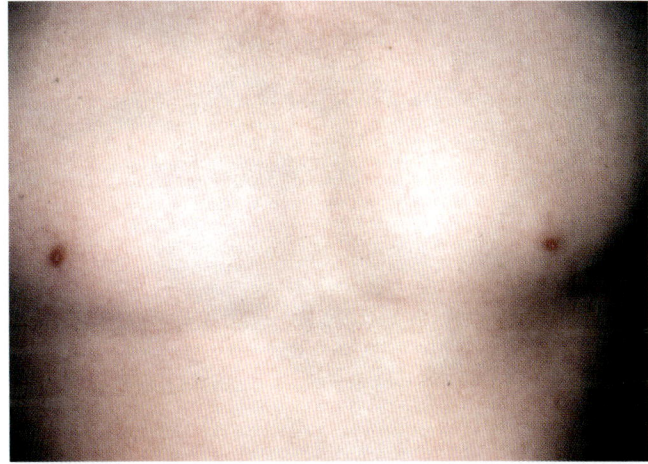

Fig. 27.104 Hypohidrotic X-linked ectodermal dysplasia.

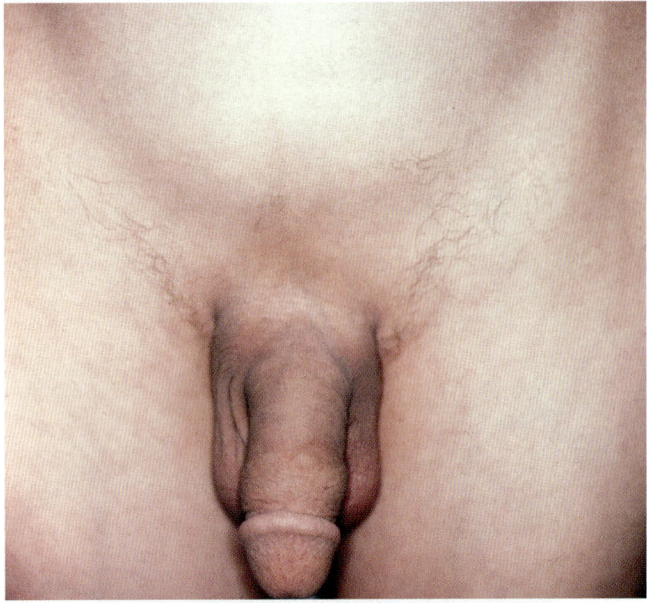

Fig. 27.105 Hypohidrotic X-linked ectodermal dysplasia.

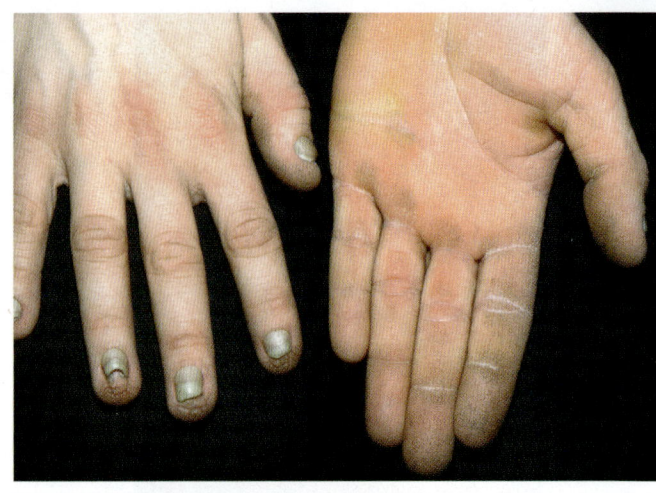

Fig. 27.106 Hidrotic ectodermal dysplasia.

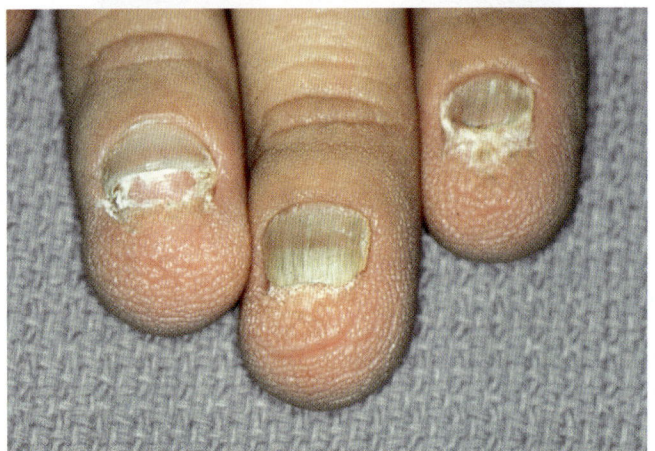

Fig. 27.107 Hidrotic ectodermal dysplasia.

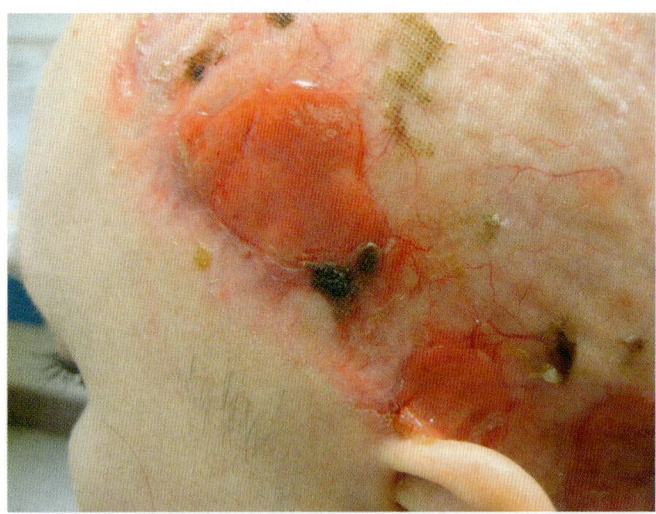

Fig. 27.108 Ankyloblepharon-ectodermal dysplasia-clefting

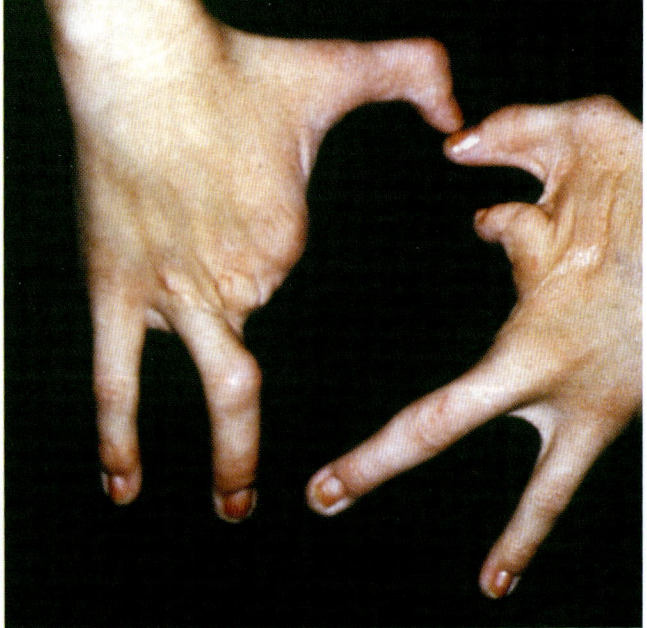

Fig. 27.109 Ectrodactyly ectodermal dysplasia-clefting.

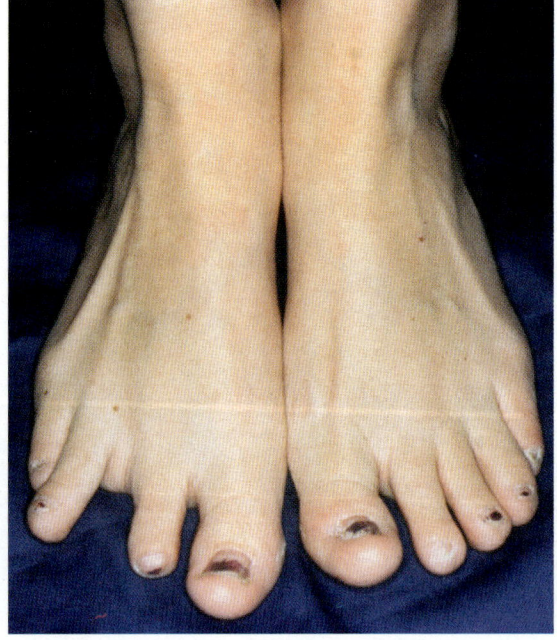

Fig. 27.110 Ectrodactyly ectodermal dysplasia-clefting.

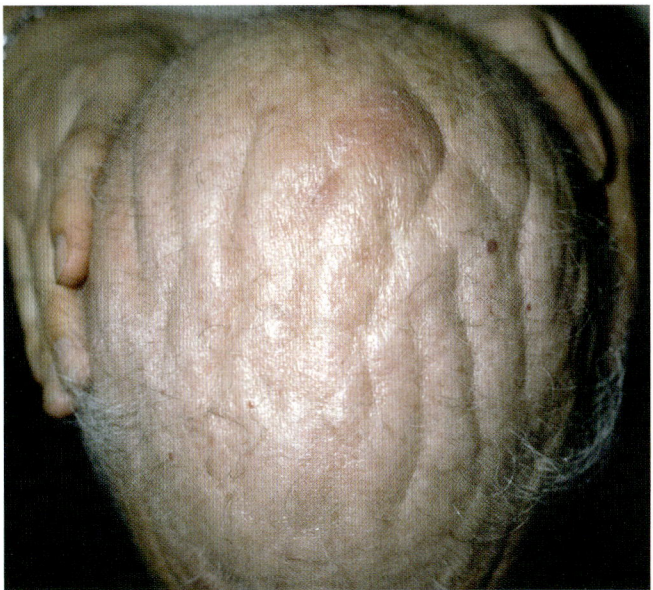

Fig. 27.111 Cutis verticis gyrata.

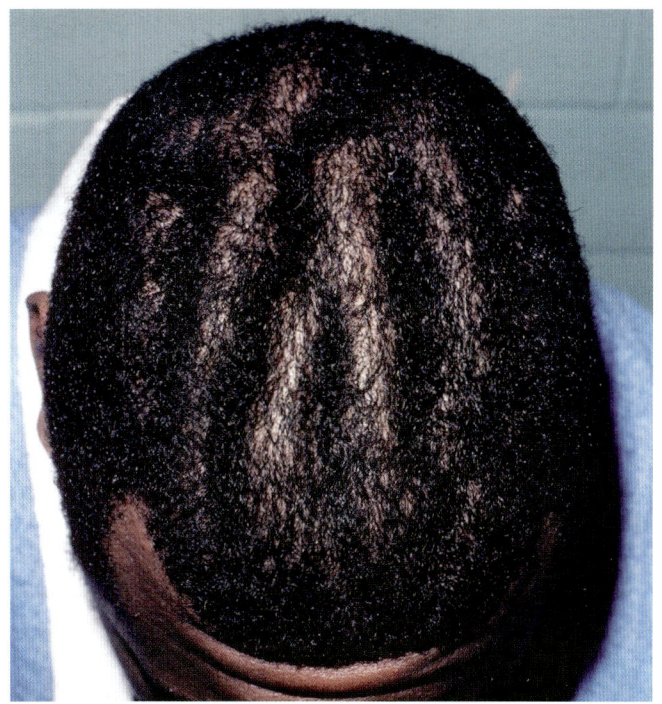

Fig. 27.112 Cutis verticis gyrata. *Courtesy Steven Binnick, MD.*

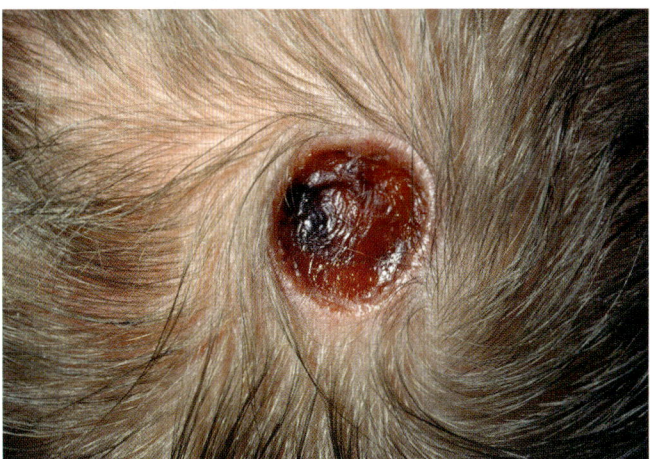

Fig. 27.113 Aplasia cutis congenita.

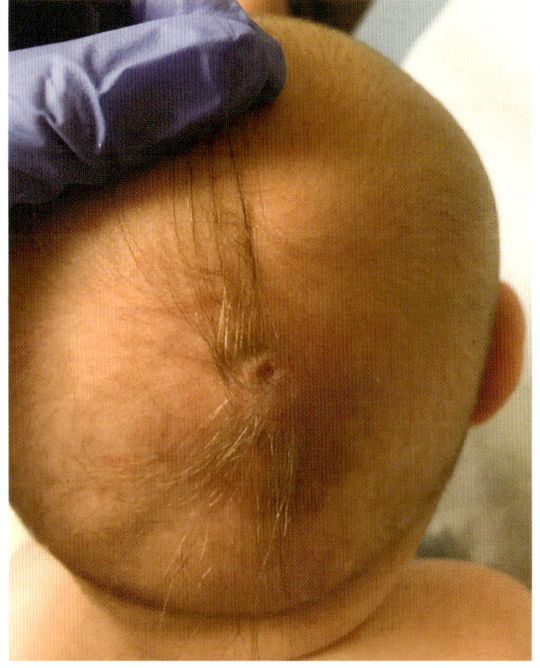

Fig. 27.114 Aplasia cutis congenita with hair collar sign.

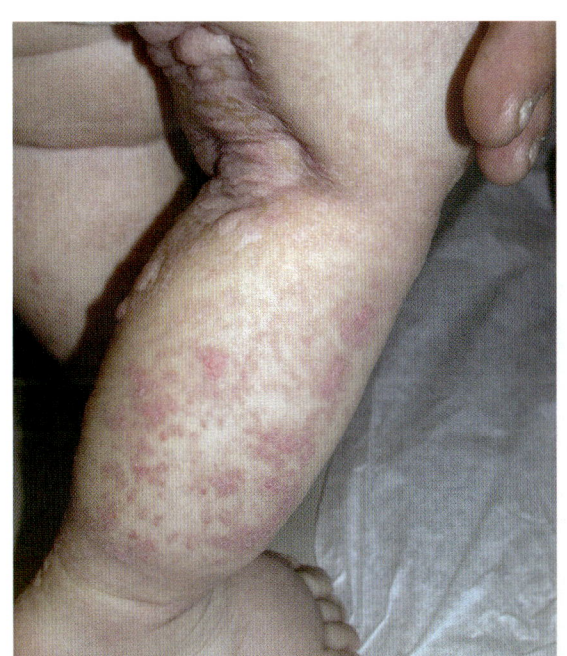

Fig. 27.115 Goltz syndrome. *Courtesy Paul Honig, MD.*

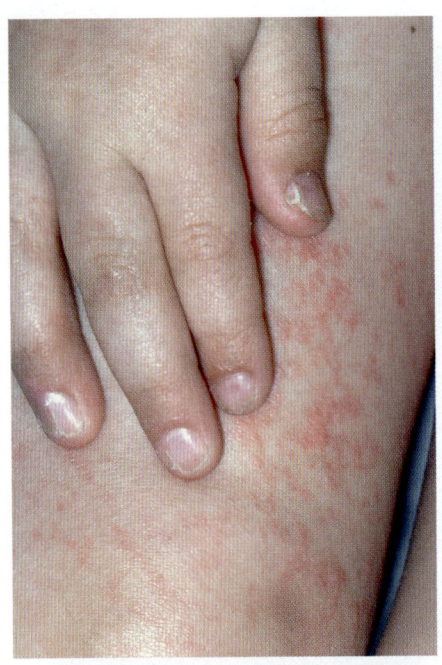

Fig. 27.116 Goltz syndrome.

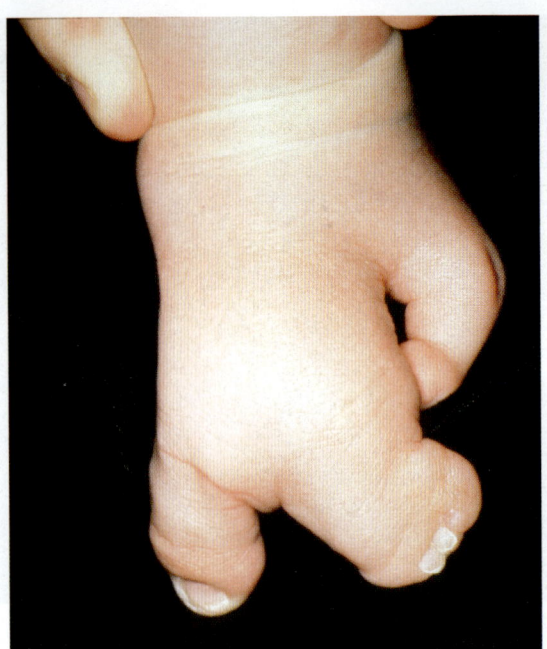

Fig. 27.117 Goltz syndrome.

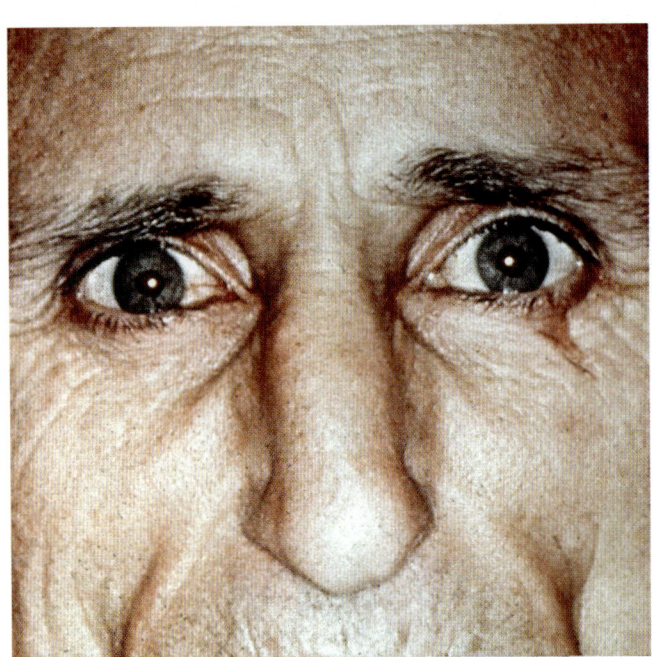

Fig. 27.118 Werner syndrome.

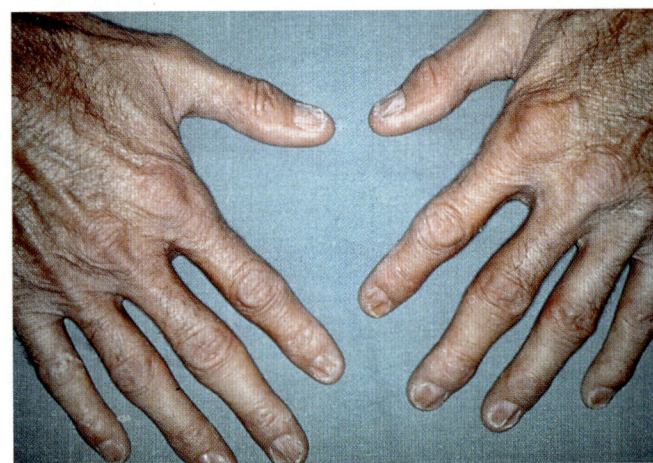

Fig. 27.119 Werner syndrome.

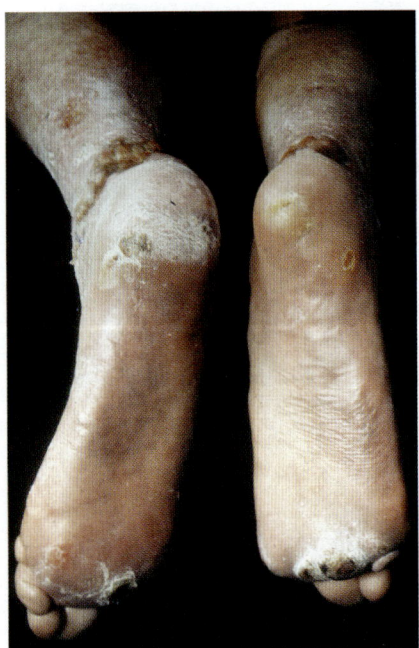

Fig. 27.120 Werner syndrome.

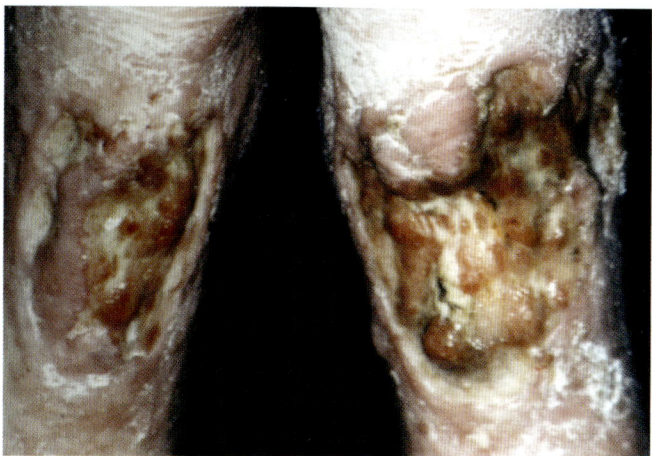

Fig. 27.121 Werner syndrome.

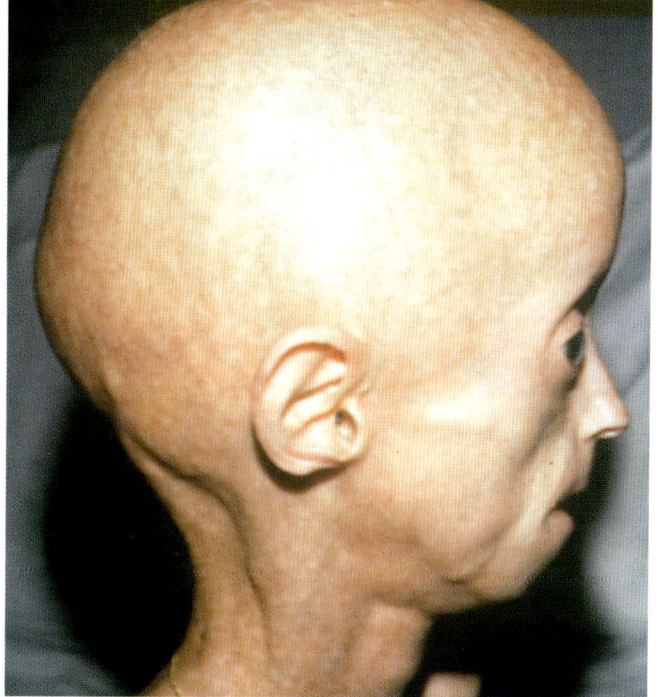

Fig. 27.122 Progeria.

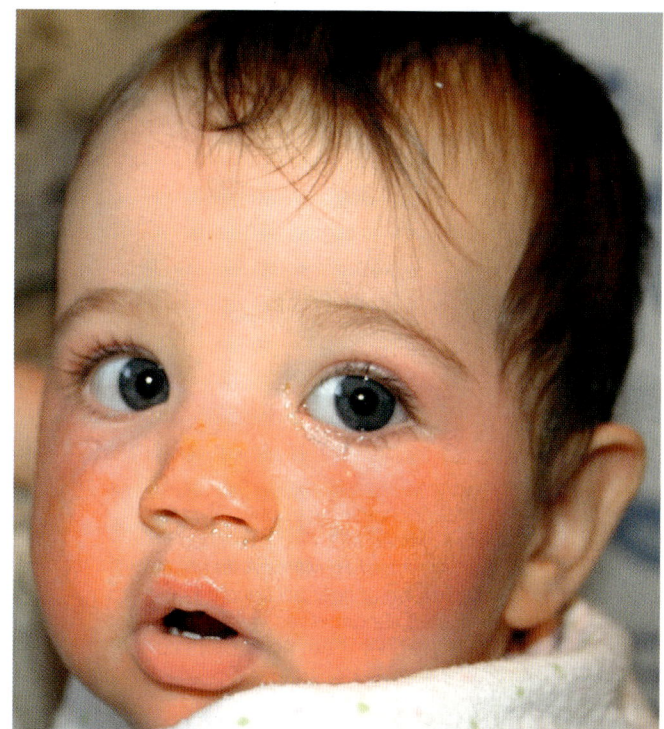

Fig. 27.123 Xeroderma pigmentosum. *Courtesy Kenneth Kraemer, MD. First published in Bradford PT, Goldstein AM, Tamura D, et al. Cancer and neurologic degeneration in xeroderma pigmentosum. J Med Genet 2011;48:168–176.*

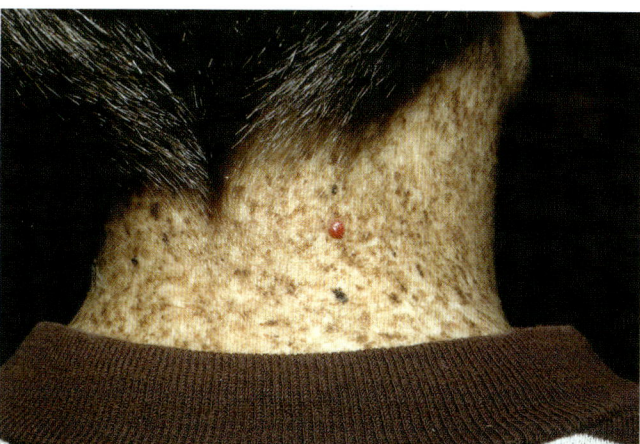

Fig. 27.124 Xeroderma pigmentosum. *Courtesy The University of Utah and Oregon Health Sciences University Leonard Swinyer MD image collection.*

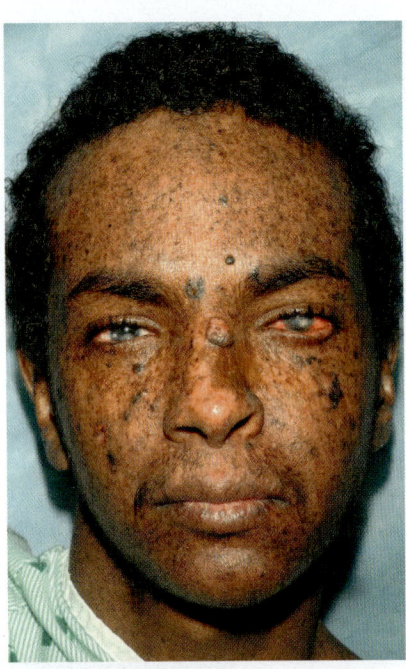

Fig. 27.125 Xeroderma pigmentosum. *Courtesy Kenneth Kraemer, MD. First published in Bradford PT, Goldstein AM, Tamura D, et al. Cancer and neurologic degeneration in xeroderma pigmentosum.* J Med Genet 2011;48: 168–176.

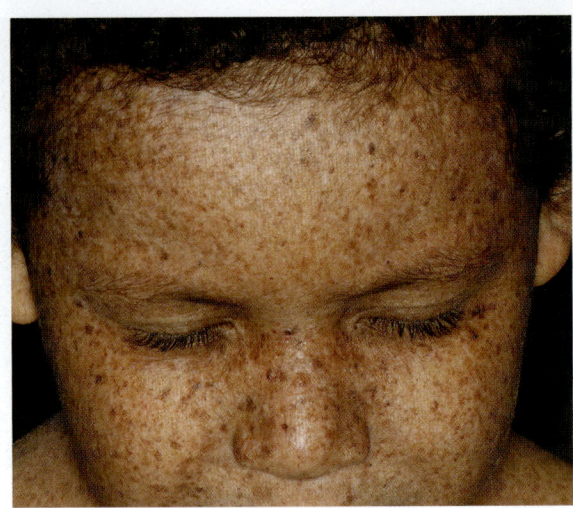

Fig. 27.126 Xeroderma pigmentosum.

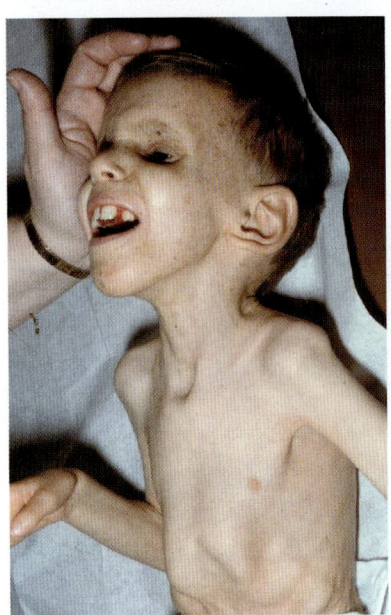

Fig. 27.127 Cockayne syndrome. *Courtesy Kenneth Kraemer, MD. First published in Lindenbaum Y, Dickson DW, Rosenbaum P, et al. Xeroderma pigmentosum/Cockayne syndrome (XP/CS) complex.* Eur J Child Neurol 2001;5:225–242.

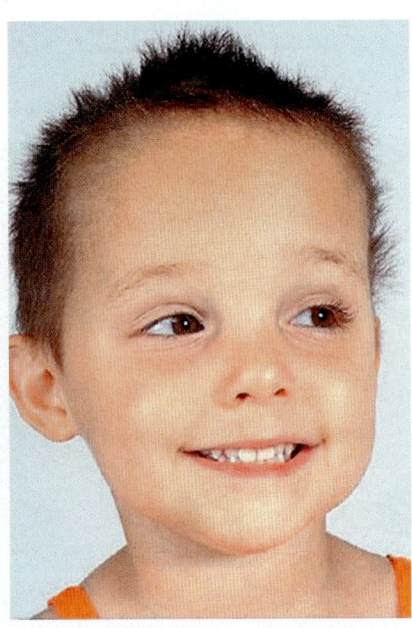

Fig. 27.129 Trichothiodystrophy. *Courtesy Kenneth Kraemer, MD. First published in Liang C, Kraemer KH, Morris A, et al. Characterization of tiger tail banding and hair shaft abnormalities in trichothiodystrophy* J Am Acad Dermatol 2005;52:224–232.

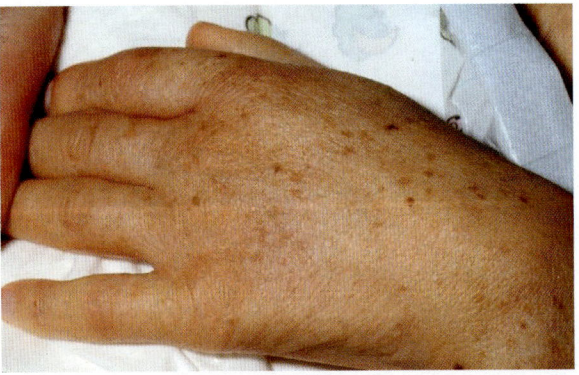

Fig. 27.128 Cockayne-xeroderma pigmentosum syndrome complex. *Courtesy Kenneth Kraemer, MD. First published in Lindenbaum Y, Dickson DW, Rosenbaum P, et al. Xeroderma pigmentosum/Cockayne syndrome (XP/CS) complex.* Eur J Child Neurol 2001;5:225–242.

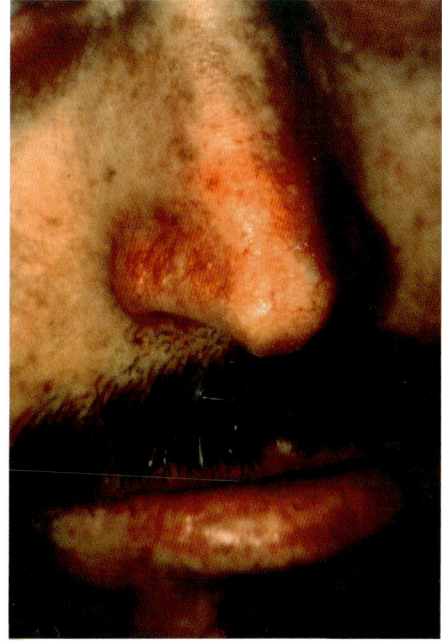

Fig. 27.130 Bloom syndrome.

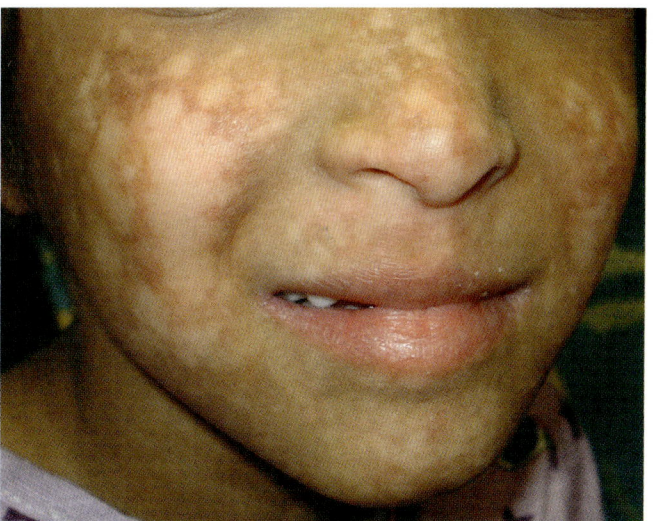

Fig. 27.131 Rothmund-Thomson syndrome.

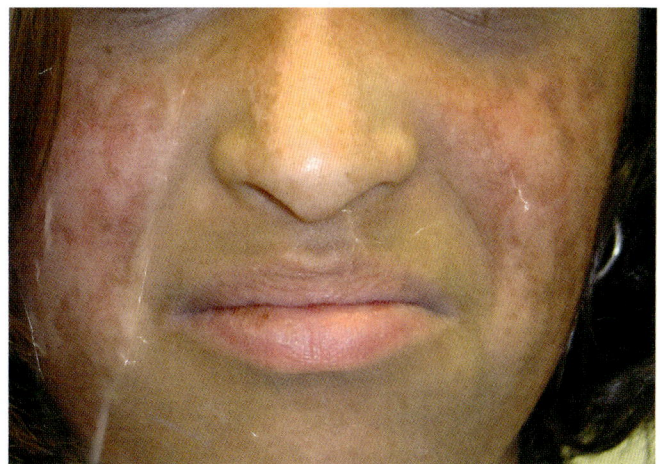

Fig. 27.132 Rothmund-Thomson syndrome.

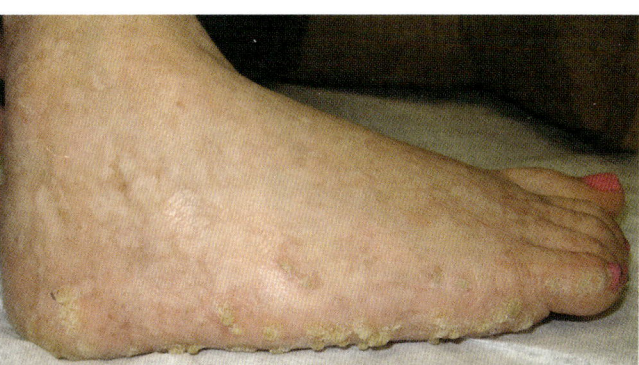

Fig. 27.133 Rothmund-Thomson syndrome.

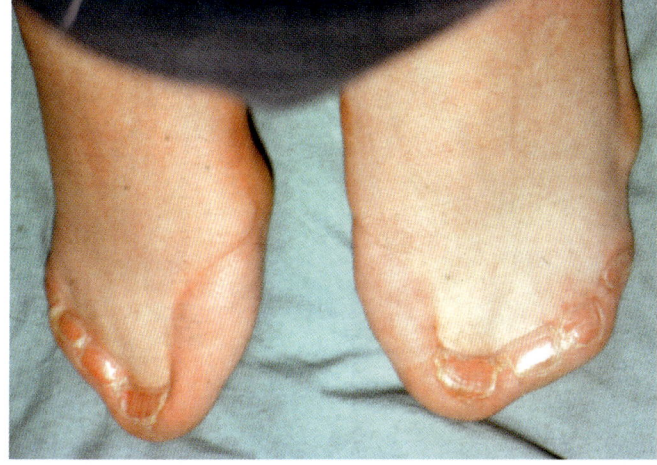

Fig. 27.134 Apert syndrome.

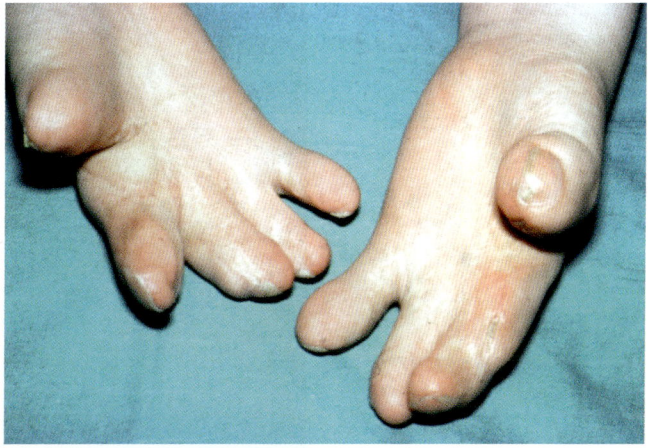

Fig. 27.135 Apert syndrome.

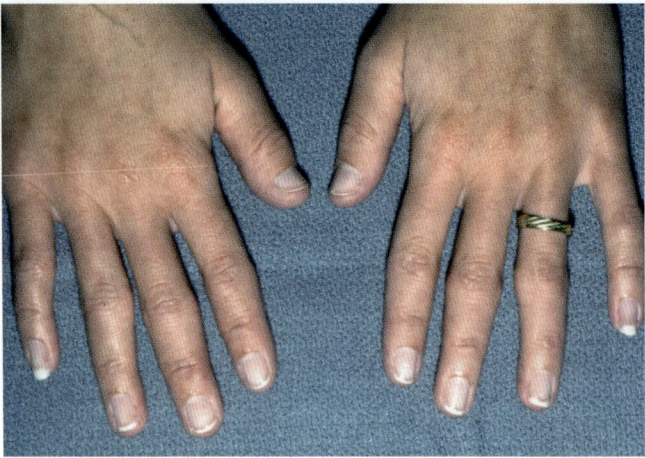

Fig. 27.136 Trichorhinophalangeal syndrome.

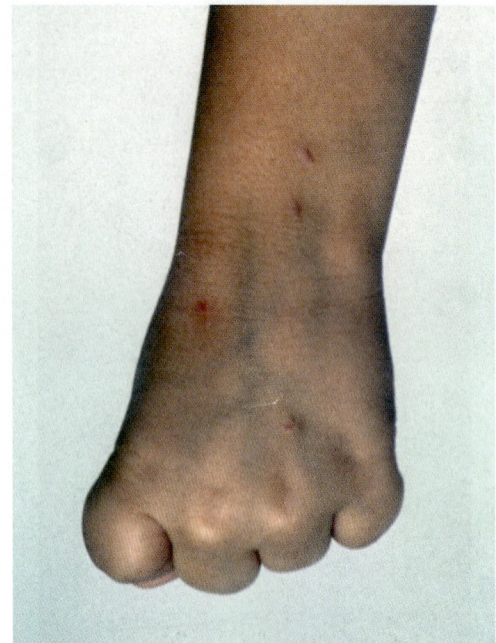

Fig. 27.137 Trichorhinophalangeal syndrome.

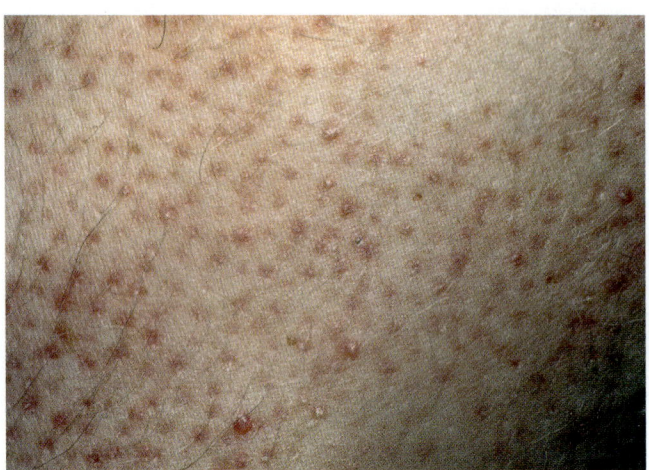

Fig. 27.138 Keratosis pilaris.

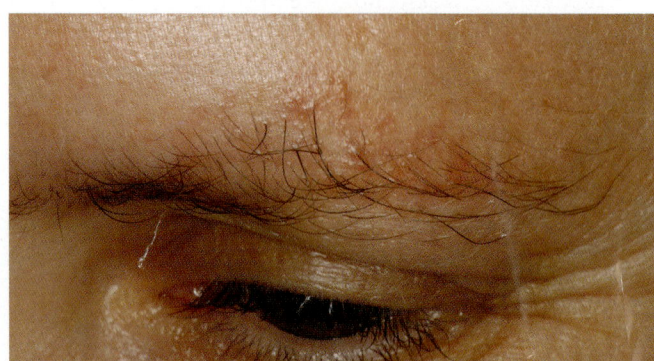

Fig. 27.139 Ulerythema ophrogenes.

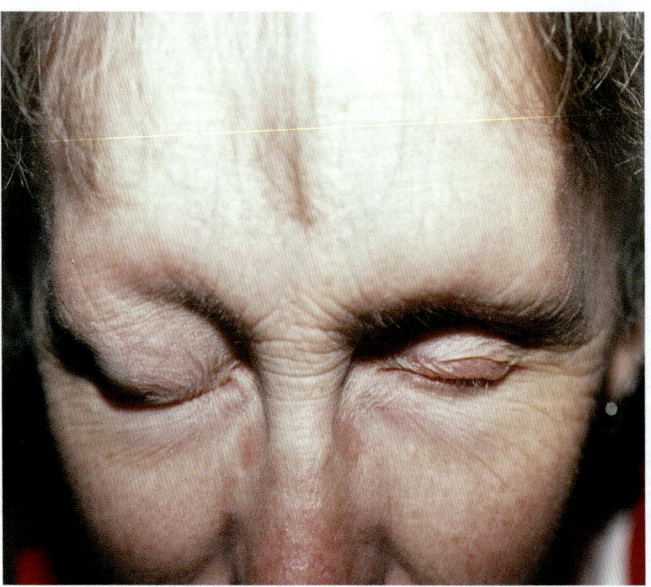

Fig. 27.140 Keratosis follicularis spinulosa decalvans.

Dermal and Subcutaneous Tumors 28

Vascular tumors range from red to blue, depending on the degree of vascular stasis and deoxygenation of hemoglobin. When associated with thrombosis or consumptive coagulopathy, the lesions often become hard and tender. The clinician should attempt to distinguish vascular proliferative lesions from vascular malformations, as the former tend to respond to beta blockers, whereas the latter do not. Malformations include nevus flammeus, salmon patch, nevus anemicus, and cutis marmorata telangiectatica congenita. Some vascular malformations are associated with overgrowth of surrounding tissues and can lead to considerable morbidity. This portion of the atlas will focus on the clinical findings of dermal tumors, including fibrous and vascular proliferations, as well as growths, in addition to those composed of muscles, nerves, and fatty tissue.

A biopsy may be required for the definitive diagnosis of dermal neoplasms, but the color, morphology, and distribution of the lesions can often lead to an accurate clinical diagnosis. Dermatofibromas present as firm, pink-to brown dermal nodules with overlying epidermal acanthosis imparting a dull or velvety appearance to the skin. A characteristic dimpling sign occurs when the surrounding skin is compressed laterally. Granular cell tumors tend to be larger, but are accompanied by a similar velvety or verrucous appearance of the overlying skin. In contrast, dermatofibrosarcoma protuberans presents with a multinodular appearance with overlying epidermal atrophy imparting a taught, glossy appearance to the skin. All of these tumors are quite firm to palpation in contrast to the soft rubbery or gelatinous feel of a neurofibroma.

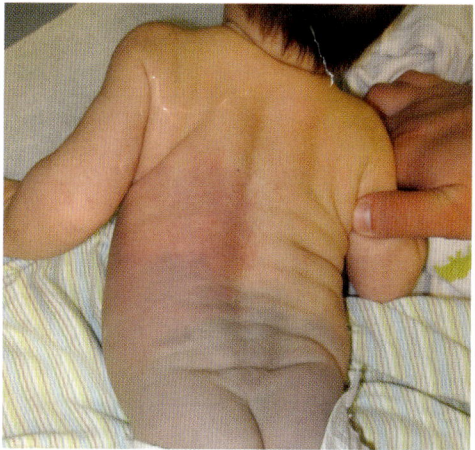

Fig. 28.1 Phacomatosis pigmentovascularis. *Courtesy Department of Dermatology, Keio University School of Medicine, Tokyo, Japan.*

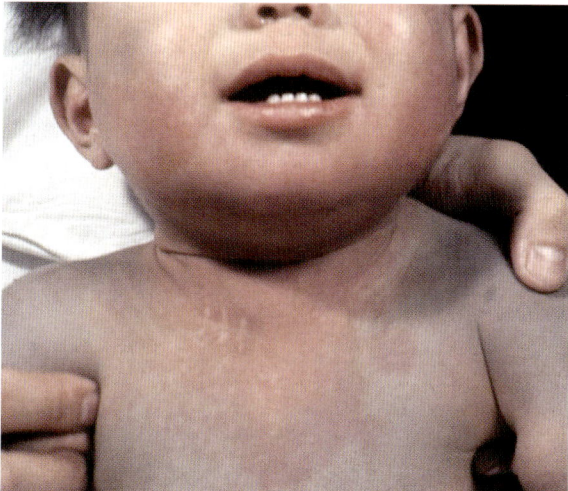

Fig. 28.2 Phacomatosis pigmentovascularis.

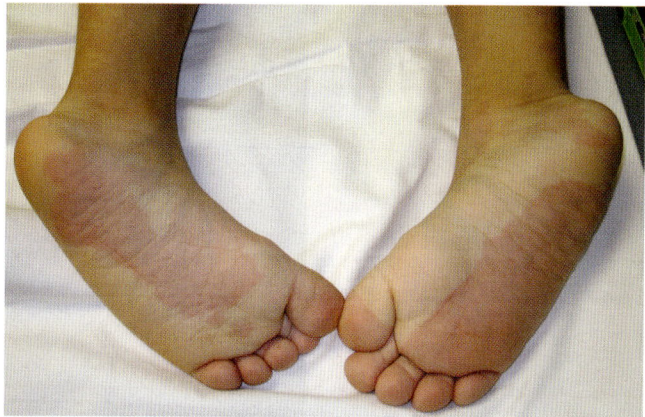

Fig. 28.3 PIK3CA-related segmental overgrowth syndrome.

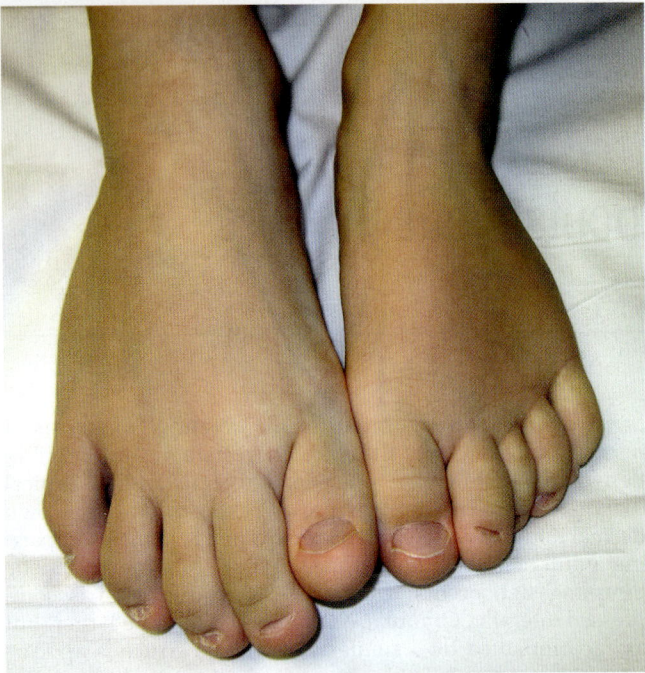

Fig. 28.4 PIK3CA-related segmental overgrowth syndrome.

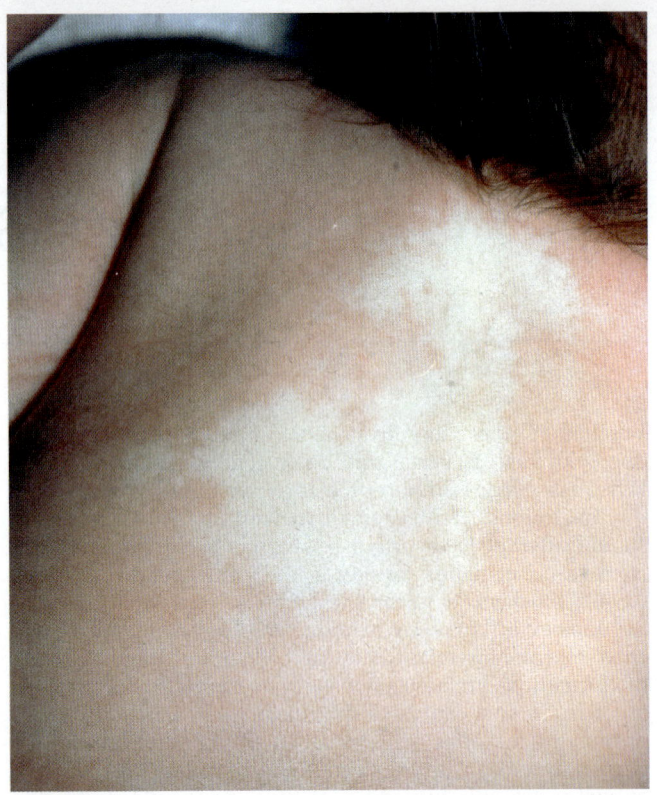

Fig. 28.5 Nevus anemicus.

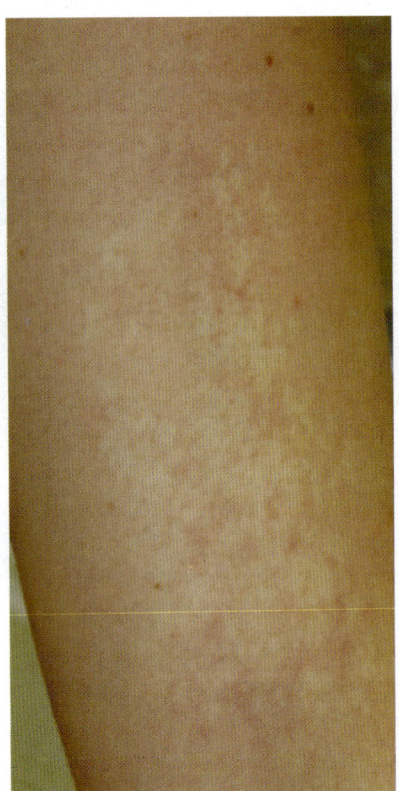

Fig. 28.6 Nevus anemicus in a patient with neurofibromatosis.

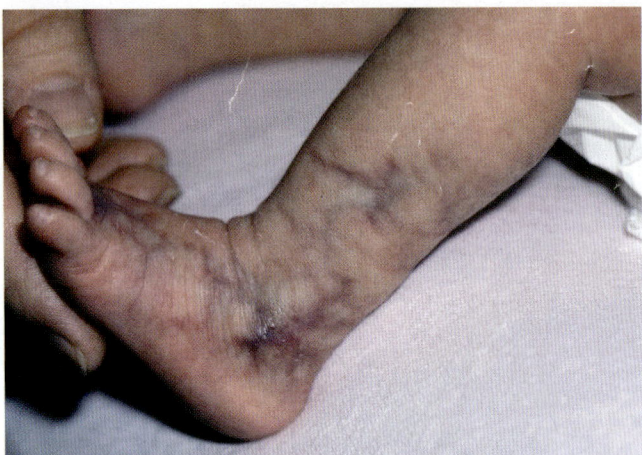

Fig. 28.7 Cutis marmorata telangiectatica congenita. *Courtesy Paul Honig, MD.*

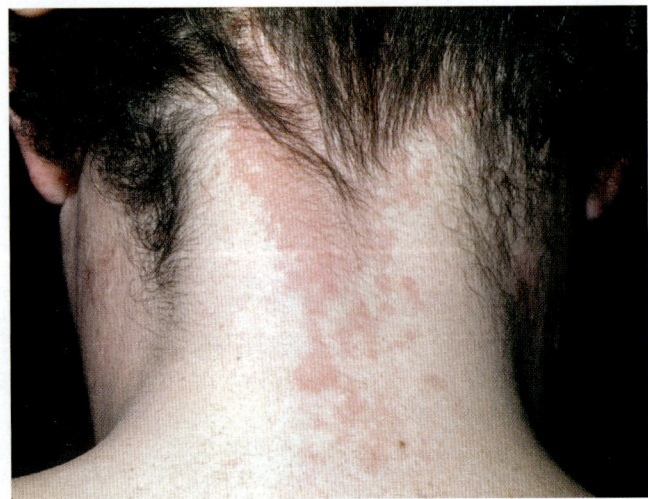

Fig. 28.8 Nevus simplex. *Courtesy Steven Binnick, MD.*

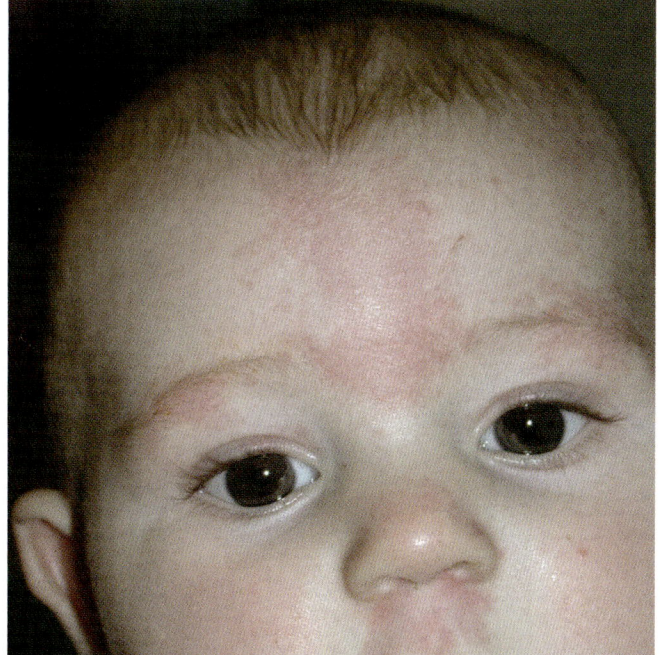

Fig. 28.9 Nevus simplex.

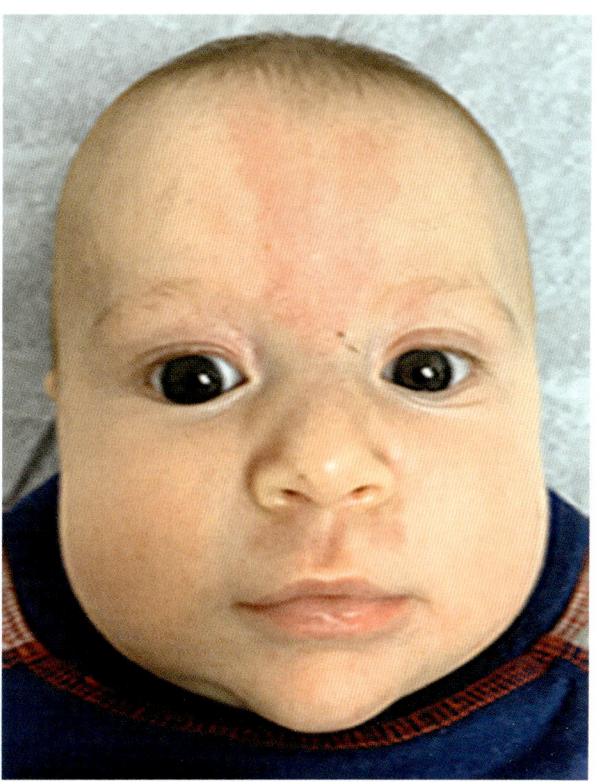

Fig. 28.10 Nevus simplex.

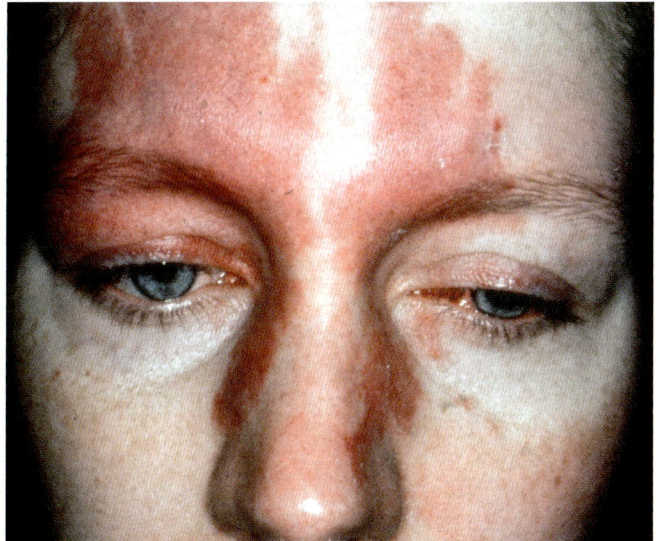

Fig. 28.11 Capillary malformation (port-wine stain) with Sturge-Weber syndrome.

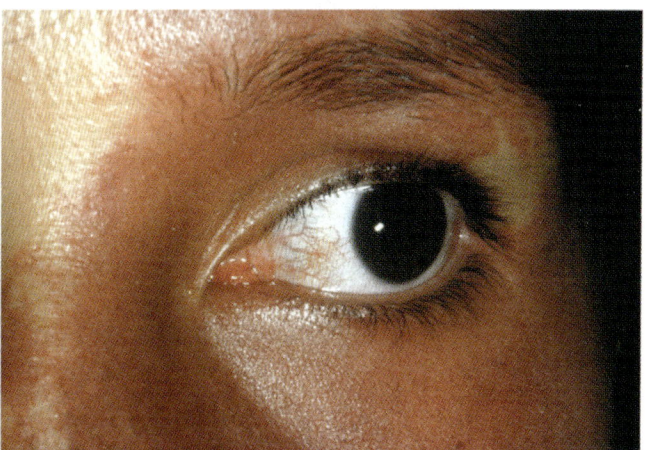

Fig. 28.12 Capillary malformation (port-wine stain) with Sturge-Weber syndrome.

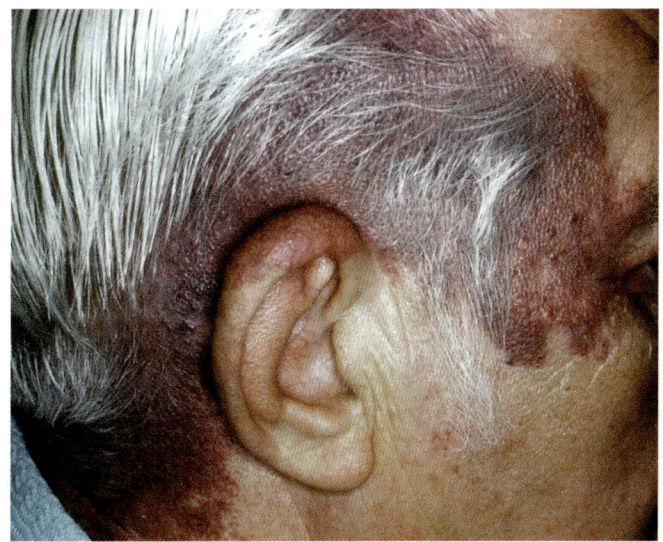

Fig. 28.13 Capillary malformation (port-wine stain).

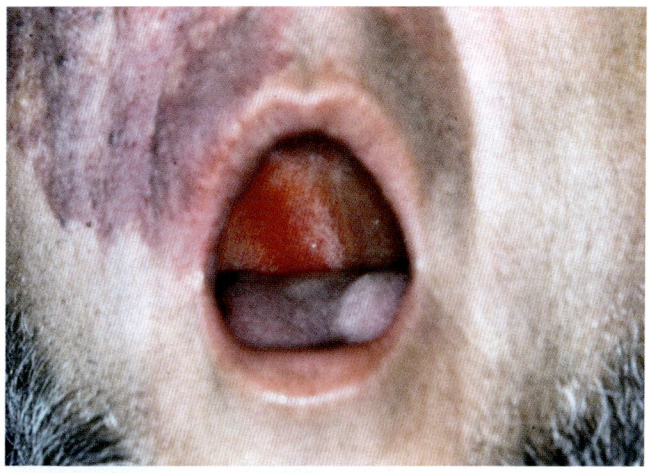

Fig. 28.14 Capillary malformation (port-wine stain).

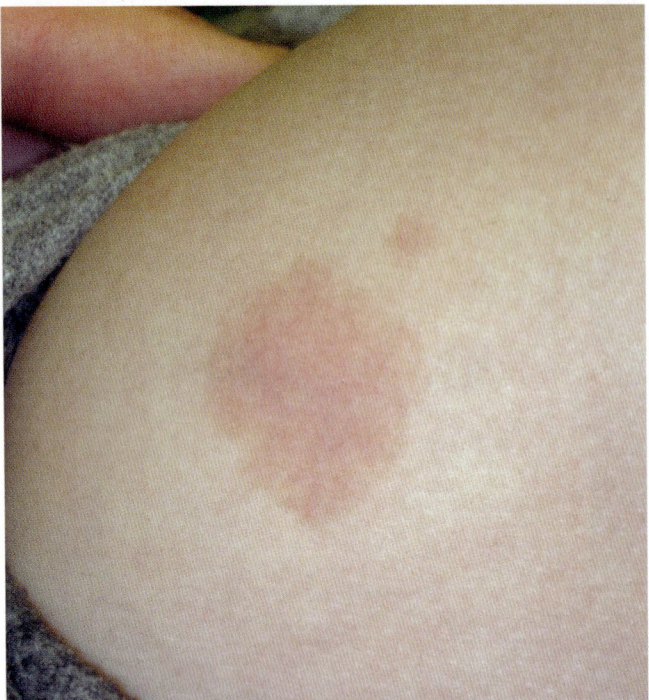

Fig. 28.15 RASA1-associated capillary malformation-arteriovenous malformation syndrome.

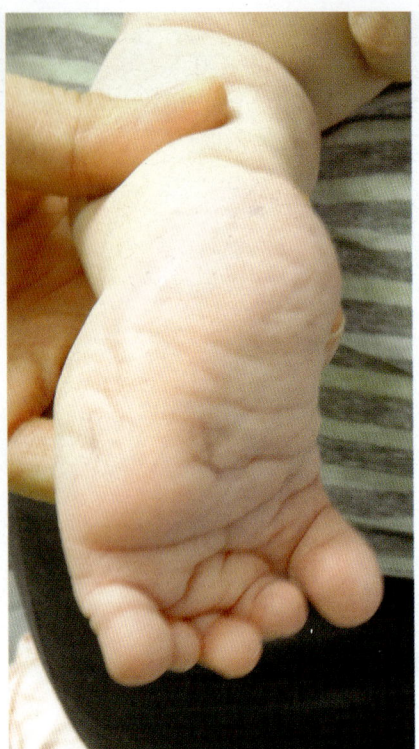

Fig. 28.16 CLOVES syndrome.

Fig. 28.17 Cavernous venous malformation.

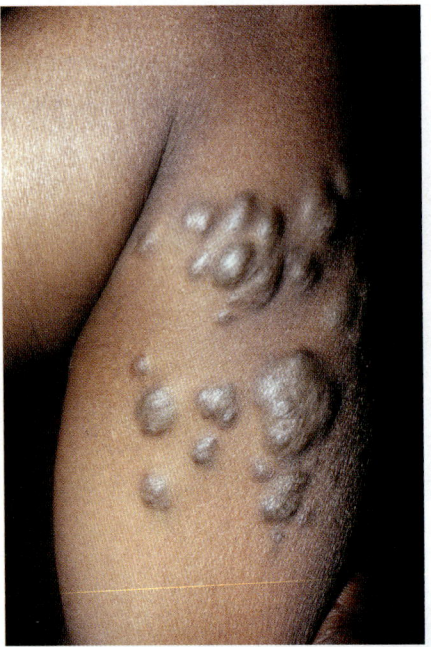

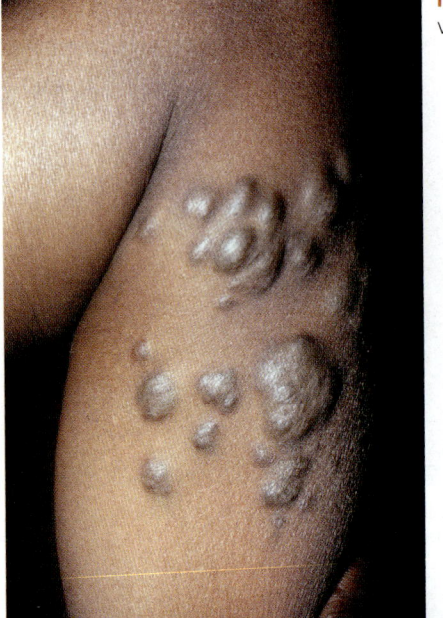

Fig. 28.18 Cavernous venous malformation.

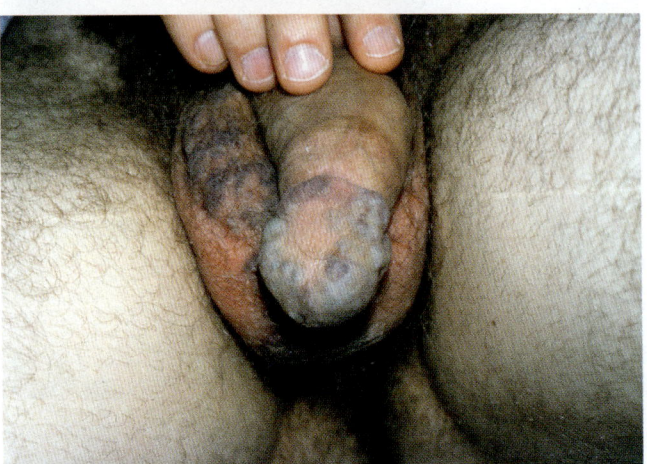

Fig. 28.19 Venous malformation.

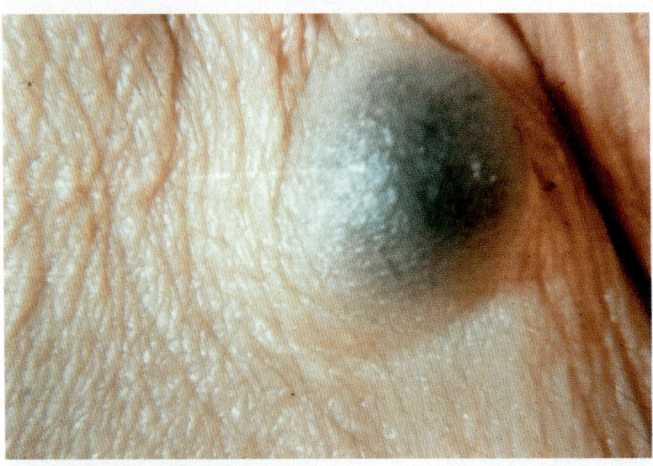

Fig. 28.20 Blue rubber bleb syndrome.

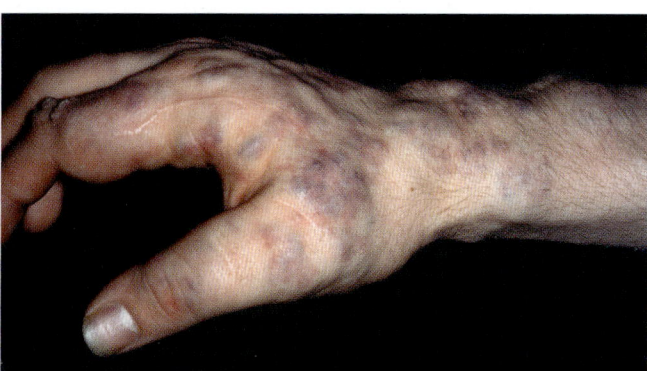

Fig. 28.21 Maffucci syndrome.

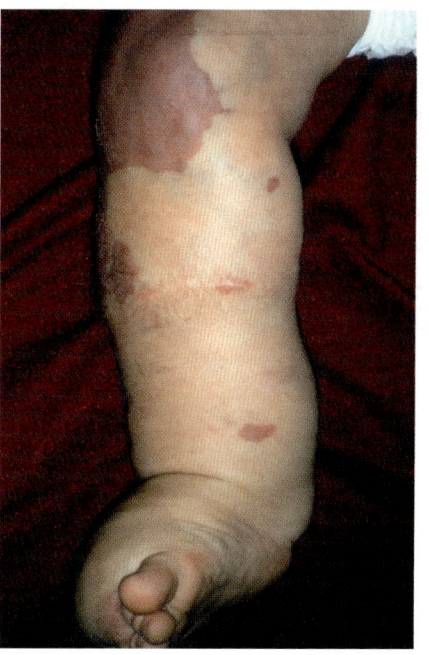

Fig. 28.22 Klippel-Trenaunay syndrome.

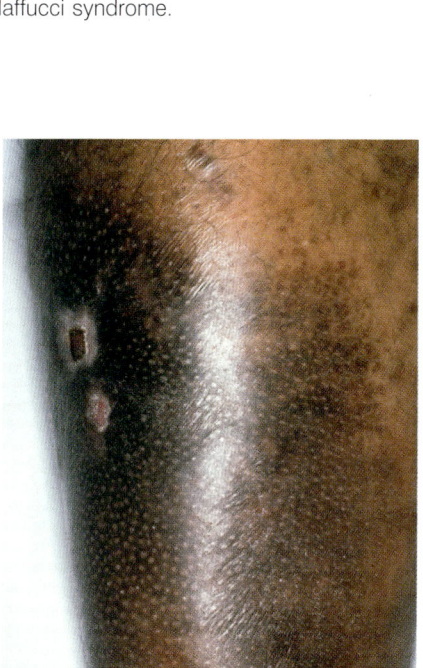

Fig. 28.23 Arteriovenous fistula.

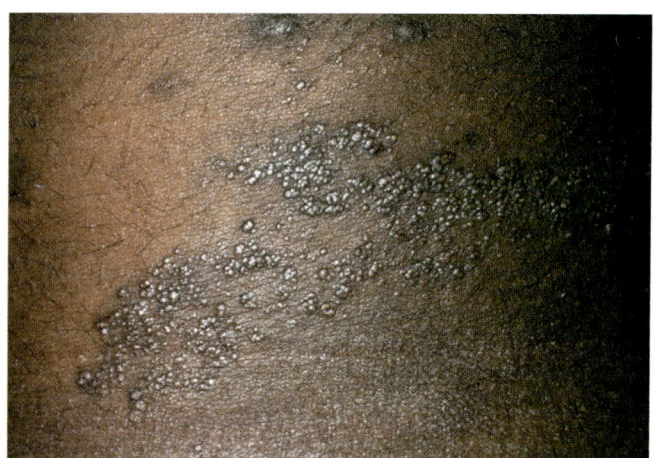

Fig. 28.24 Microcystic lymphatic malformation.

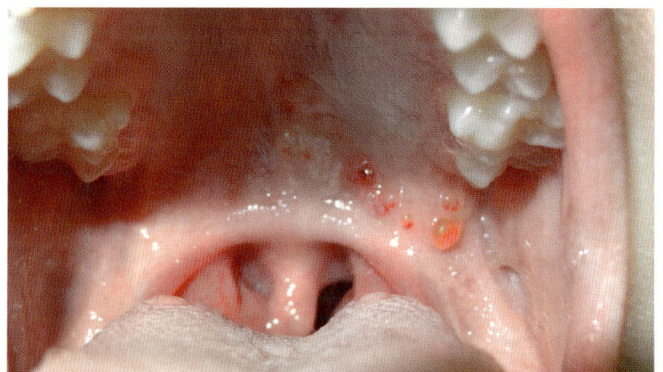

Fig. 28.25 Oral lymphatic malformation.

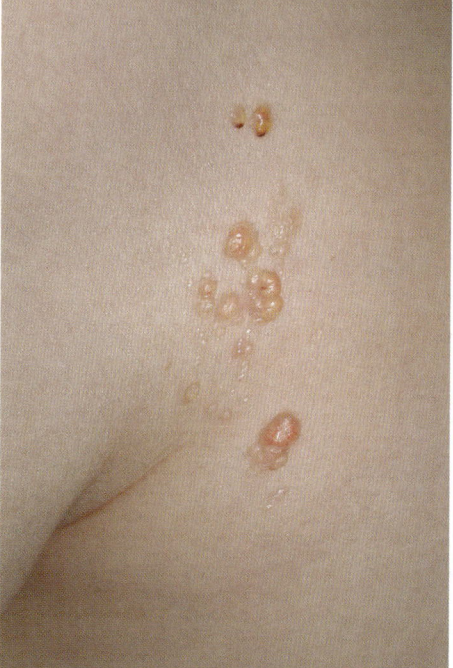

Fig. 28.26 Superficial lymphatic malformation.

Dermal and Subcutaneous Tumors

409

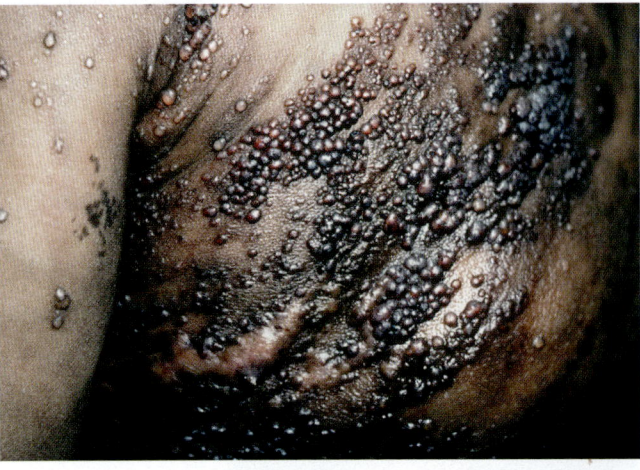

Fig. 28.27 Venolymphatic malformation. *Courtesy Ken Greer, MD.*

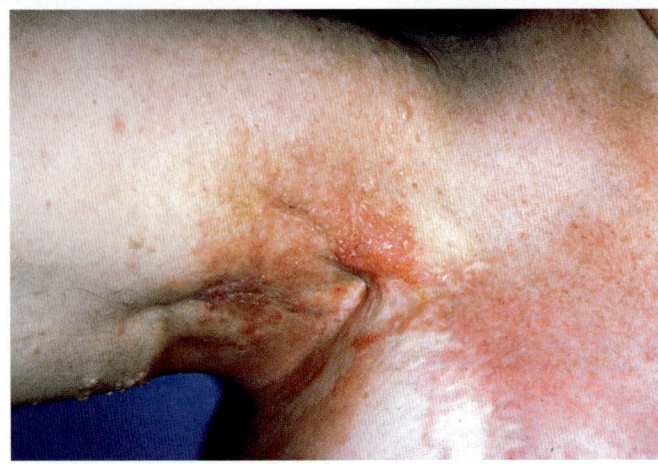

Fig. 28.28 Acquired lymphangiectasia after surgery and radiation therapy for breast cancer. Redness is irritation from chylous discharge.

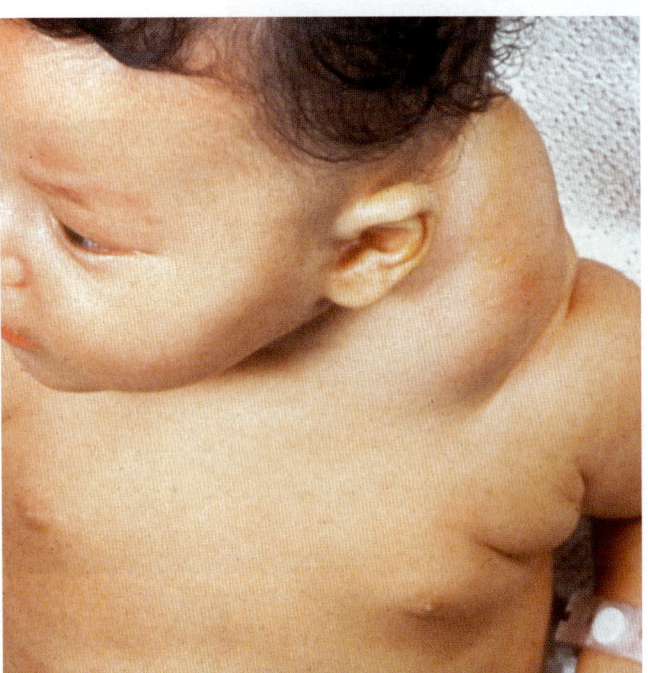

Fig. 28.29 Deep lymphatic malformation.

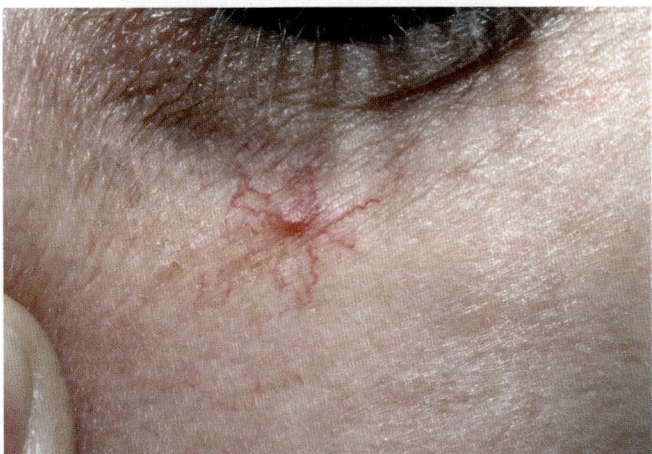

Fig. 28.30 Spider angioma. *Courtesy Steven Binnick, MD.*

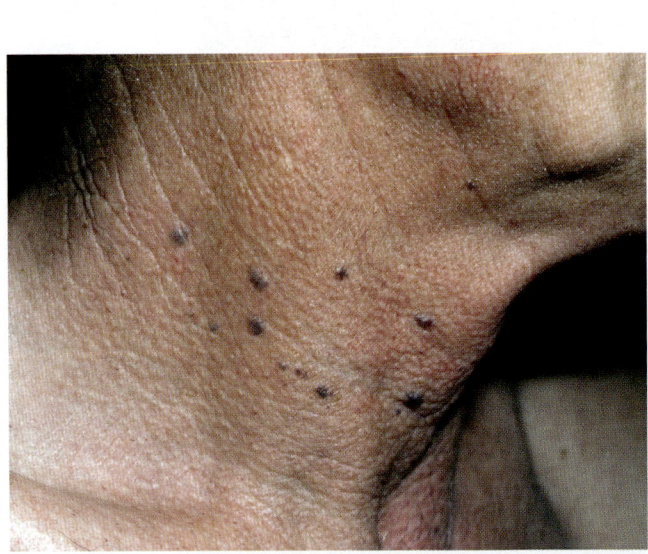

Fig. 28.31 Venous lakes. *Courtesy Ken Greer, MD.*

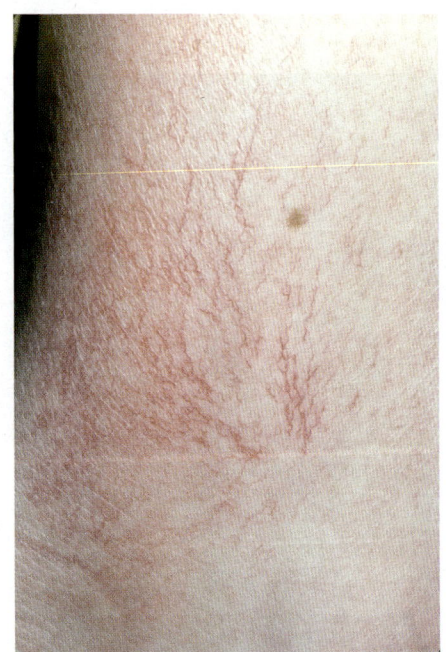

Fig. 28.32 Generalized essential telangiectasia. *Courtesy Steven Binnick, MD.*

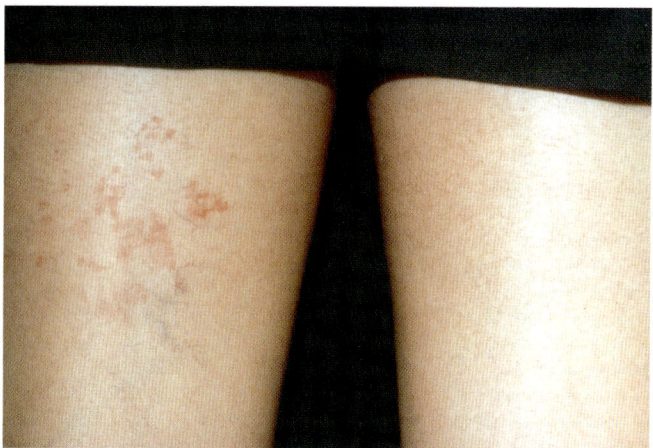

Fig. 28.33 Unilateral nevoid telangiectasia.

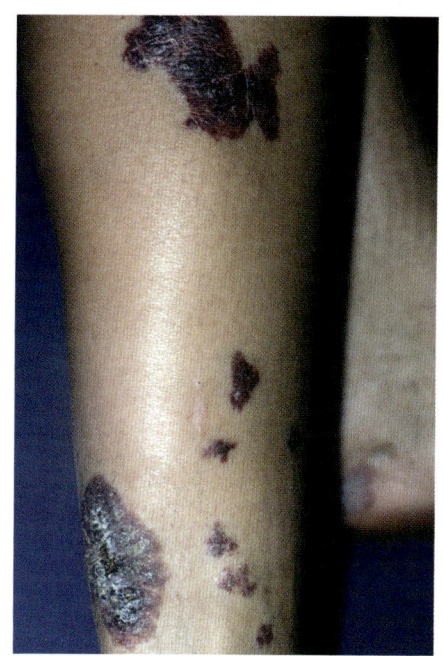

Fig. 28.34 Angiokeratoma circumscriptum. *Courtesy Steven Binnick, MD.*

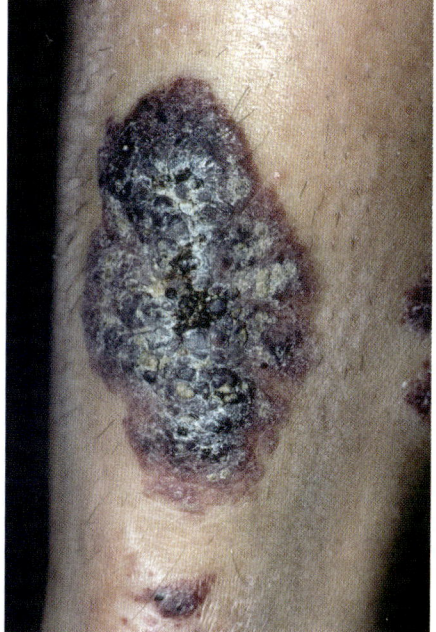

Fig. 28.35 Angiokeratoma circumscriptum. *Courtesy Steven Binnick, MD.*

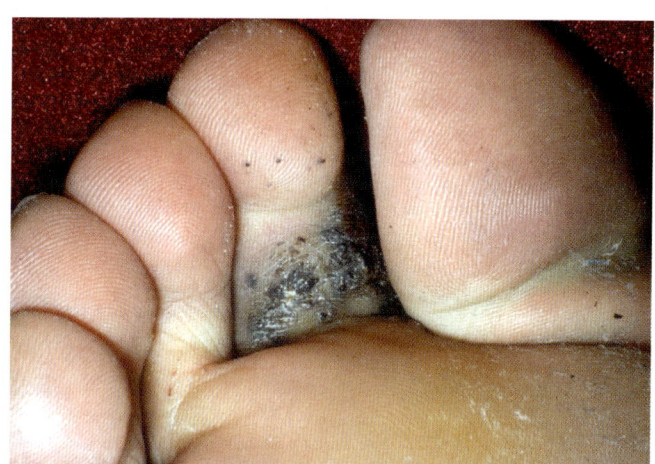

Fig. 28.36 Angiokeratoma of Mibelli.

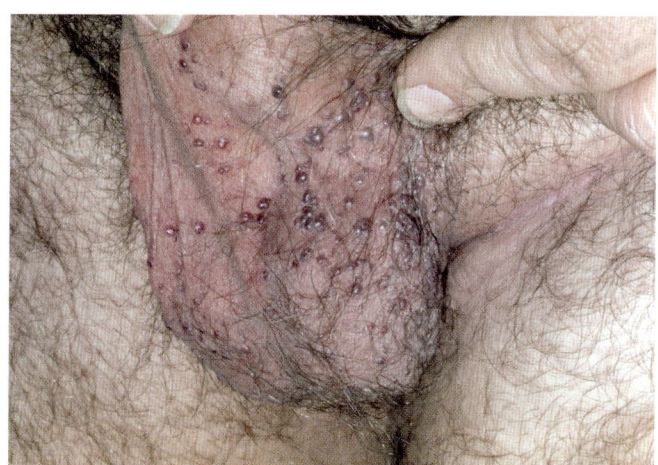

Fig. 28.37 Angiokeratoma of Fordyce.

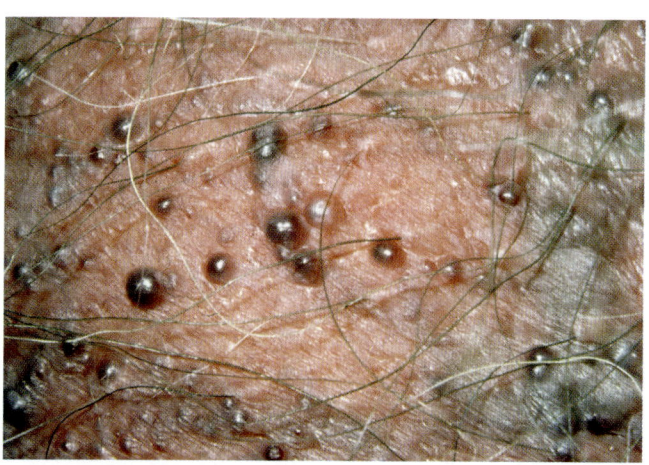

Fig. 28.38 Angiokeratoma of Fordyce.

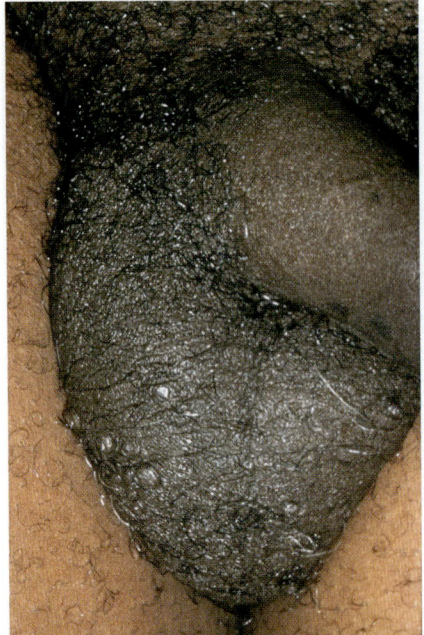

Fig. 28.39 Angiokeratoma of Fordyce.

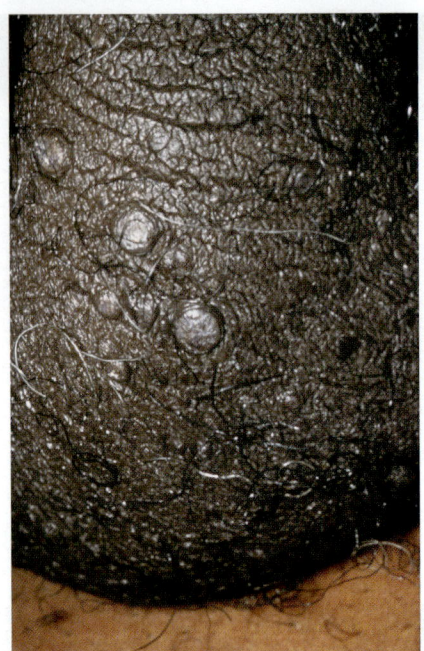

Fig. 28.40 Angiokeratoma of Fordyce.

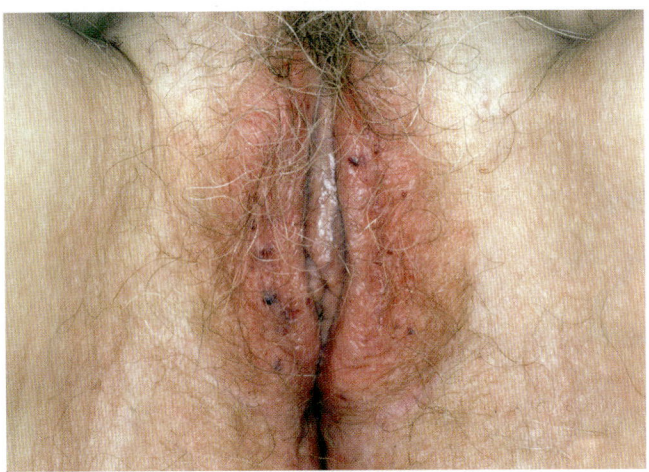

Fig. 28.41 Angiokeratoma of Fordyce.

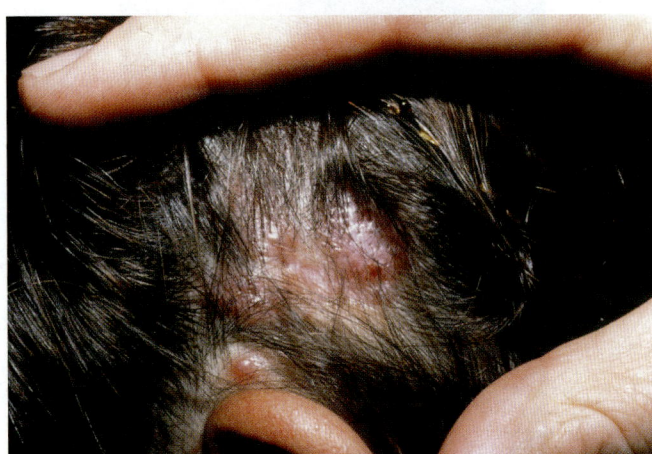

Fig. 28.42 Angiolymphoid hyperplasia with eosinophilia.

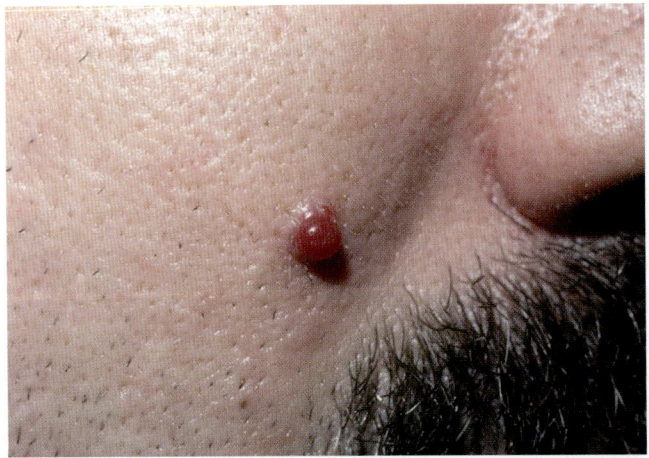

Fig. 28.43 Pyogenic granuloma. *Courtesy Steven Binnick, MD.*

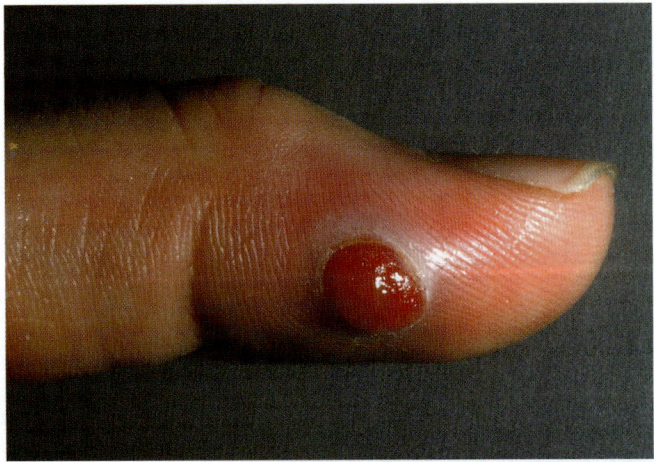

Fig. 28.44 Pyogenic granuloma. *Courtesy The University of Utah and Oregon Health Sciences University Leonard Swinyer MD image collection.*

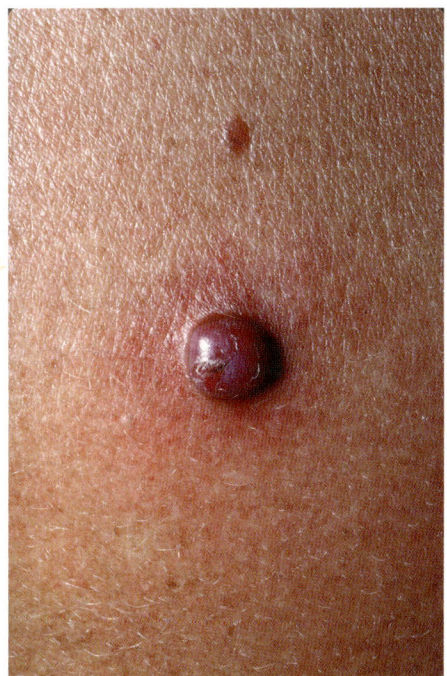

Fig. 28.45 Pyogenic granuloma. *Courtesy The University of Utah and Oregon Health Sciences University Leonard Swinyer MD image collection.*

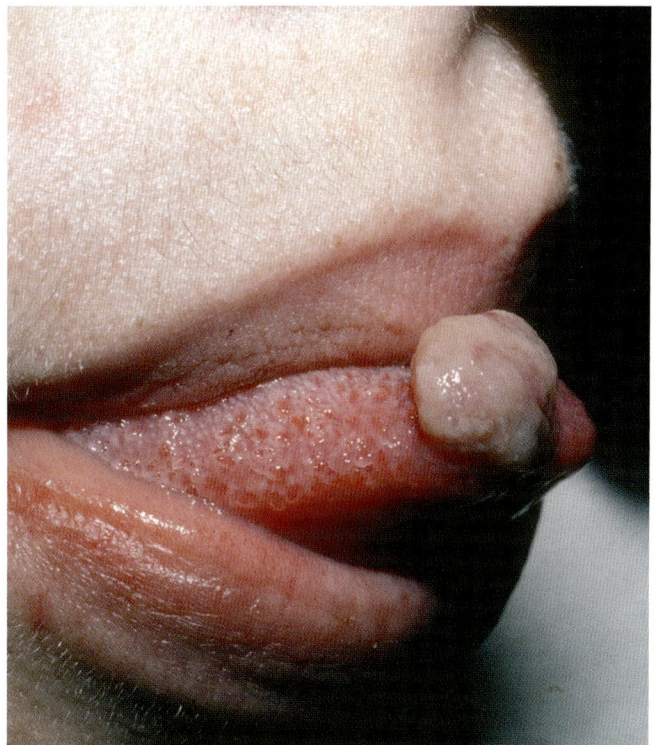

Fig. 28.46 Pyogenic granuloma. *Courtesy Steven Binnick, MD.*

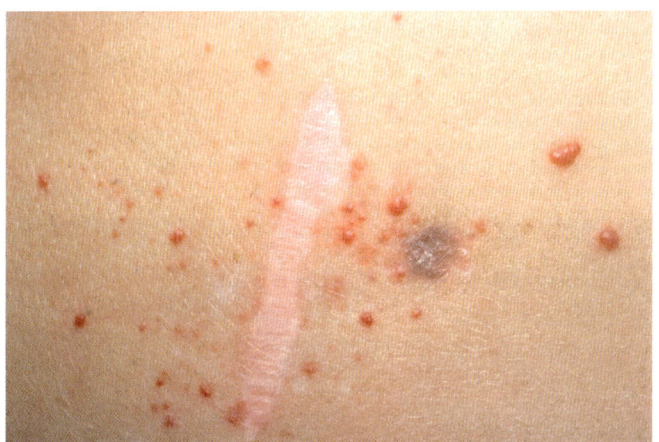

Fig. 28.47 Recurrent pyogenic granulomas with satellite lesions.

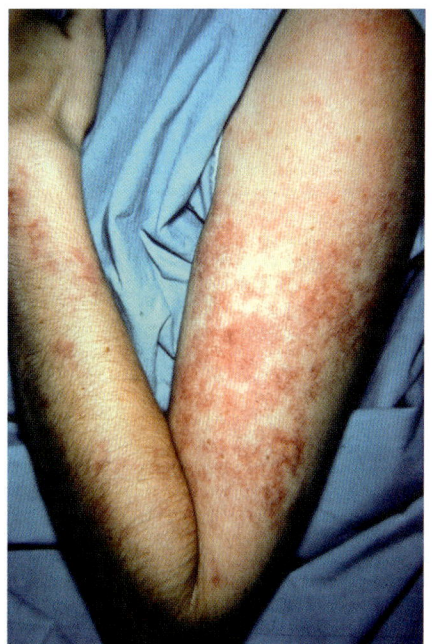

Fig. 28.48 Angioma serpiginosum.

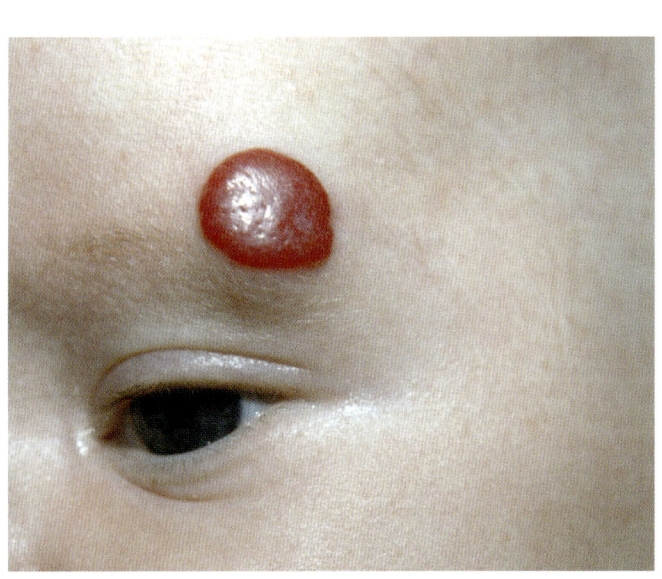

Fig. 28.49 Infantile hemangioma. *Courtesy Steven Binnick, MD.*

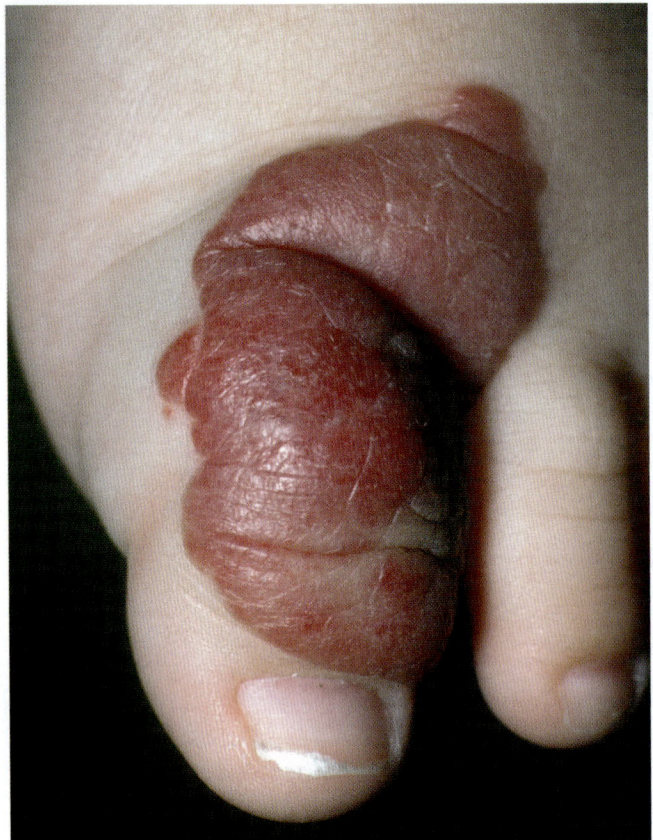

Fig. 28.50 Infantile hemangioma.

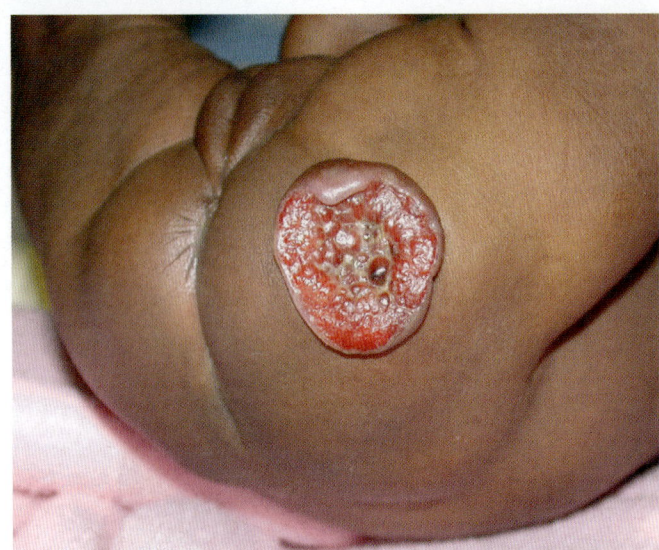

Fig. 28.51 Infantile hemangioma with ulceration.

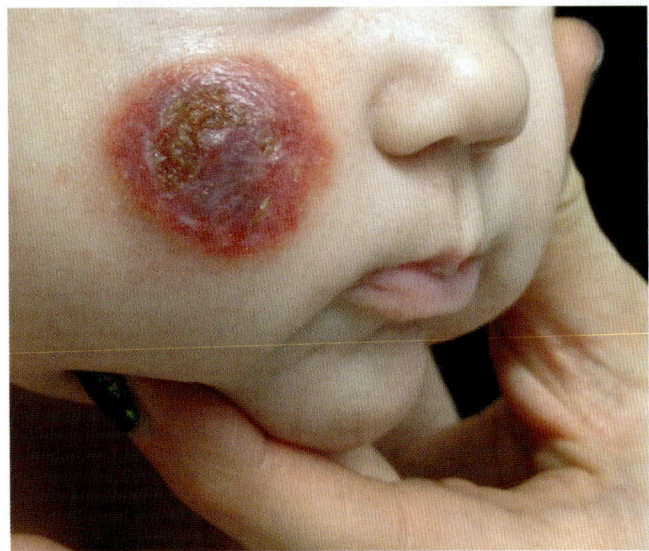

Fig. 28.52 Infantile hemangioma with ulceration.

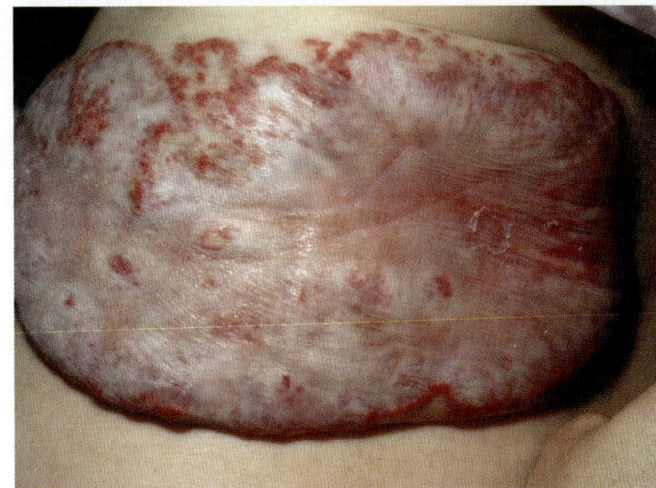

Fig. 28.53 Involuting infantile hemangioma.

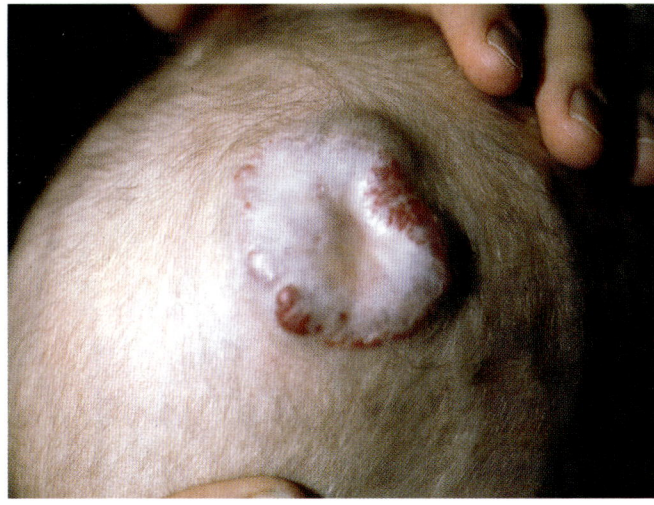

Fig. 28.54 Involuting infantile hemangioma.

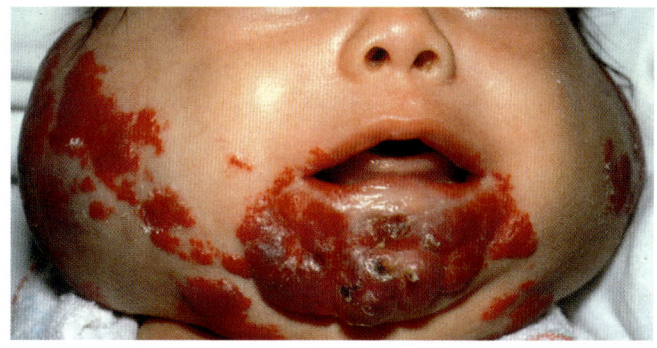

Fig. 28.55 PHACE syndrome.

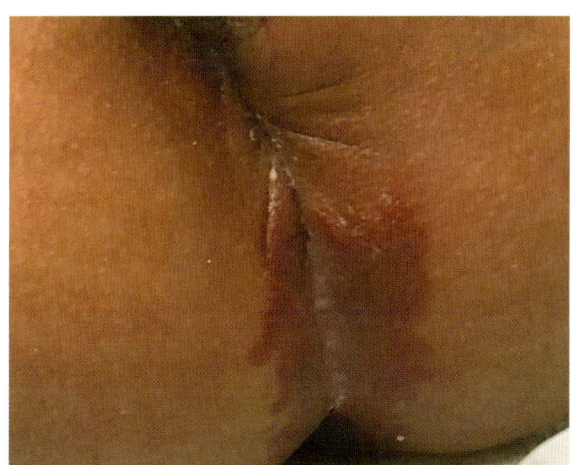

Fig. 28.56 Linear perianal hemangioma associated with LUMBAR syndrome.

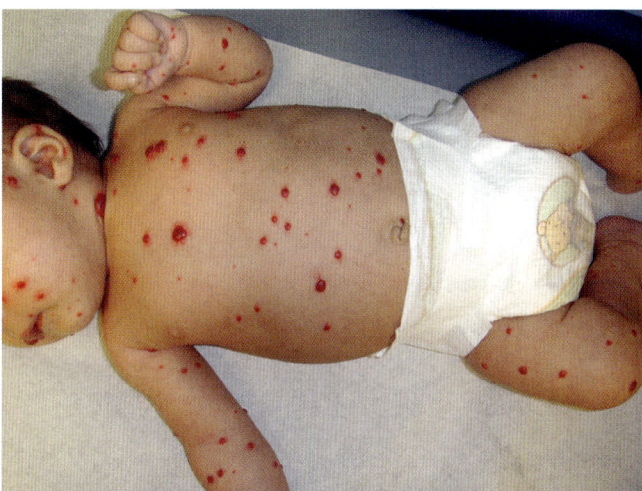

Fig. 28.57 Diffuse neonatal hemangiomatosis.

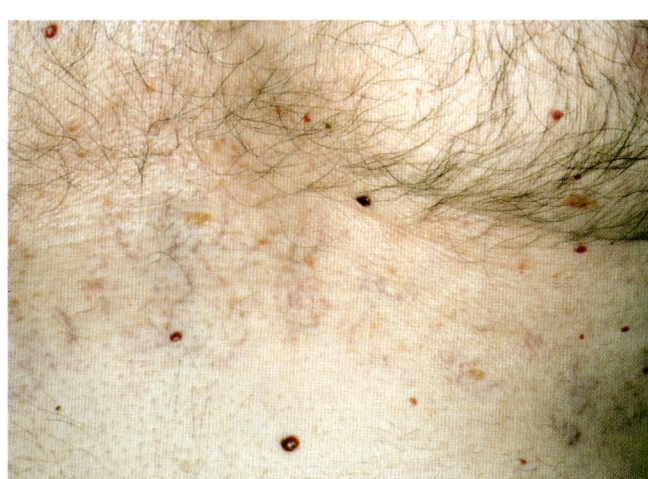

Fig. 28.58 Cherry angiomas and costal fringe telangiectases.

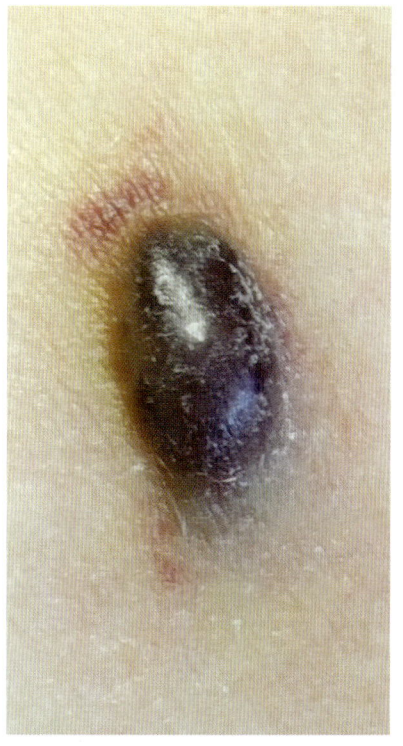

Fig. 28.59 Targetoid hemosiderotic hemangioma. *Courtesy Dr. Rui Carlos Taveres Bello.*

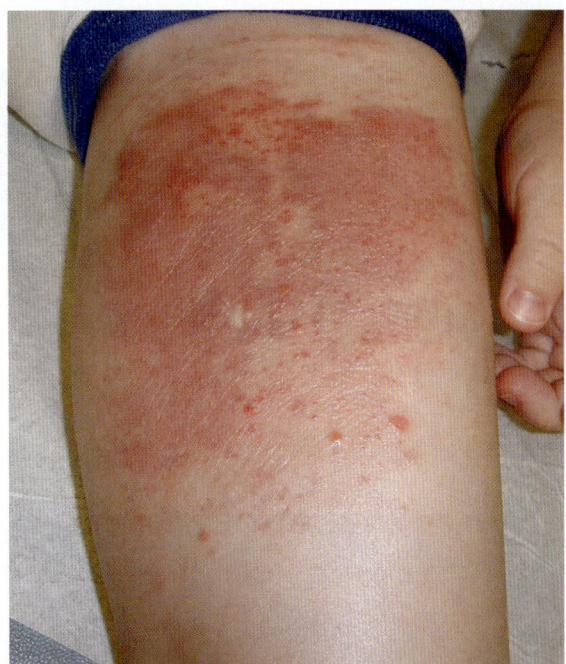

Fig. 28.60 Tufted angioma.

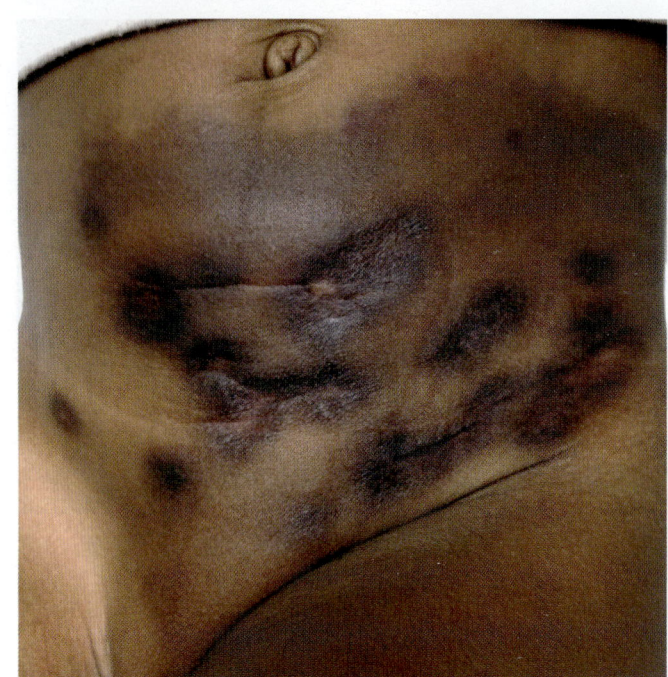

Fig. 28.61 Kaposiform hemangioendothelioma.

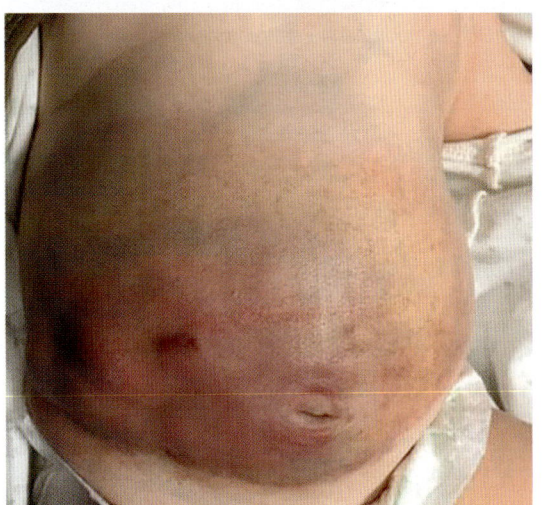

Fig. 28.62 Kasabach-Merritt syndrome.

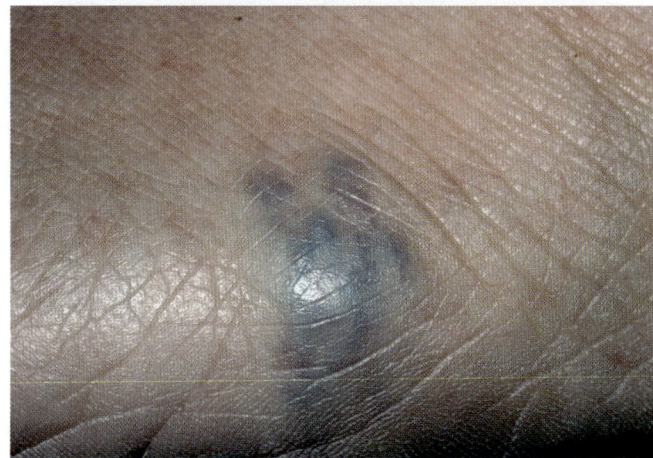

Fig. 28.63 Glomangioma.

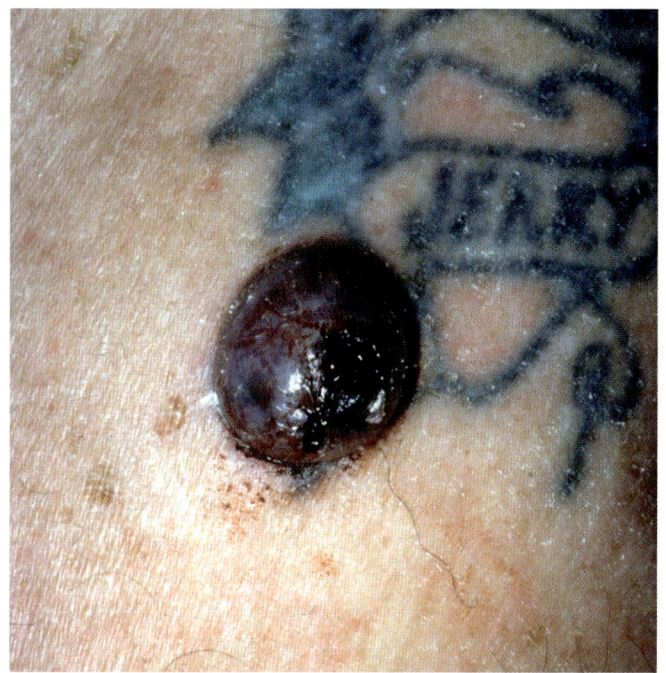

Fig. 28.64 Glomangioma.

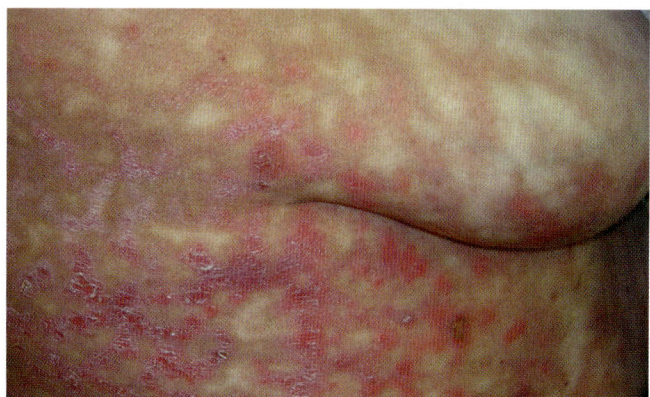

Fig. 28.65 Diffuse dermal angiomatosis.

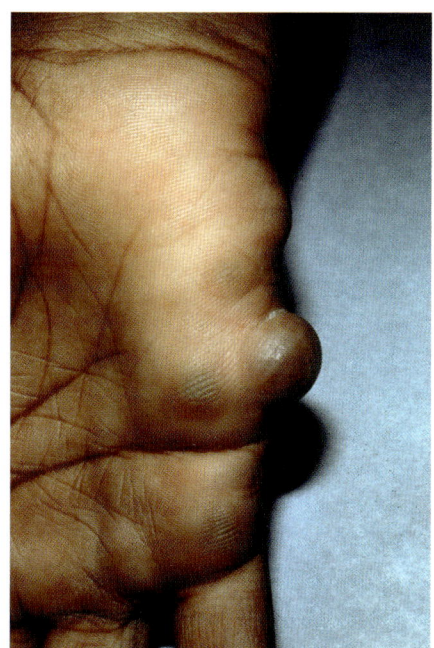

Fig. 28.66 Spindle cell hemangioma.

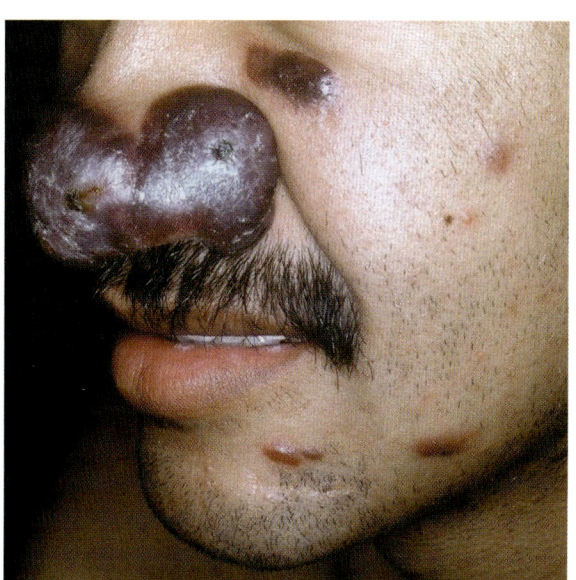

Fig. 28.67 Kaposi sarcoma in an HIV-infected patient.

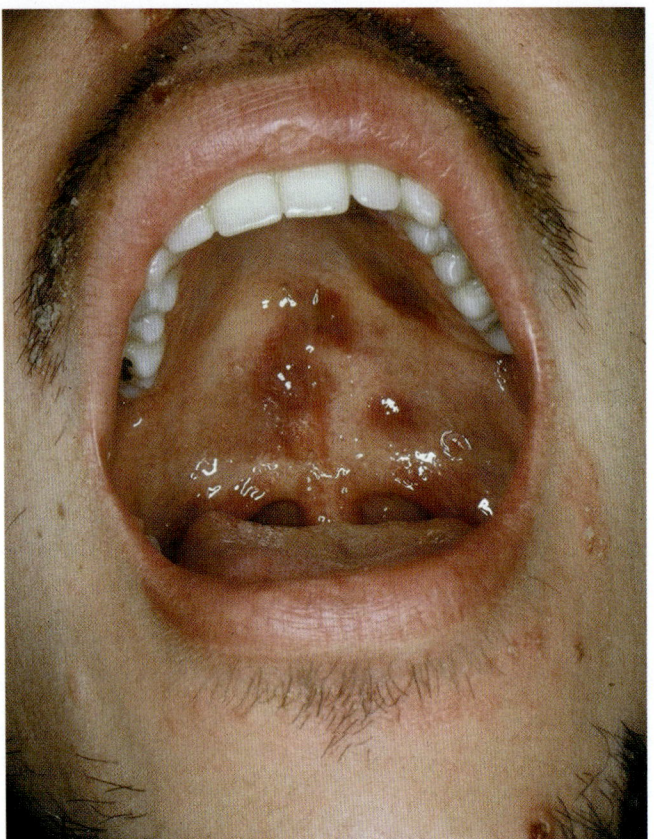

Fig. 28.68 Kaposi sarcoma in an HIV-infected patient; the palate is commonly involved.

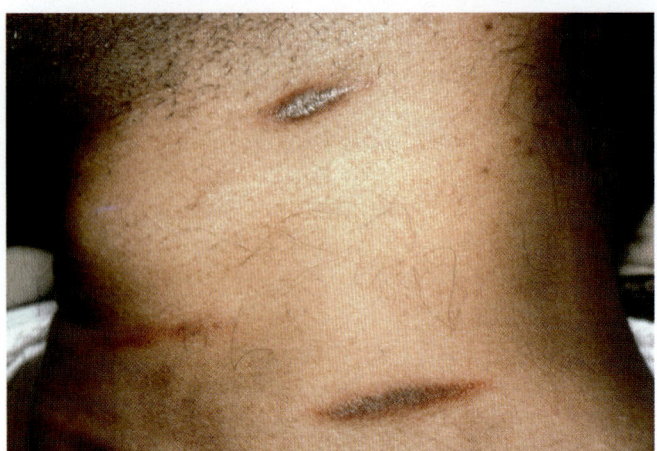

Fig. 28.69 Kaposi sarcoma in an HIV-infected patient; the linear elongated lesions along skin lines are characteristic.

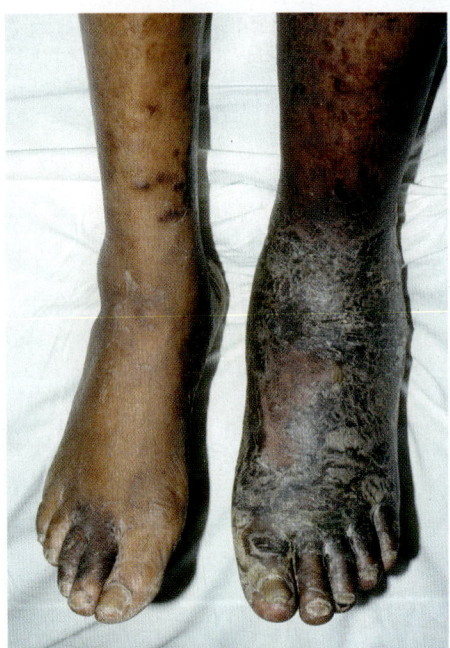

Fig. 28.70 Kaposi sarcoma in an HIV-infected patient. *Courtesy Steven Binnick, MD.*

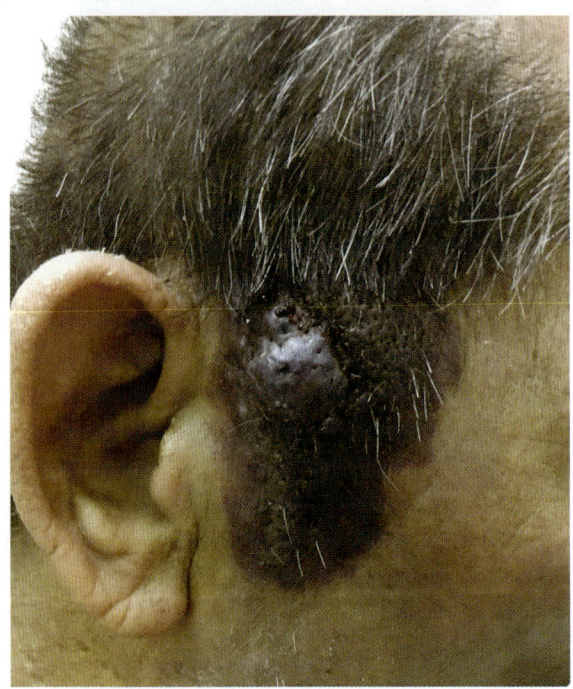

Fig. 28.71 Angiosarcoma. *Courtesy Dr. Yi-Shuan Sheen.*

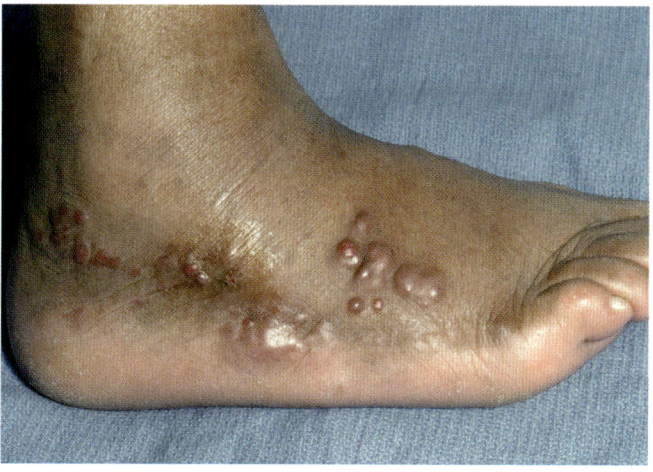

Fig. 28.72 Angiosarcoma.

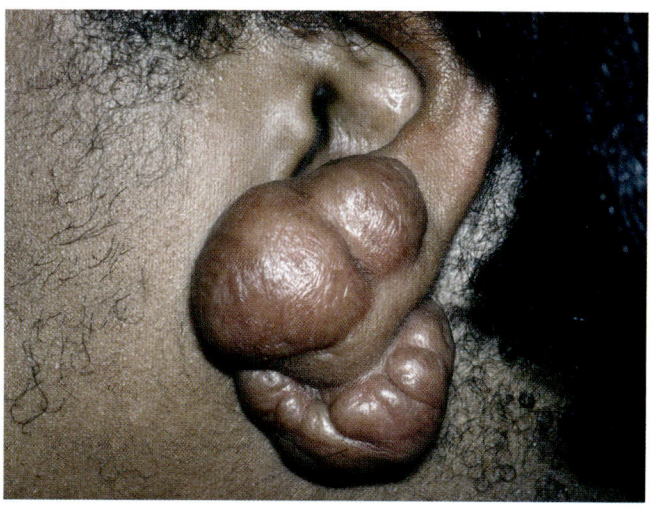

Fig. 28.73 Keloid. *Courtesy Steven Binnick, MD.*

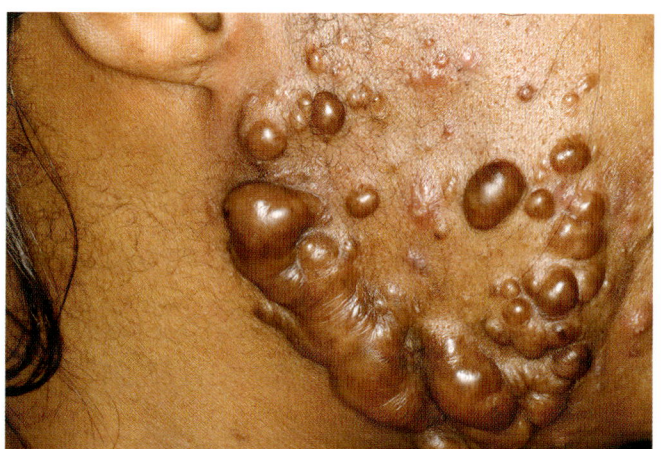

Fig. 28.74 Keloids.

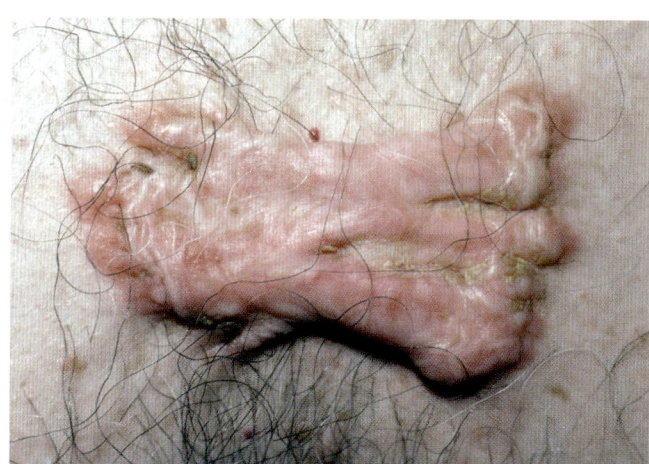

Fig. 28.75 Keloid. *Courtesy Steven Binnick, MD.*

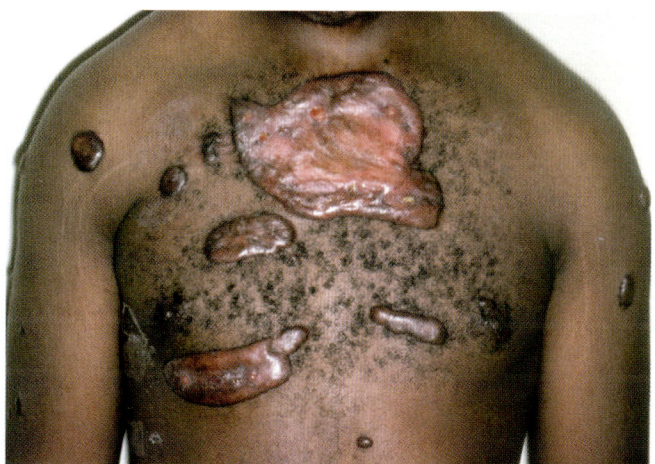

Fig. 28.76 Ulcerated keloids.

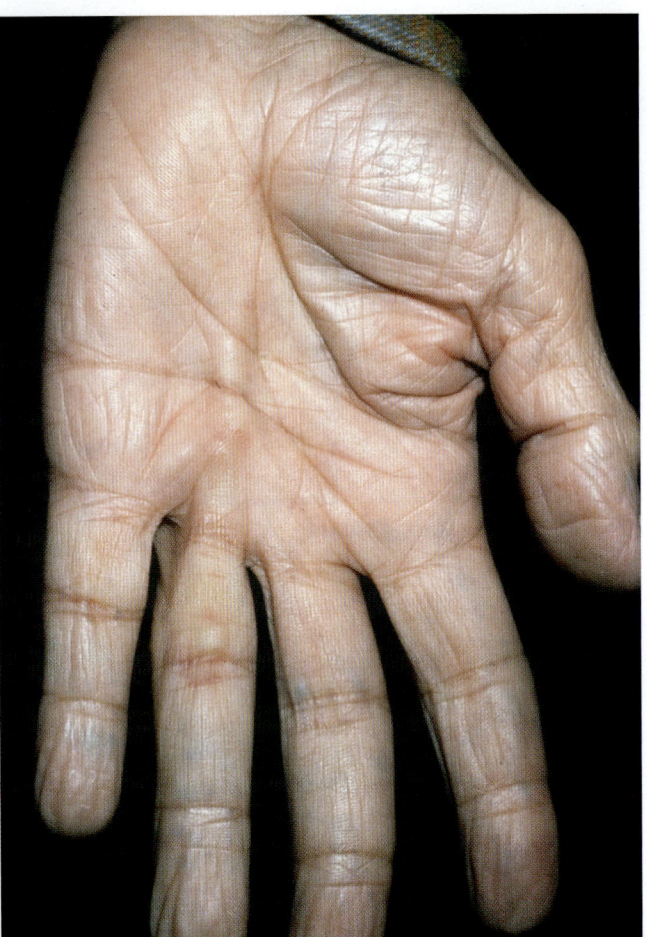

Fig. 28.77 Dupuytren contracture.

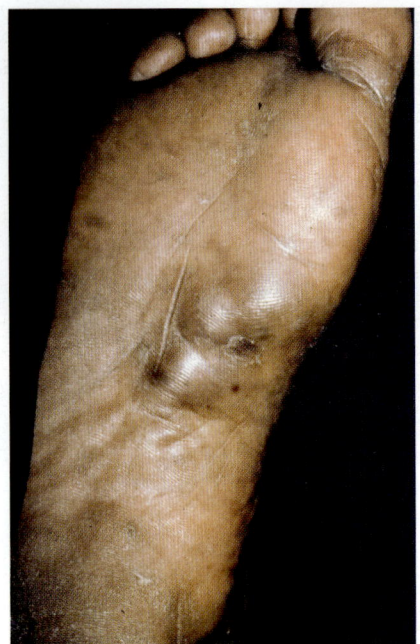

Fig. 28.78 Plantar fibromatosis.

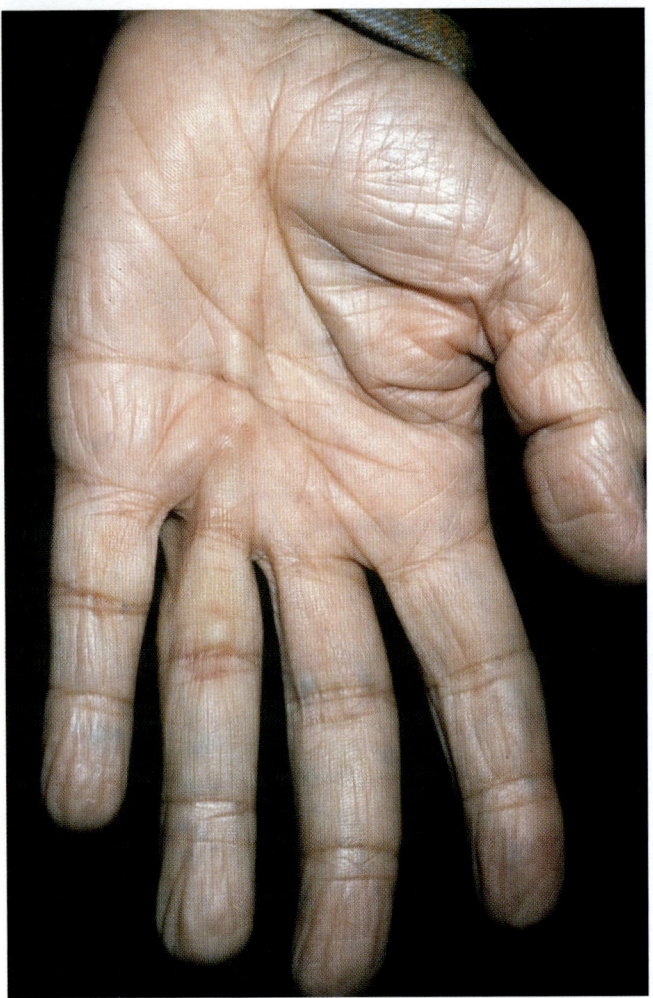

Fig. 28.79 Knuckle pads. *Courtesy Curt Samlaska, MD.*

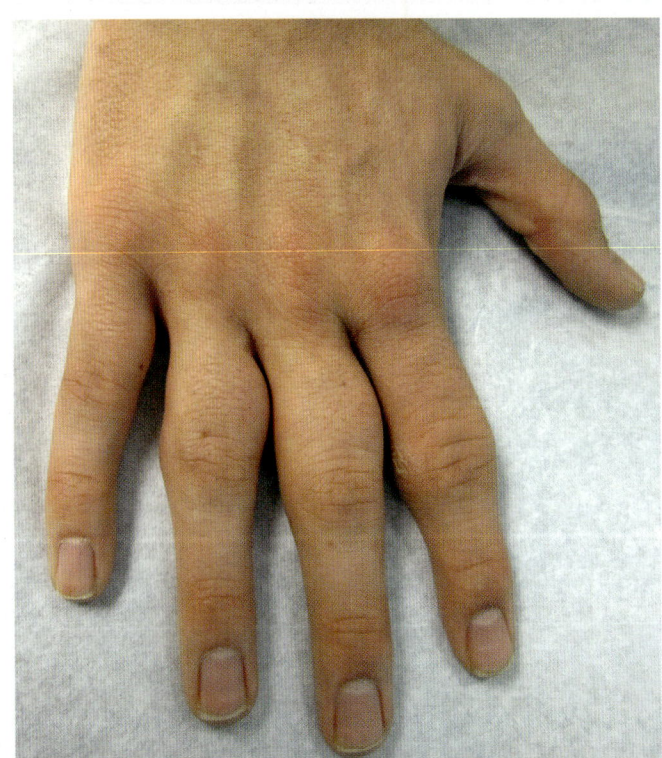

Fig. 28.80 Pachydermodactyly.

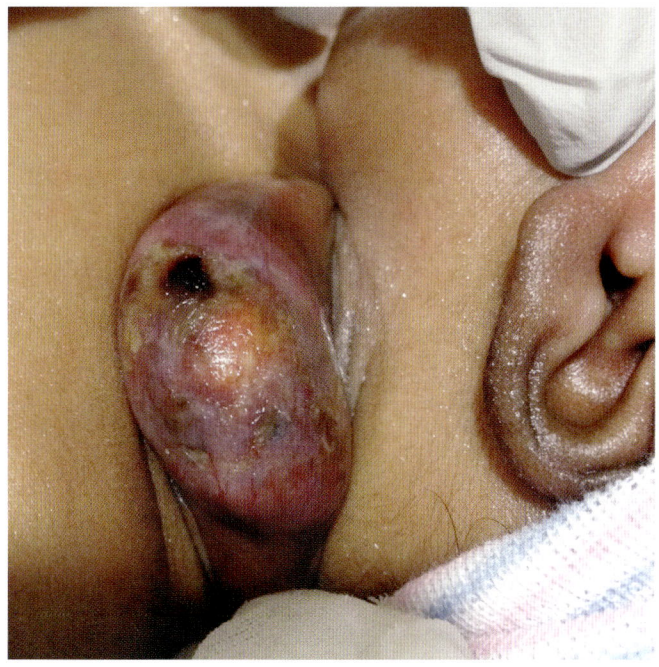

Fig. 28.81 Solitary congenital myofibroma.

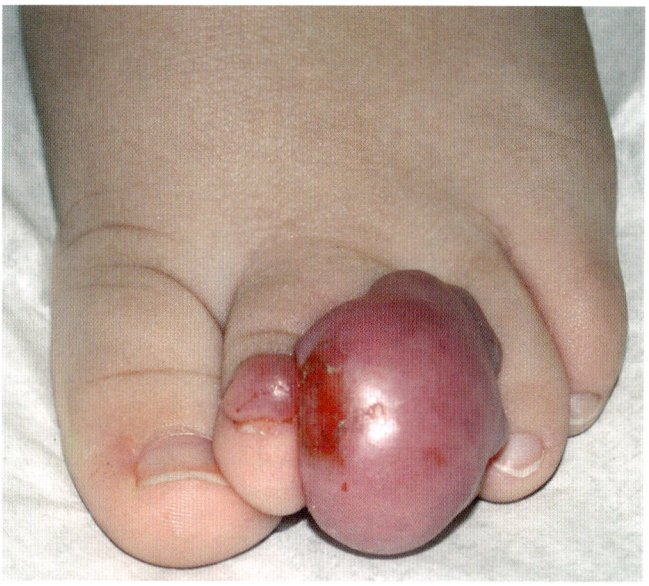

Fig. 28.82 Infantile digital fibromas.

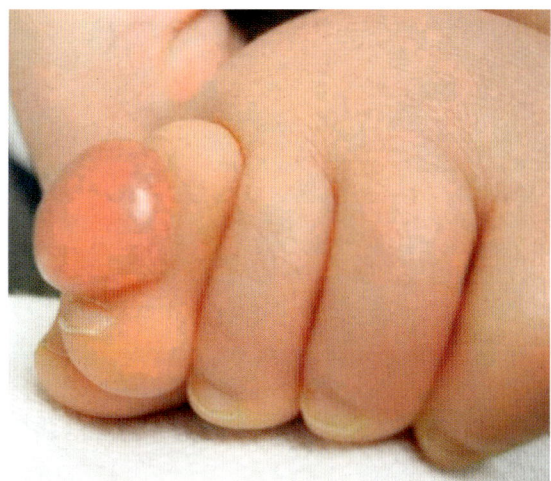

Fig. 28.83 Infantile digital fibromas. *Courtesy Sheilagh Maguiness, MD.*

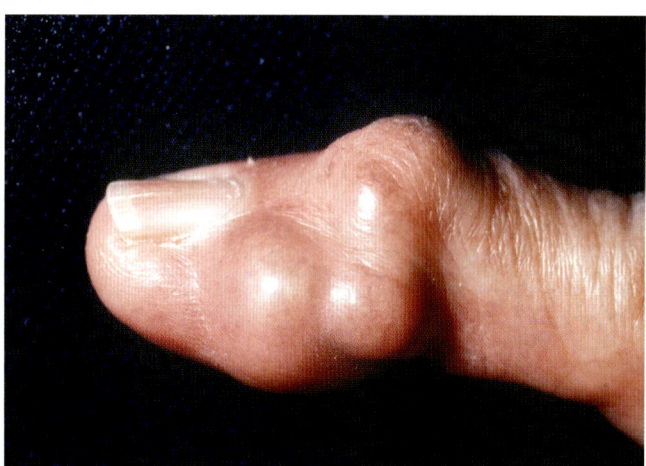

Fig. 28.84 Giant cell tumor of the tendon sheath.

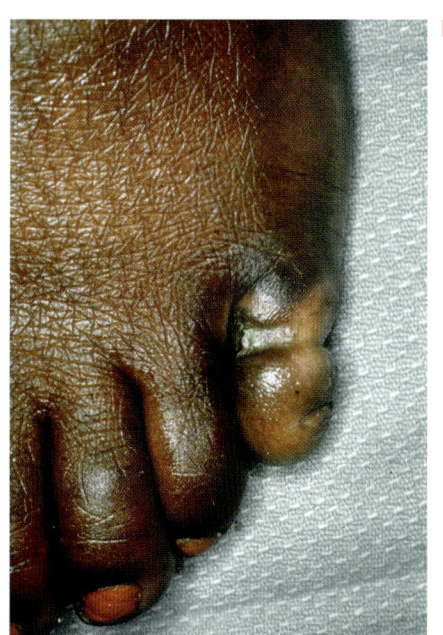

Fig. 28.85 Ainhum.

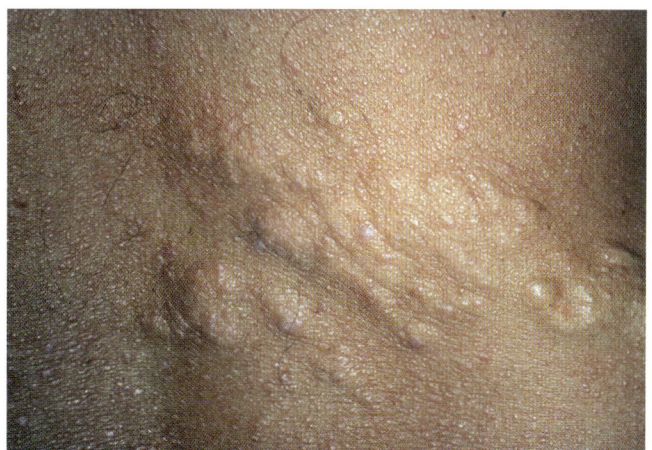

Fig. 28.86 Connective tissue nevus.

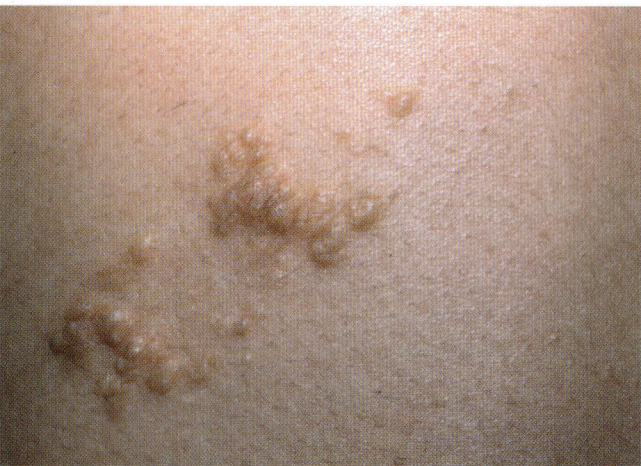

Fig. 28.87 Connective tissue nevus.

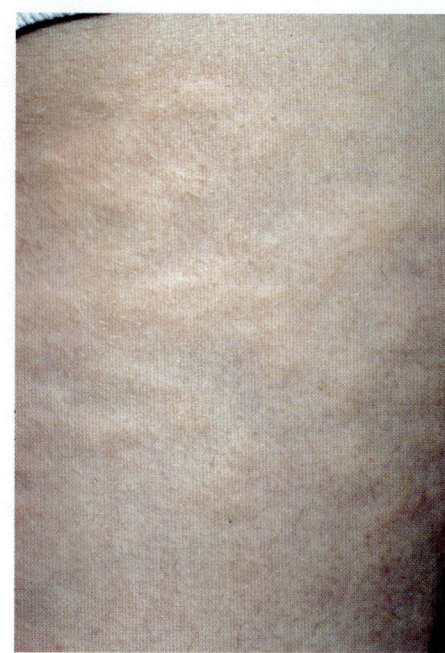

Fig. 28.88 Buschke-Ollendorff syndrome.

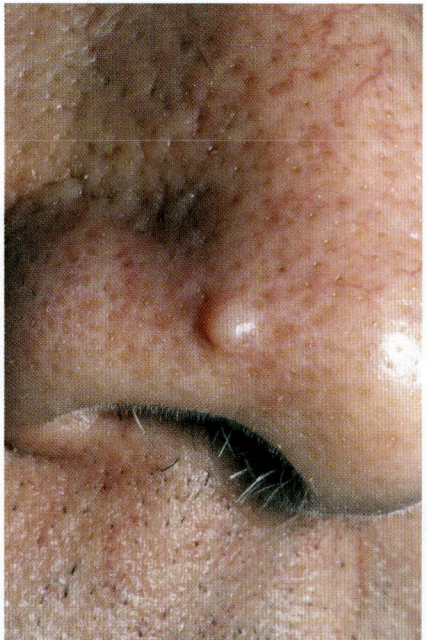

Fig. 28.89 Fibrous papule of the nose. *Courtesy Curt Samlaska, MD.*

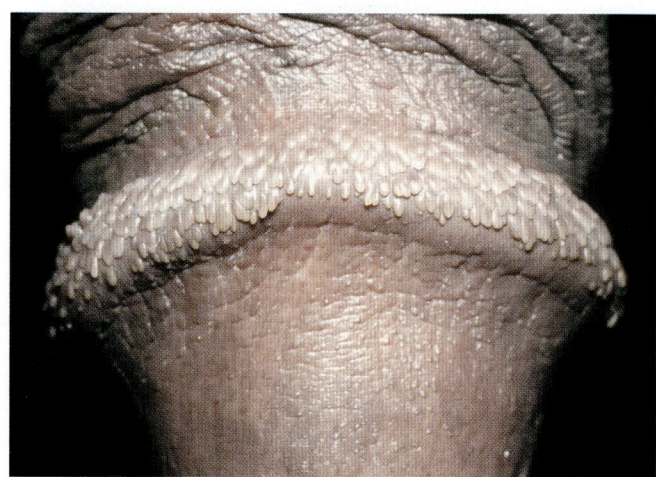

Fig. 28.90 Pearly penile papules.

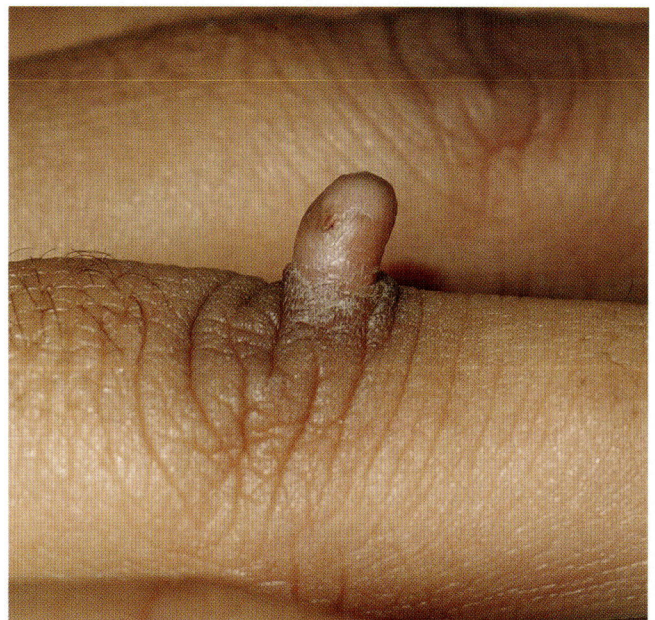

Fig. 28.91 Acquired digital fibrokeratoma. *Courtesy Debabrata Bandyopadhyay.*

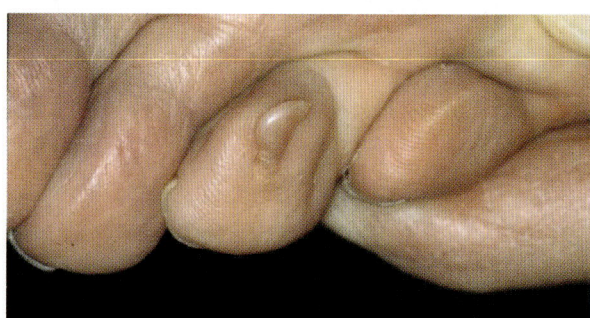

Fig. 28.92 Acquired digital fibrokeratoma.

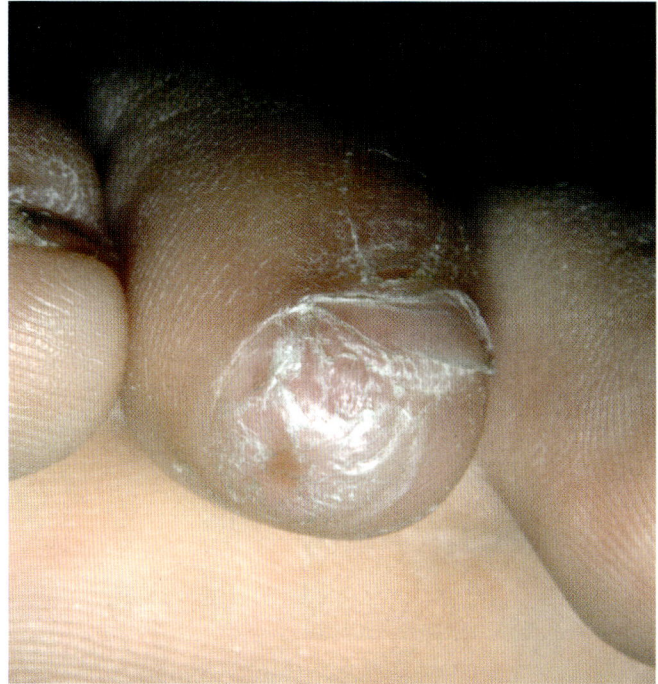

Fig. 28.93 Subungual exostosis. *Courtesy Curt Samlaska, MD.*

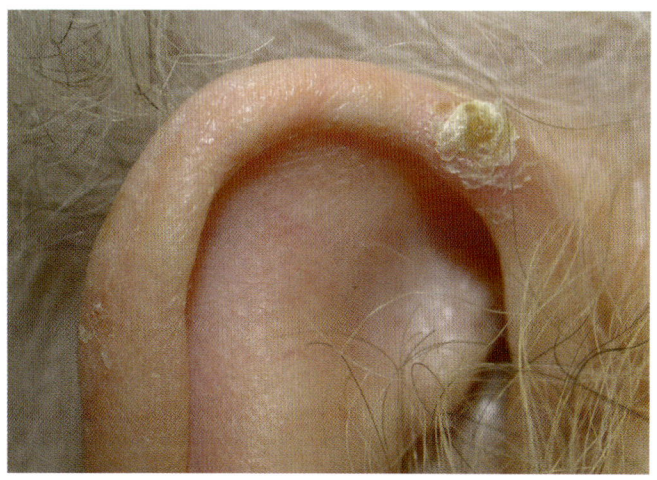

Fig. 28.94 Chondrodermatitis nodularis chronica helices.

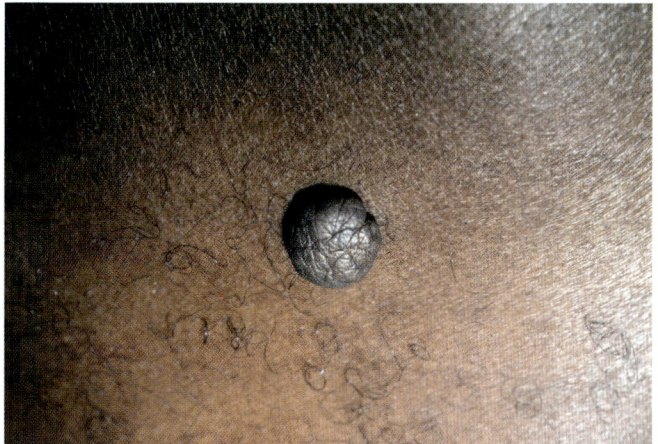

Fig. 28.95 Skin tag. *Courtesy Steven Binnick, MD.*

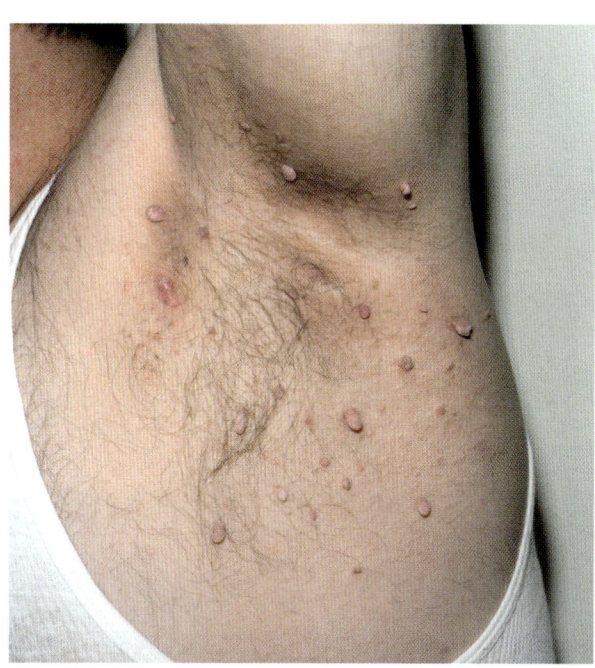

Fig. 28.96 Skin tags. *Courtesy Steven Binnick, MD.*

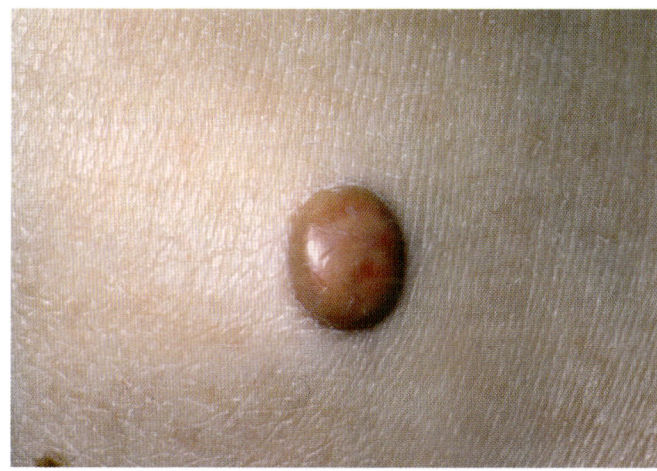

Fig. 28.97 Dermatofibroma. *Courtesy Steven Binnick, MD.*

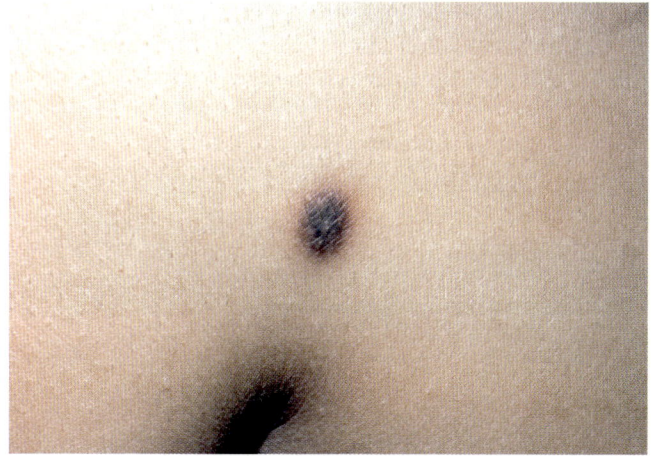

Fig. 28.98 Dermatofibroma. *Courtesy Steven Binnick, MD.*

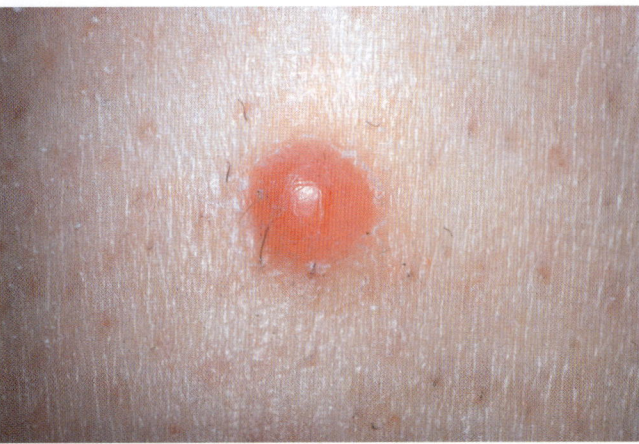

Fig. 28.99 Dermatofibroma.

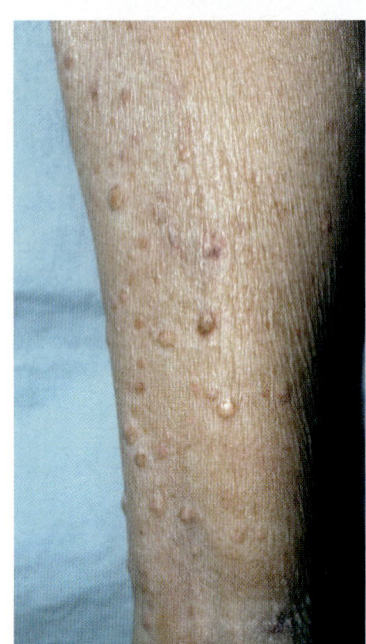

Fig. 28.100 Multiple dermatofibromas. *Courtesy Ken Greer, MD.*

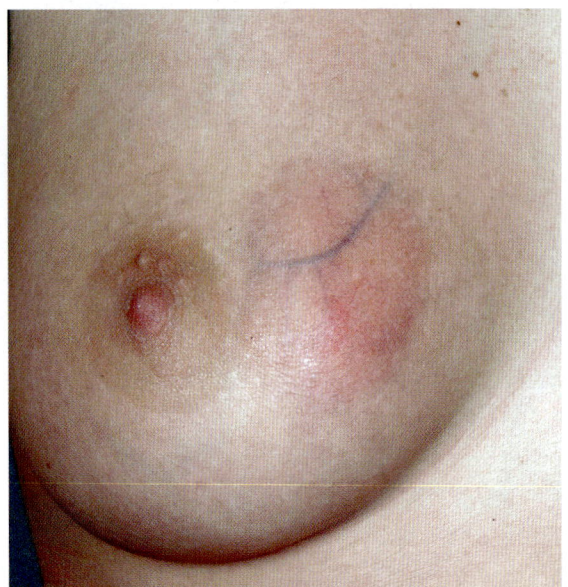

Fig. 28.101 Dermal dendrocyte hamartoma.

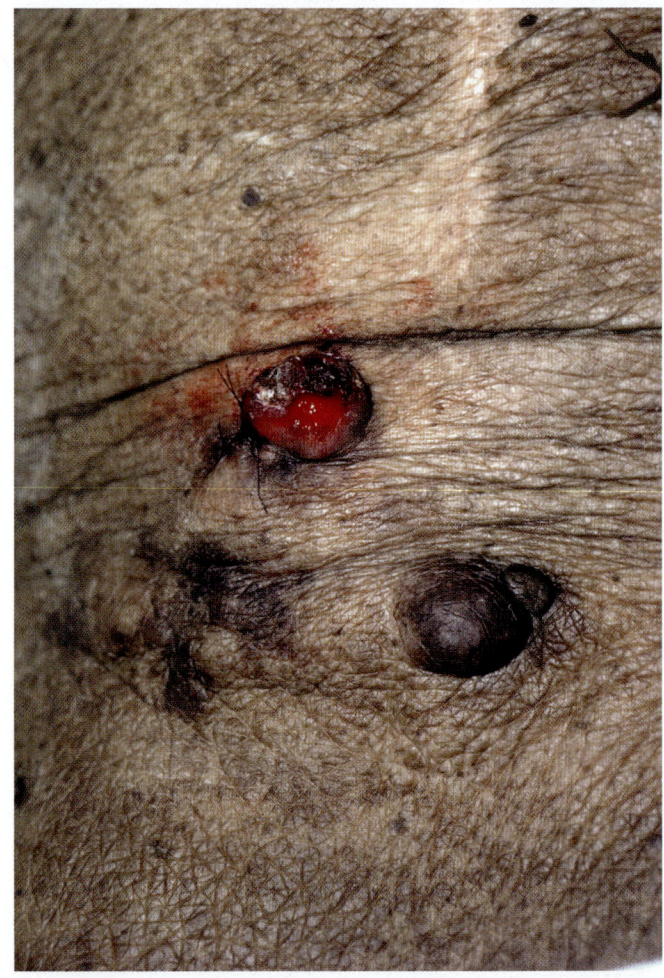

Fig. 28.102 Dermatofibroma sarcoma protuberans. *Courtesy Ken Greer, MD.*

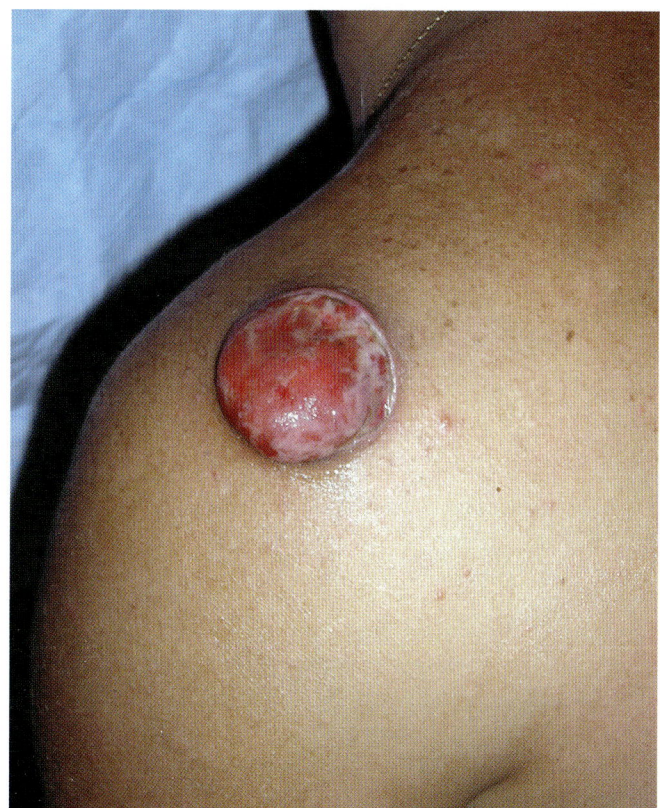

Fig. 28.103 Dermatofibroma sarcoma protuberans. *Courtesy Chris Miller, MD.*

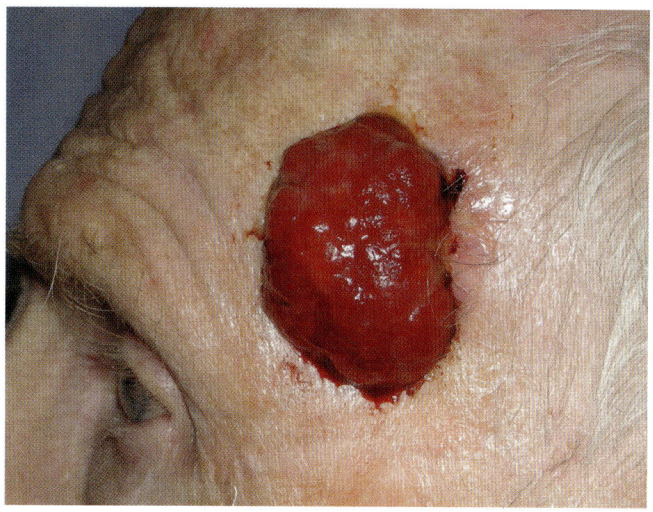

Fig. 28.104 Atypical fibroxanthoma. *Courtesy Chris Miller, MD.*

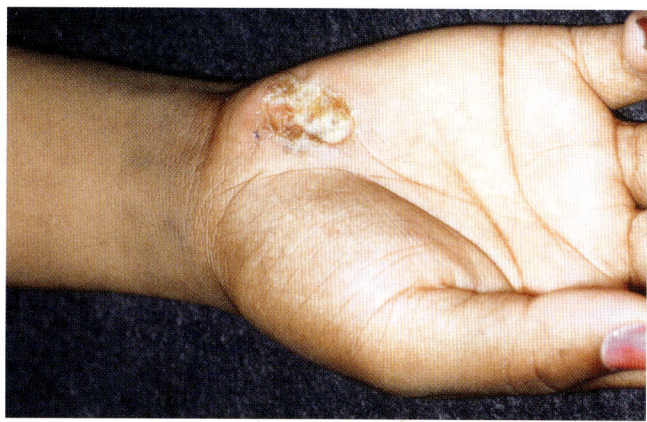

Fig. 28.106 Epithelioid sarcoma.

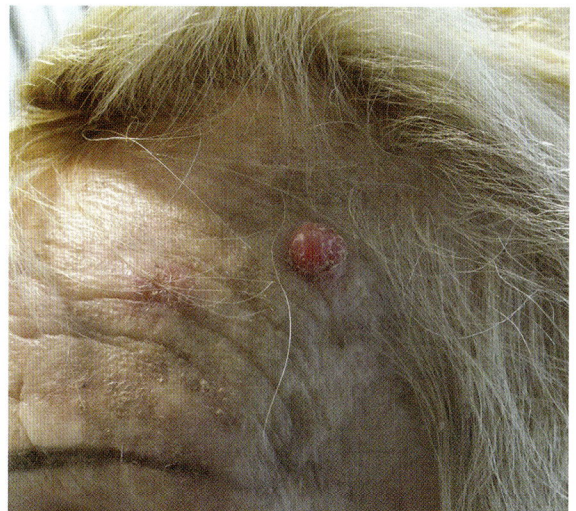

Fig. 28.105 Atypical fibroxanthoma. *Courtesy Dr. Rui Carlos Taveres Bello.*

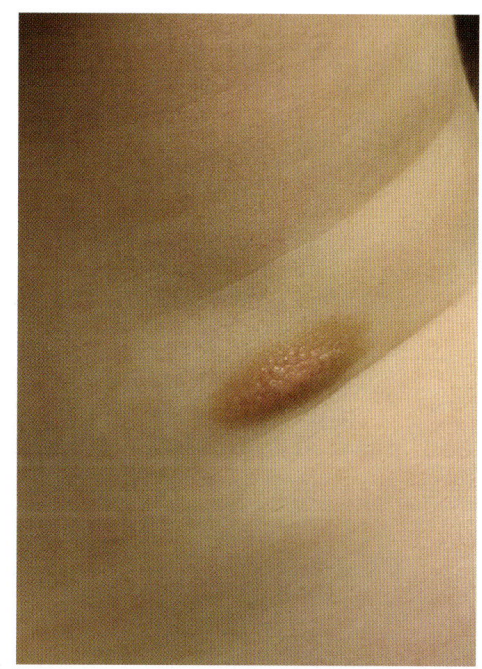

Fig. 28.107 Solitary mastocytoma.

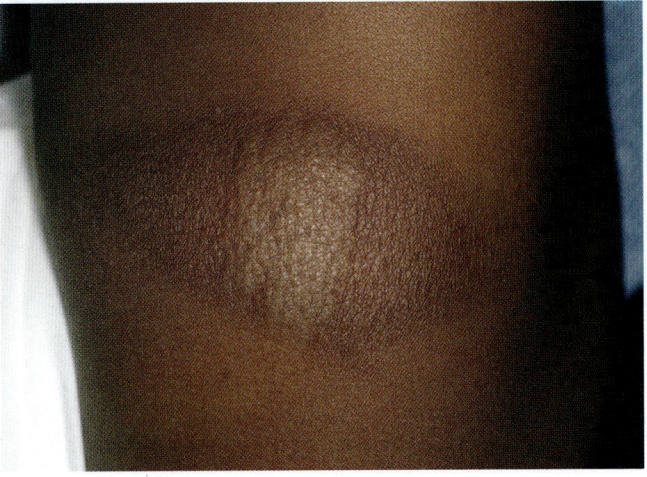

Fig. 28.108 Darier sign in mastocytoma. *Courtesy Steven Binnick, MD.*

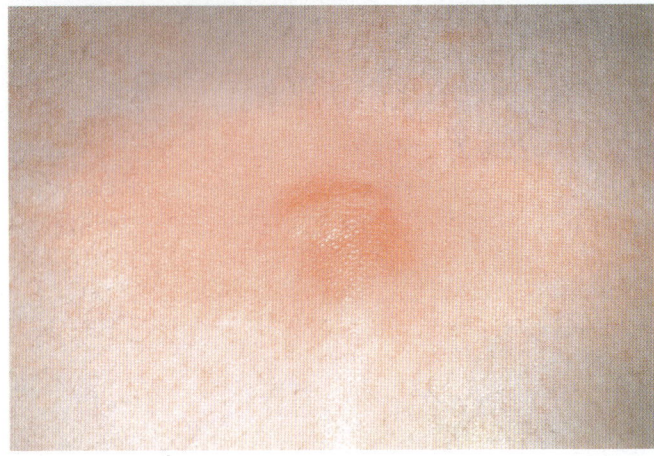

Fig. 28.109 Darier sign in mastocytoma. *Courtesy Steven Binnick, MD.*

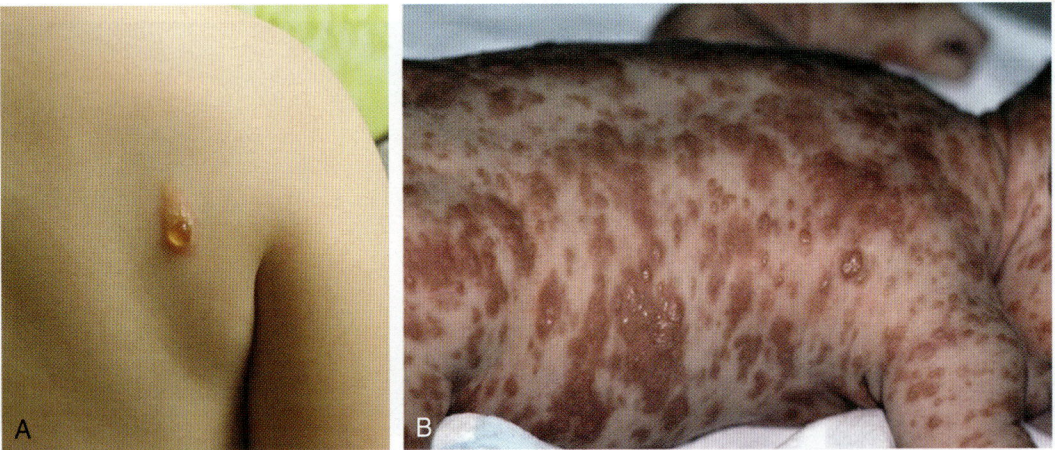

Fig. 28.110 (A) and (B) Bullous mastocytosis. *Courtesy Steven Binnick, MD.*

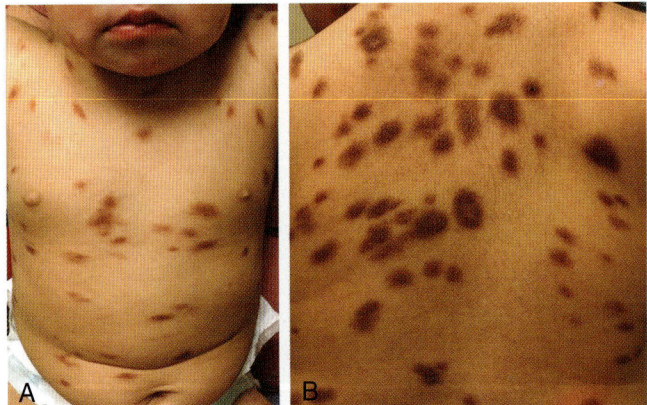

Fig. 28.111 (A) and (B) Urticaria pigmentosa.

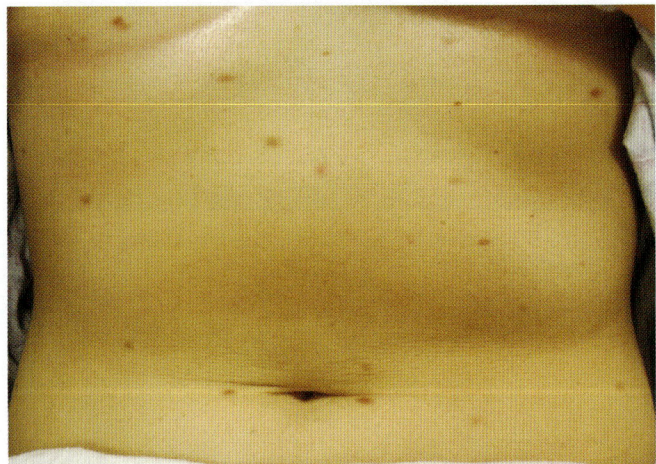

Fig. 28.112 Mastocytosis.

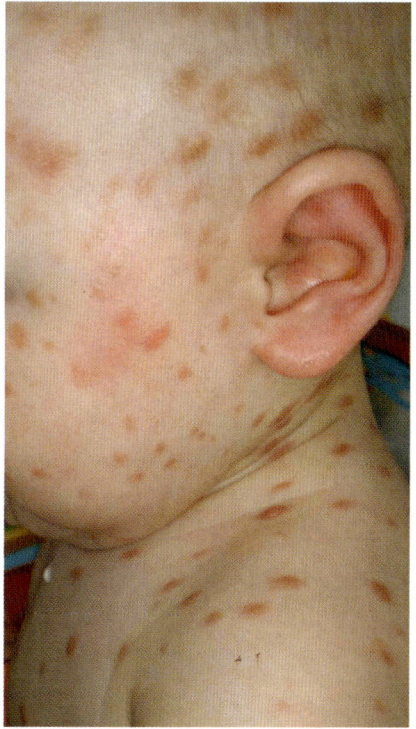

Fig. 28.113 Urticaria pigmentosa.

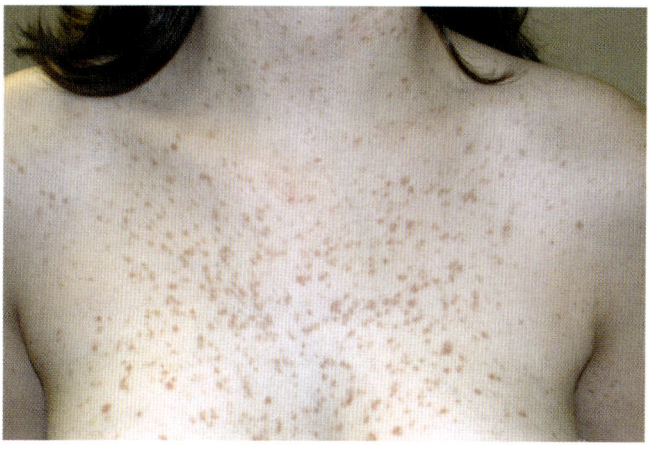

Fig. 28.114 Mastocytosis.

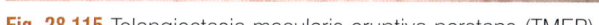

Fig. 28.115 Telangiectasia macularis eruptiva perstans (TMEP).

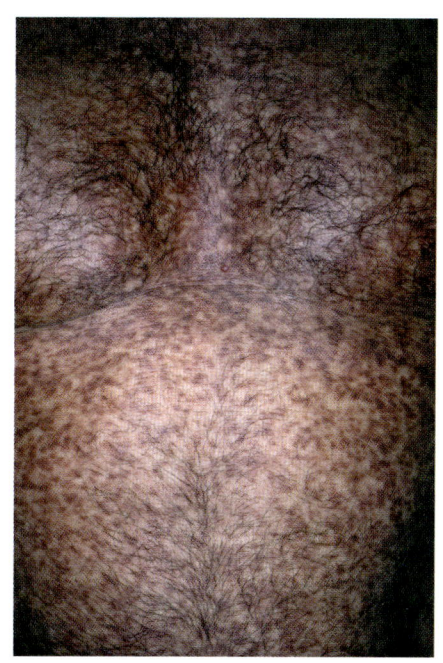

Fig. 28.116 Generalized adult mastocytosis.

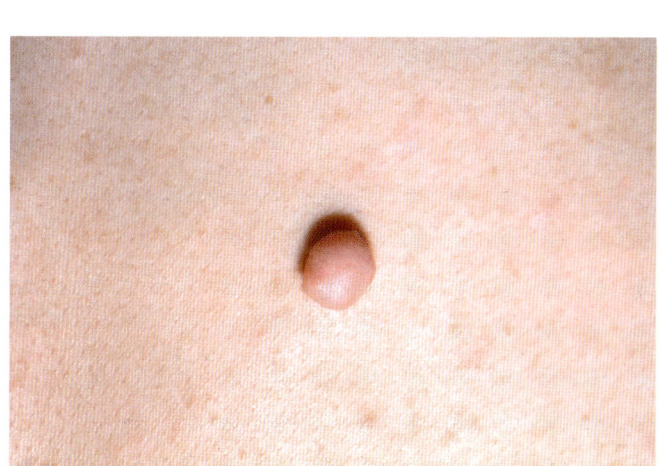

Fig. 28.117 Solitary neurofibroma. *Courtesy Steven Binnick, MD.*

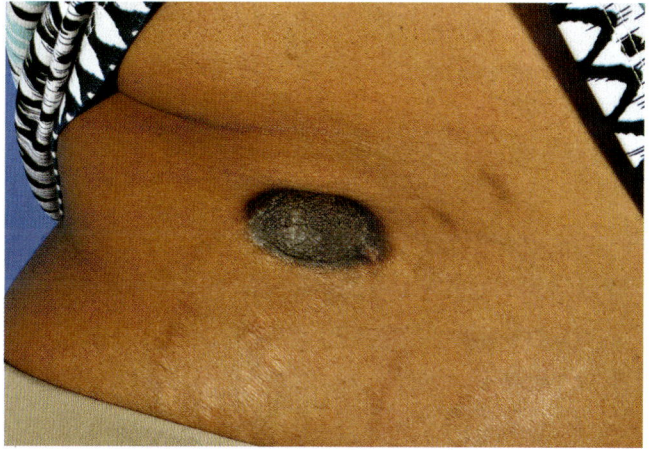

Fig. 28.118 Granular cell tumor. *Courtesy Curt Samlaska, MD.*

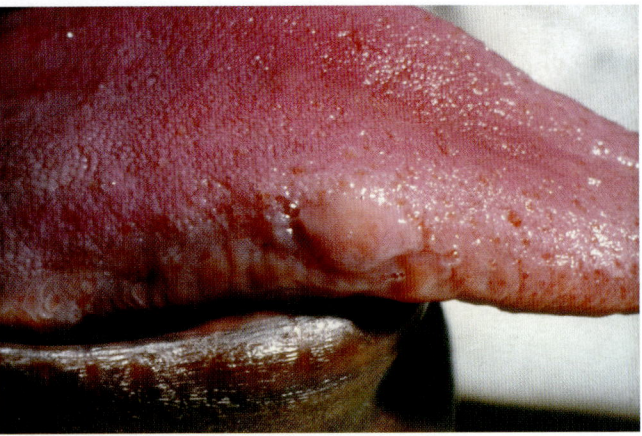

Fig. 28.119 Granular cell tumor.

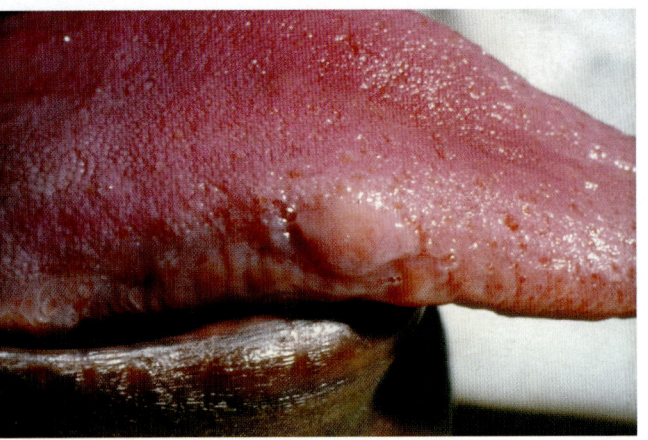

Fig. 28.120 Multiple granular cell tumor.

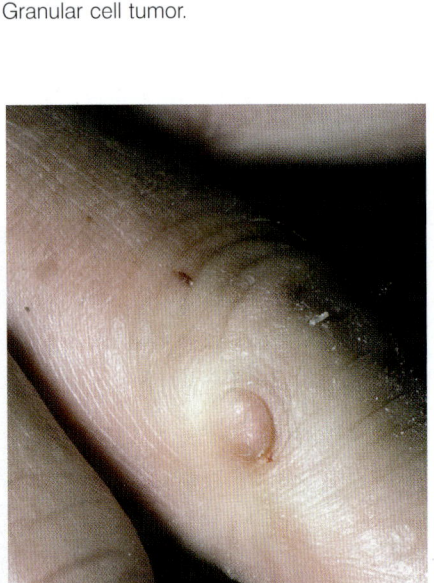

Fig. 28.121 Neuroma.

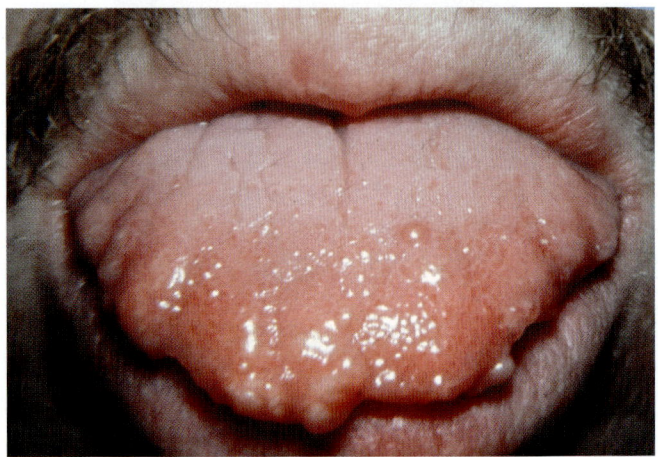

Fig. 28.122 Multiple mucosal neuroma syndrome.

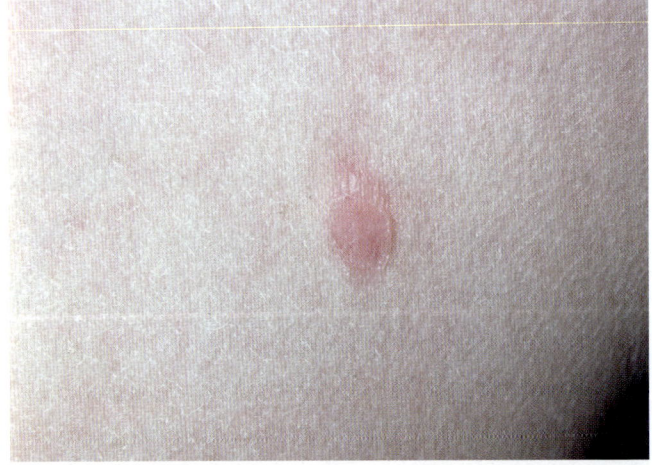

Fig. 28.123 Neurilemmoma.

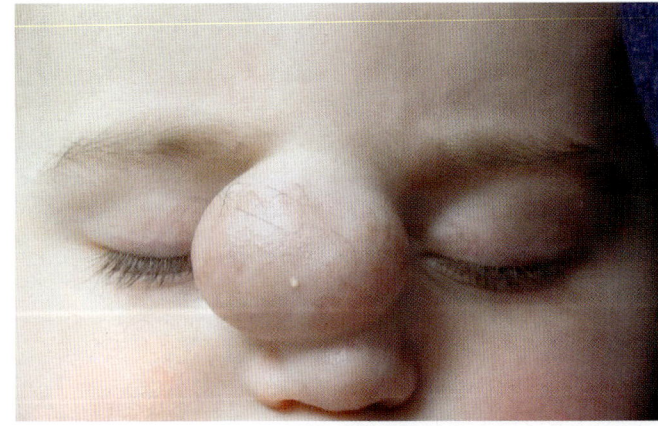

Fig. 28.124 Nasal glioma. *Courtesy Scott Bartlett, MD.*

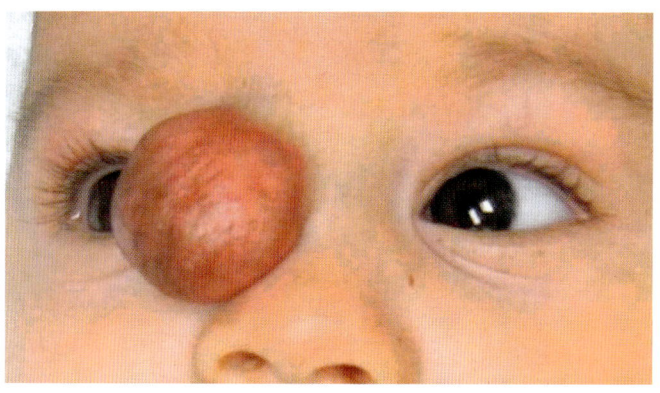

Fig. 28.125 Encephalocele. *Courtesy Scott Bartlett, MD.*

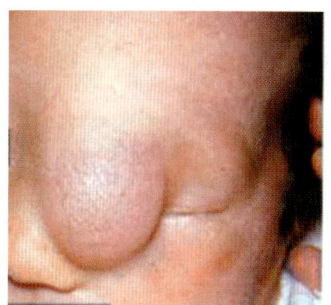

Fig. 28.126 Encephalocele.

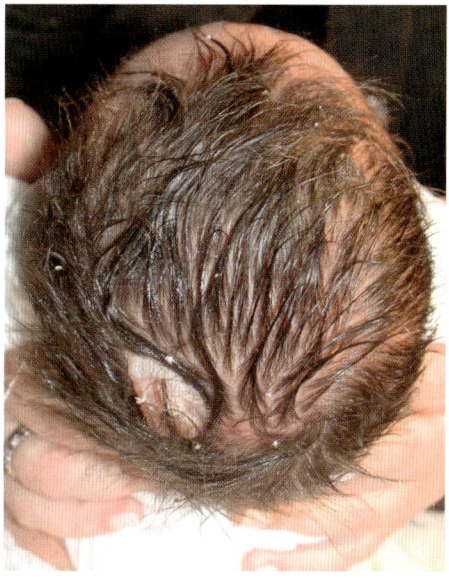

Fig. 28.127 Encephalocele. *Courtesy Paul Honig, MD.*

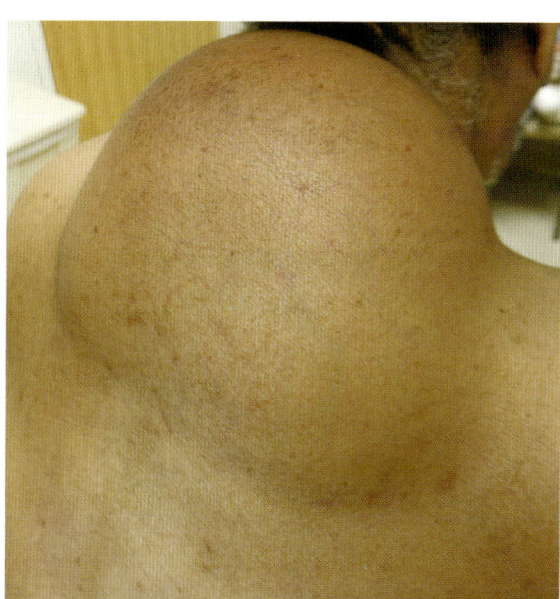

Fig. 28.128 Lipoma.

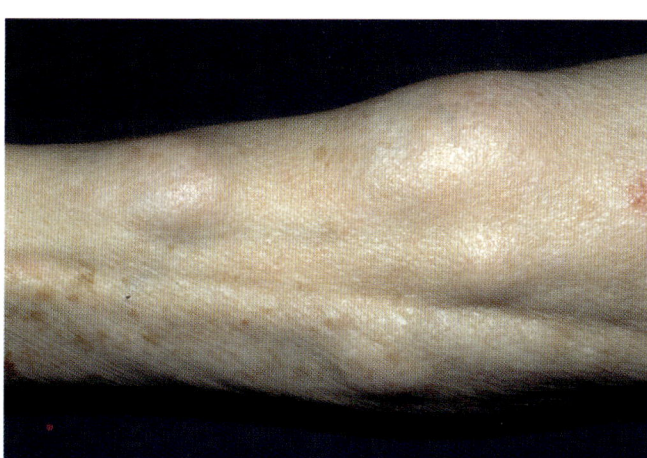

Fig. 28.129 Multiple lipomas.

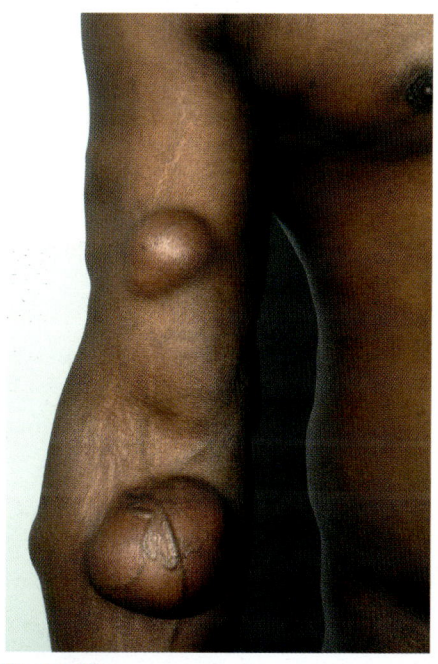

Fig. 28.130 Multiple lipomas.

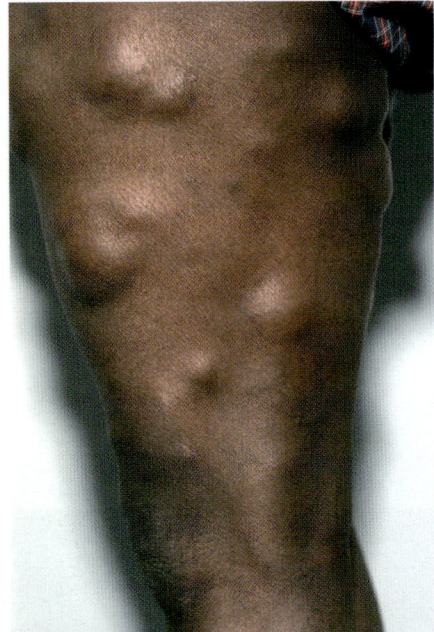

Fig. 28.131 Multiple lipomas.

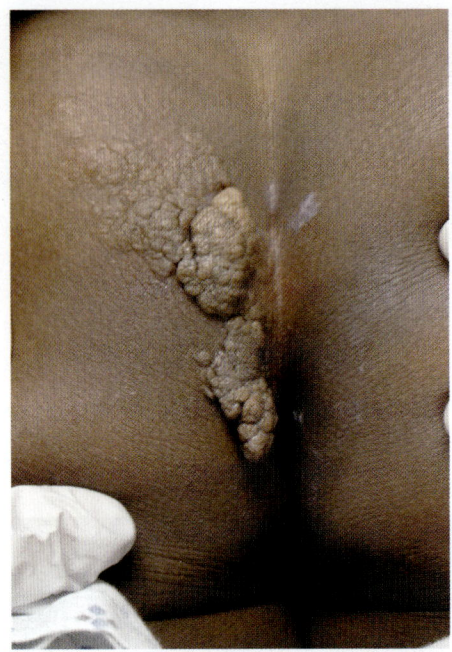

Fig. 28.132 Nevus lipomatosis superficialis.

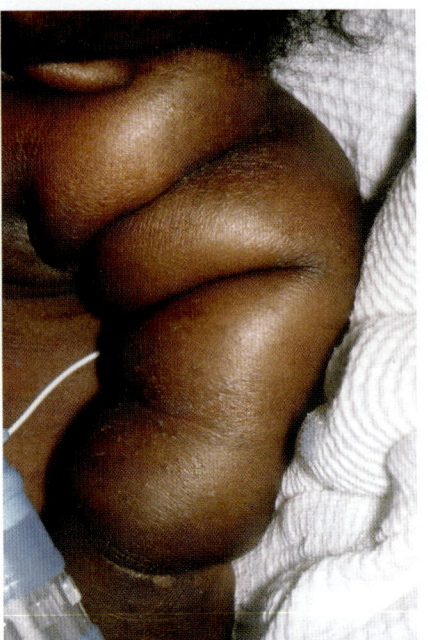

Fig. 28.133 Michelin tire baby.

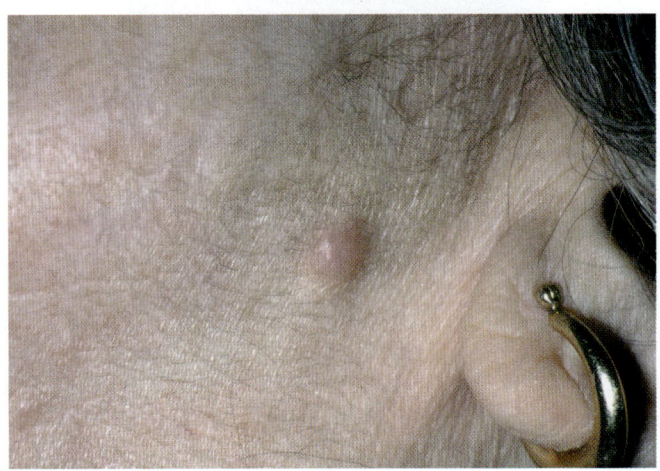

Fig. 28.134 Leiomyoma. *Courtesy Steven Binnick, MD.*

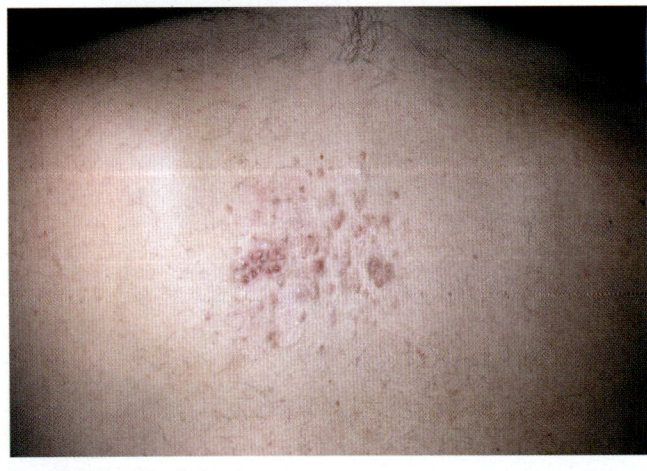

Fig. 28.135 Multiple leiomyomas.

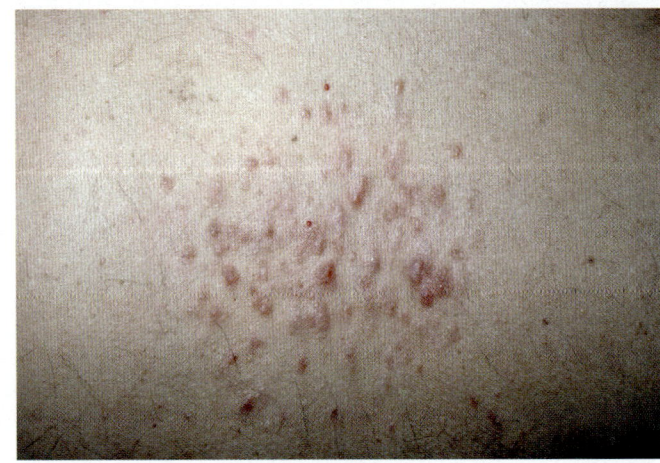

Fig. 28.136 Multiple leiomyomas. *Courtesy Steven Binnick, MD.*

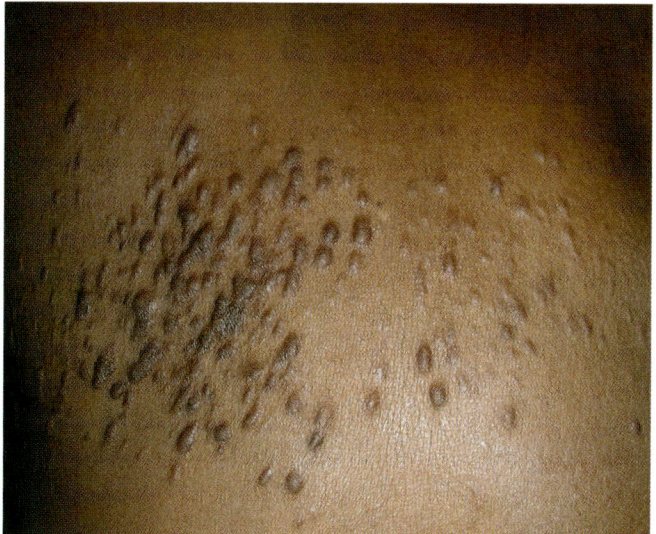

Fig. 28.137 Multiple leiomyomas. *Courtesy Debabrata Bandyopadhyay.*

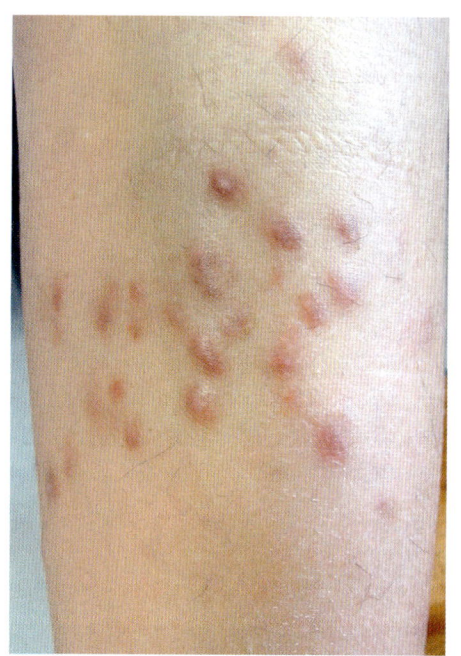

Fig. 28.138 Multiple leiomyomas.

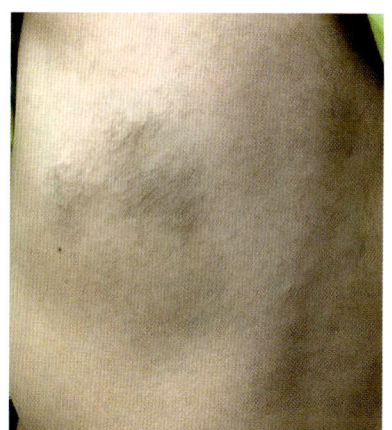

Fig. 28.139 Smooth muscle hamartoma.

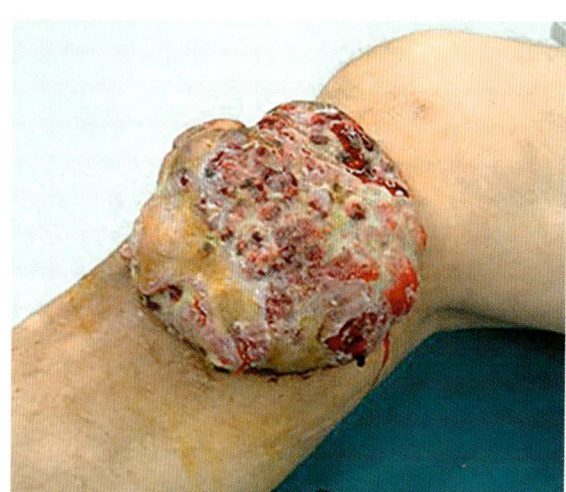

Fig. 28.140 Leiomyosarcoma.

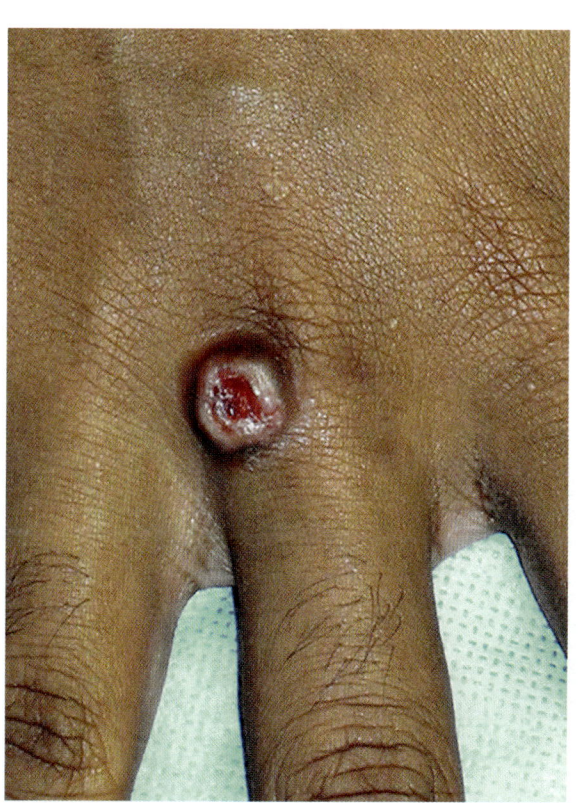

Fig. 28.141 Leiomyosarcoma. *Courtesy Chris Miller, MD.*

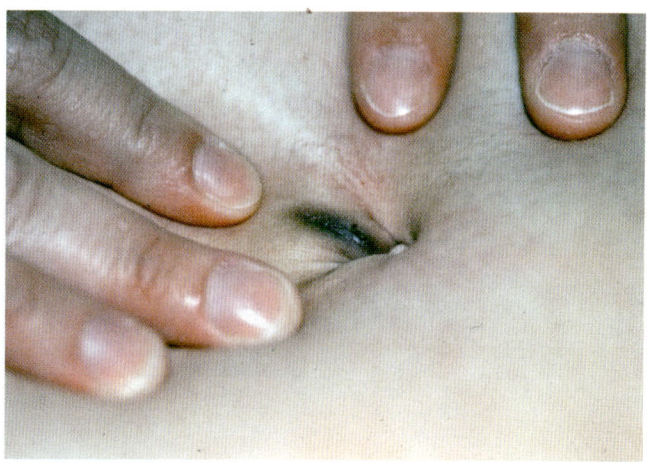

Fig. 28.142 Cutaneous endometriosis. *Courtesy Scott Norton, MD.*

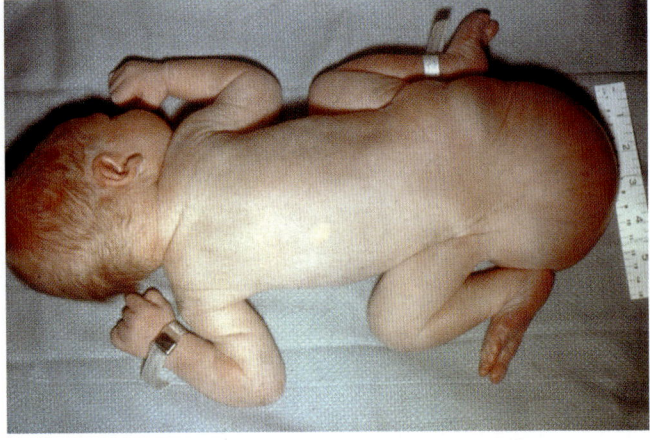

Fig. 28.143 Teratoma.

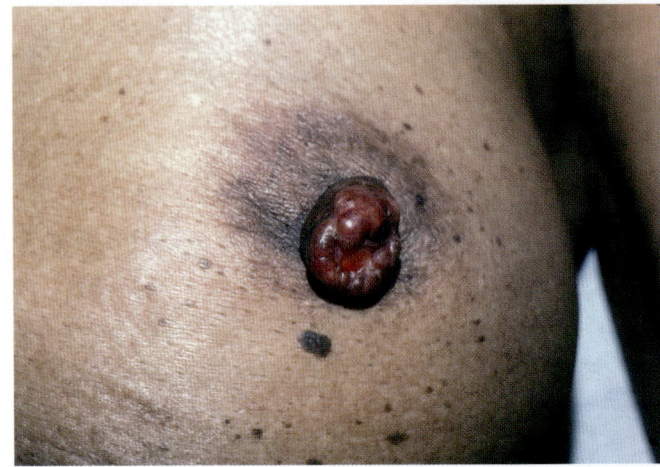

Fig. 28.144 Ductal breast cancer. *Courtesy Steven Binnick, MD.*

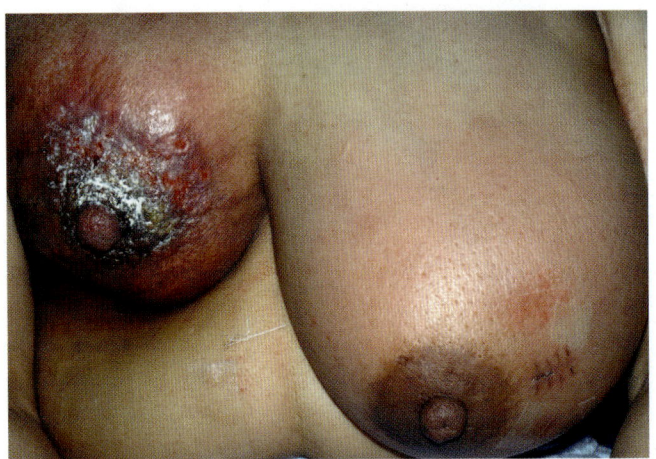

Fig. 28.145 Inflammatory breast cancer.

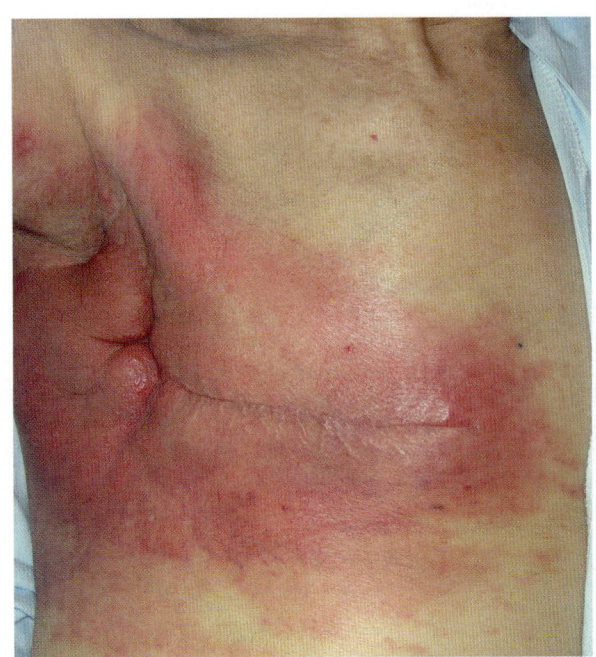

Fig. 28.146 Carcinoma erysipeloides.

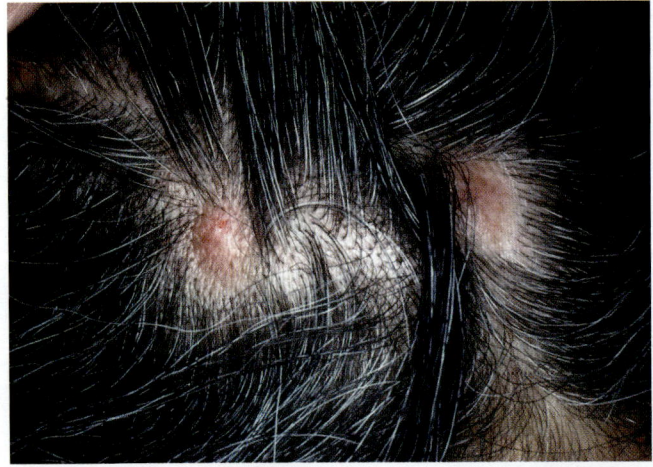

Fig. 28.147 Alopecia neoplastica (breast cancer).

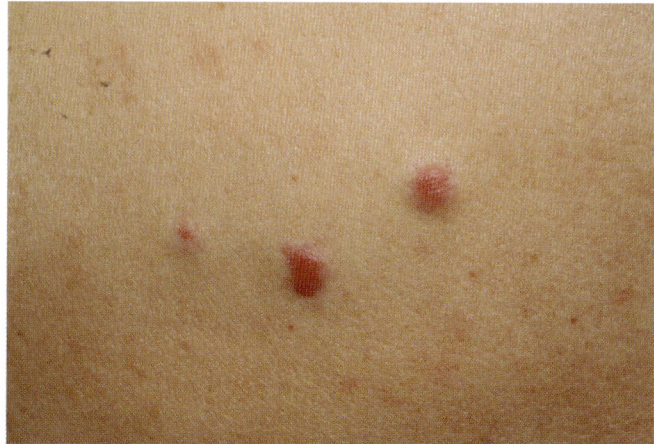

Fig. 28.148 Metastatic cholangiocarcinoma. *Courtesy Yung-Tsu Cho, MD.*

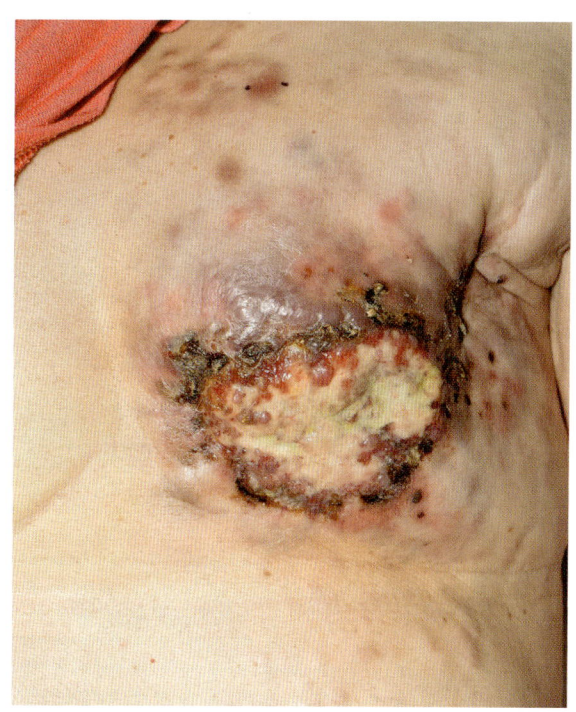

Fig. 28.149 Metastatic breast cancer. *Courtesy National Cheng Kung University, Taiwan.*

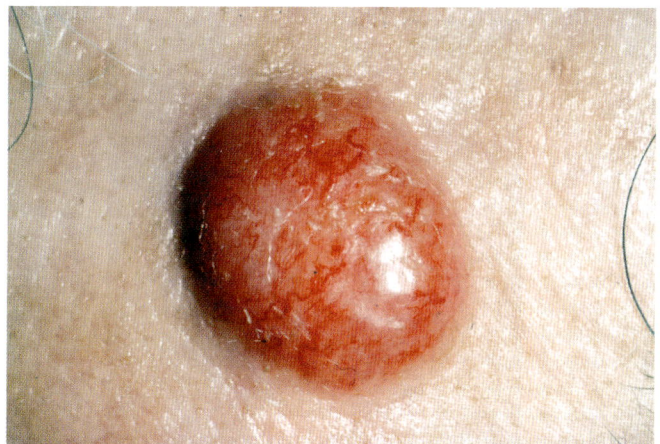

Fig. 28.150 Lung cancer metastasis.

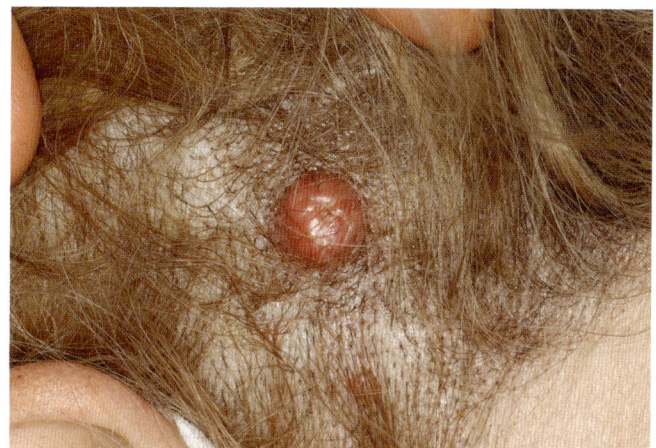

Fig. 28.151 Metastatic renal cell carcinoma.

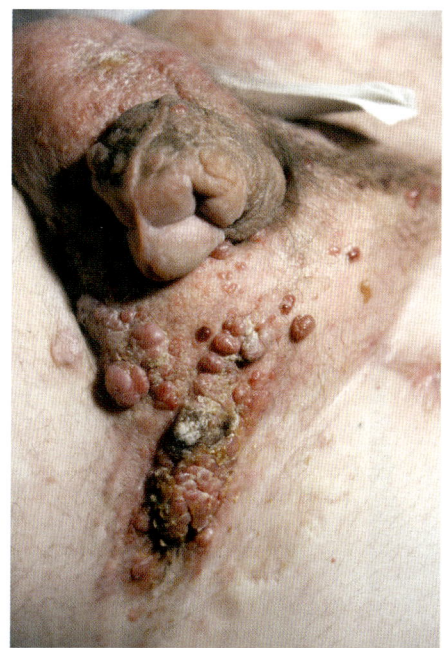

Fig. 28.152 Prostate cancer metastases.

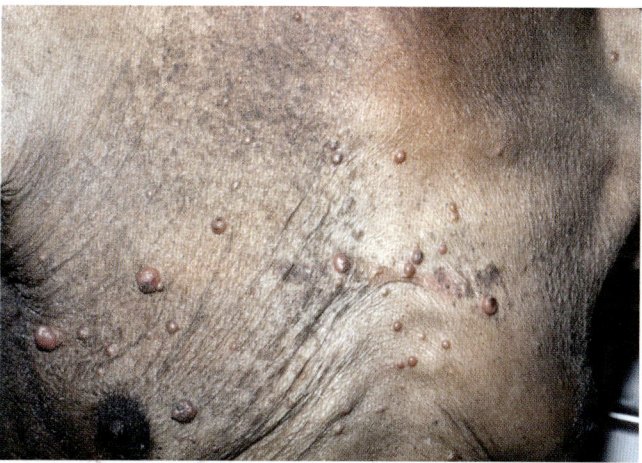

Fig. 28.153 Prostate cancer metastases.

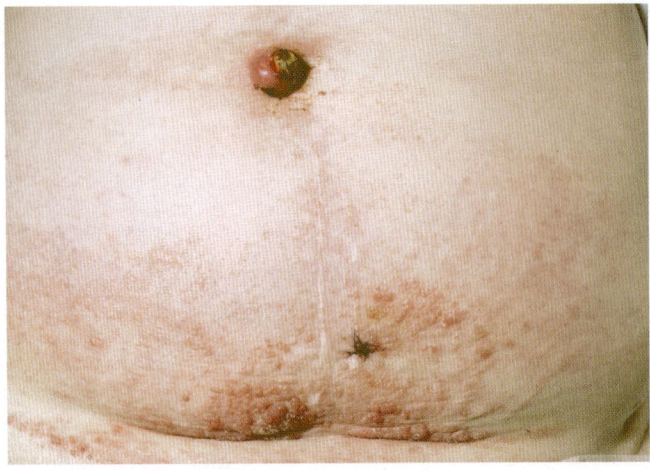

Fig. 28.154 Uterine cancer metastases (Sister Mary Joseph nodule).

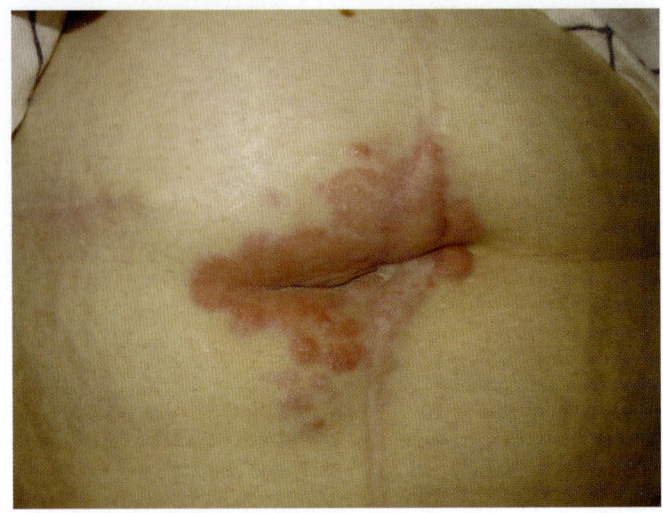

Fig. 28.155 Metastatic adenocarcinoma of the ileum.

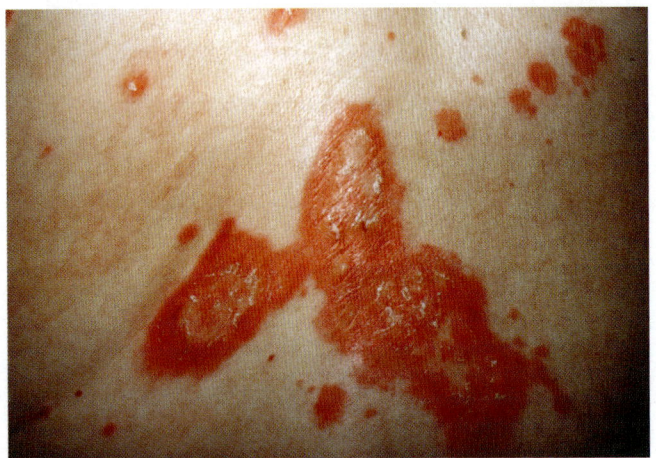

Fig. 28.156 Glucagonoma.

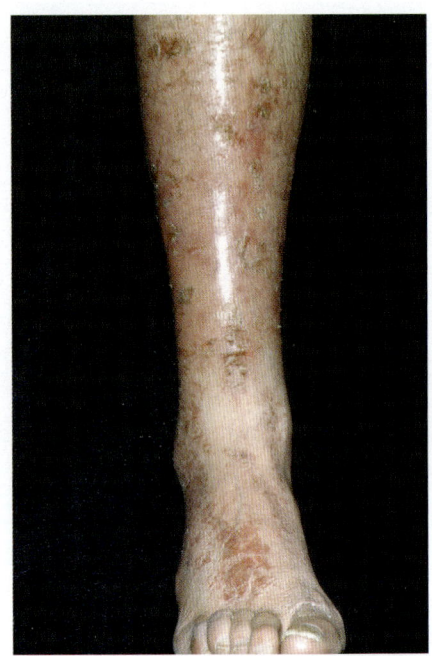

Fig. 28.157 Glucagonoma.

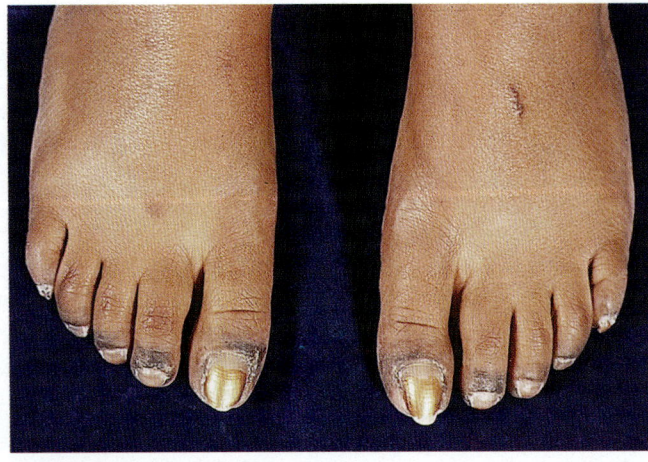

Fig. 28.158 Bazex syndrome.

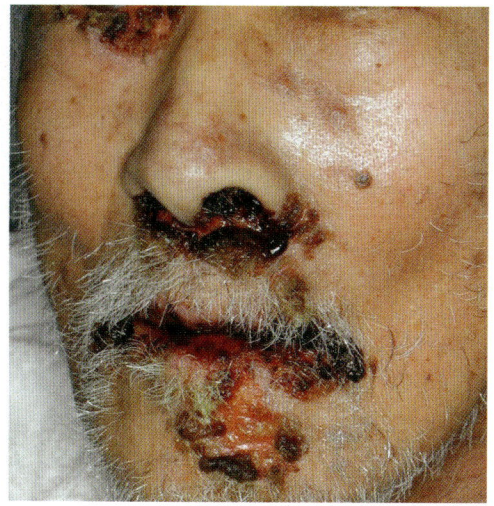

Fig. 28.159 Paraneoplastic pemphigus. *Courtesy Department of Dermatology, Keio University School of Medicine, Tokyo, Japan.*

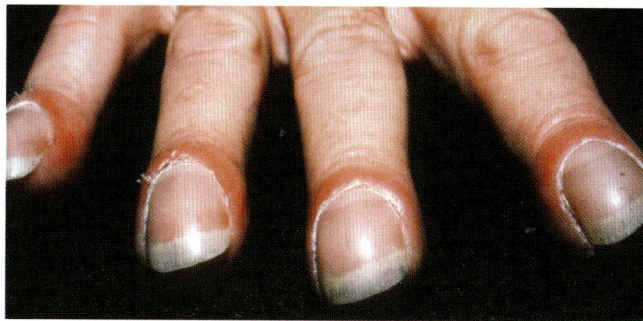

Fig. 28.160 Hypertrophic osteoarthropathy from lung cancer.

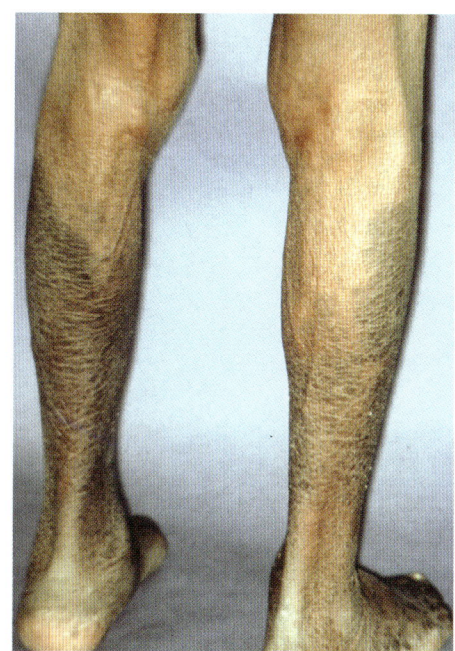

Fig. 28.161 Acquired ichthyosis in a patient with myeloma.

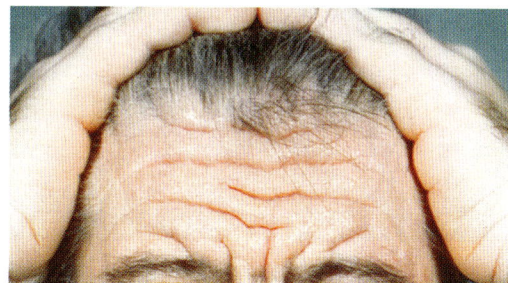

Fig. 28.162 Pachydermoperiostosis secondary to cancer.

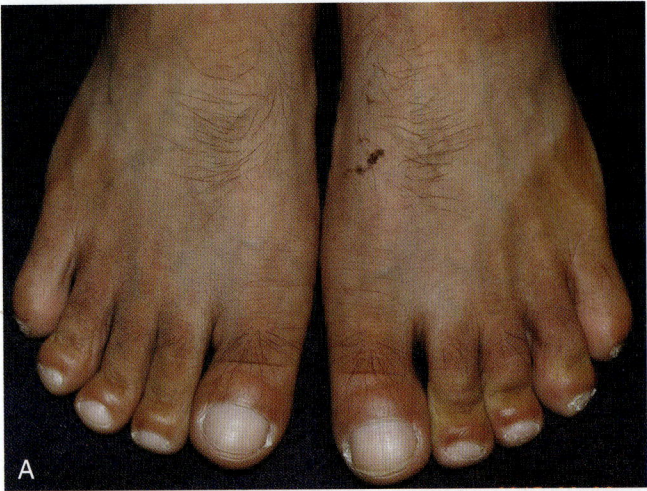
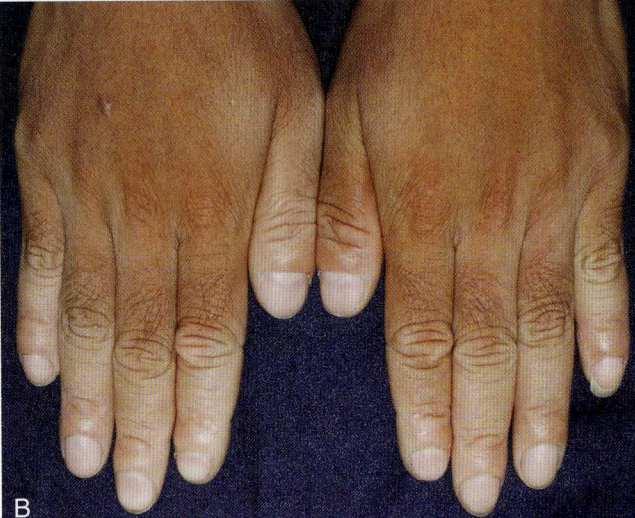

Fig. 28.163 (A) and (B) Pachydermoperiostosis. *Courtesy National Cheng Kung University, Taiwan.*

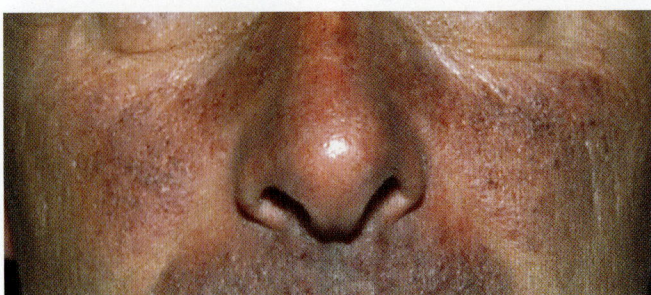

Fig. 28.164 Carcinoid syndrome.

Epidermal Nevi, Neoplasms, and Cysts 29

Epidermal neoplasms commonly present with hyperkeratosis, acanthosis, or papillomatosis. These may manifest clinically as a cutaneous horn, scale, palpable induration, a velvety or filiform appearance, or a smooth lesion raised above the surrounding skin surface. As an example, epidermal nevi tend to be raised and linear in configuration, following Blaschko lines. They may be hyperpigmented, hypopigmented, fleshy, or keratotic in appearance.

Cysts and dermal epithelial neoplasms displace the overlying skin and may produce overlying atrophy, erythema, or telangiectasia. The presence of tumor-associated vascularity lends a red or blue appearance, depending on the speed of blood flow and oxygen saturation of the blood. The presence of cytoplasm lends a yellow appearance due to carotenoids dissolved in the aqueous phase of cytoplasm. A brown appearance most commonly relates to melanin within the epithelial cells and underlying dermis, but can also be a result of dermal hemosiderin or lipofuscin deposition. Lipofuscin dissolved in apocrine sweat often lends a blue appearance to portions of sweat gland tumors as a result of diffraction of light (the Tyndall effect). Sebaceous elements lend a yellow or orange appearance. An appreciation of the color, morphology, and distribution of the lesions will help the physician narrow the differential diagnosis.

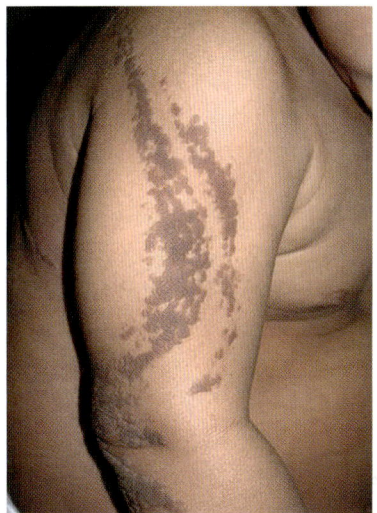

Fig. 29.2 Epidermal nevus.

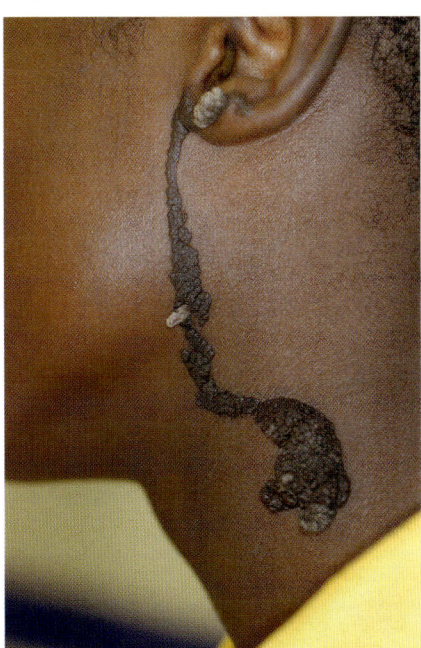

Fig. 29.1 Epidermal nevus.

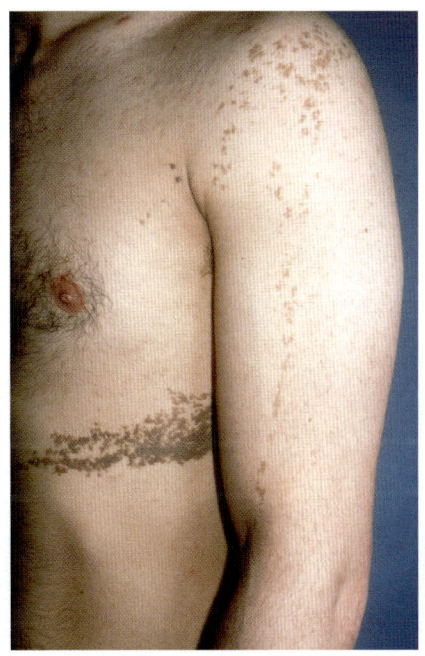

Fig. 29.3 Epidermal nevus.

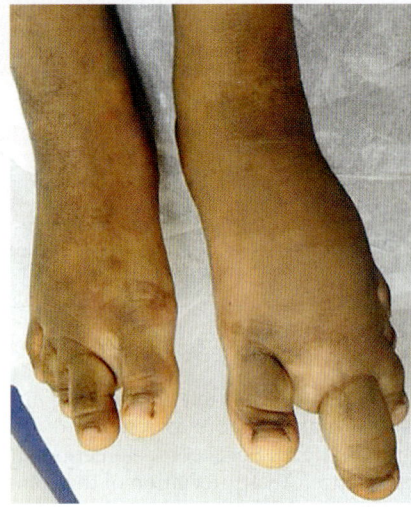

Fig. 29.4 CLOVE syndrome.

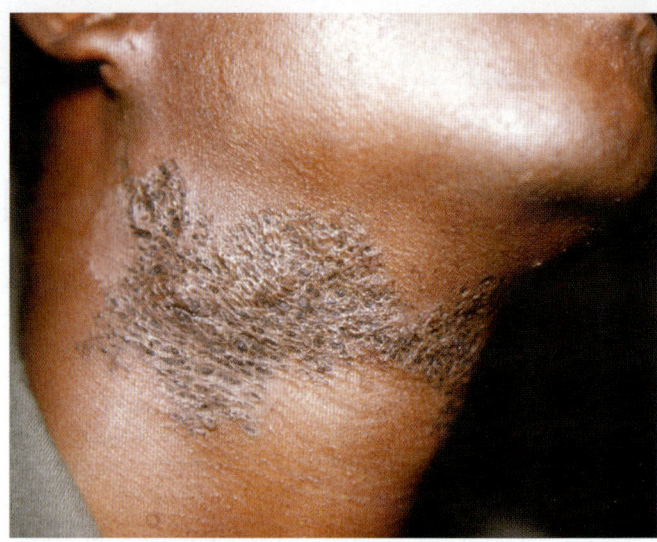

Fig. 29.5 Nevus comedonicus.

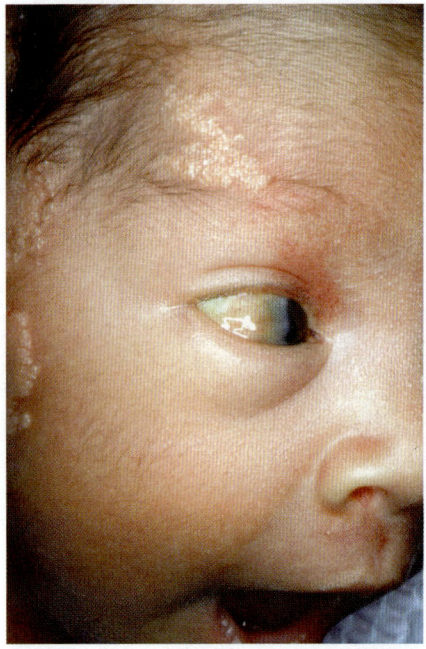

Fig. 29.6 Schimmelpenning syndrome with a lipodermoid of the conjunctiva.

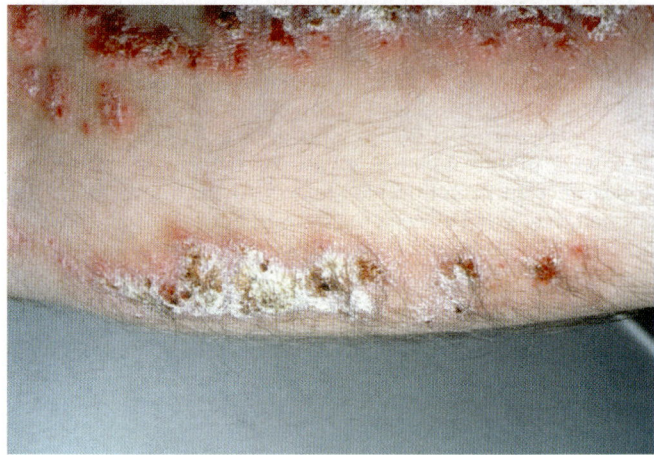

Fig. 29.7 Inflammatory linear verrucous epidermal nevus.

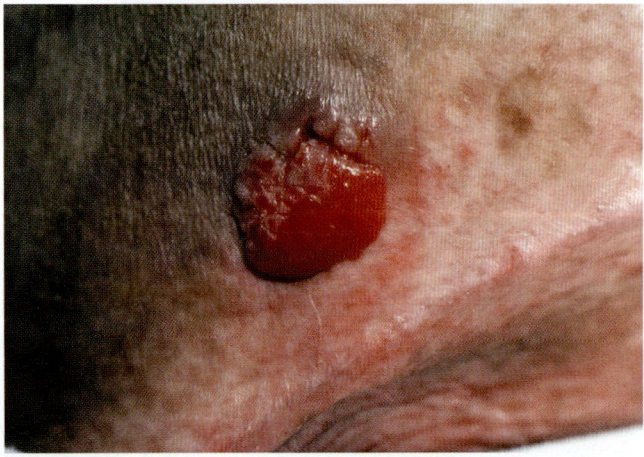

Fig. 29.8 Clear cell acanthoma. *Courtesy Ken Greer, MD.*

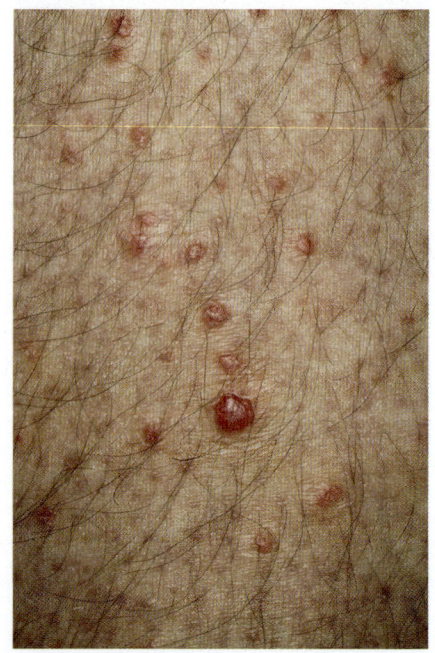

Fig. 29.9 Multiple clear cell acanthomas.

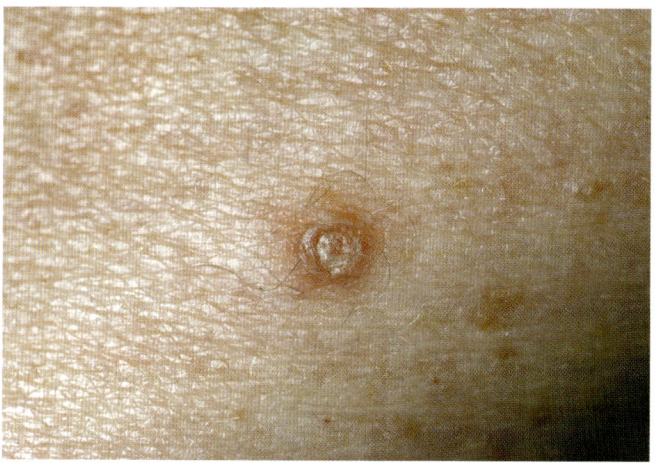

Fig. 29.10 Warty dyskeratomas.

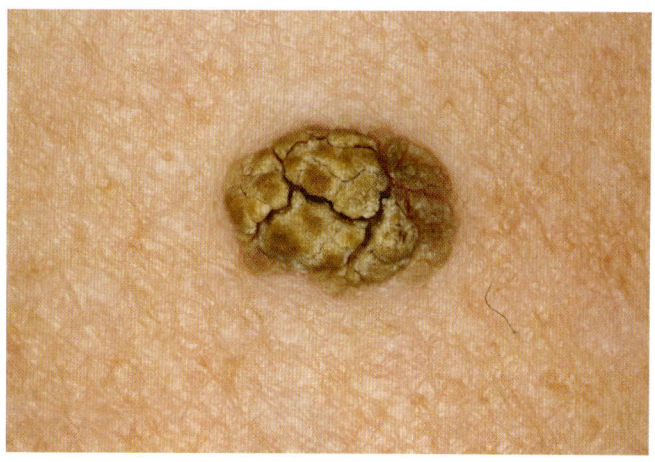

Fig. 29.11 Seborrheic keratosis.

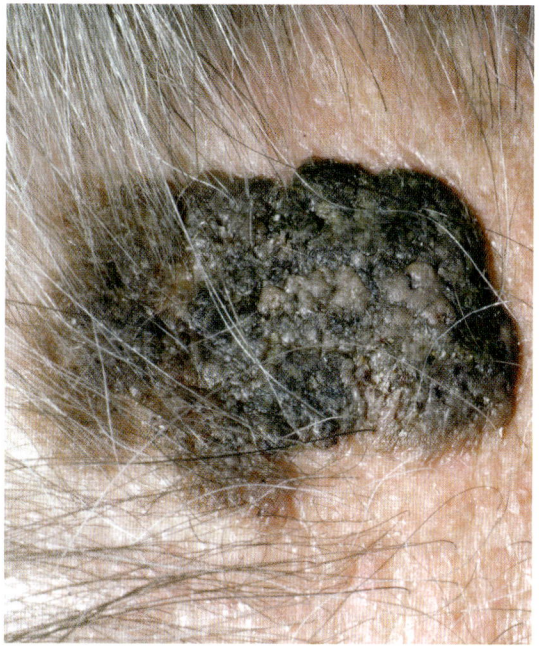

Fig. 29.12 Seborrheic keratosis. *Courtesy Steven Binnick, MD.*

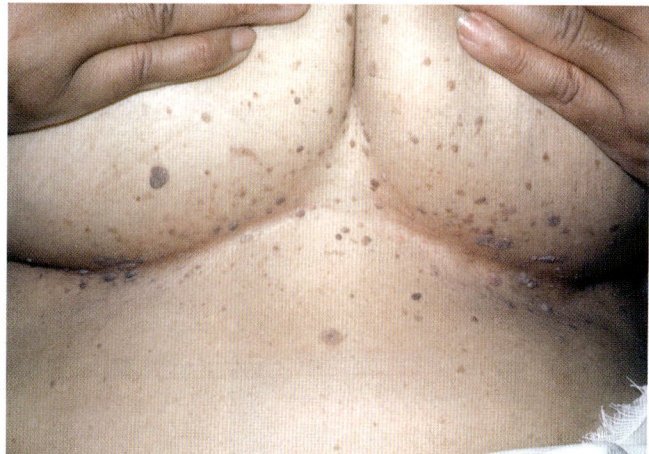

Fig. 29.13 Seborrheic keratosis. *Courtesy Steven Binnick, MD.*

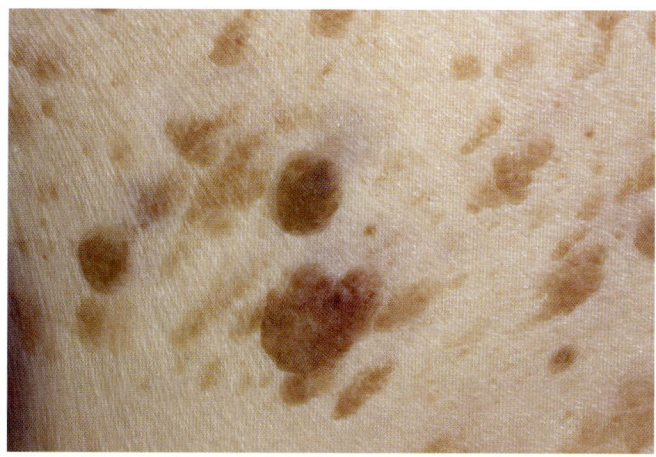

Fig. 29.14 Seborrheic keratosis.

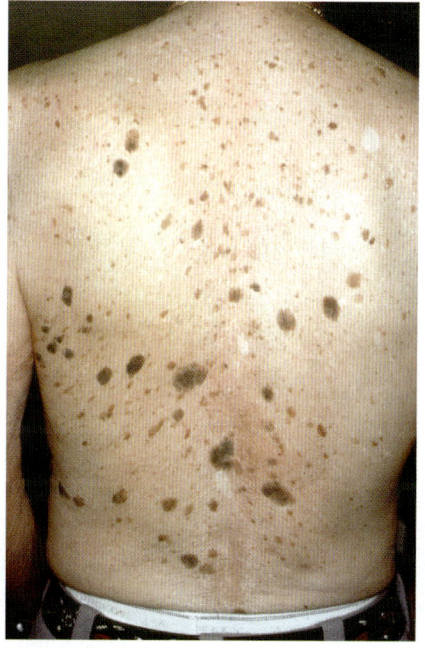

Fig. 29.15 Seborrheic keratosis.

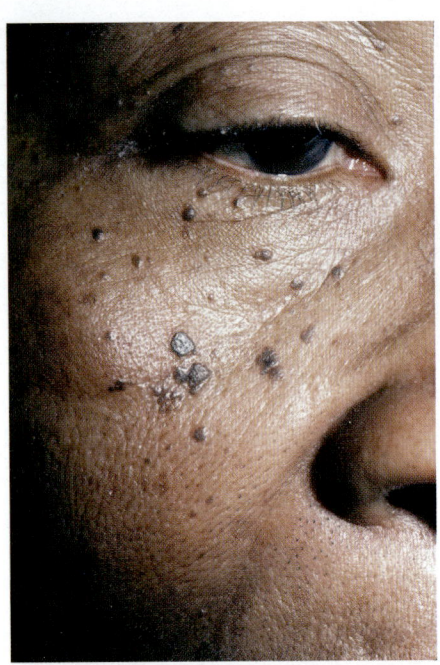

Fig. 29.16 Dermatosis papulosa nigra. *Courtesy Steven Binnick, MD.*

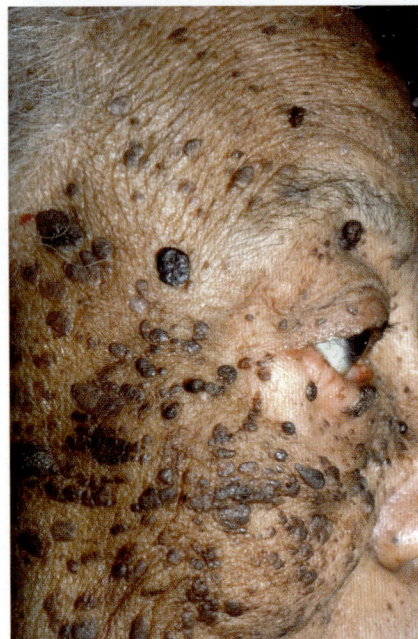

Fig. 29.17 Dermatosis papulosa nigra.

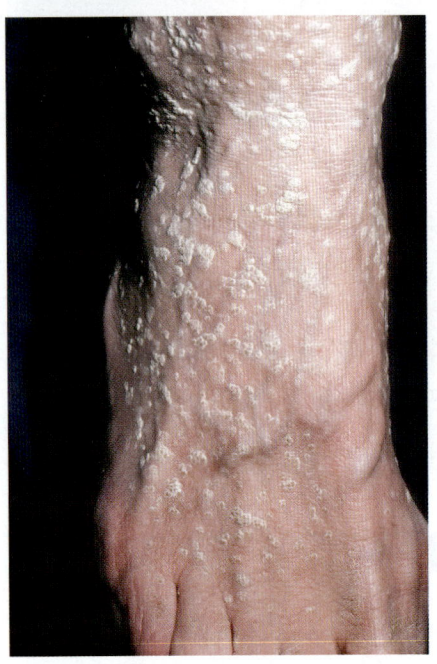

Fig. 29.18 Stucco keratosis.

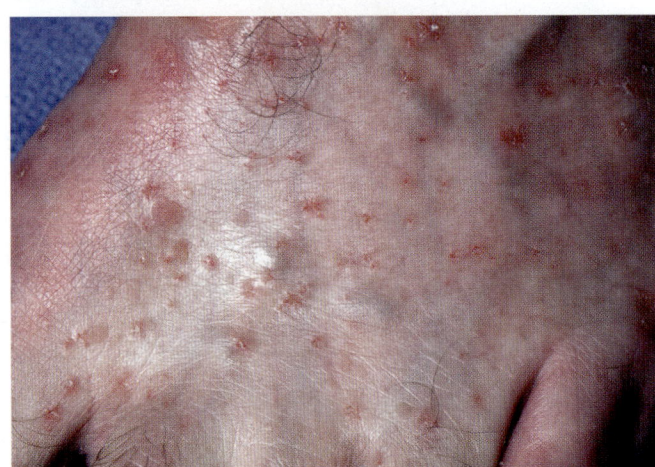

Fig. 29.19 Flegel disease.

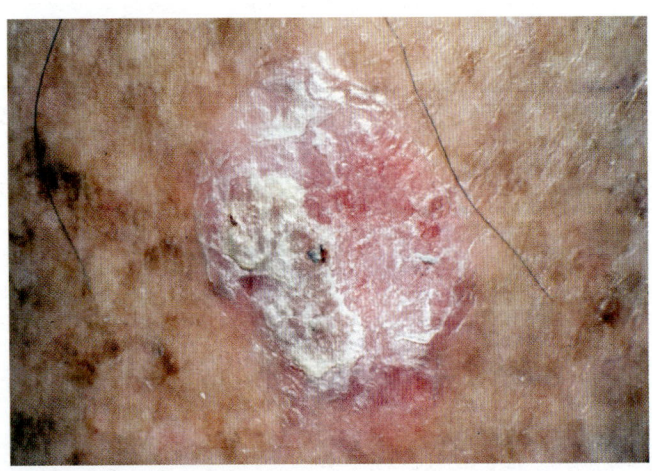

Fig. 29.20 Benign lichenoid keratosis.

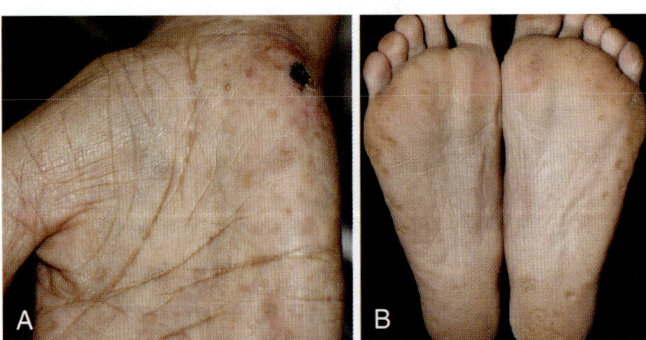

Fig. 29.21 (A) Arsenical keratoses, palm. (B) Arsenical keratoses, soles. *Courtesy National Cheng Kung University, Taiwan.*

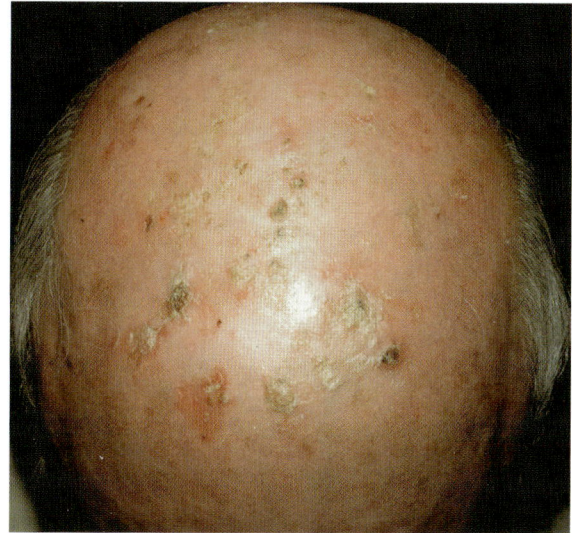

Fig. 29.22 Actinic keratoses. *Courtesy The University of Utah and Oregon Health Sciences University Leonard Swinyer MD image collection.*

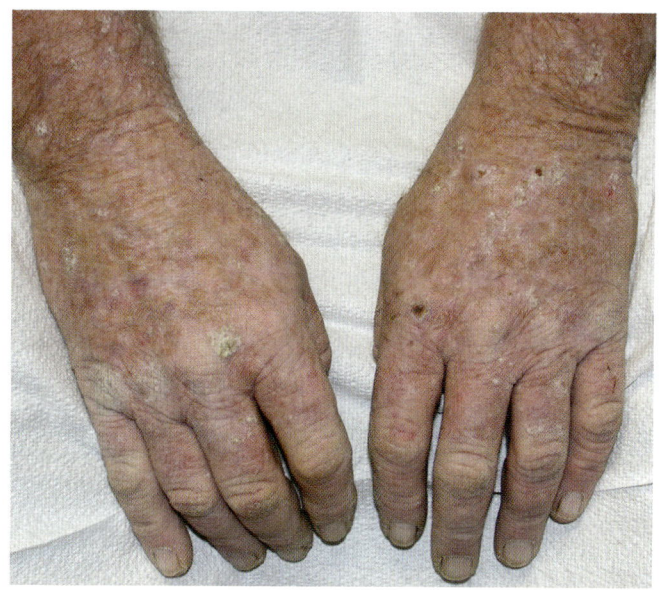

Fig. 29.23 Actinic keratoses.

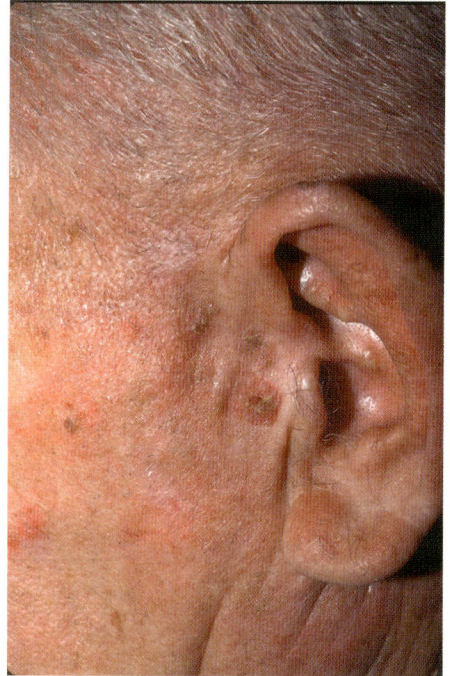

Fig. 29.24 Actinic keratoses in vitiliginous skin. *Courtesy The University of Utah and Oregon Health Sciences University Leonard Swinyer MD image collection.*

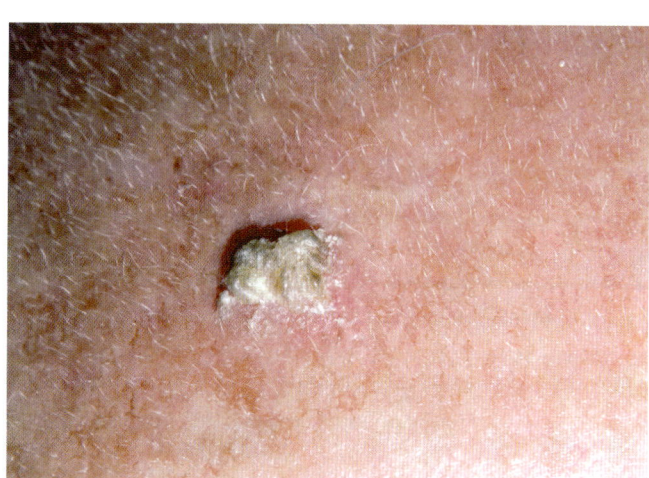

Fig. 29.25 Hypertrophic actinic keratosis.

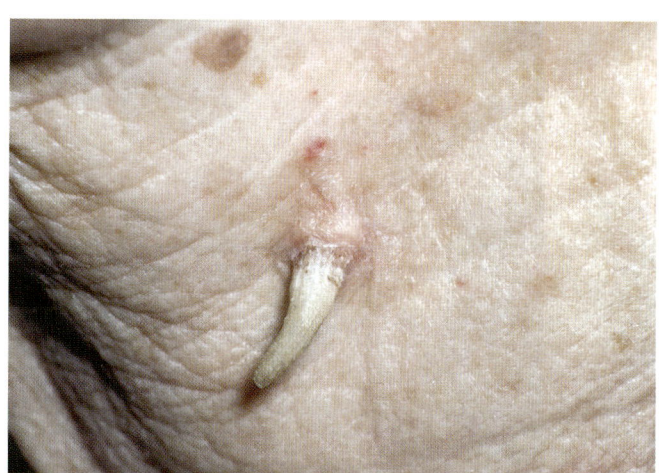

Fig. 29.26 Cutaneous horn. *Courtesy Steven Binnick, MD.*

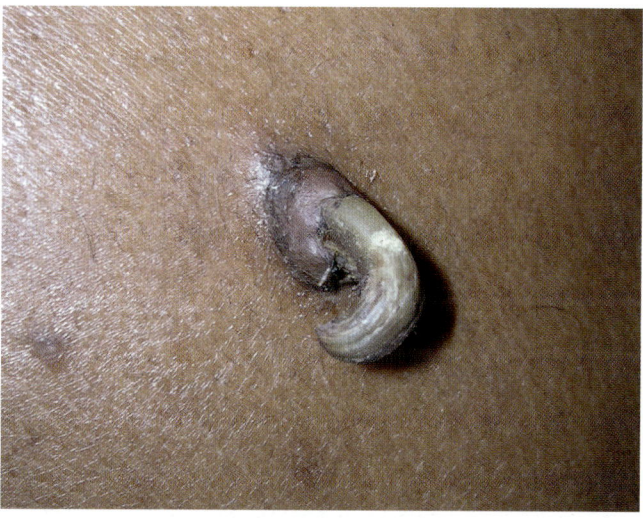

Fig. 29.27 Cutaneous horn. *Courtesy Debabrata Bandyopadhyay.*

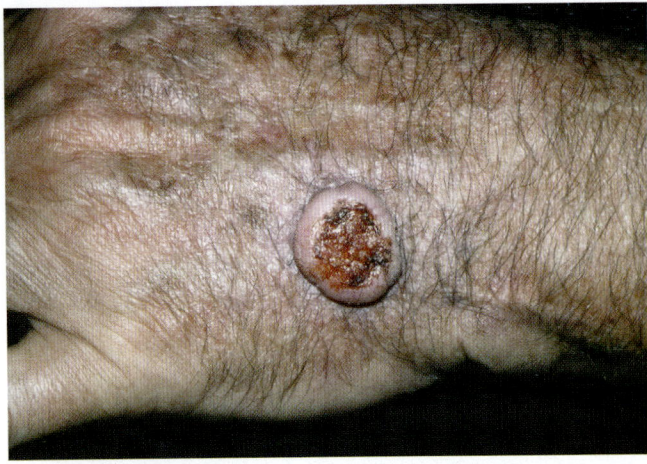

Fig. 29.28 Keratoacanthoma. *Courtesy Curt Samlaska, MD.*

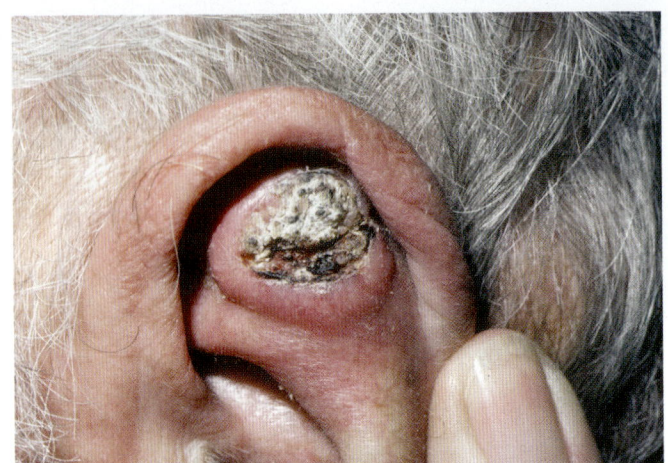

Fig. 29.29 Keratoacanthoma. *Courtesy Steven Binnick, MD.*

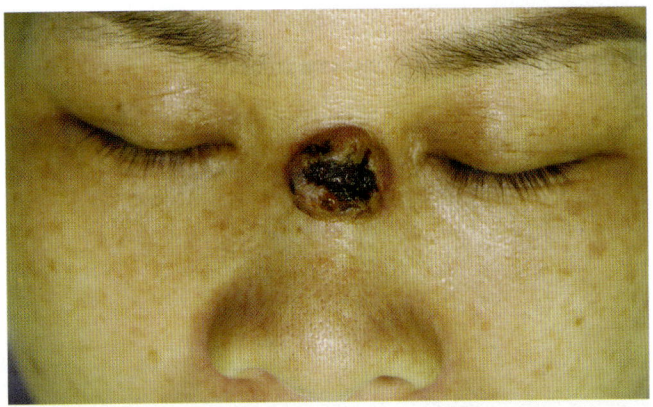

Fig. 29.30 Keratoacanthoma. *Courtesy Dr. Yi-Shaun Sheen.*

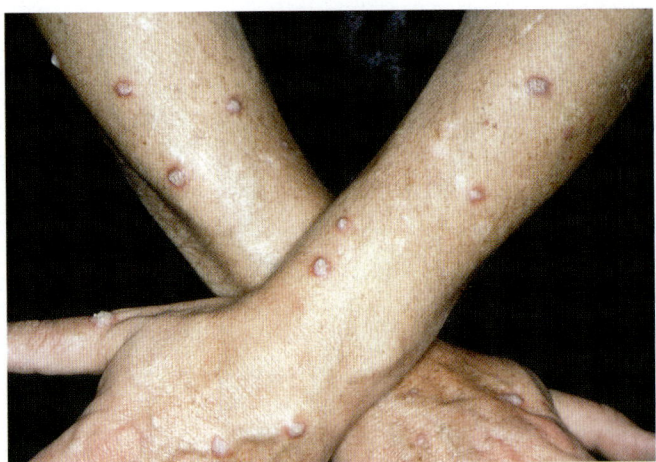

Fig. 29.31 Multiple keratoacanthomas.

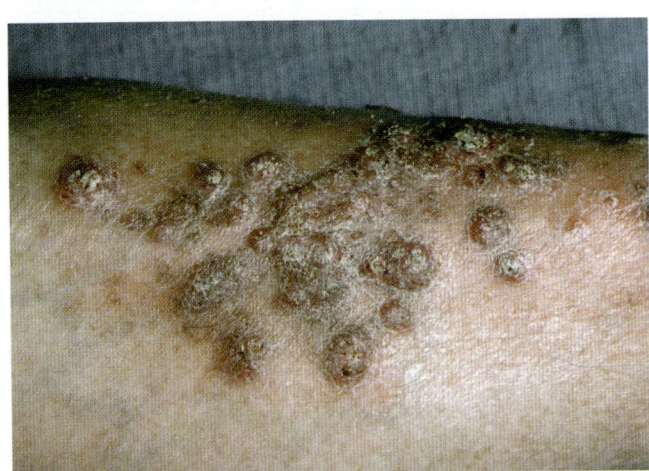

Fig. 29.32 Eruptive keratoacanthoma.

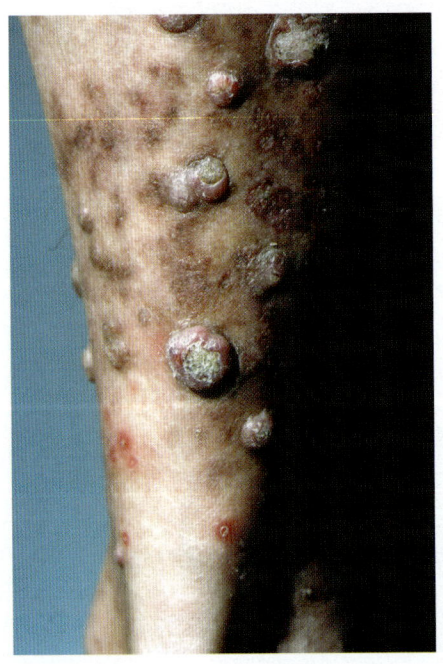

Fig. 29.33 Eruptive keratoacanthoma.

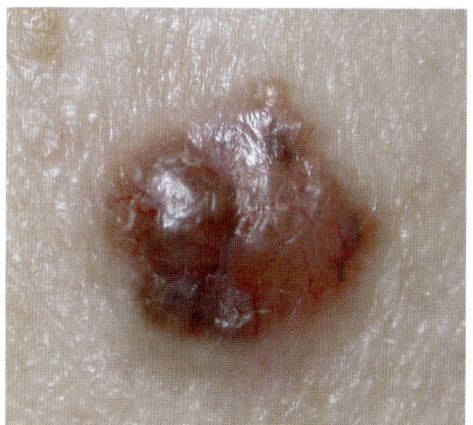

Fig. 29.34 Basal cell carcinoma.

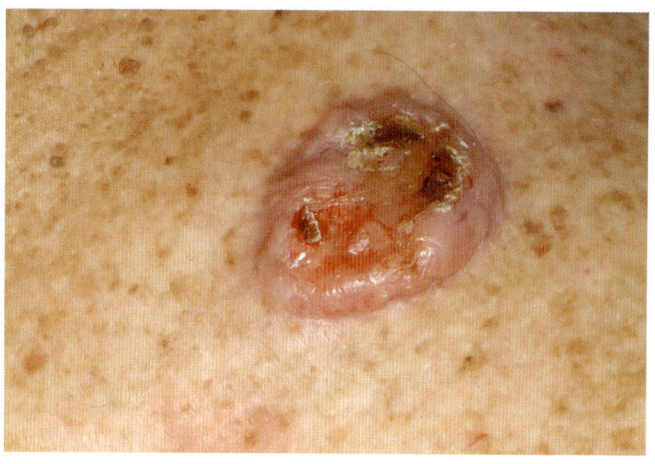

Fig. 29.35 Basal cell carcinoma.

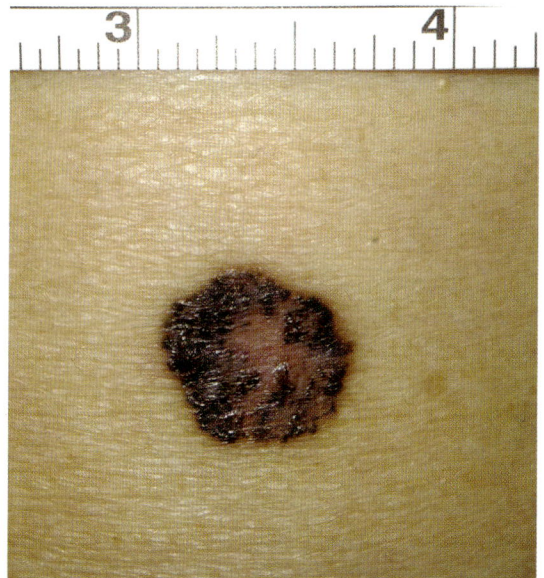

Fig. 29.36 Basal cell carcinoma. *Courtesy Dr. Yi-Shuan Sheen.*

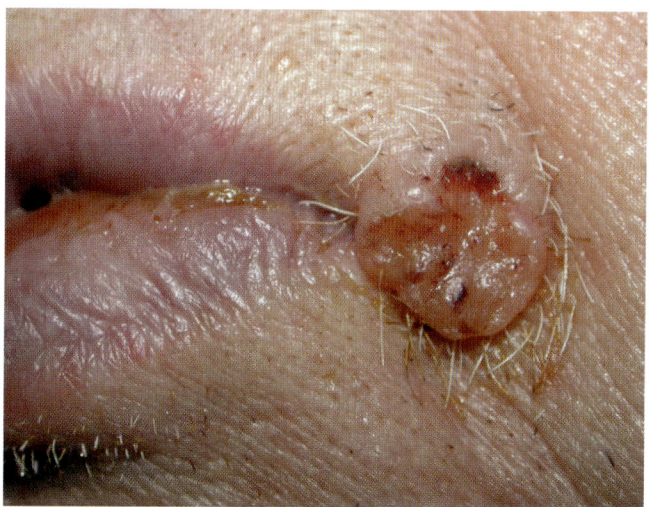

Fig. 29.37 Basal cell carcinoma.

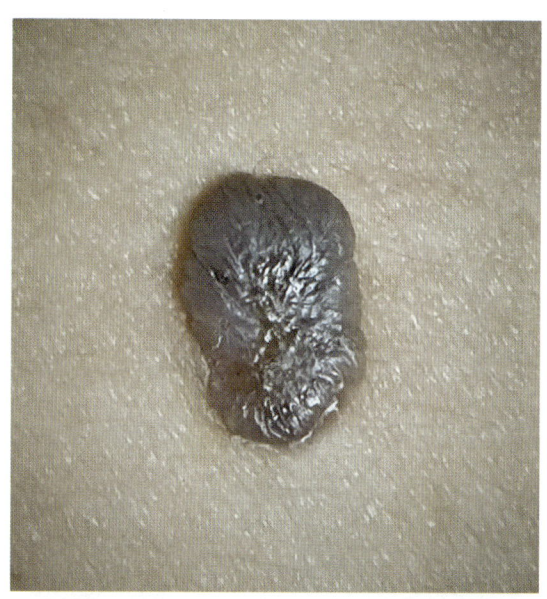

Fig. 29.38 Fibroepithelioma of Pinkus. *Courtesy Dr. Rui Carlos Taveres Bello.*

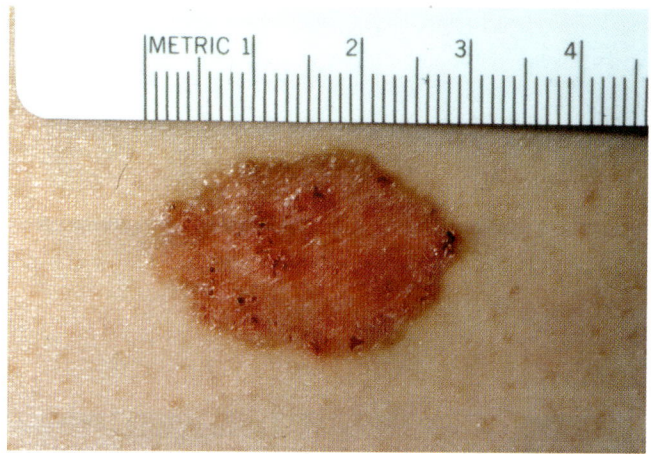

Fig. 29.39 Superficial basal cell carcinoma.

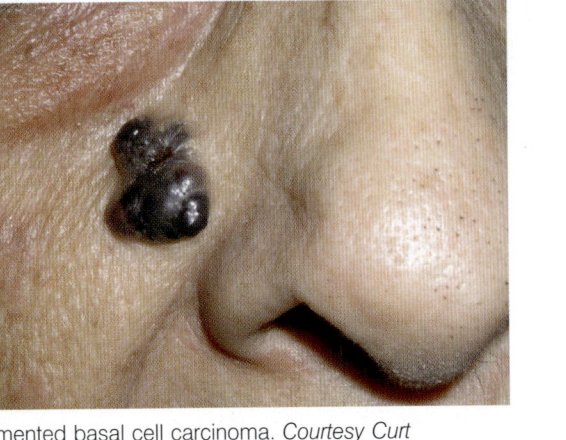

Fig. 29.40 Pigmented basal cell carcinoma. *Courtesy Curt Samlaska, MD.*

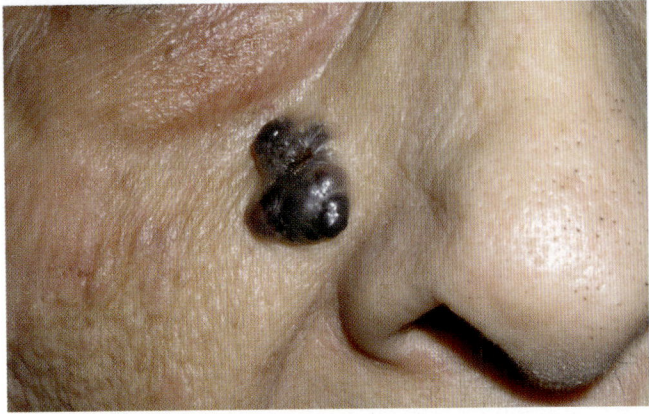

Fig. 29.41 Pigmented basal cell carcinoma. *Courtesy Debabrata Bandyopadhyay, MD.*

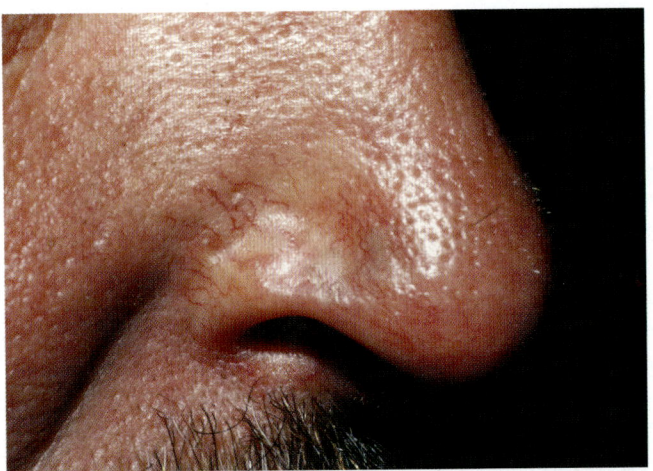

Fig. 29.42 Morpheaform basal cell carcinoma. *Courtesy Steven Binnick, MD.*

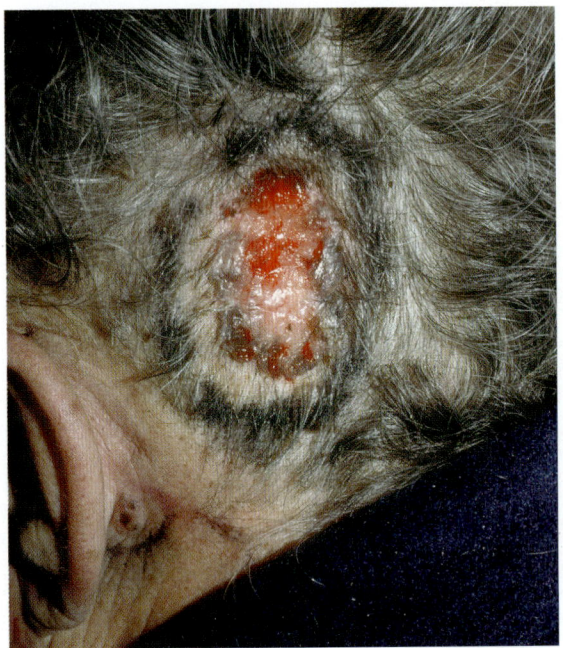

Fig. 29.43 Basal cell carcinoma.

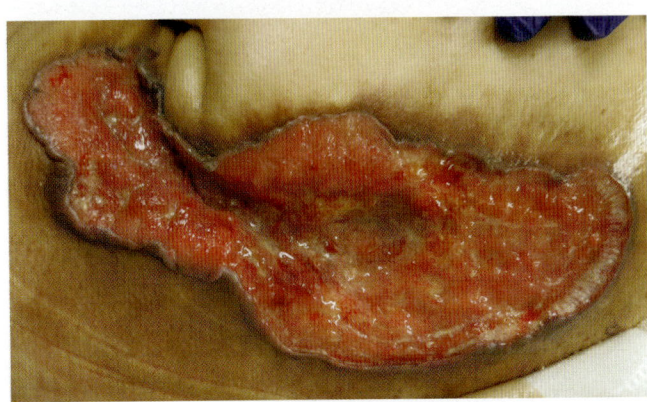

Fig. 29.44 Large basal cell carcinoma.

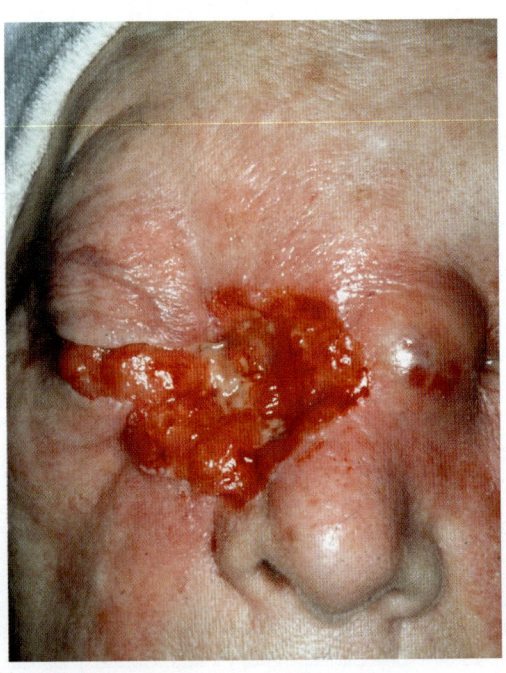

Fig. 29.45 Aggressive basal cell carcinoma.

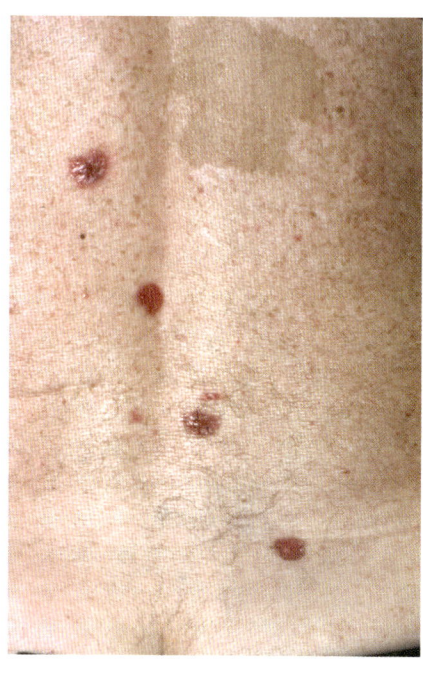

Fig. 29.46 Multiple basal cell carcinomas in a radiation site. *Courtesy Steven Binnick, MD.*

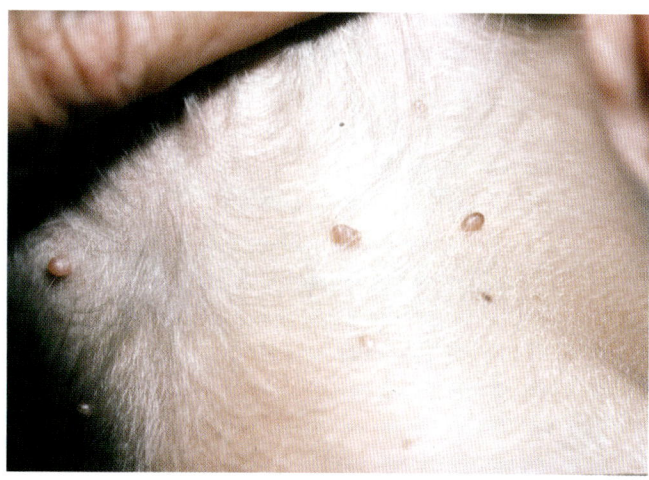

Fig. 29.47 Basal cell nevus syndrome with skin tag–like basal cell carcinomas. *Courtesy Ken Greer, MD.*

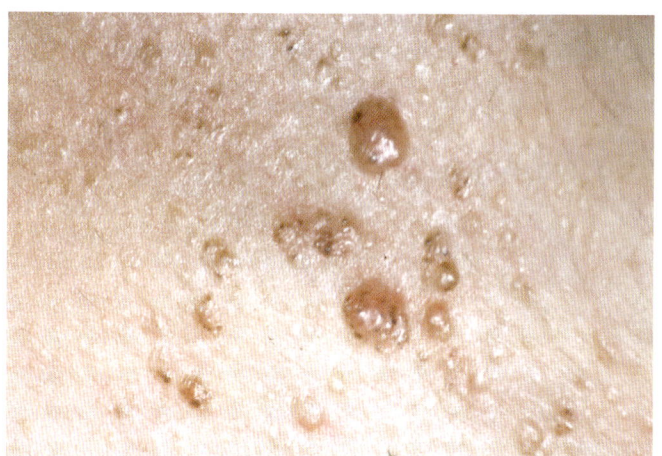

Fig. 29.48 Basal cell nevus syndrome. *Courtesy Steven Binnick, MD.*

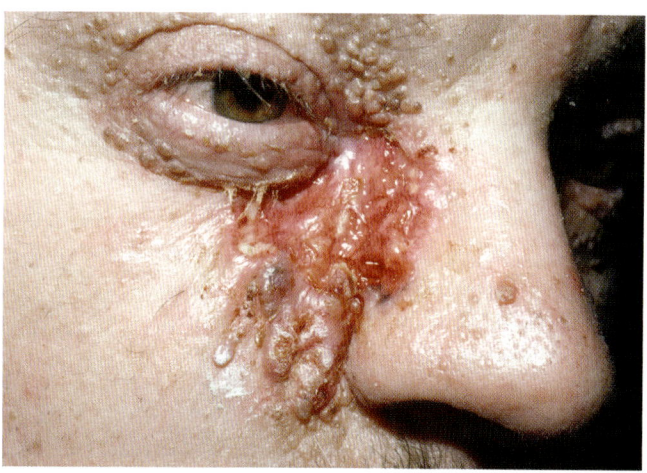

Fig. 29.49 Basal cell nevus syndrome. *Courtesy Steven Binnick, MD.*

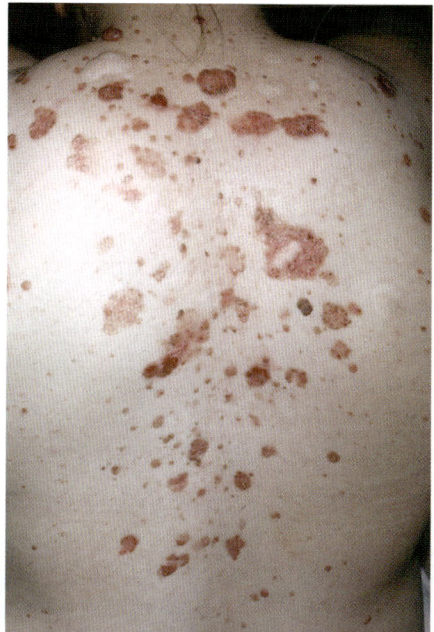

Fig. 29.50 Basal cell nevus syndrome. *Courtesy Steven Binnick, MD.*

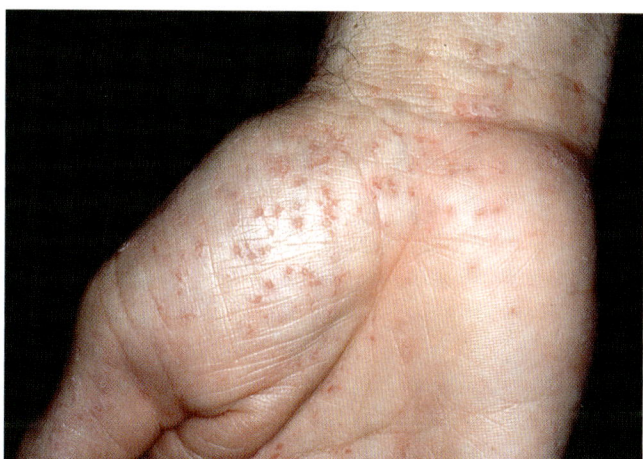

Fig. 29.51 Palmar pits in basal cell nevus syndrome.

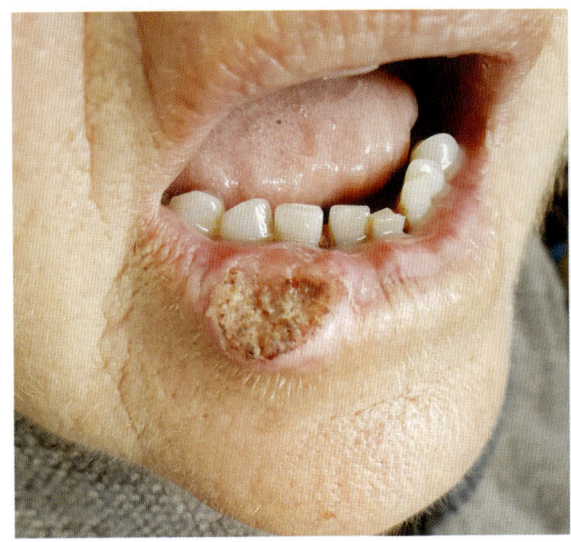

Fig. 29.52 Squamous cell carcinoma of the lip. *Courtesy Dr. Rui Carlos Taveres Bello.*

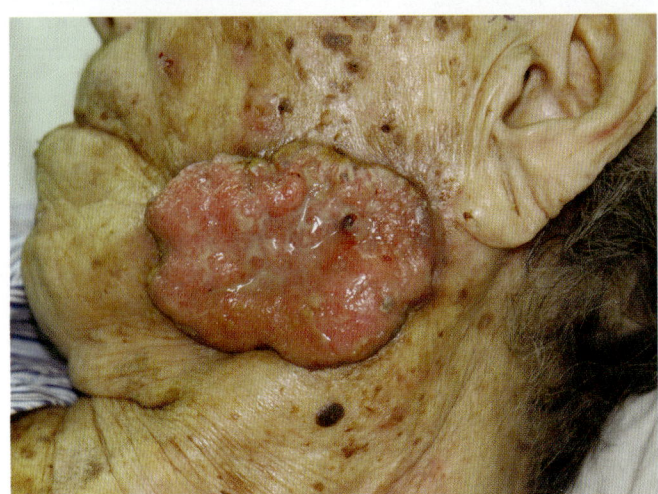

Fig. 29.53 Squamous cell carcinoma. *Courtesy Dr. Yi-Shuan Sheen.*

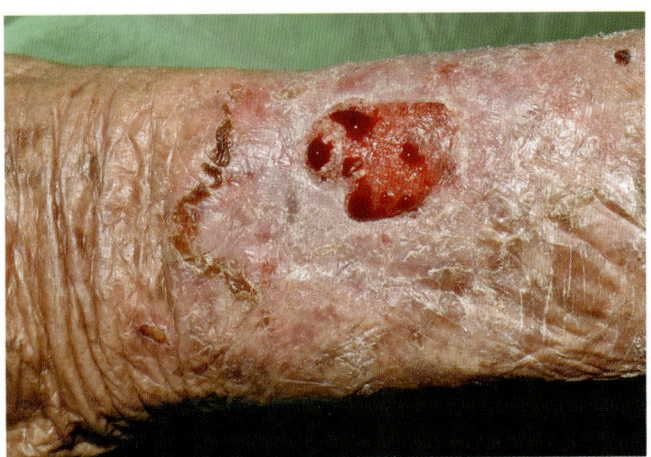

Fig. 29.54 Squamous cell carcinoma of the dorsal forearm. *Courtesy Dr. Yi-Shuan Sheen.*

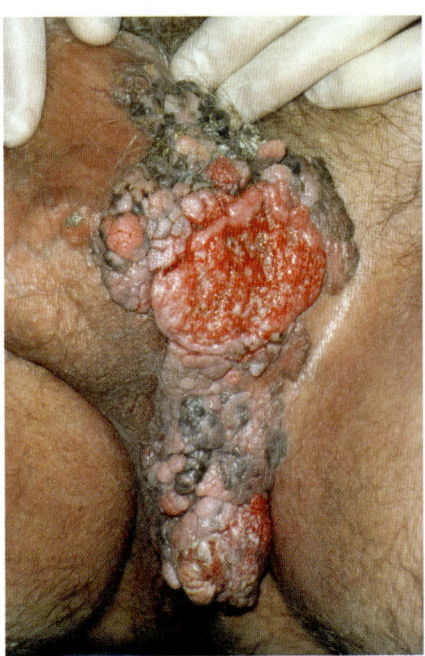

Fig. 29.55 Squamous cell carcinoma.

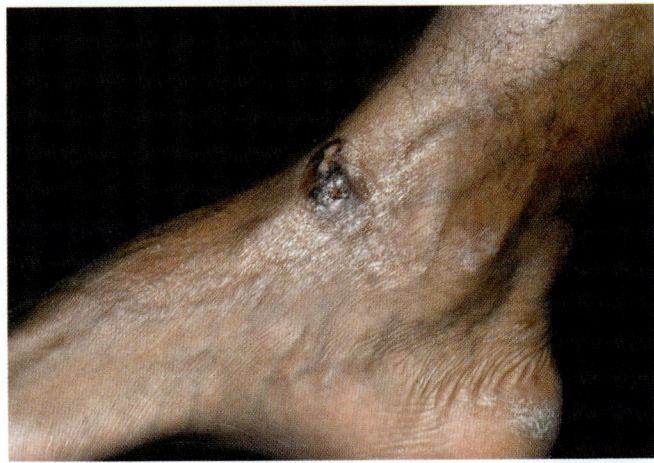

Fig. 29.56 Squamous cell carcinoma. *Courtesy Shyam Verma, MBBS, DVD.*

Fig. 29.57 Squamous cell carcinoma in an African American patient. *Courtesy Steven Binnick, MD.*

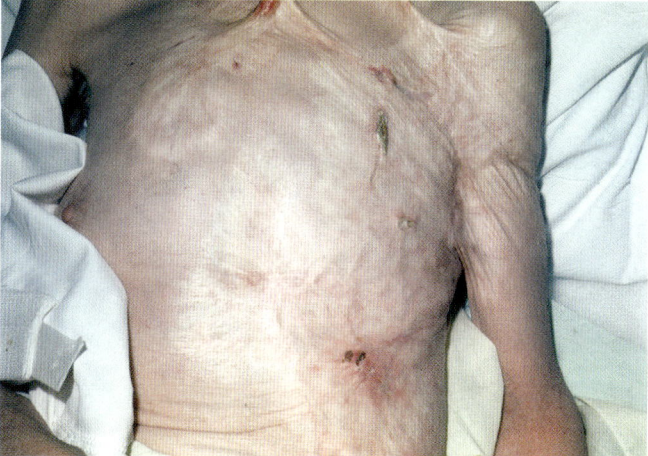

Fig. 29.58 Squamous cell carcinoma in a burn scar. *Courtesy Steven Binnick, MD.*

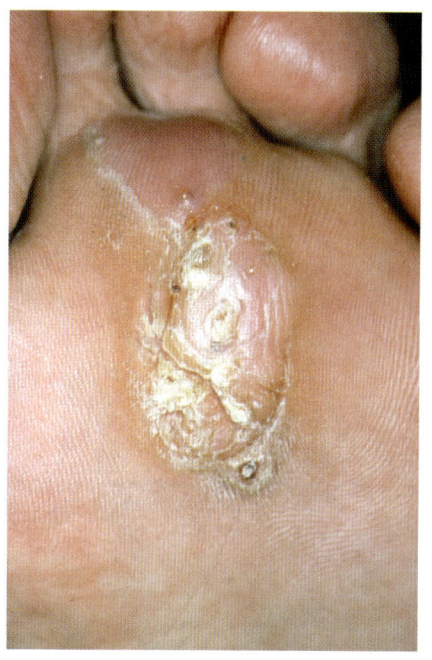

Fig. 29.59 Verrucous carcinoma.

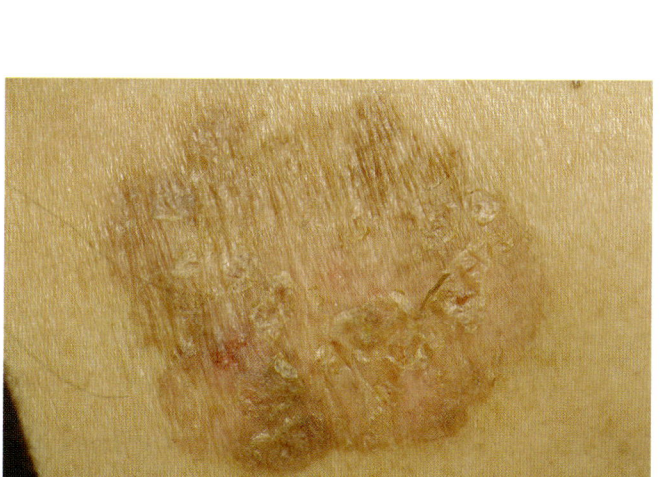

Fig. 29.60 Bowen disease. *Courtesy Yung-Tsu Cho, MD.*

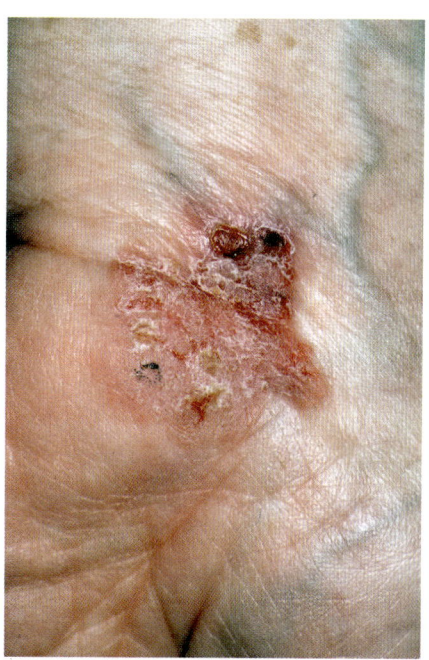

Fig. 29.61 Bowen disease. *Courtesy Steven Binnick, MD.*

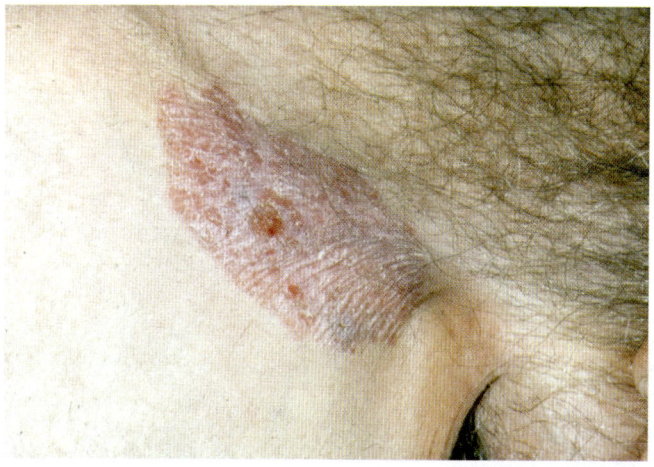

Fig. 29.62 Bowen disease.

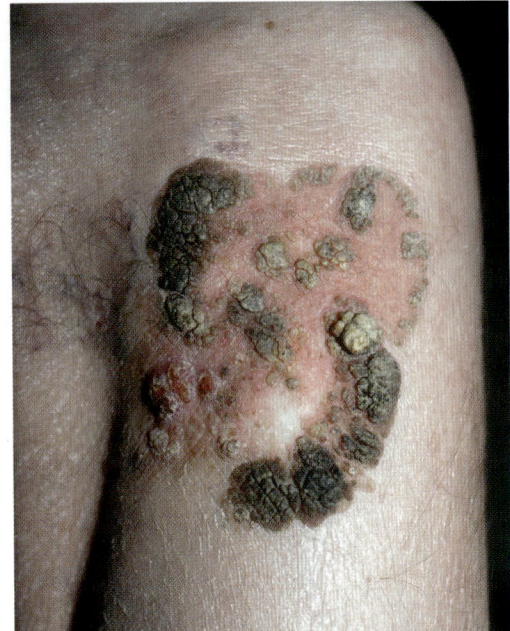

Fig. 29.63 Bowen disease with squamous cell carcinoma.

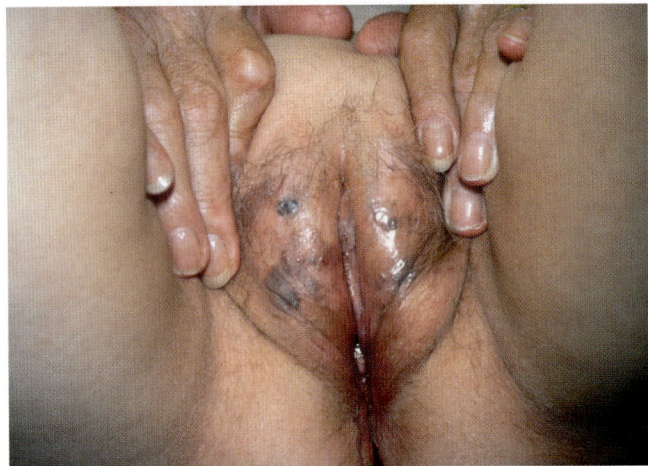

Fig. 29.65 Pigmented multicentric Bowen disease.

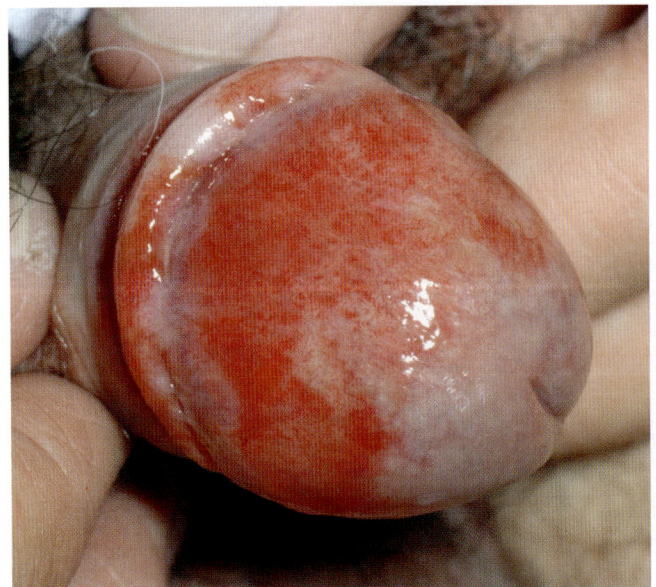

Fig. 29.67 Zoon balanitis.

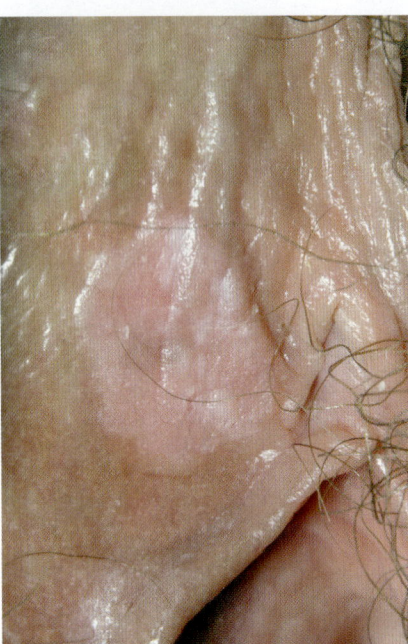

Fig. 29.64 Bowen disease.

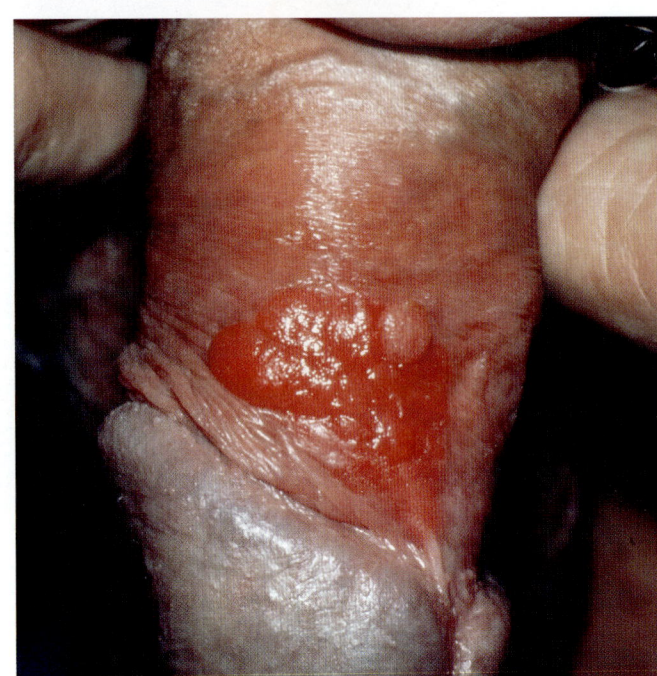

Fig. 29.66 Erythroplasia of Queyrat.

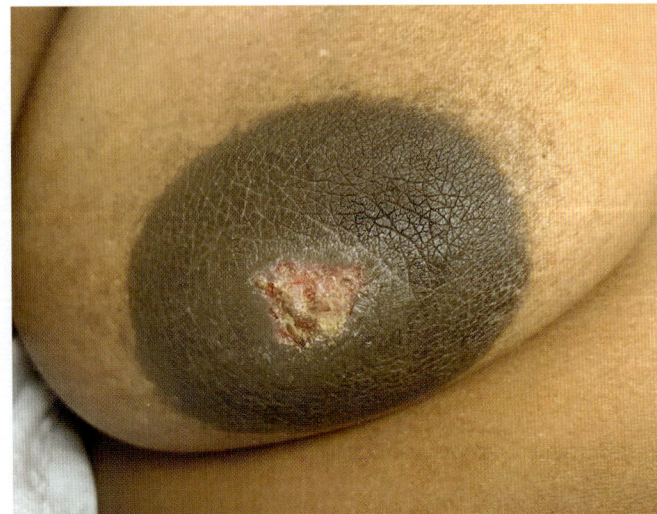

Fig. 29.68 Paget disease of the breast.

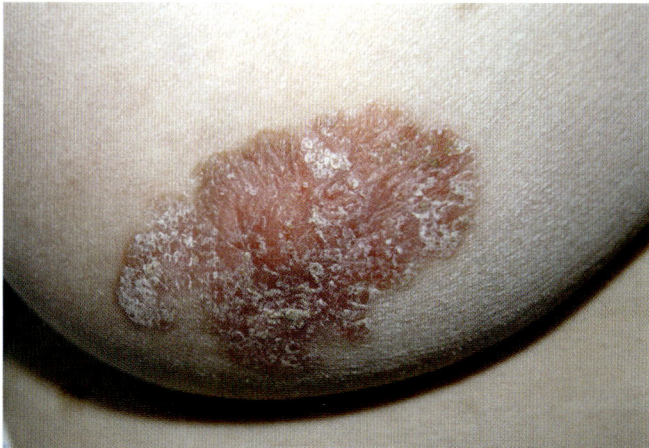

Fig. 29.69 Paget disease of the breast. *Courtesy Steven Binnick, MD.*

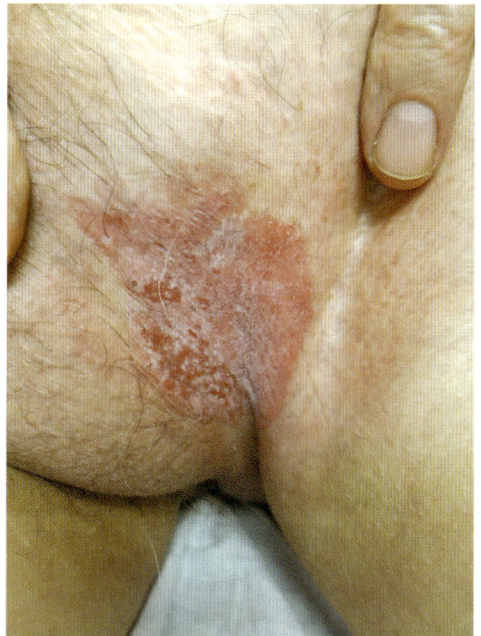

Fig. 29.71 Extramammary Paget disease.

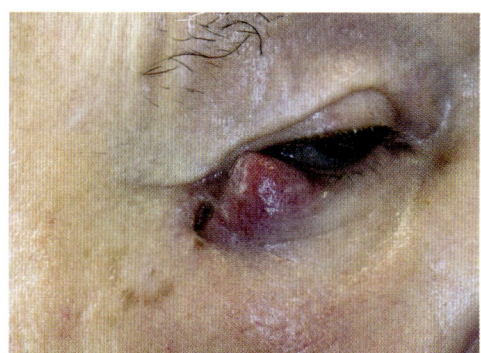

Fig. 29.73 Merkel cell carcinoma. *Courtesy Chris Miller, MD.*

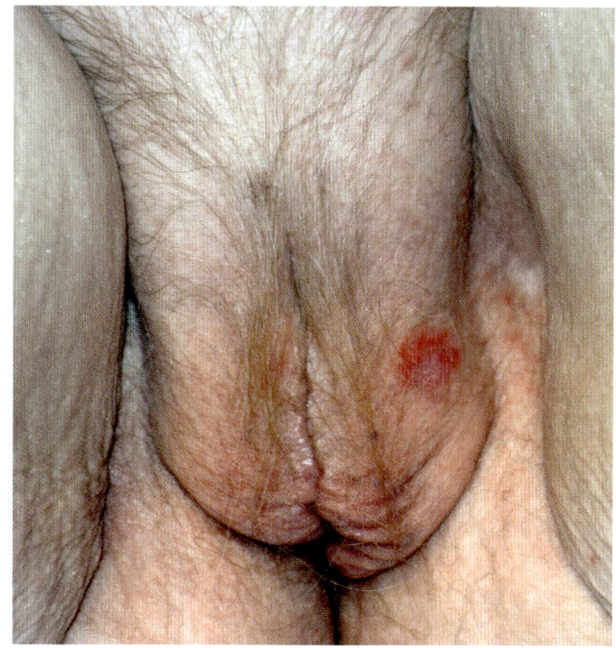

Fig. 29.70 Extramammary Paget disease. *Courtesy Steven Binnick, MD.*

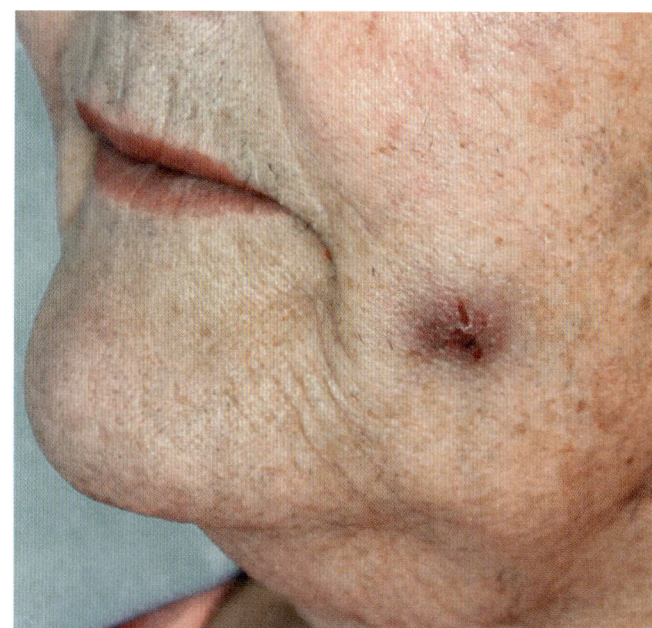

Fig. 29.72 Merkel cell carcinoma. *Courtesy Thuzar Shin, MD, PhD.*

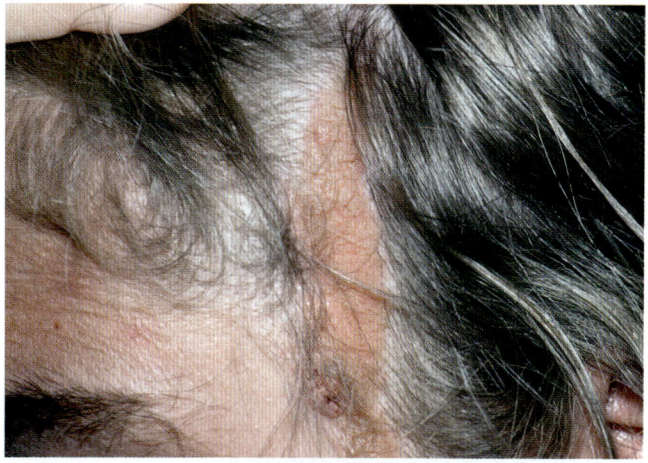

Fig. 29.74 Nevus sebaceous. *Courtesy Steven Binnick, MD.*

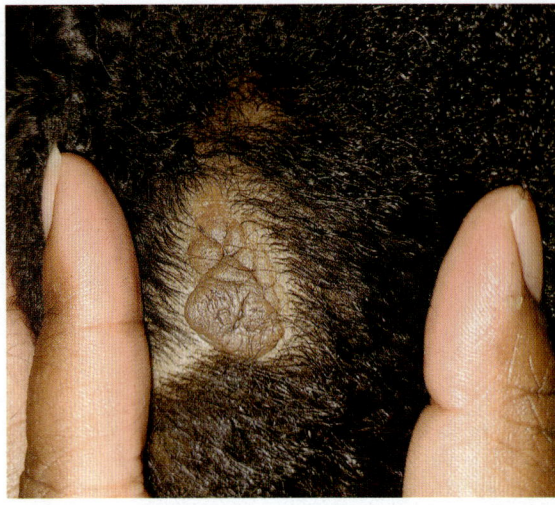

Fig. 29.75 Nevus sebaceous.

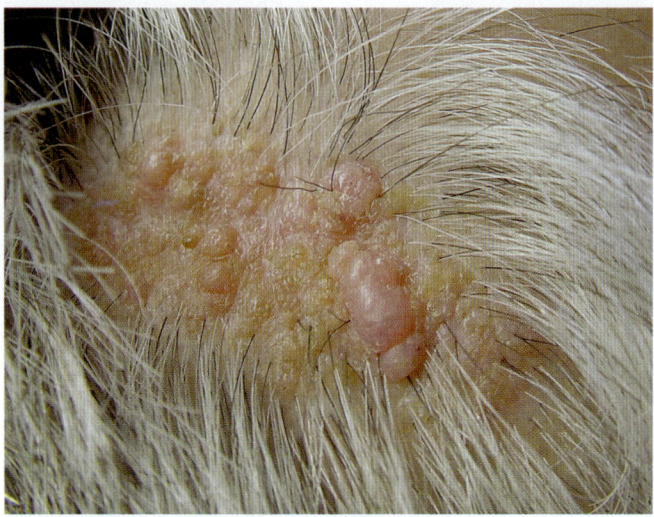

Fig. 29.76 Desmoplastic trichilemmoma arising in a nevus sebaceous of the scalp. *Courtesy Dr. Rui Carlos Taveres Bello.*

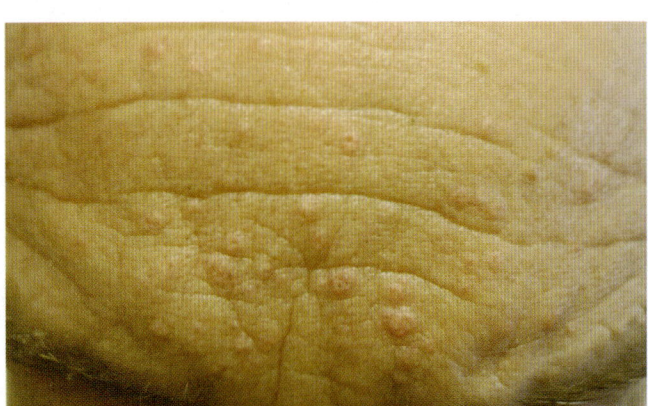

Fig. 29.77 Sebaceous hyperplasia.

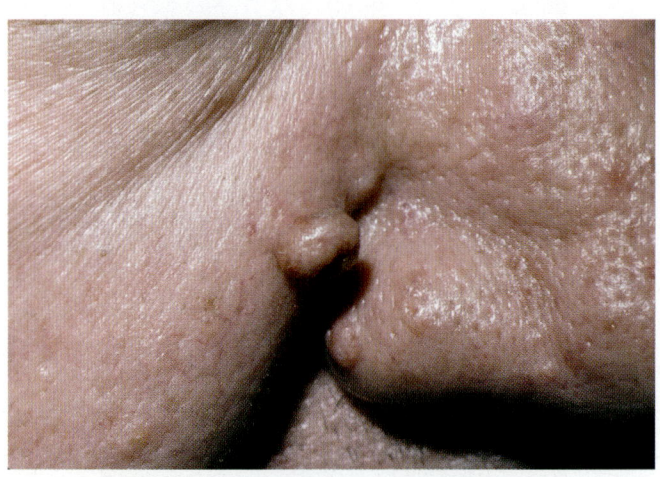

Fig. 29.78 Sebaceous adenomas of Muir Torre syndrome. *Courtesy Steven Binnick, MD.*

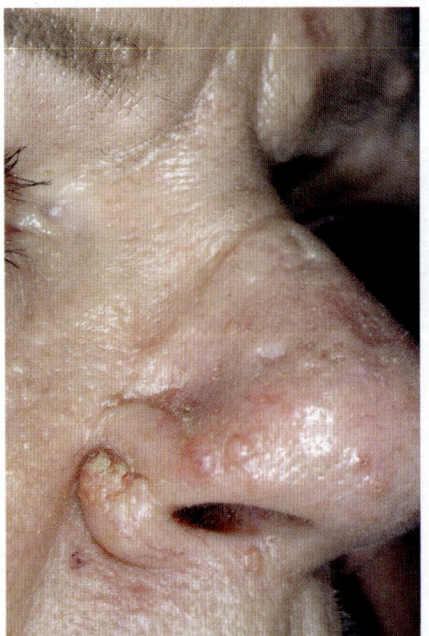

Fig. 29.79 Sebaceous adenomas of Muir Torre syndrome.

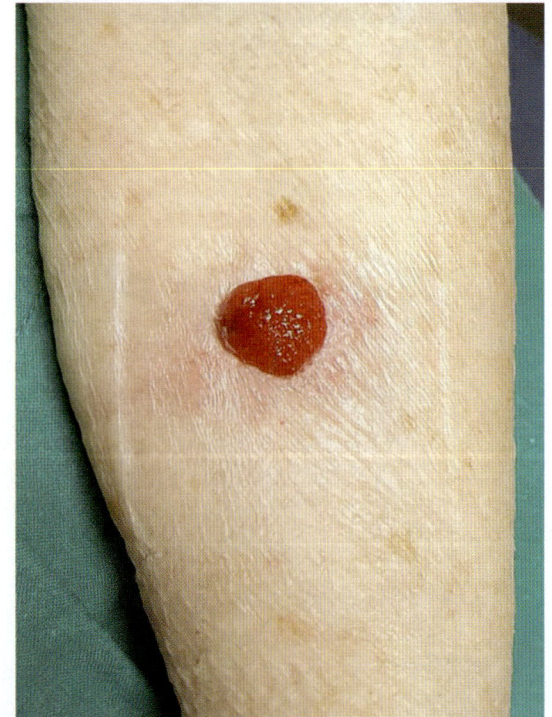

Fig. 29.80 Sebaceous carcinoma. *Courtesy Dr. Rui Carlos Taveres Bello.*

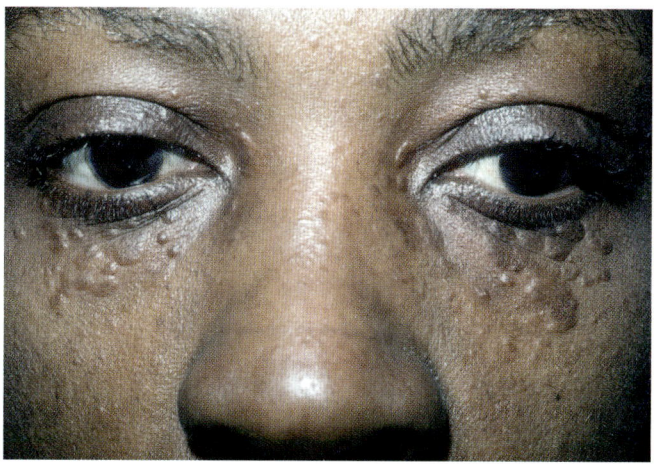

Fig. 29.81 Syringomas. *Courtesy Steven Binnick, MD.*

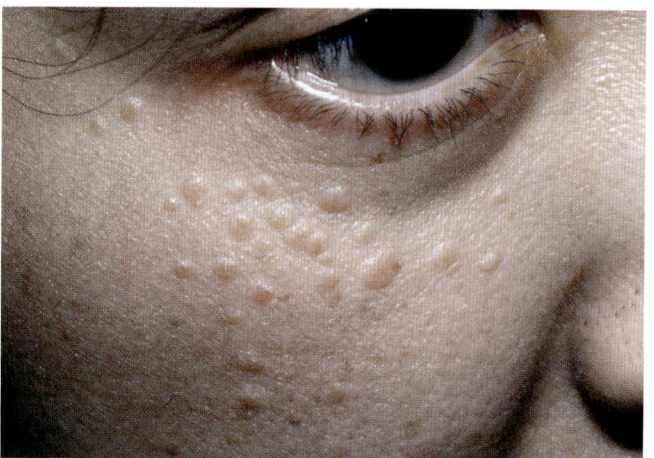

Fig. 29.82 Syringomas. *Courtesy Steven Binnick, MD.*

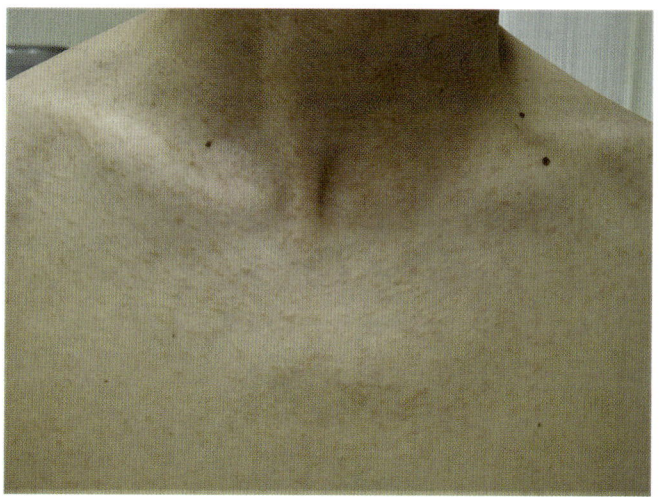

Fig. 29.83 Eruptive syringomas. *Courtesy Dr. Rui Carlos Taveres Bello.*

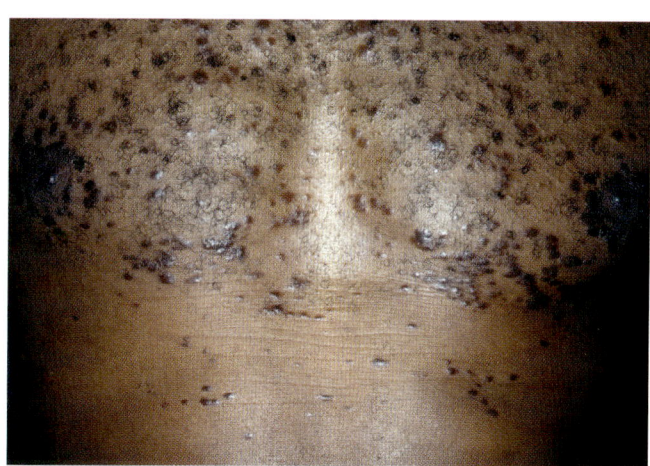

Fig. 29.84 Syringomas.

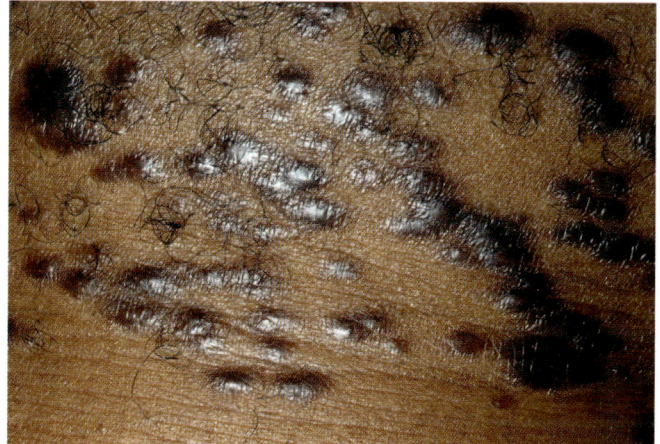

Fig. 29.85 Syringomas.

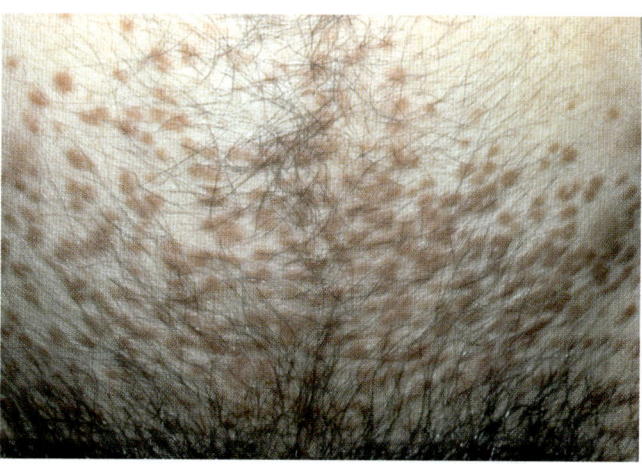

Fig. 29.86 Syringomas.

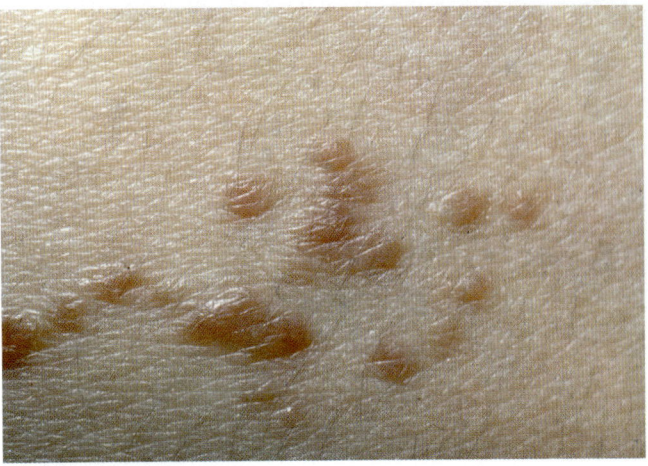

Fig. 29.87 Syringomas.

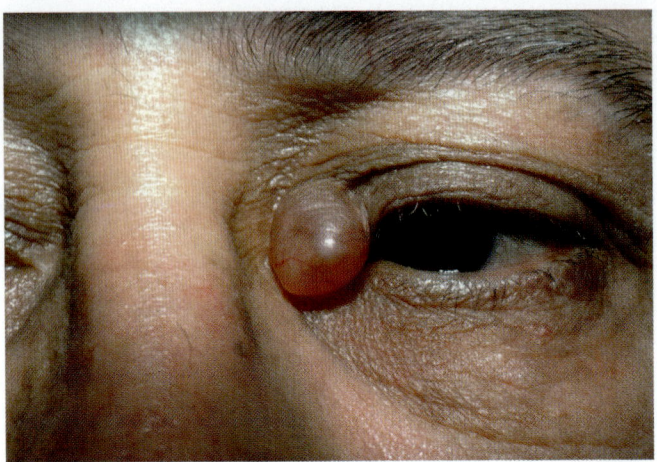

Fig. 29.88 Hidrocystoma.

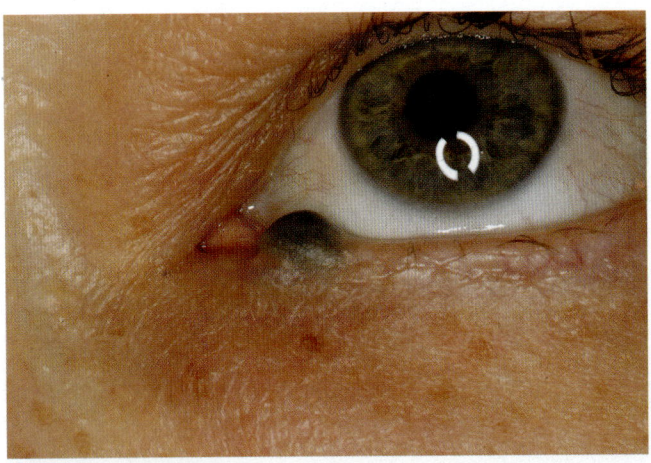

Fig. 29.89 Hidrocystoma.

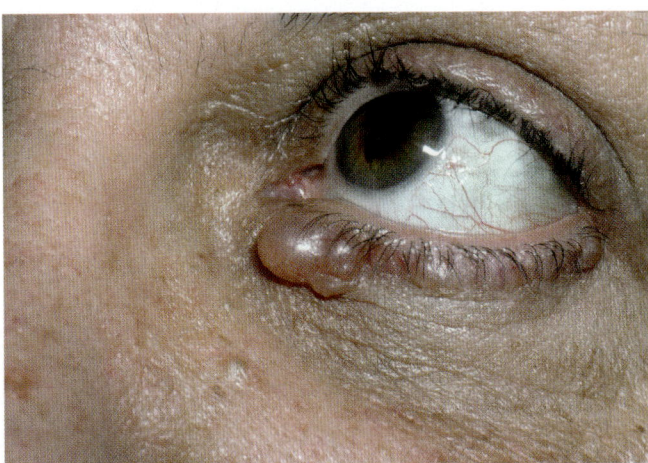

Fig. 29.90 Hidrocystoma. *Courtesy Steven Binnick, MD.*

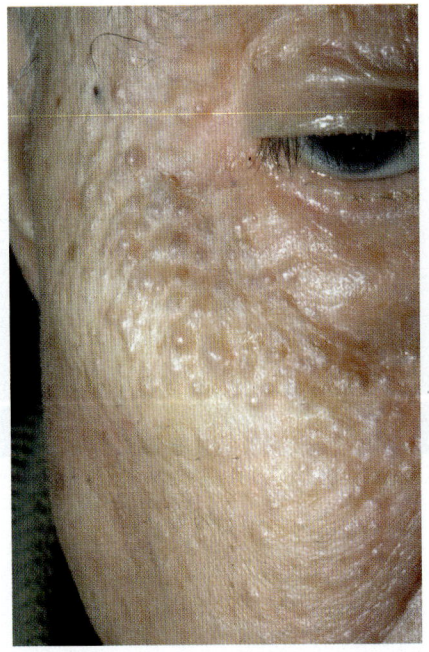

Fig. 29.91 Multiple hidrocystomas.

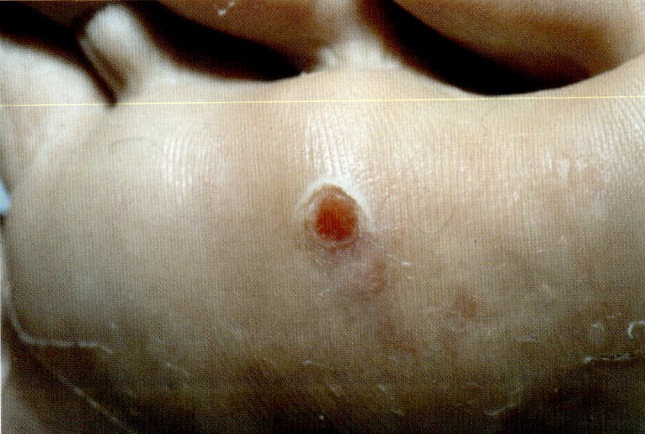

Fig. 29.92 Eccrine poroma.

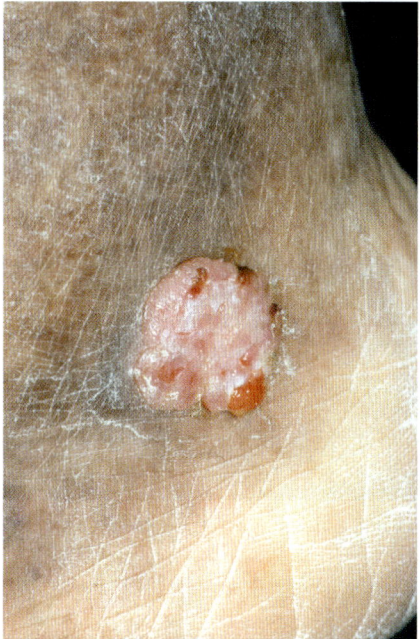

Fig. 29.93 Eccrine poroma.

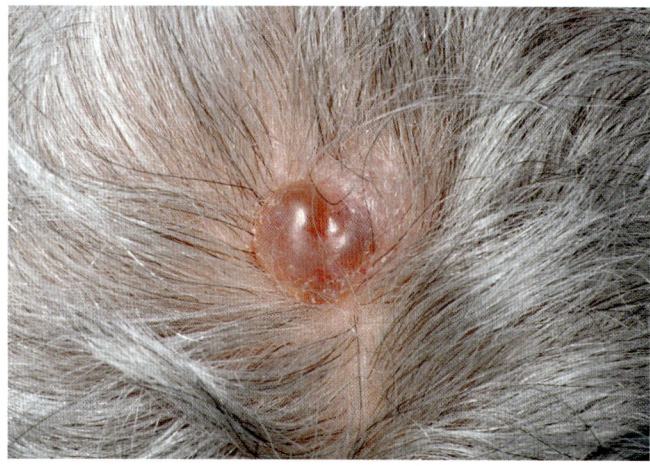

Fig. 29.94 Nodular hidradenoma. *Courtesy Steven Binnick, MD.*

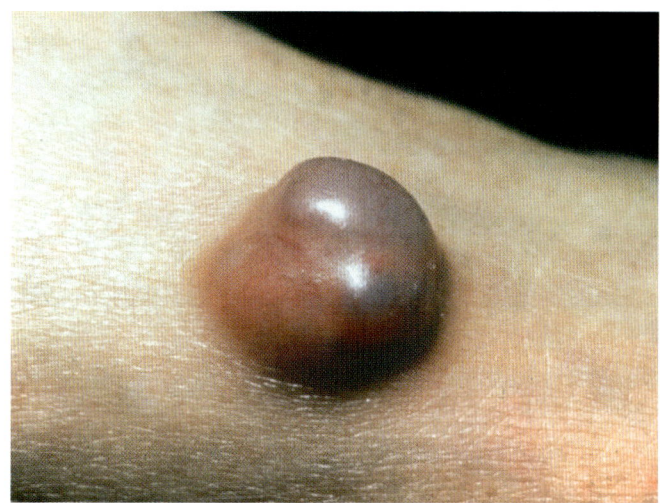

Fig. 29.95 Eccrine acrospiroma.

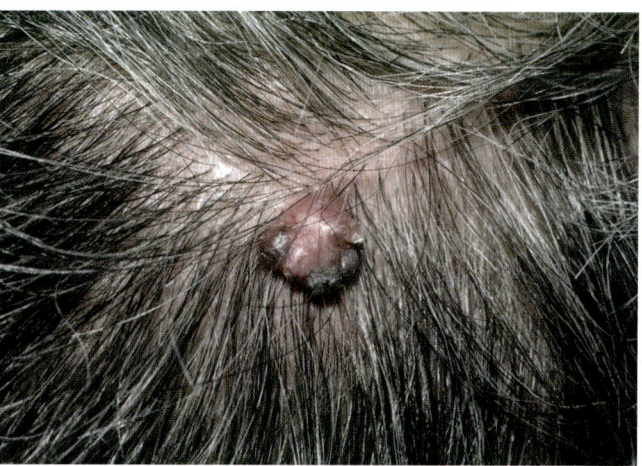

Fig. 29.96 Eccrine spiradenoma. *Courtesy Steven Binnick, MD.*

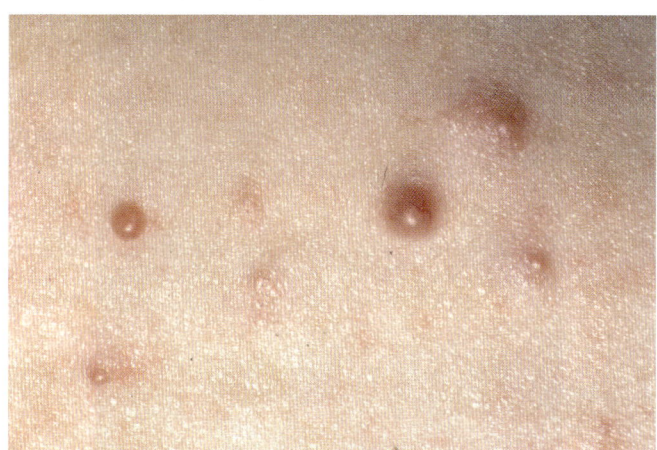

Fig. 29.97 Multiple acrospiromas. *Courtesy Steven Binnick, MD.*

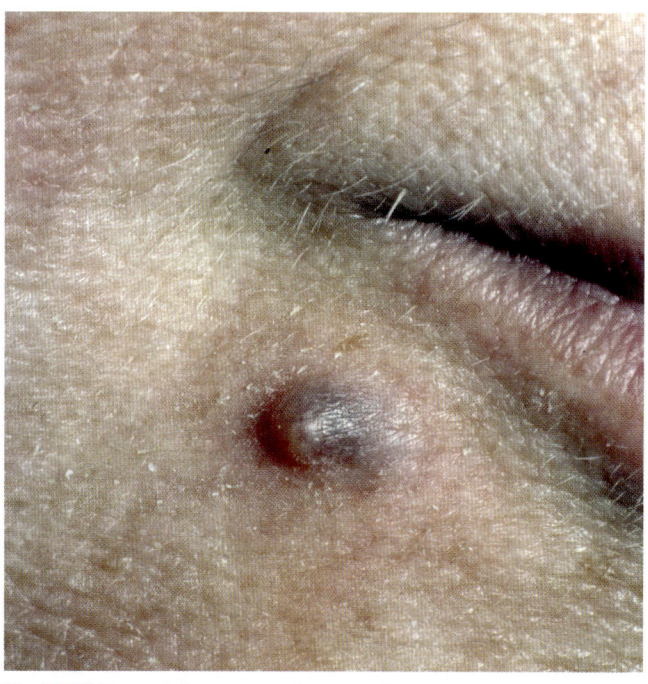

Fig. 29.98 Dermal duct tumor. *Courtesy Steven Binnick, MD.*

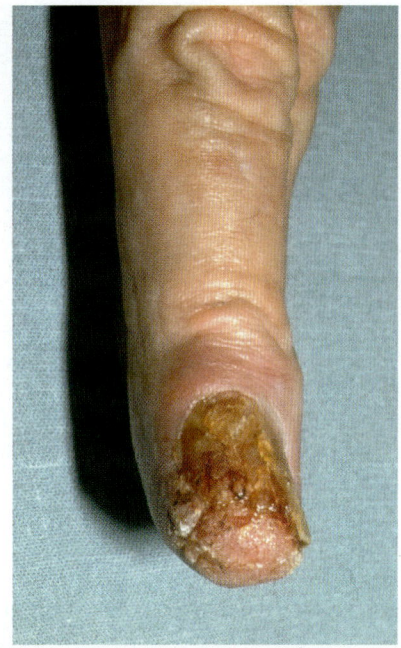

Fig. 29.99 Eccrine porocarcinoma.

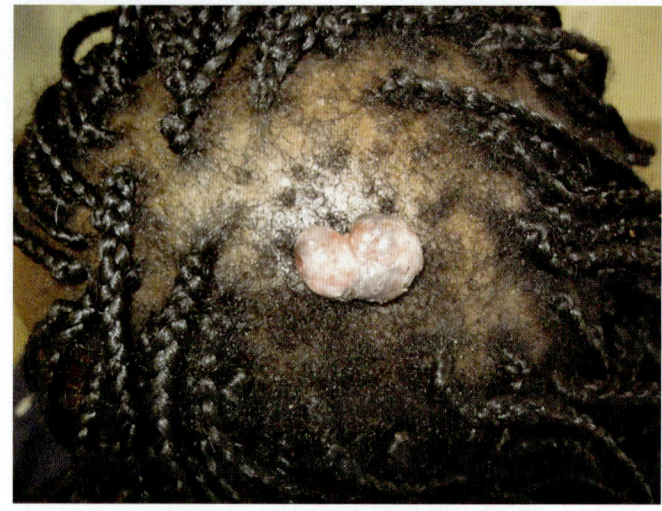

Fig. 29.100 Eccrine porocarcinoma. *Courtesy Chris Miller, MD.*

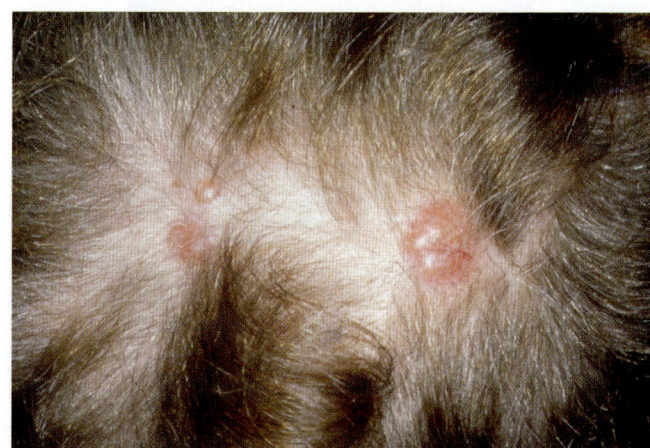

Fig. 29.102 Multiple cylindromas.

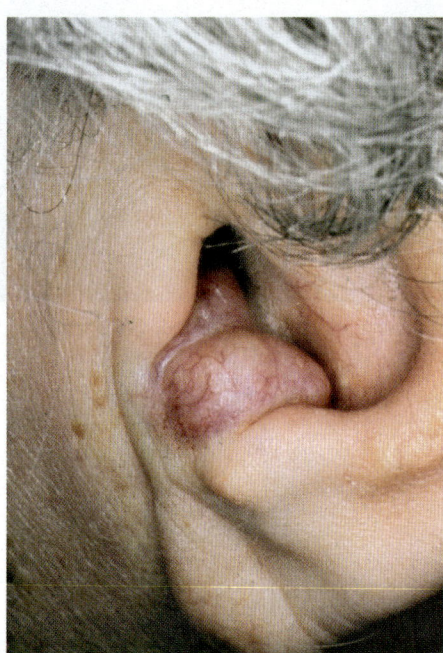

Fig. 29.101 Cylindroma.

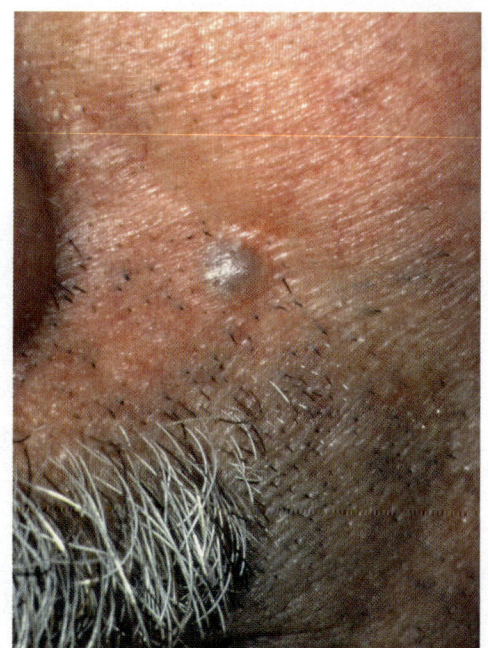

Fig. 29.103 Chondroid syringoma.

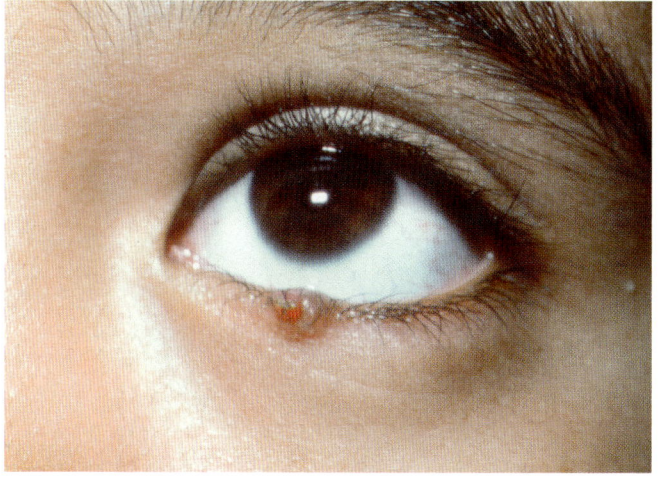

Fig. 29.104 Syringocystadenoma papilliferum.

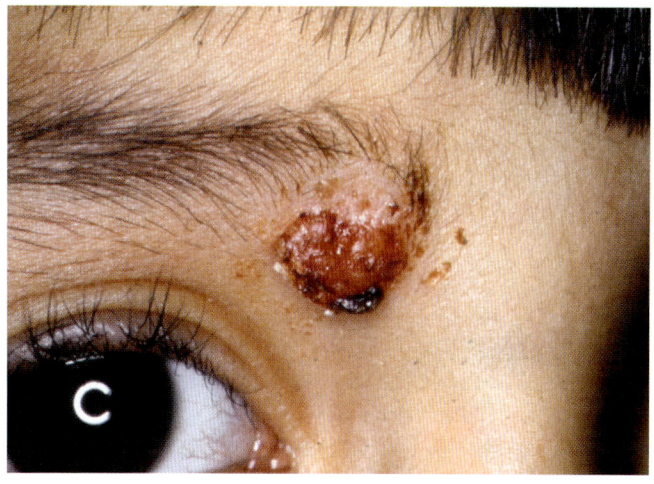

Fig. 29.105 Syringocystadenoma papilliferum.

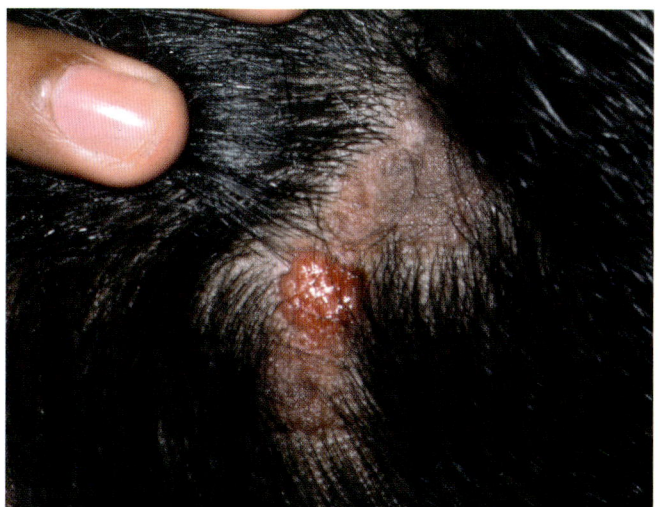

Fig. 29.106 Syringocystadenoma papilliferum in nevus sebaceous. *Courtesy Steven Binnick, MD.*

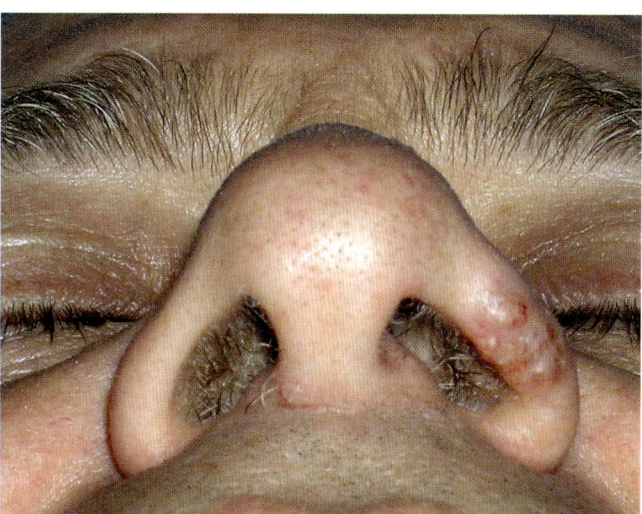

Fig. 29.107 Microcystic adnexal carcinoma. *Courtesy Chris Miller, MD.*

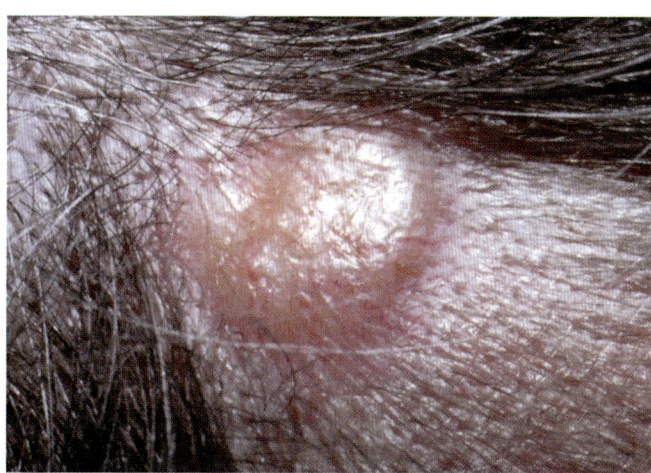

Fig. 29.108 Eccrine carcinoma.

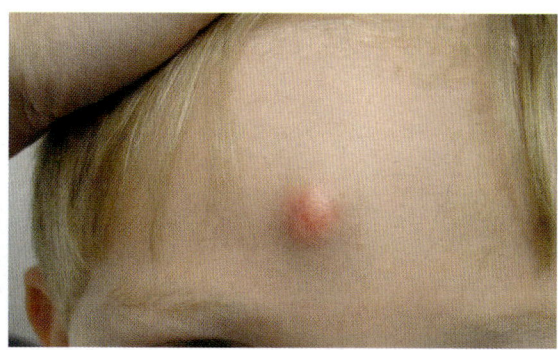

Fig. 29.109 Pilomatricoma. *Courtesy Scott Bartlett, MD.*

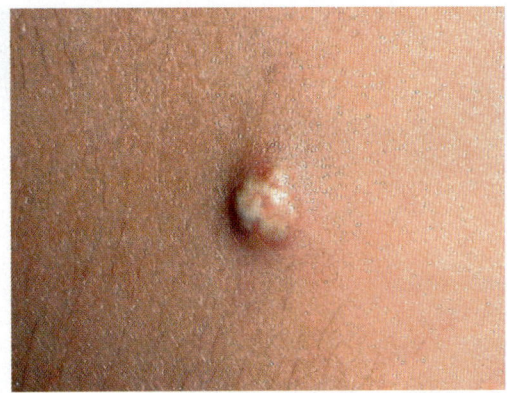

Fig. 29.110 Pilomatricoma.

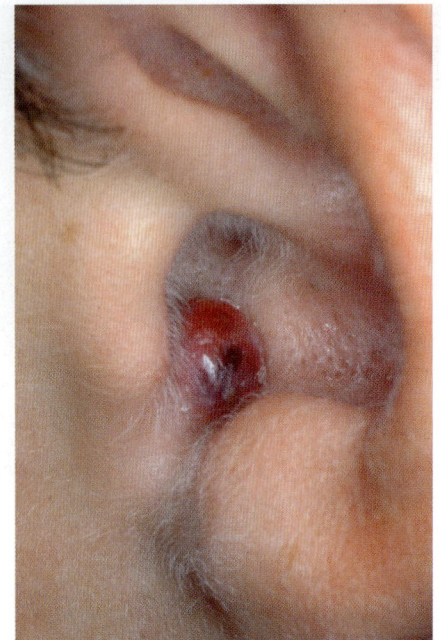

Fig. 29.111 Pilomatricoma. *Courtesy Curt Samlaska, MD.*

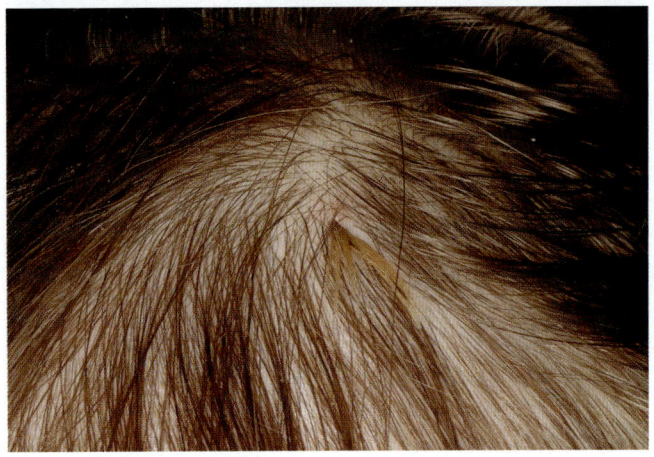

Fig. 29.112 Trichofolliculoma.

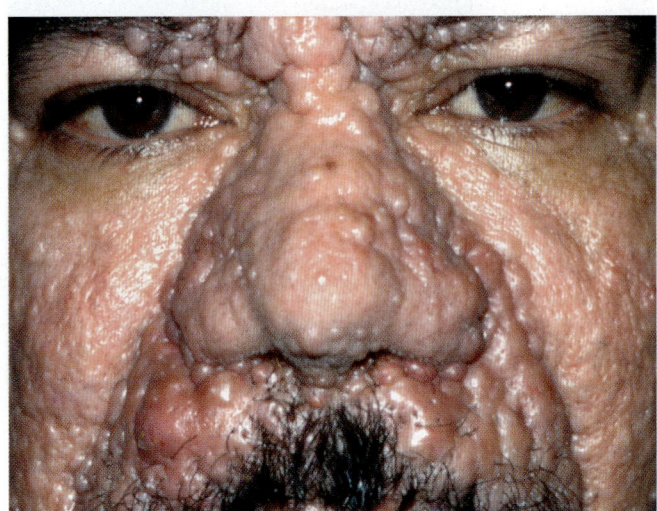

Fig. 29.113 Brooke-Spiegler syndrome.

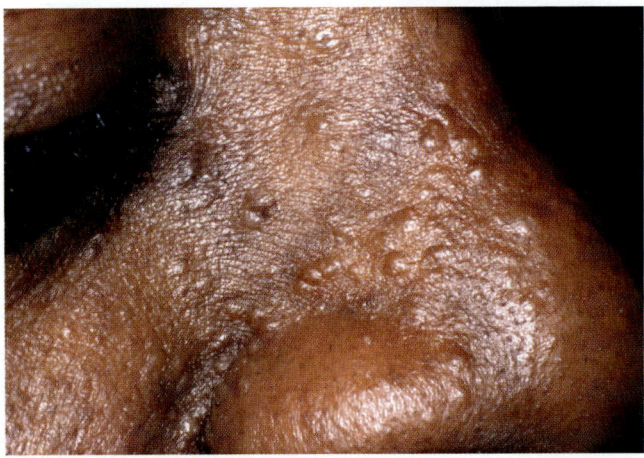

Fig. 29.114 Brooke-Spiegler syndrome.

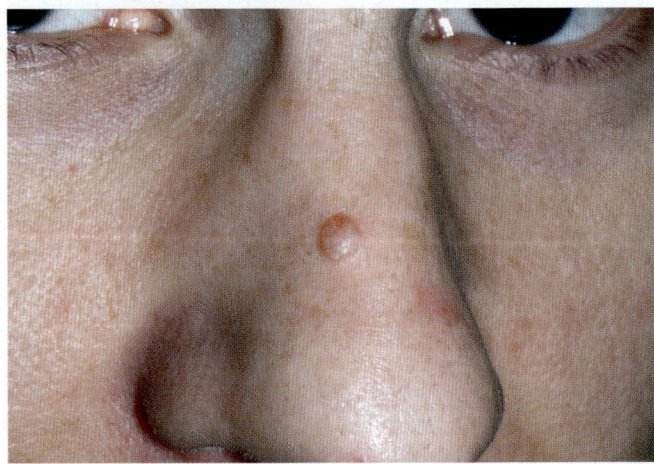

Fig. 29.115 Solitary trichoepithelioma.

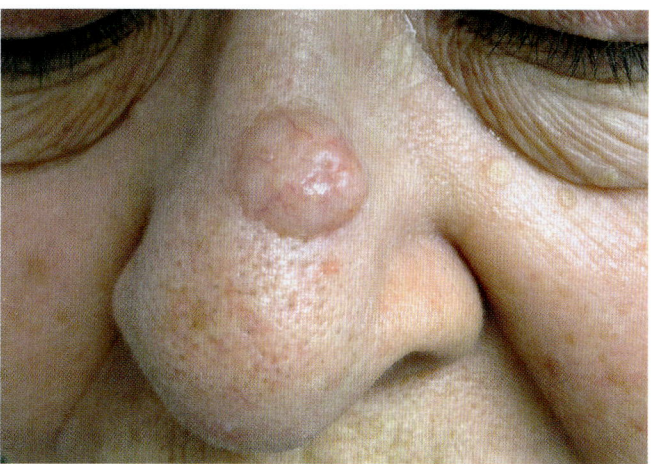

Fig. 29.116 Giant trichoepithelioma. *Courtesy Patrick Carrington, MD.*

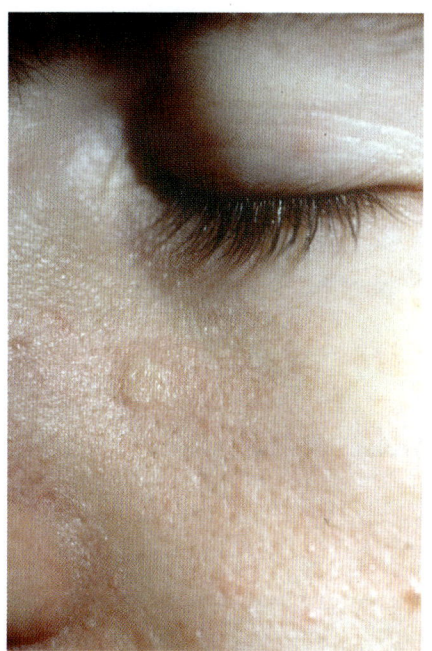

Fig. 29.117 Desmoplastic trichoepithelioma.

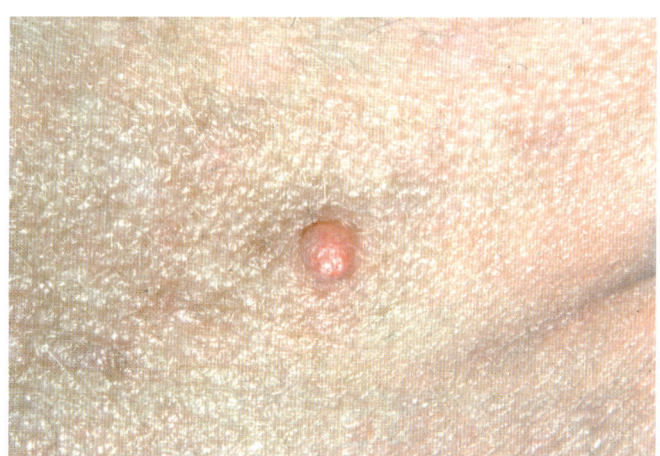

Fig. 29.118 Solitary trichilemmoma.

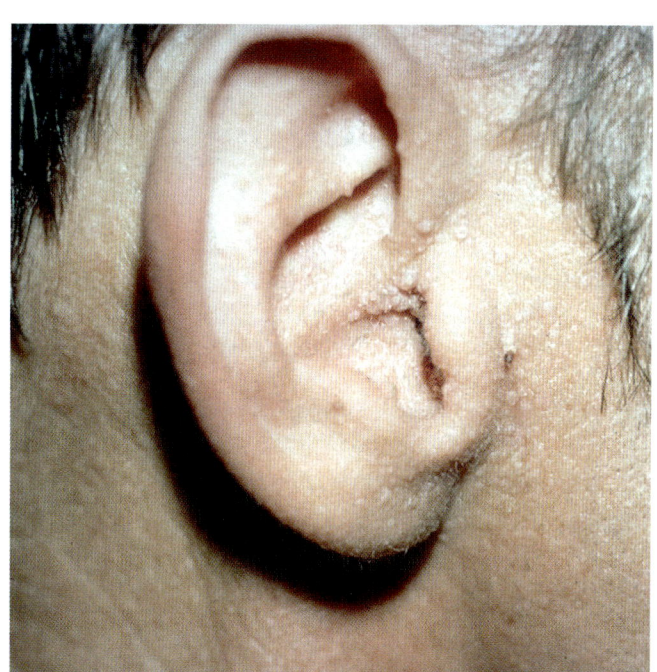

Fig. 29.119 Cowden syndrome.

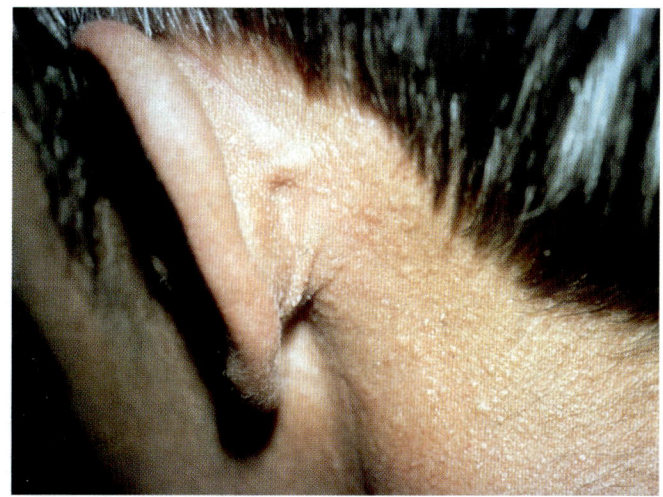

Fig. 29.120 Cowden syndrome.

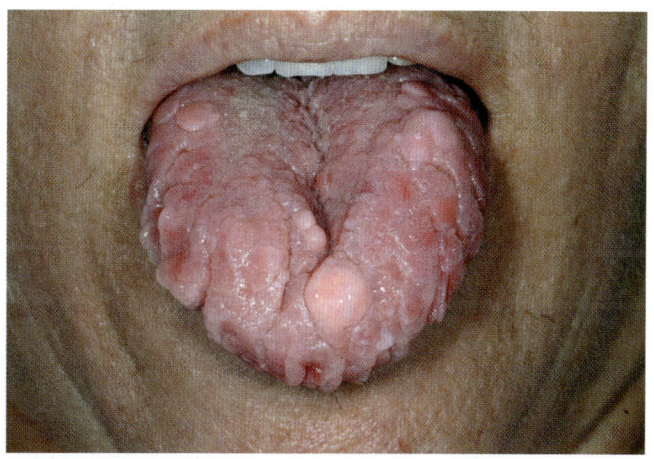

Fig. 29.121 Oral papillomas in Cowden syndrome.

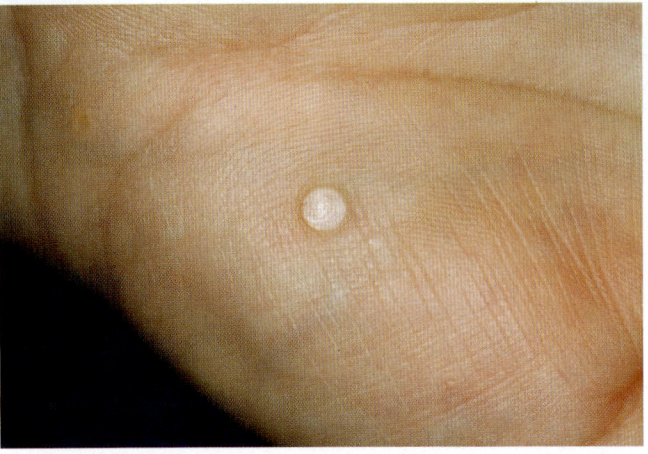

Fig. 29.122 Sclerotic fibroma.

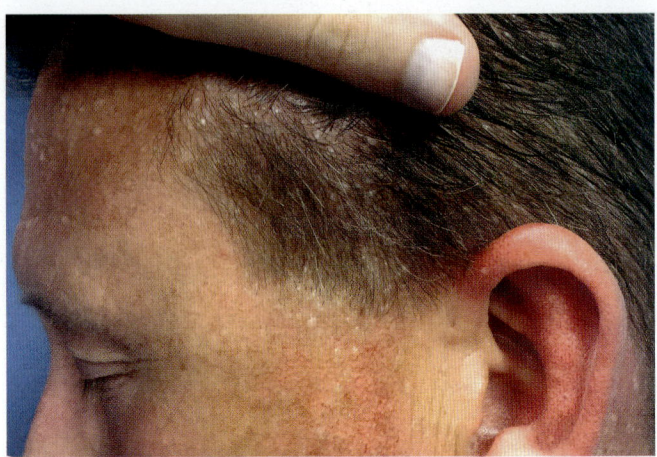

Fig. 29.123 Birt-Hogg-Dubé syndrome.

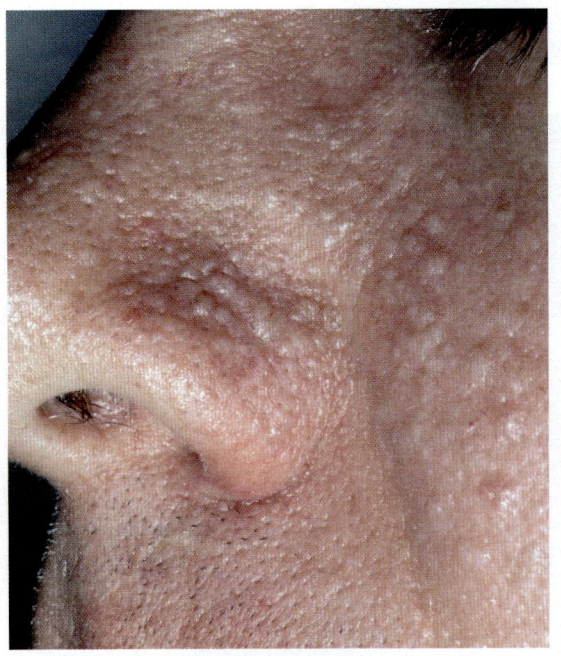

Fig. 29.124 Birt-Hogg-Dubé syndrome.

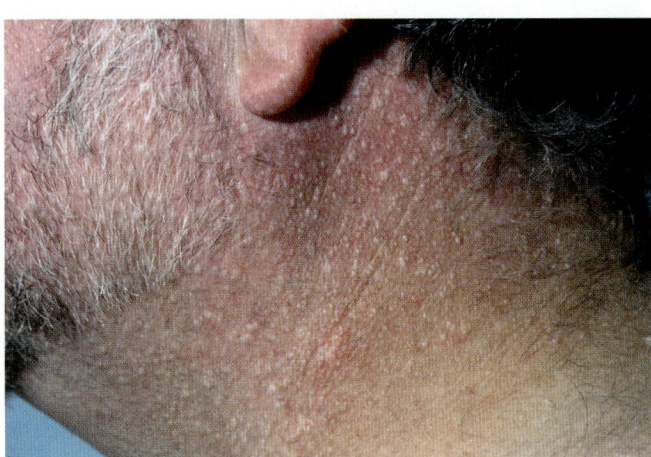

Fig. 29.125 Birt-Hogg-Dubé syndrome.

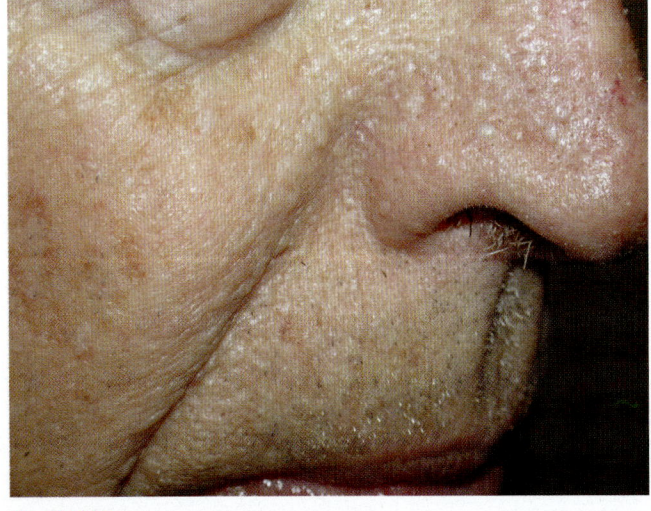

Fig. 29.126 Birt-Hogg-Dubé syndrome.

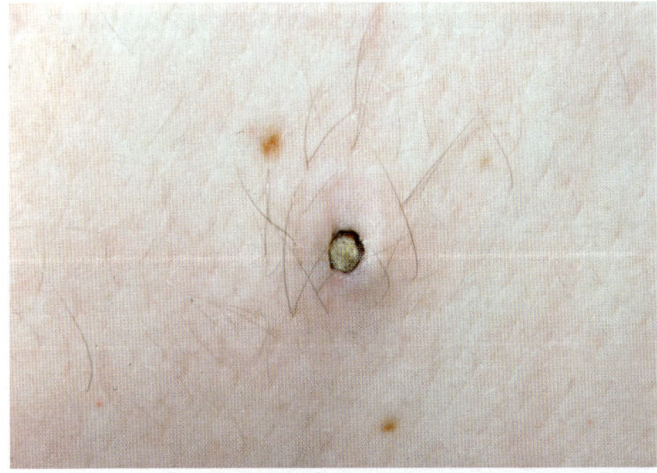

Fig. 29.127 Pore of Winer.

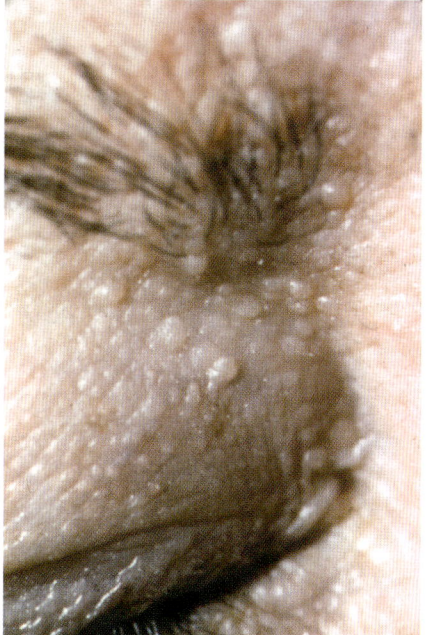

Fig. 29.128 Basaloid follicular hamartoma.

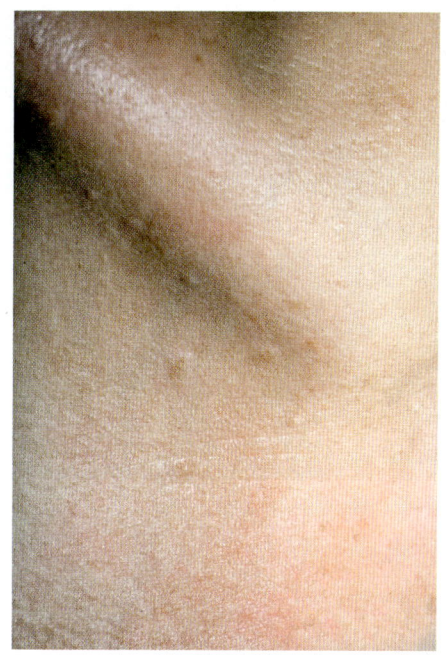

Fig. 29.129 Tumor of the follicular infundibulum.

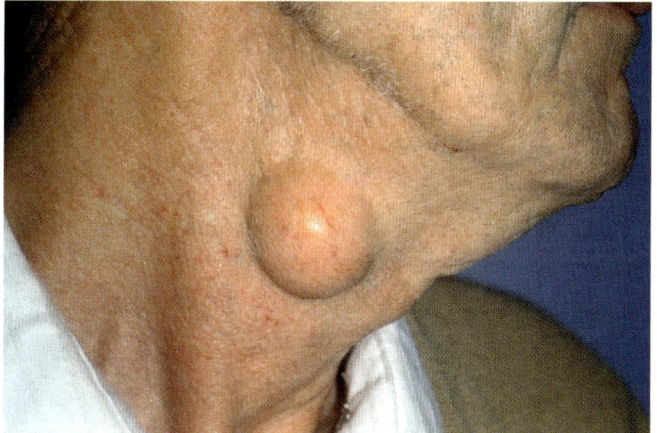

Fig. 29.130 Epidermal inclusion cyst.

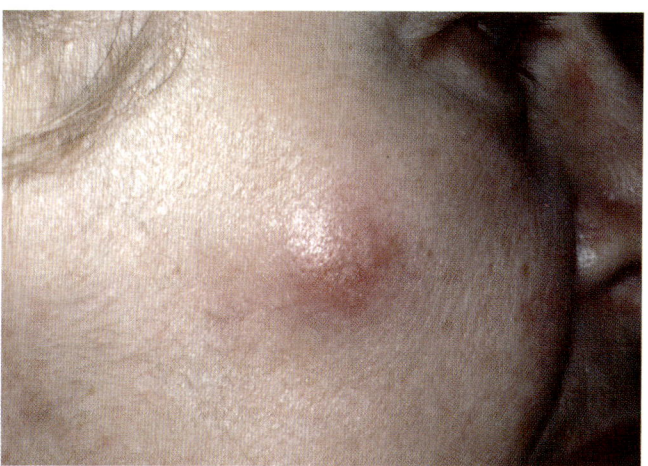

Fig. 29.131 Inflamed epidermal inclusion cyst. *Courtesy Steven Binnick, MD.*

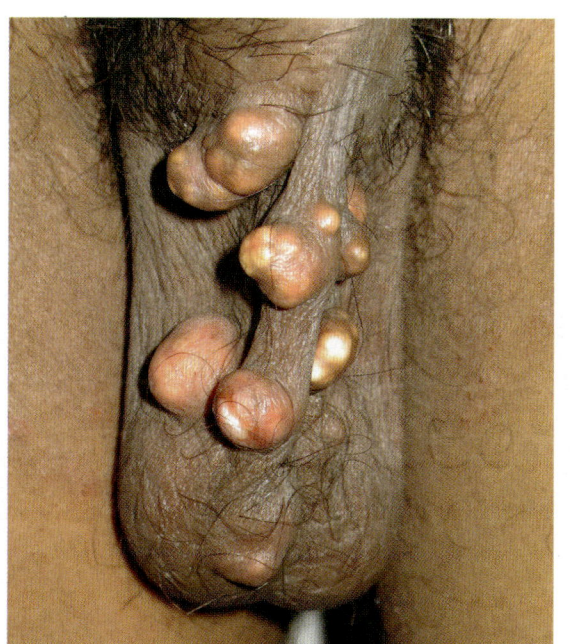

Fig. 29.132 Scrotal cysts.

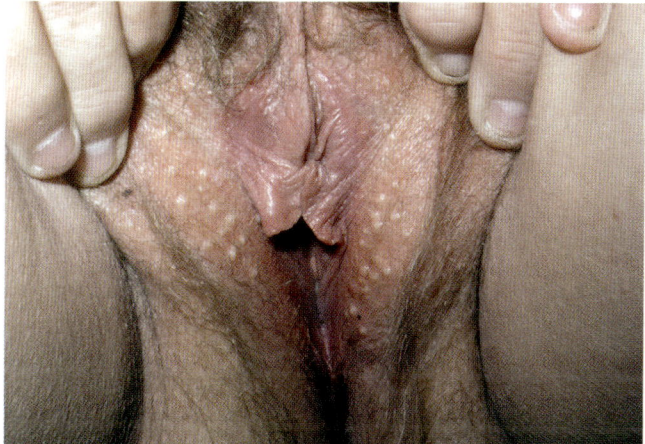

Fig. 29.133 Labial cysts. *Courtesy Steven Binnick, MD.*

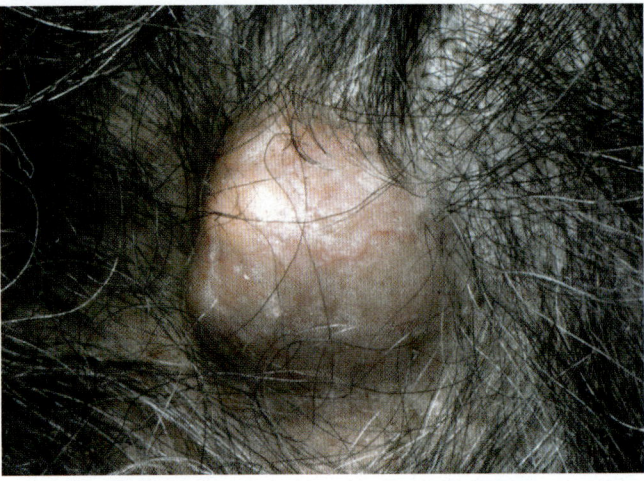

Fig. 29.134 Pilar cyst.

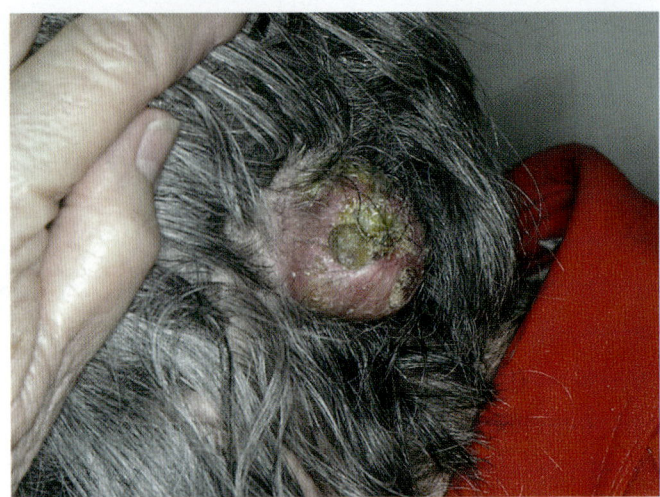

Fig. 29.135 Proliferating pilar cyst.

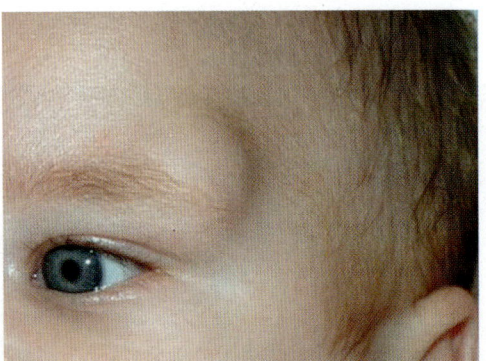

Fig. 29.136 Dermoid cyst. *Courtesy Scott Bartlett, MD.*

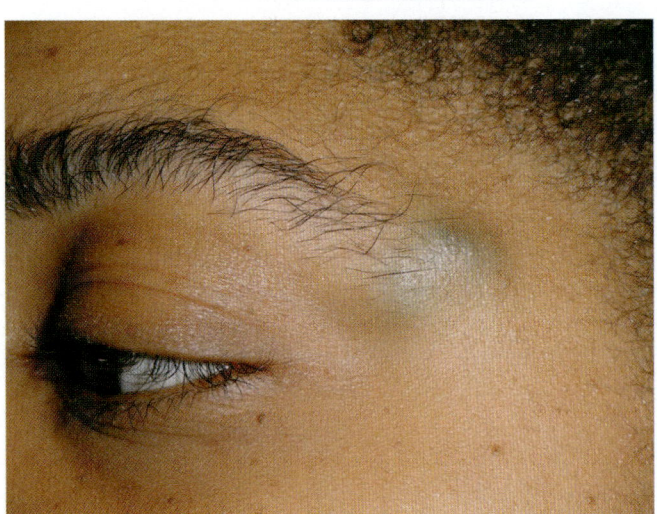

Fig. 29.137 Dermoid cyst. *Courtesy Scott Norton, MD.*

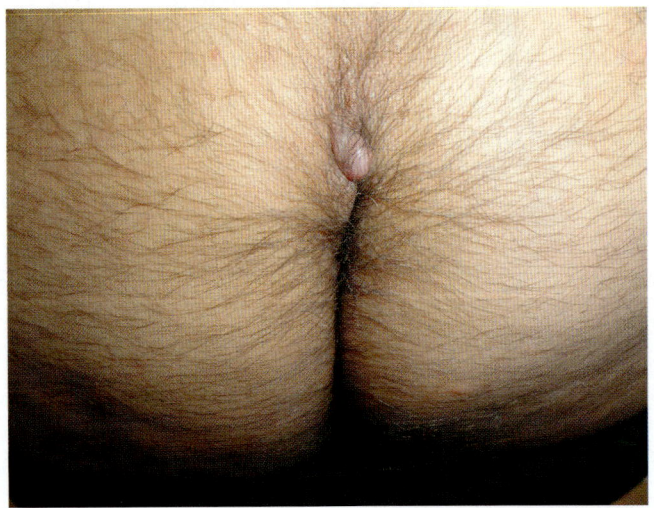

Fig. 29.138 Pilonidal cyst. *Courtesy Scott Norton, MD.*

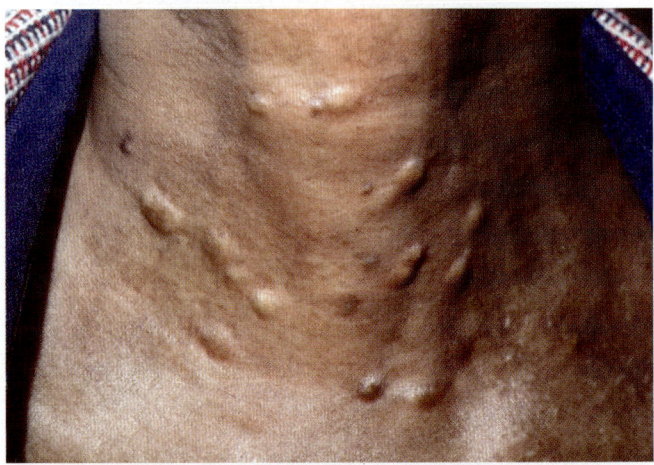

Fig. 29.139 Steatocystoma multiplex. *Courtesy Steven Binnick, MD.*

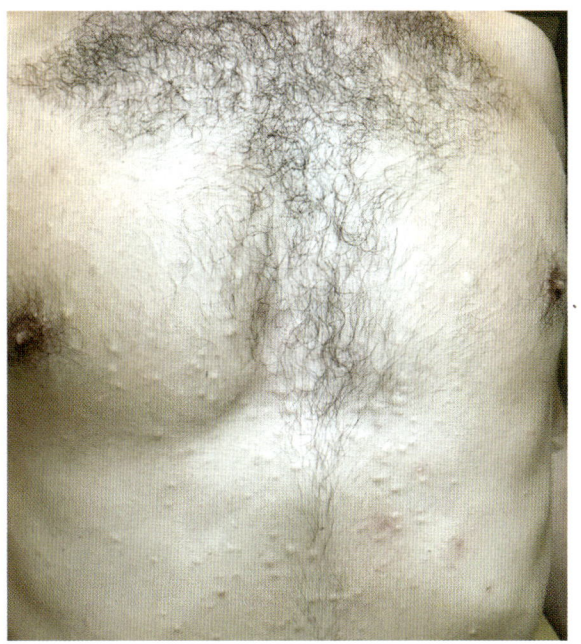

Fig. 29.140 Steatocystoma multiplex.

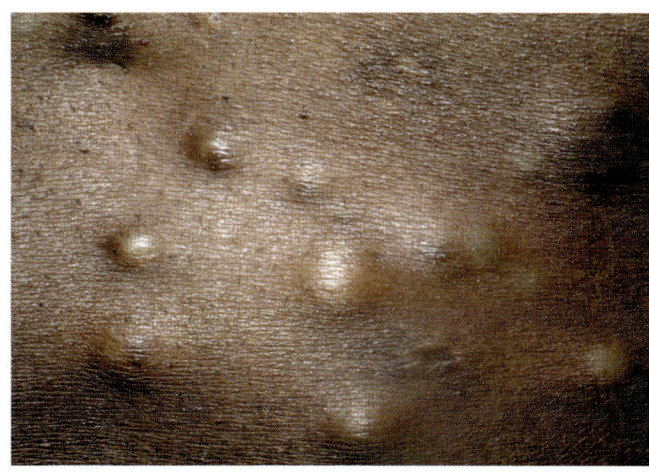

Fig. 29.141 Steatocystoma multiplex. *Courtesy Steven Binnick, MD.*

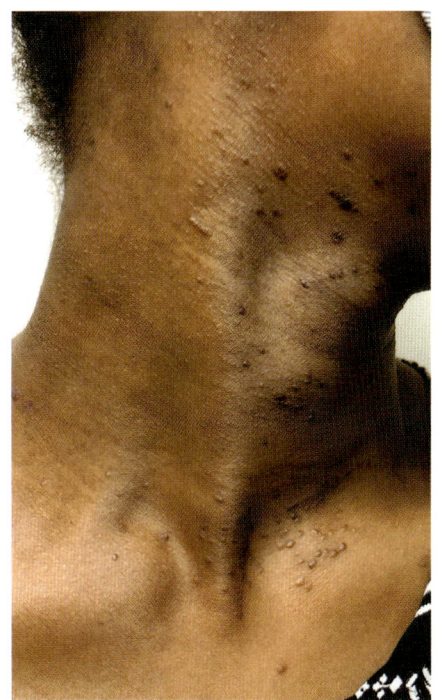

Fig. 29.142 Eruptive vellus hair cysts.

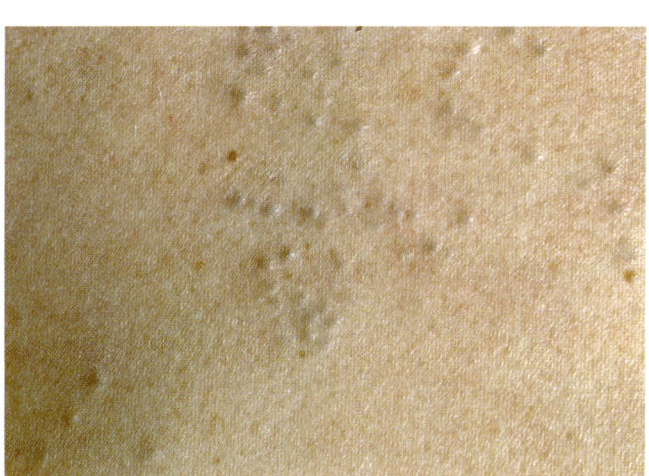

Fig. 29.143 Eruptive vellus hair cysts.

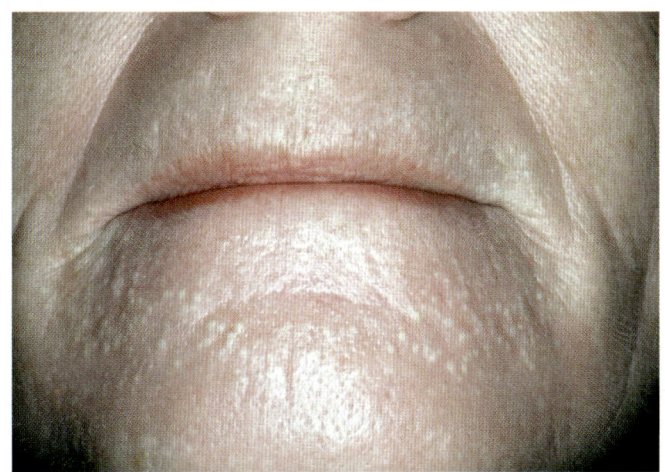

Fig. 29.144 Milia. *Courtesy Steven Binnick, MD.*

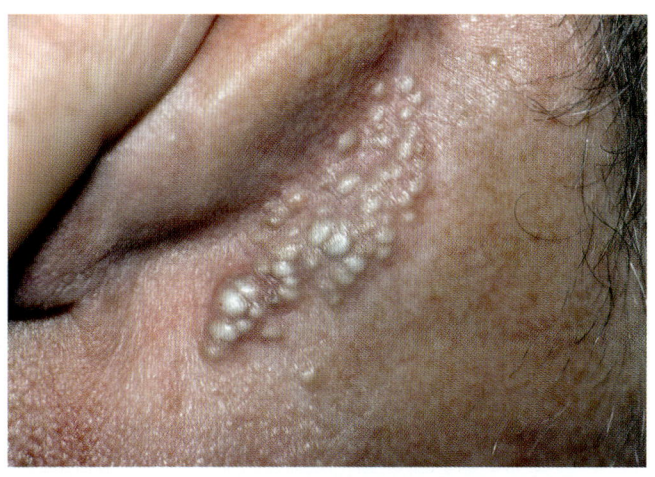

Fig. 29.145 Milia en plaque. *Courtesy Steven Binnick, MD.*

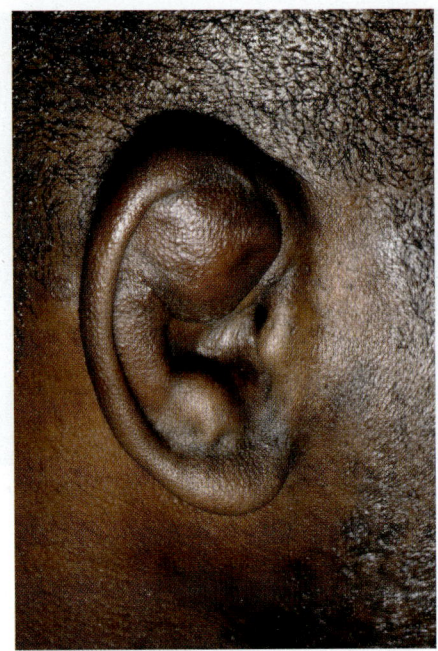

Fig. 29.146 Auricular pseudocyst.

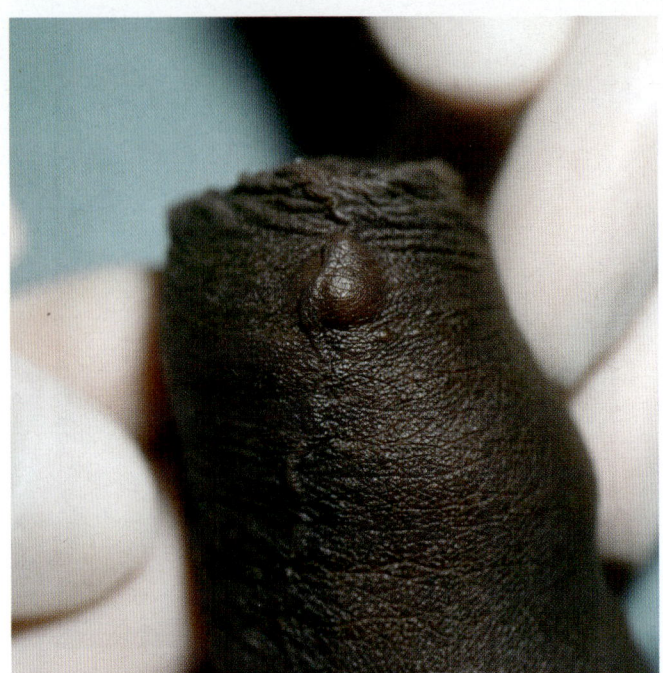

Fig. 29.147 Median raphe cyst. *Courtesy Shyam Verma, MBBS, DVD.*

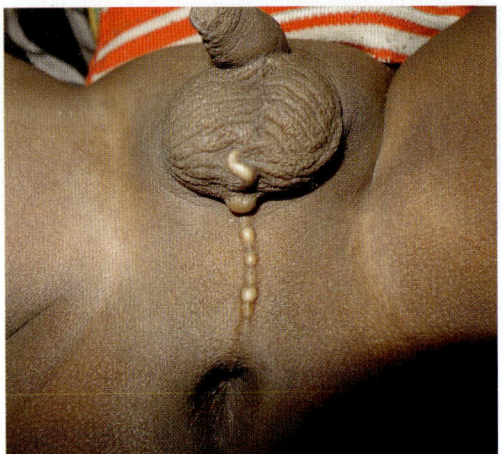

Fig. 29.148 Median raphe cyst. *Courtesy Debabrata Bandyopadhyay.*

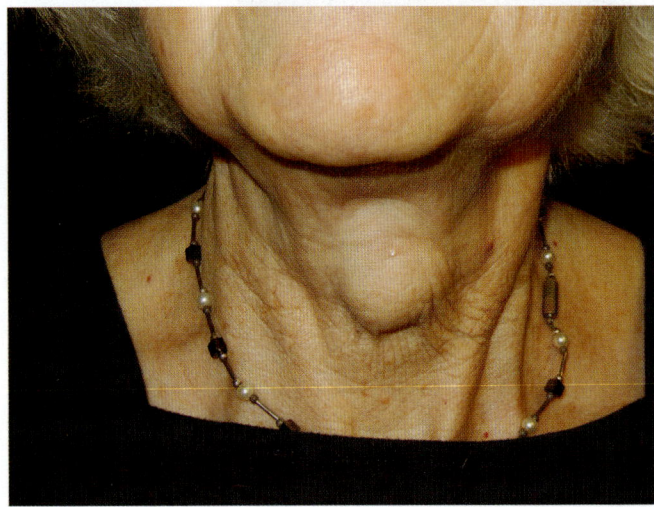

Fig. 29.149 Thyroglossal duct cyst.

Melanocytic Nevi and Neoplasms 30

The evaluation of pigmented lesions is one of the most important skill sets in dermatology. The incidence of melanoma continues to increase, and early diagnosis plays a critical role in reducing mortality, morbidity, and the cost of health care. Melanocytic lesions may be distributed anywhere on the body, and certain lesions, such as the so-called *zosteriform lentiginous nevus* follow a segmental blaschkoid distribution, suggesting genetic mosaicism. Most benign lesions are round to oval, relatively small, evenly pigmented, and stable in appearance. In contrast, malignant lesions are often asymmetric with an irregular border, uneven pigmentation, larger diameter, and evolve over time. It should be noted that these concepts apply mainly to primary lesions, as metastatic lesions are often spherical and symmetric in all dimensions. The "ABCDs" of melanoma are a useful tool for education of the lay public, but only serve to identify some lesions of potential concern. They often miss amelanotic, symmetric, and evenly pigmented tumors and do not substitute for a dermatologist's global assessment of the lesion. They should never be used as the sole criteria for biopsy or for referral to a dermatologist.

Dermoscopy allows the physician to see lesion characteristics not visible on routine examination, and confocal microscopy offers the potential for in vivo microscopic imaging of some lesions. Ultimately, though, careful visual examination of the patient's skin remains the key initial step in identifying lesions of concern.

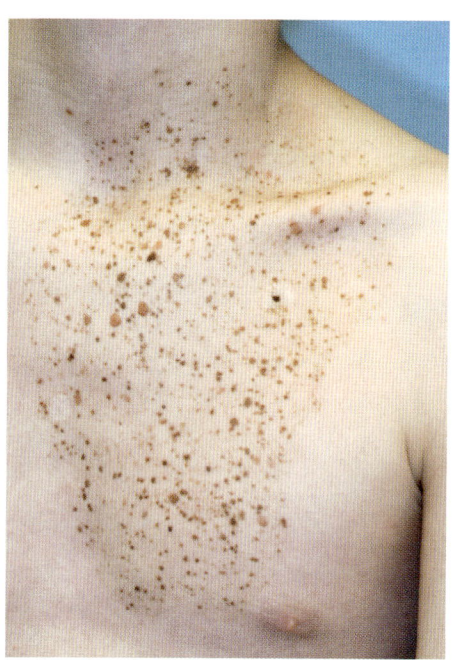

Fig. 30.2 Large nevus spilus.

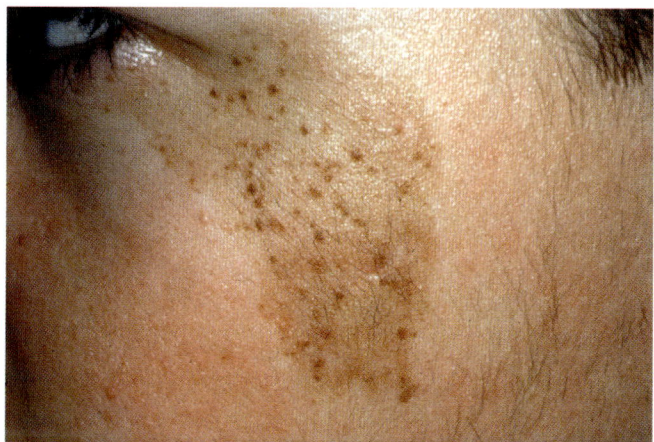

Fig. 30.1 Nevus spilus.

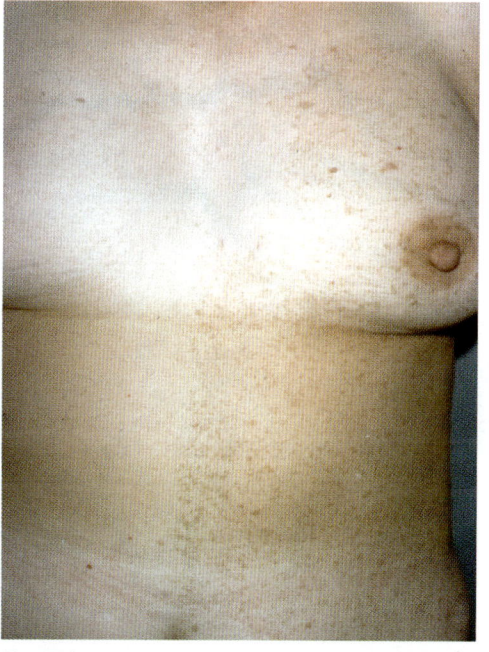

Fig. 30.3 Widespread unilateral nevus spilus.

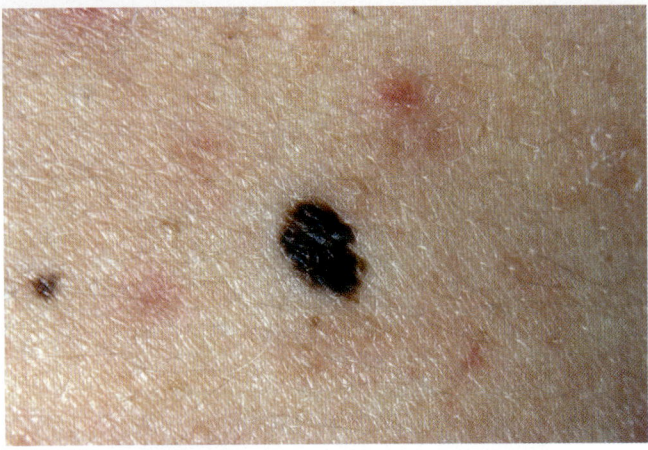

Fig. 30.4 Lentigo simplex.

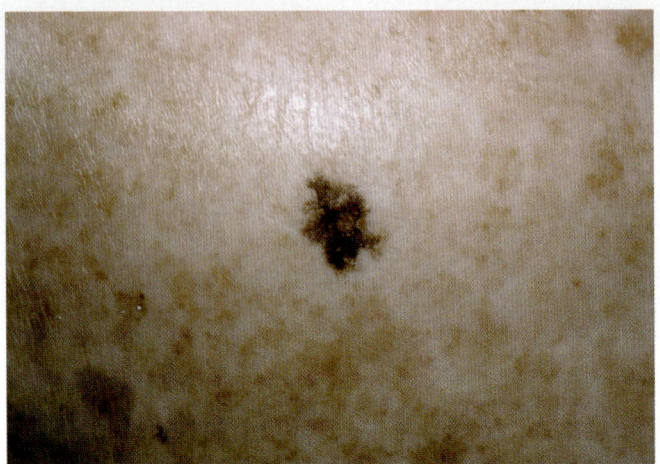

Fig. 30.5 Ink spot lentigo. *Courtesy Steven Binnick, MD.*

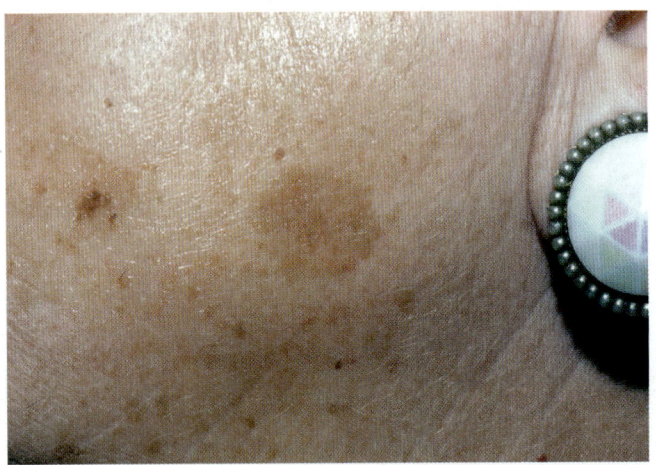

Fig. 30.6 Solar lentigo. *Courtesy Steven Binnick, MD.*

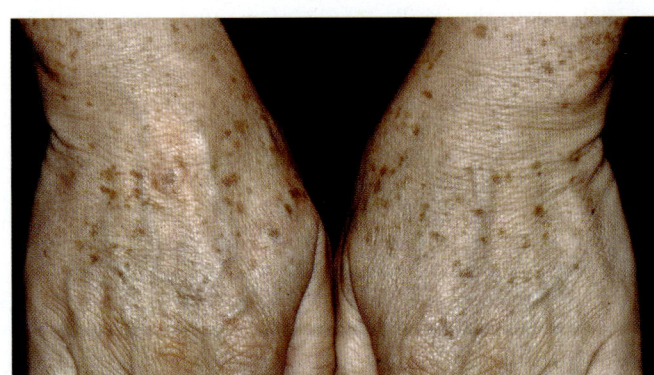

Fig. 30.7 Solar lentigines.

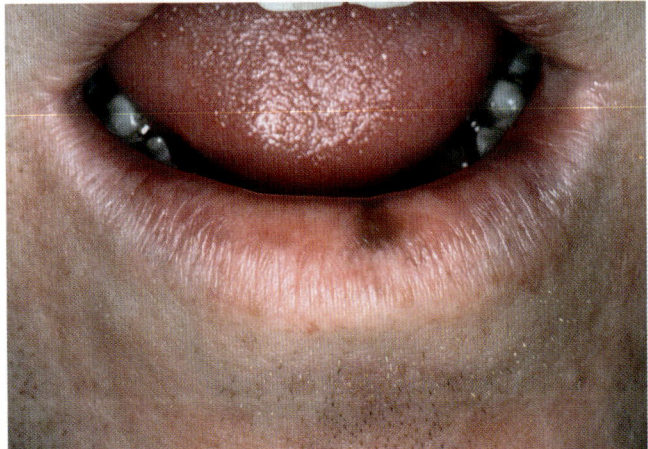

Fig. 30.8 Labial melanotic macule. *Courtesy Steven Binnick, MD.*

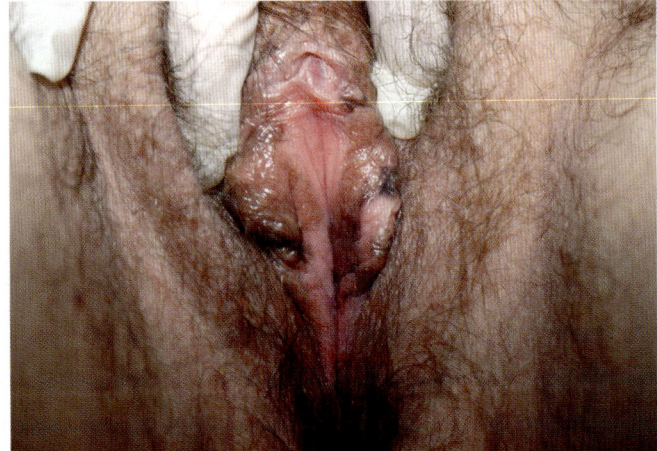

Fig. 30.9 Vulvar melanosis.

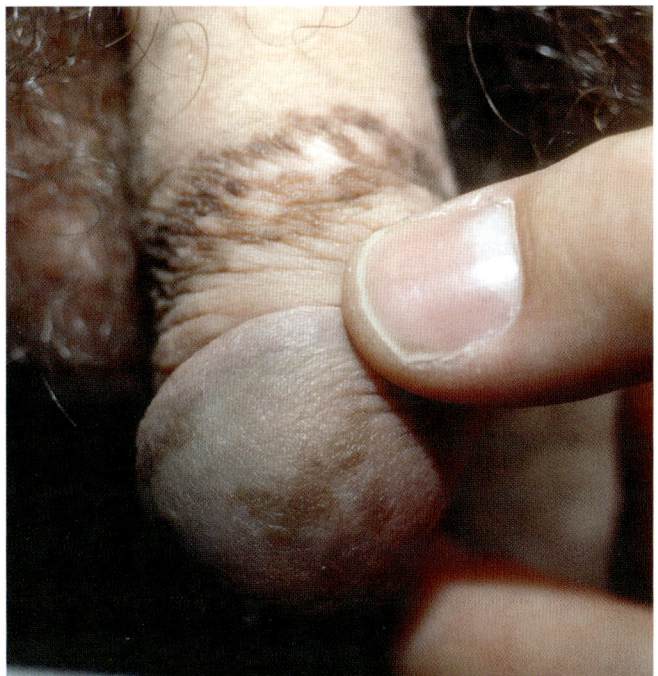
Fig. 30.10 Penile melanosis.

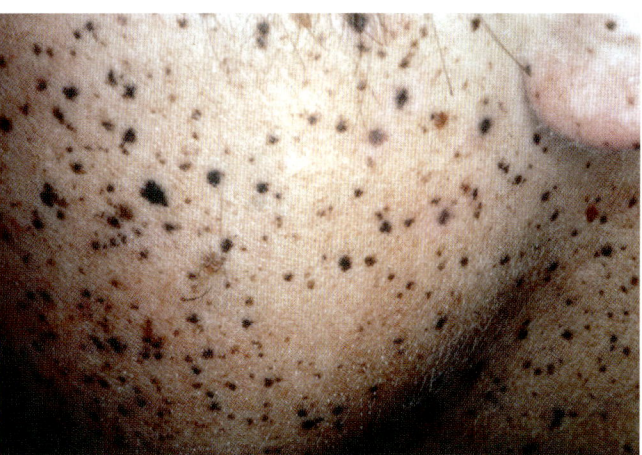
Fig. 30.11 Lentigines in LEOPARD syndrome.

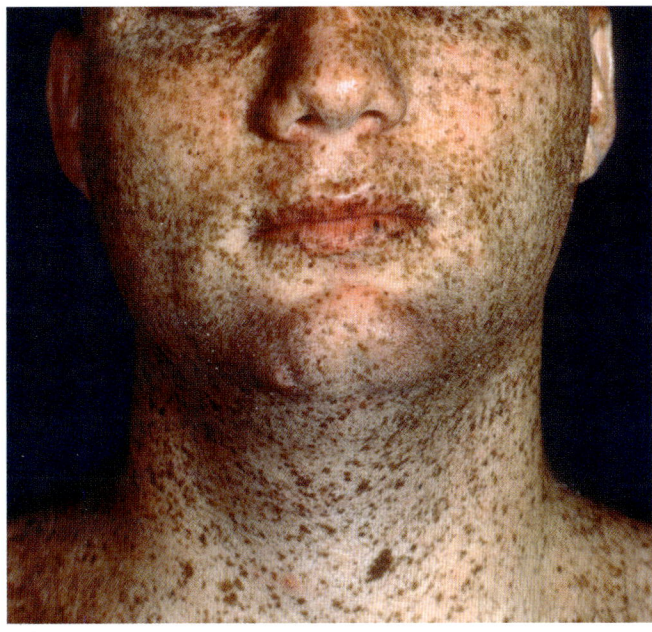
Fig. 30.12 Generalized lentiginosis.

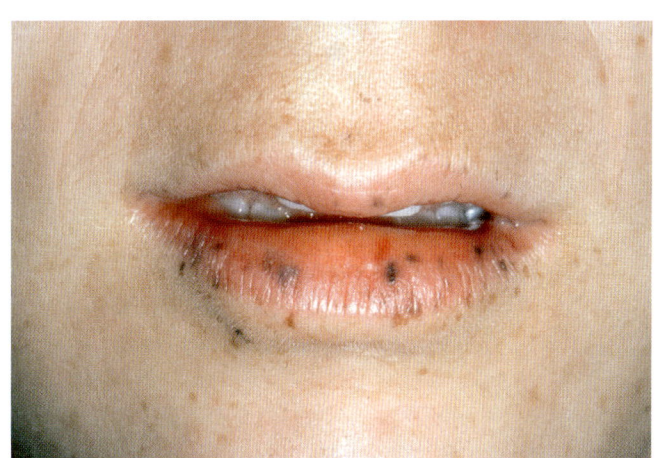
Fig. 30.13 Carney syndrome.

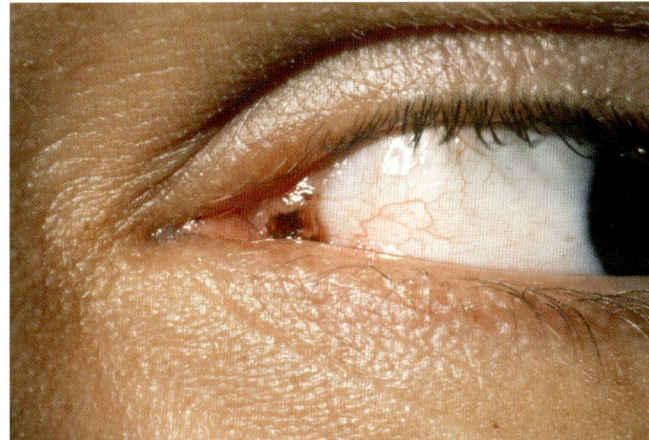
Fig. 30.14 Carney syndrome.

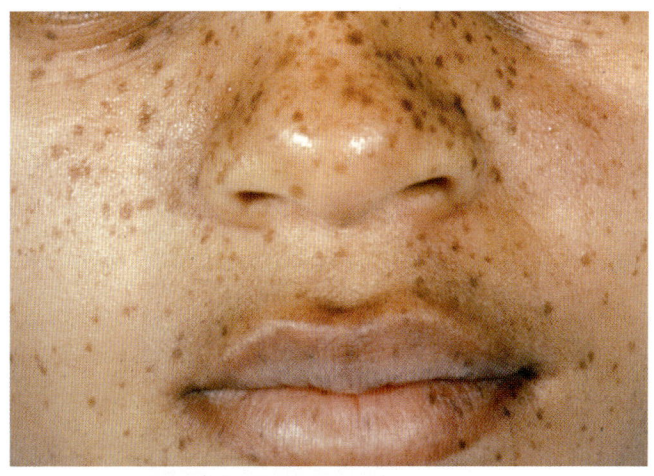
Fig. 30.15 Inherited patterned lentiginosis.

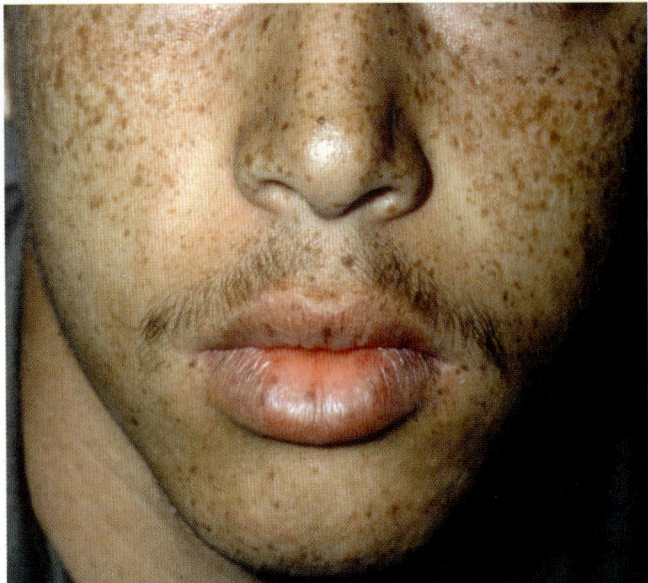

Fig. 30.16 Inherited patterned lentiginosis.

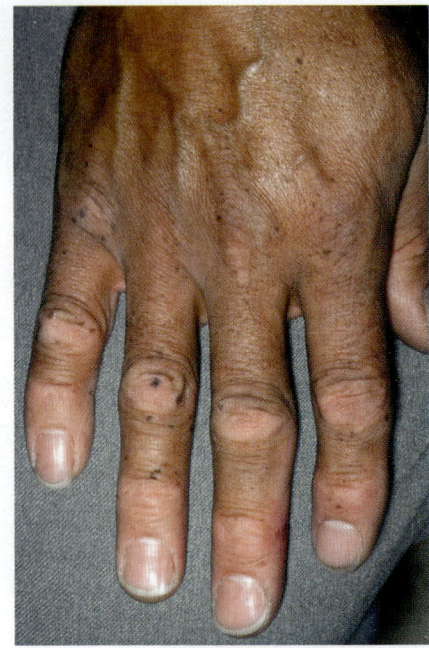

Fig. 30.17 Inherited patterned lentiginosis.

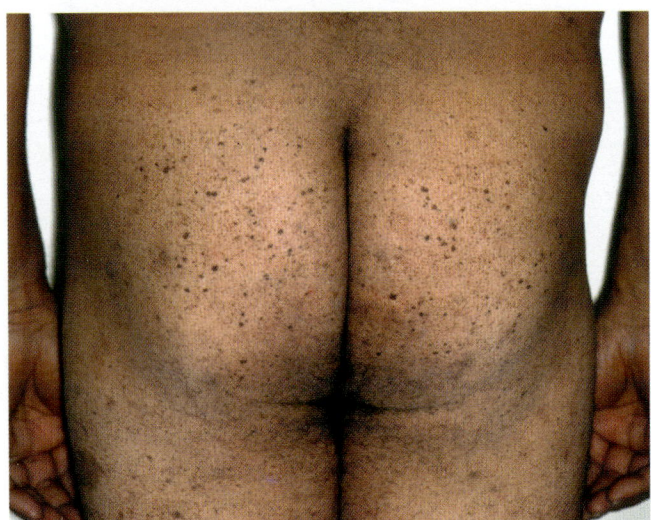

Fig. 30.18 Inherited patterned lentiginosis.

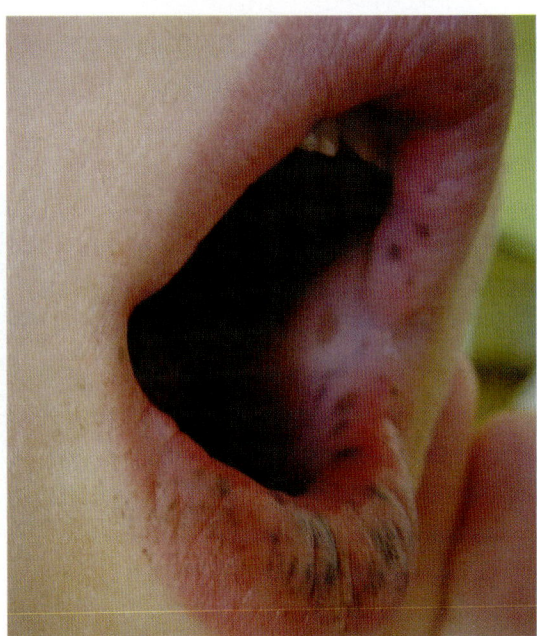

Fig. 30.19 Peutz-Jeghers syndrome. *Courtesy Dr. Rui Carlos Taveres Bello.*

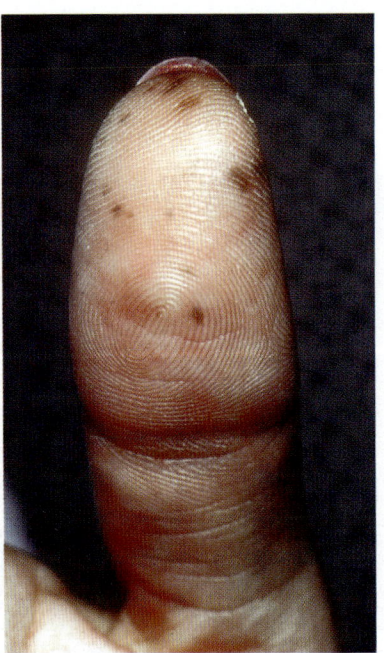

Fig. 30.20 Peutz-Jeghers syndrome.

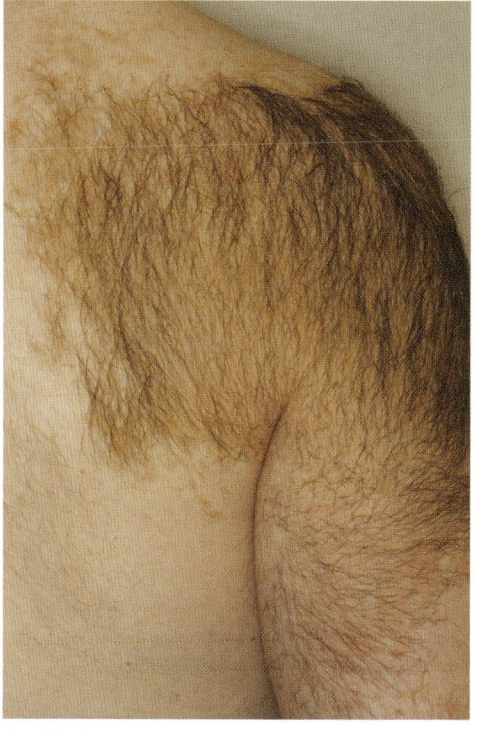

Fig. 30.21 Becker nevus.

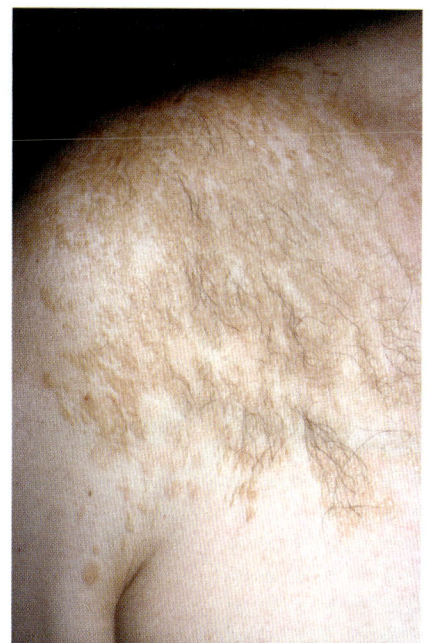

Fig. 30.22 Becker nevus.

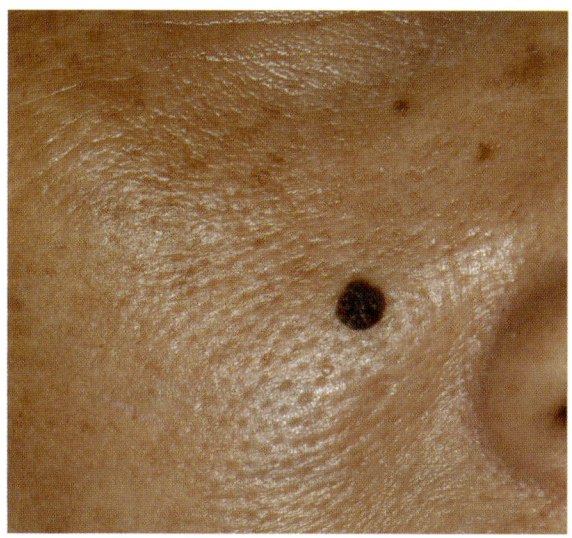

Fig. 30.23 Melanoacanthoma. *Courtesy National Cheng Kung University, Taiwan.*

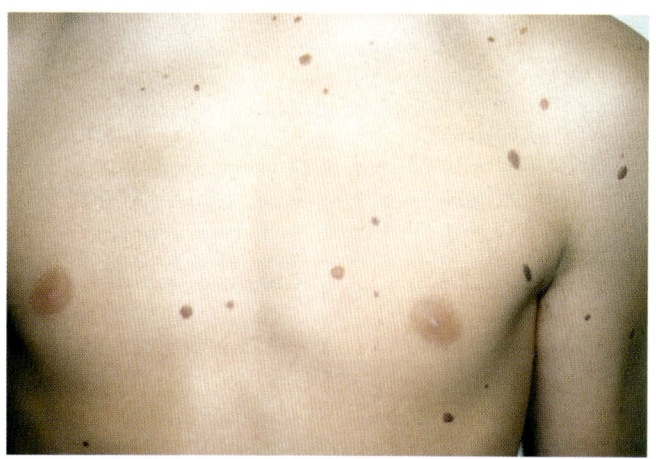

Fig. 30.24 Junctional nevi.

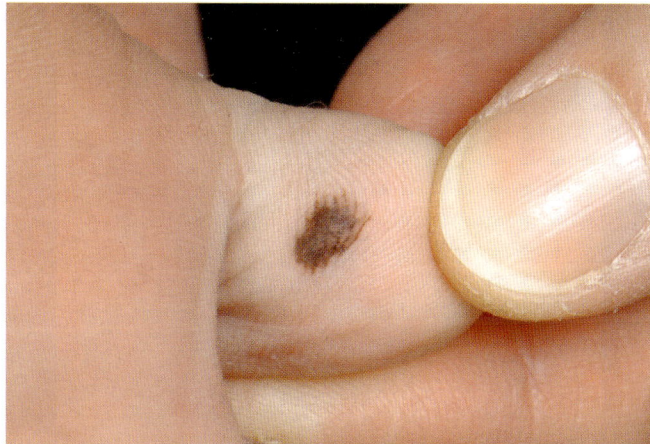

Fig. 30.25 Junctional acral nevus.

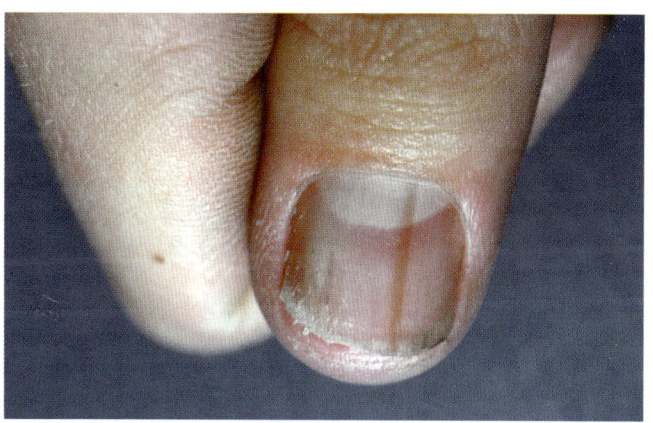

Fig. 30.26 Longitudinal melanonychia secondary to a junctional nevus.

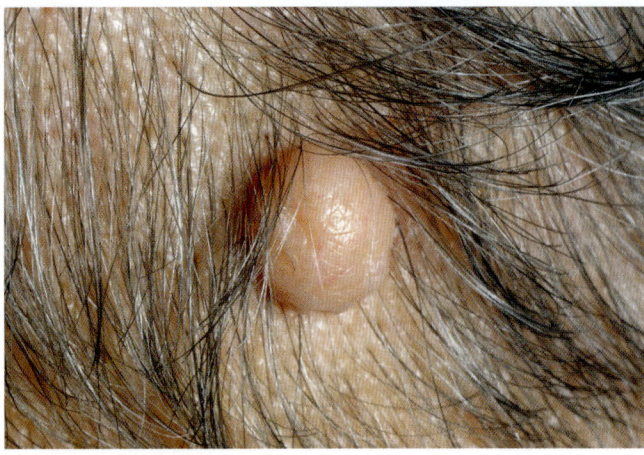

Fig. 30.27 Intradermal nevi.

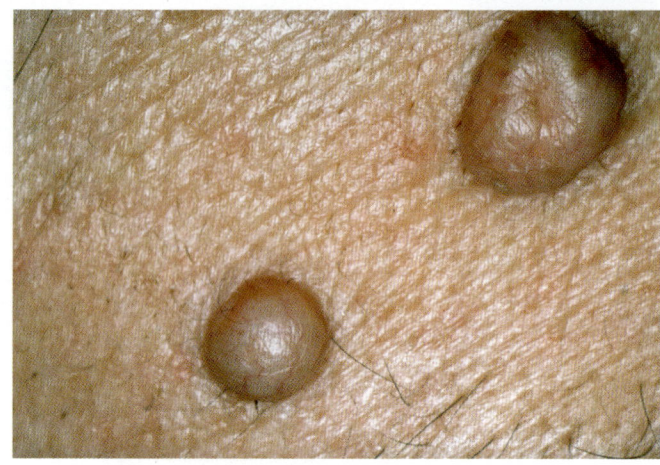

Fig. 30.28 Intradermal nevi.

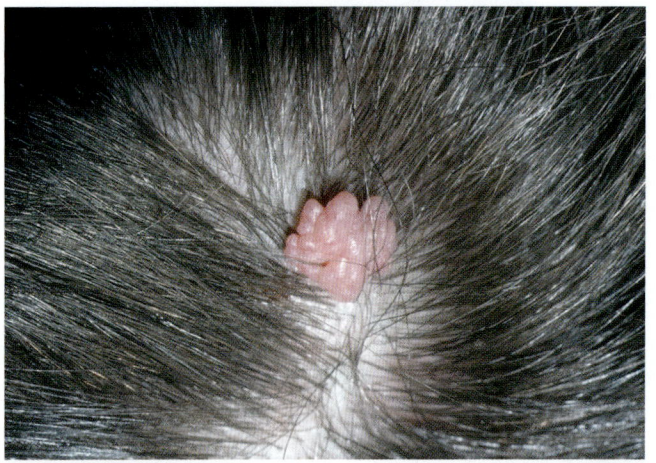

Fig. 30.29 Nevus.

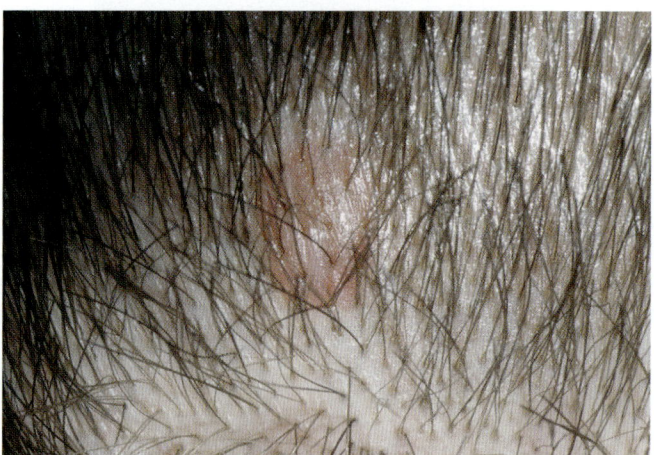

Fig. 30.30 Nevus.

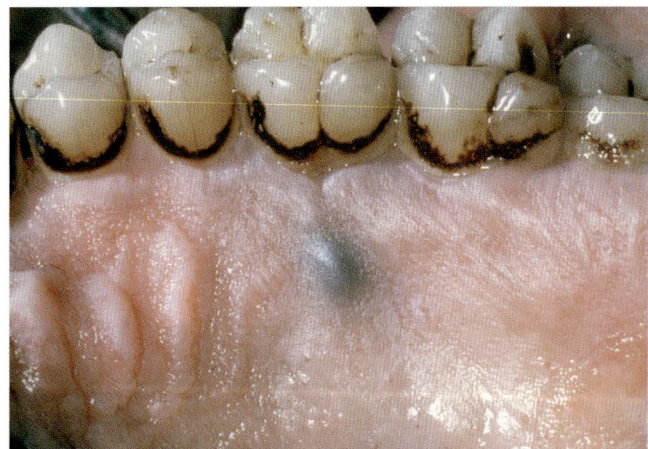

Fig. 30.31 Oral blue nevus.

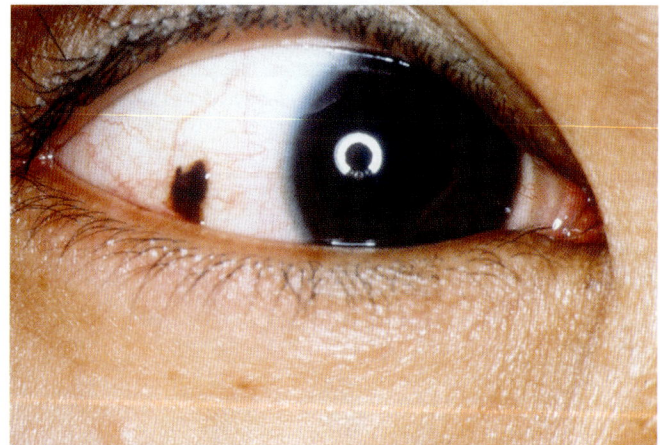

Fig. 30.32 Ocular nevus.

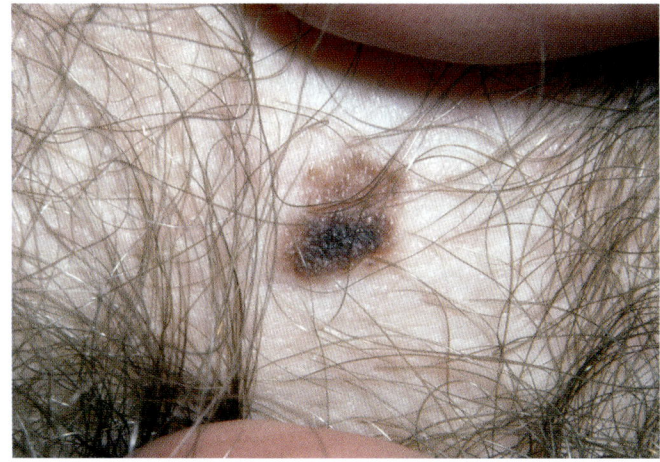

Fig. 30.33 Large variably pigmented nevus in genital area of a woman.

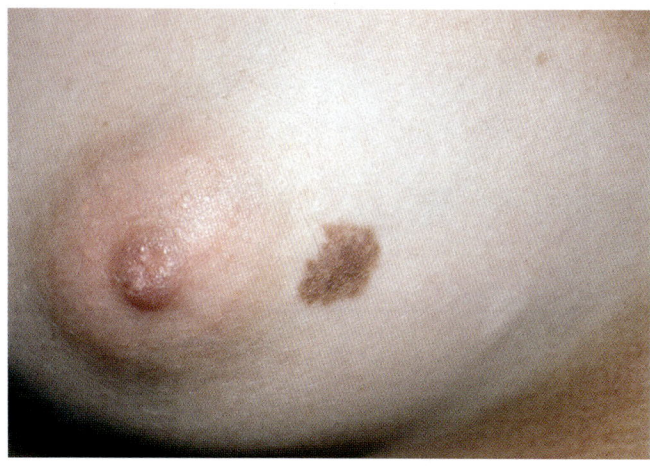

Fig. 30.34 Large irregular nevus on the breast of a woman. Often nevi in such estrogen-dependent sites are larger. *Courtesy Steven Binnick, MD.*

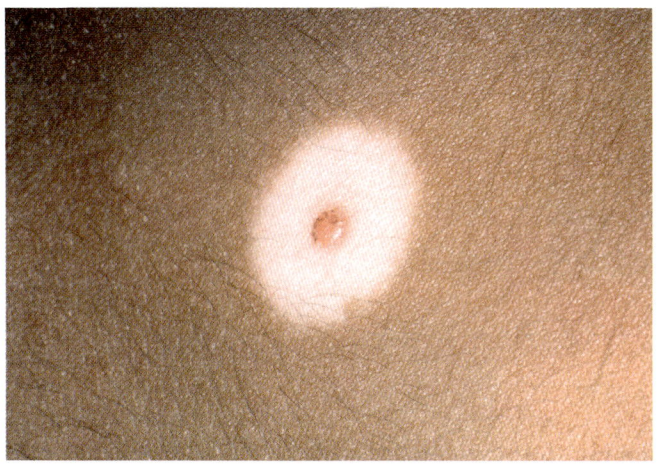

Fig. 30.35 Halo nevus. *Courtesy Steven Binnick, MD.*

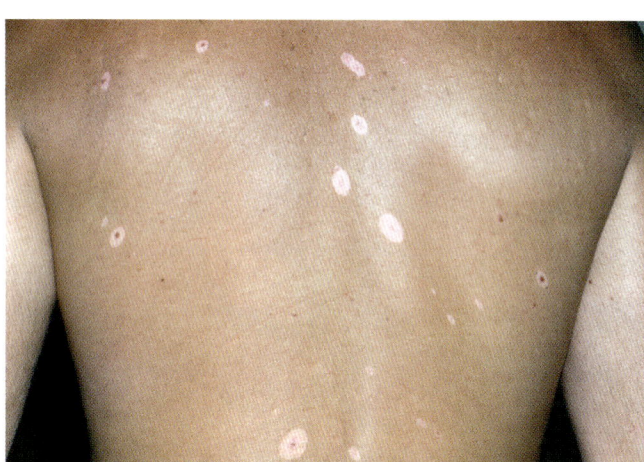

Fig. 30.36 Halo nevi. *Courtesy Steven Binnick, MD.*

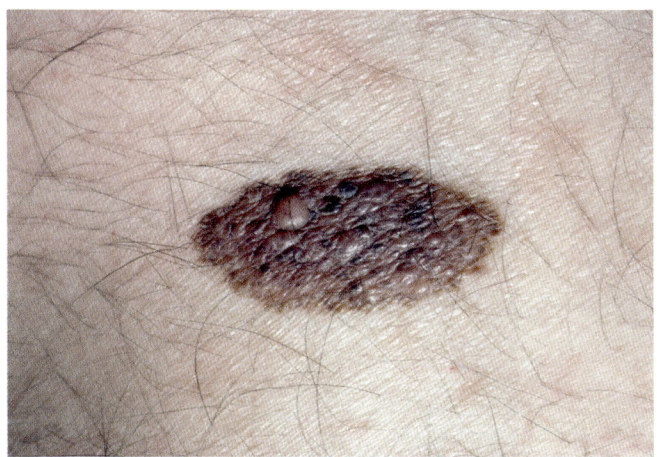

Fig. 30.37 Congenital nevus. *Courtesy Steven Binnick, MD.*

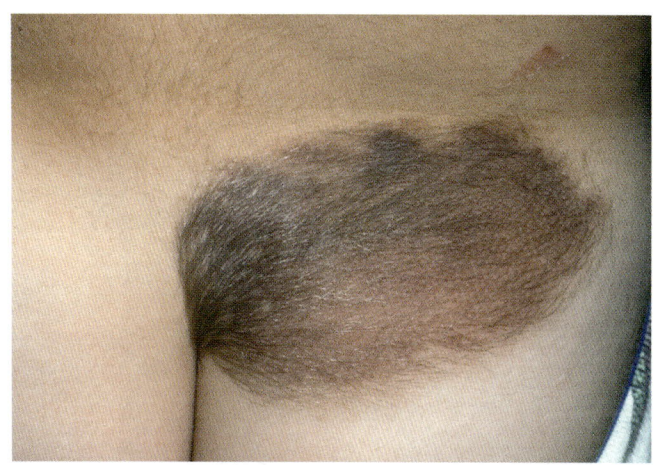

Fig. 30.38 Congenital nevus. *Courtesy Steven Binnick, MD.*

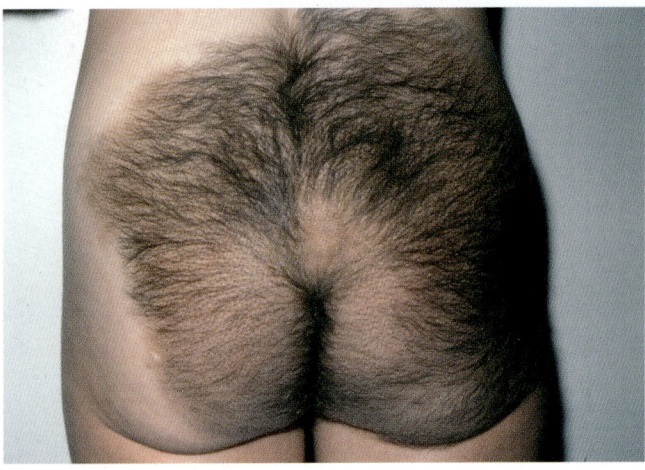

Fig. 30.39 Congenital nevus. *Courtesy Steven Binnick, MD.*

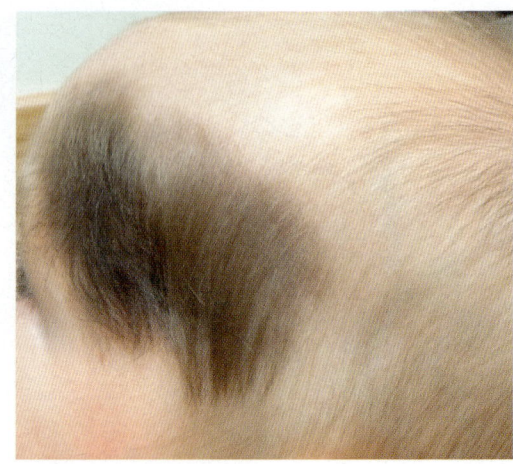

Fig. 30.40 Congenital nevus. Note thick hair within the nevus.

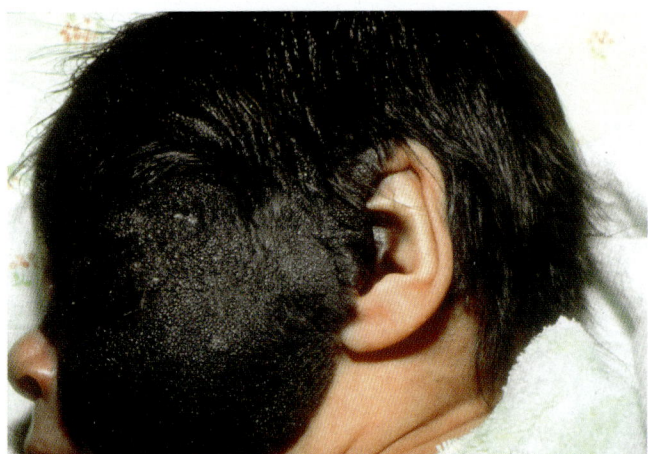

Fig. 30.41 Congenital nevus.

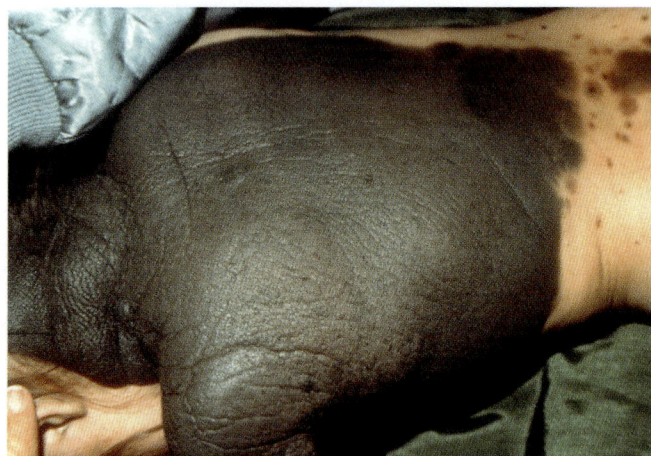

Fig. 30.42 Congenital nevus.

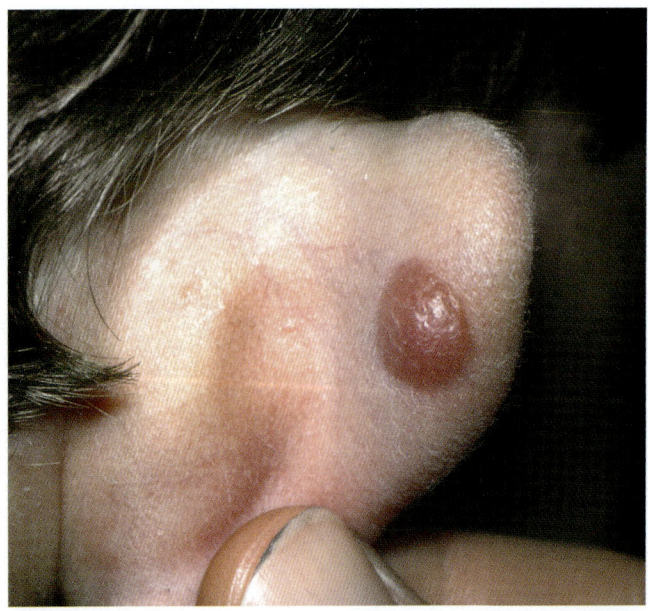

Fig. 30.43 Spitz nevus. *Courtesy Steven Binnick, MD.*

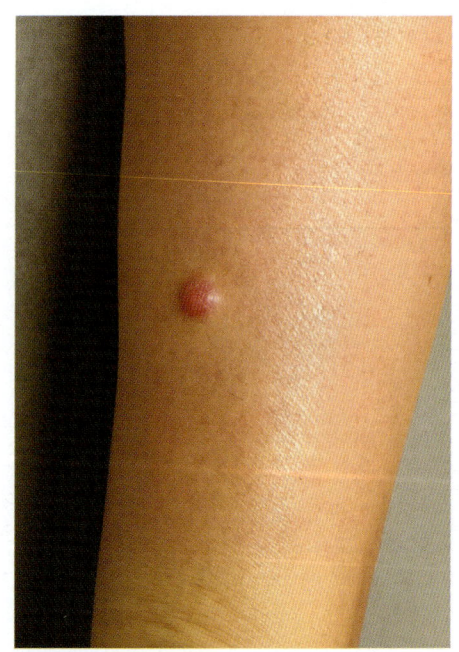

Fig. 30.44 Atypical Spitz nevus.

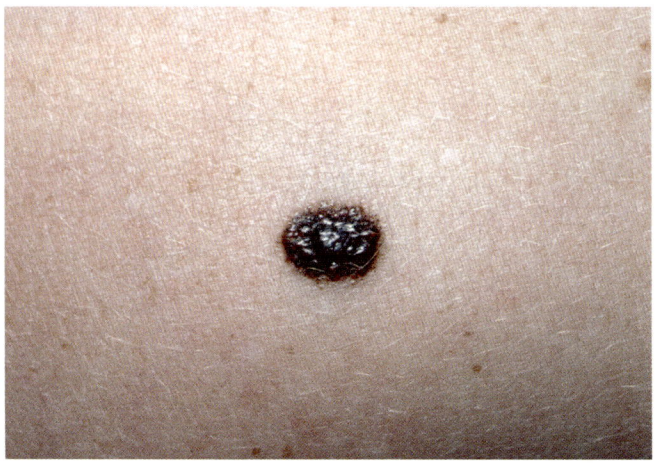

Fig. 30.45 Spitz nevus. *Courtesy Curt Samlaska, MD.*

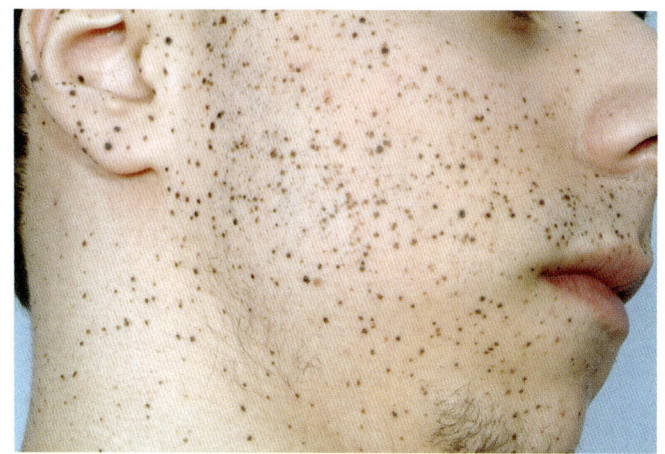

Fig. 30.46 Spindle cell nevi.

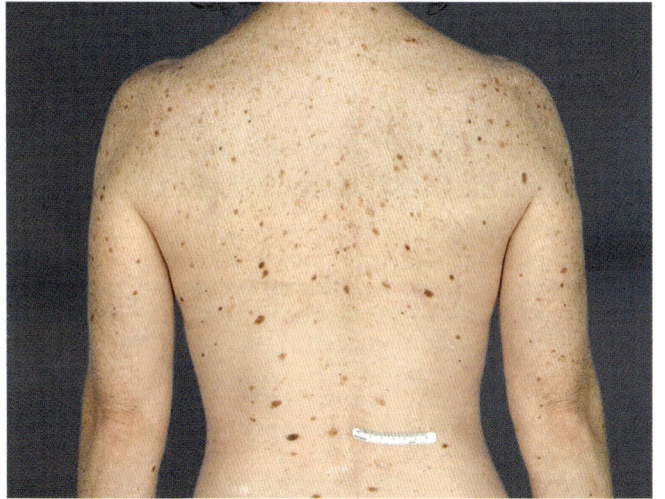

Fig. 30.47 Patient with a CDKN2A mutation. This patient had many melanomas and a positive family history of melanoma. *Courtesy Ellen Kim, MD.*

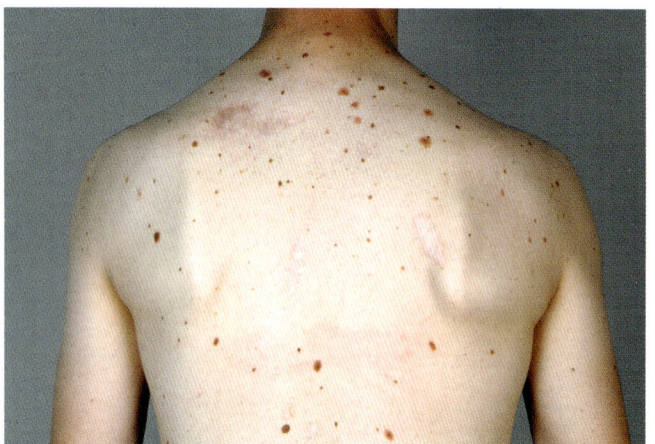

Fig. 30.48 Dysplastic nevi. *Courtesy Michael Ming, MD.*

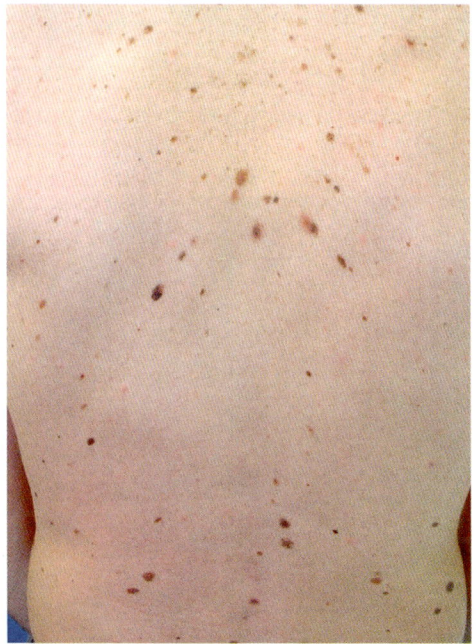

Fig. 30.49 Dysplastic nevi.

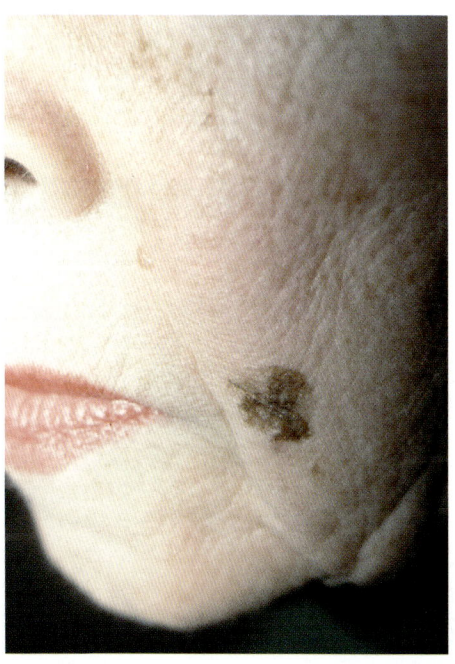

Fig. 30.50 Lentigo maligna.

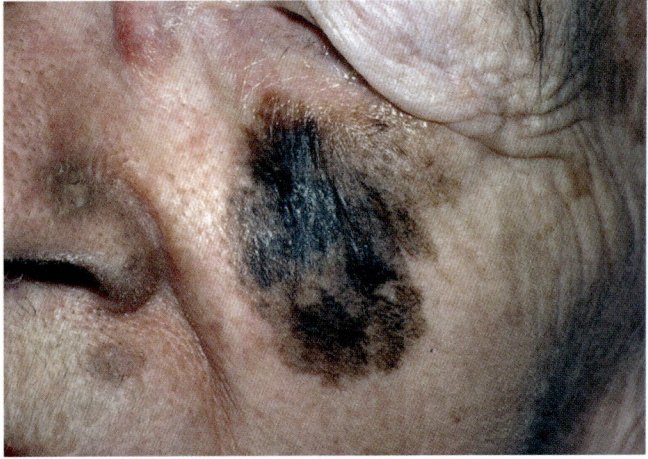

Fig. 30.51 Lentigo maligna. *Courtesy Steven Binnick, MD.*

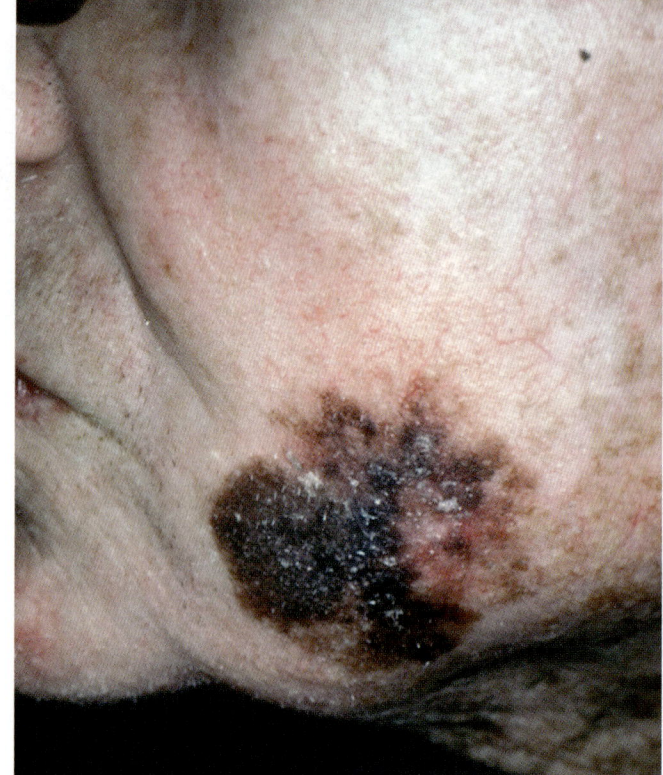

Fig. 30.52 Lentigo maligna melanoma.

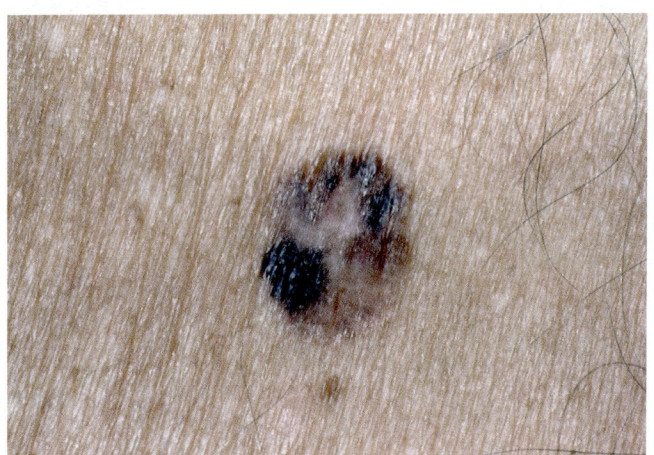

Fig. 30.53 Superficial spreading melanoma. *Courtesy Steven Binnick, MD.*

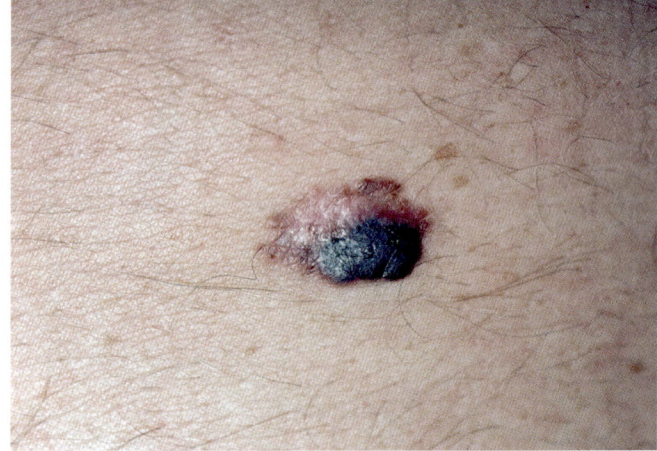

Fig. 30.54 Superficial spreading melanoma. *Courtesy Steven Binnick, MD.*

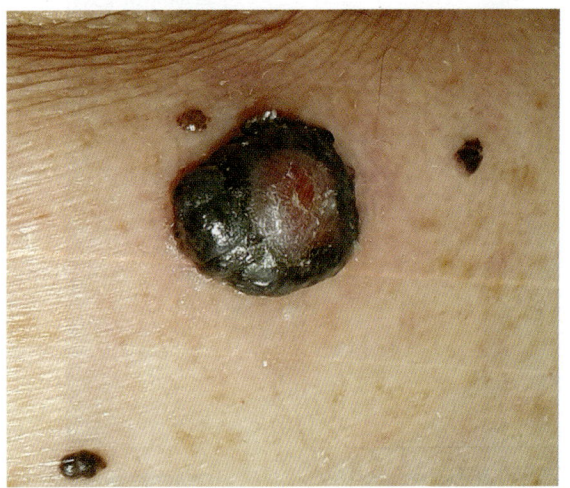

Fig. 30.55 Melanoma with satellitosis. *Courtesy Dr. Rui Carlos Taveres Bello.*

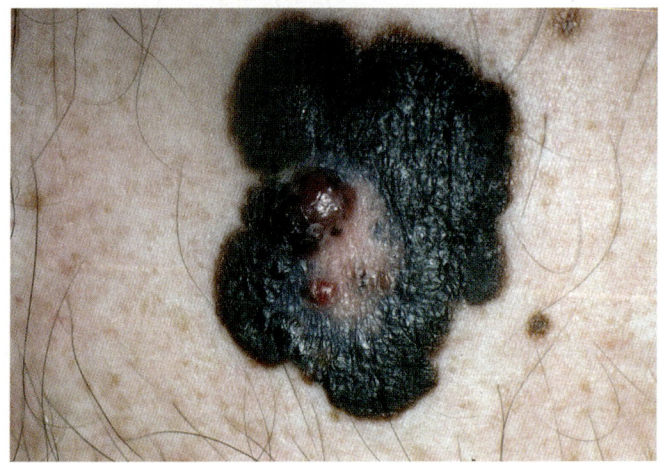

Fig. 30.56 Superficial spreading melanoma. *Courtesy Steven Binnick, MD.*

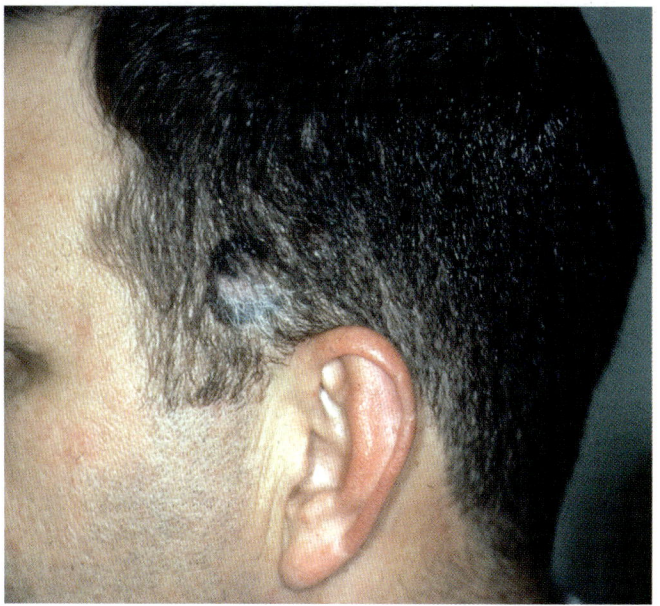

Fig. 30.57 Superficial spreading melanoma.

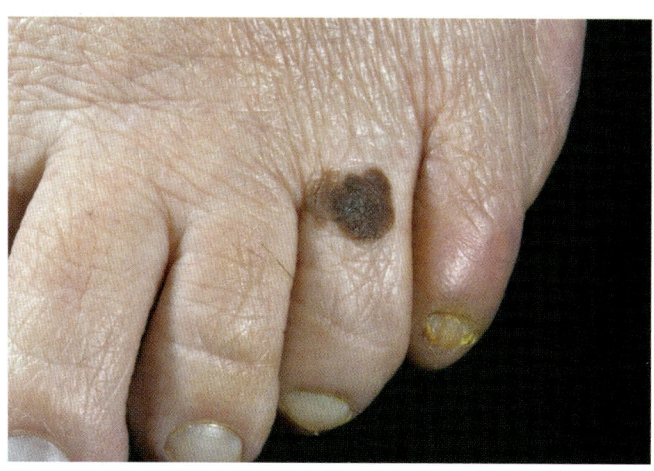

Fig. 30.58 Acral melanoma. *Courtesy Curt Samlaska, MD.*

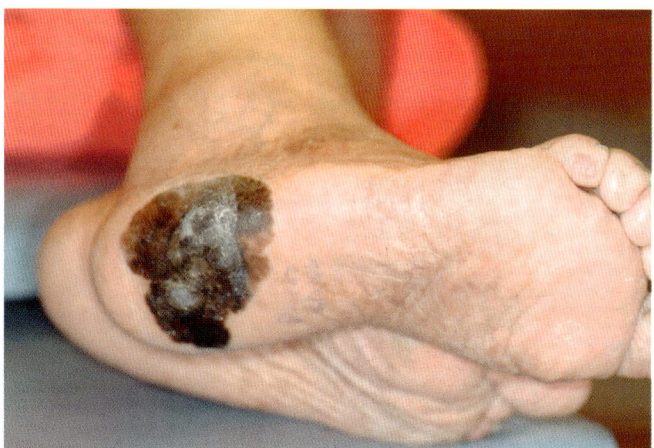

Fig. 30.59 Acral melanoma. *Courtesy Chris Miller, MD.*

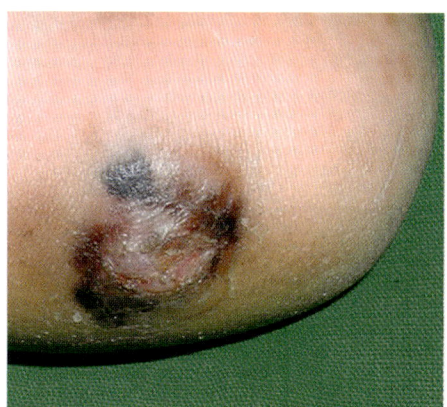

Fig. 30.60 Acral melanoma. *Courtesy Shyam Verma, MBBS, DVD.*

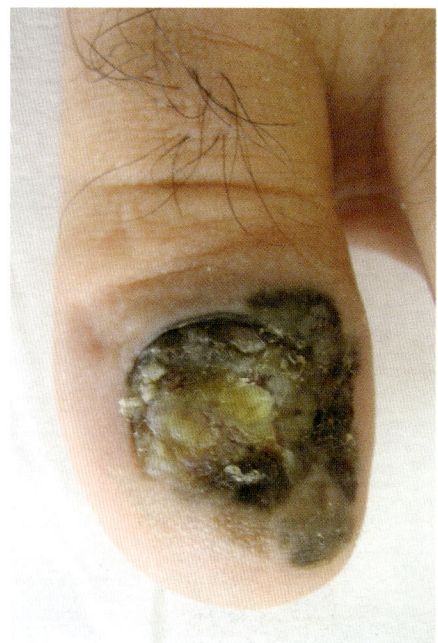

Fig. 30.61 Acral melanoma.

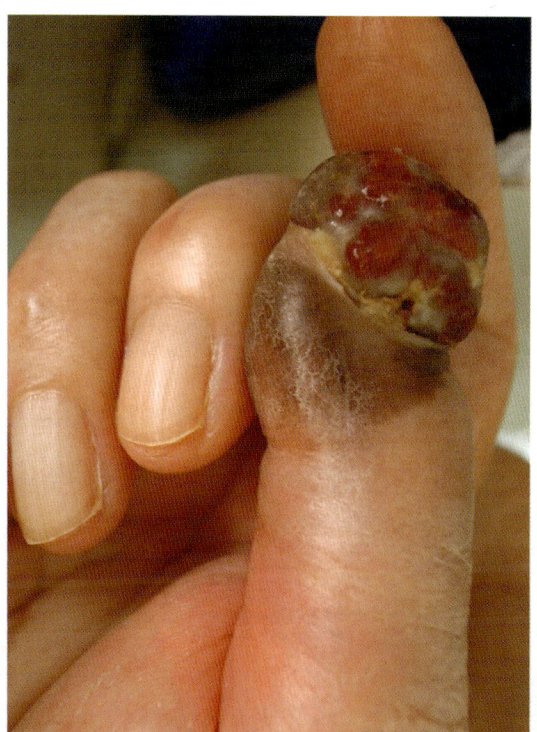

Fig. 30.62 Acral lentiginous melanoma. *Courtesy Yung-Tsu Cho, MD.*

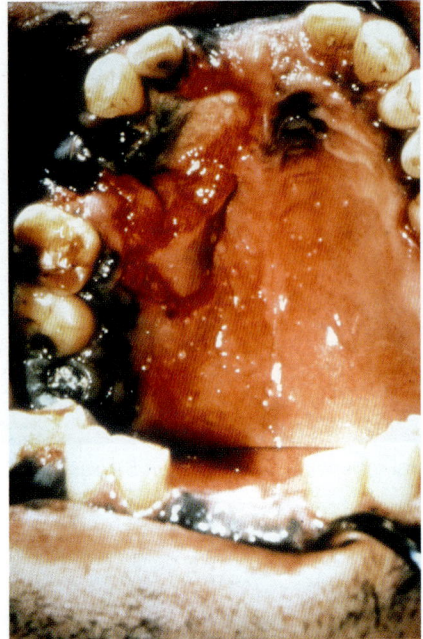

Fig. 30.63 Oral melanoma.

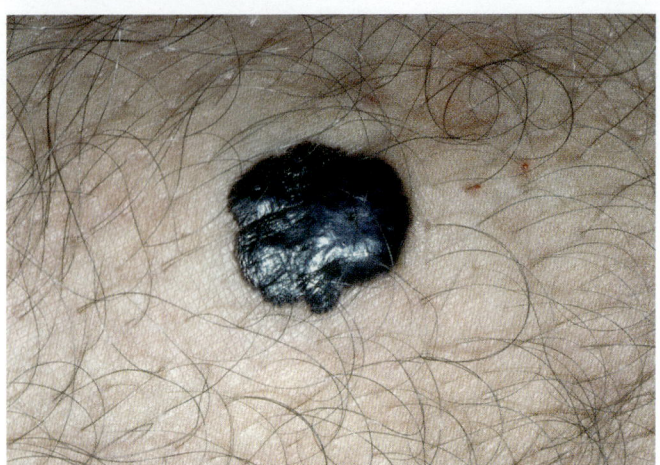

Fig. 30.64 Nodular melanoma. *Courtesy Curt Samlaska, MD.*

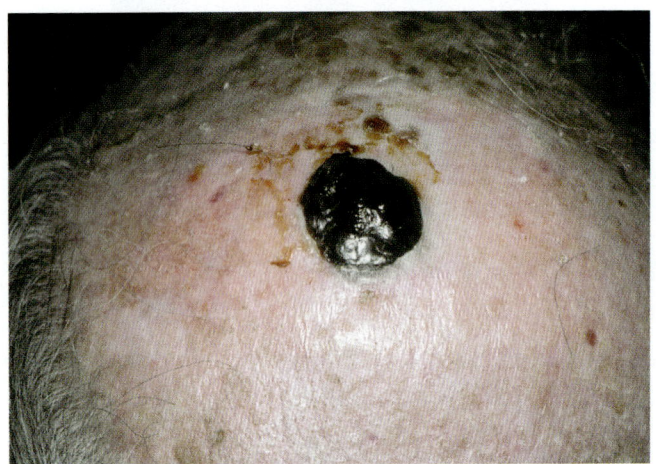

Fig. 30.65 Nodular melanoma. *Courtesy Steven Binnick, MD.*

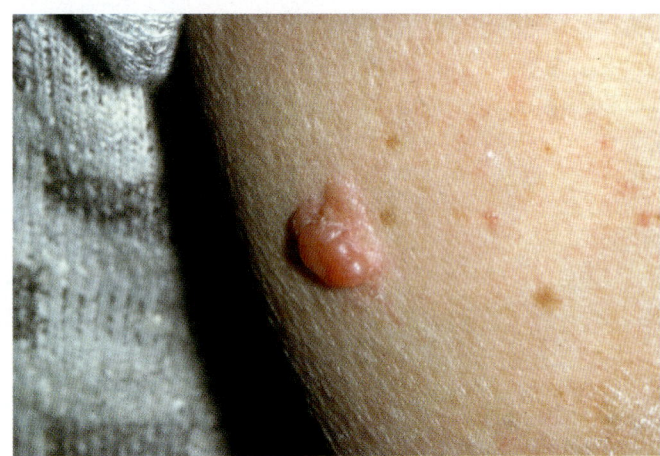

Fig. 30.66 Amelanotic melanoma.

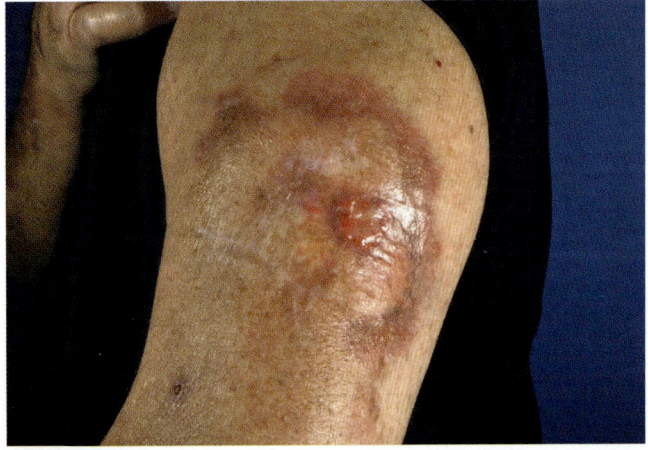

Fig. 30.67 Amelanotic melanoma within a morphea lesion. *Courtesy Curt Samlaska, MD.*

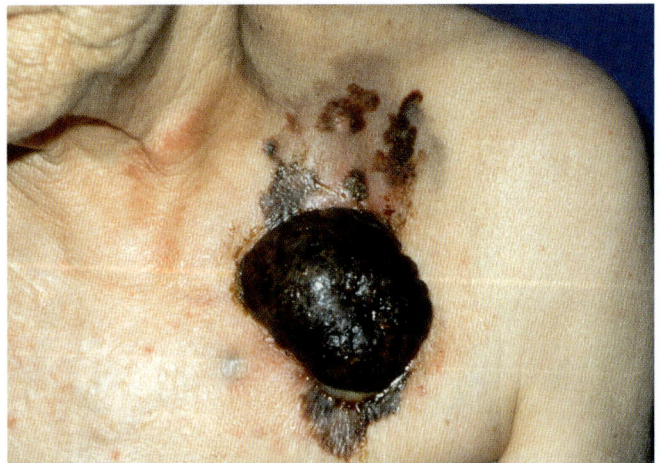

Fig. 30.68 Large melanoma.

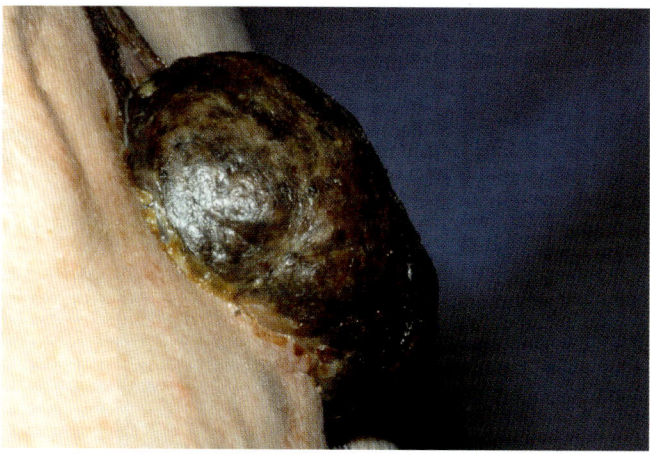

Fig. 30.69 Large melanoma.

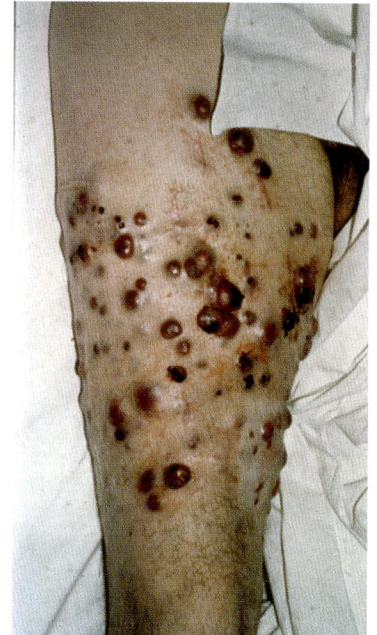

Fig. 30.70 Satellite metastases from melanoma.

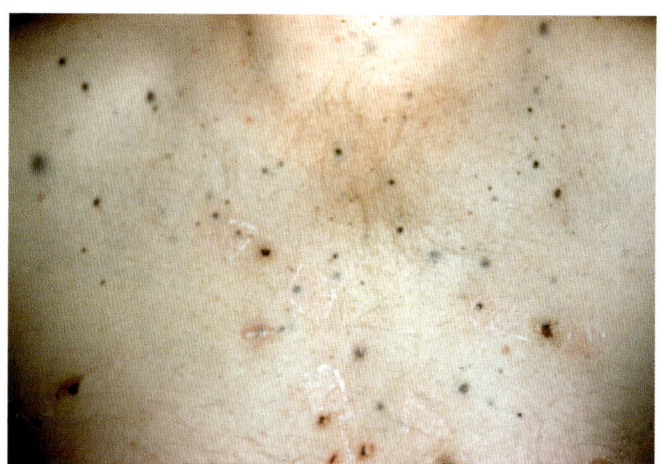

Fig. 30.71 Metastatic melanoma.

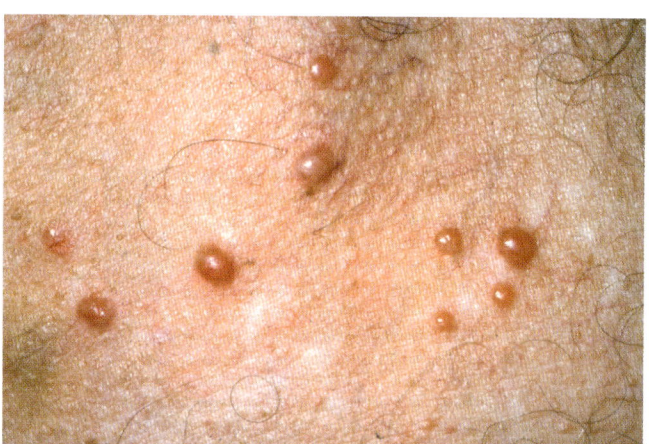

Fig. 30.72 Metastatic amelanotic melanoma.

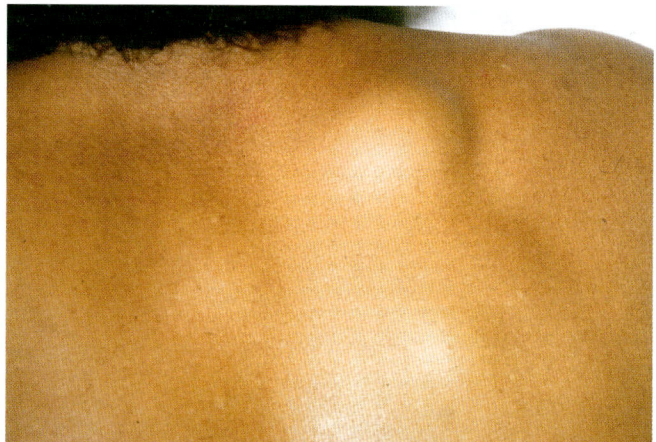

Fig. 30.73 Metastatic melanoma.

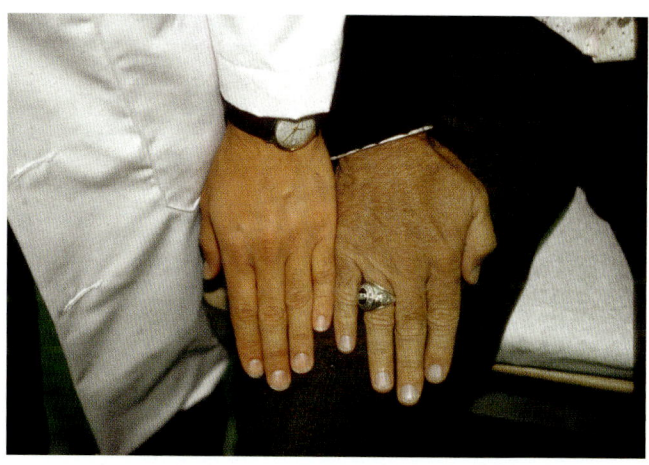

Fig. 30.74 Diffuse melanosis in metastatic melanoma; dark hand compared with normal.

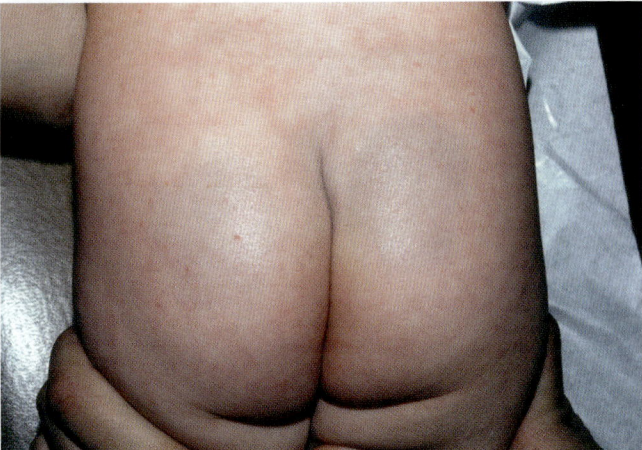

Fig. 30.75 Dermal melanocytosis. *Courtesy Steven Binnick, MD.*

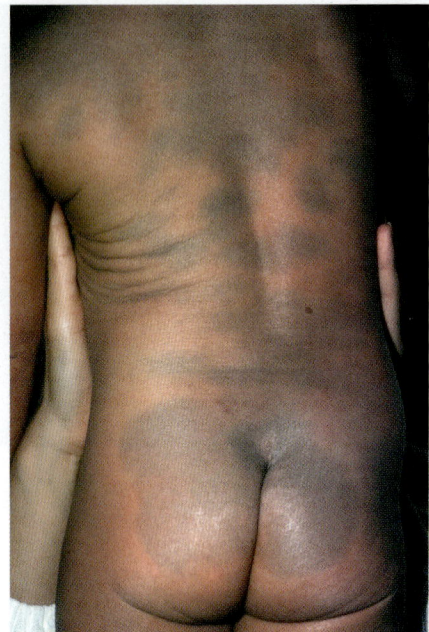

Fig. 30.76 Dermal melanocytosis. *Courtesy Steven Binnick, MD.*

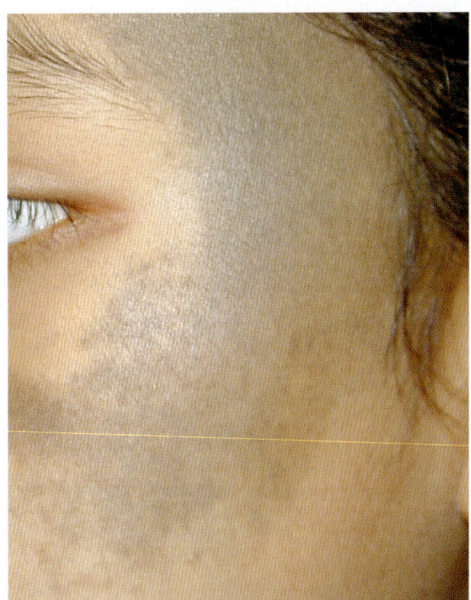

Fig. 30.77 Nevus of Ota. *Courtesy Vasanop Vachiramon, MD.*

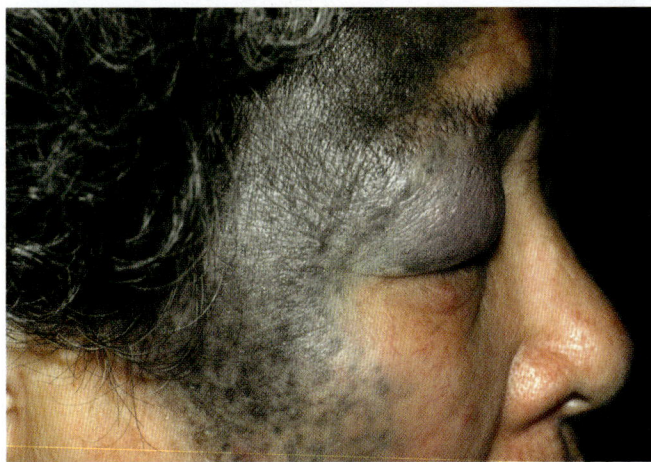

Fig. 30.78 Nevus of Ota. *Courtesy Steven Binnick, MD.*

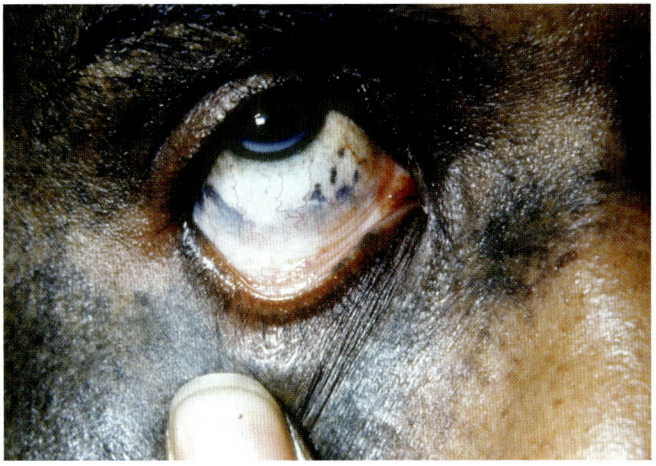

Fig. 30.79 Nevus of Ota.

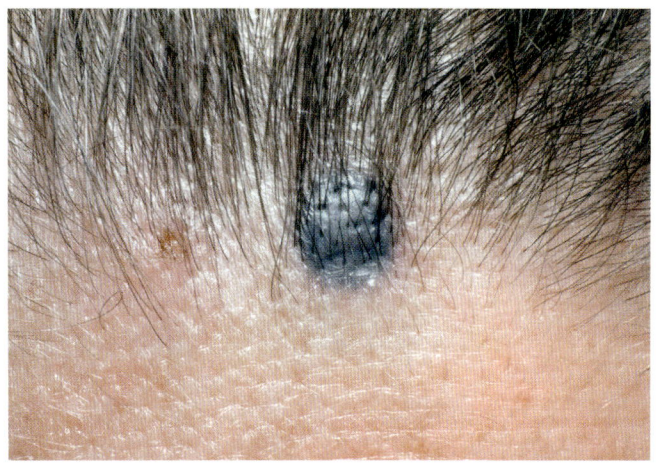

Fig. 30.80 Blue nevus.

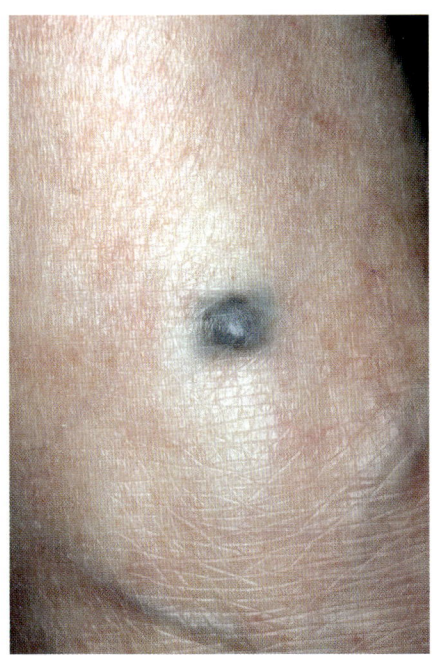

Fig. 30.81 Blue nevus.

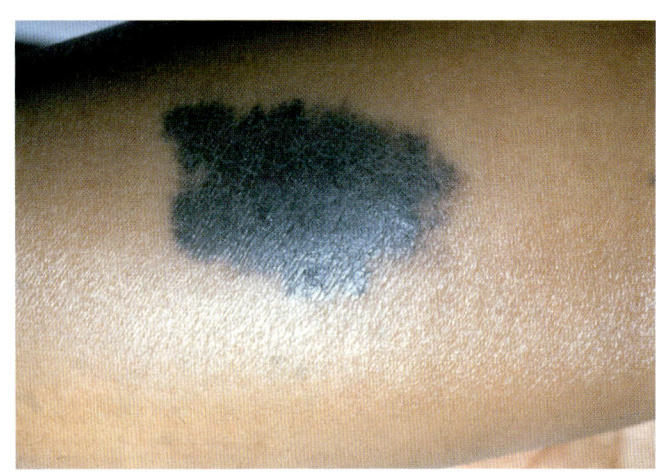

Fig. 30.82 Congenital blue nevus.

Macrophage/Monocyte Disorders 31

This chapter includes granulomatous and histiocytic conditions that are either localized to the skin or can involve the skin as part of a systemic disease. Many will require a skin biopsy to confirm the diagnosis and direct further workup and treatment.

One common granulomatous condition included here is granuloma annulare (GA), a skin condition that typically presents on frictional sites, such as the dorsal feet, forearms, or legs, with skin-colored papules or nodules that form a ring. Other forms of GA can be more difficult to diagnosis, such as the perforating or deep (subcutaneous) forms. Sarcoidosis is another granulomatous condition with skin manifestations in the setting of what is a chronic systemic disease. Skin findings in sarcoidosis can vary and include papules, annular GA-like plaques, ichthyosiform patches, and nodules at site of tattoos. Screening for systemic involvement is essential when sarcoidosis is suspected because it can affect almost every organ in the body.

Histiocytic conditions are featured as well, including juvenile xanthogranulomas (JXG), Langerhans cell histiocytosis (LCH), and rarer conditions such as multicentric reticulohistiocytosis. JXG is a common pediatric condition most commonly limited to the skin in the form of a yellow/orange, smooth papule or nodule. LCH has more varied clinical presentations depending on the age and degree of systemic involvement. Common skin manifestations include erosive, red patches in the folds with petechiae; red-brown papules that can become crusted; xanthomatous nodules; and in adults acneiform eruption on the chest and back.

This portion of the atlas contains images of diseases due to macrophages and monocytes, including granulomatous and histiocytic conditions.

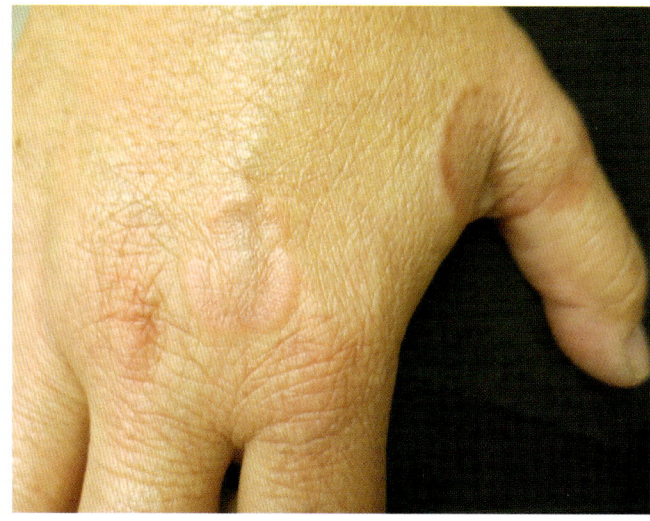

Fig. 31.2 Granuloma annulare.

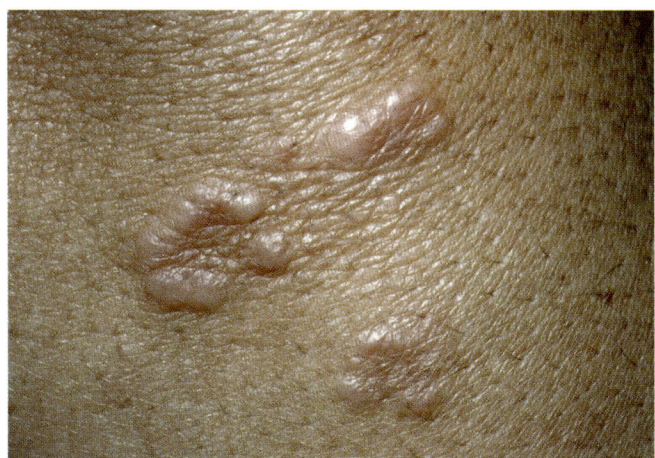

Fig. 31.1 Granuloma annulare.

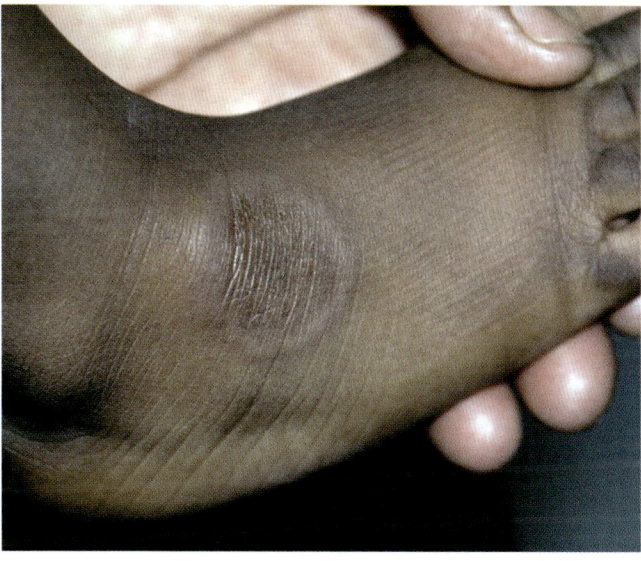

Fig. 31.3 Granuloma annulare. *Courtesy Paul Honig, MD.*

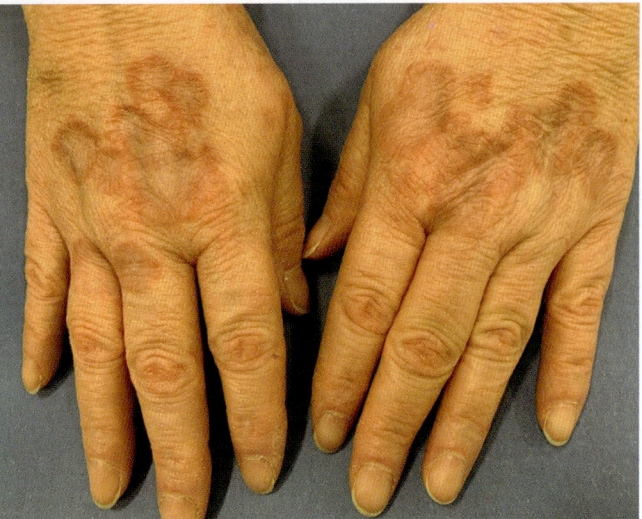

Fig. 31.4 Granuloma annulare.

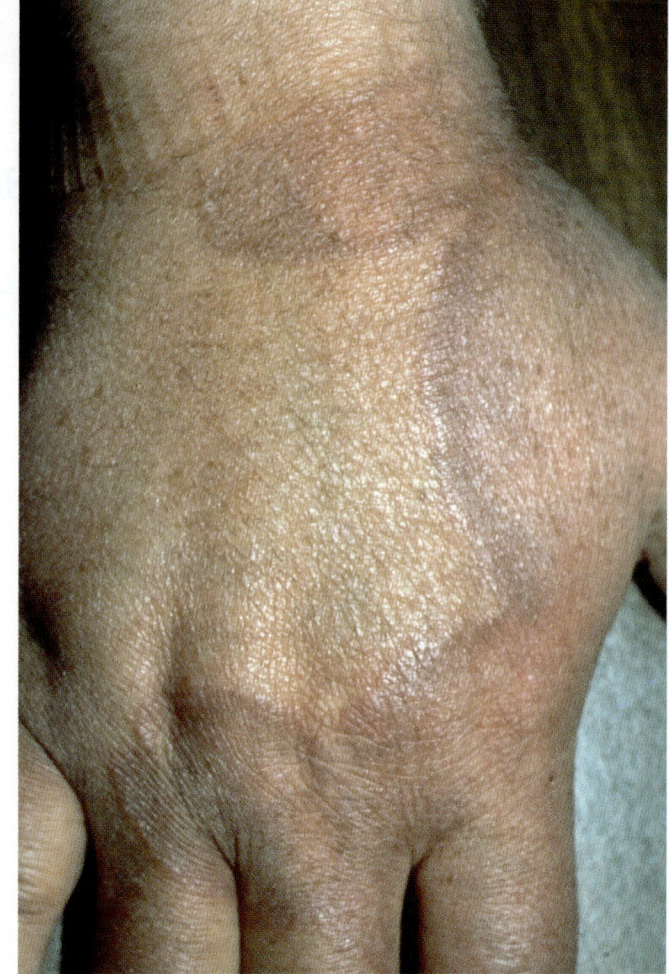

Fig. 31.5 Granuloma annulare.

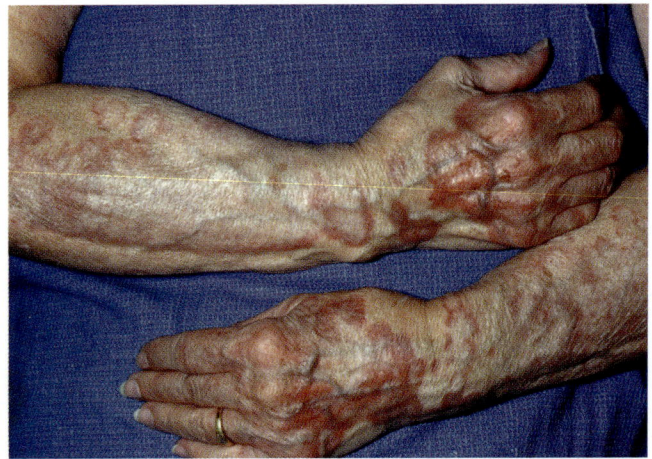

Fig. 31.6 Granuloma annulare.

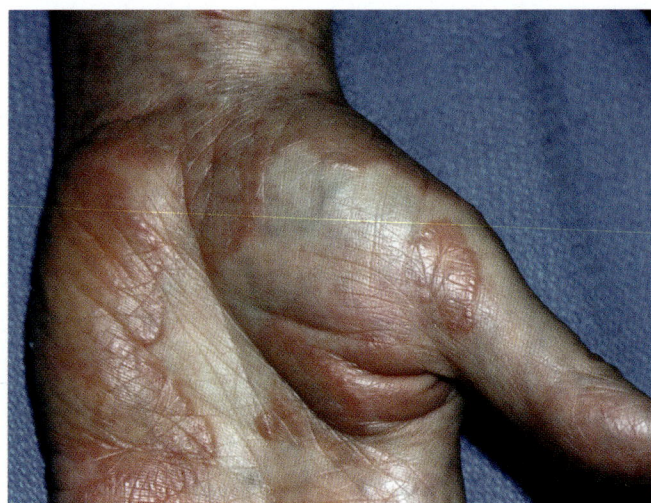

Fig. 31.7 Granuloma annulare.

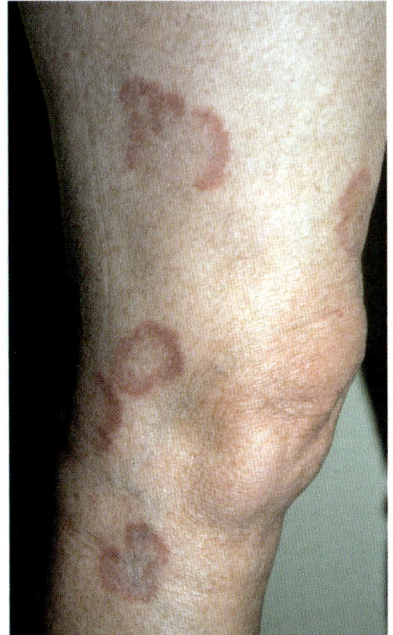

Fig. 31.8 Granuloma annulare.

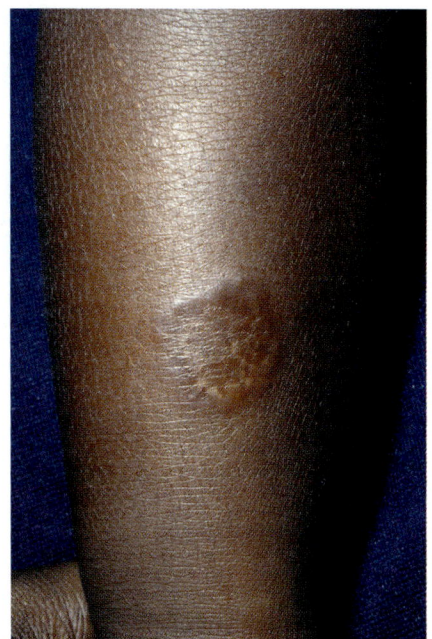

Fig. 31.9 Granuloma annulare.

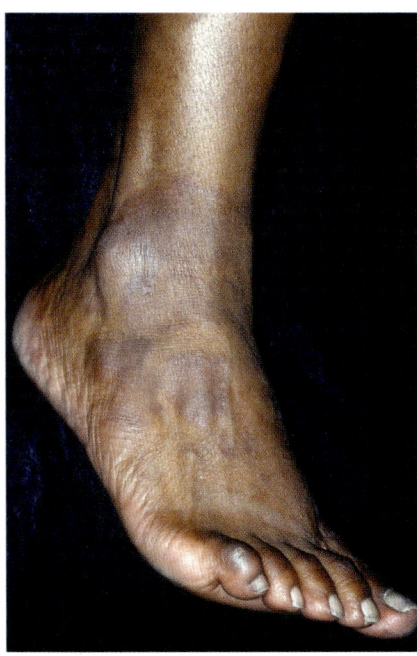

Fig. 31.10 Granuloma annulare.

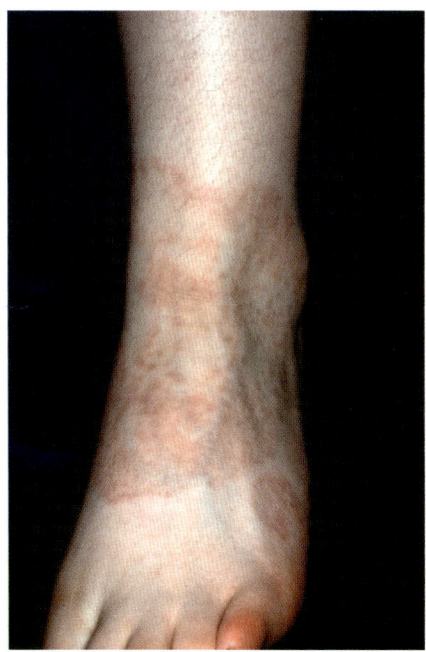

Fig. 31.11 Granuloma annulare.

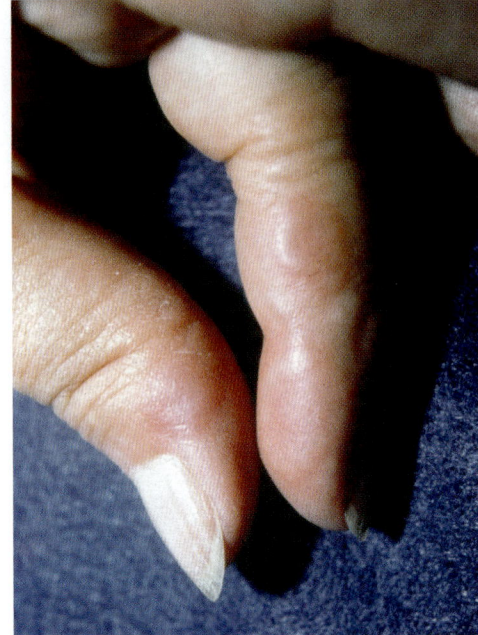

Fig. 31.12 Granuloma annulare.

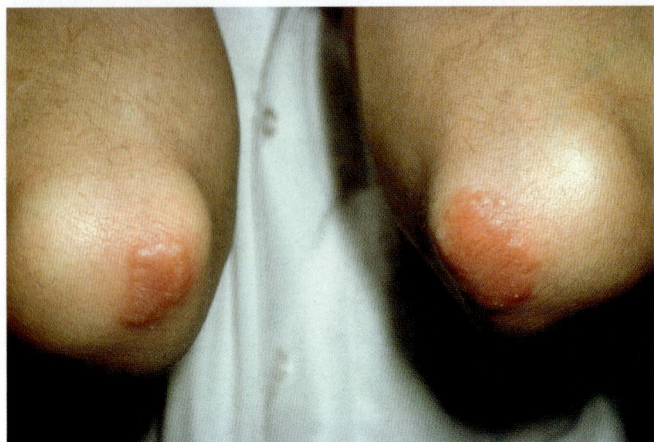

Fig. 31.13 Granuloma annulare.

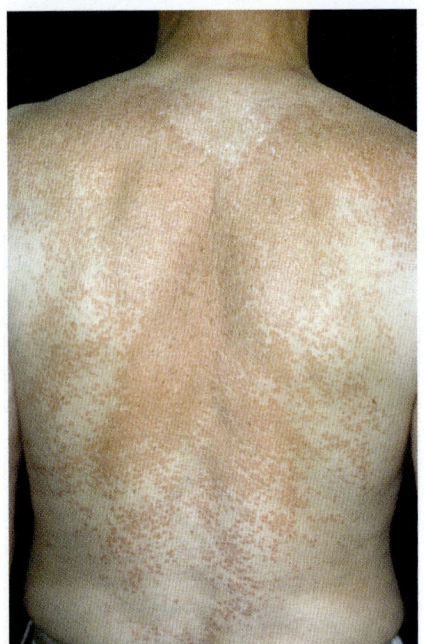

Fig. 31.14 Disseminated granuloma annulare.

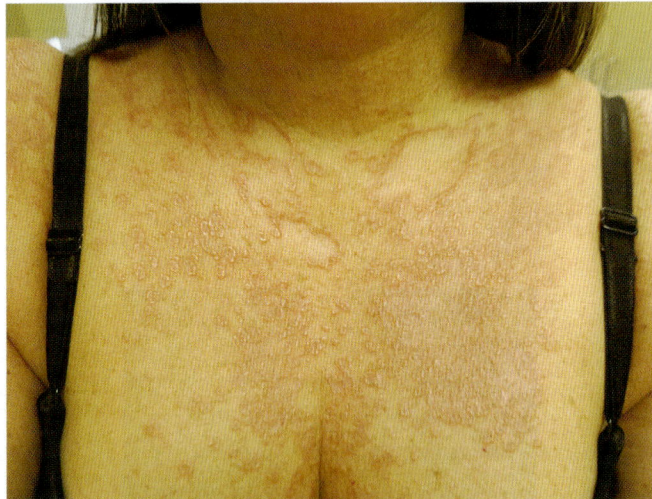

Fig. 31.15 Disseminated granuloma annulare.

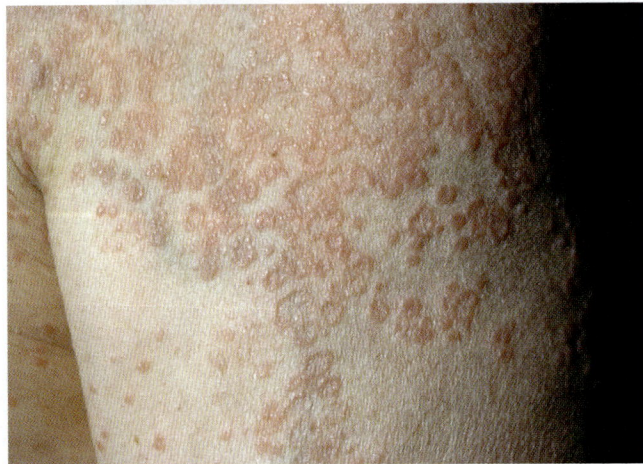

Fig. 31.16 Disseminated granuloma annulare.

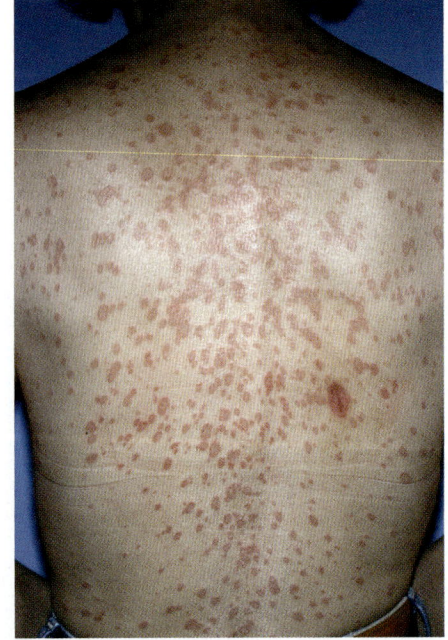

Fig. 31.17 Disseminated granuloma annulare. *Courtesy Curt Samlaska, MD.*

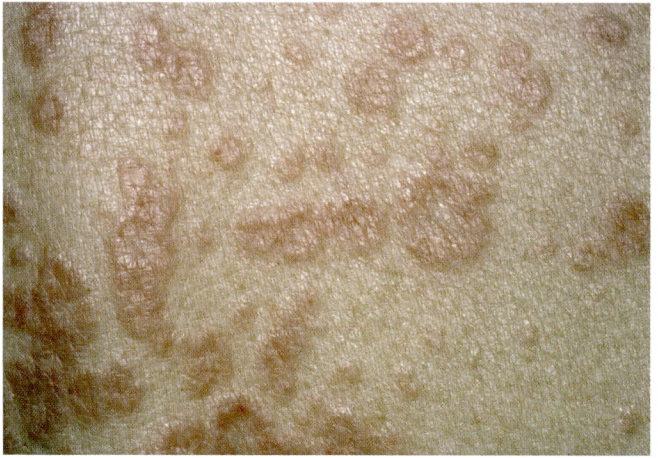

Fig. 31.18 Disseminated granuloma annulare. *Courtesy Curt Samlaska, MD.*

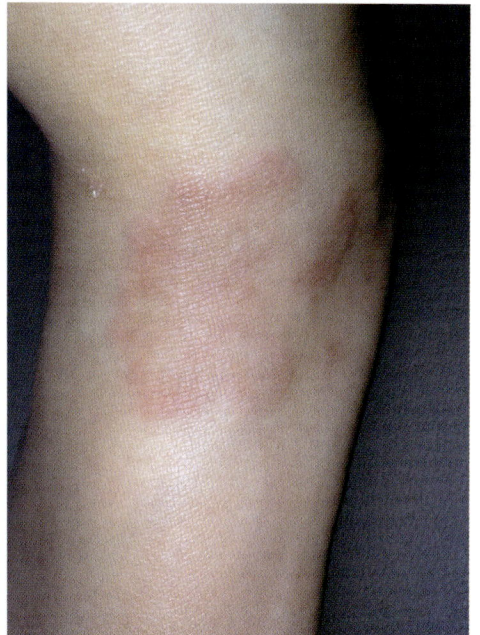

Fig. 31.19 Granuloma annulare.

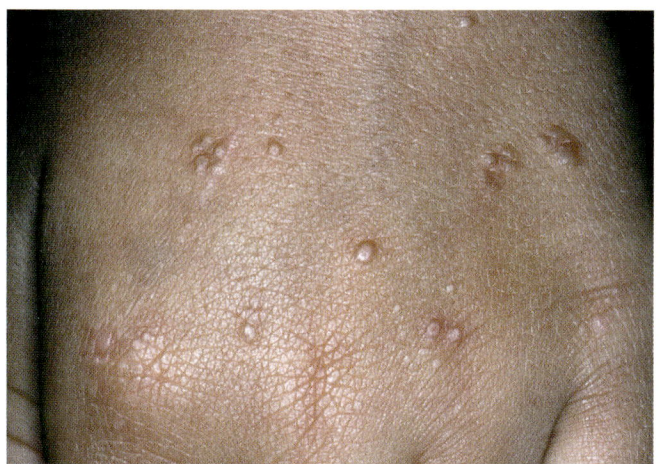

Fig. 31.20 Perforating granuloma annulare. *Courtesy Curt Samlaska, MD.*

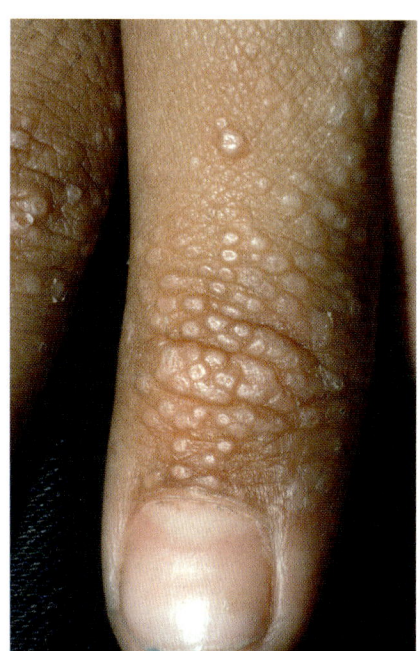

Fig. 31.21 Perforating granuloma annulare. *Courtesy Curt Samlaska, MD.*

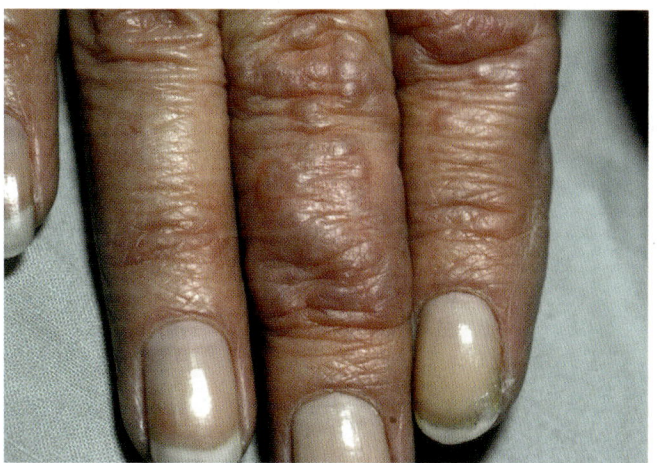

Fig. 31.22 Deep granuloma annulare. *Courtesy Ken Greer, MD.*

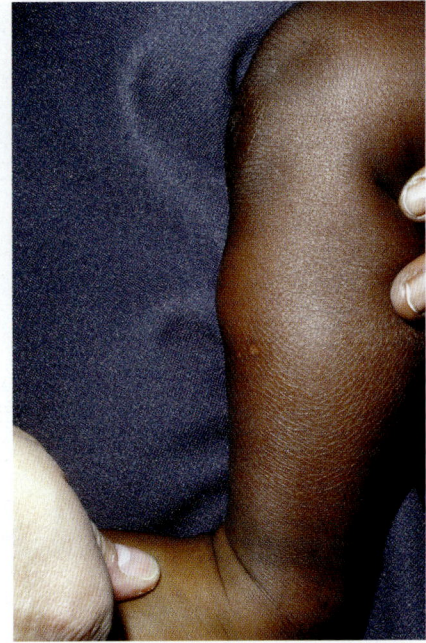

Fig. 31.23 Subcutaneous granuloma annulare.

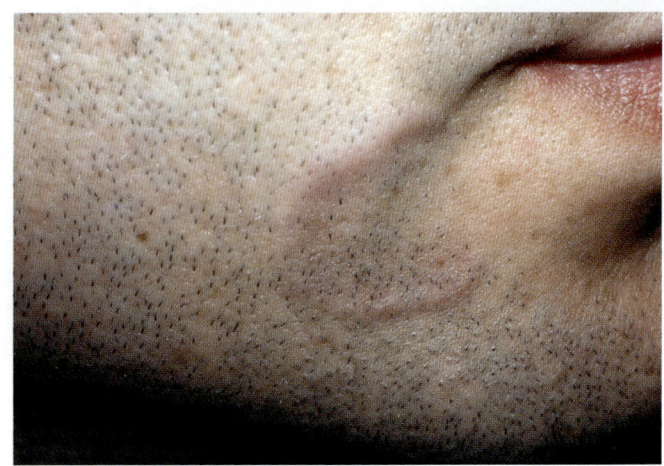

Fig. 31.24 Facial granuloma annulare. *Courtesy Steven Binnick, MD.*

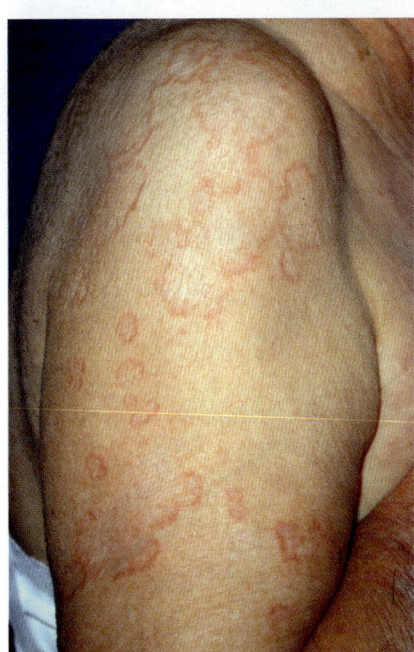

Fig. 31.25 Annular elastolytic granuloma.

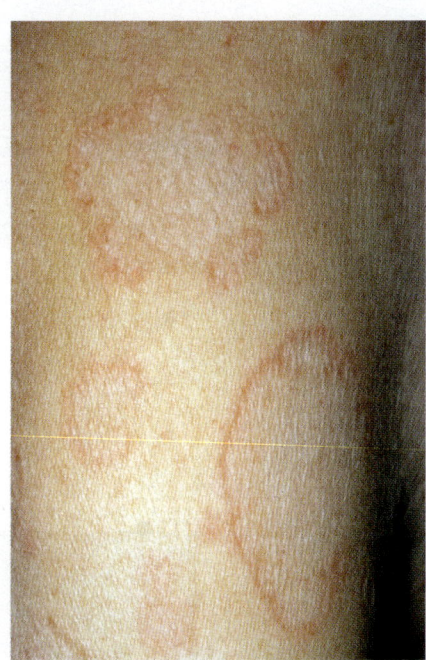

Fig. 31.26 Annular elastolytic granuloma.

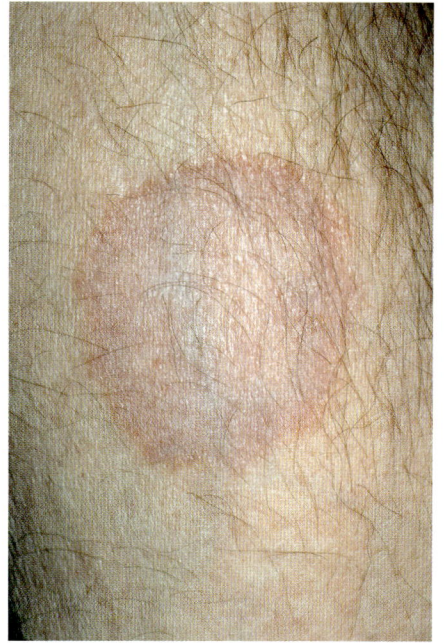

Fig. 31.27 Annular elastolytic granuloma. *Courtesy Curt Samlaska, MD.*

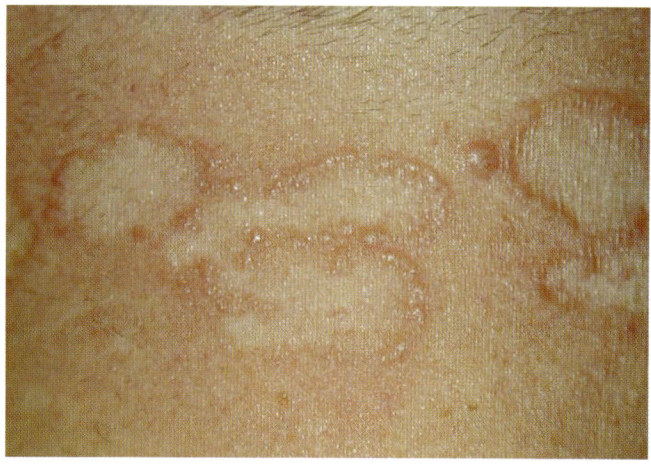

Fig. 31.28 Actinic granuloma.

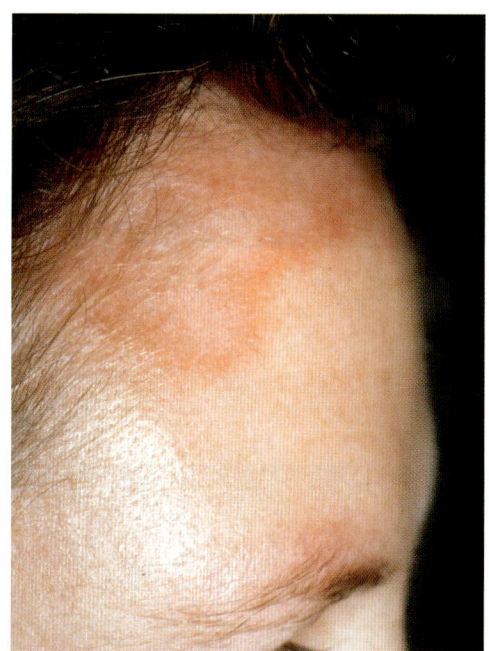

Fig. 31.29 Miescher granuloma.

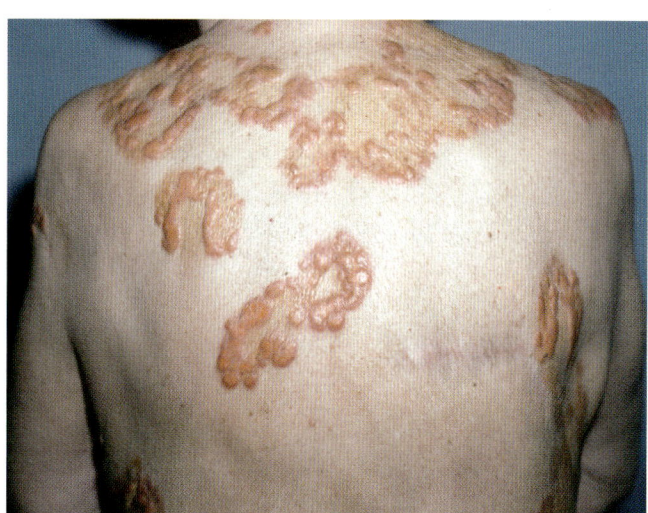

Fig. 31.30 Necrobiotic xanthogranuloma.

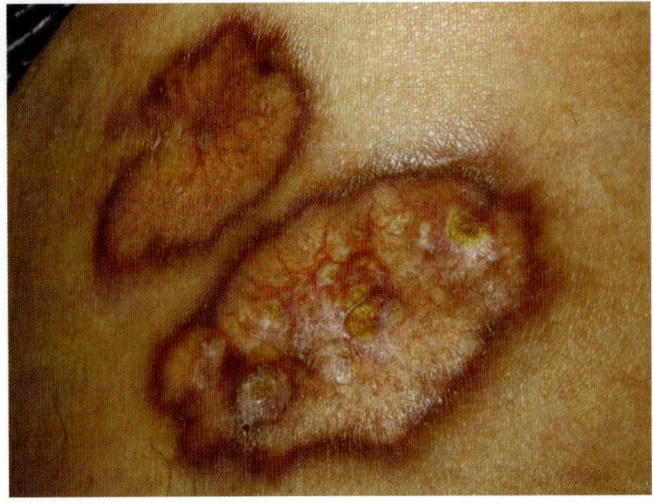

Fig. 31.31 Necrobiotic xanthogranuloma. *Courtesy Yung-Tsu Cho, MD.*

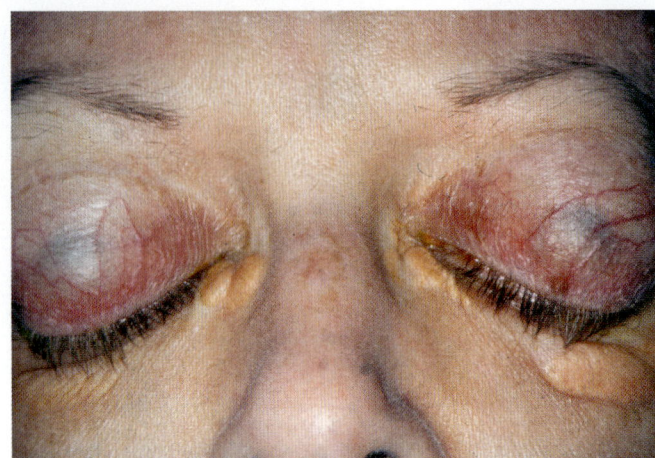

Fig. 31.32 Necrobiotic xanthogranuloma with upper and lower eyelid involvement.

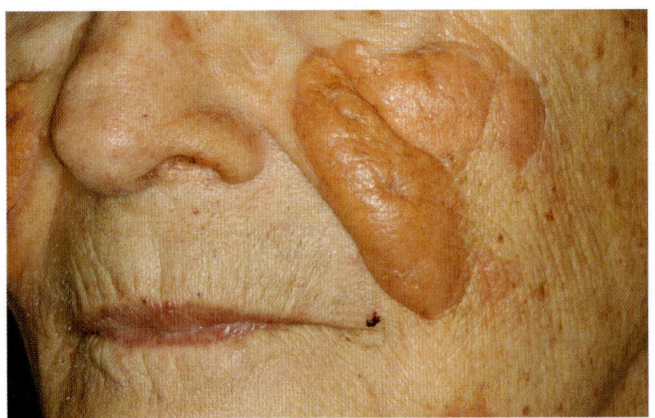

Fig. 31.33 Necrobiotic xanthogranuloma.

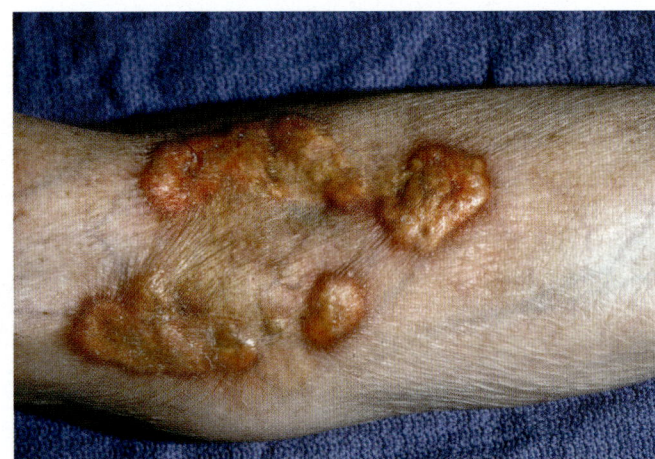

Fig. 31.34 Necrobiotic xanthogranuloma.

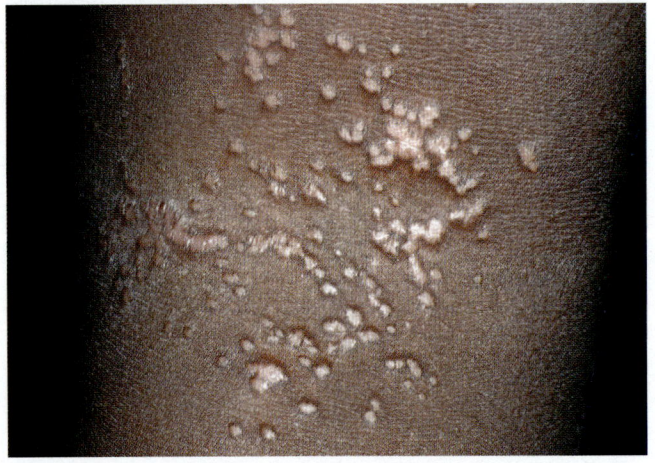

Fig. 31.35 Papular sarcoidosis. *Courtesy Steven Binnick, MD.*

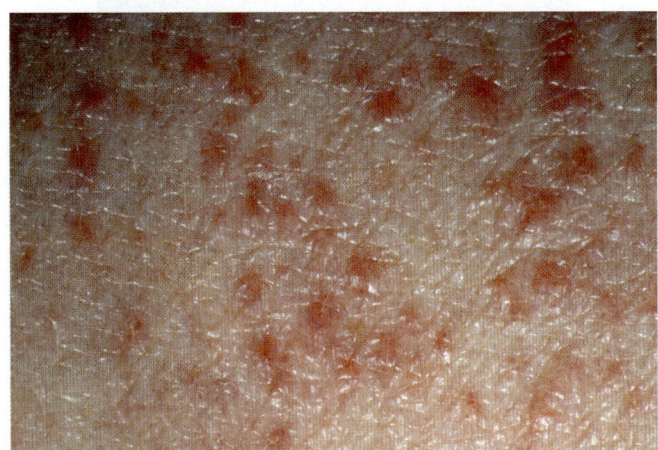

Fig. 31.36 Papular sarcoidosis.

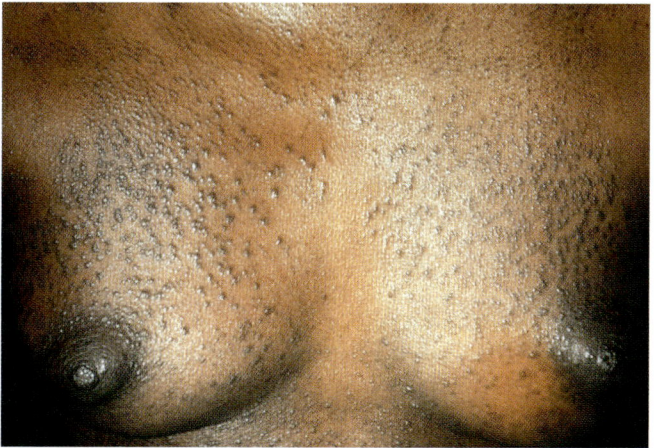

Fig. 31.37 Papular sarcoidosis.

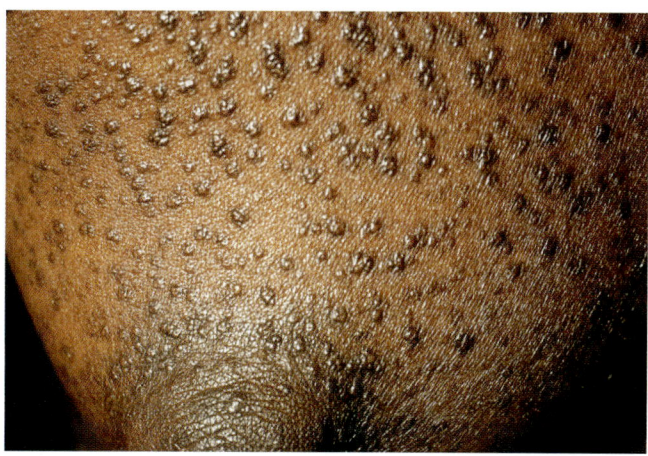

Fig. 31.38 Papular sarcoidosis.

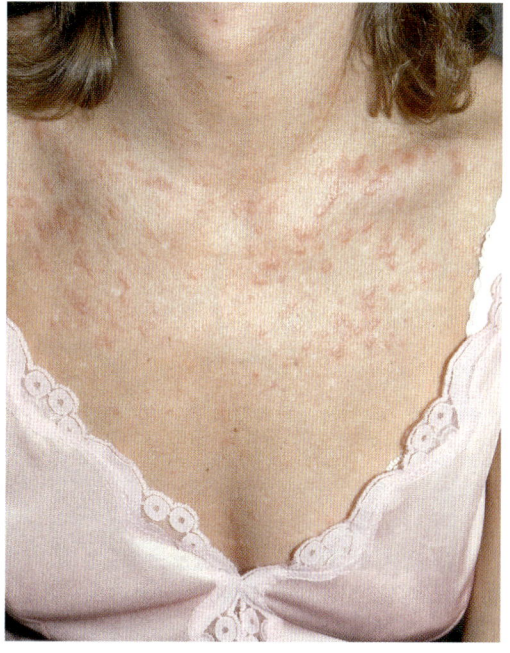

Fig. 31.39 Papular sarcoidosis.

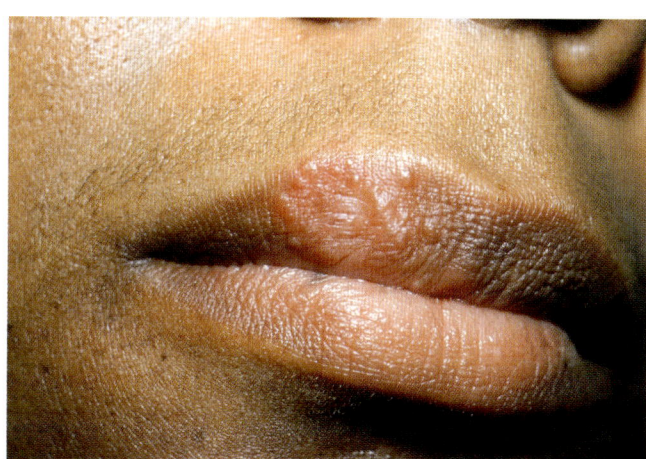

Fig. 31.40 Papular sarcoidosis.

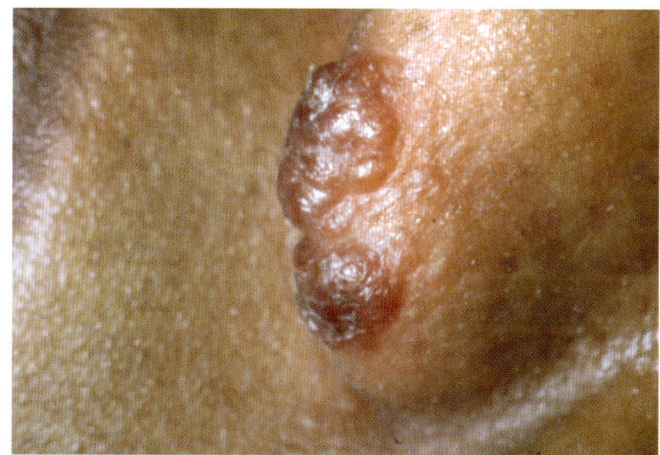

Fig. 31.41 Nodular sarcoidosis.

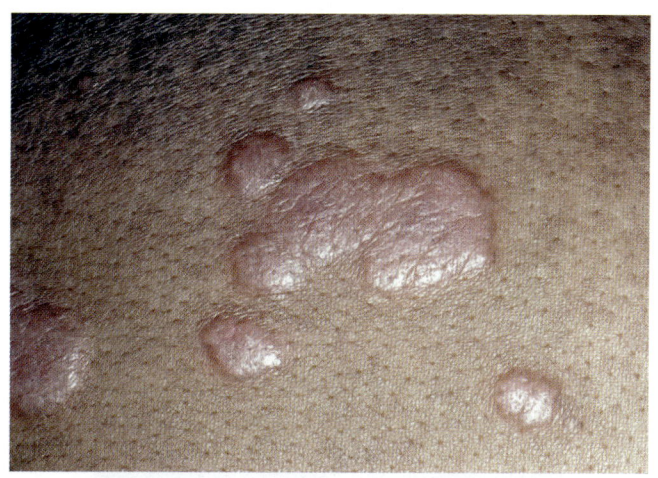

Fig. 31.42 Plaque sarcoidosis. *Courtesy Steven Binnick, MD.*

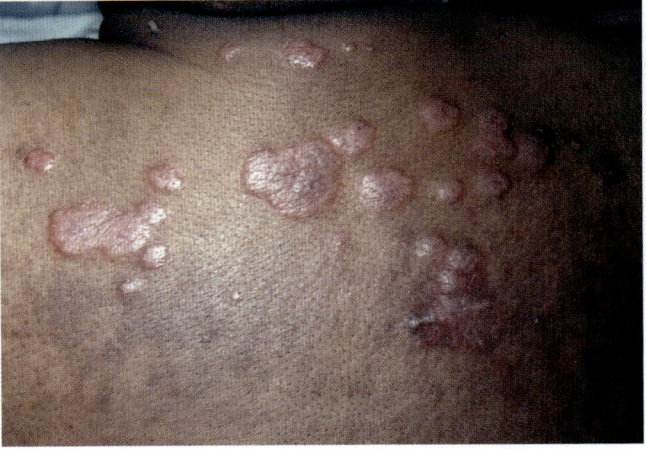

Fig. 31.43 Plaque sarcoidosis. *Courtesy Steven Binnick, MD.*

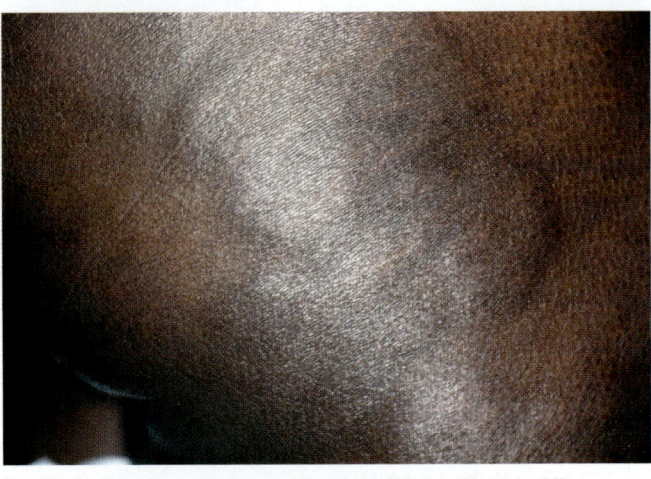

Fig. 31.44 Plaque sarcoidosis. *Courtesy Steven Binnick, MD.*

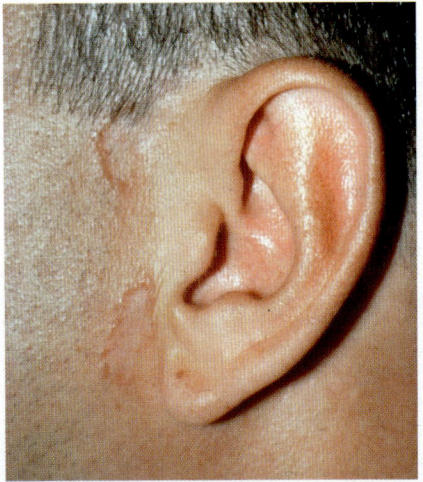

Fig. 31.45 Annular sarcoidosis.

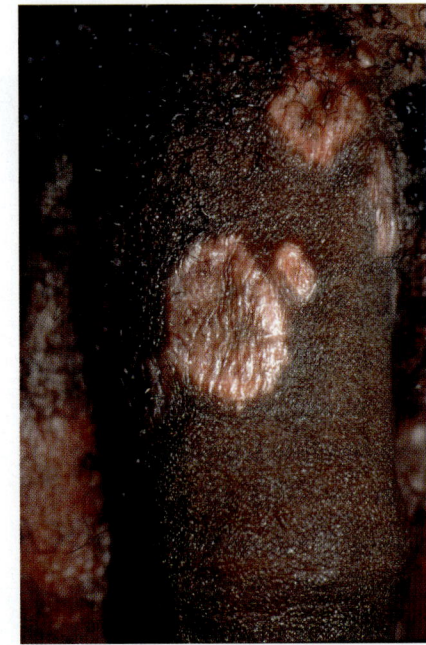

Fig. 31.46 Annular genital sarcoid.

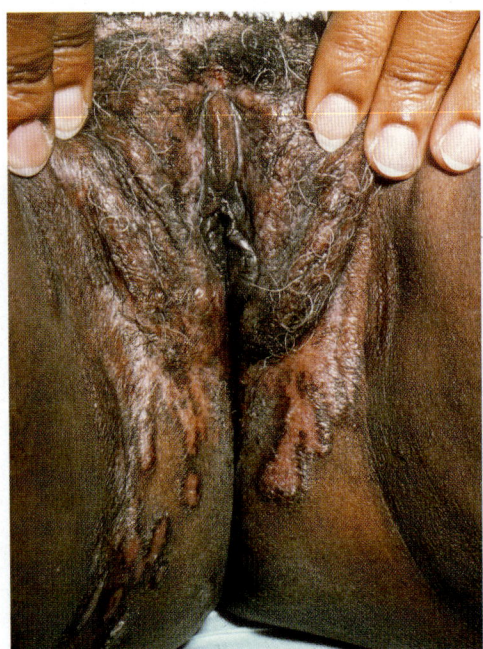

Fig. 31.47 Genital sarcoidosis.

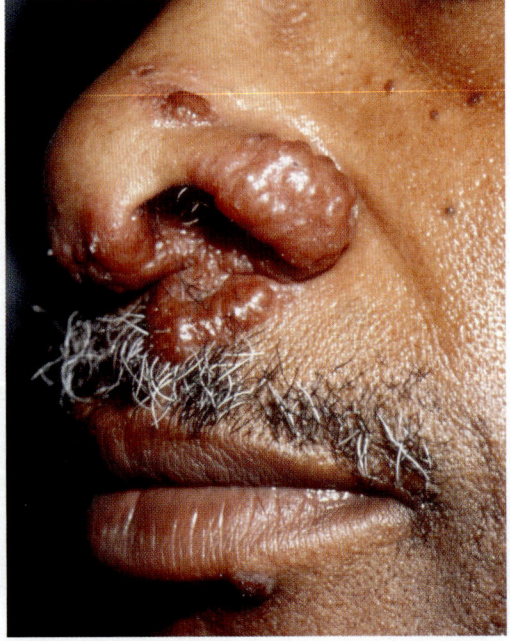

Fig. 31.48 Lupus pernio.

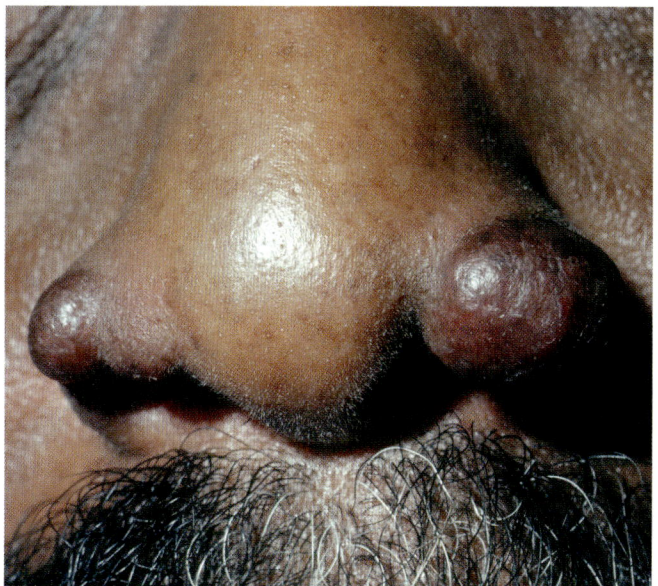

Fig. 31.49 Lupus pernio. *Courtesy Steven Binnick, MD.*

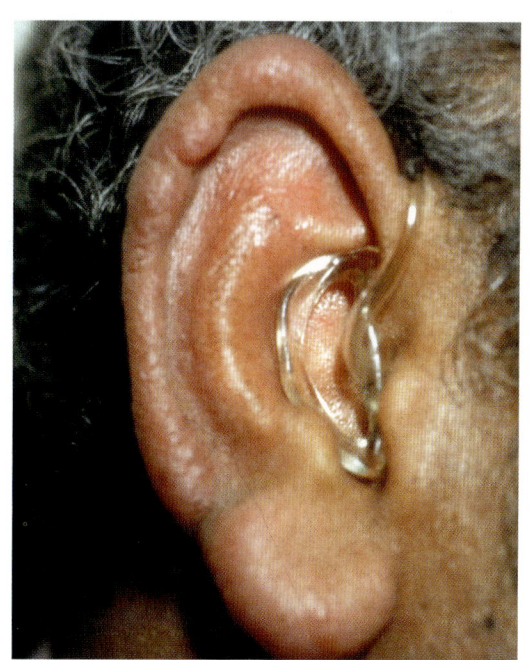

Fig. 31.50 Lupus pernio.

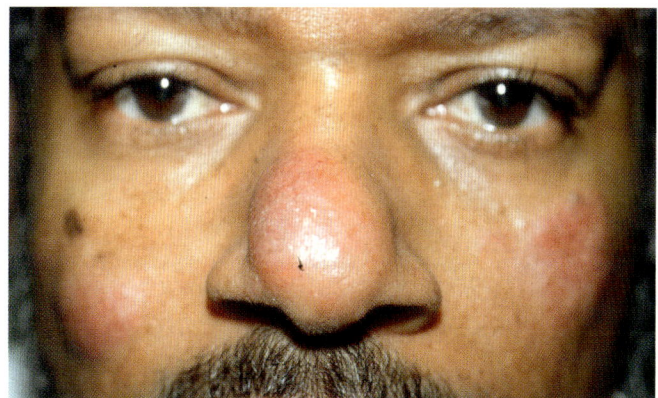

Fig. 31.51 Lupus pernio.

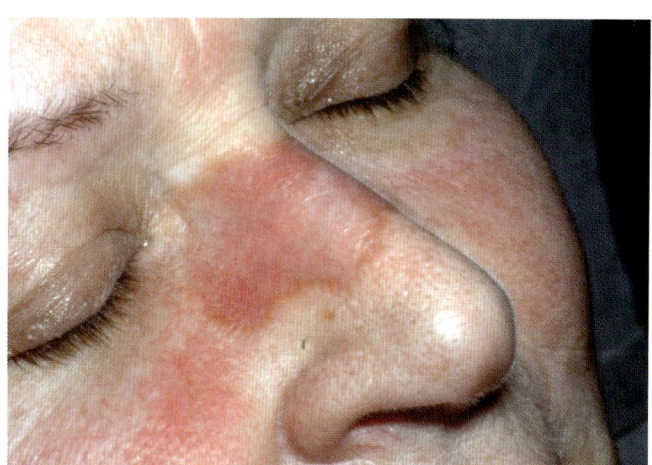

Fig. 31.52 Lupus pernio. *Courtesy Steven Binnick, MD.*

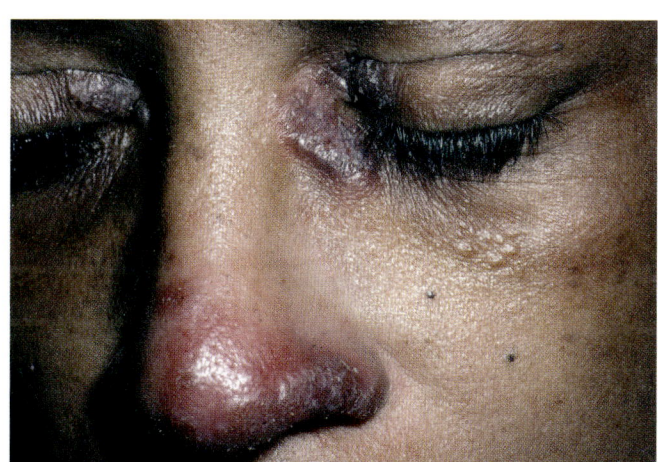

Fig. 31.53 Lupus pernio. *Courtesy Steven Binnick, MD.*

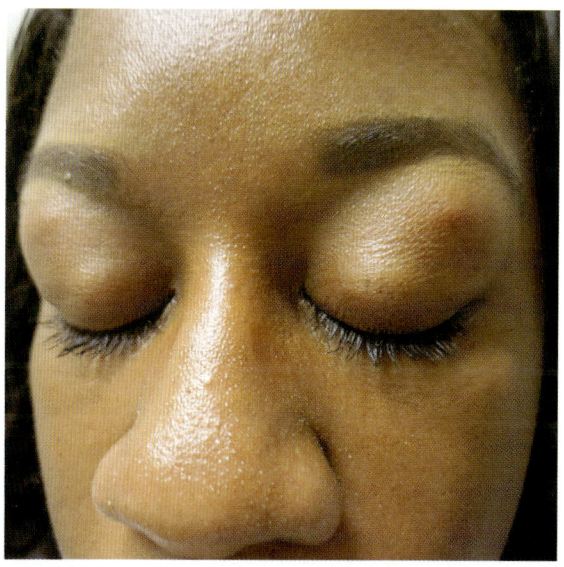

Fig. 31.54 Exocrine gland swelling in sarcoidosis.

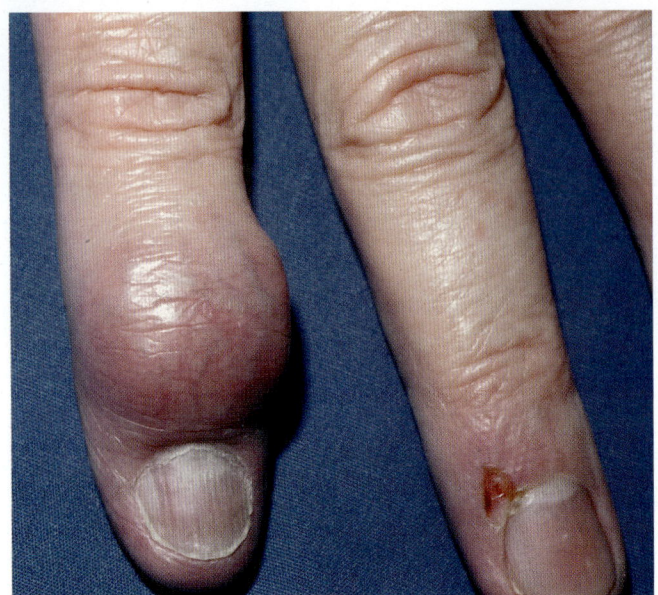

Fig. 31.55 Digital sarcoidosis. *Courtesy Steven Binnick, MD.*

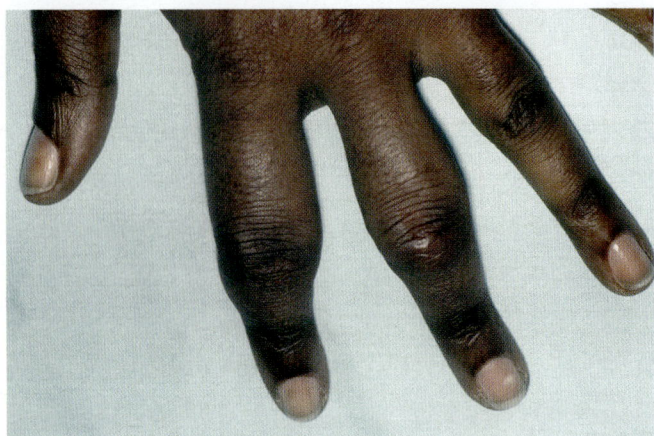

Fig. 31.56 Osseous sarcoidosis. *Courtesy Steven Binnick, MD.*

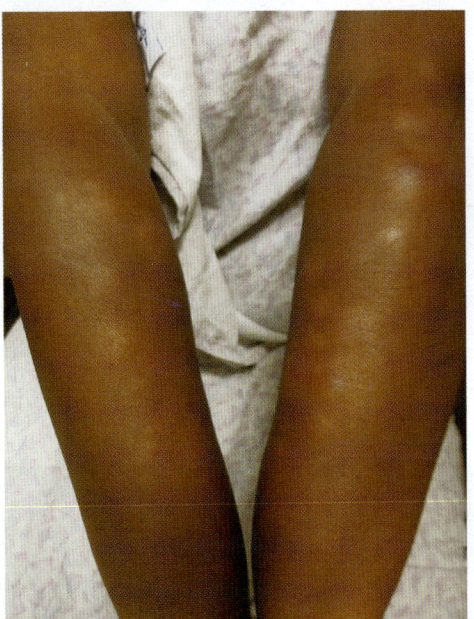

Fig. 31.57 Hypopigmentation overlying subcutaneous sarcoidosis.

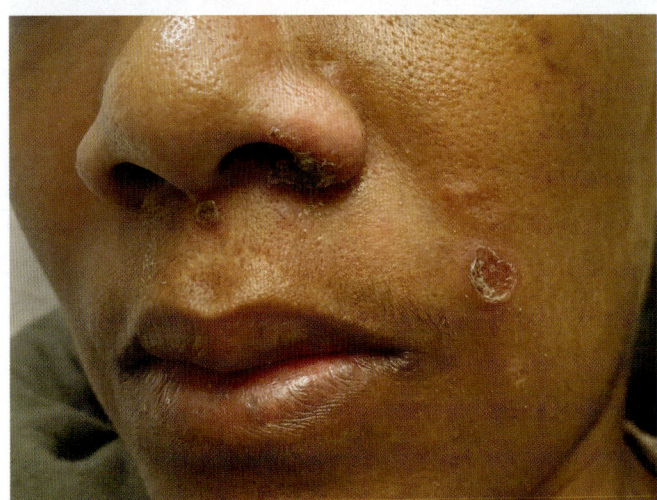

Fig. 31.58 Ulcerative sarcoidosis.

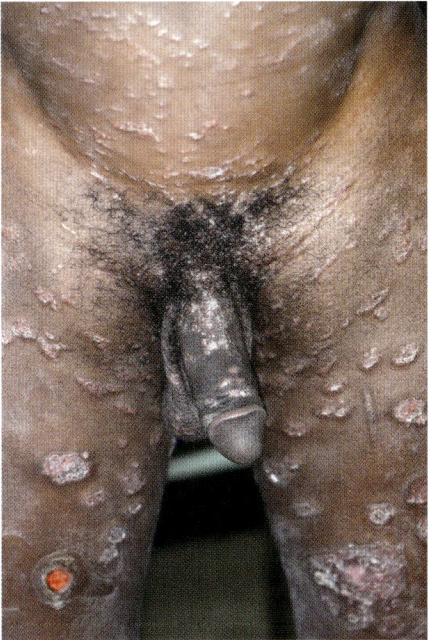

Fig. 31.59 Ulcerative sarcoidosis.

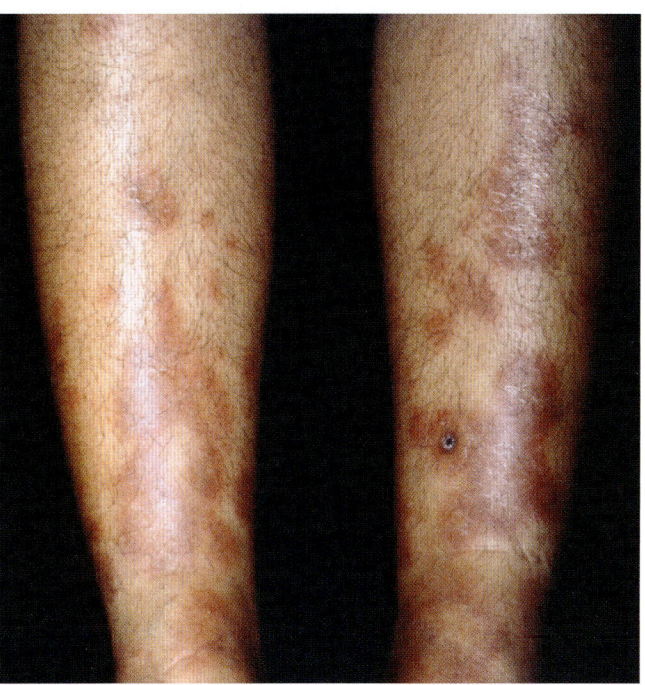

Fig. 31.60 Erythema nodosum–like sarcoidosis. Biopsy was granulomatous.

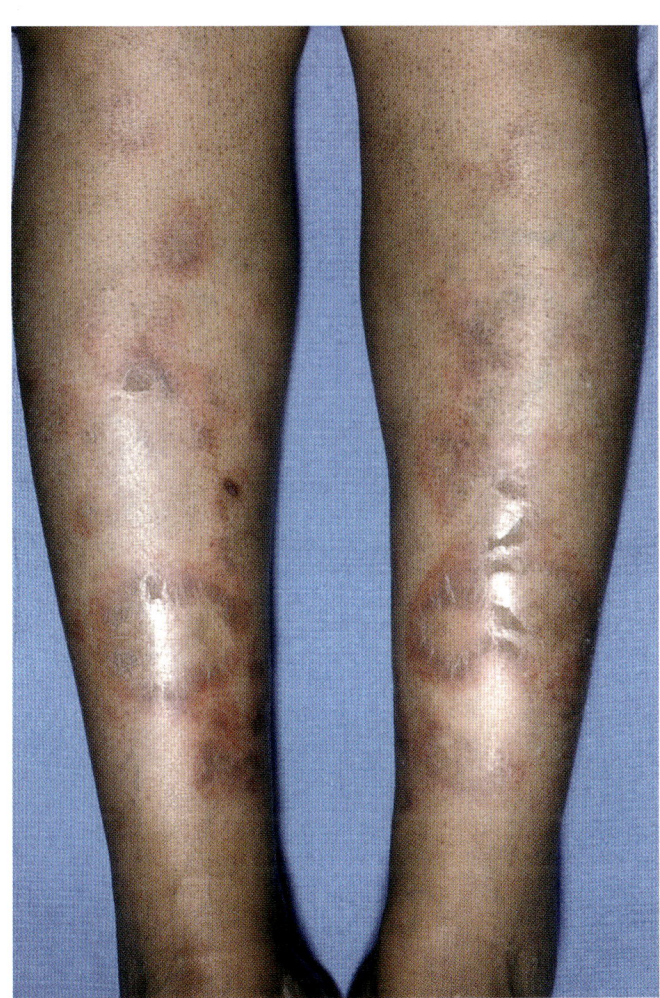

Fig. 31.61 Sarcoidosis.

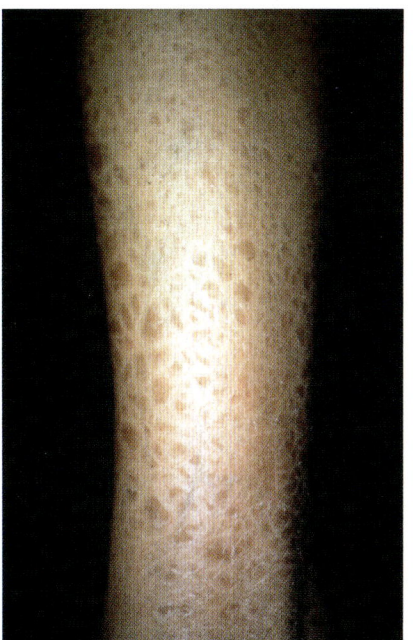

Fig. 31.62 Ichthyosiform sarcoidosis. *Courtesy Steven Binnick, MD.*

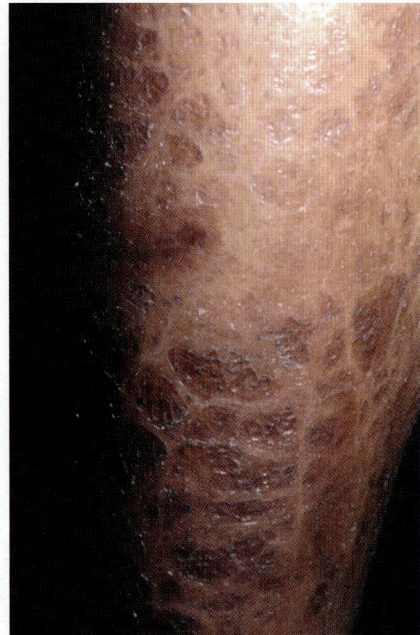

Fig. 31.63 Ichthyosiform sarcoidosis.

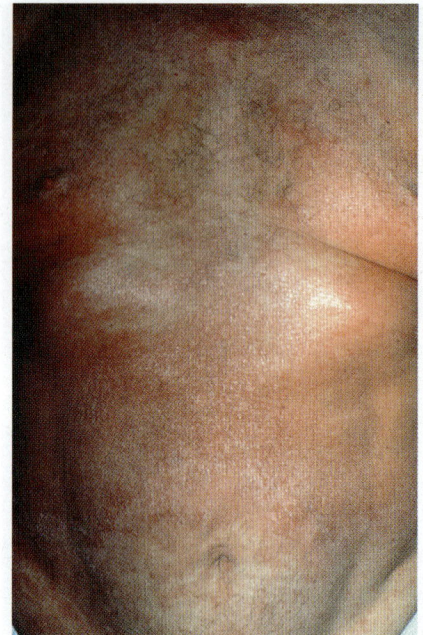

Fig. 31.64 Erythrodermic sarcoidosis.

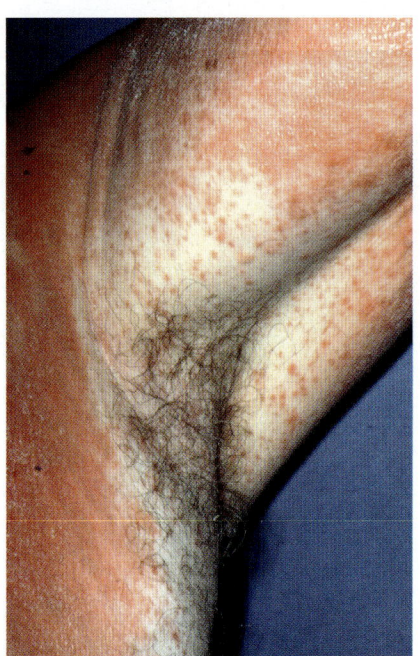

Fig. 31.65 Erythrodermic sarcoidosis.

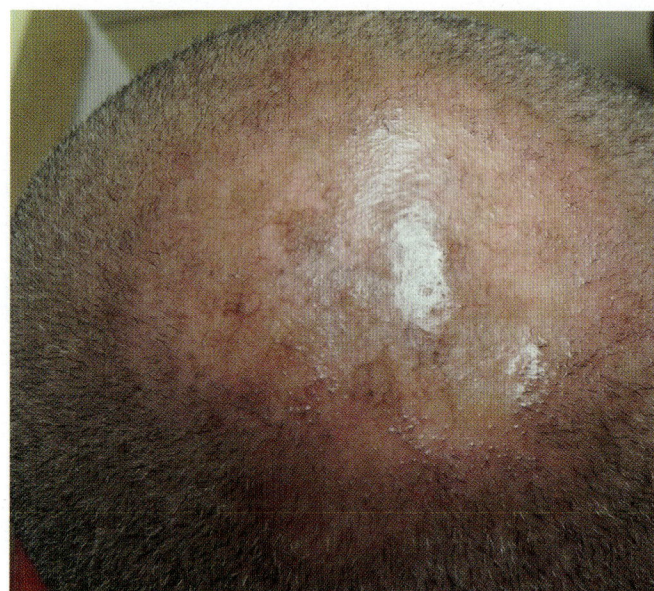

Fig. 31.66 Alopecia in sarcoidosis. *Courtesy Misha Rosenbach, MD.*

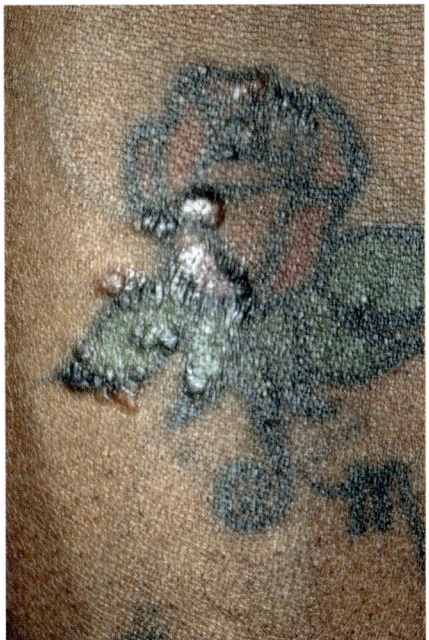

Fig. 31.67 Sarcoid in a tattoo.

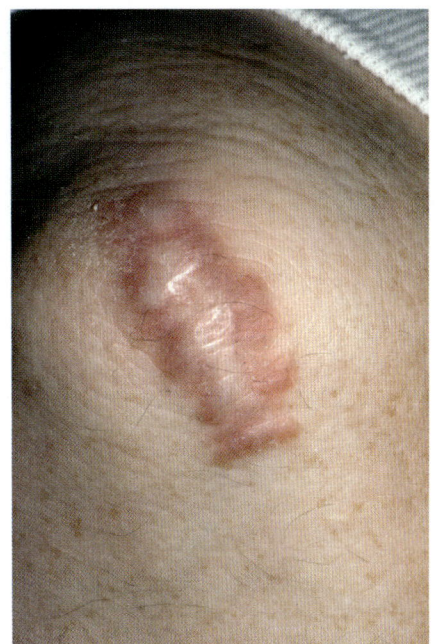

Fig. 31.68 Scar sarcoidosis. *Courtesy Steven Binnick, MD.*

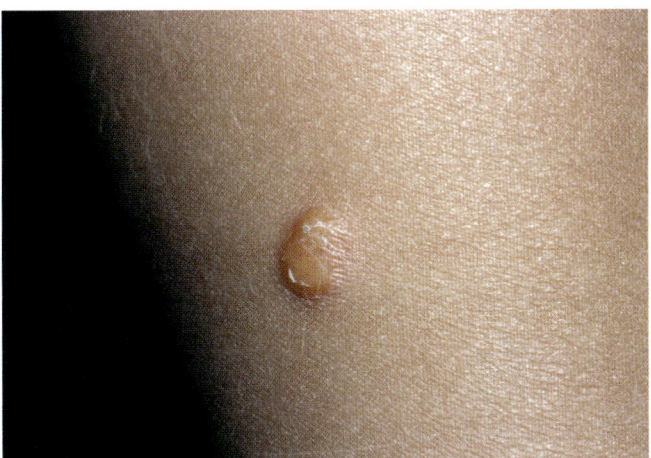

Fig. 31.69 Juvenile xanthogranuloma. *Courtesy Curt Samlaska, MD.*

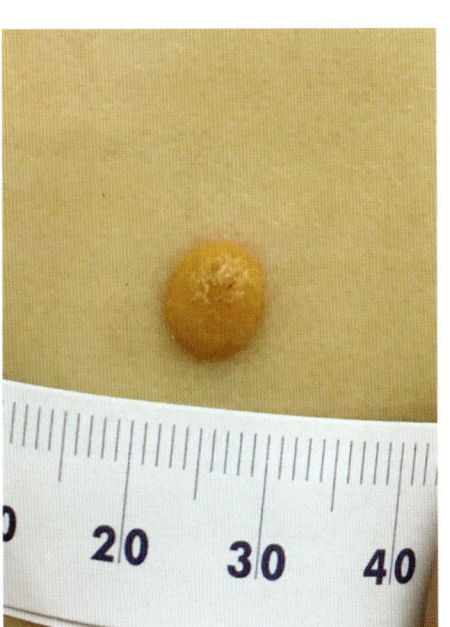

Fig. 31.71 Juvenile xanthogranuloma. *Courtesy National Taiwan University Hospital.*

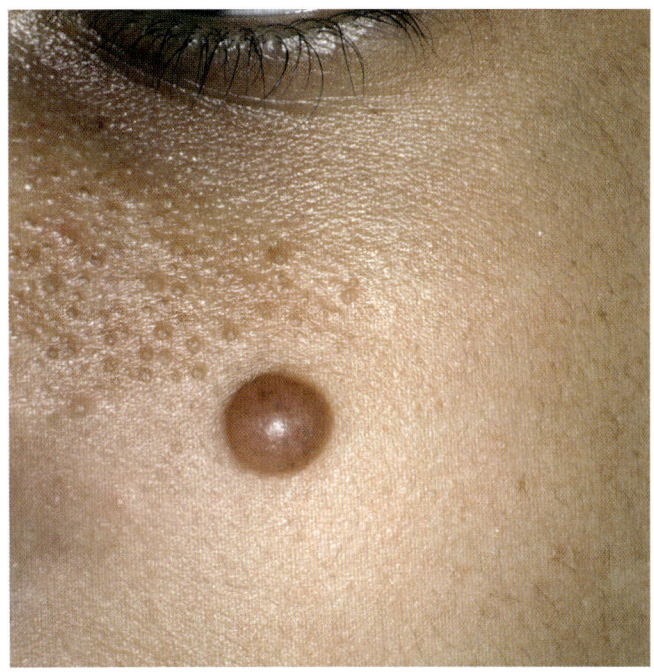

Fig. 31.70 Juvenile xanthogranuloma. *Courtesy Steven Binnick, MD.*

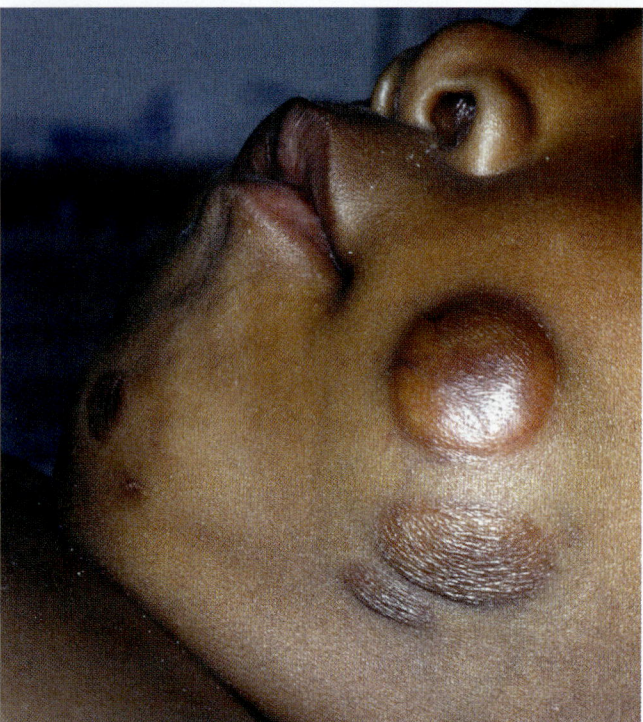

Fig. 31.72 Large juvenile xanthogranuloma.

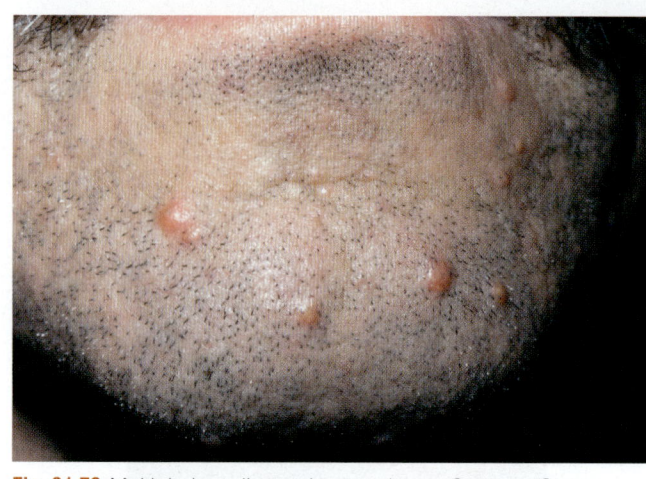

Fig. 31.73 Multiple juvenile xanthogranuloma. *Courtesy Steven Binnick, MD.*

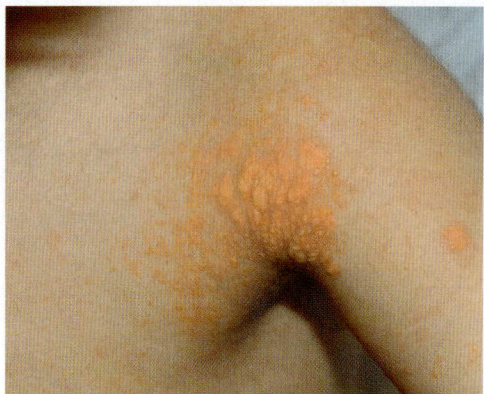

Fig. 31.74 Juvenile xanthogranulomatous plaque. *Courtesy Scott Norton, MD.*

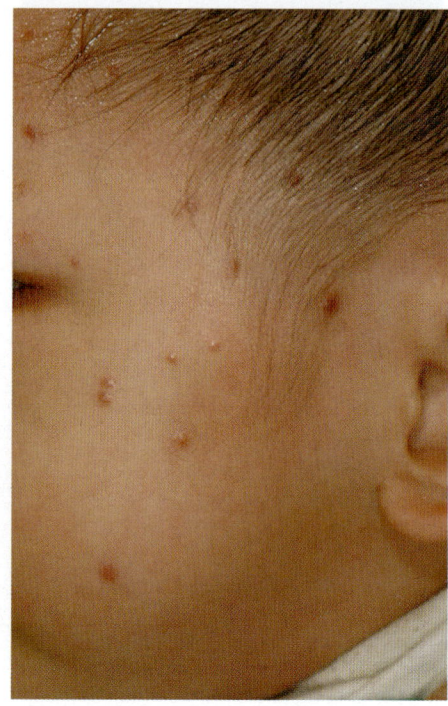

Fig. 31.75 Benign cephalic histiocytosis. *Courtesy Kaohsiung Chang Gang Memorial Hospital, Taiwan.*

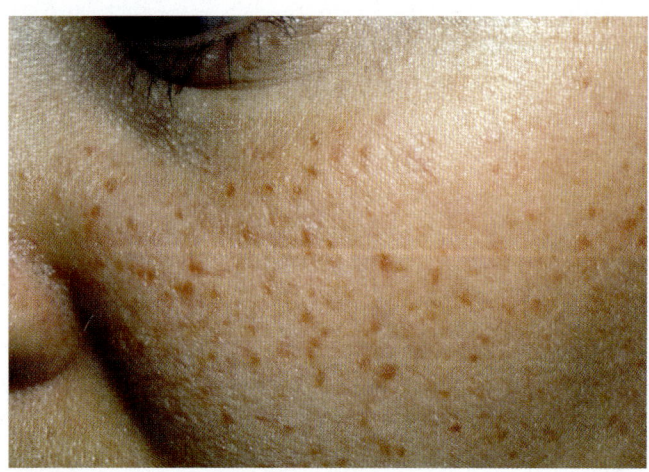

Fig. 31.76 Generalized eruptive histiocytomas.

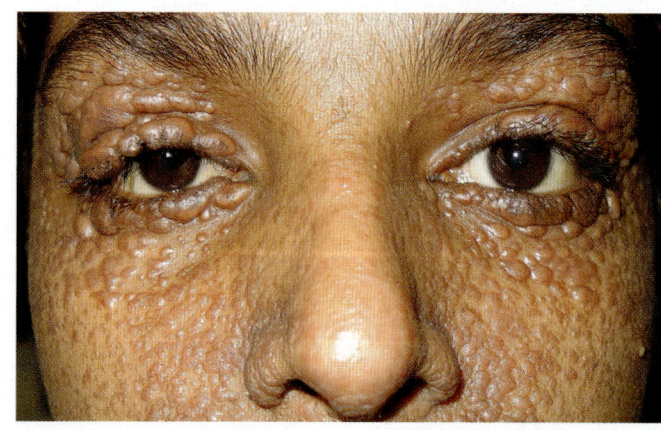

Fig. 31.77 Xanthoma disseminatum. *Courtesy Debabrata Bandyopadhyay, MD.*

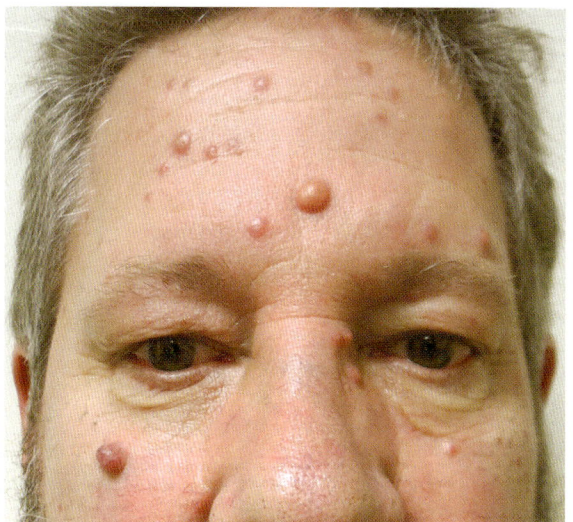

Fig. 31.78 Progressive nodular histiocytosis.

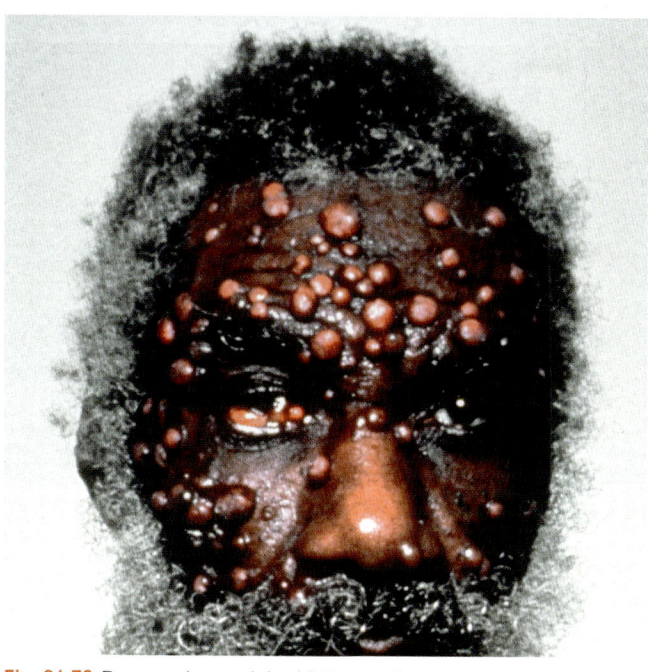

Fig. 31.79 Progressive nodular histiocytosis.

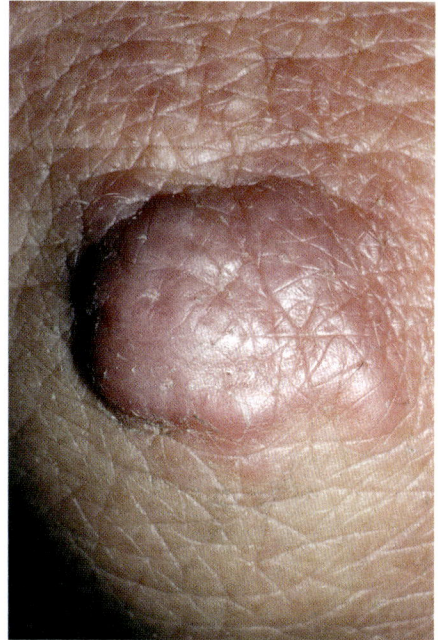

Fig. 31.80 Reticulohistiocytoma. *Courtesy Steven Binnick, MD.*

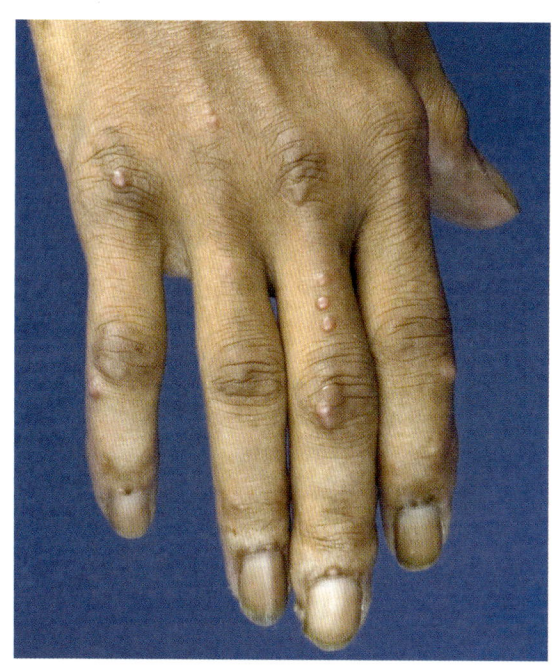

Fig. 31.81 Multicentric reticulohistiocytosis.

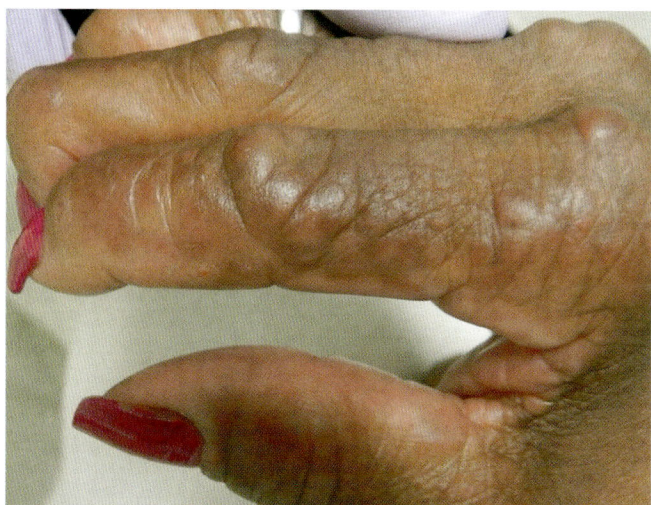

Fig. 31.82 Multicentric reticulohistiocytosis.

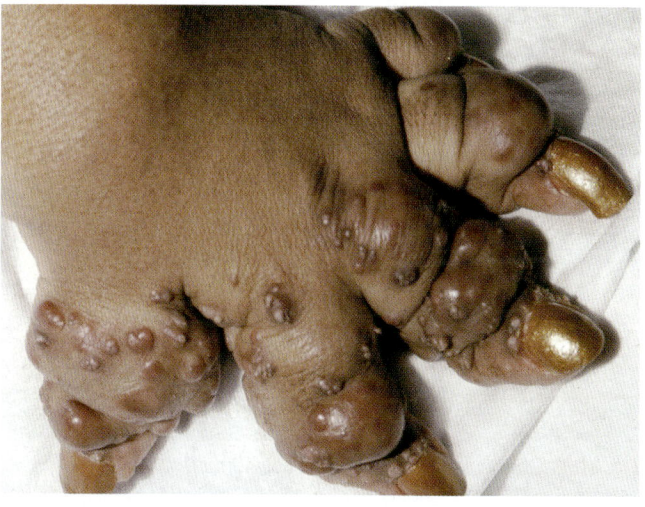

Fig. 31.83 Multicentric reticulohistiocytosis.

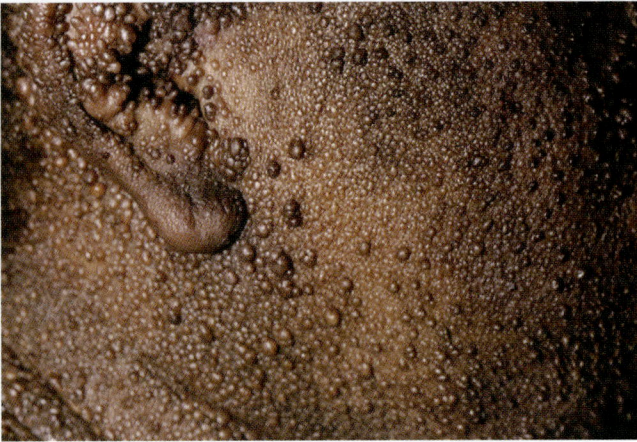

Fig. 31.84 Multicentric reticulohistiocytosis.

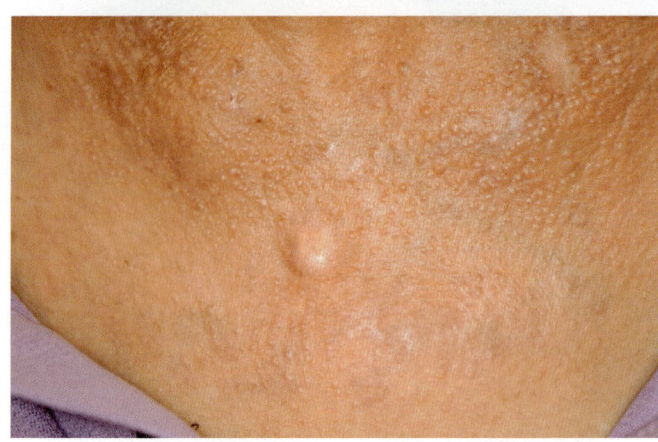

Fig. 31.85 Multicentric reticulohistiocytosis. *Courtesy Kaohsiung Chang Gang Memorial Hospital, Taiwan.*

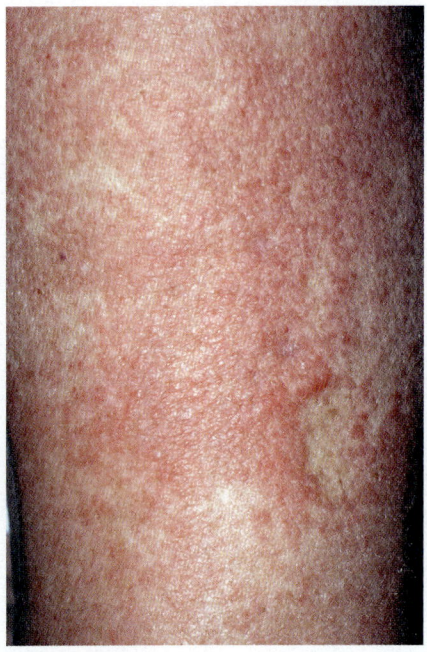

Fig. 31.86 Multicentric reticulohistiocytosis. *Courtesy Steven Binnick, MD.*

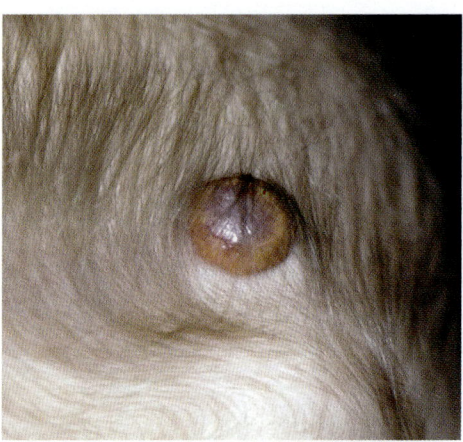

Fig. 31.87 Congenital self-healing histiocytosis. *Courtesy Paul Honig, MD.*

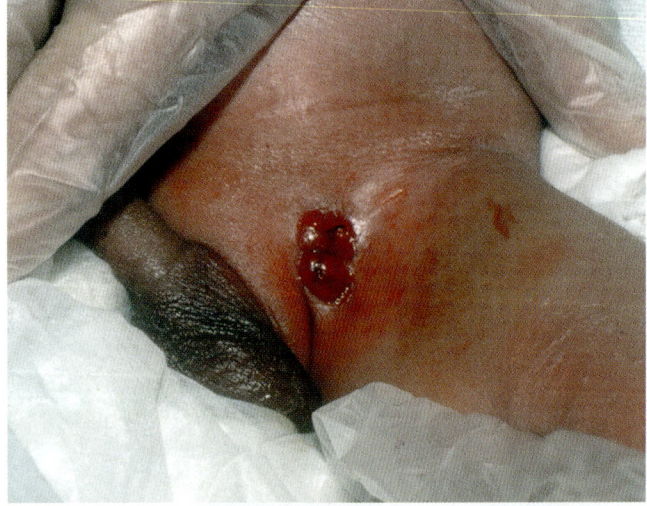

Fig. 31.88 Congenital self-healing histiocytomas.

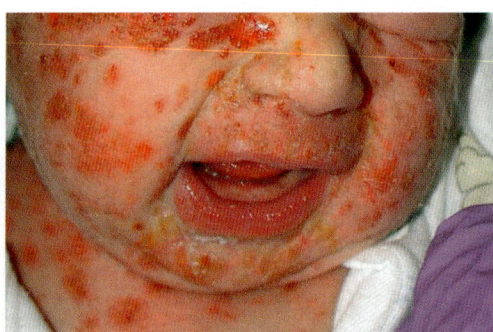

Fig. 31.89 Congenital Langerhans cell histiocytosis.

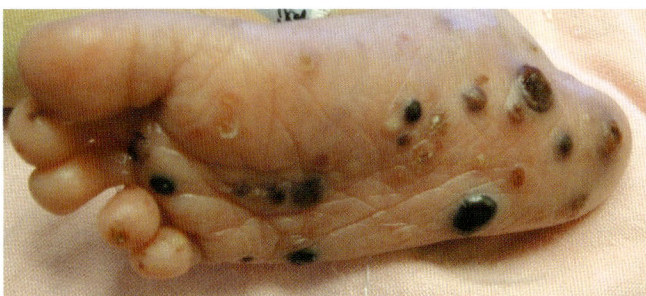

Fig. 31.90 Langerhans cell histiocytosis. *Courtesy Kaohsiung Chang Gang Memorial Hospital, Taiwan.*

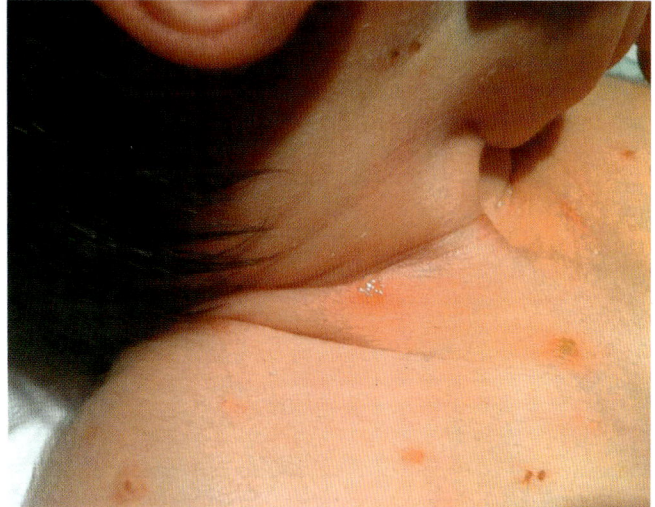

Fig. 31.91 Congenital Langerhans cell histiocytosis. *Courtesy Sheilagh Maguiness, MD.*

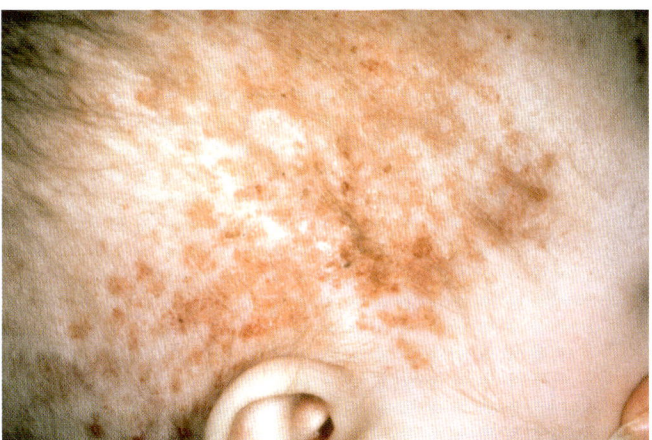

Fig. 31.92 Langerhans cell histiocytosis.

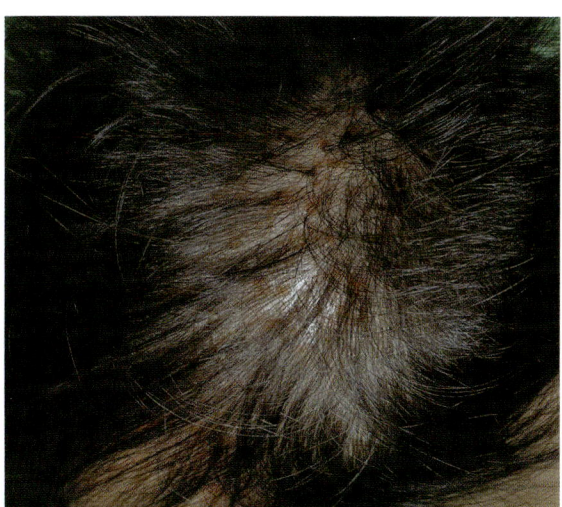

Fig. 31.93 Langerhans cell histiocytosis. *Courtesy National Cheng Kung University, Taiwan.*

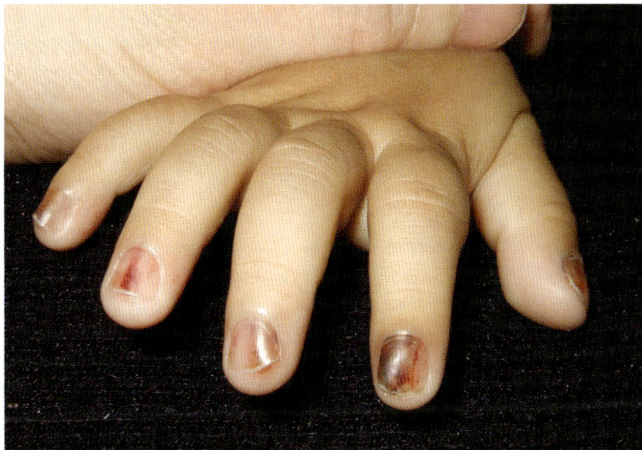

Fig. 31.94 Nail involvement with Langerhans cell histiocytosis. *Courtesy National Taiwan University Hospital.*

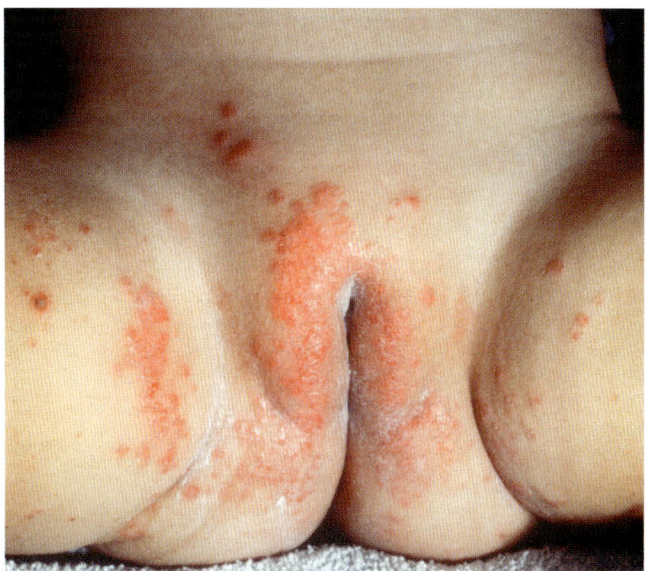

Fig. 31.95 Langerhans cell histiocytosis.

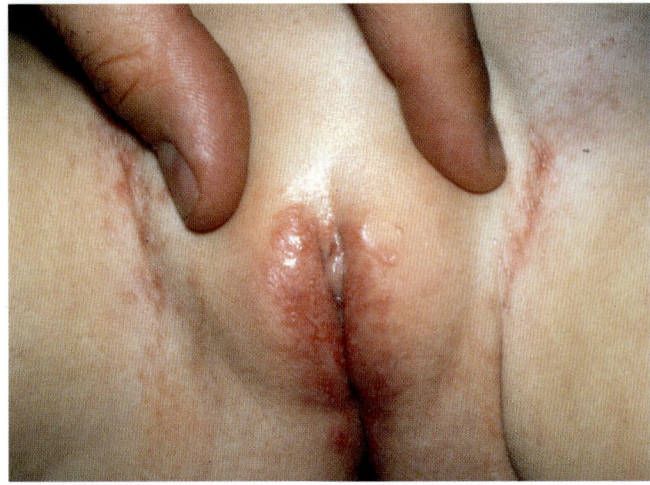

Fig. 31.96 Langerhans cell histiocytosis.

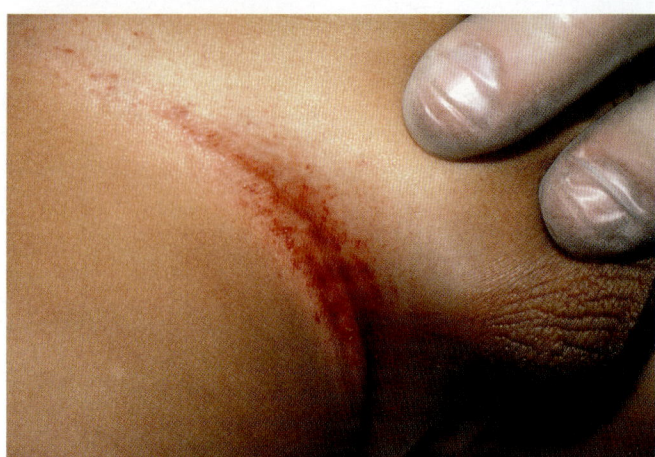

Fig. 31.97 Langerhans cell histiocytosis.

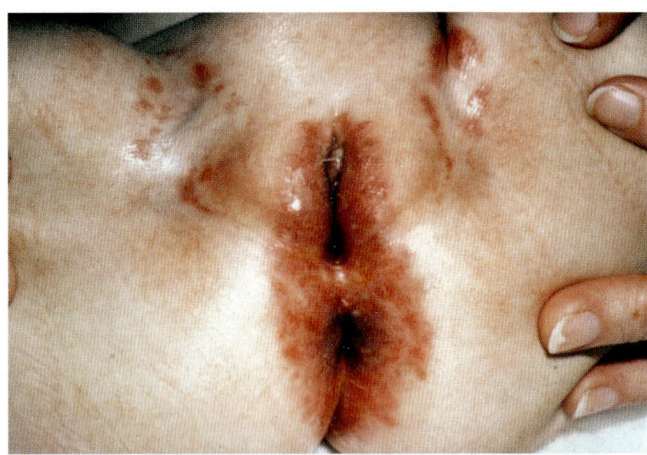

Fig. 31.98 Langerhans cell histiocytosis.

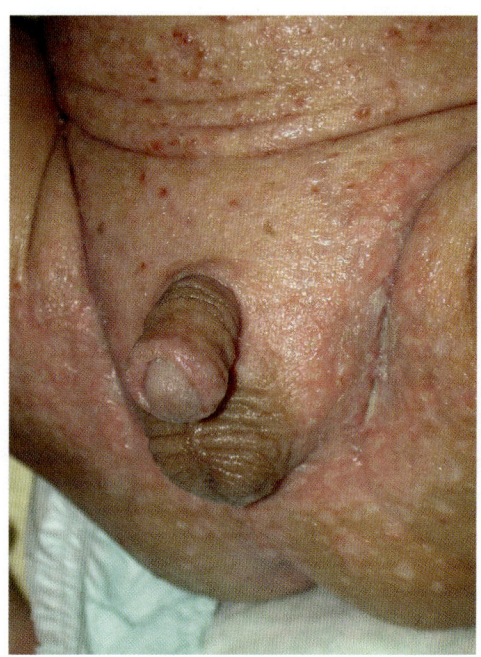

Fig. 31.99 Langerhans cell histiocytosis.

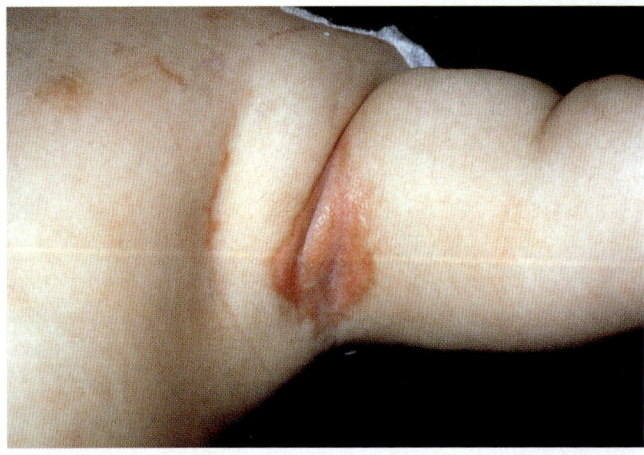

Fig. 31.100 Langerhans cell histiocytosis.

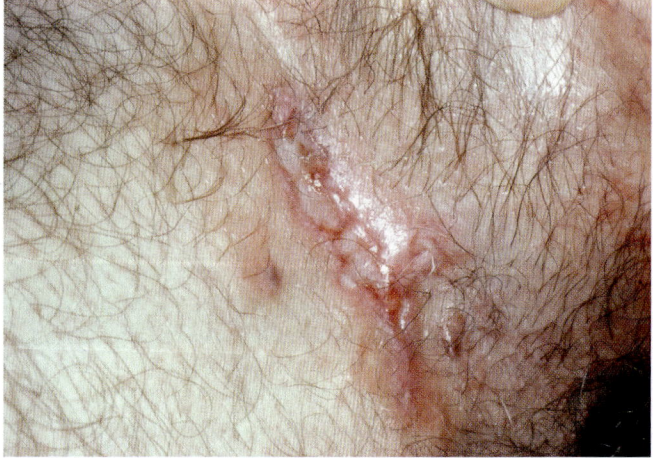

Fig. 31.101 Adult Langerhans cell histiocytosis.

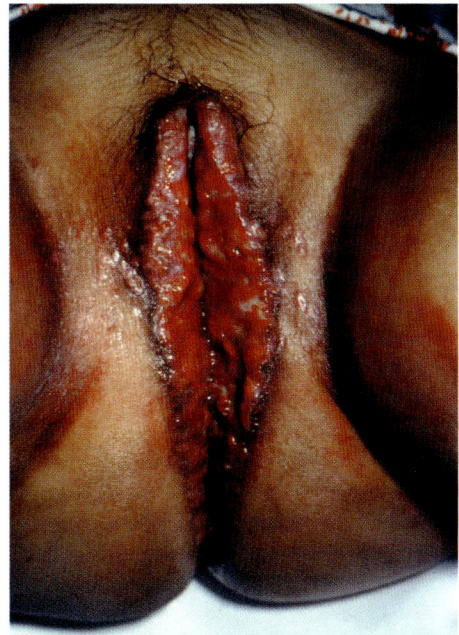

Fig. 31.102 Adult Langerhans cell histiocytosis.

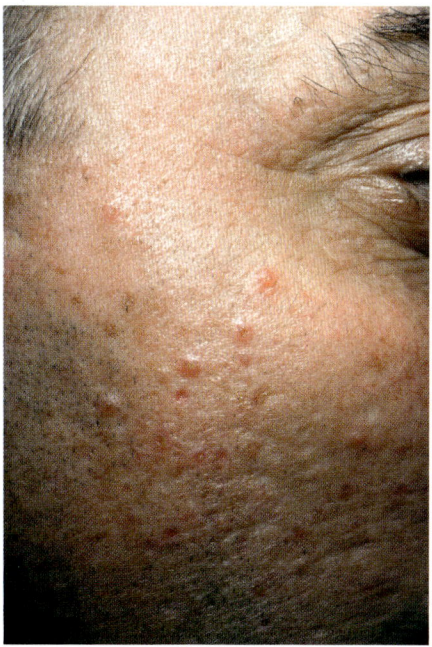

Fig. 31.103 Adult Langerhans cell histiocytosis.

Cutaneous Lymphoid Hyperplasia, Cutaneous T-Cell Lymphoma, Other Malignant Lymphomas, and Allied Diseases

32

The evaluation of lymphoid neoplasms typically requires clinicopathological correlation, and classification often requires panels of immunostains. This section of the atlas will focus on the clinical appearance of cutaneous lymphomas that should prompt the physician to perform a biopsy. The distribution and morphology of the lesion are also helpful in classification of the neoplasm to ensure optimal therapy.

Mycosis fungoides commonly involve the trunk, buttocks, and proximal extremities. The lesions tend to be larger than 5 cm in diameter with a poikilodermatous appearance (mottled, hyperpigmentation and hypopigmentation, atrophy, and telangiectasia). B-cell lymphomas commonly present as plum-colored nodules with a smooth, shiny surface. Discrete nodules on the head and neck, trunk, or proximal extremities; arcuate lesions and nodules on the trunk; taught, shiny nodules on the lower extremities; and multinodular lesions on the legs are all seen in the wide variety of lymphoid neoplasms in this chapter. The lesions of lymphomatoid papulosis are often papulonecrotic, erupt in crops, and resolve spontaneously. Leukemias and myelomas often appear as skin-colored to purple papules and nodules, at times with accompanying hemorrhage into the lesions. This portion of the atlas will focus on the cutaneous manifestations of lymphoid proliferations.

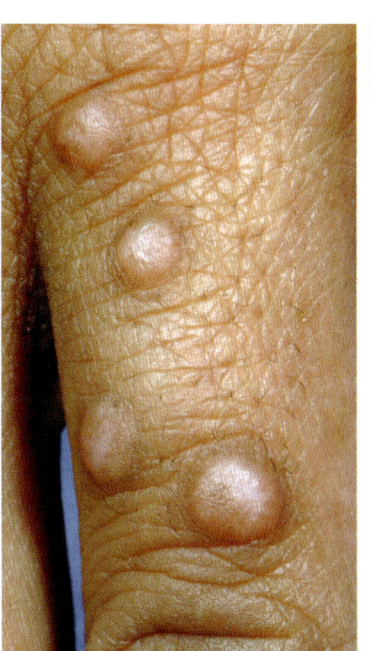

Fig. 32.1 Cutaneous lymphoid hyperplasia, nodular B-cell pattern.

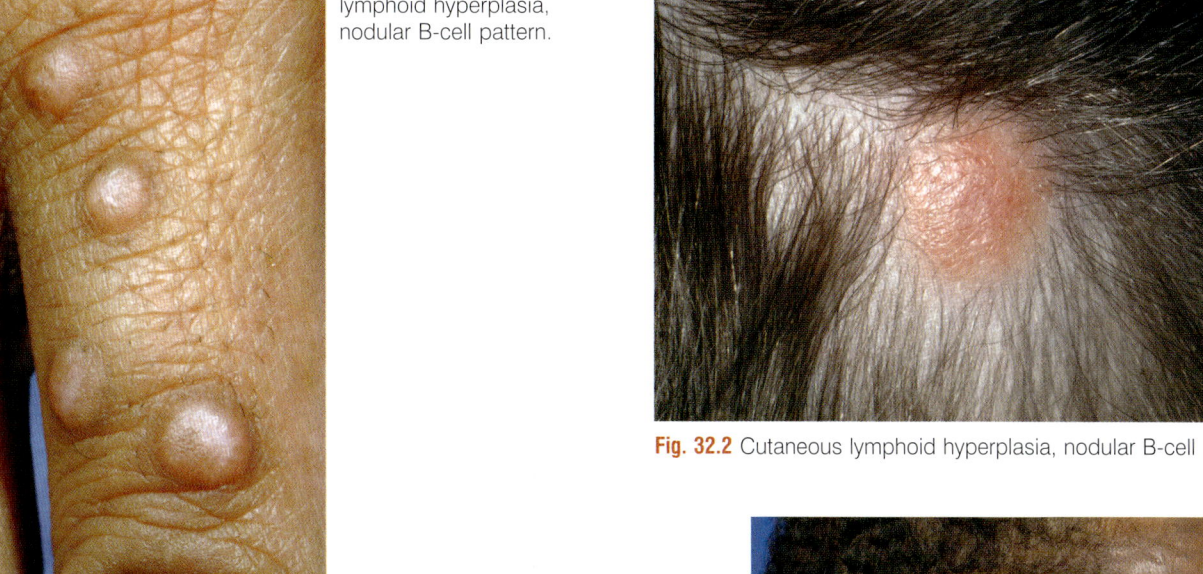

Fig. 32.2 Cutaneous lymphoid hyperplasia, nodular B-cell pattern.

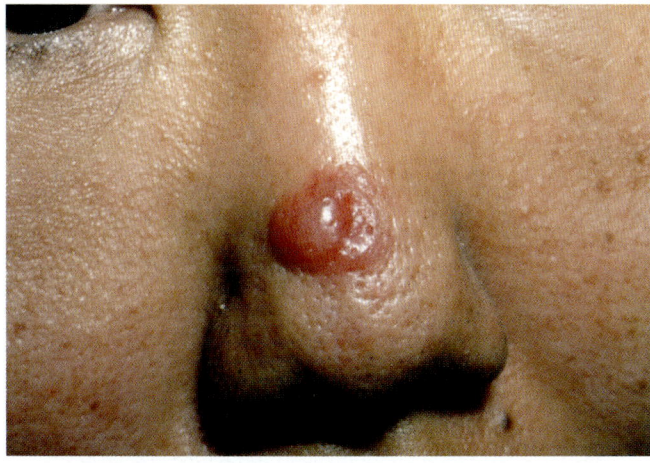

Fig. 32.3 Cutaneous lymphoid hyperplasia, nodular B-cell pattern.

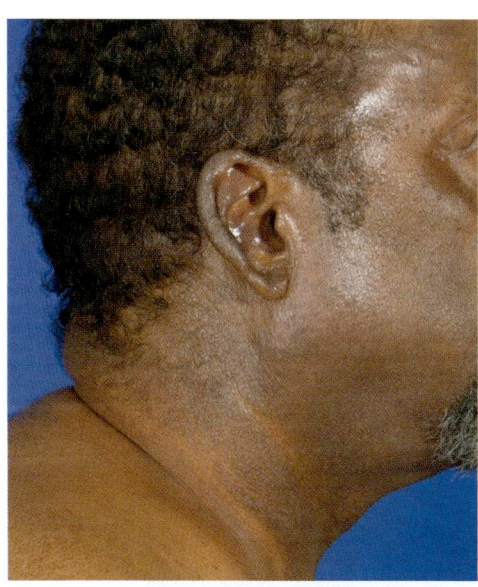

Fig. 32.4 Cutaneous lymphoid hyperplasia, bandlike T-cell pattern.

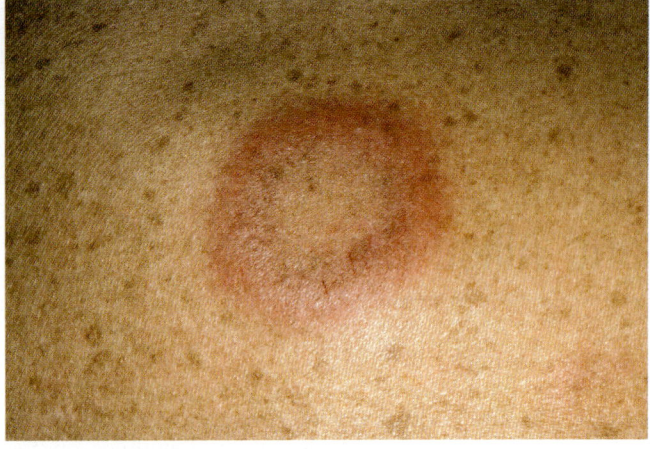
Fig. 32.5 Jessner lymphocytic infiltrate of the skin.

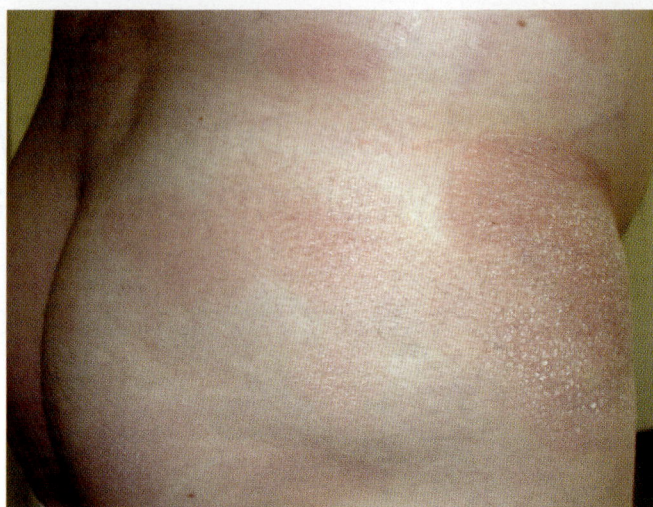
Fig. 32.6 Mycosis fungoides, patch stage.

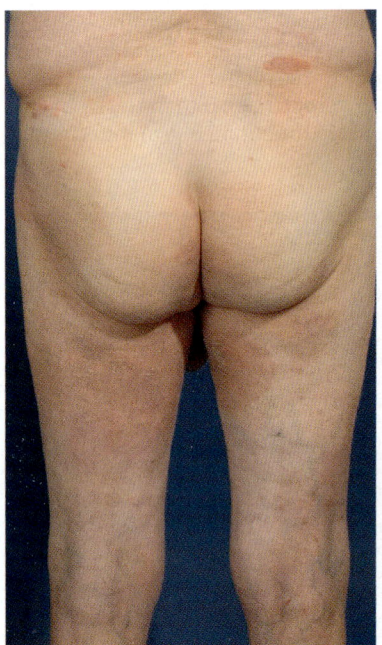
Fig. 32.7 Mycosis fungoides, patch stage.

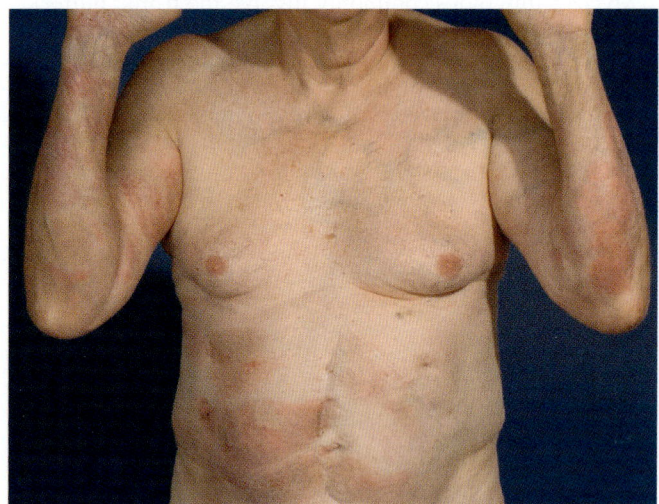
Fig. 32.8 Mycosis fungoides, patch stage.

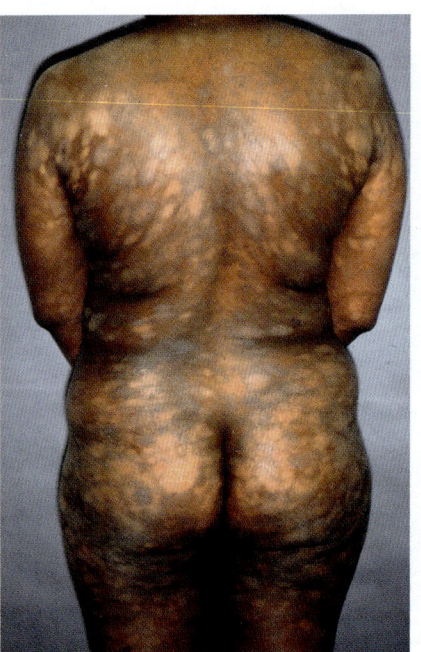
Fig. 32.9 Mycosis fungoides, patch stage.

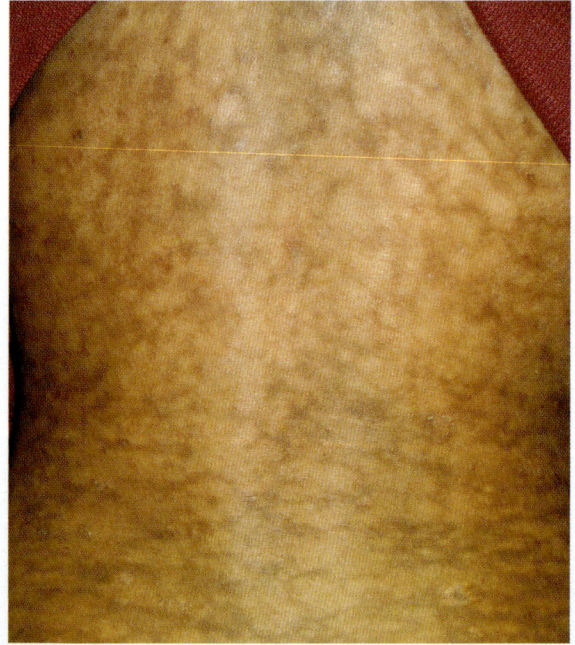
Fig. 32.10 Hypopigmented mycosis fungoides in a child.

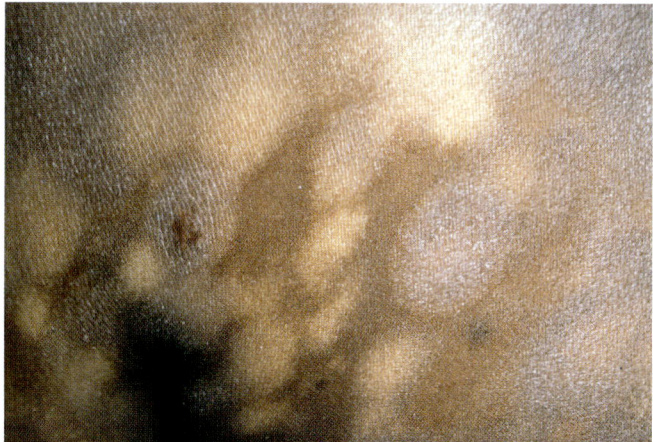

Fig. 32.11 Mycosis fungoides, patch stage.

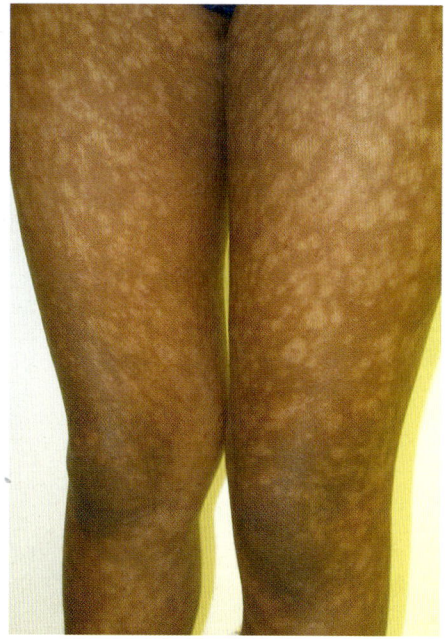

Fig. 32.12 Hypopigmented mycosis fungoides in a child.

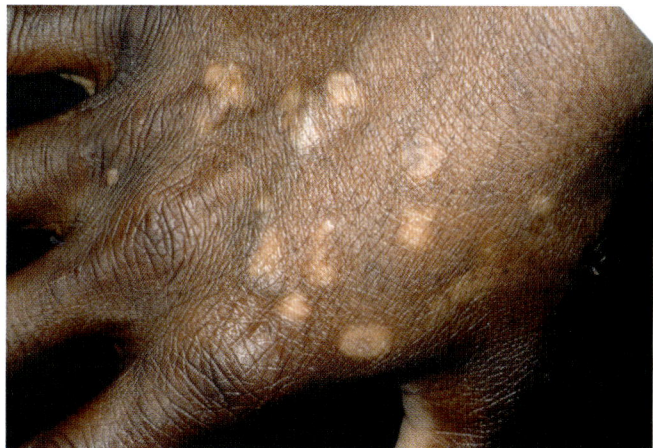

Fig. 32.13 Mycosis fungoides, patch stage.

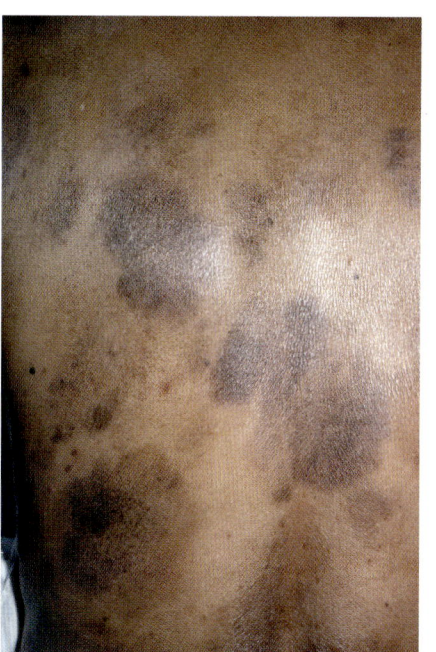

Fig. 32.14 Mycosis fungoides, patch stage.

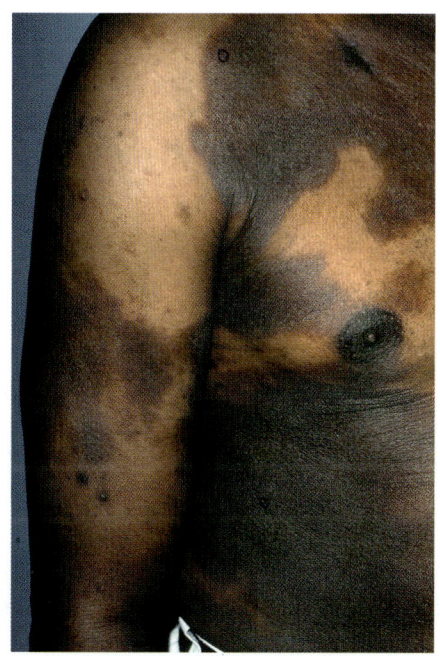

Fig. 32.15 Mycosis fungoides, patch stage.

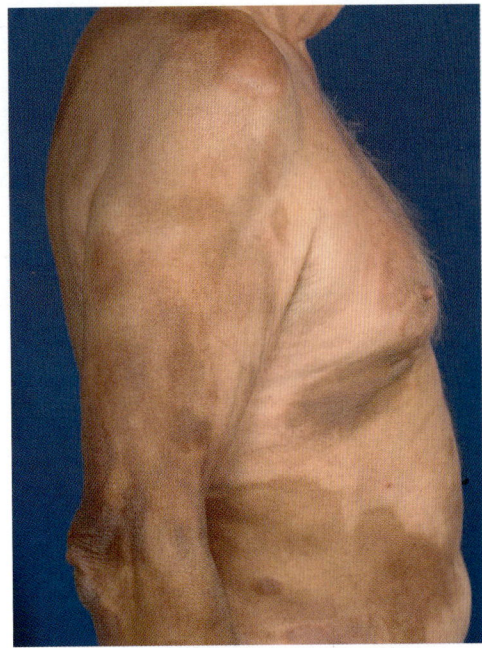

Fig. 32.16 Mycosis fungoides, patch stage.

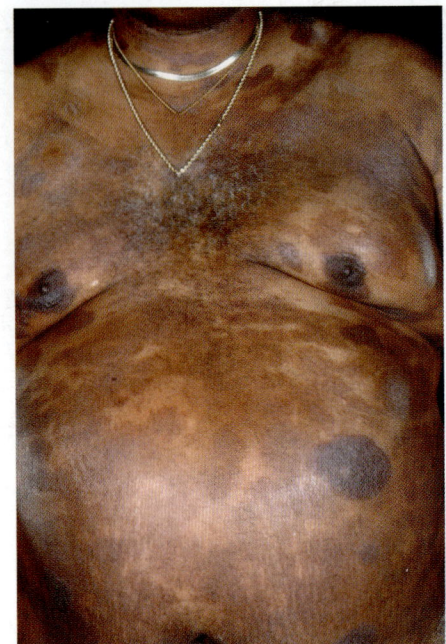

Fig. 32.17 Mycosis fungoides, patch stage. *Courtesy Scott Norton, MD.*

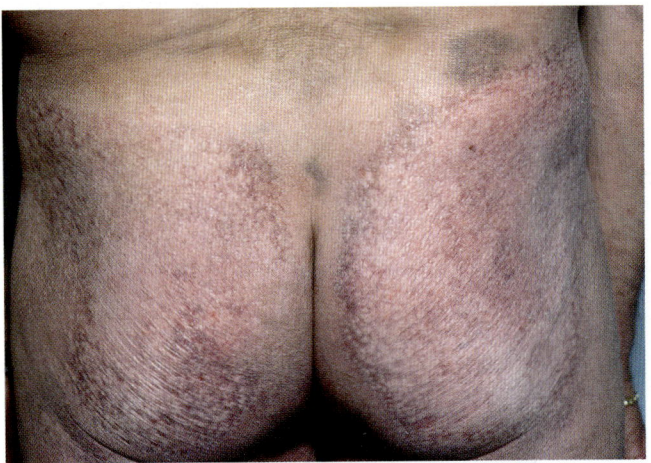

Fig. 32.18 Mycosis fungoides, patch stage with poikiloderma.

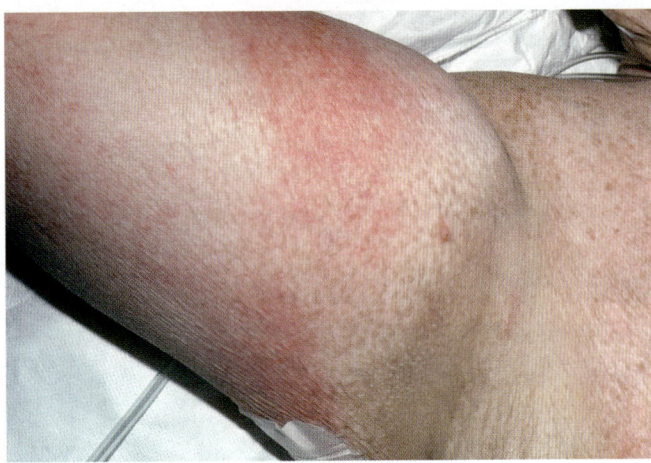

Fig. 32.19 Mycosis fungoides, patch stage with poikiloderma. *Courtesy Steven Binnick, MD.*

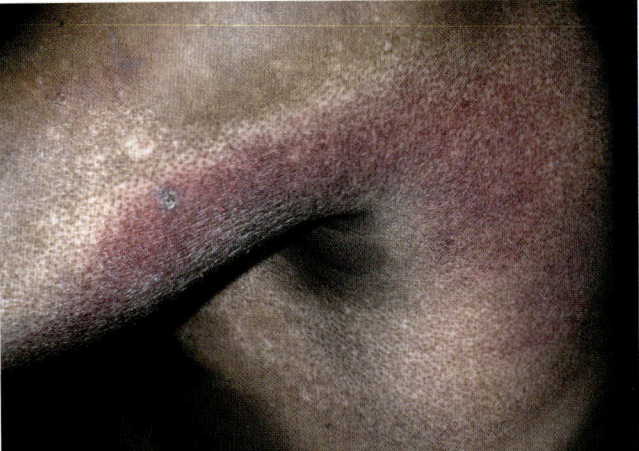

Fig. 32.20 Mycosis fungoides, patch stage with poikiloderma. *Courtesy Steven Binnick, MD.*

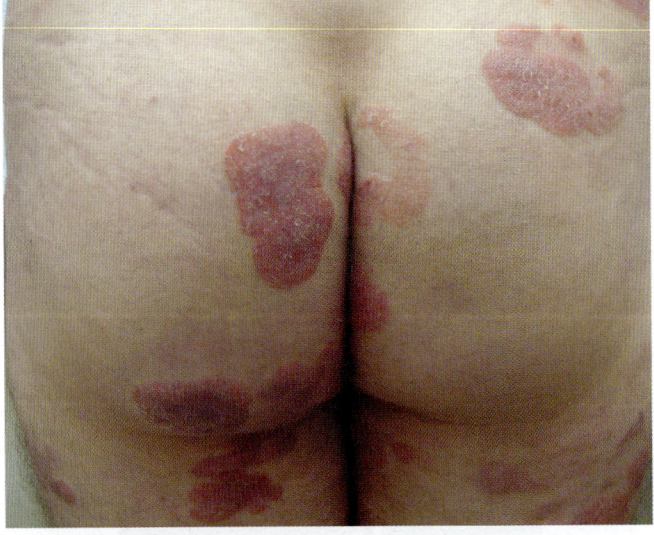

Fig. 32.21 Mycosis fungoides, plaque stage.

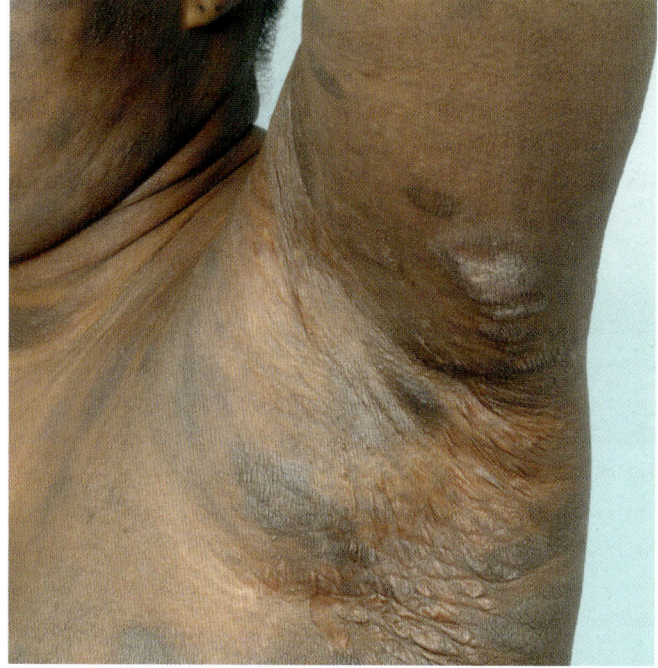

Fig. 32.22 Mycosis fungoides, plaque stage.

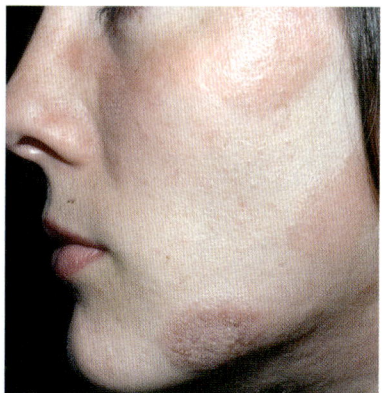

Fig. 32.24 Mycosis fungoides, plaque stage. *Courtesy Steven Binnick, MD.*

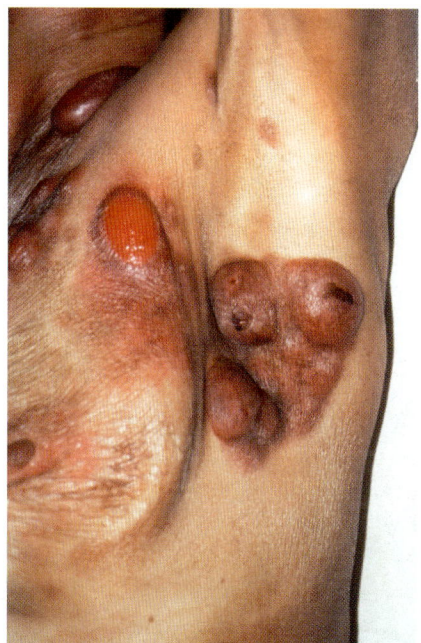

Fig. 32.26 Mycosis fungoides, tumor stage.

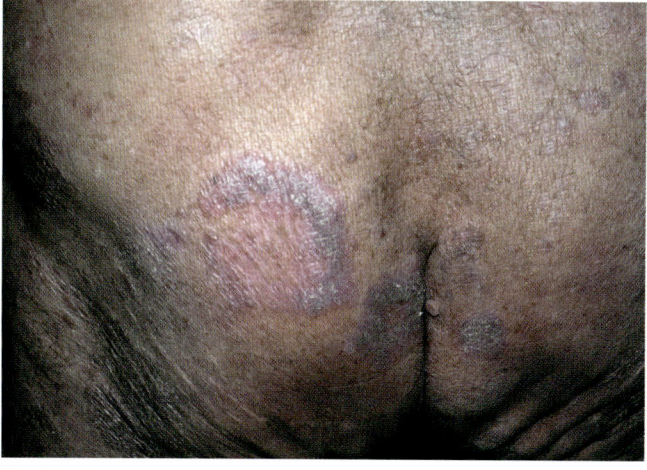

Fig. 32.23 Mycosis fungoides, plaque stage. *Courtesy Steven Binnick, MD.*

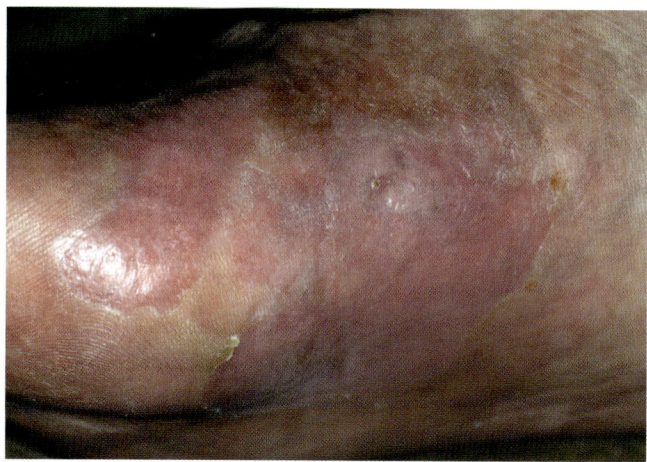

Fig. 32.25 Mycosis fungoides, plaque stage. *Courtesy Steven Binnick, MD.*

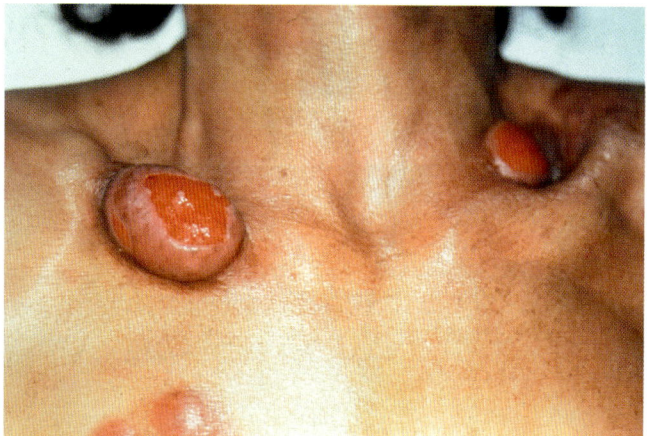

Fig. 32.27 Mycosis fungoides, tumor stage.

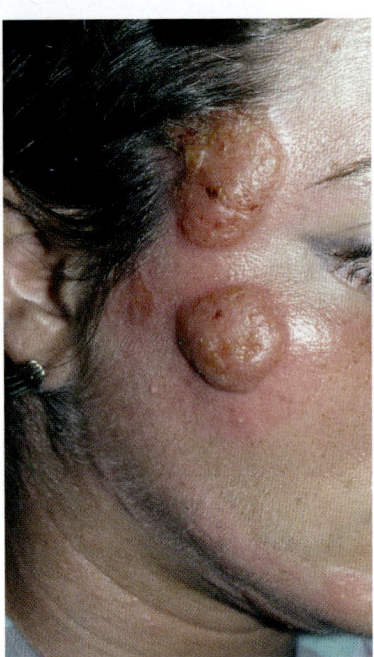

Fig. 32.28 Mycosis fungoides, tumor stage. *Courtesy Steven Binnick, MD.*

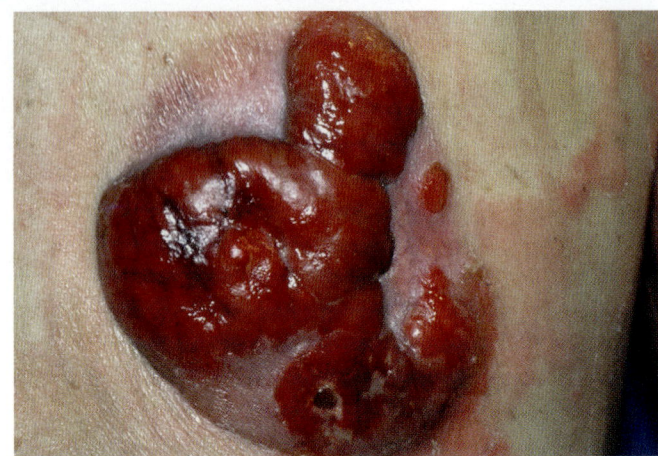

Fig. 32.29 Mycosis fungoides, tumor stage.

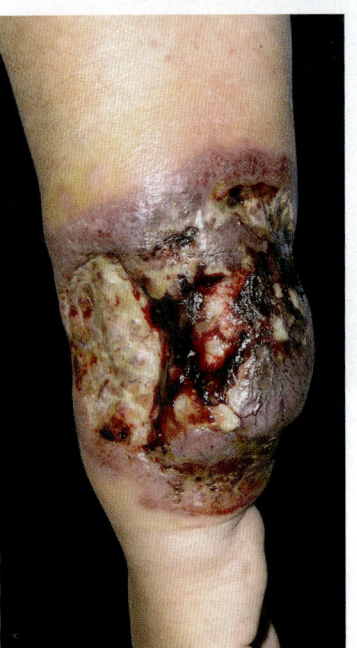

Fig. 32.30 Mycosis fungoides, tumor stage. *Courtesy Maria Hicks, MD.*

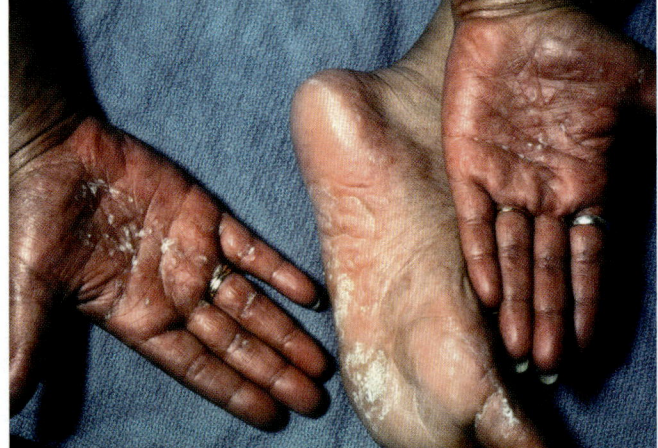

Fig. 32.31 Palmar plantar mycosis fungoides.

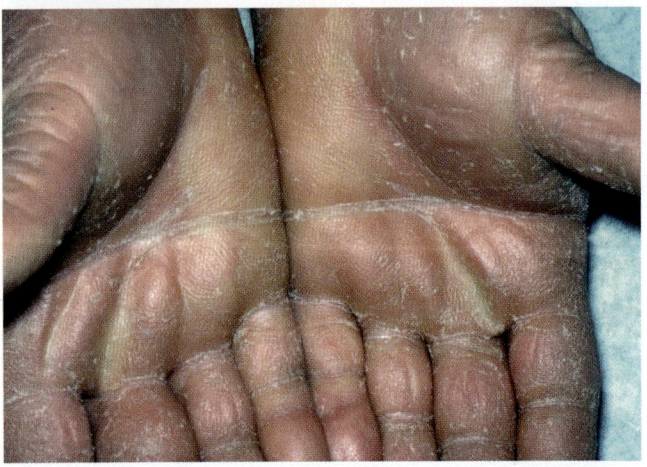

Fig. 32.32 Palmar plantar mycosis fungoides. *Courtesy Steven Binnick, MD.*

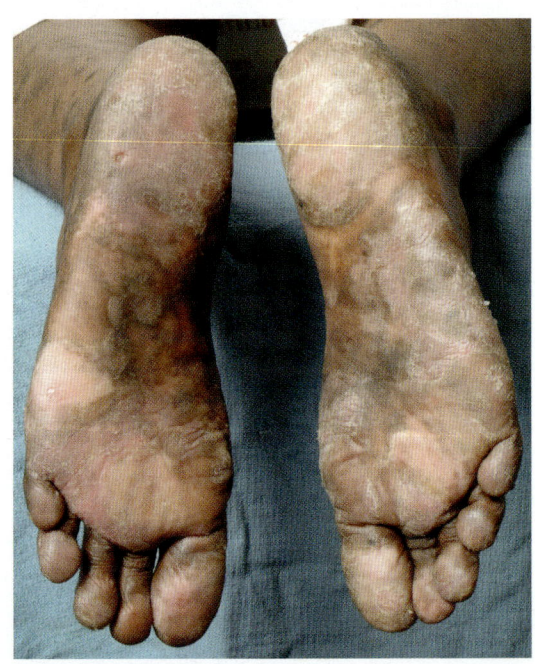

Fig. 32.33 Palmar plantar mycosis fungoides.

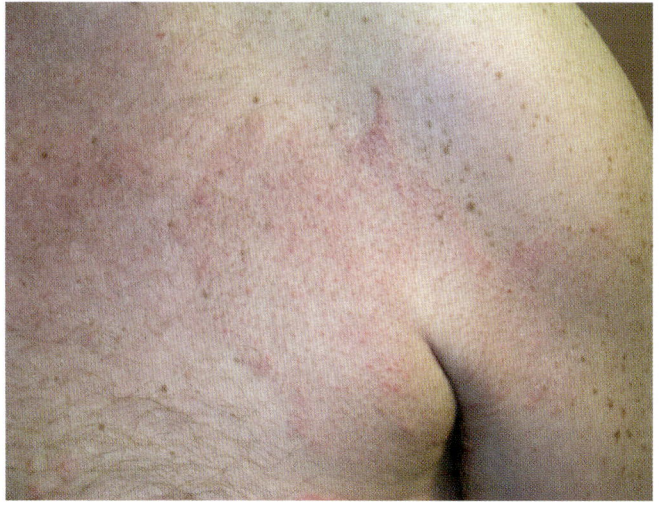

Fig. 32.34 Alopecia mucinosa associated with mycosis fungoides. *Courtesy Ellen Kim, MD.*

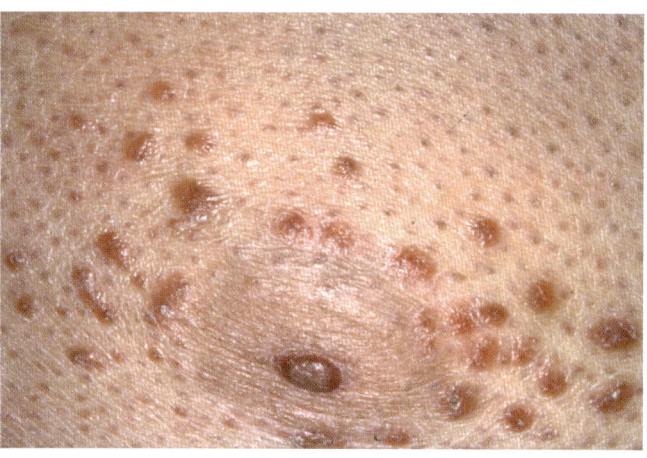

Fig. 32.35 Follicular mycosis fungoides.

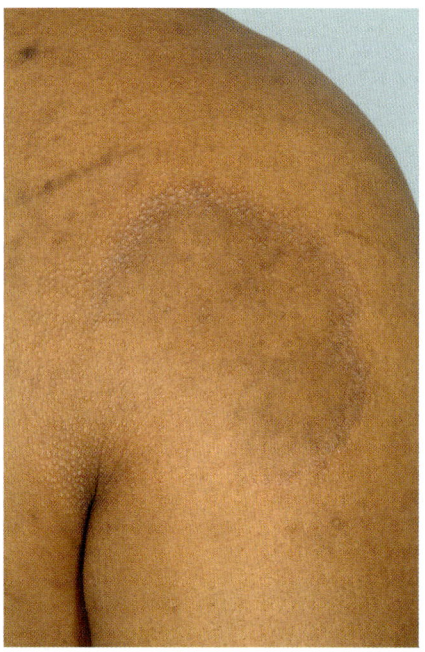

Fig. 32.36 Follicular mycosis fungoides. *Courtesy Ellen Kim, MD.*

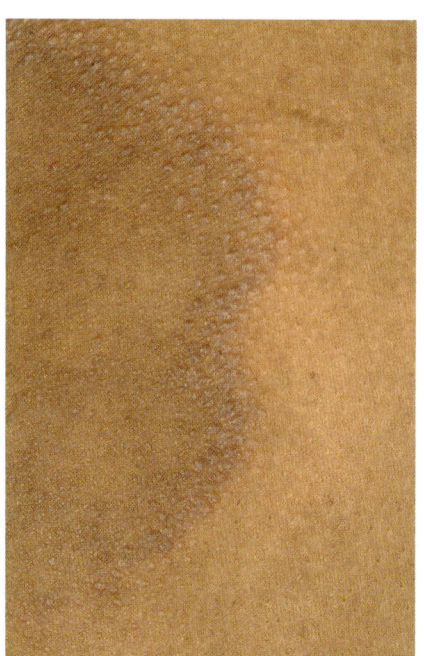

Fig. 32.37 Follicular mycosis fungoides. *Courtesy Ellen Kim, MD.*

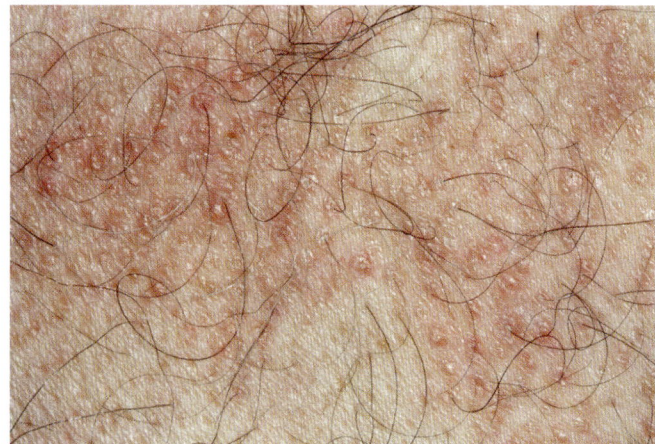

Fig. 32.38 Follicular mycosis fungoides. *Courtesy Alain Rook, MD.*

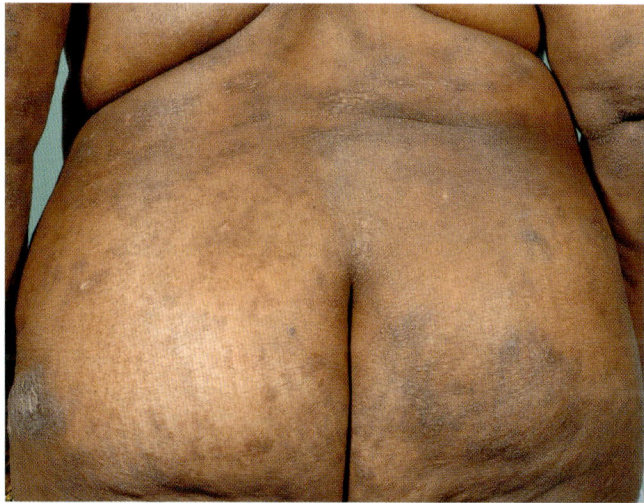

Fig. 32.39 Follicular mycosis fungoides with large cell transformation. *Courtesy Alain Rook, MD.*

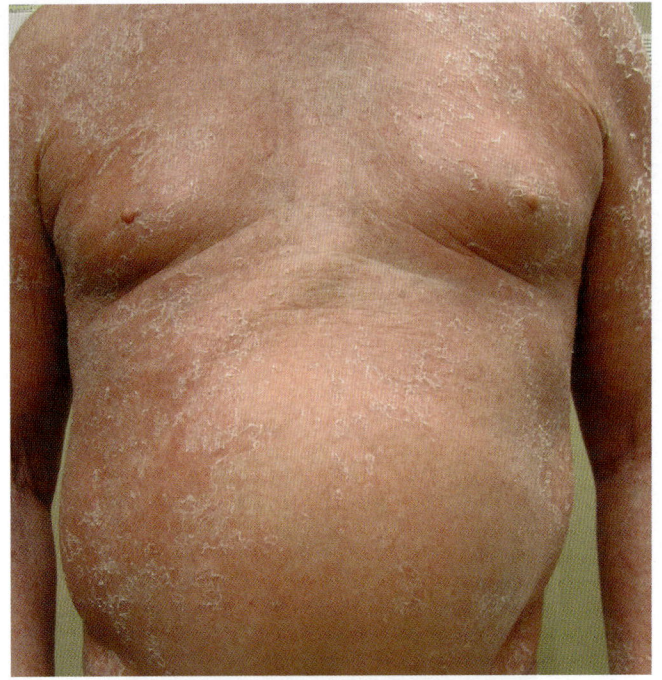

Fig. 32.40 Sézary syndrome. *Courtesy Alain Rook, MD.*

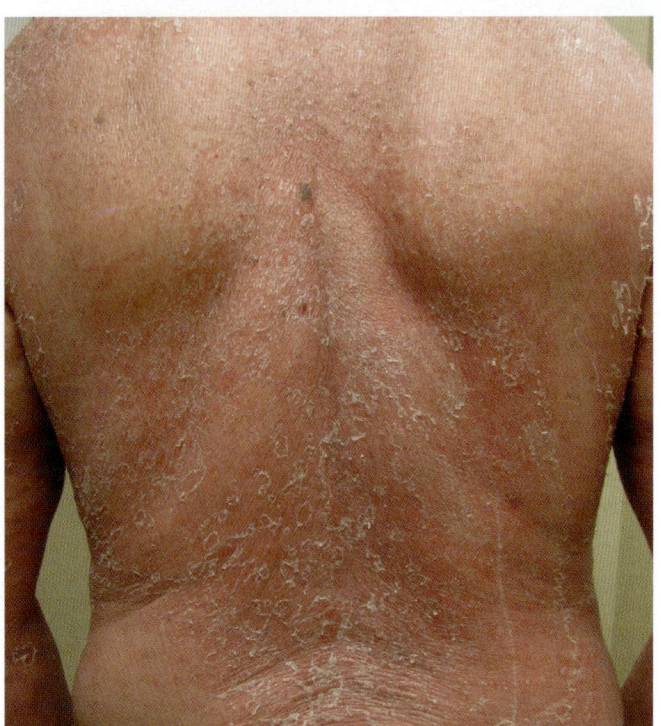

Fig. 32.41 Sézary syndrome. *Courtesy Alain Rook, MD.*

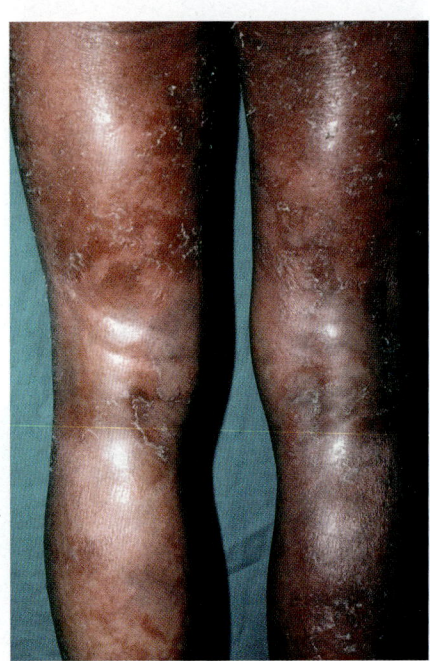

Fig. 32.42 Sézary syndrome. *Courtesy Ken Greer, MD.*

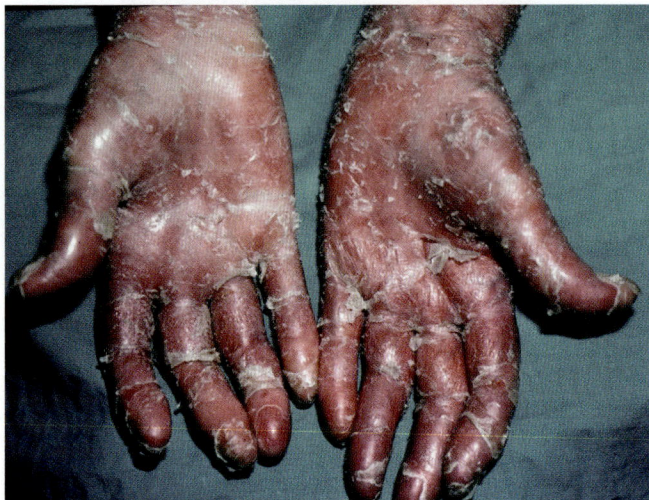

Fig. 32.43 Sézary syndrome. *Courtesy Ken Greer, MD.*

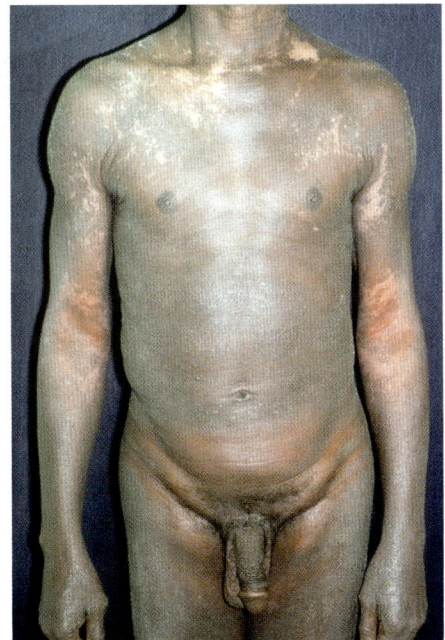

Fig. 32.44 Sézary syndrome.

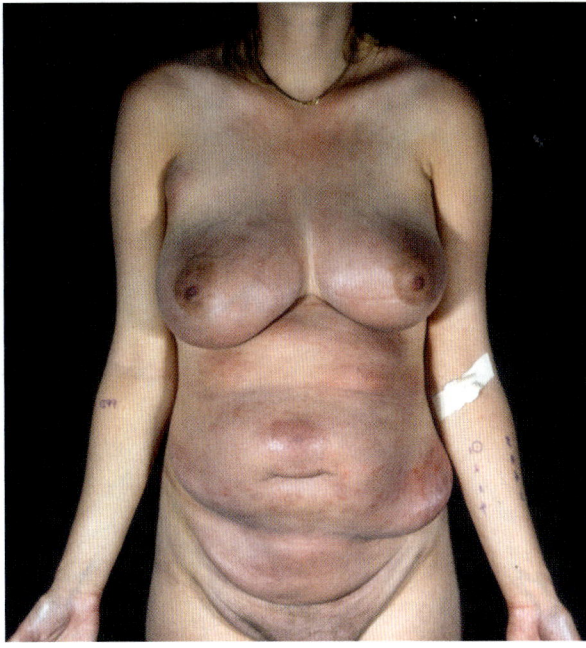

Fig. 32.45 Granulomatous slack skin.

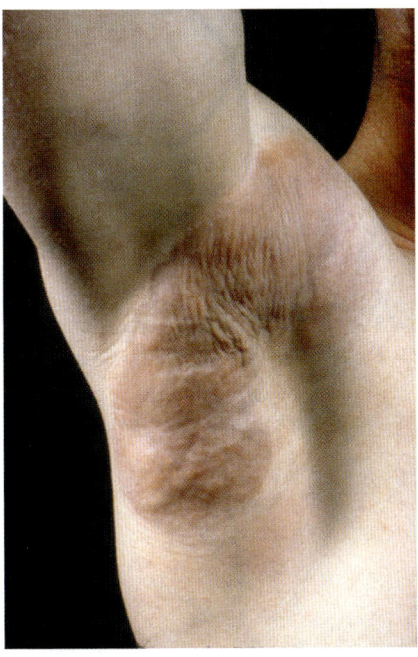

Fig. 32.46 Granulomatous slack skin.

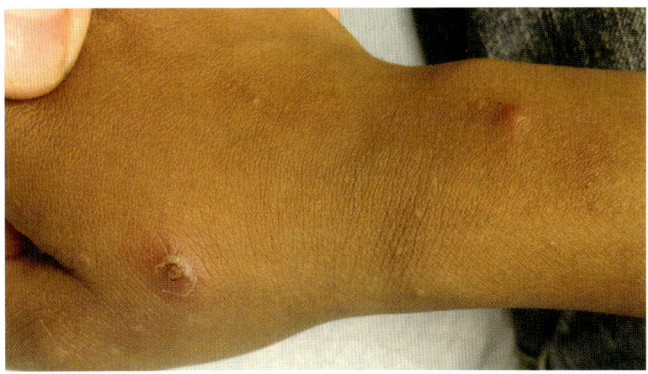

Fig. 32.47 Lymphomatoid papulosis.

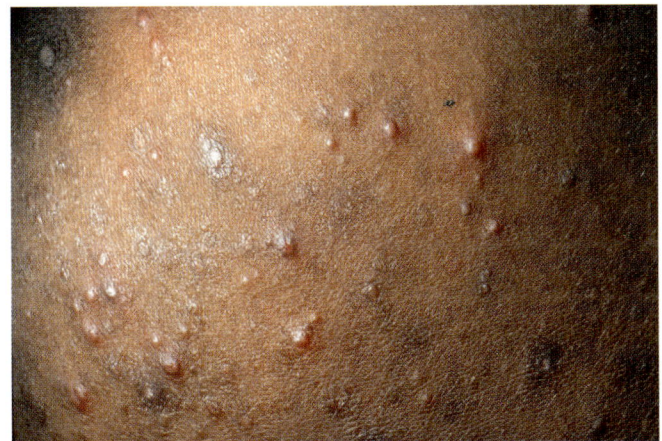

Fig. 32.48 Lymphomatoid papulosis.

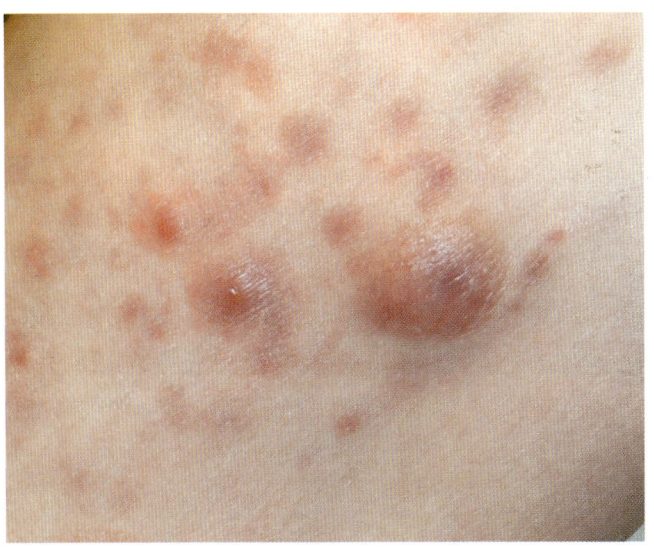

Fig. 32.49 Lymphomatoid papulosis. *Courtesy Alain Rook, MD.*

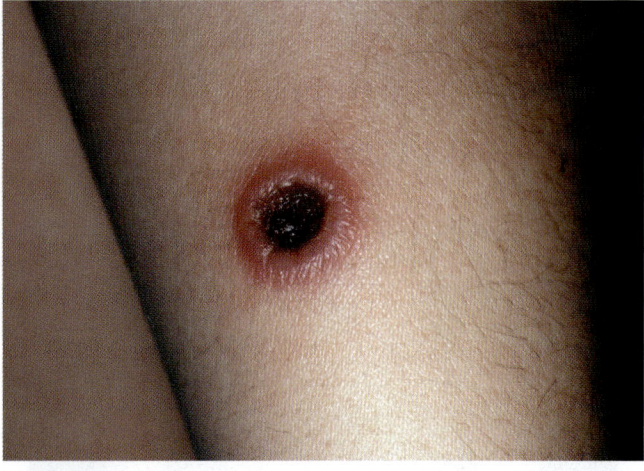

Fig. 32.50 Lymphomatoid papulosis. *Courtesy Steven Binnick, MD.*

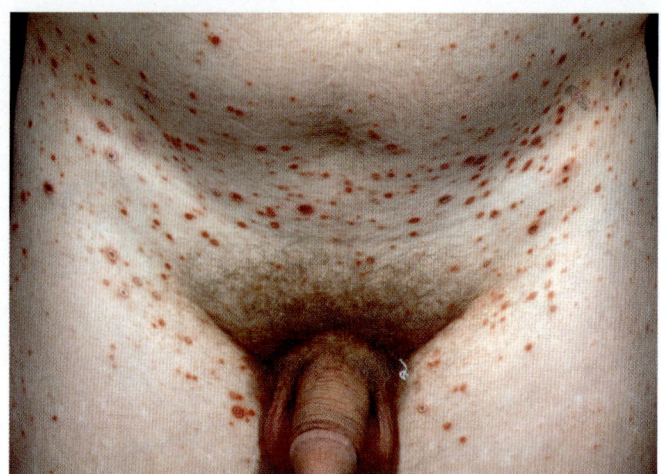

Fig. 32.51 Pityriasis lichenoides et varioliformis acuta.

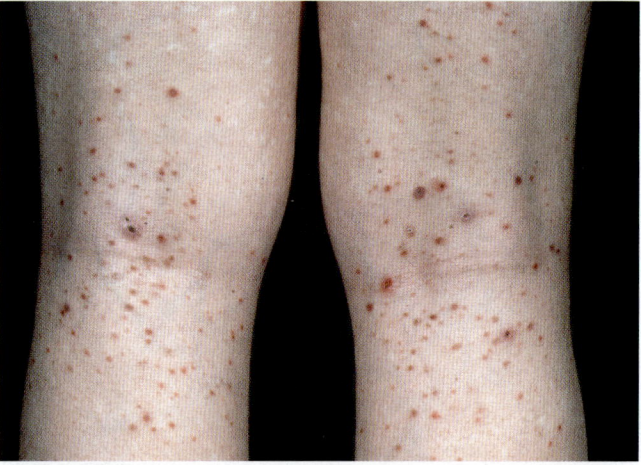

Fig. 32.52 Pityriasis lichenoides et varioliformis acuta.

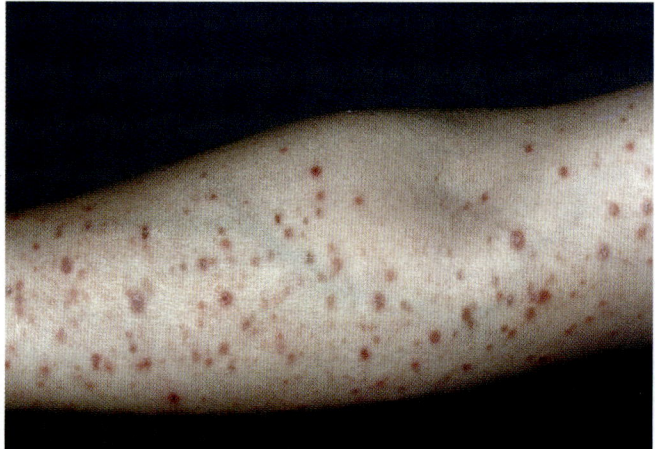

Fig. 32.53 Pityriasis lichenoides et varioliformis acuta.

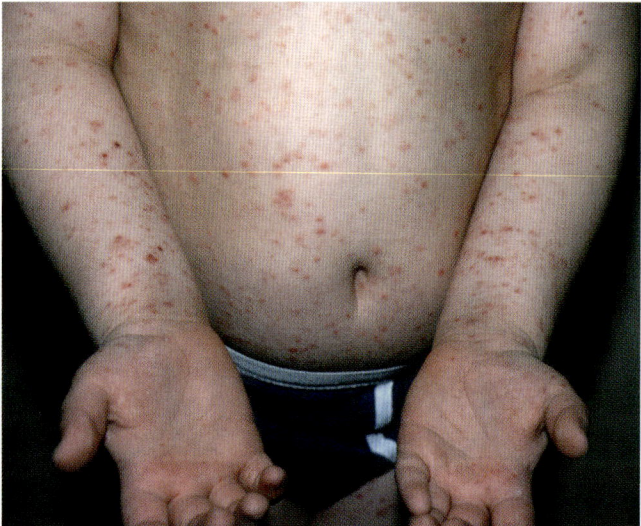

Fig. 32.54 Pityriasis lichenoides et varioliformis acuta. *Courtesy Steven Binnick, MD.*

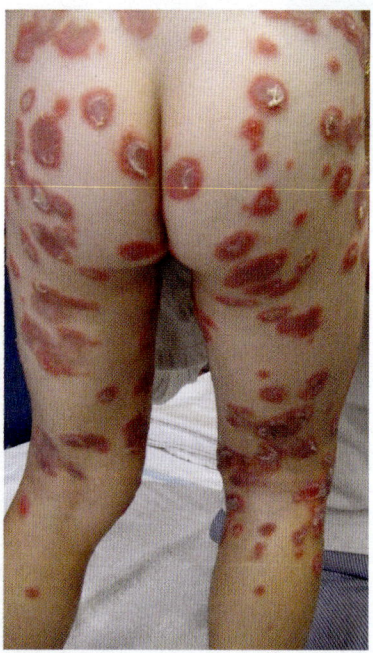

Fig. 32.55 Ulceronecrotic Mucha-Habermann disease.

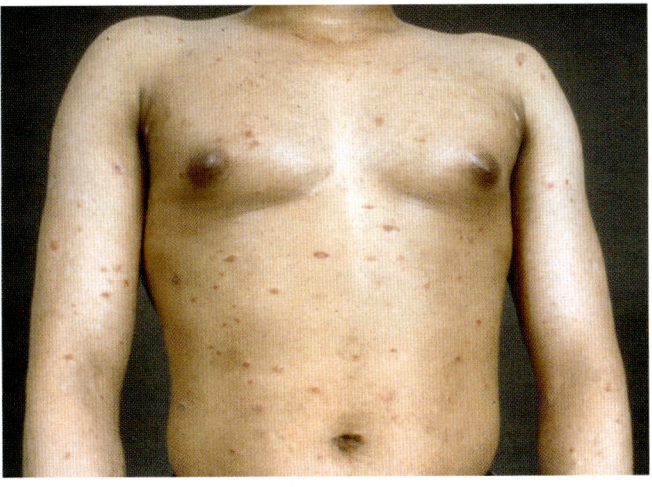

Fig. 32.56 Pityriasis lichenoides chronica.

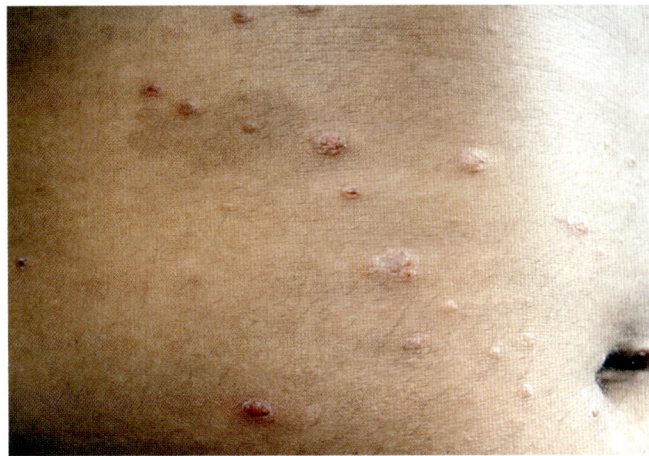

Fig. 32.57 Pityriasis lichenoides chronica.

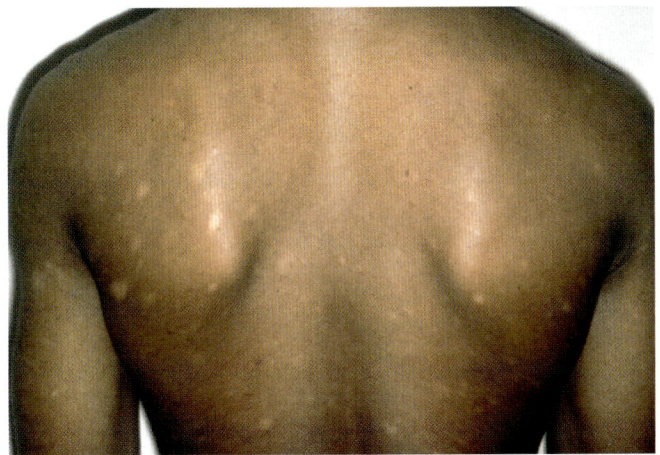

Fig. 32.58 Pityriasis lichenoides chronica.

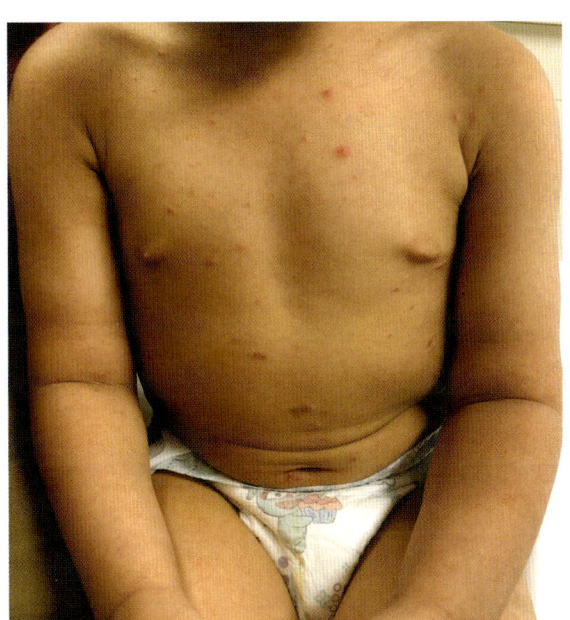

Fig. 32.59 Pityriasis lichenoides chronica.

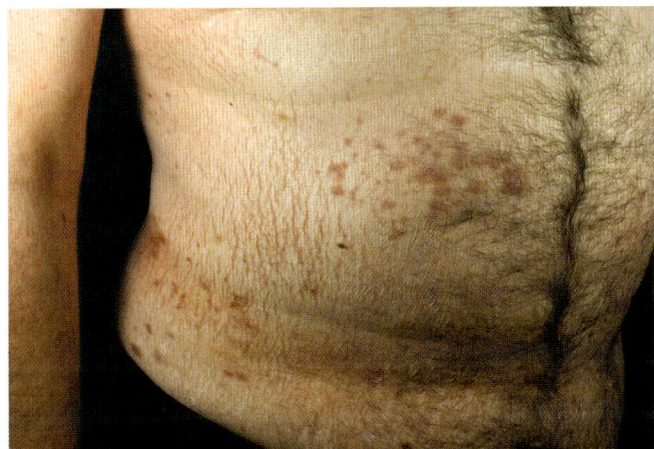

Fig. 32.60 Anaplastic large cell lymphoma with acquired ichthyosis. *Courtesy Curt Samlaska MD.*

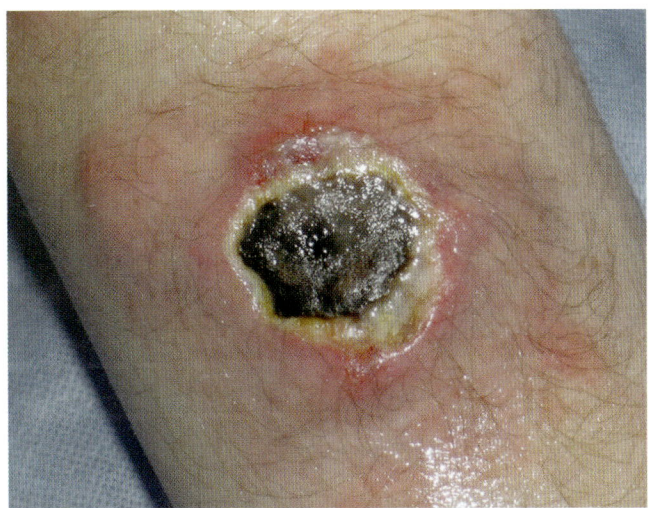

Fig. 32.61 CD30+ anaplastic T-cell lymphoma. *Courtesy Alain Rook, MD.*

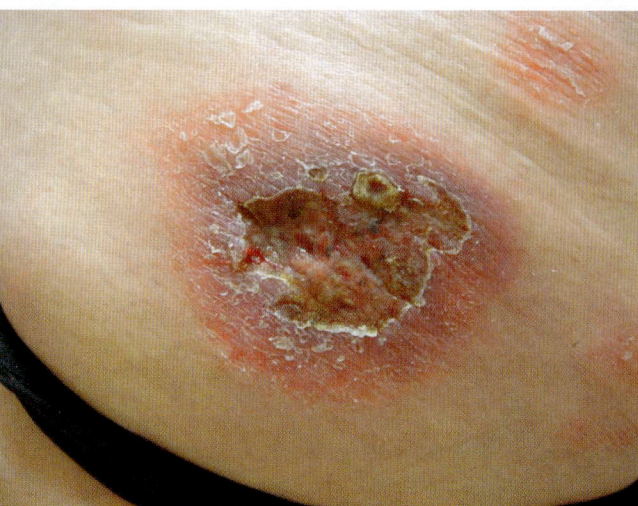

Fig. 32.62 Gamma-delta T-cell lymphoma. *Courtesy Ellen Kim, MD.*

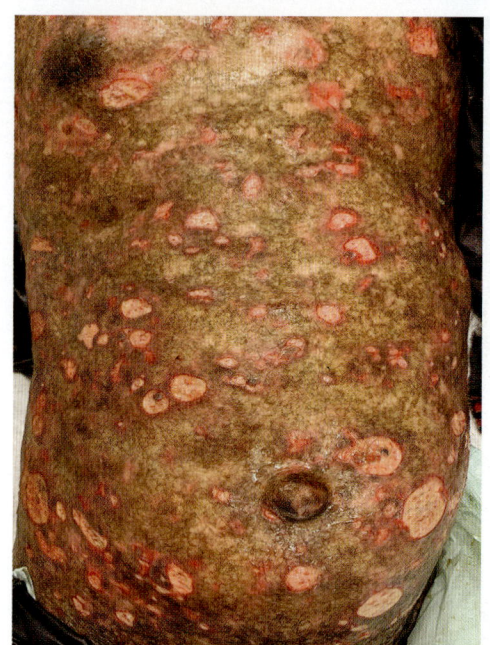

Fig. 32.63 Primary cutaneous aggressive epidermotropic CD8+ T-cell lymphoma.

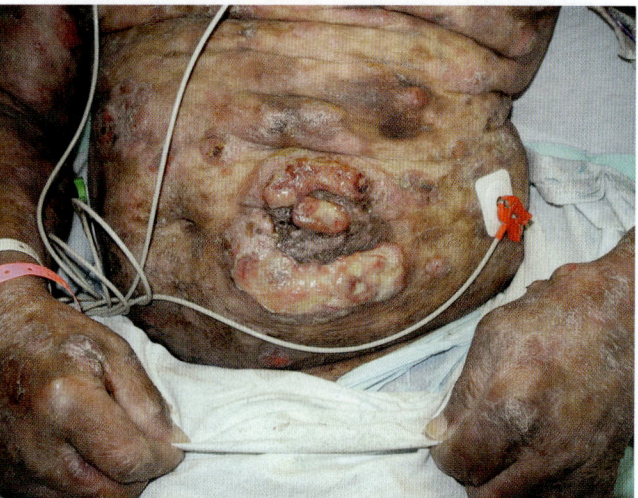

Fig. 32.64 Gamma-delta T-cell lymphoma. *Courtesy Alain Rook, MD.*

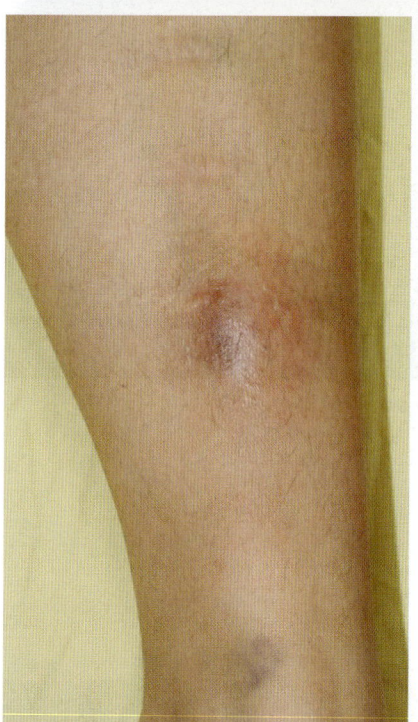

Fig. 32.65 Subcutaneous panniculitis-like T-cell lymphoma. *Courtesy Yung-Tsu Cho, MD.*

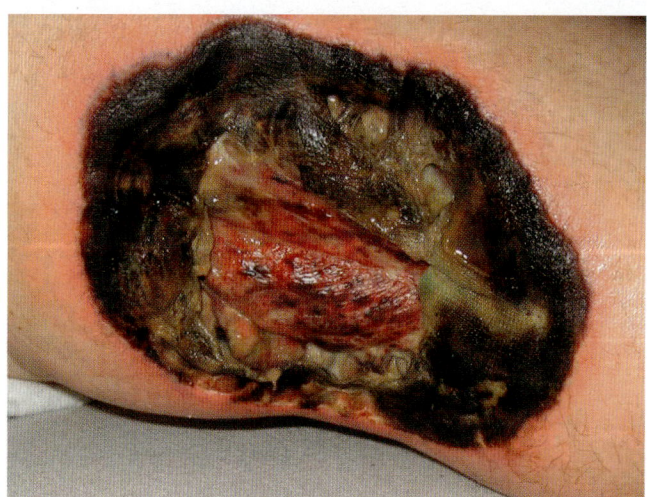

Fig. 32.66 Natural killer T-cell lymphoma. *Courtesy Alain Rook, MD.*

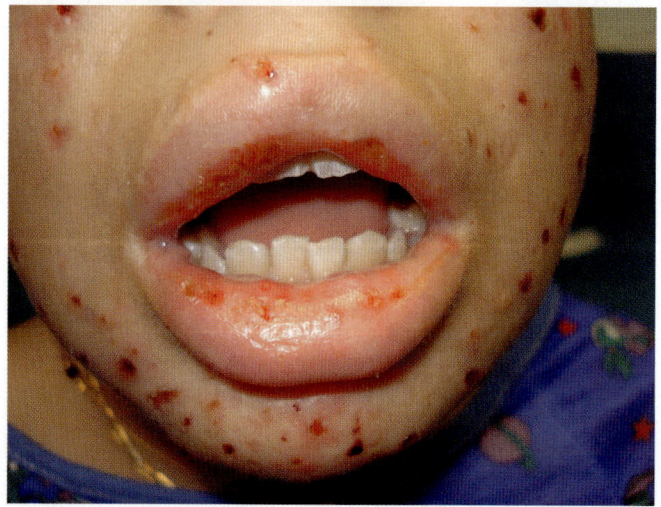

Fig. 32.67 Hydroa vacciniforme–like natural killer T-cell lymphoma.

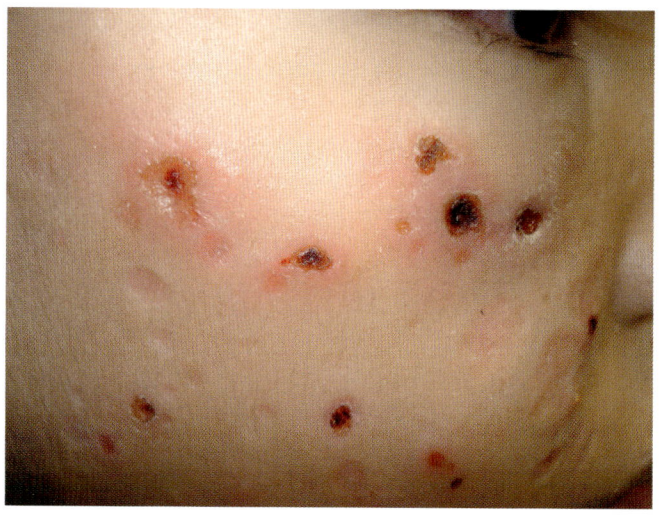

Fig. 32.68 Hydroa vacciniforme–like natural killer T-cell lymphoma.

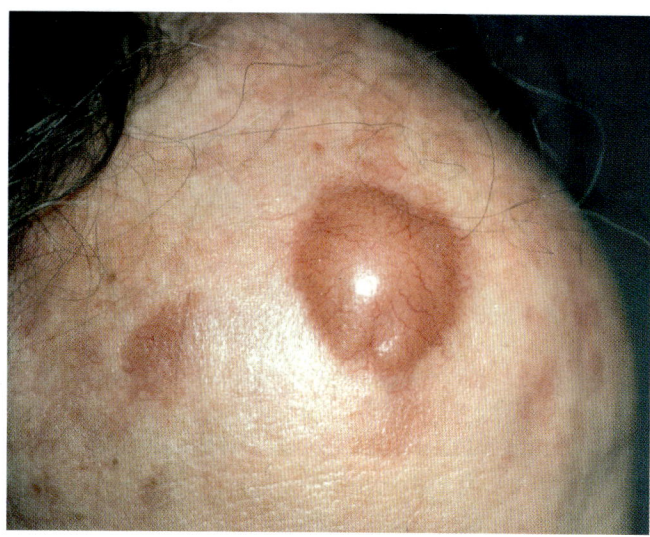

Fig. 32.69 B-cell lymphoma.

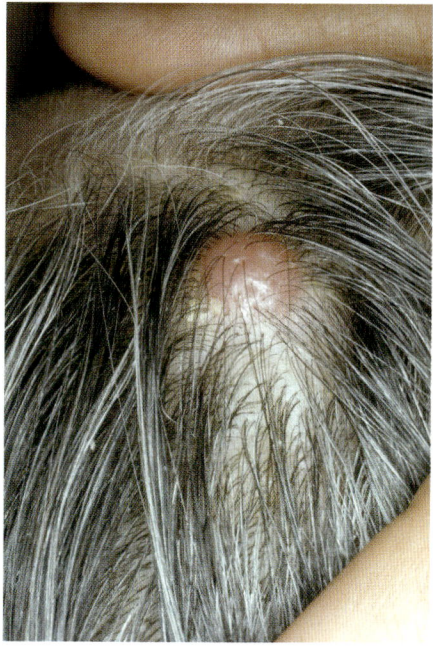

Fig. 32.70 B-cell lymphoma.

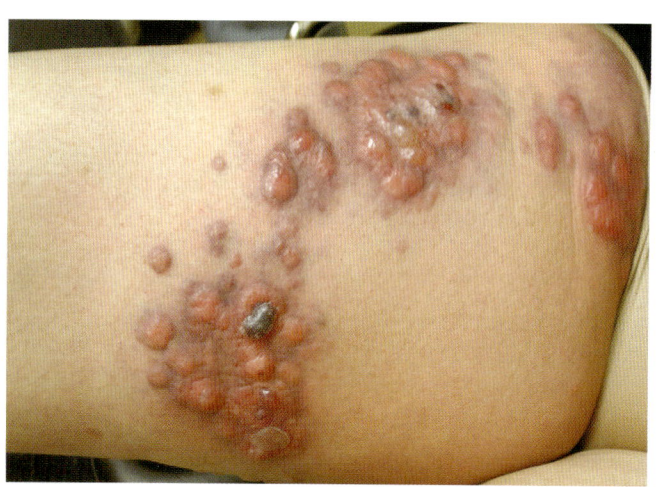

Fig. 32.71 Mantle cell lymphoma.

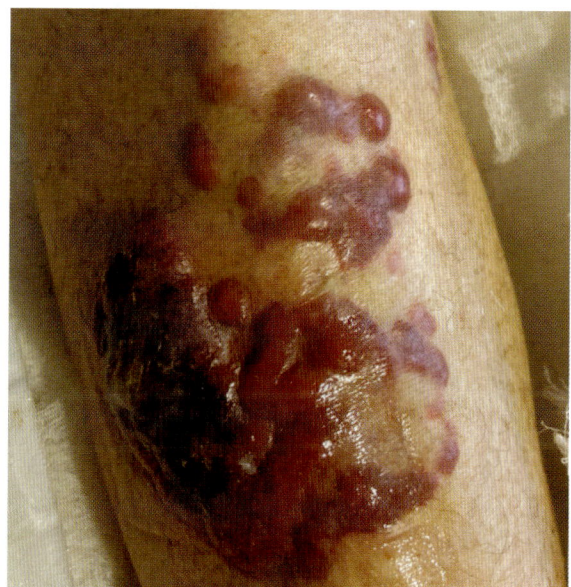

Fig. 32.72 Diffuse large B-cell lymphoma.

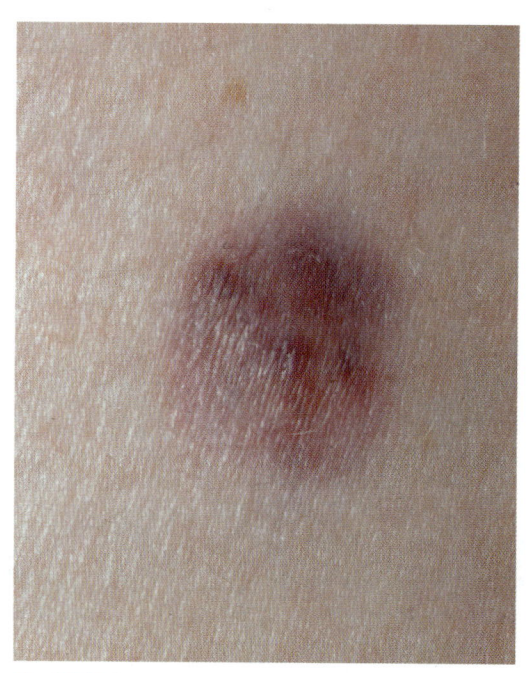

Fig. 32.73 Secondary cutaneous lymphoma.

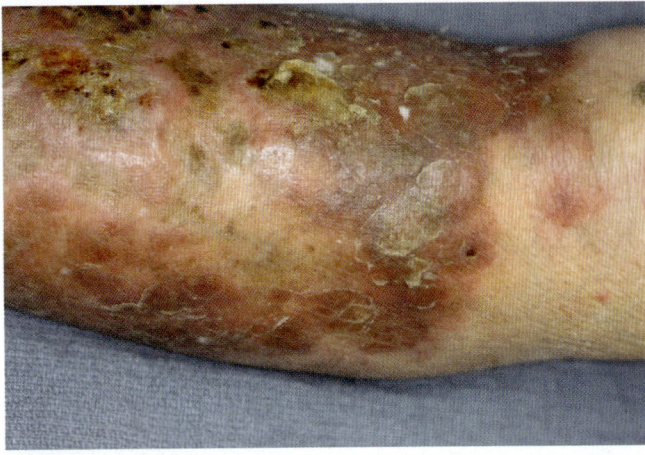

Fig. 32.74 B-cell lymphoma, leg type.

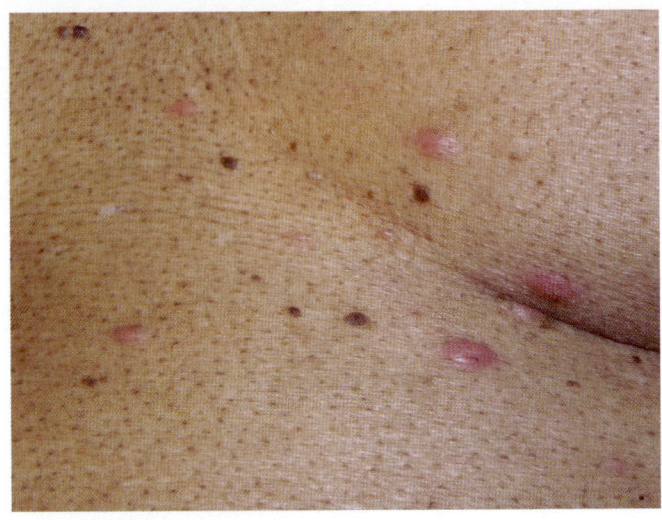

Fig. 32.75 Plasmacytomas.

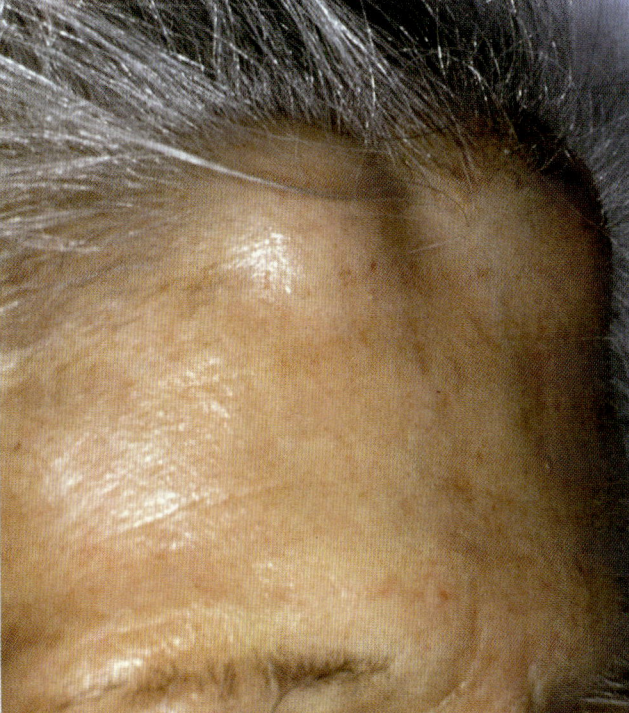

Fig. 32.76 Plasmacytomas.

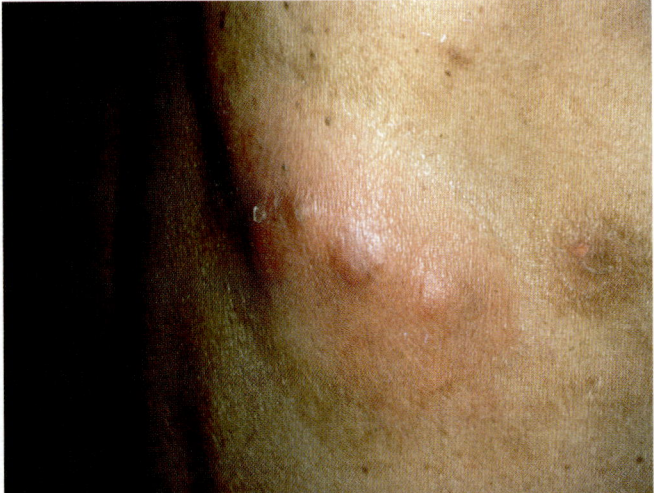

Fig. 32.77 Malignant histiocytosis.

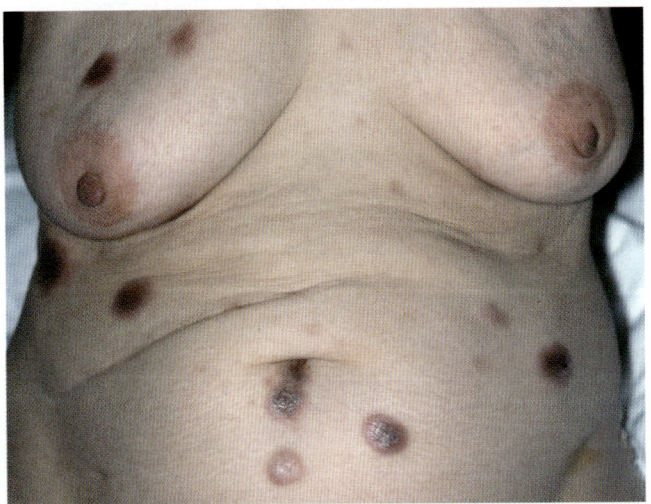

Fig. 32.78 Acute myelomonocytic leukemia cutis.

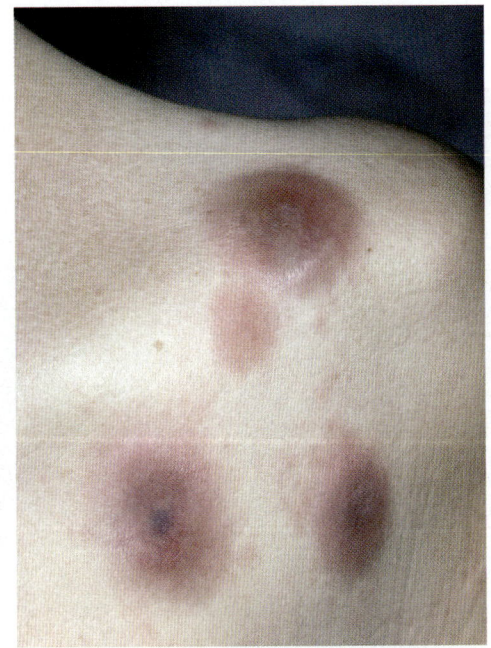

Fig. 32.79 Acute myelomonocytic leukemia cutis.

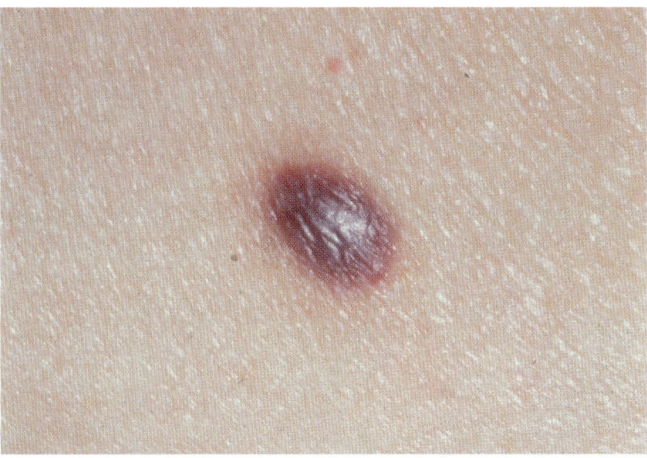

Fig. 32.80 Leukemia cutis.

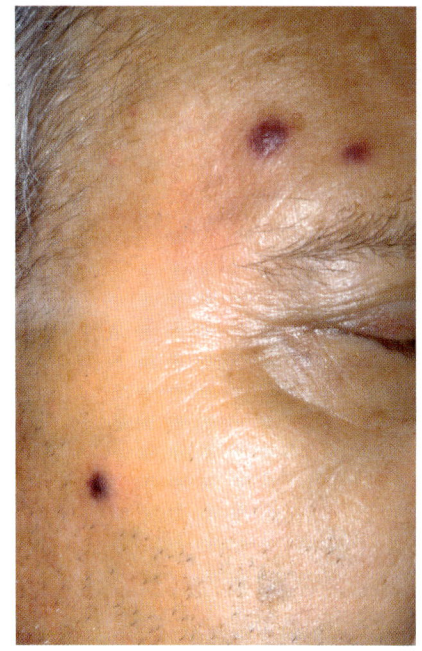

Fig. 32.81 Acute myelogenous leukemia cutis.

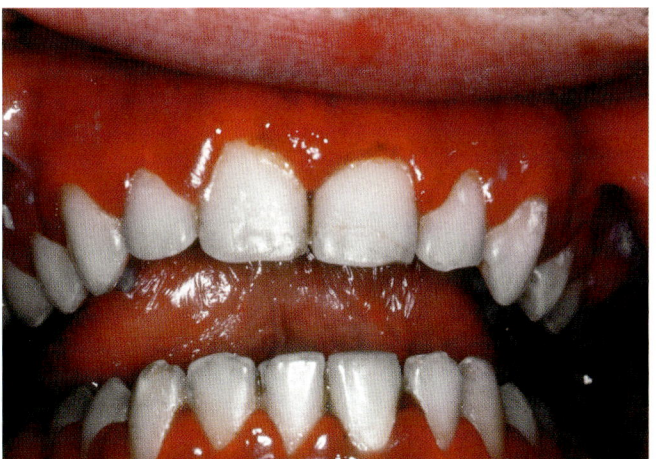

Fig. 32.82 Acute myelomonocytic leukemia.

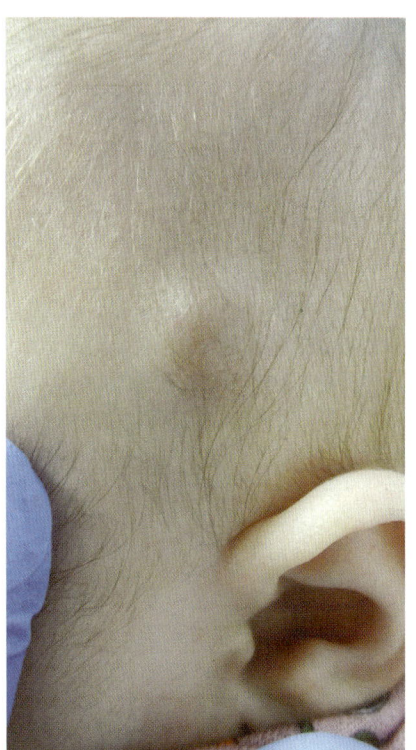

Fig. 32.83 Acute myelogenous leukemia cutis.

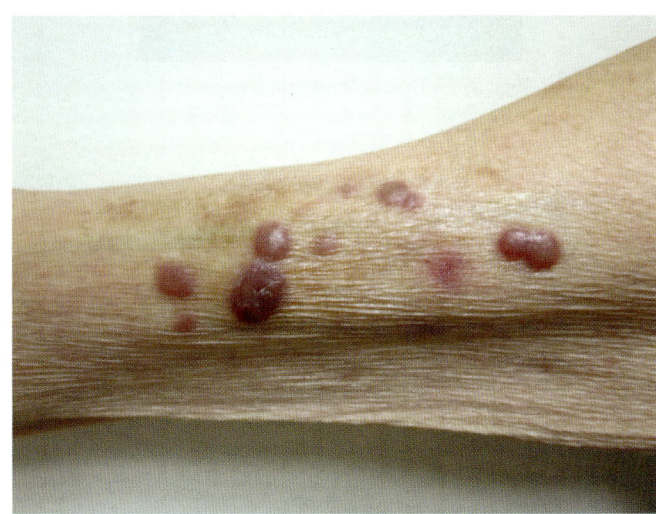

Fig. 32.84 Leukemia cutis. *Courtesy Robert Micheletti, MD.*

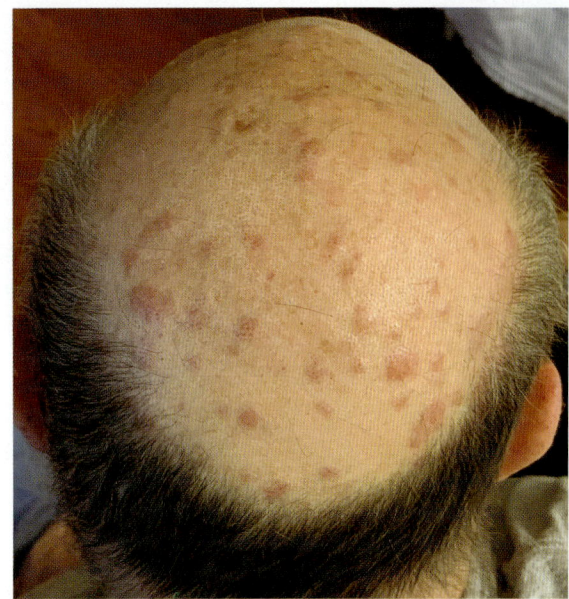

Fig. 32.85 Leukemia cutis.

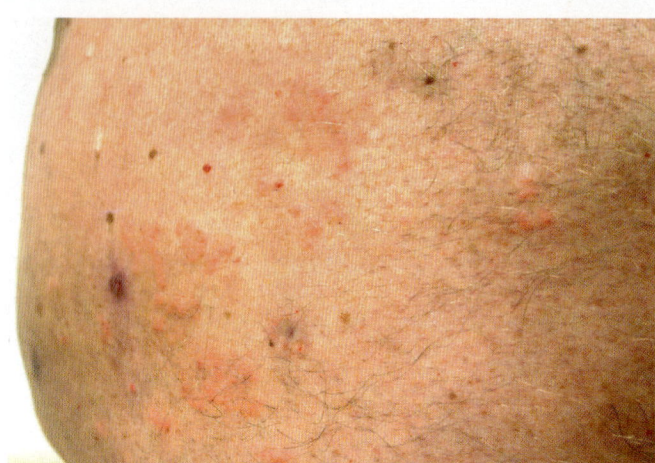

Fig. 32.86 Hypereosinophilic syndrome. *Courtesy John Stanley, MD.*

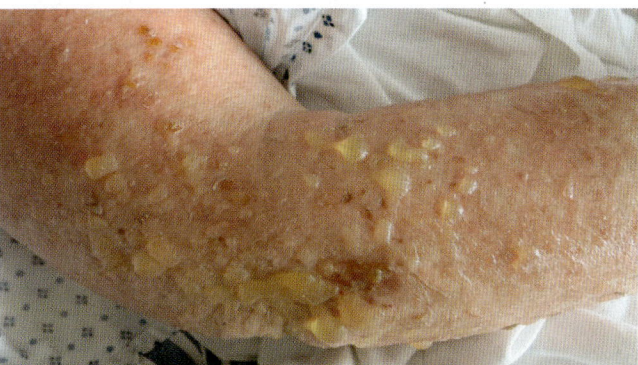

Fig. 32.87 Angioimmunoblastic T-cell lymphoma.

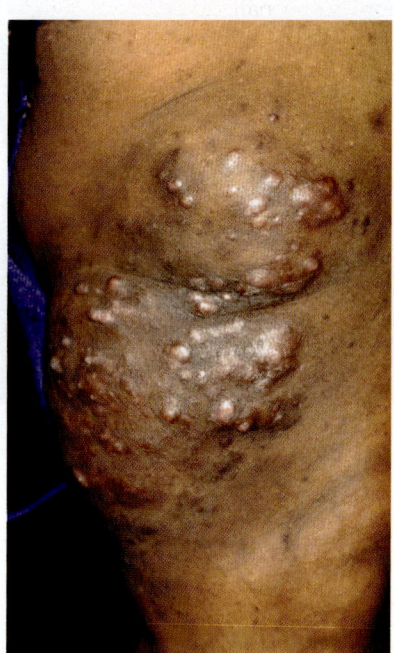

Fig. 32.88 Rosai-Dorfman disease.

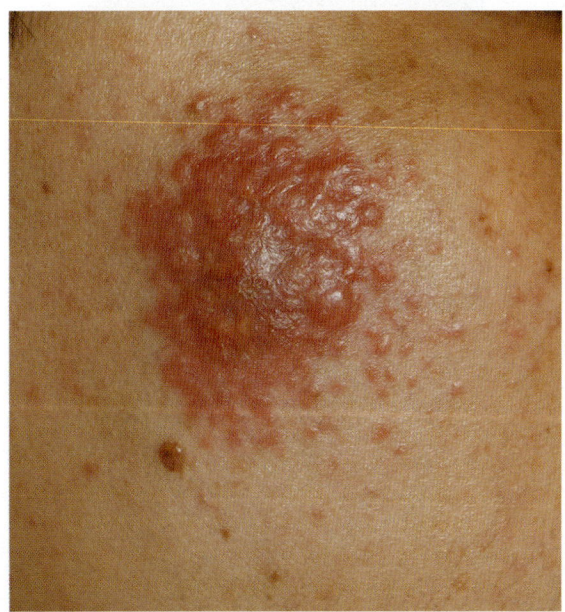

Fig. 32.89 Rosai-Dorfman disease. *Courtesy National Cheng Kung University, Taiwan.*

Diseases of Skin Appendages 33

The field of dermatology includes diseases of both skin and the skin appendages, namely hair, sweat glands, and nails. A great variety of conditions affect the skin appendages, and some are isolated to the hair, nail, or sweat glands, whereas some are found in the setting of a more widespread cutaneous or systemic disease.

Diseases of the hair include alopecia, hirsutism, and those affecting the hair color and hair shaft. Evaluation of these conditions includes a directed history along with evaluation of the scalp, eyebrows, eyelashes, and body hair. Beyond a biopsy of the affected region to assess the hair follicles, bedside tests such as the pull test and tug test help investigate the integrity of the hair follicles and shafts, respectively.

Examination of the nail units includes inspection of the nail plate, nail folds, and cuticles, as well as the nail bed and lunula. Like hair conditions, some nail conditions are isolated to the nail, such as melanonychia, and others are associated with more widespread disease. Some nail findings can be a clue to an underlying skin condition, such as the pitting seen in psoriasis, whereas other nail findings can be associated with systemic diseases such as half-and-half nails with proximal white discoloration that can be seen in patients with kidney disease. Still other nail conditions can be secondary to medications or trauma.

Lastly, sweat glands include the widespread eccrine glands and more localized apocrine variant predominantly found in the axillae and groin. This portion of the atlas will provide images of those conditions involving the skin appendages, including the hair, sweat glands, and nails.

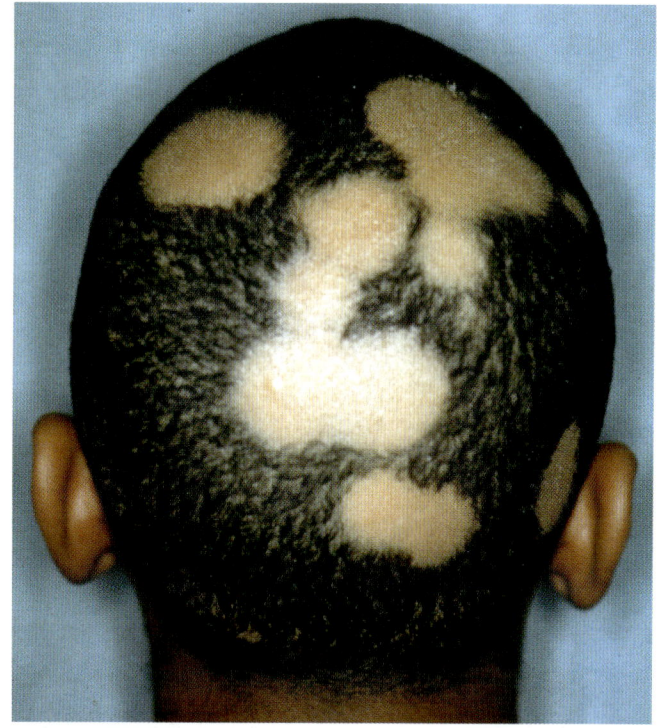

Fig. 33.2 Alopecia areata.

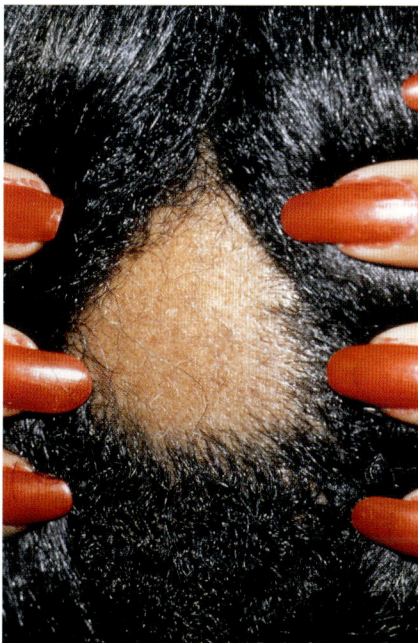

Fig. 33.1 Alopecia areata.

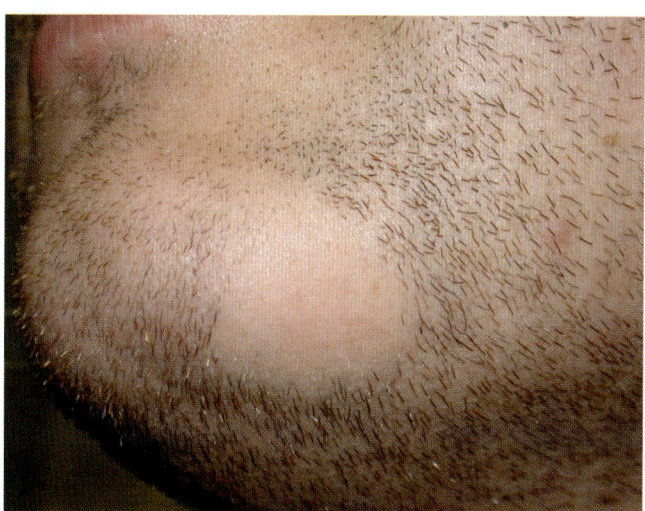

Fig. 33.3 Alopecia areata of the beard.

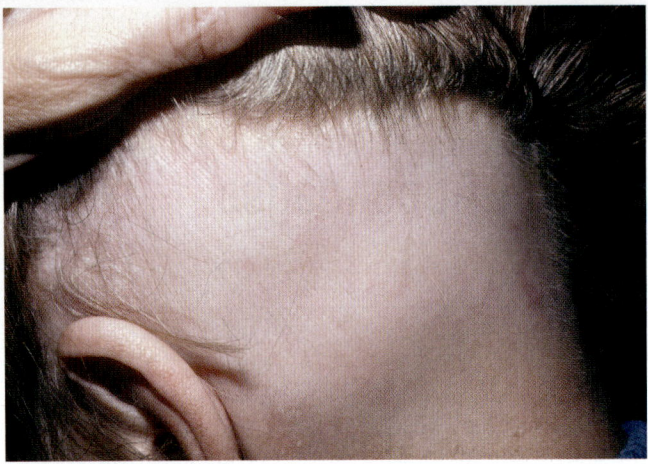

Fig. 33.4 Ophiasis type of alopecia areata. *Courtesy Steven Binnick, MD.*

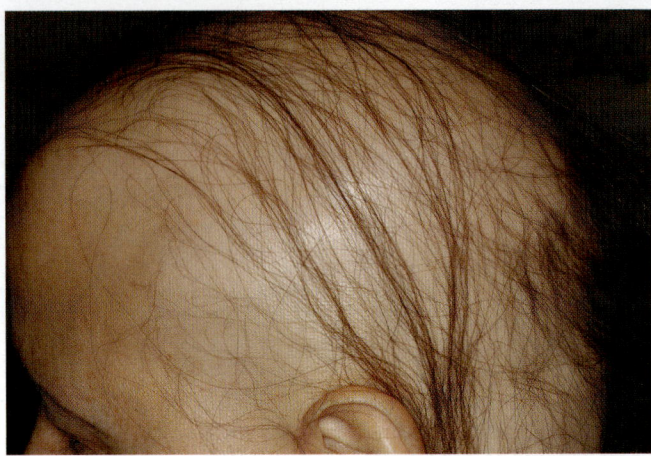

Fig. 33.5 Alopecia areata.

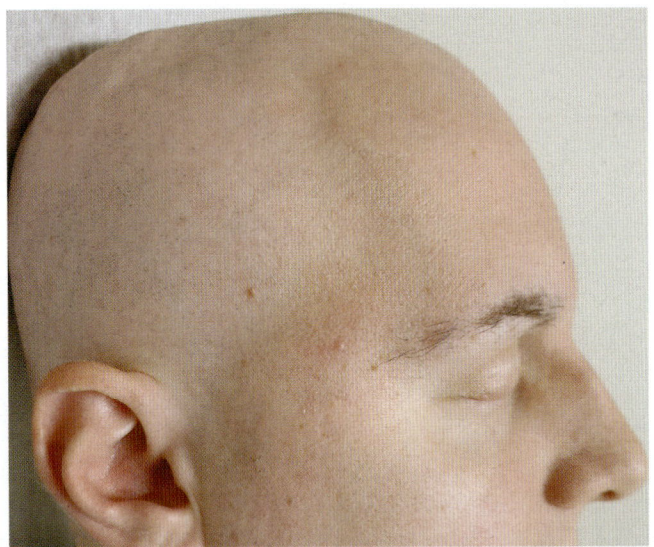

Fig. 33.6 Alopecia totalis.

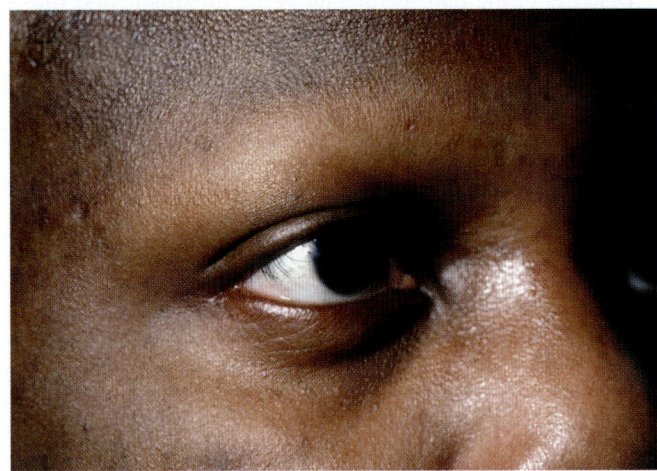

Fig. 33.7 Alopecia universalis.

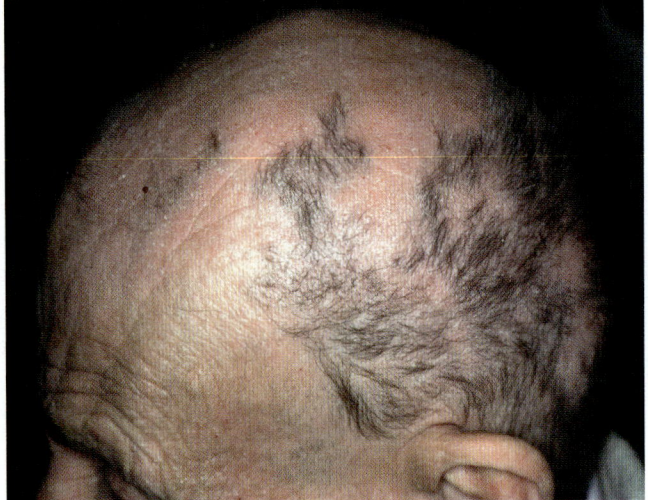

Fig. 33.8 Recurrent alopecia areata in an atopic patient.

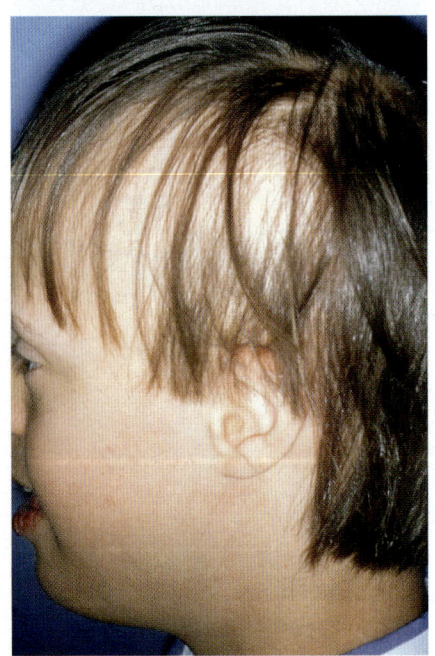

Fig. 33.9 Alopecia areata in a patient with Down syndrome.

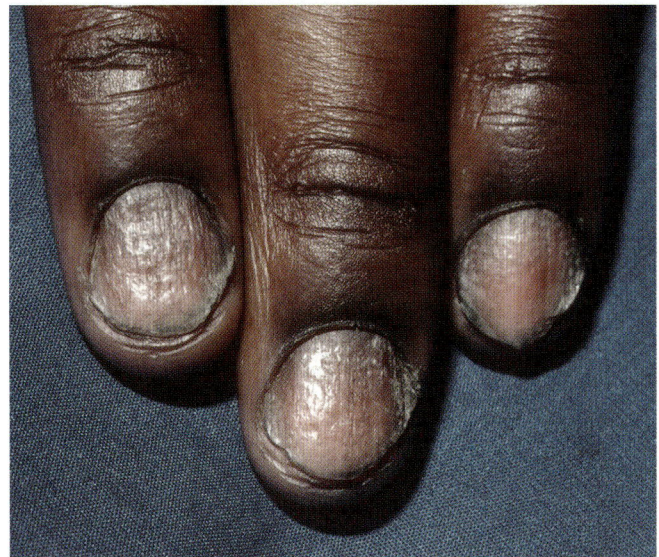

Fig. 33.10 Nails of a patient with alopecia areata. *Courtesy Steven Binnick, MD.*

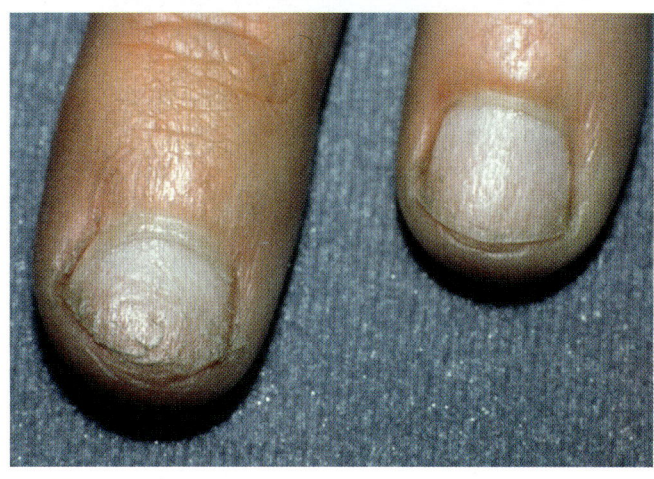

Fig. 33.11 Nails of a patient with alopecia areata. *Courtesy Steven Binnick, MD.*

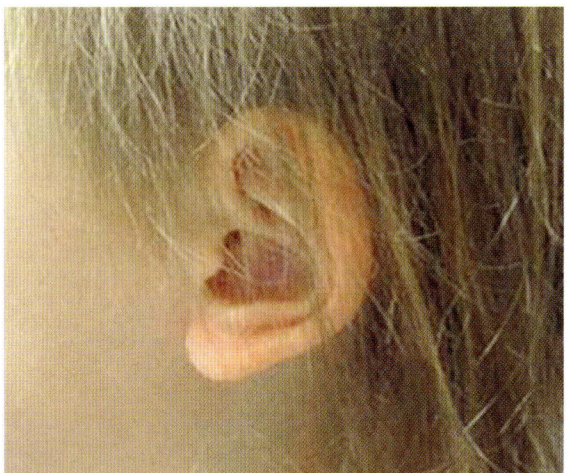

Fig. 33.12 Loose anagen hair syndrome.

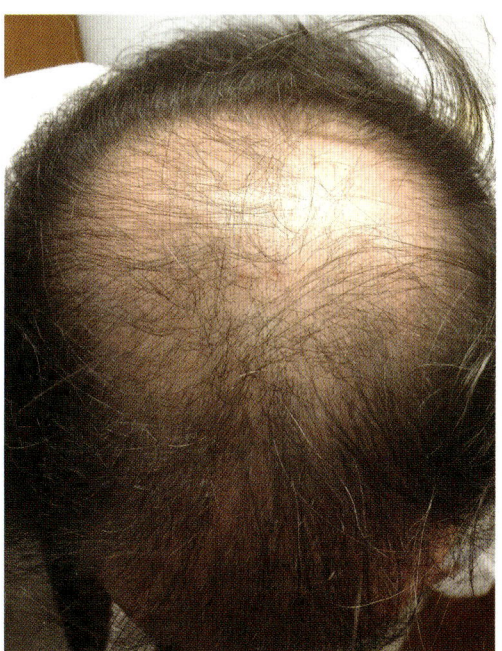

Fig. 33.13 Androgenetic alopecia in a man. *Courtesy Len Sperling, MD.*

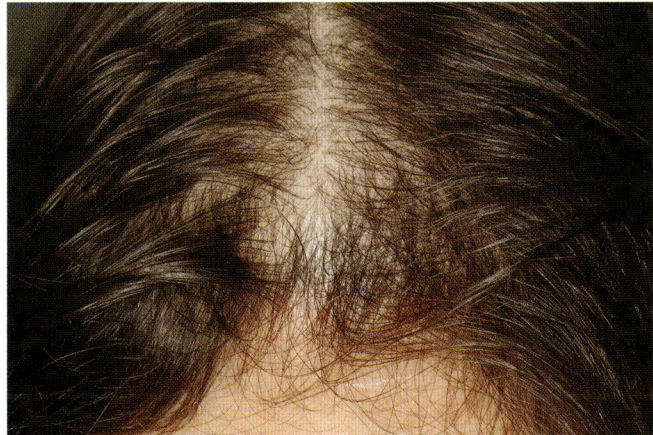

Fig. 33.14 Androgenetic alopecia with a widened central part.

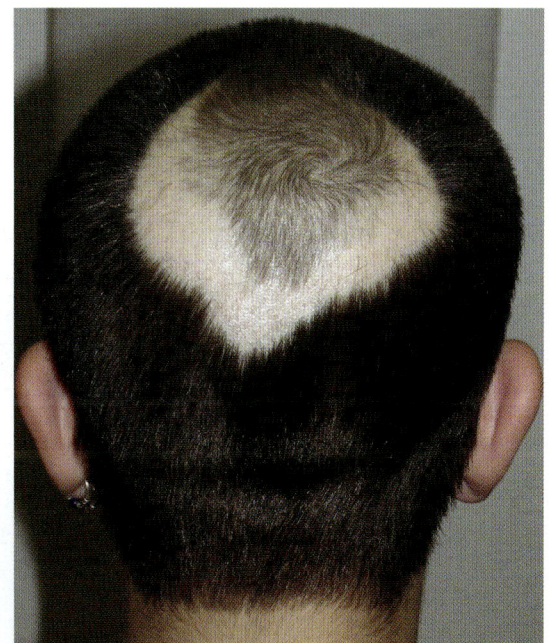

Fig. 33.15 Trichotillosis.

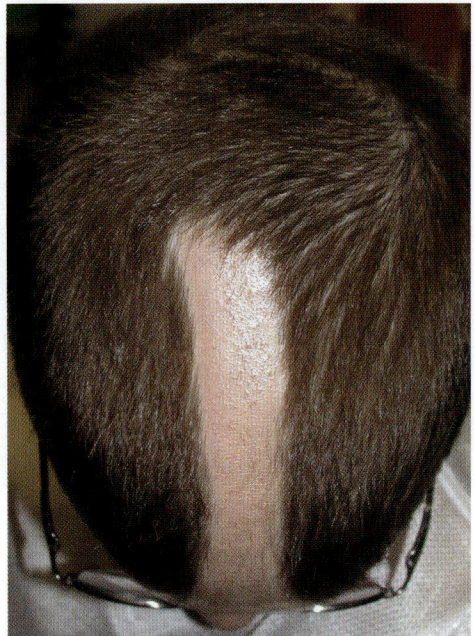

Fig. 33.16 Trichotillosis.

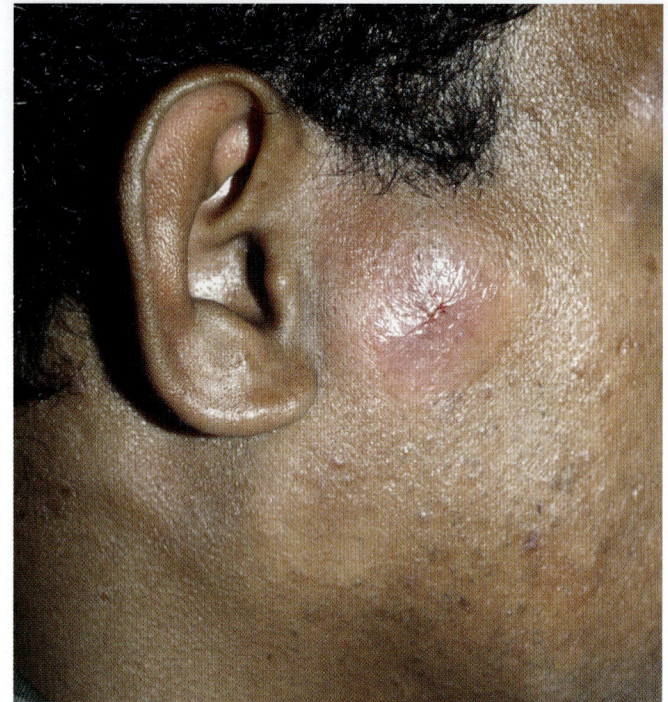

Fig. 33.17 Alopecia mucinosa.

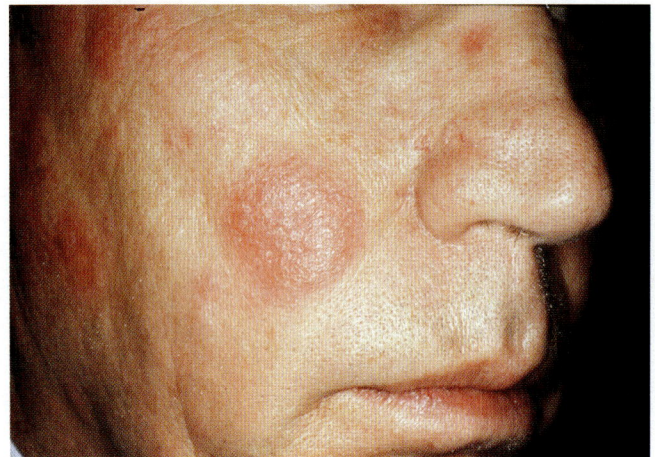

Fig. 33.18 Alopecia mucinosa.

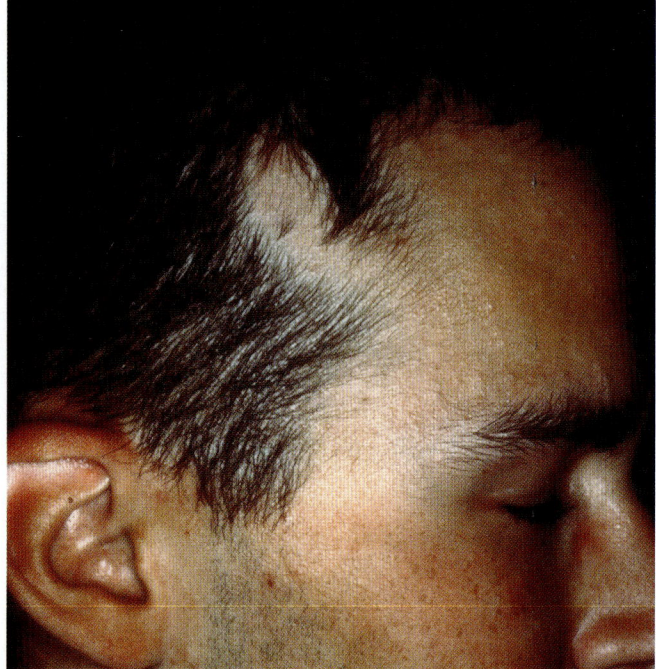

Fig. 33.19 Congenital triangular alopecia.

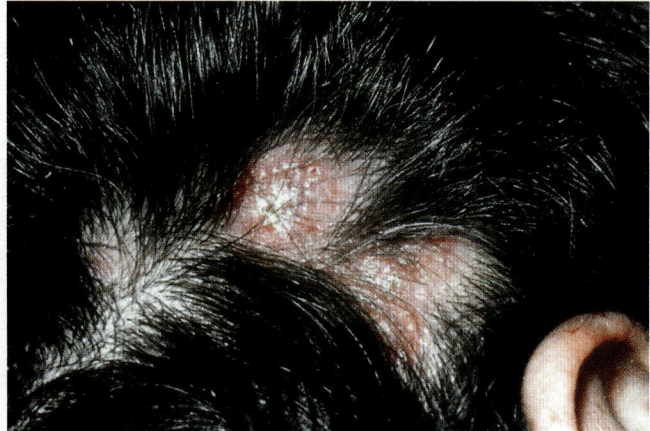

Fig. 33.20 Discoid lupus of the scalp.

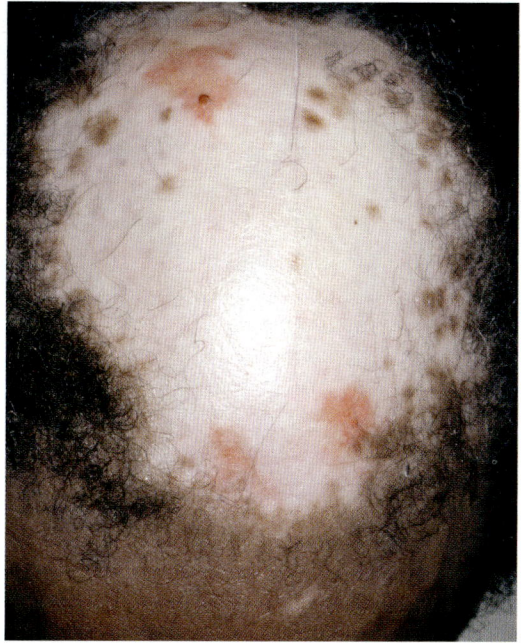

Fig. 33.21 Scarring alopecia secondary to discoid lupus erythematosus. *Courtesy Steven Binnick, MD.*

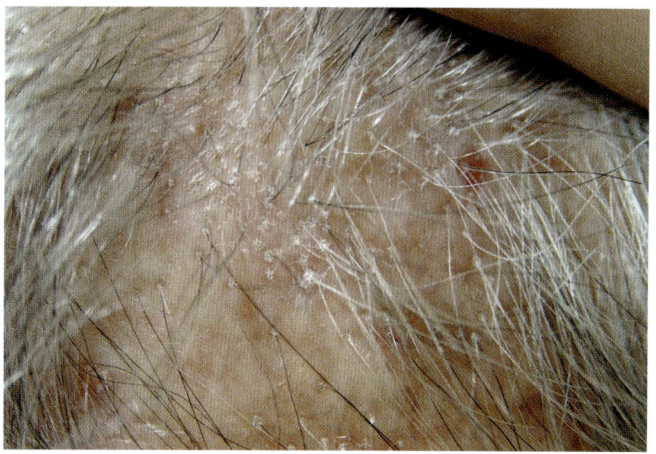

Fig. 33.22 Lichen planopilaris.

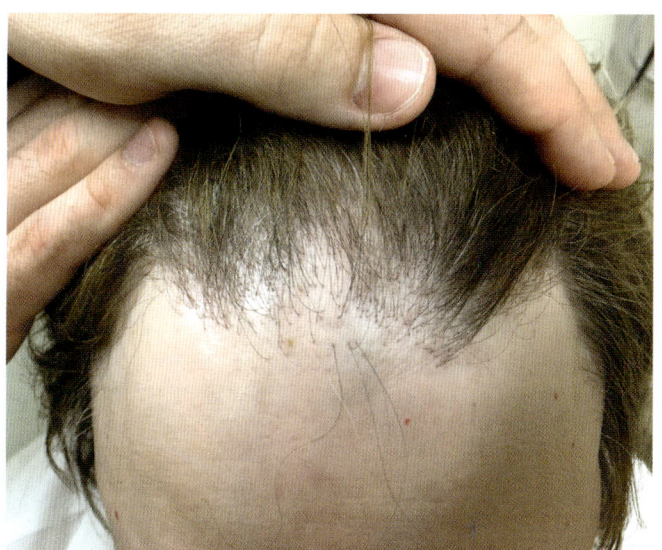

Fig. 33.23 Frontal fibrosing alopecia. *Courtesy Len Sperling, MD.*

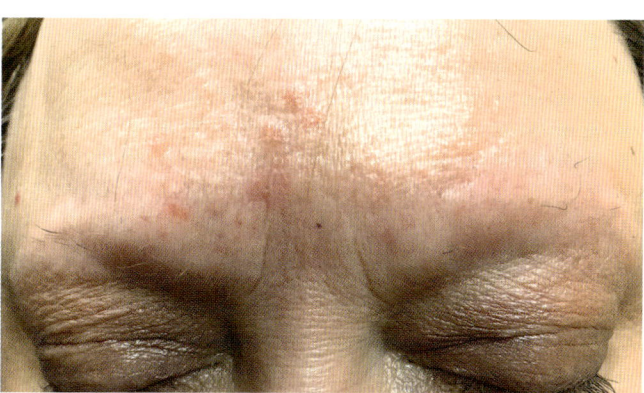

Fig. 33.24 Frontal fibrosing alopecia.

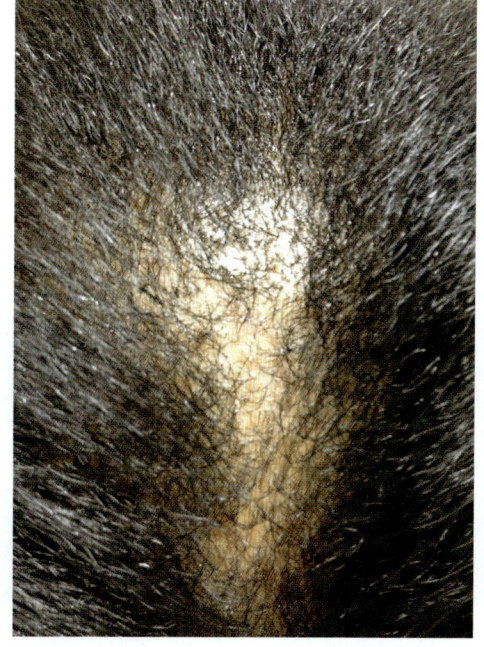

Fig. 33.25 Central centrifugal cicatricial alopecia. *Courtesy Len Sperling, MD.*

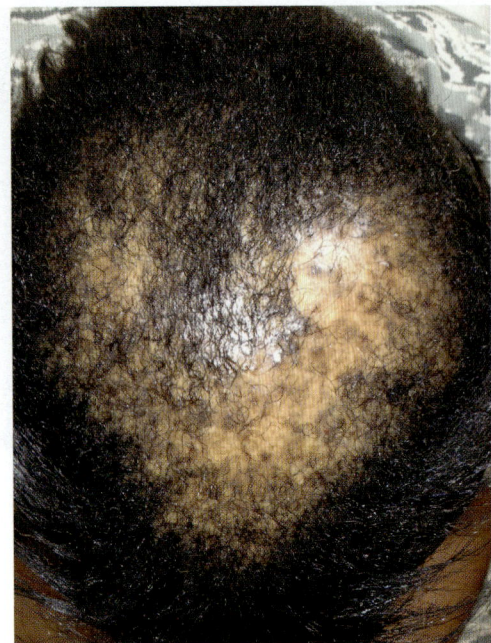

Fig. 33.26 Central centrifugal cicatricial alopecia. *Courtesy Len Sperling, MD.*

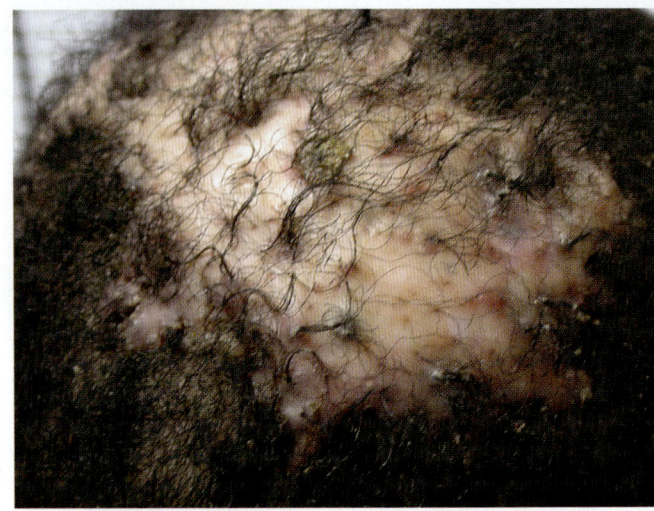

Fig. 33.27 Folliculitis decalvans.

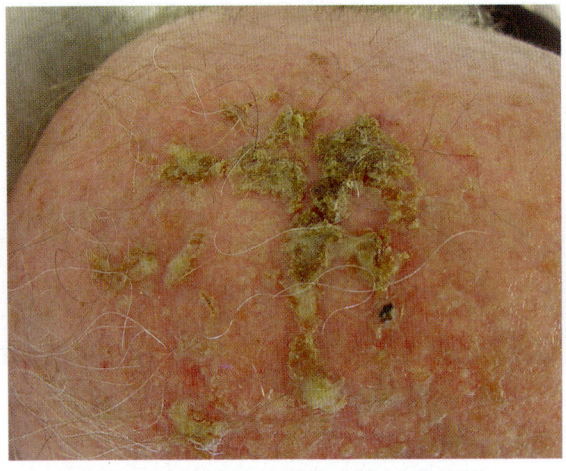

Fig. 33.28 Erosive pustular dermatosis of the scalp. *Courtesy Dr. Rui Carlos Taveres Bello.*

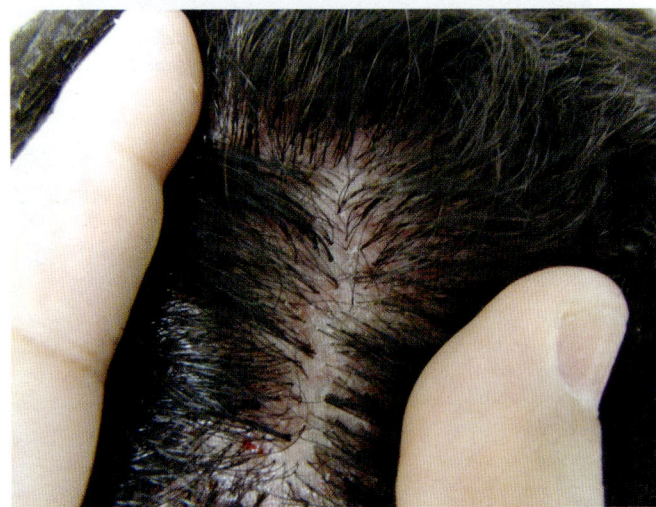

Fig. 33.29 Tufted folliculitis.

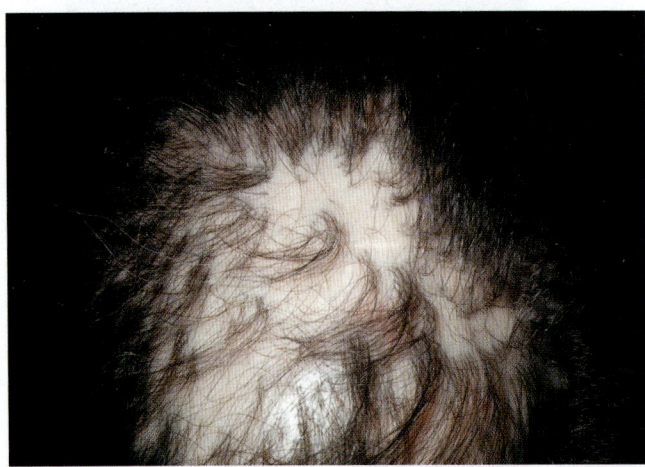

Fig. 33.30 Pseudopelade of Brocq. *Courtesy Steven Binnick, MD.*

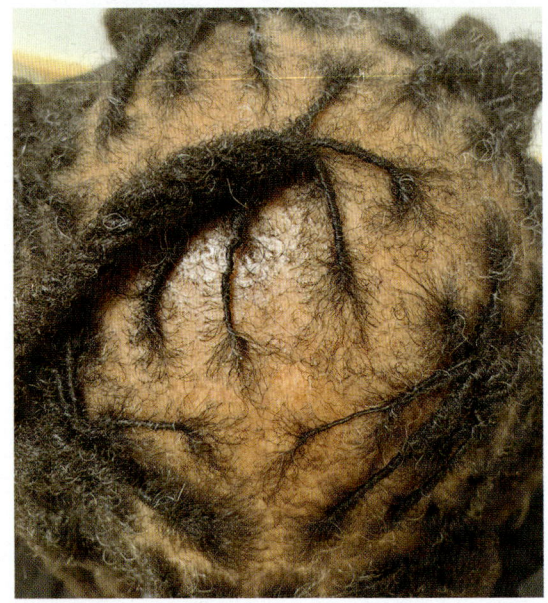

Fig. 33.31 Traction alopecia.

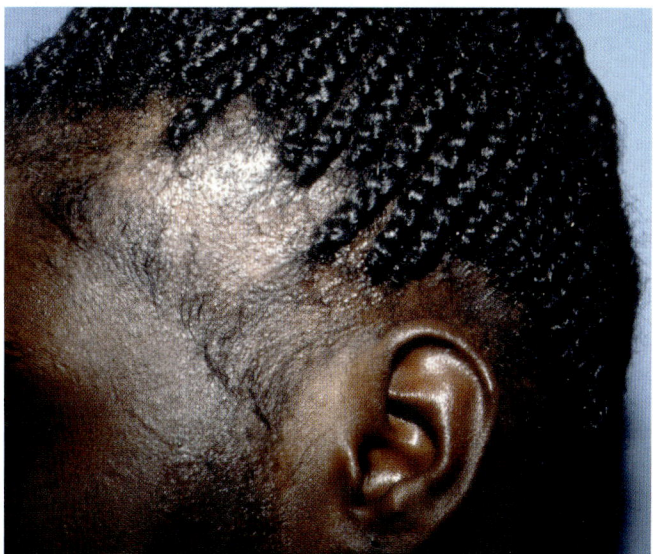

Fig. 33.32 Traction alopecia.

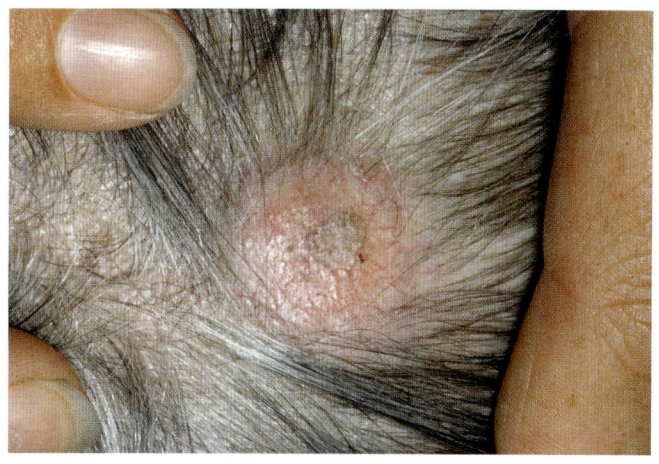

Fig. 33.33 Alopecia neoplastica from metastatic breast cancer.

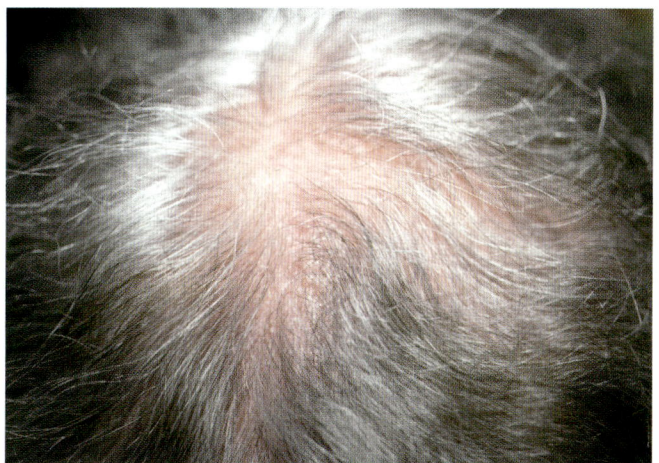

Fig. 33.34 Keratosis follicularis spinulosa decalvans. *Courtesy Steven Binnick, MD.*

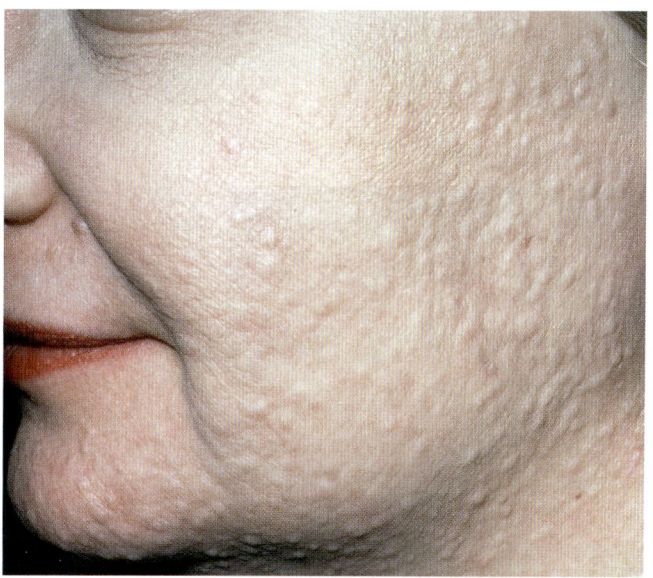

Fig. 33.35 Atrichia with papular lesions. *Courtesy Steven Binnick, MD.*

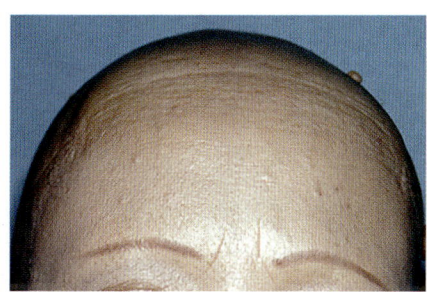

Fig. 33.36 Atrichia with papular lesions.

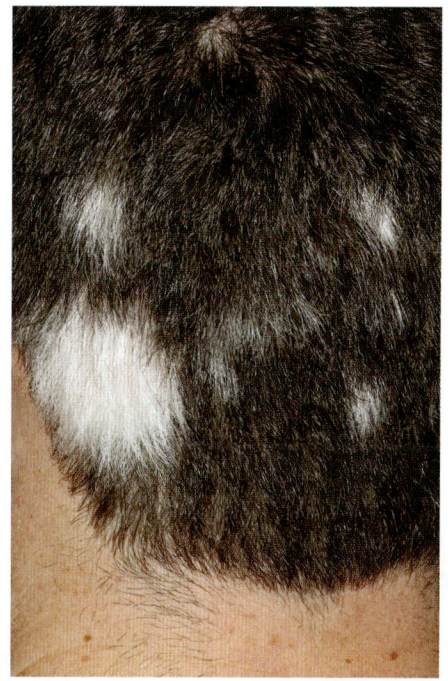

Fig. 33.37 Poliosis.

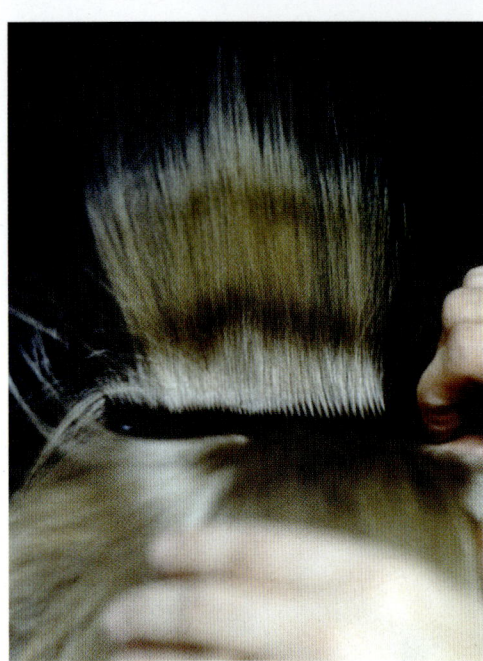

Fig. 33.38 Flag sign.

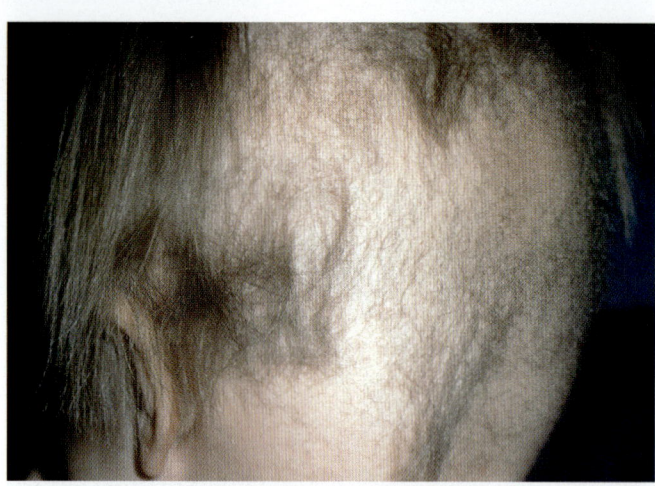

Fig. 33.39 Pili torti. *Courtesy Curt Samlaska, MD.*

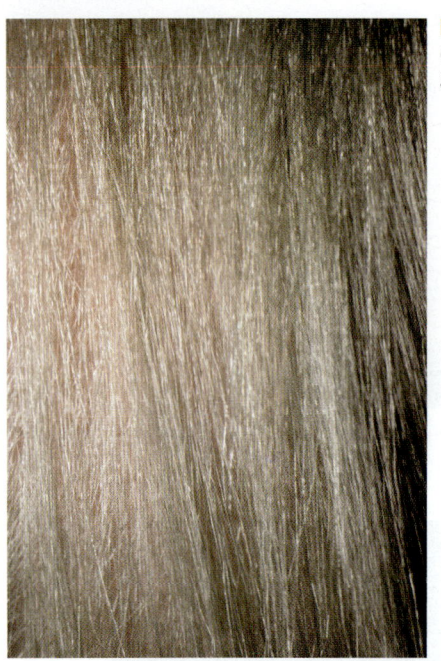

Fig. 33.40 Pili torti. *Courtesy Curt Samlaska, MD.*

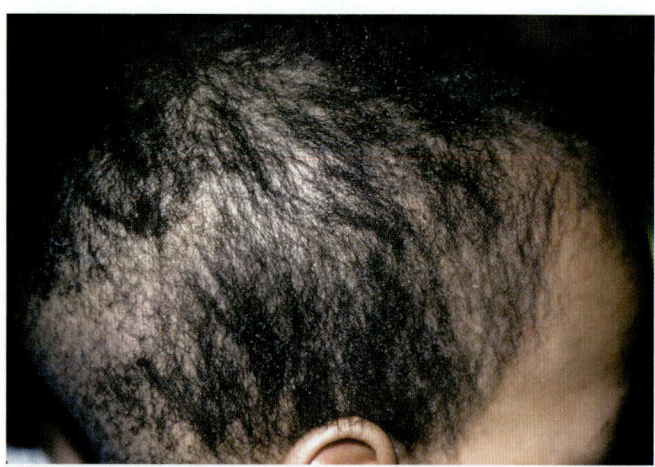

Fig. 33.41 Menkes kinky hair syndrome. *Courtesy Paul Honig, MD.*

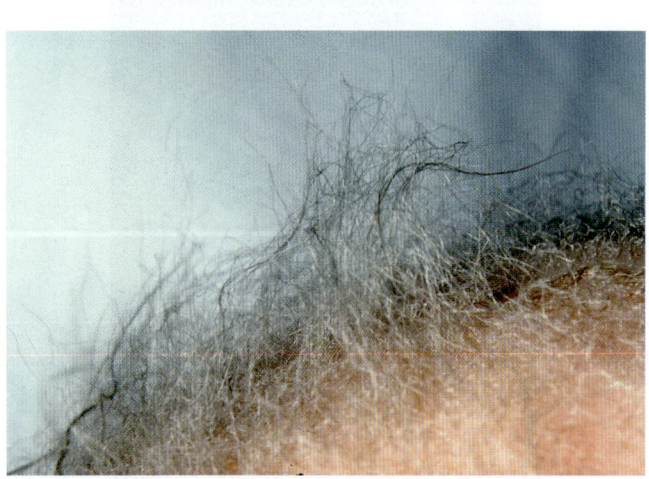

Fig. 33.42 Menkes kinky hair syndrome.

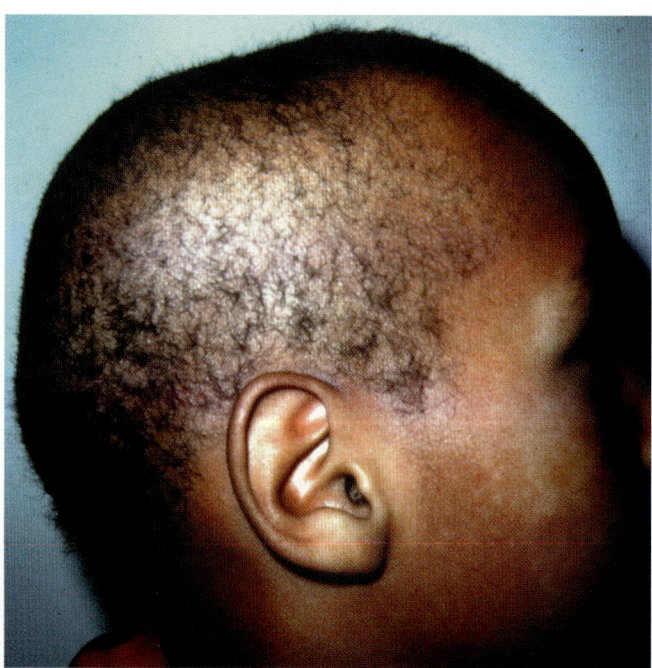

Fig. 33.43 Proximal trichorrhexis nodosa.

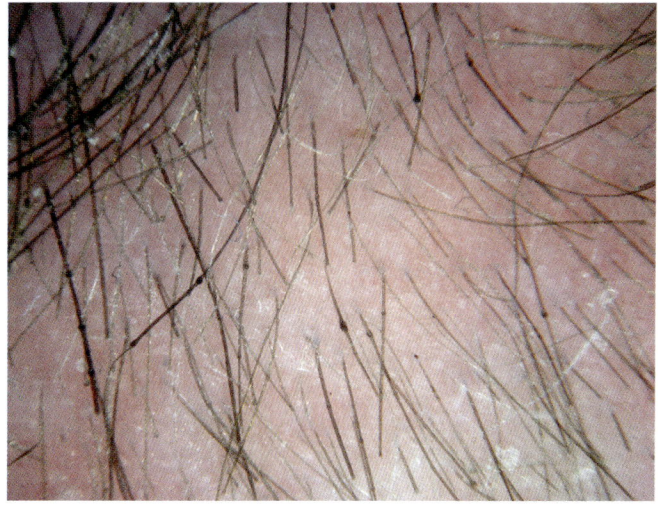

Fig. 33.44 Trichorrhexis invaginata in Netherton syndrome.

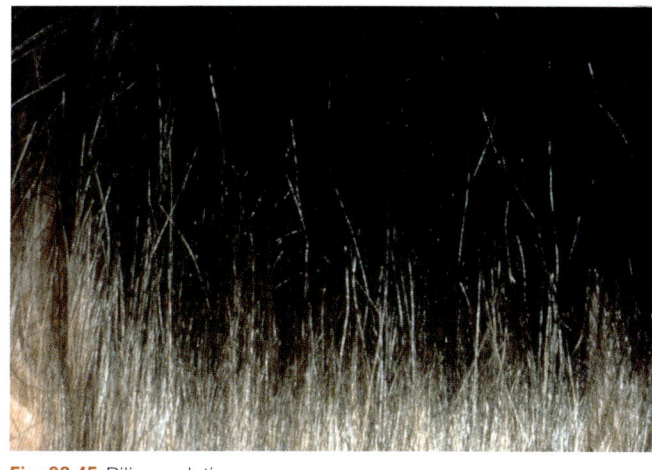

Fig. 33.45 Pili annulati.

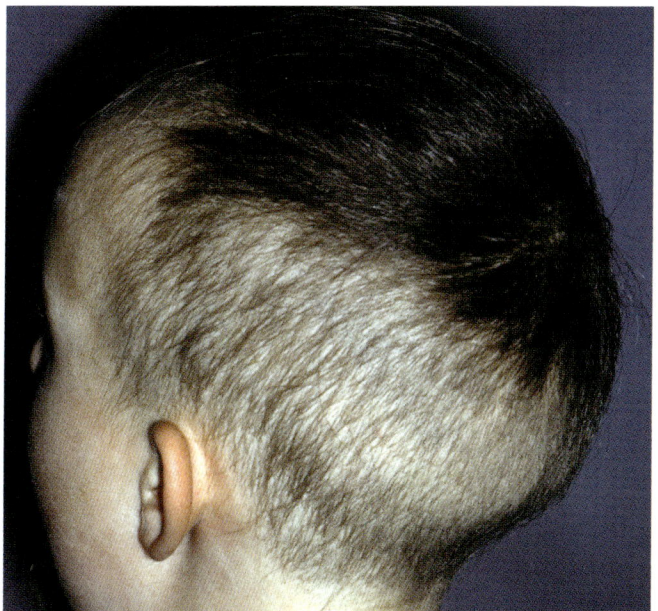

Fig. 33.46 Monilethrix.

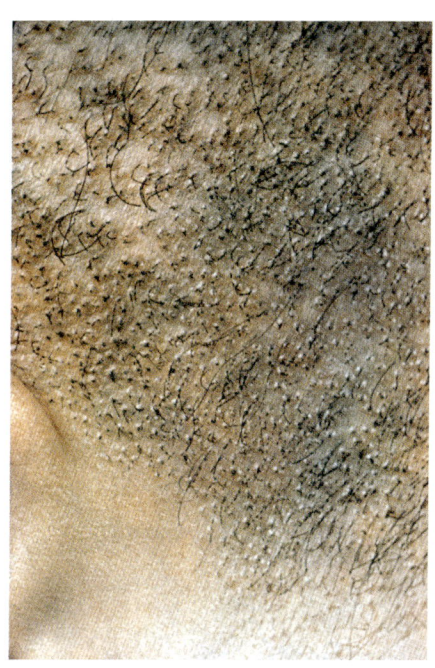

Fig. 33.47 Monilethrix.

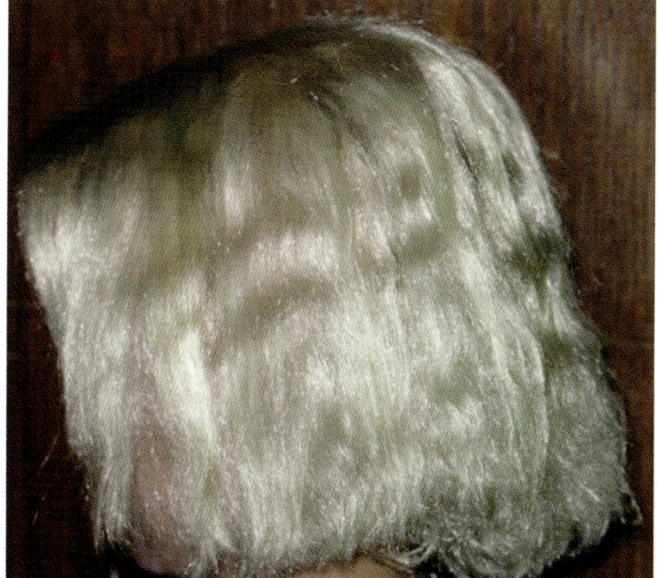

Fig. 33.48 Uncombable hair syndrome. *Courtesy Paul Honig, MD.*

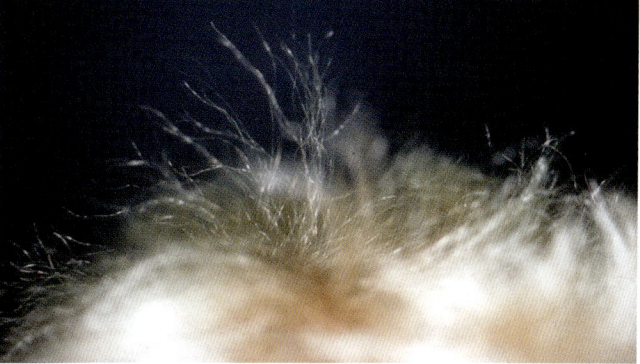

Fig. 33.49 Uncombable hair syndrome.

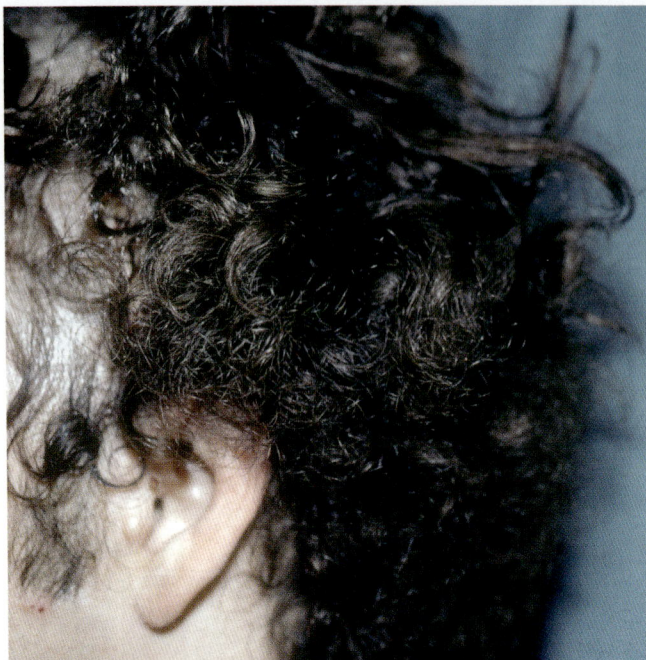

Fig. 33.50 Progressive kinking of the hair. *Courtesy Ken Greer, MD.*

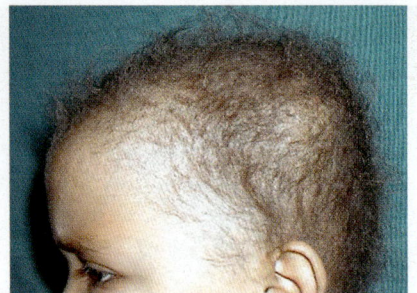

Fig. 33.51 Wooly hair.

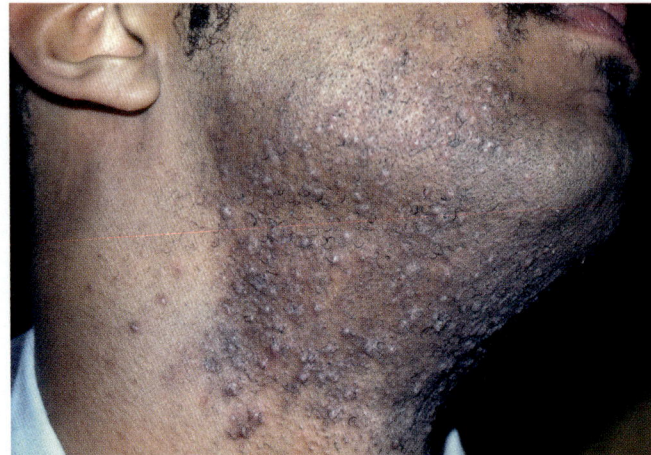

Fig. 33.53 Pseudofolliculitis barbae. *Courtesy Steven Binnick, MD.*

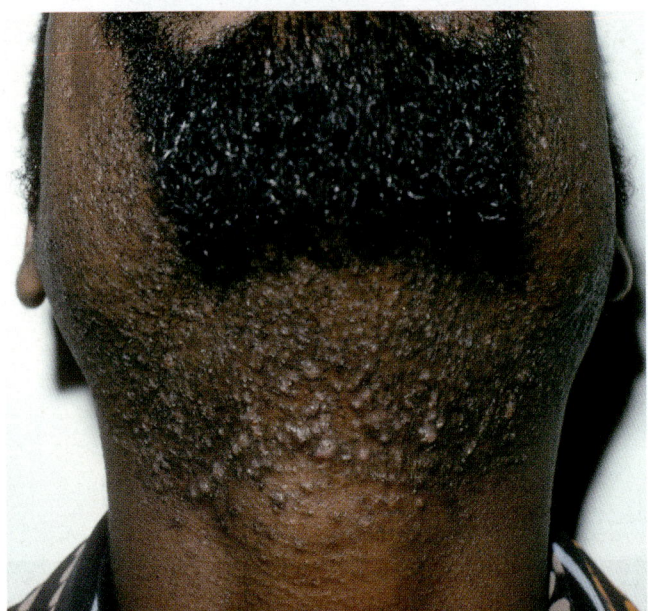

Fig. 33.52 Pseudofolliculitis barbae. *Courtesy Steven Binnick, MD.*

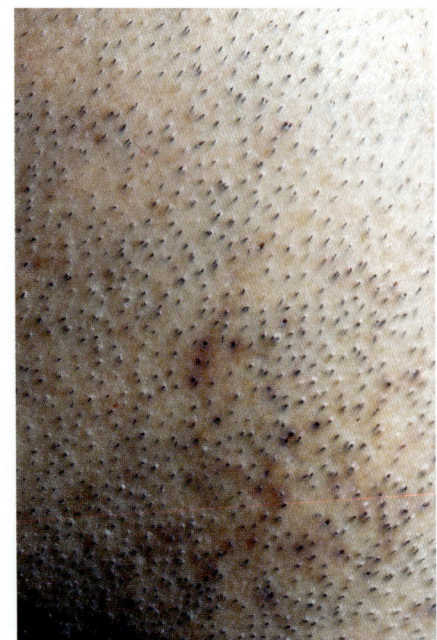

Fig. 33.54 Pili multigemini.

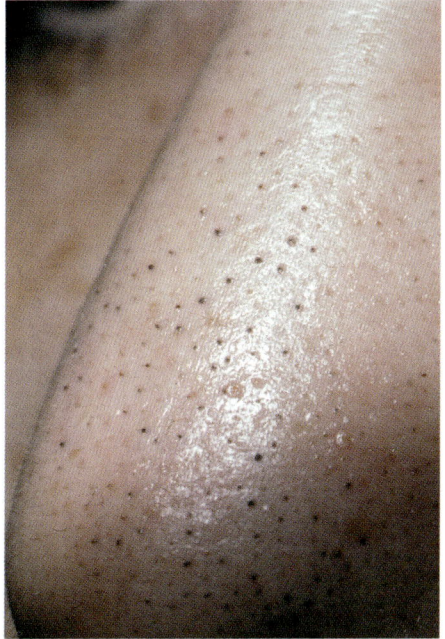

Fig. 33.55 Trichostasis spinulosa. *Courtesy Steven Binnick, MD.*

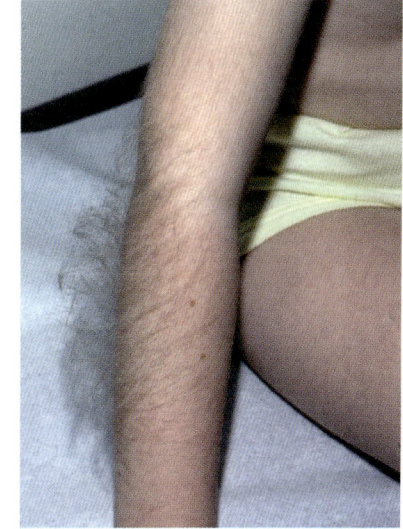

Fig. 33.56 Hypertrichosis cubiti. *Courtesy Paul Honig, MD.*

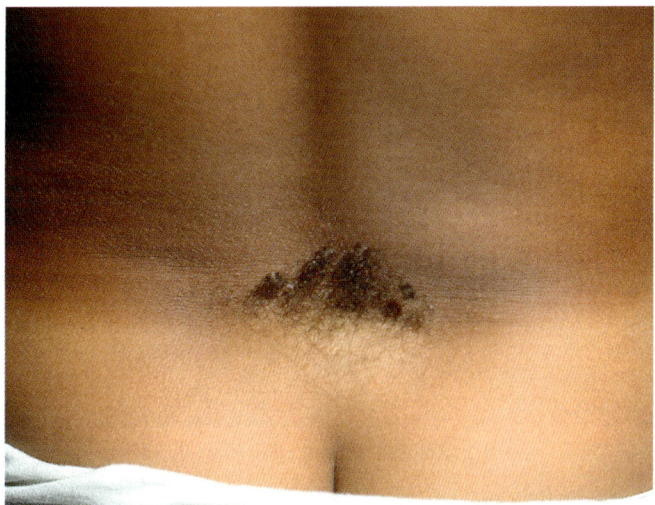

Fig. 33.57 Localized hypertrichosis over the sacrum with a lipoma and underlying tethered cord.

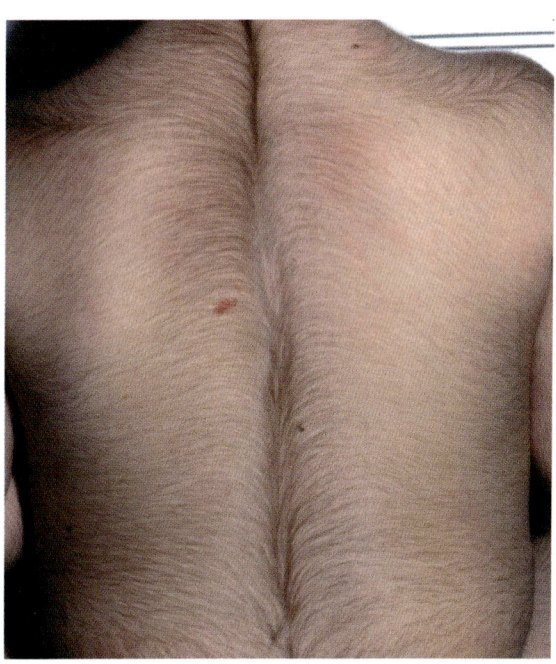

Fig. 33.58 Hypertrichosis from minoxidil. *Courtesy Paul Honig, MD.*

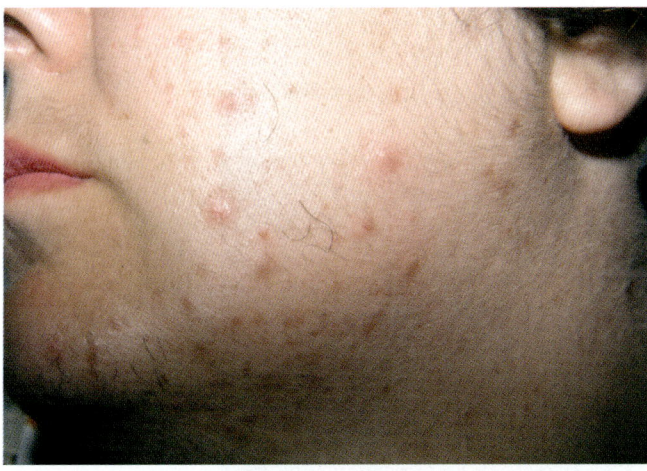

Fig. 33.59 Hirsutism and acne. *Courtesy Steven Binnick, MD.*

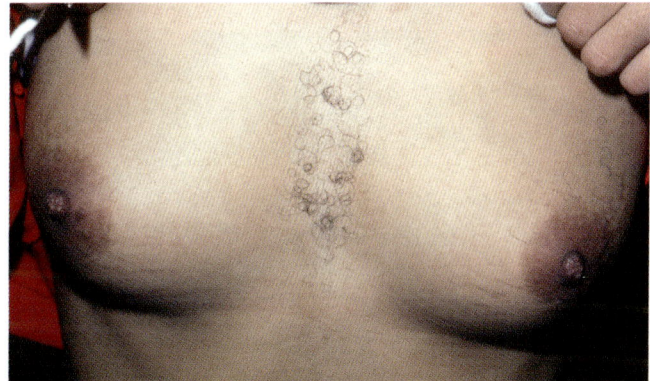

Fig. 33.60 Hirsutism. *Courtesy Steven Binnick, MD.*

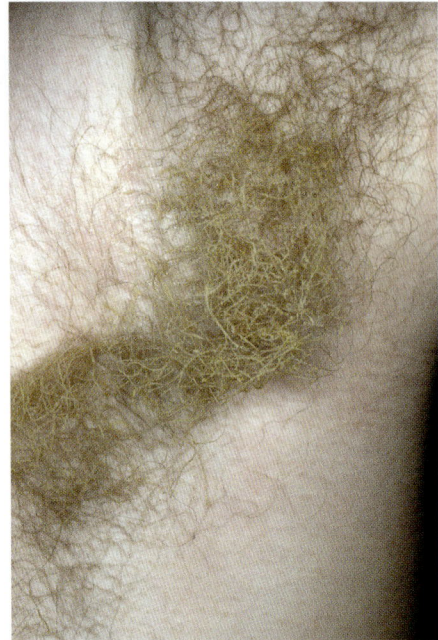

Fig. 33.61 Trichomycosis axillaris. *Courtesy Steven Binnick, MD.*

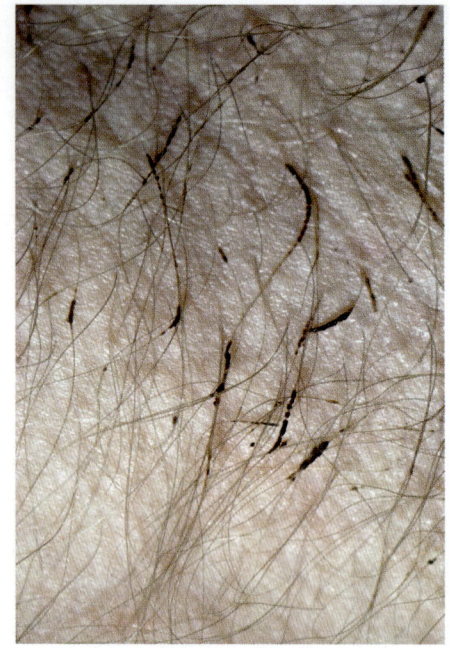

Fig. 33.62 Trichomycosis axillaris.

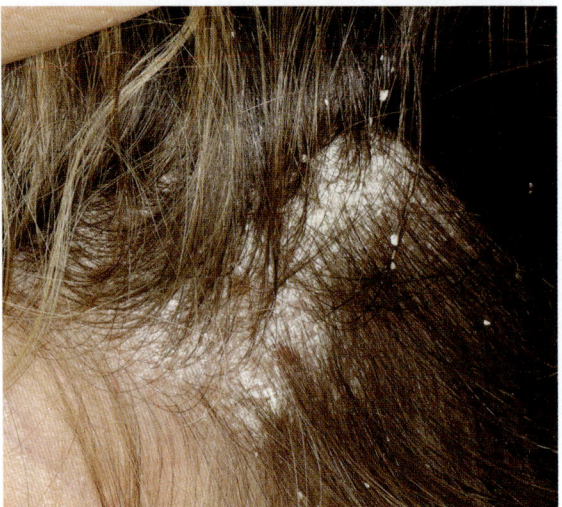

Fig. 33.63 Tinea amiantacea.

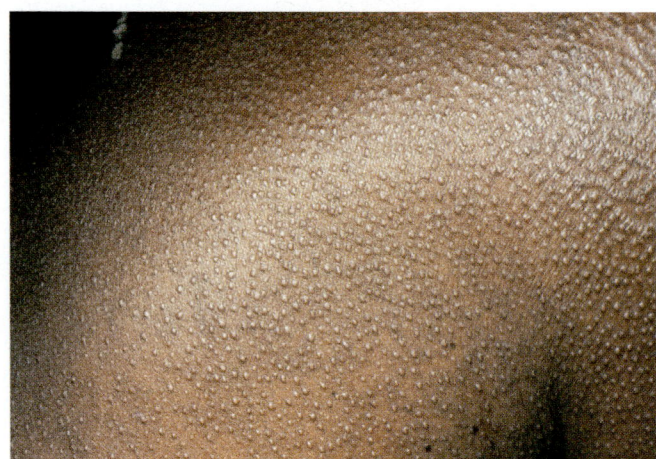

Fig. 33.64 Disseminate and recurrent infundibulofolliculitis.

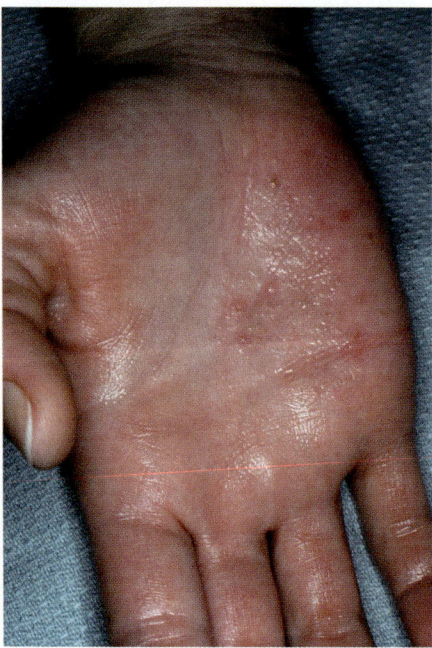

Fig. 33.66 Palmar hyperhidrosis.

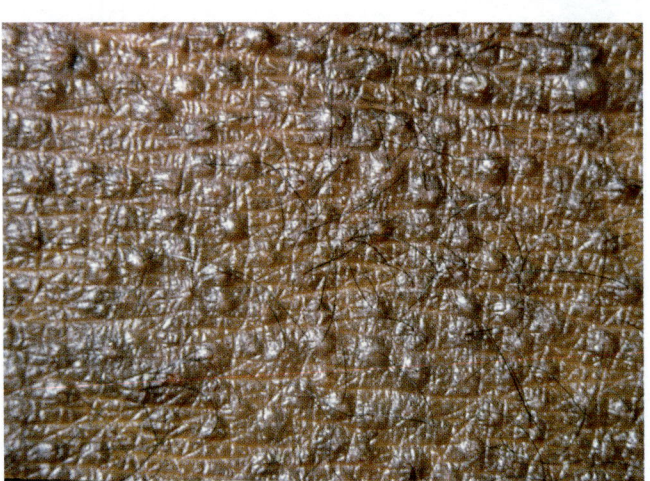

Fig. 33.65 Disseminate and recurrent infundibulofolliculitis.

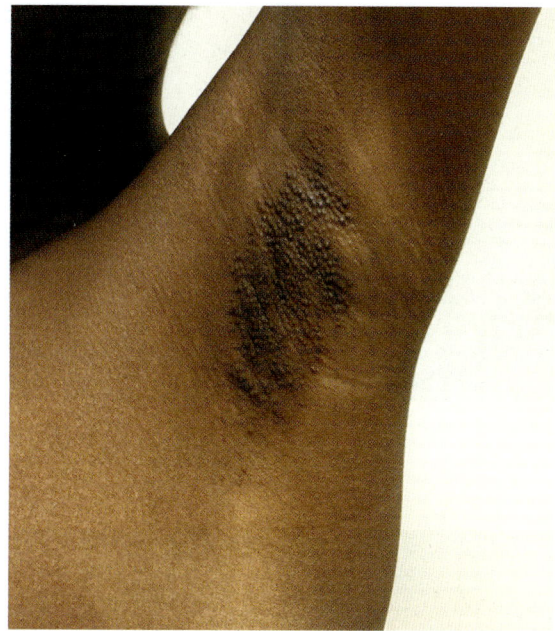

Fig. 33.67 Fox-Fordyce disease.

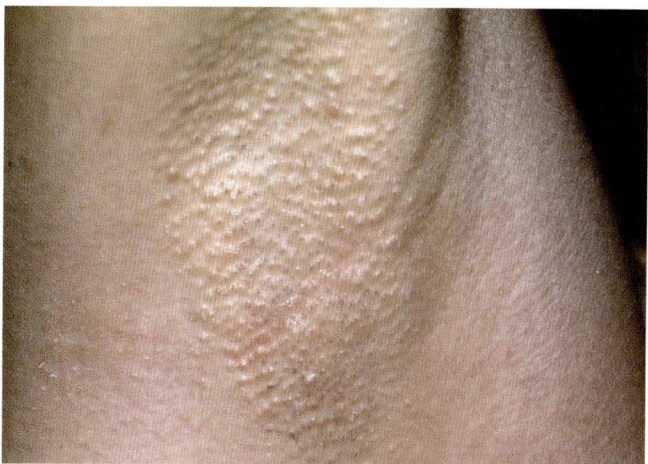

Fig. 33.68 Fox-Fordyce disease. *Courtesy Steven Binnick, MD.*

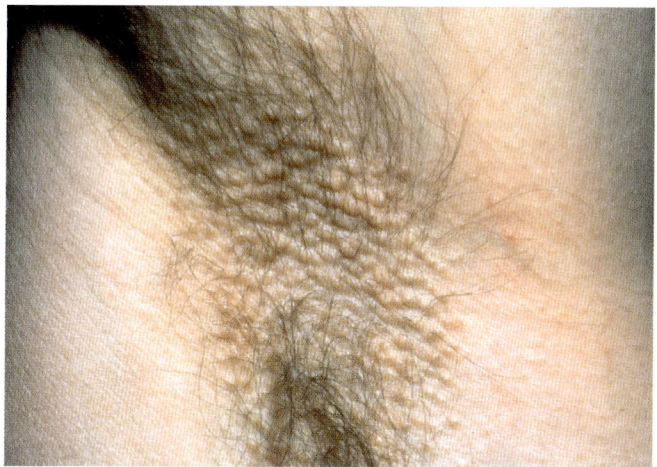

Fig. 33.69 Fox-Fordyce disease with xanthomatous change.

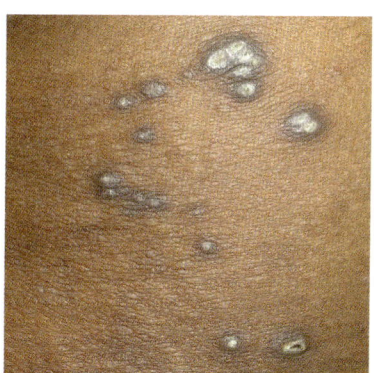

Fig. 33.70 Perforating disorder of renal failure. *Courtesy Scott Norton, MD.*

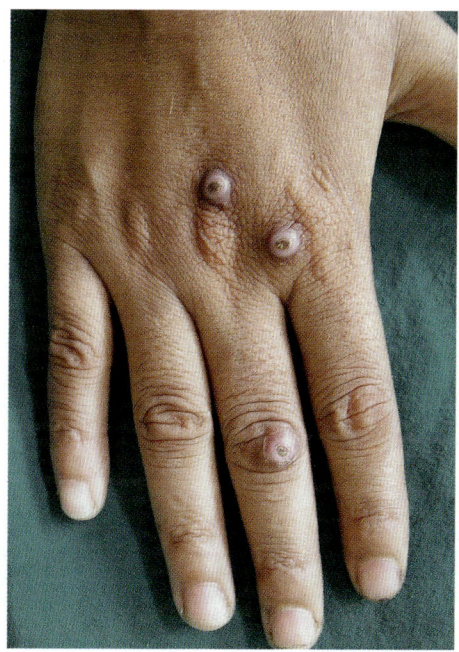

Fig. 33.71 Reactive perforating collagenosis.

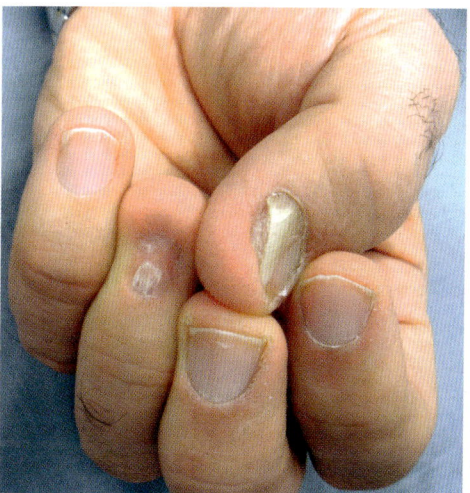

Fig. 33.72 Nail lichen planus. *Courtesy Adam Rubin, MD.*

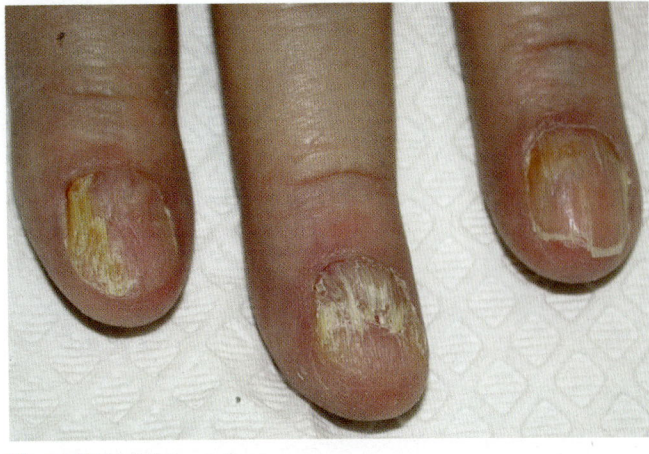

Fig. 33.73 Nail lichen planus.

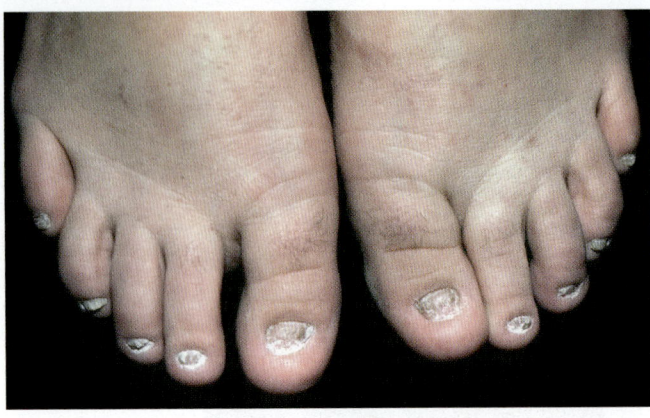

Fig. 33.74 Nail lichen planus.

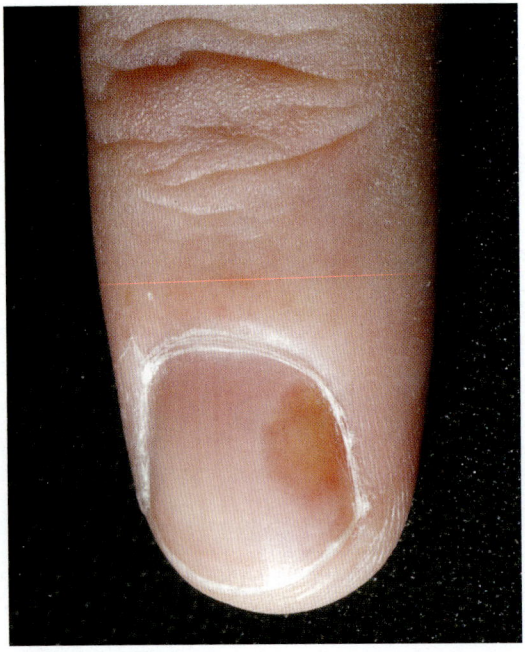

Fig. 33.75 Oil spot in a psoriatic nail.

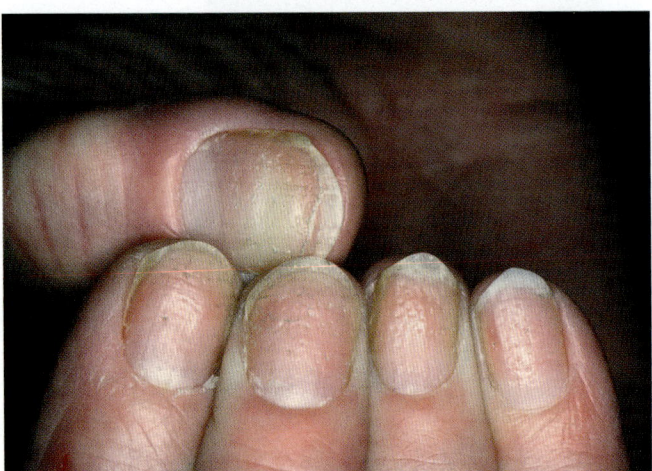

Fig. 33.76 Nail pits in psoriatic nails.

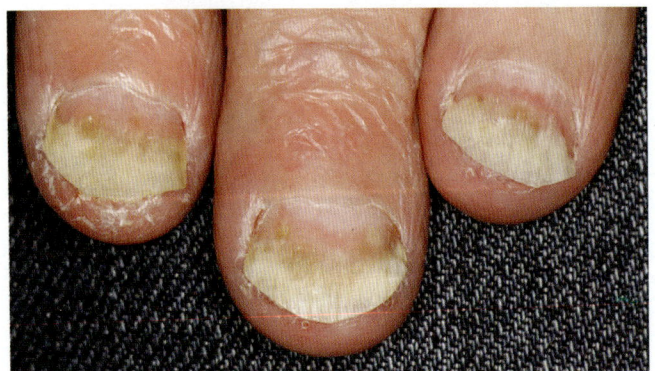

Fig. 33.77 Psoriatic nails.

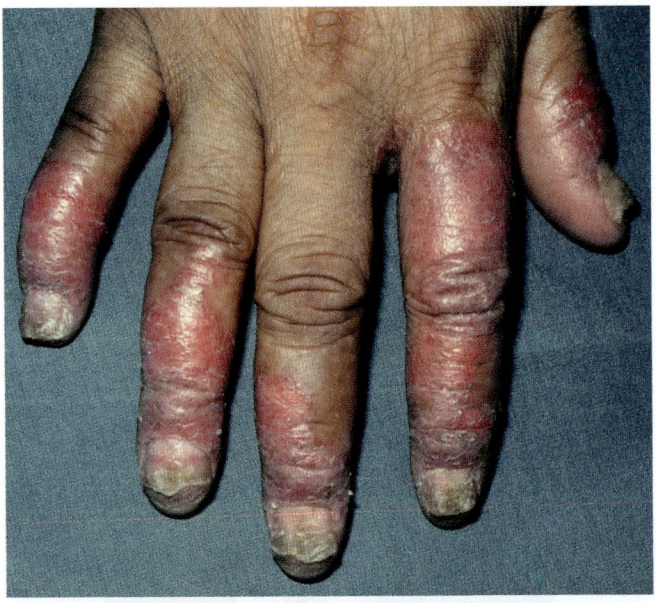

Fig. 33.78 Nail psoriasis in a patient with psoriatic arthritis.

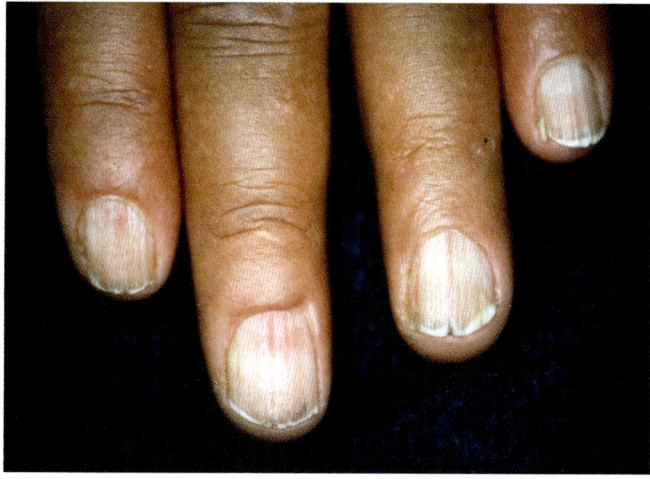

Fig. 33.79 Darier disease of the nail.

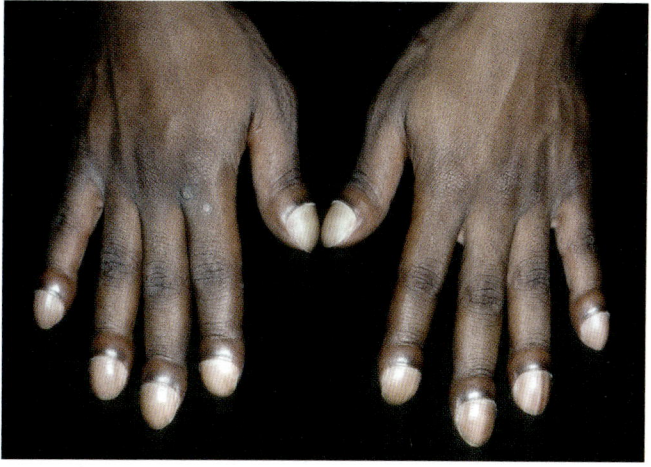

Fig. 33.80 Clubbing.

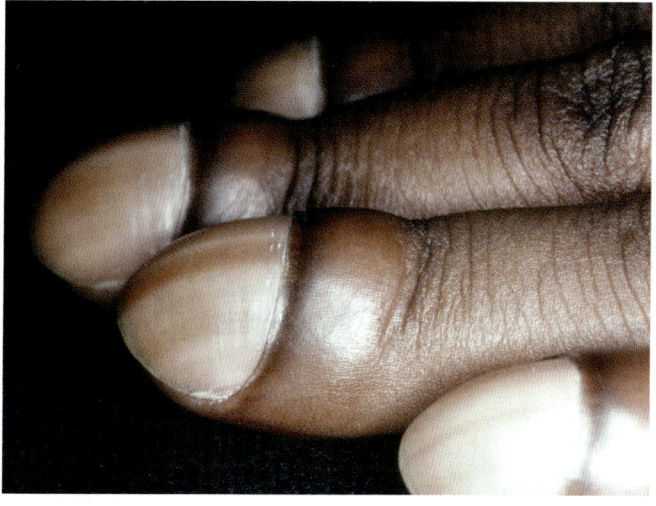

Fig. 33.81 Clubbing.

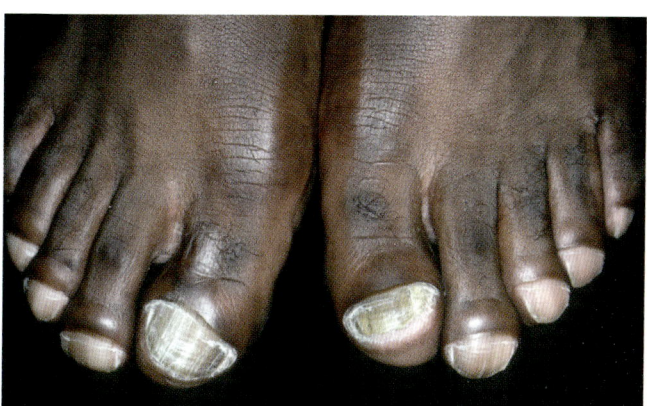

Fig. 33.82 Clubbing.

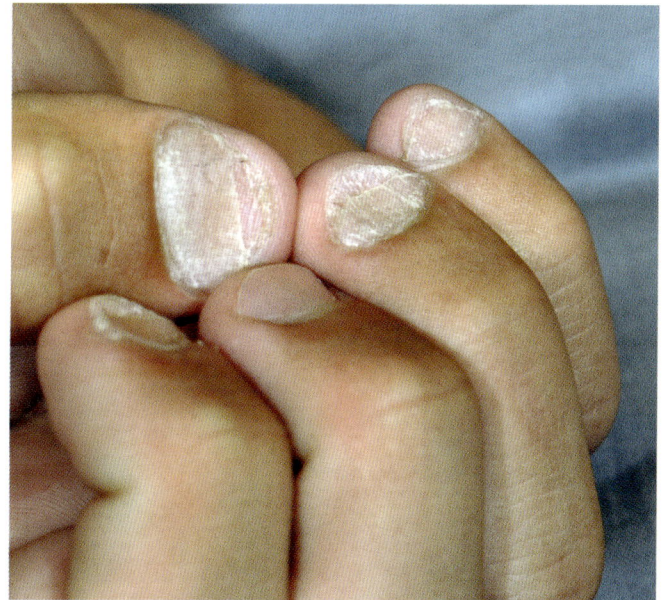

Fig. 33.83 Koilonychia with trachyonychia. *Courtesy Adam Rubin, MD.*

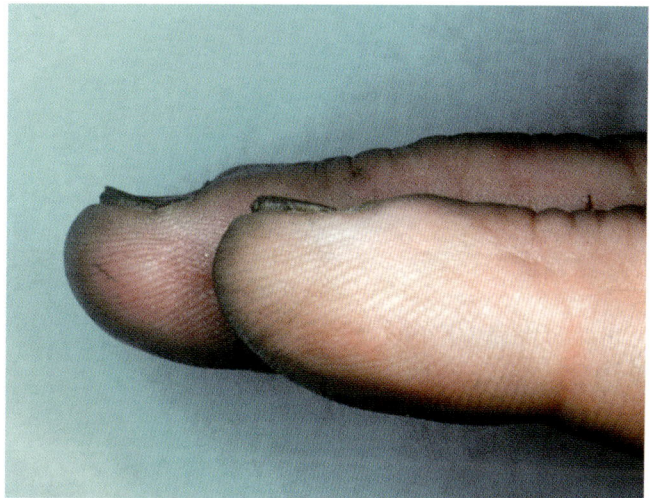

Fig. 33.84 Koilonychia.

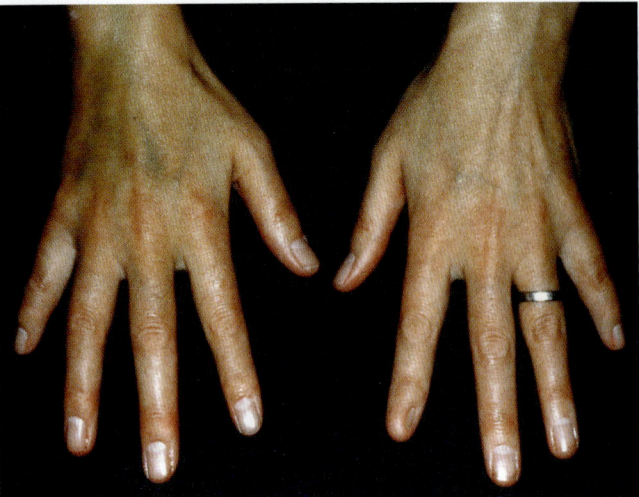

Fig. 33.85 Congenital onychodysplasia of the index finger.

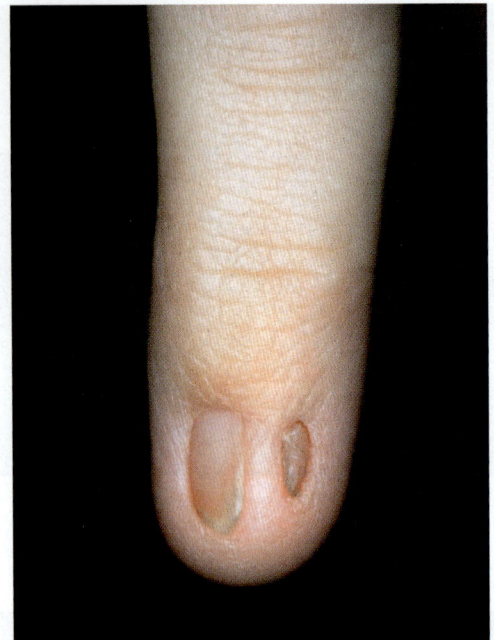

Fig. 33.86 Congenital onychodysplasia of the index finger.

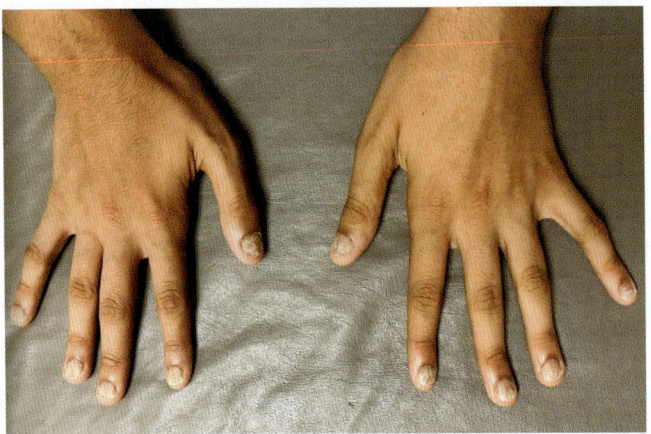

Fig. 33.87 Trachyonychia.

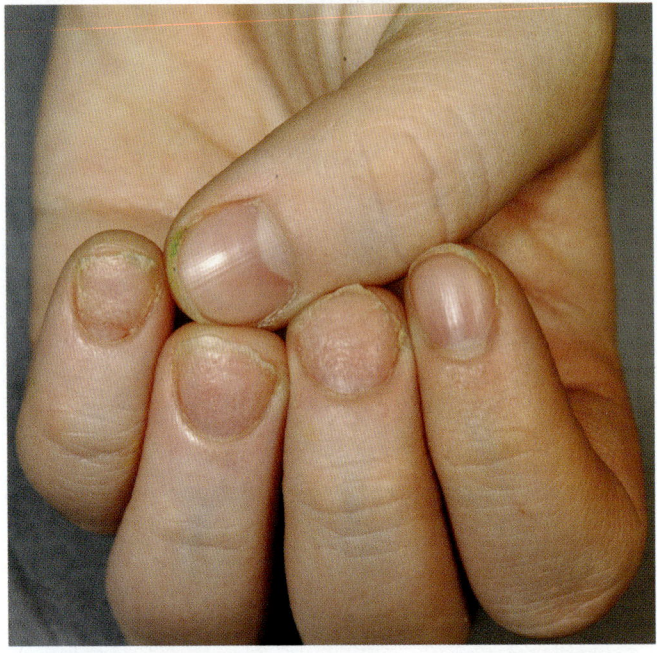

Fig. 33.88 Trachyonychia. *Courtesy Adam Rubin, MD.*

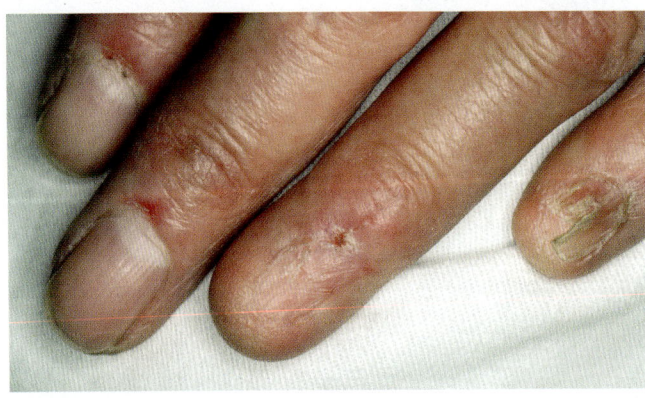

Fig. 33.89 Anonychia.

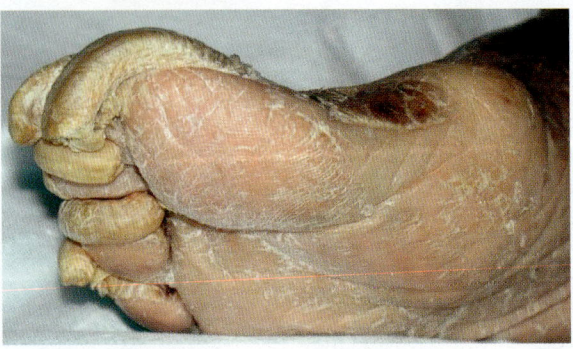

Fig. 33.90 Onychogryphosis. *Courtesy Scott Norton, MD.*

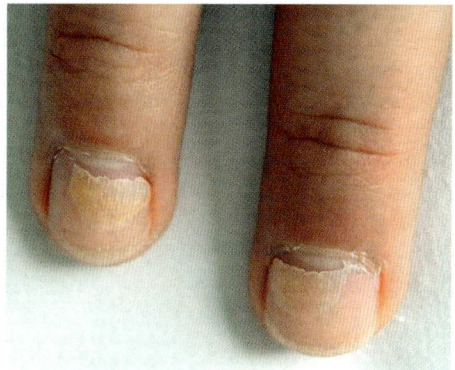

Fig. 33.91 Onychomadesis after hand-foot-mouth disease.

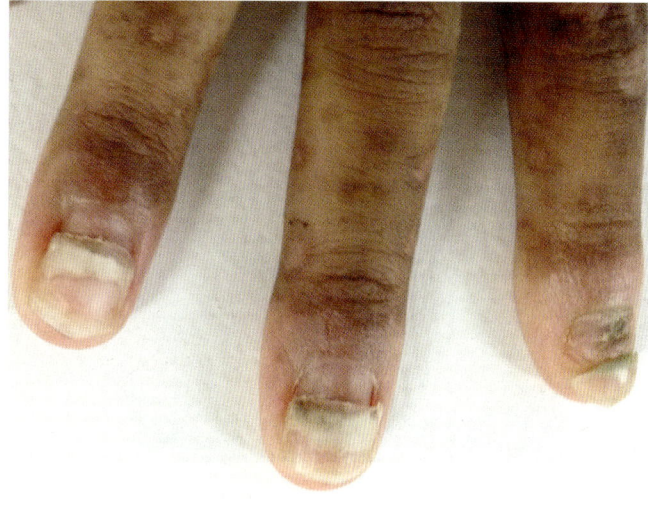

Fig. 33.92 Onychomadesis after toxic epidermal necrolysis.

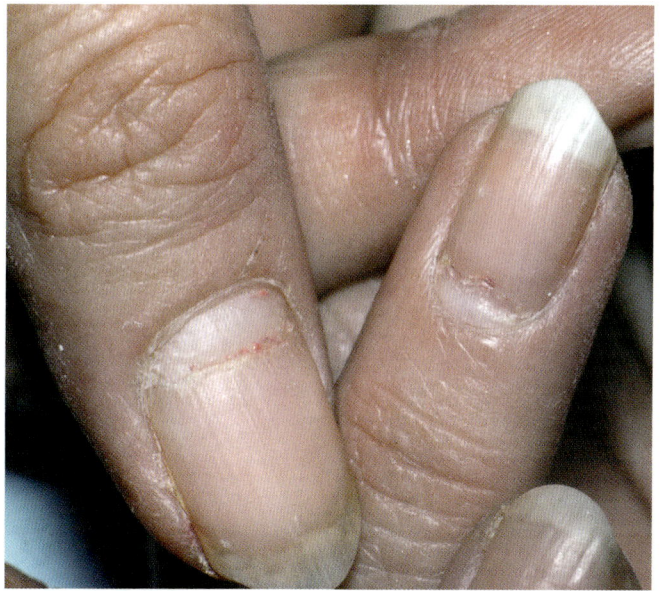

Fig. 33.93 Beau lines. *Courtesy Steven Binnick, MD.*

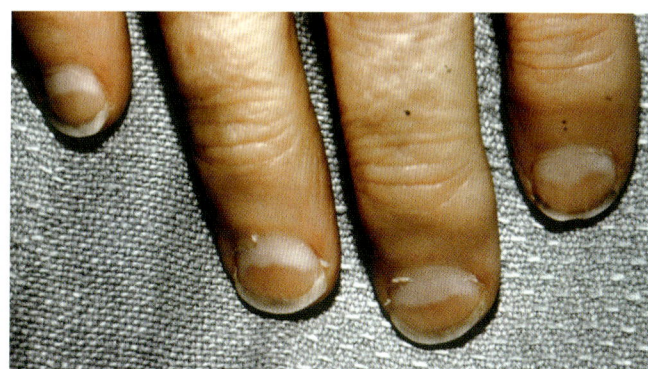

Fig. 33.94 Half-and-half nails.

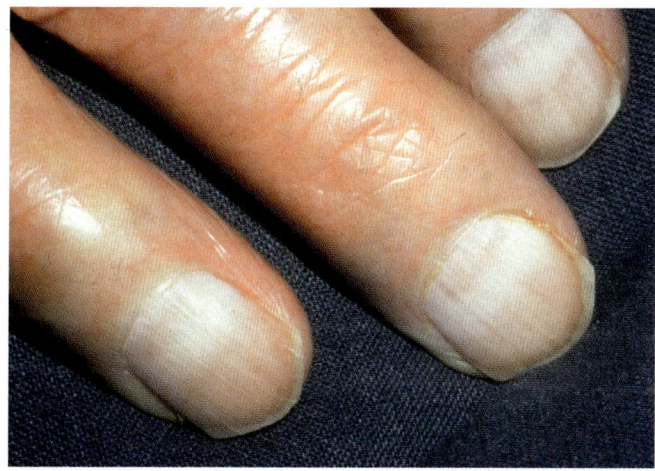

Fig. 33.95 Muehrcke lines.

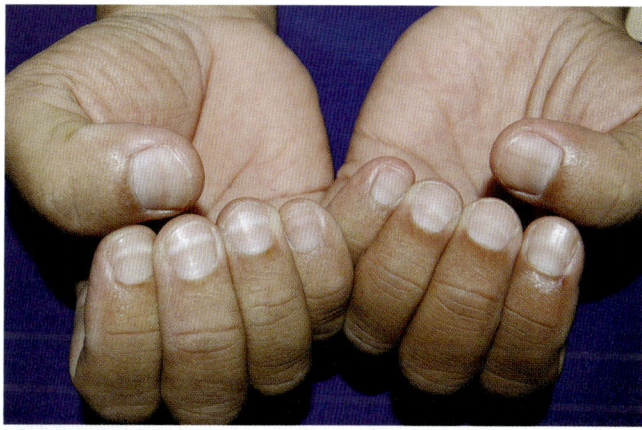

Fig. 33.96 Mee lines. *Courtesy National Cheng Kung University, Taiwan.*

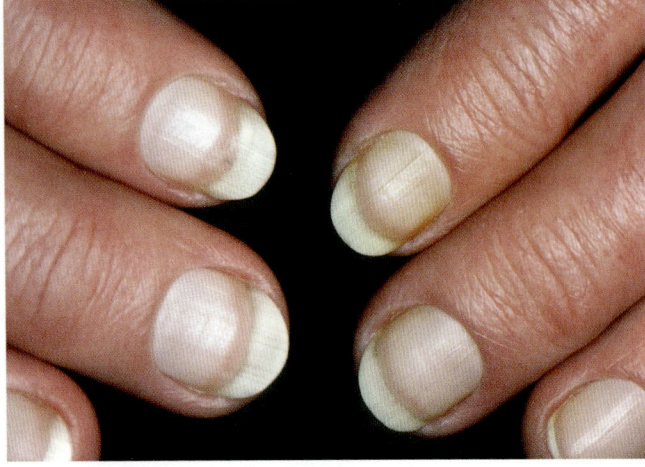

Fig. 33.97 Terry nails.

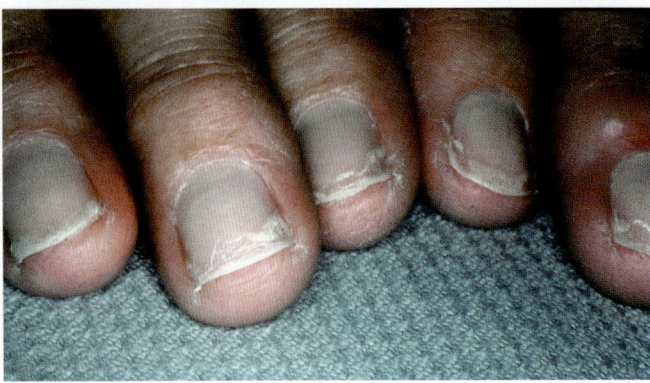

Fig. 33.98 Onychoschizia.

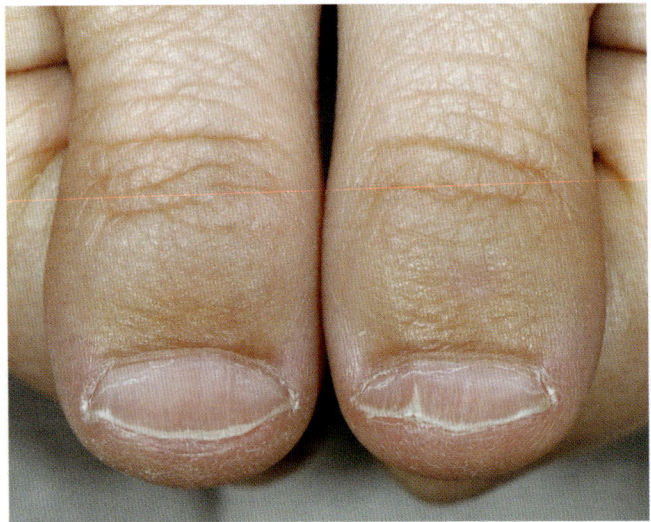

Fig. 33.99 Racquet nails. *Courtesy Adam Rubin, MD.*

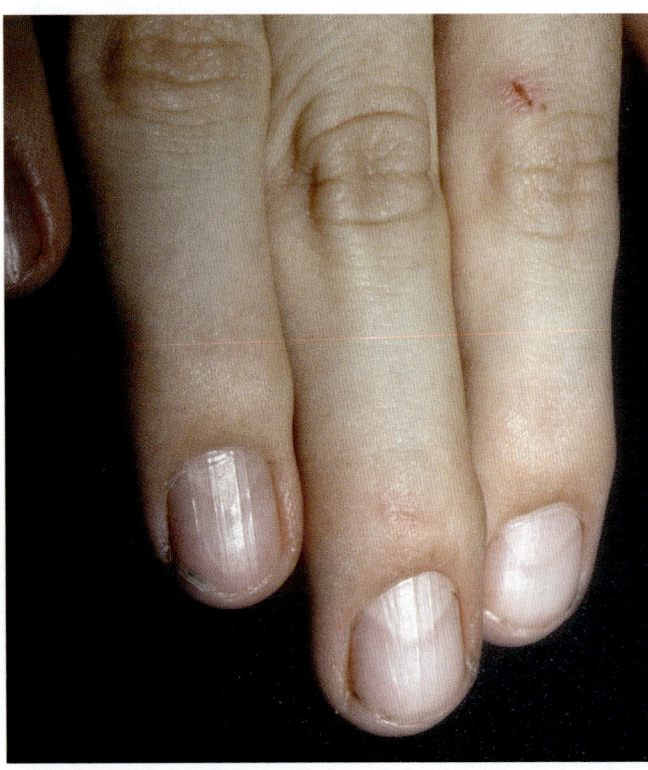

Fig. 33.100 Nail patella syndrome. Note triangular lunulae.

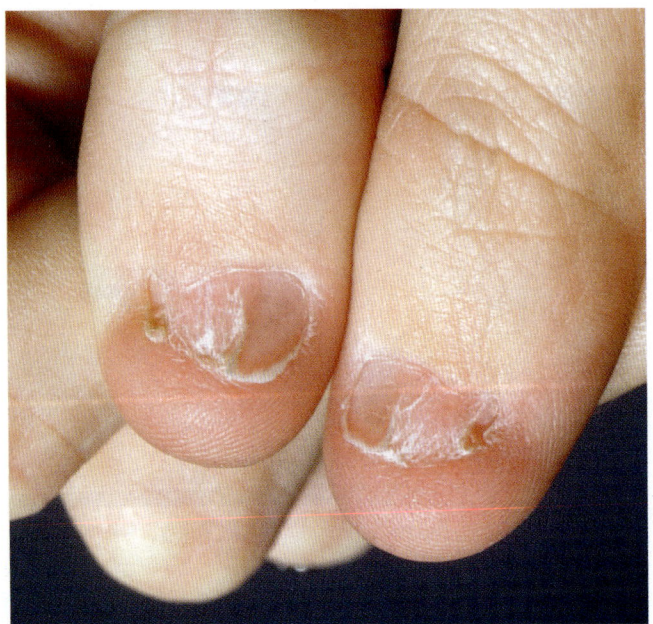

Fig. 33.101 Nail patella syndrome with nail dystrophy.

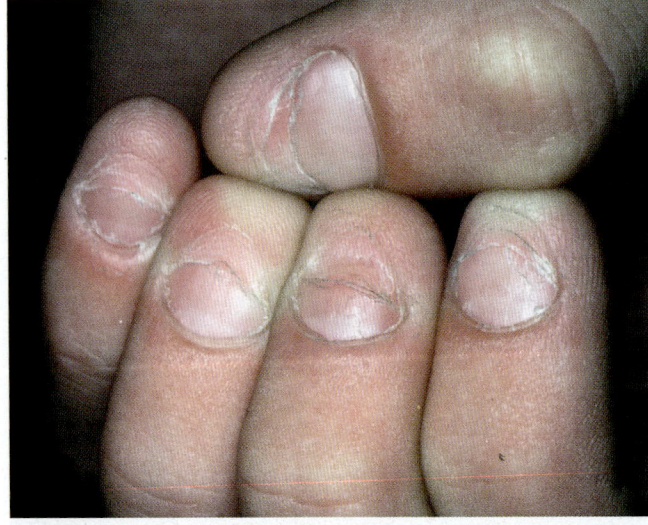

Fig. 33.102 Onychophagia.

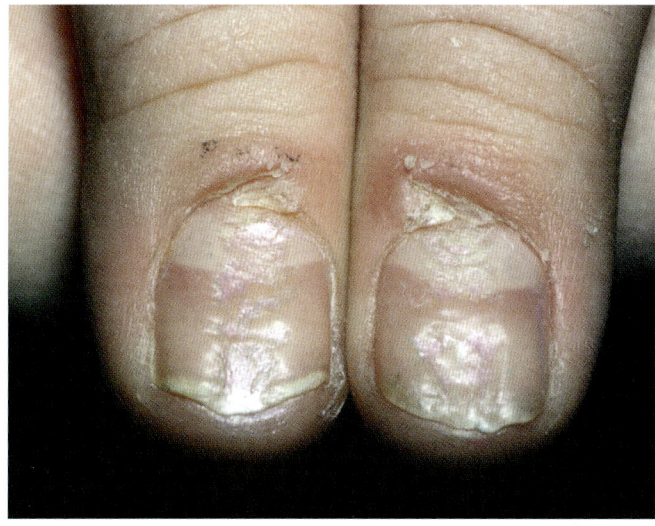

Fig. 33.103 Nail dystrophy, with washboard nail caused by a habit of pushing back the cuticles. *Courtesy Steven Binnick, MD.*

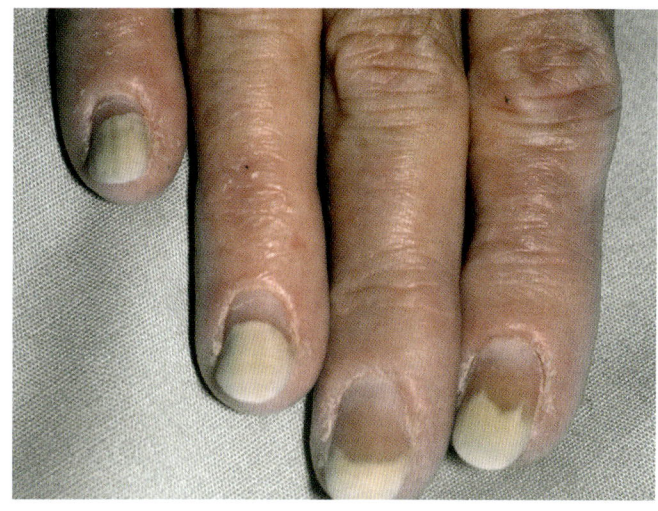

Fig. 33.104 Onycholysis. *Courtesy Steven Binnick, MD.*

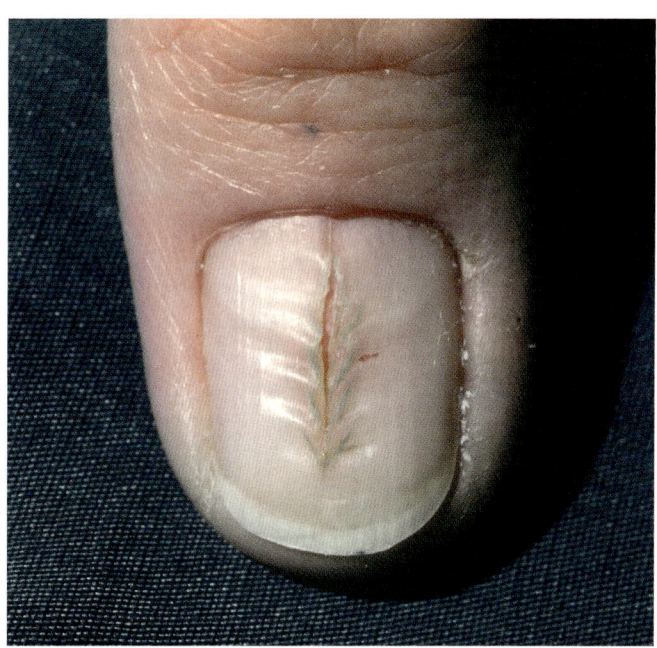

Fig. 33.105 Median nail dystrophy. *Courtesy Steven Binnick, MD.*

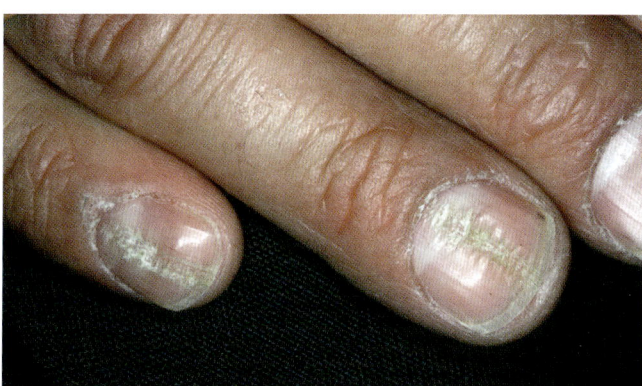

Fig. 33.106 Median nail dystrophy.

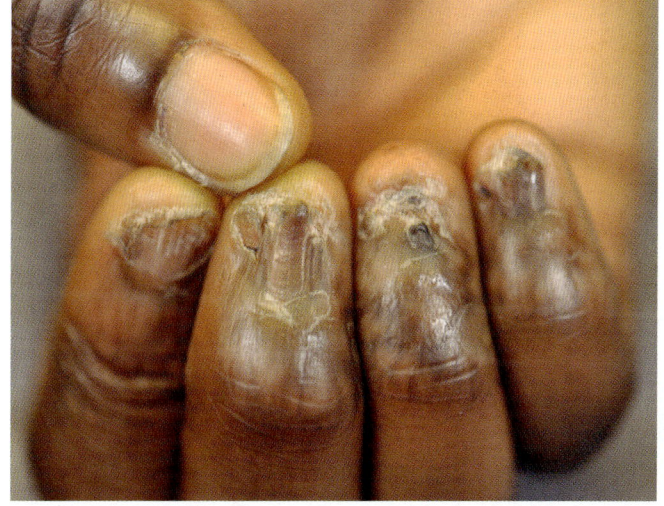

Fig. 33.107 Pterygium unguis. *Courtesy Adam Rubin, MD.*

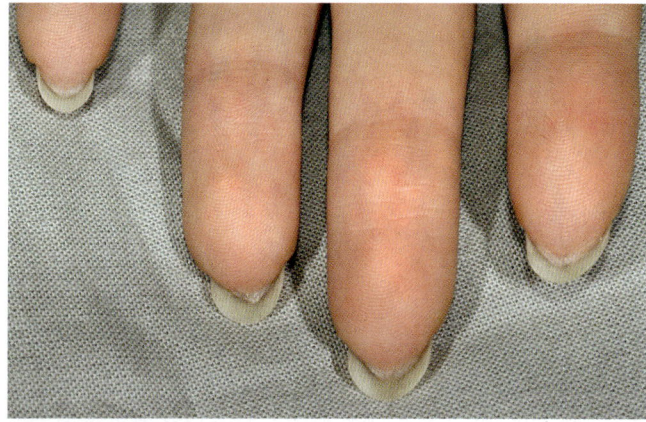

Fig. 33.108 Pterygium inversum unguis. *Courtesy Adam Rubin, MD.*

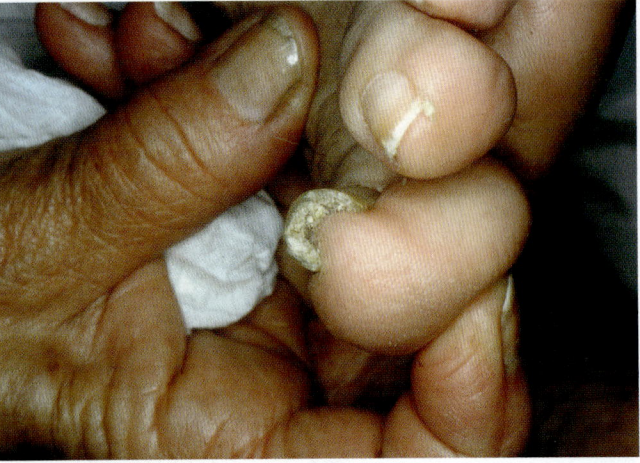

Fig. 33.109 Pincer nail.

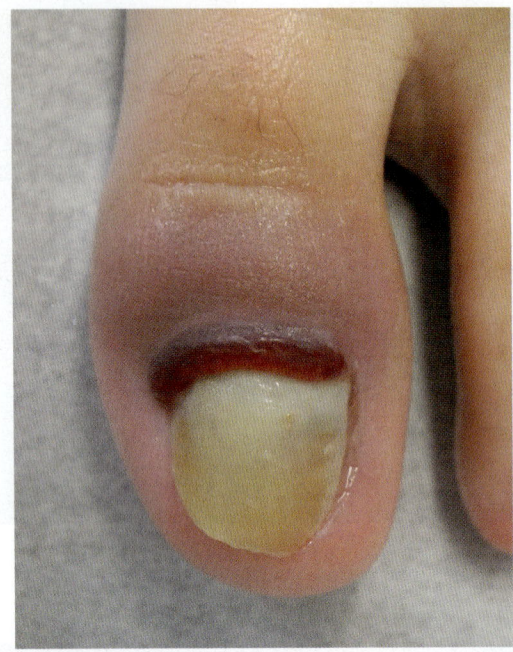

Fig. 33.110 Retronychia. *Courtesy Rui Tavares Bello, MD.*

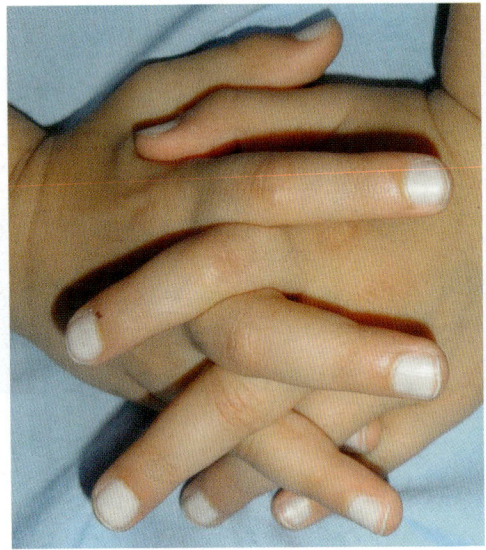

Fig. 33.111 Leukonychia. *Courtesy Scott Norton, MD.*

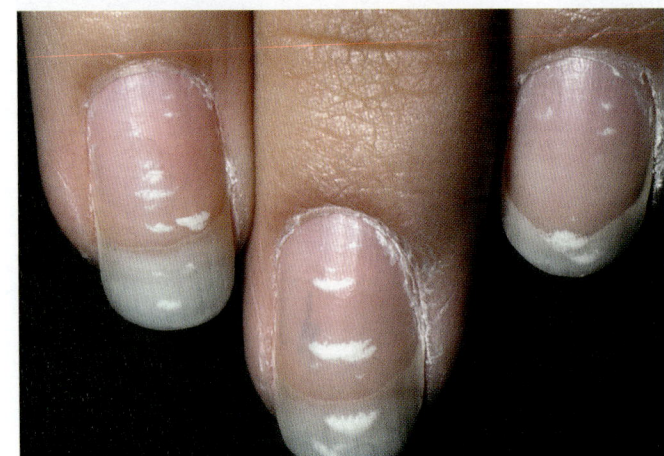

Fig. 33.112 Transverse leukonychia. *Courtesy Curt Samlaska, MD.*

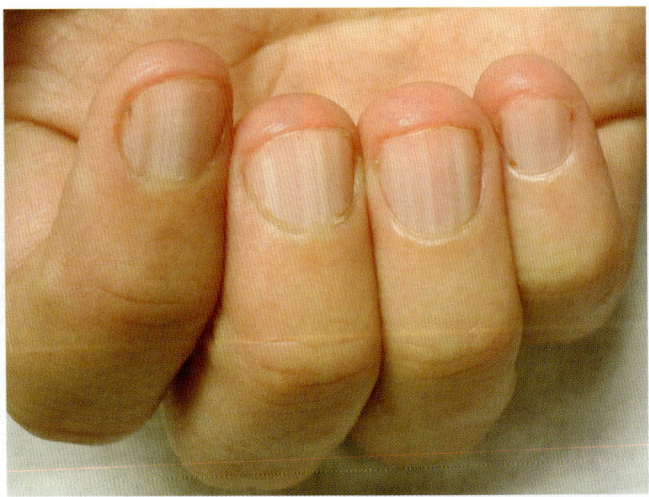

Fig. 33.113 Longitudinal erythronychia in Darier disease.

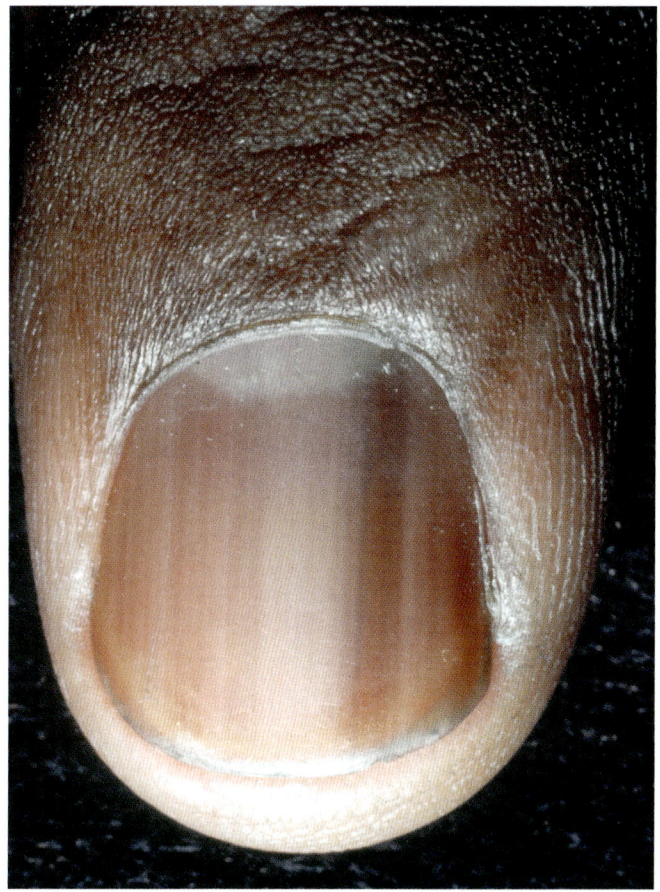

Fig. 33.114 Melanonychia striata, benign, involved multiple nails in an African American patient.

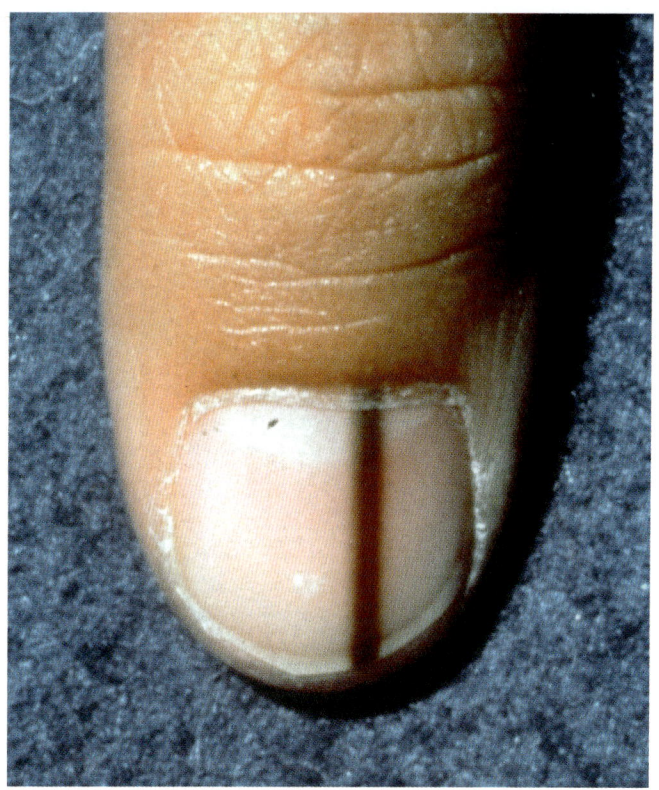

Fig. 33.115 Melanonychia striata, benign.

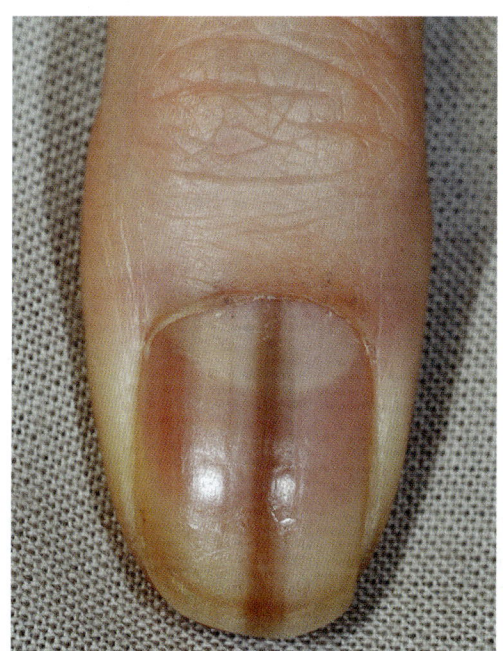

Fig. 33.116 Melanonychia striata caused by melanoma in situ. *Courtesy Adam Rubin, MD.*

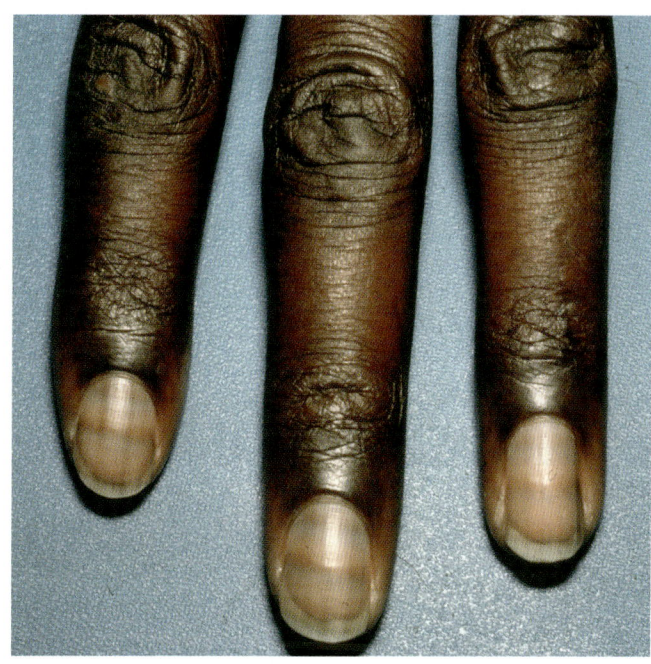

Fig. 33.117 Transverse nail bands secondary to chemotherapy.

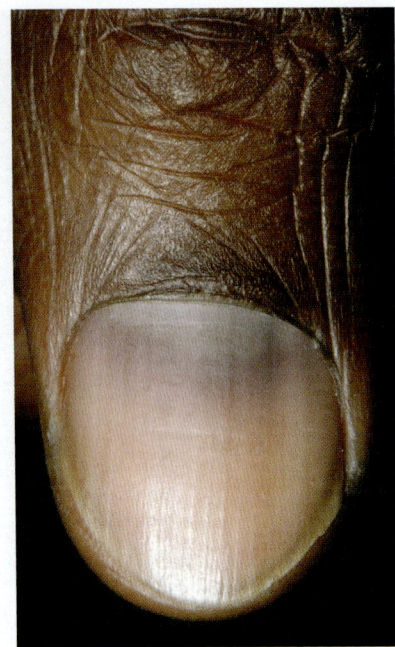

Fig. 33.118 Zidovudine pigmentation.

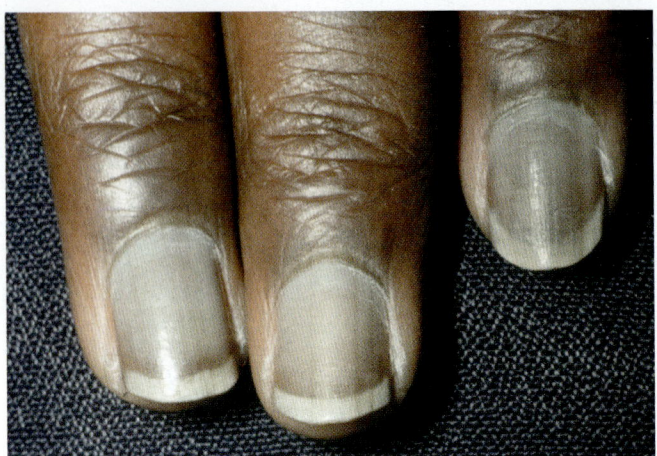

Fig. 33.119 Zidovudine pigmentation.

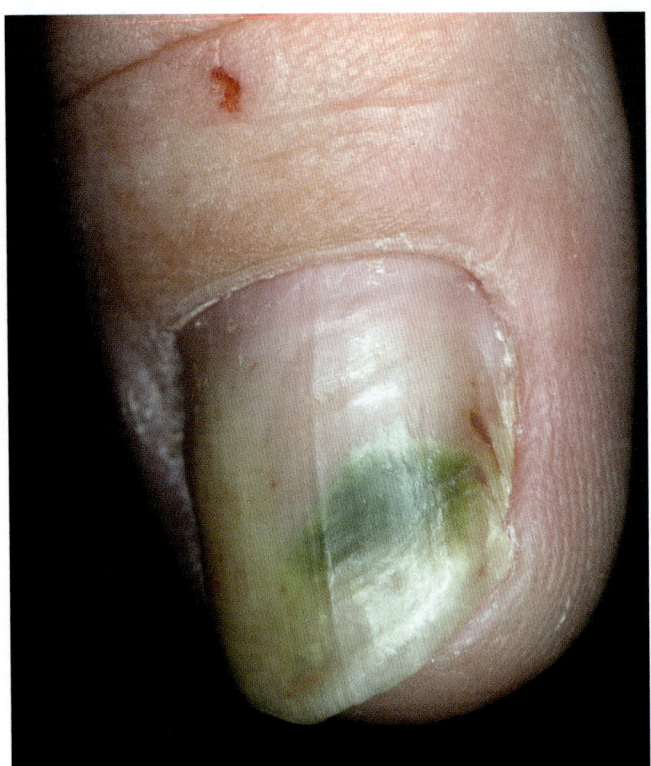

Fig. 33.120 Green nail.

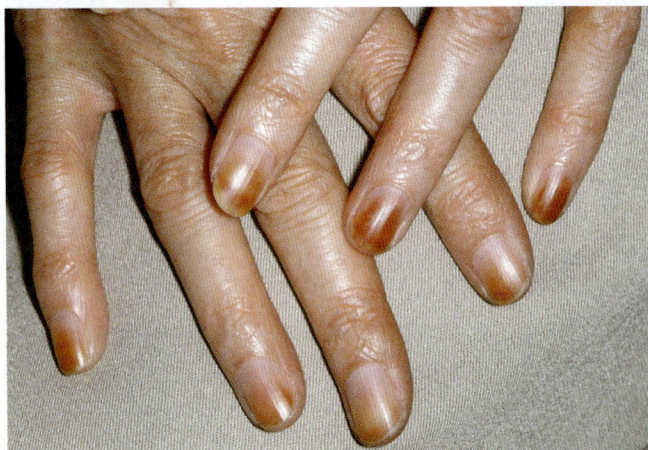

Fig. 33.121 Exogenous nail staining. Note pigment follows the curvature of the proximal and lateral nail folds.

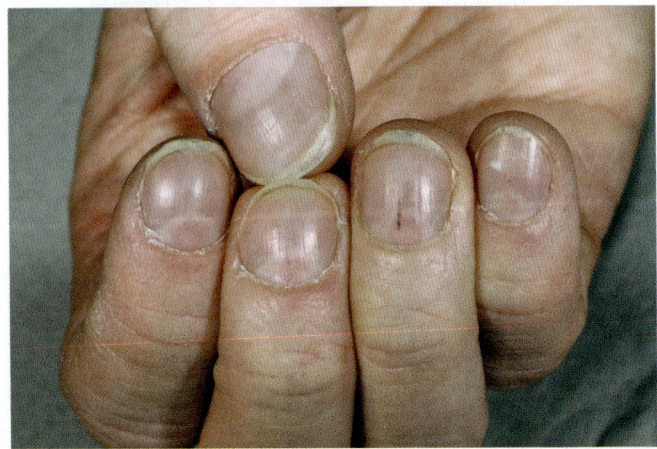

Fig. 33.122 Red lunula.

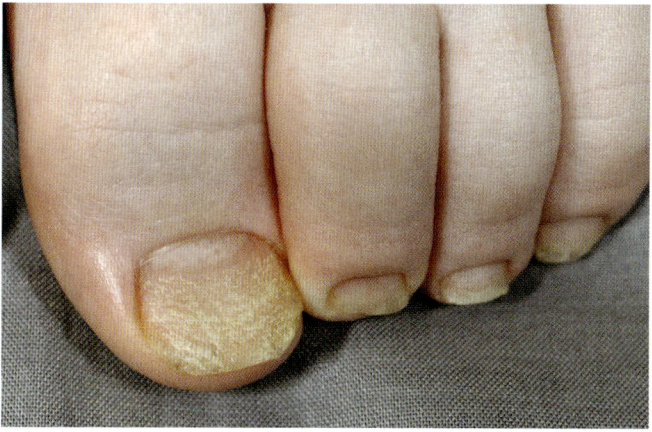

Fig. 33.123 Spotted lunula.

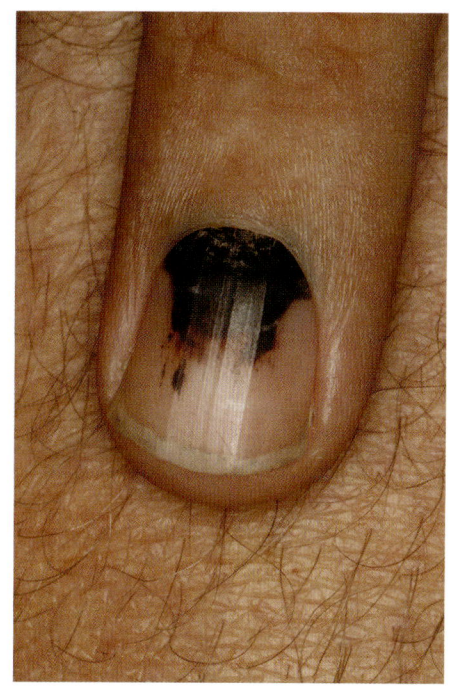

Fig. 33.124 Subungual hemorrhage.

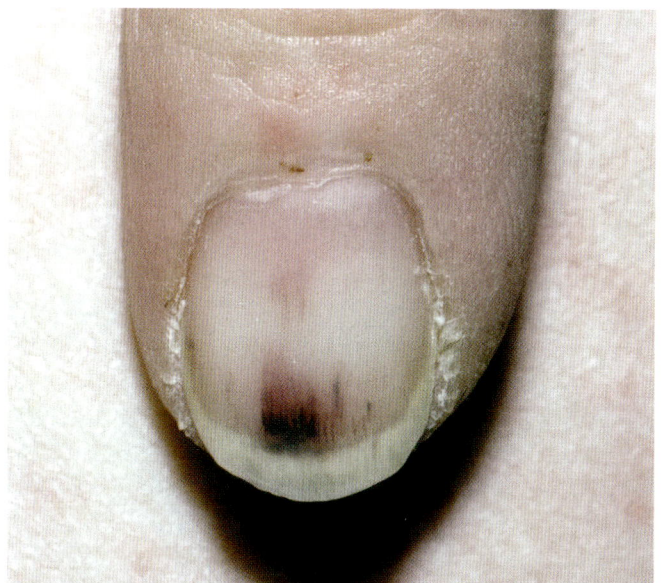

Fig. 33.125 Splinter hemorrhage. *Courtesy Steven Binnick, MD.*

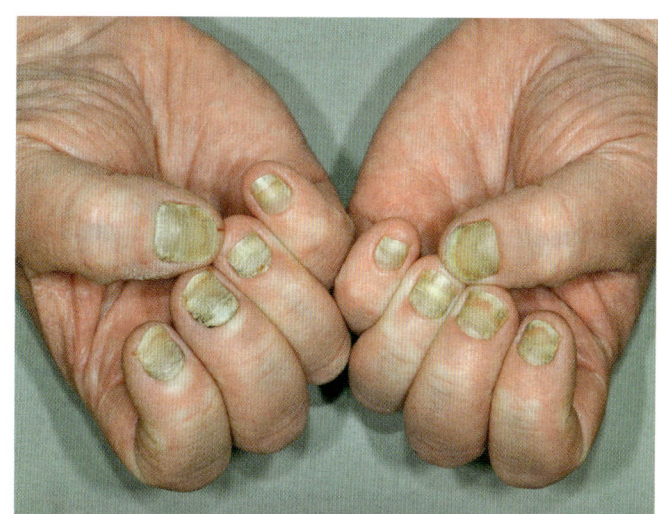

Fig. 33.126 Yellow nail syndrome. *Courtesy Adam Rubin, MD.*

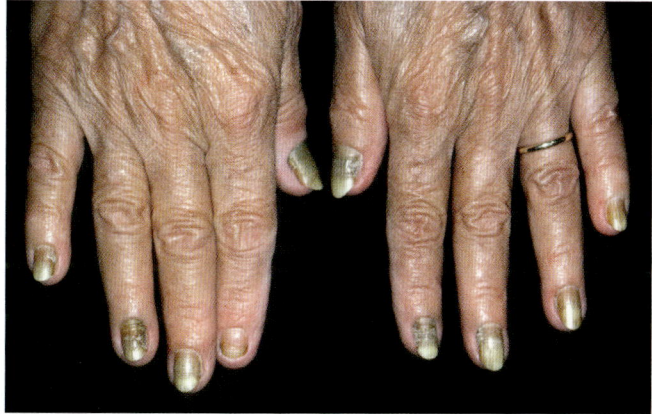

Fig. 33.127 Yellow nail syndrome.

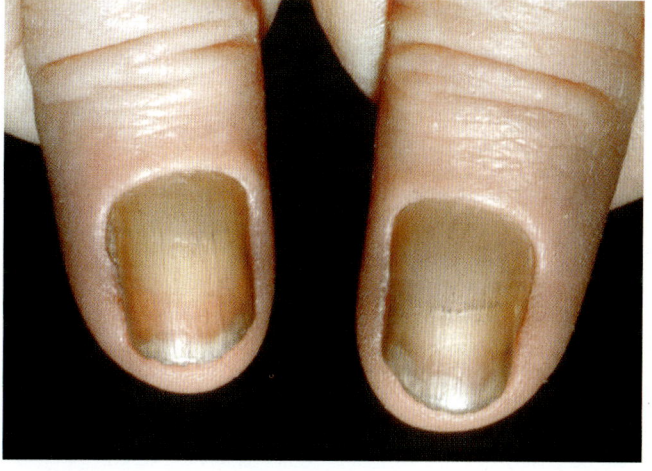

Fig. 33.128 Yellow nail syndrome.

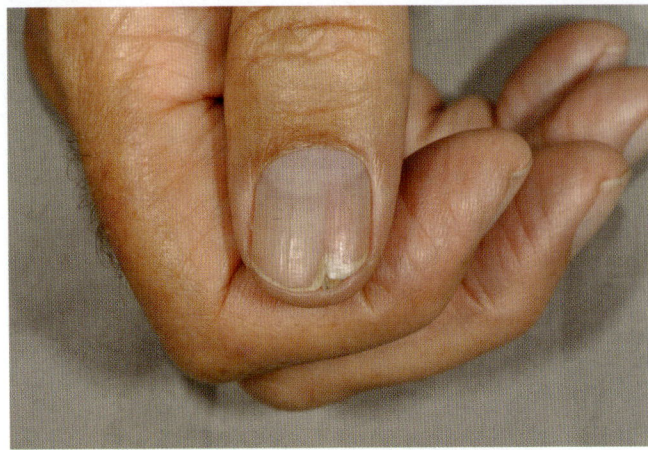

Fig. 33.129 Onychopapilloma. *Courtesy Adam Rubin, MD.*

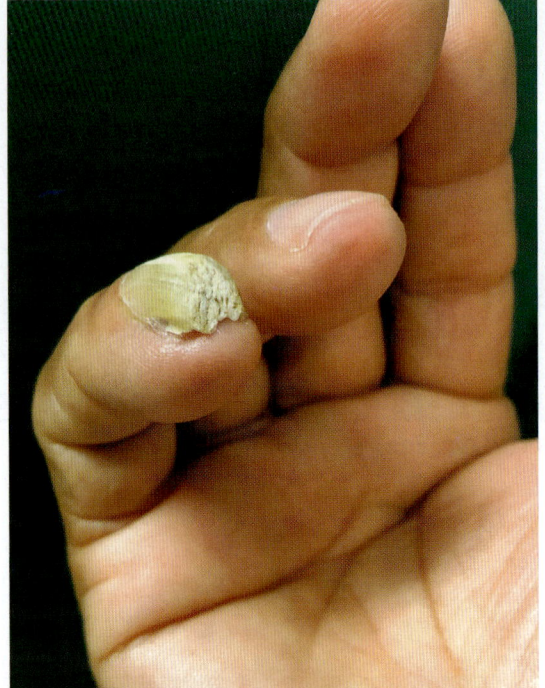

Fig. 33.130 Onychomatricoma. *Courtesy Dr. Tatiana Andrade.*

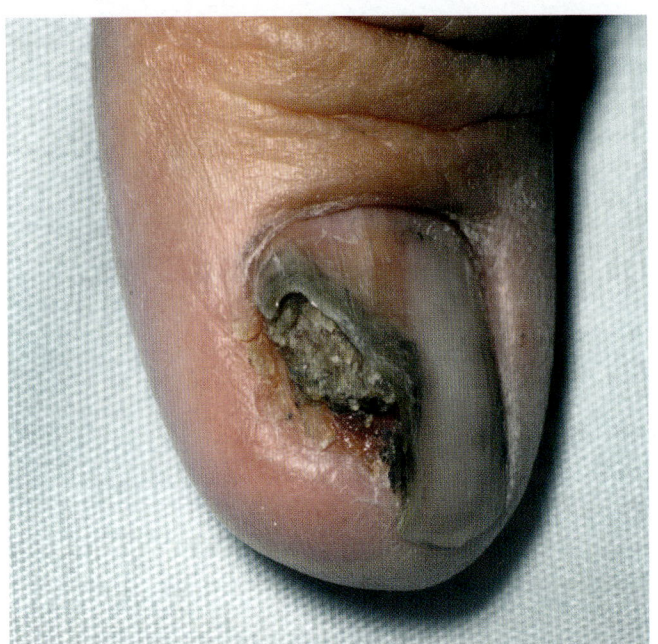

Fig. 33.131 Bowen disease of the nail bed.

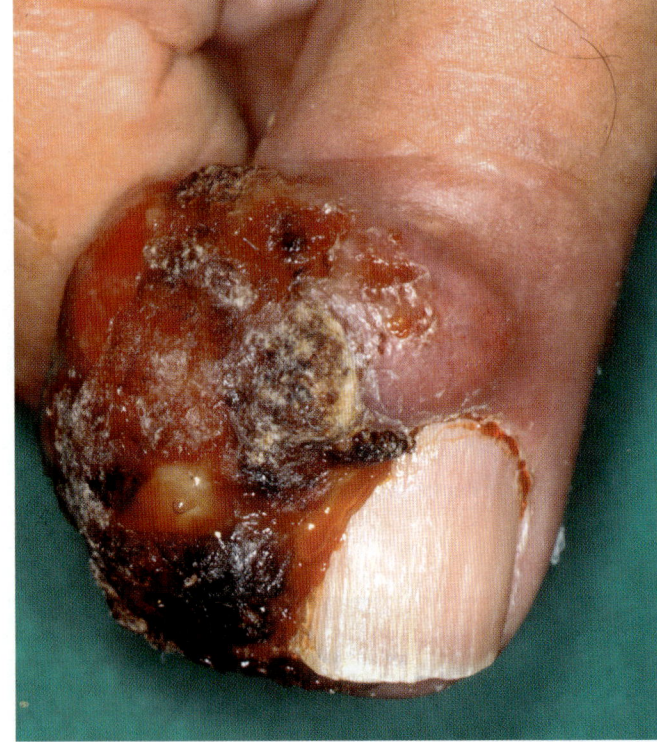

Fig. 33.132 Squamous cell carcinoma.

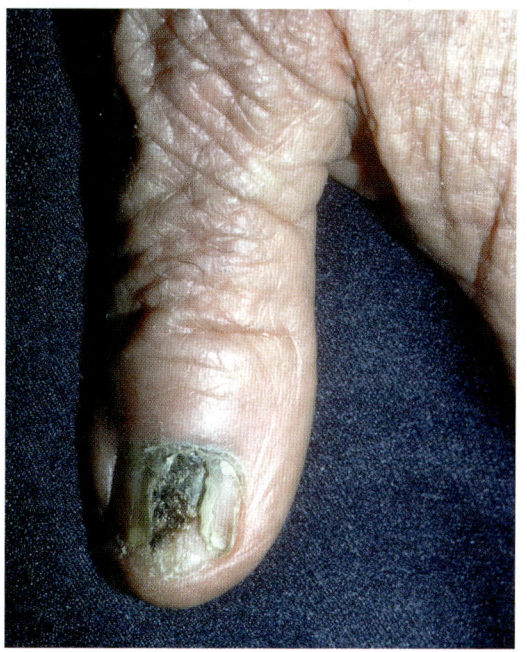

Fig. 33.133 Melanoma.

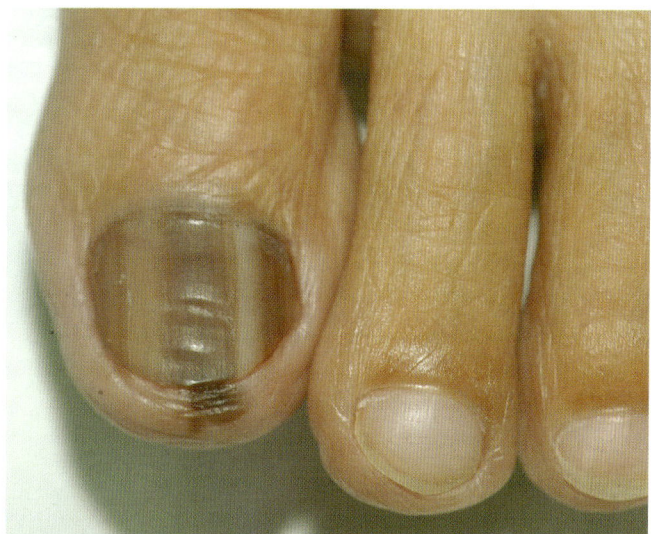

Fig. 33.134 Acral lentiginous melanoma. *Courtesy Yung-Tsu Cho, MD.*

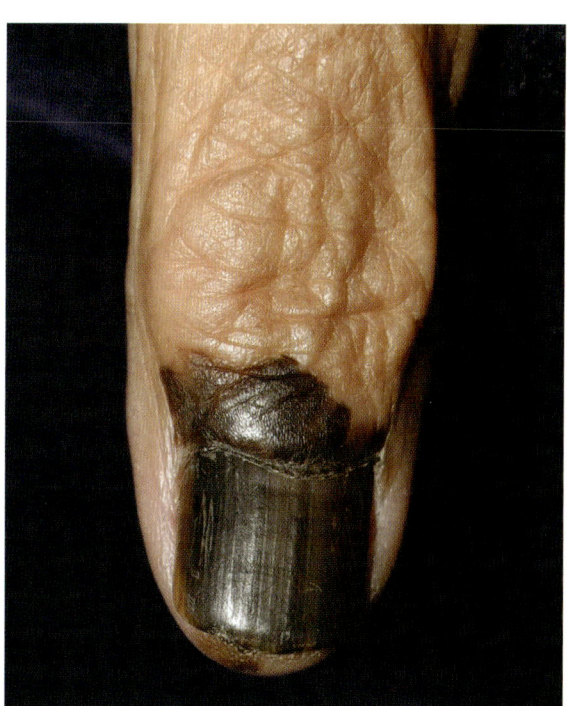

Fig. 33.135 Acral lentiginous melanoma. *Courtesy Dr. Liao, National Cheng Kung University, Taiwan.*

Diseases of Mucous Membranes 34

Diseases of the mucous membranes include those involving the lips, tongue, palate, gingiva, teeth, and the floor of the mouth. Inspection of this entire surface should be included in the full skin examination to screen for evidence of mucocutaneous conditions, such as lichen planus, and primary diseases of the mucosa, such as squamous cell carcinoma of the lip. Routine examination of these surfaces also allows one to become familiar with the spectrum of benign findings such as many forms of oral melanosis.

Primary conditions of the mucosal surfaces include changes to the tongue, such as median rhomboid glossitis or inflammation of the taste buds known as *papillitis*. Aphthous ulcers provide another example of a primary oral disease, and they are featured here with their classic round, shallow, white ulcers with surrounding bright red rims.

Many oral findings can be found in the setting of a systemic disease such as inflammatory bowel disease (IBD). In IBD there are several related mucosal diseases, including the cobblestoned appearance of the mucosa, oral ulcers, granulomatous cheilitis, and pyostomatitis vegetans. Nutritional deficiencies, fixed drug eruptions, and Behçet syndrome are examples of other systemic diseases with important mucosal findings.

This portion of the atlas includes images of many common and uncommon findings of import that may be seen upon examination of the mucosal membranes.

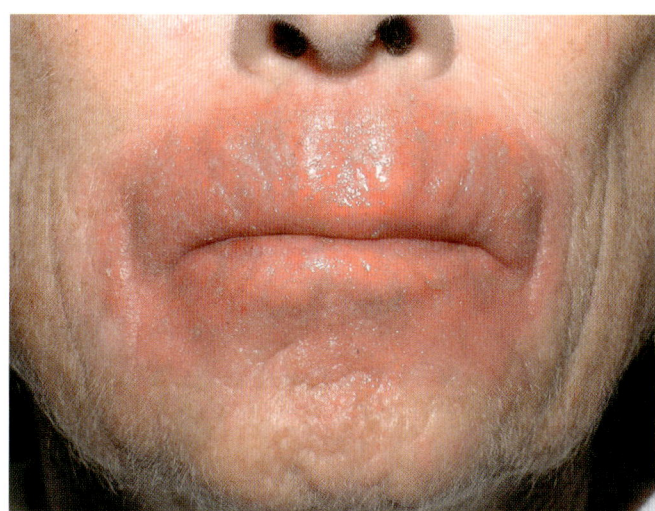

Fig. 34.1 Allergic contact cheilitis to topical steroids. *Courtesy Glen Crawford, MD.*

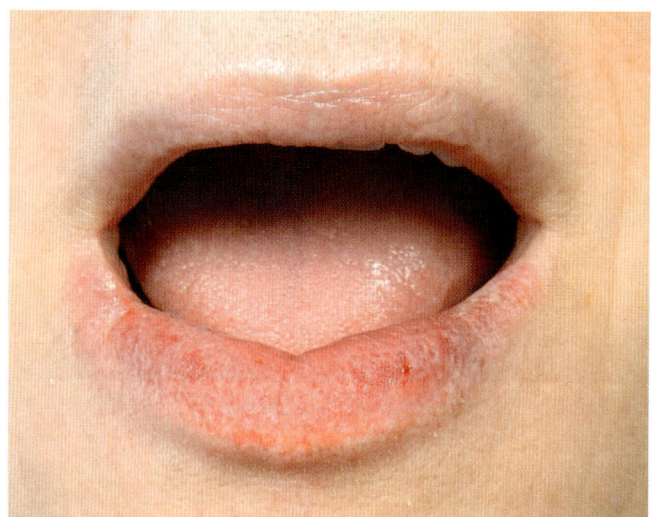

Fig. 34.2 Actinic cheilitis. *Courtesy Joseph Sobanko, MD.*

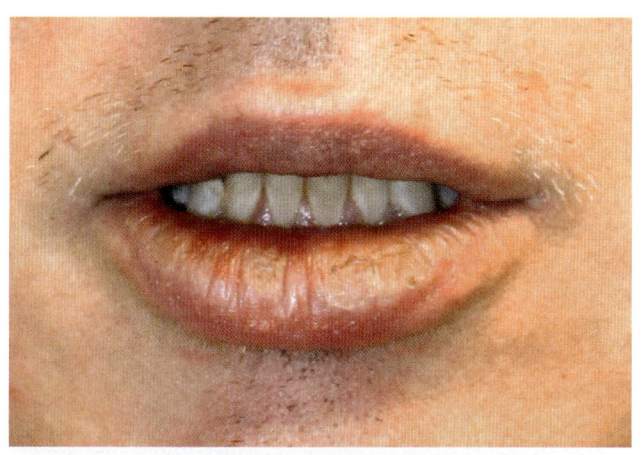

Fig. 34.3 Actinic cheilitis. *Courtesy Joseph Sobanko, MD.*

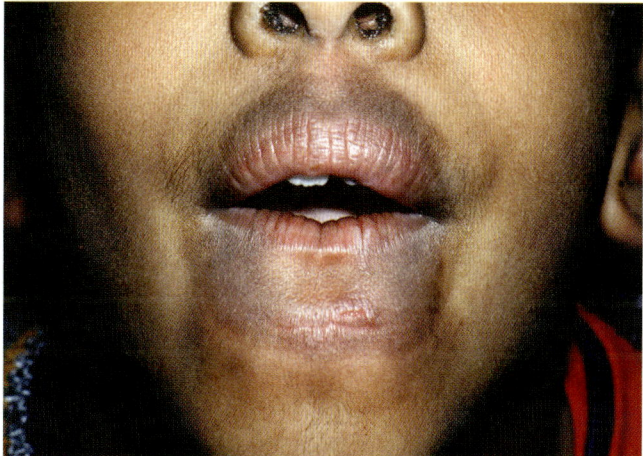

Fig. 34.4 Cheilitis secondary to lip licking. *Courtesy Steven Binnick, MD.*

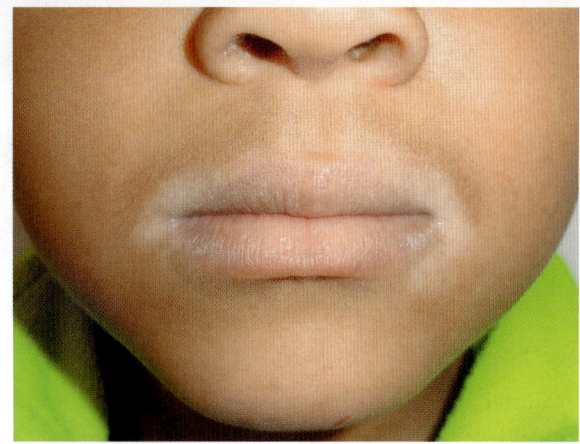

Fig. 34.5 Postinflammatory hypopigmentation secondary to lip licking. *Courtesy Scott Norton, MD.*

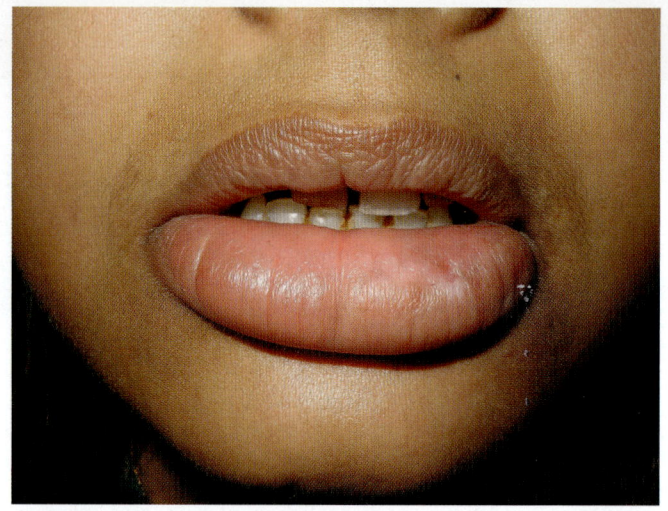

Fig. 34.6 Cheilitis glandularis. *Courtesy Debabrata Bandyopadhyay, MD.*

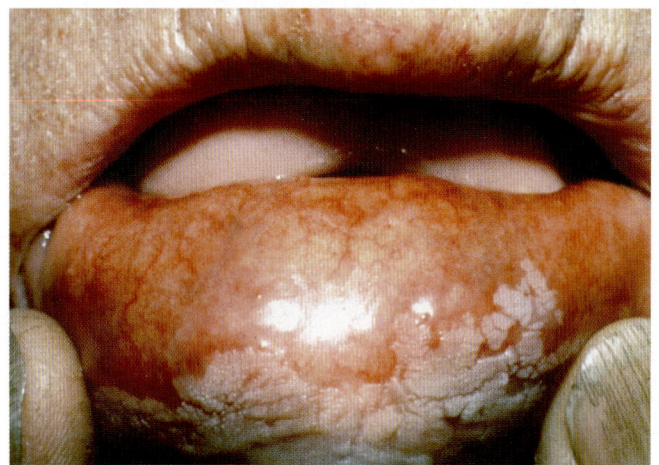

Fig. 34.7 Cheilitis glandularis with leukoplakia.

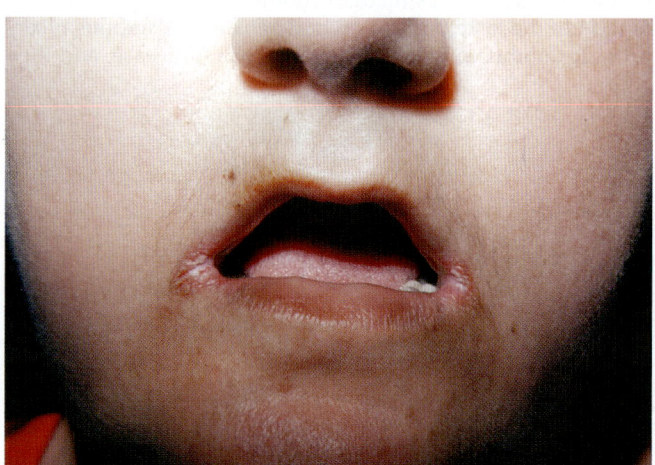

Fig. 34.8 Angular cheilitis. *Courtesy Steven Binnick, MD.*

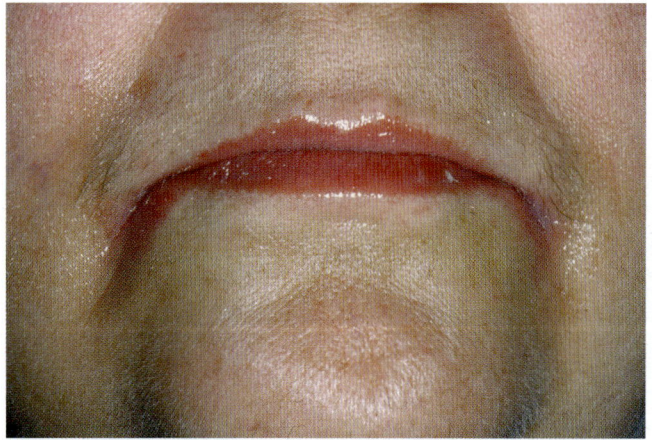

Fig. 34.9 Angular cheilitis.

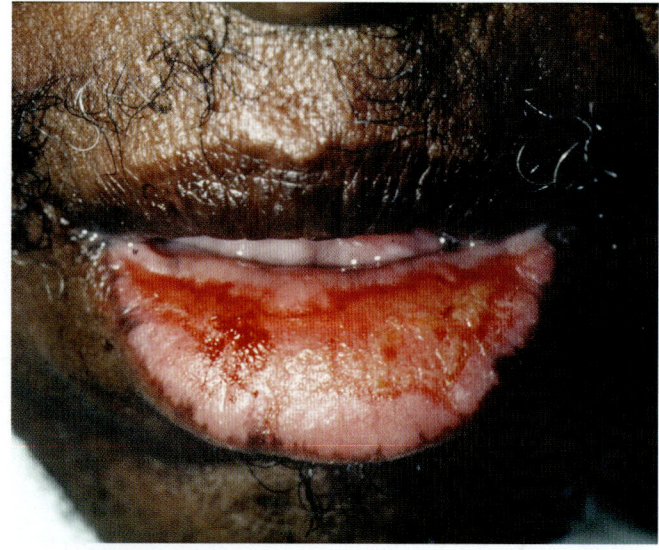

Fig. 34.10 Plasma cell cheilitis.

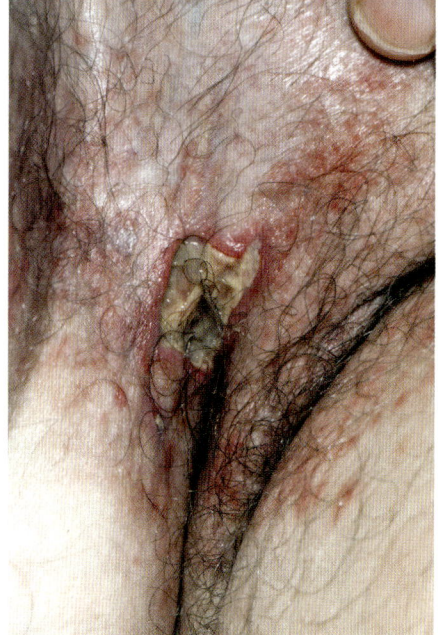

Fig. 34.11 Cutaneous Crohn disease. *Courtesy Curt Samlaska, MD.*

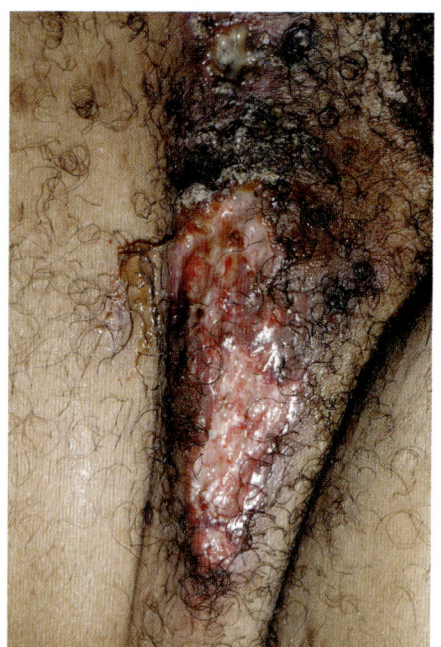

Fig. 34.12 Cutaneous Crohn disease.

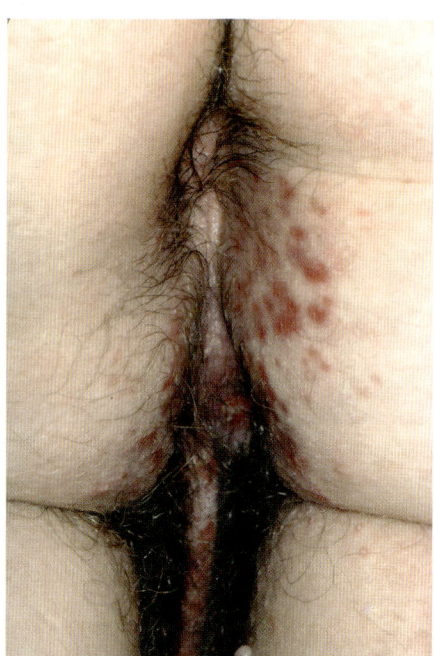

Fig. 34.13 Cutaneous Crohn disease.

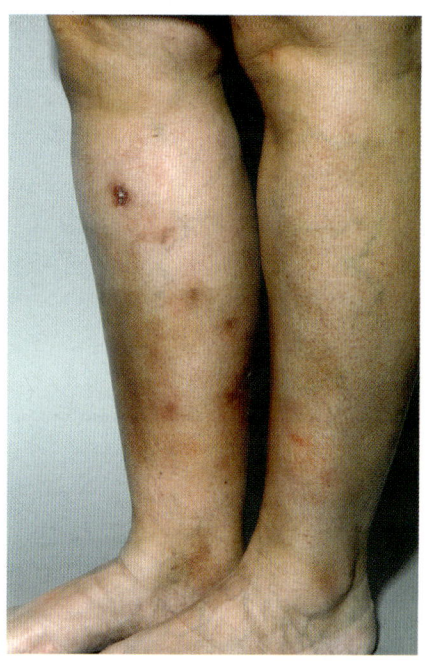

Fig. 34.14 Cutaneous Crohn disease. *Courtesy Curt Samlaska, MD.*

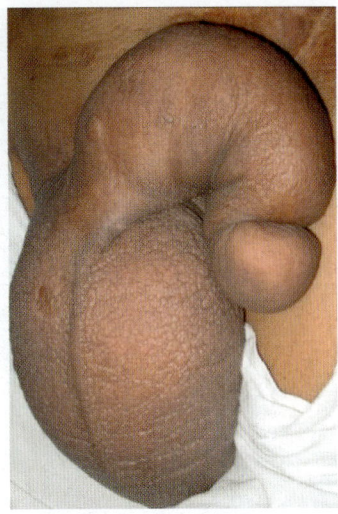

Fig. 34.15 Cutaneous Crohn disease.

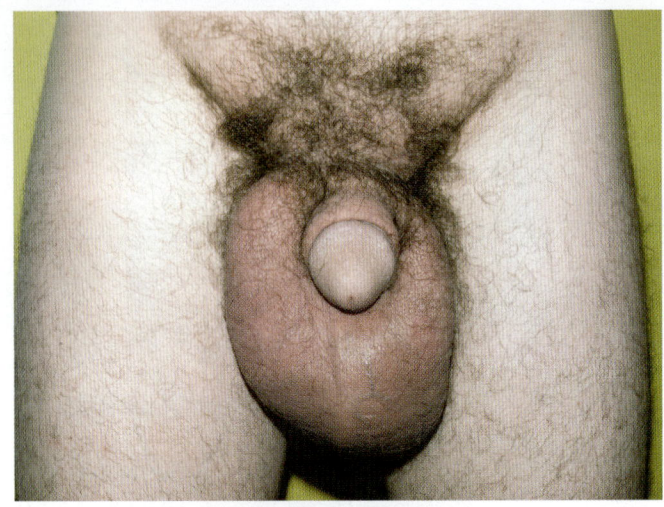

Fig. 34.16 Cutaneous Crohn disease.

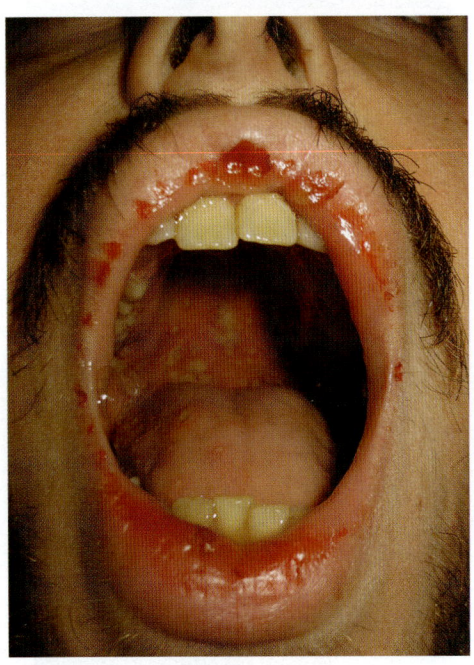

Fig. 34.17 Oral Crohn disease.

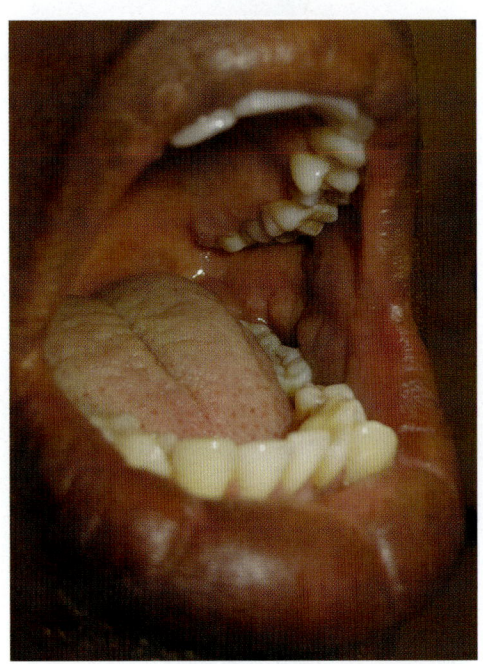

Fig. 34.18 Oral Crohn disease (granulomatous cheilitis and cobblestoning of the oral mucosa).

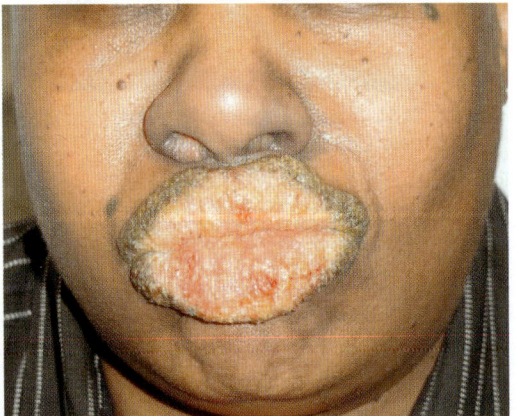

Fig. 34.19 Pyostomatitis vegetans. *Courtesy Scott Norton, MD.*

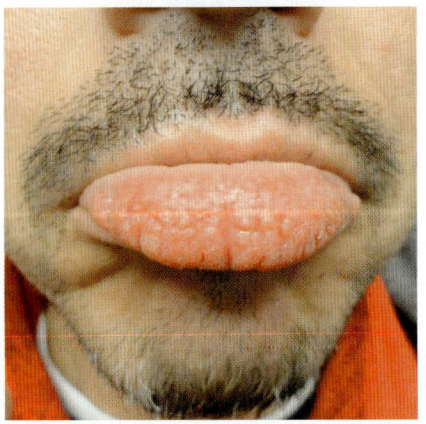

Fig. 34.20 Pyostomatitis vegetans. *Courtesy Scott Norton, MD.*

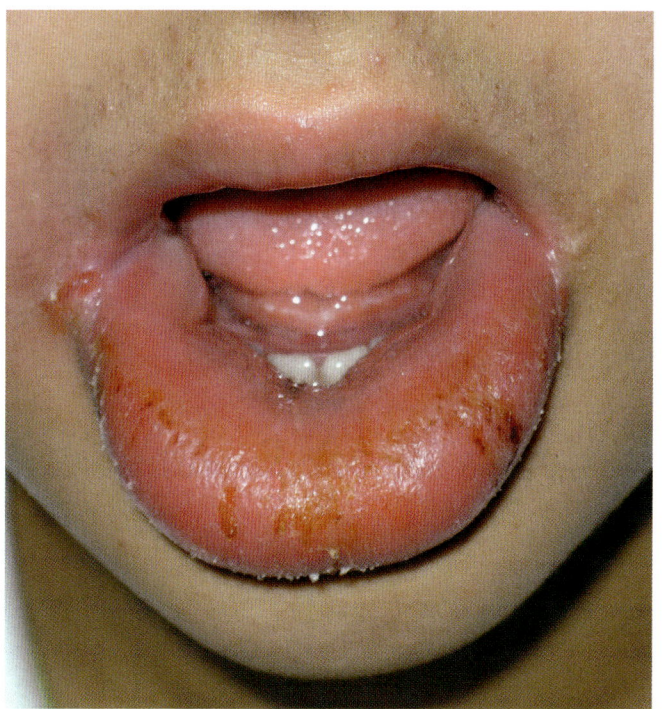

Fig. 34.21 Granulomatous cheilitis.

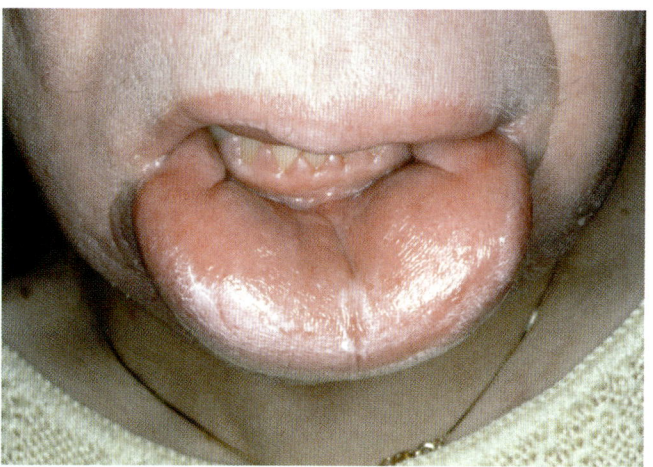

Fig. 34.22 Melkersson-Rosenthal syndrome.

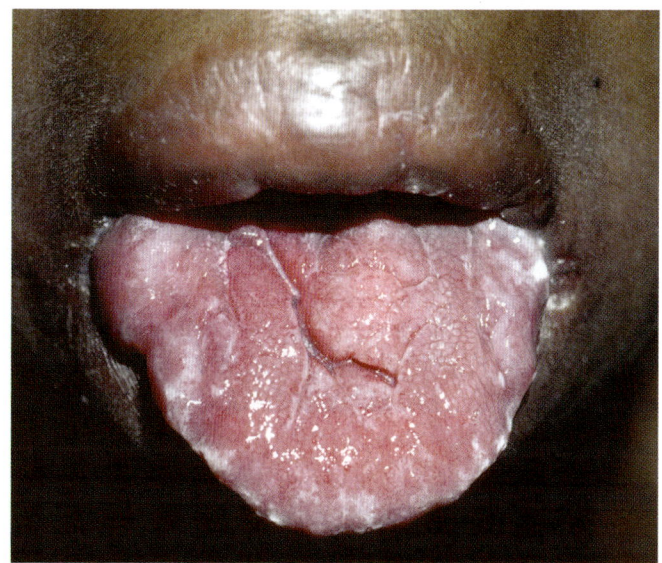

Fig. 34.23 Melkersson-Rosenthal syndrome.

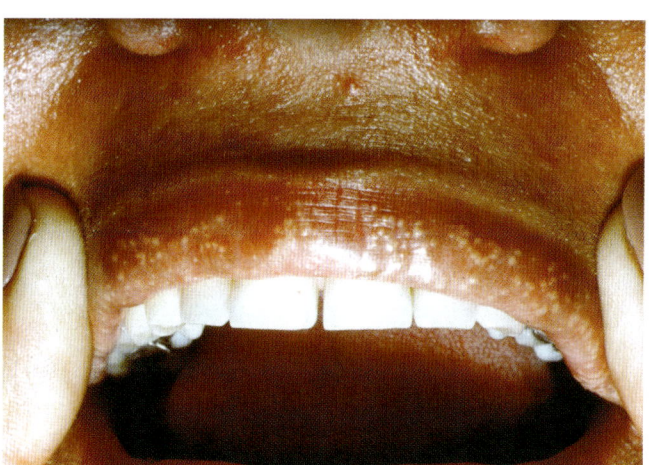

Fig. 34.24 Fordyce spots.

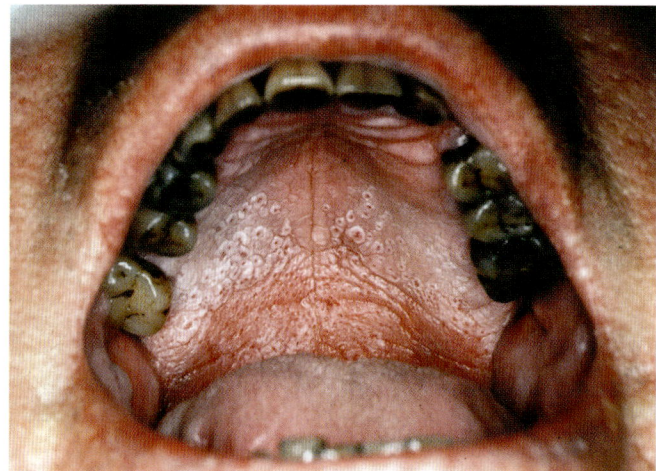

Fig. 34.25 Nicotine stomatitis. *Courtesy Ken Greer, MD.*

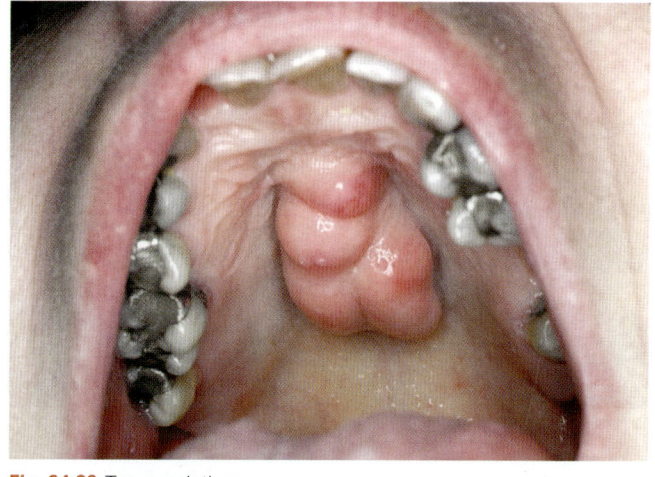

Fig. 34.26 Torus palatinus.

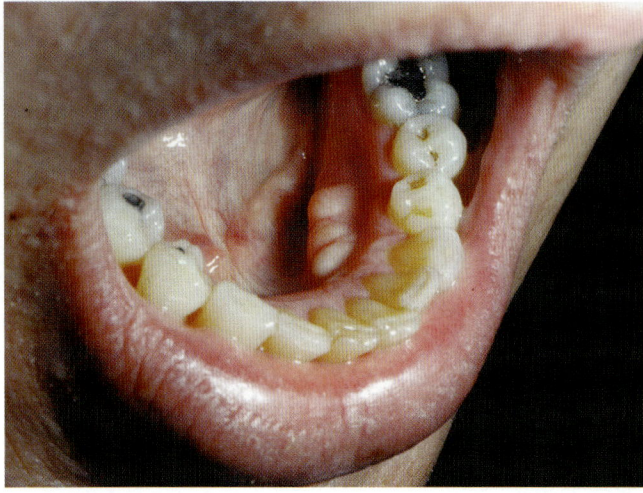

Fig. 34.27 Torus mandibularis.

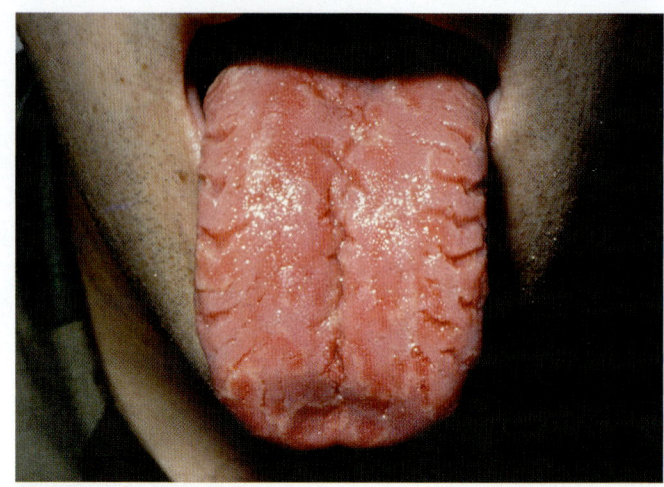

Fig. 34.28 Fissured tongue.

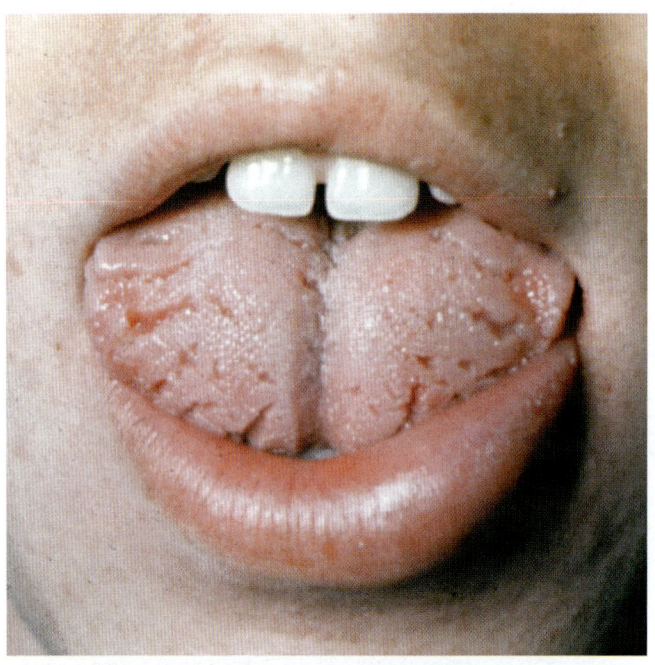

Fig. 34.29 Fissured tongue. *Courtesy Steven Binnick, MD.*

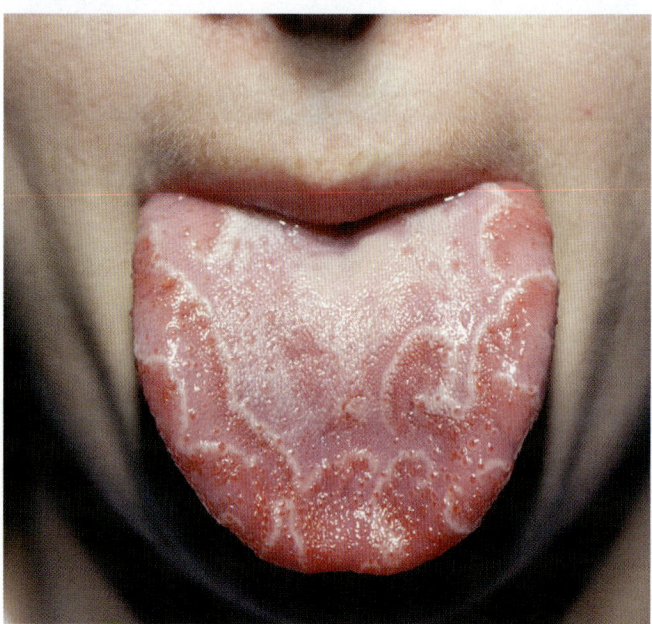

Fig. 34.30 Geographic tongue. *Courtesy Ken Greer, MD.*

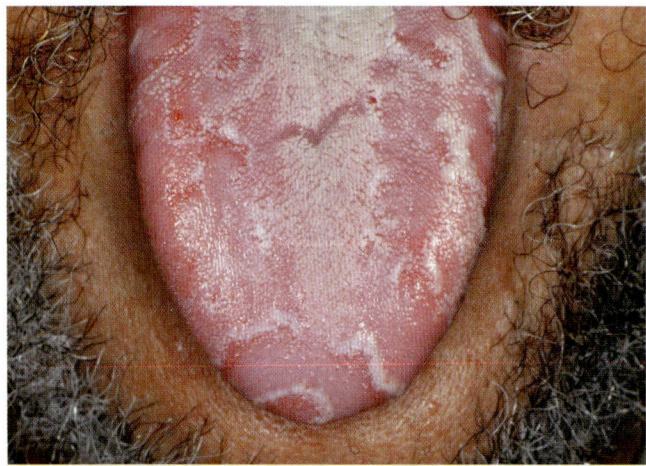

Fig. 34.31 Geographic tongue. *Courtesy Steven Binnick, MD.*

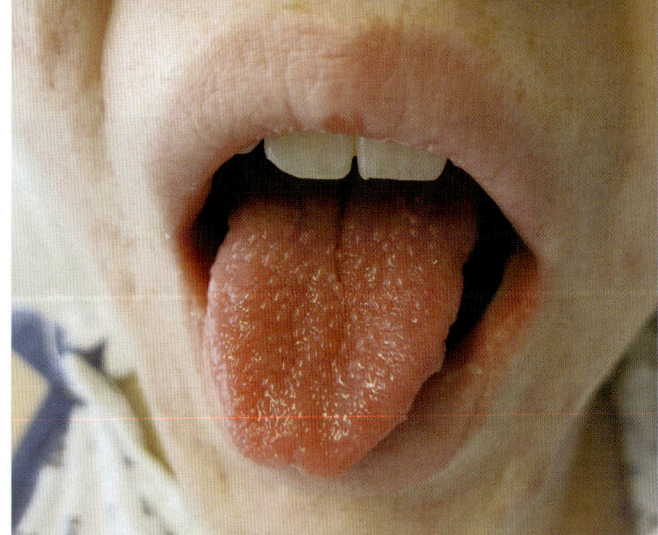

Fig. 34.32 Lingual papillitis.

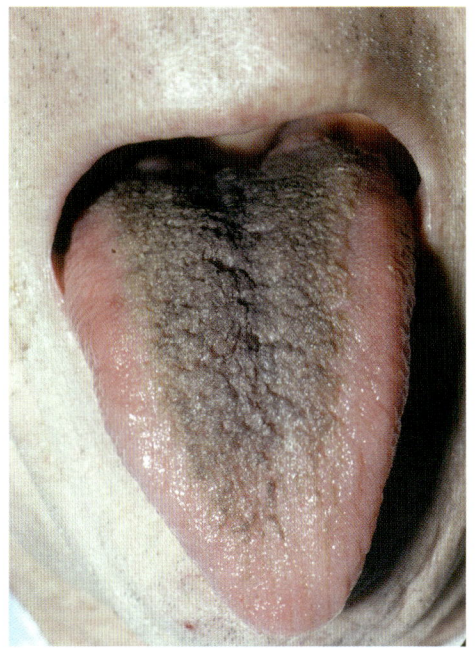

Fig. 34.33 Black hairy tongue. *Courtesy Steven Binnick, MD.*

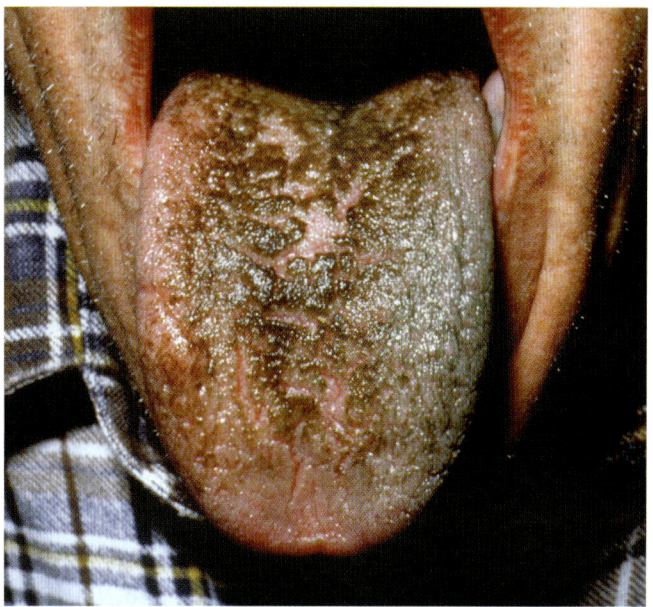

Fig. 34.34 Black hairy tongue. *Courtesy Steven Binnick, MD.*

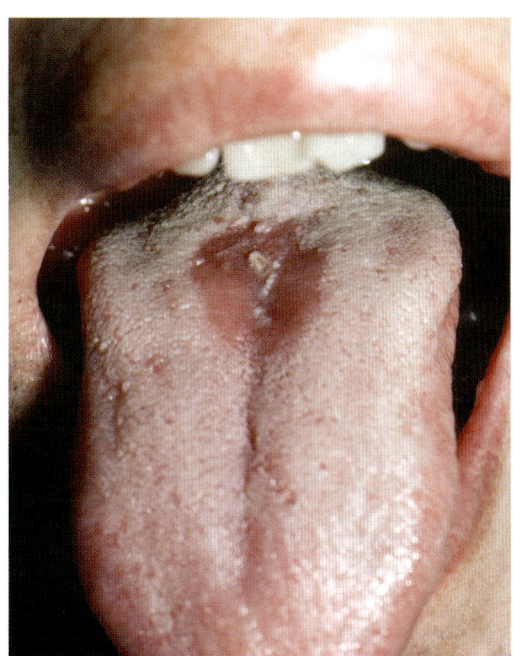

Fig. 34.35 Median rhomboid glossitis. *Courtesy Steven Binnick, MD.*

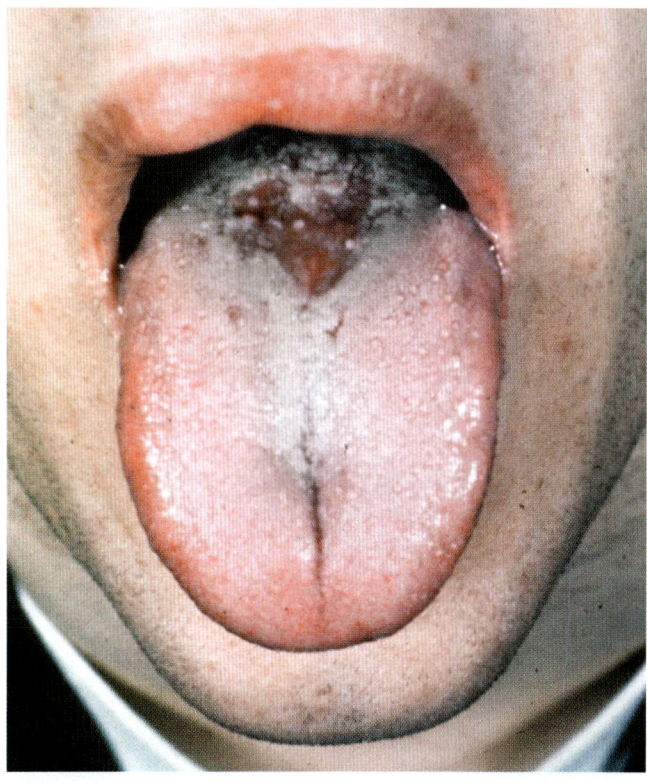

Fig. 34.36 Median rhomboid glossitis. *Courtesy Steven Binnick, MD.*

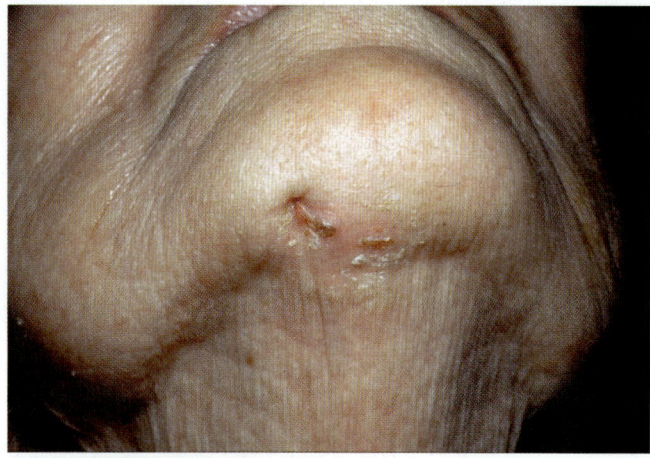

Fig. 34.37 Cutaneous dental sinus.

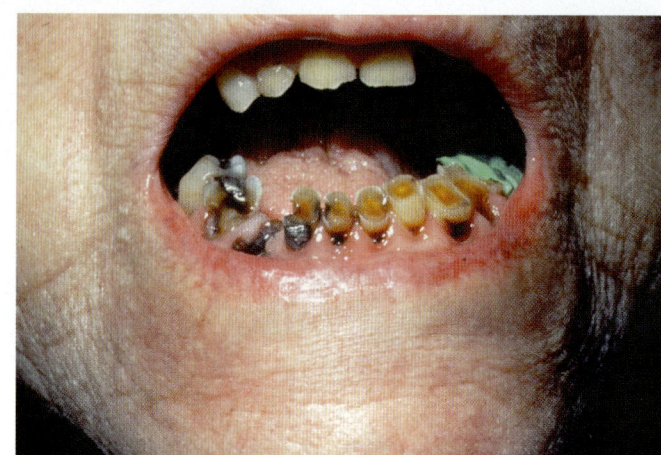

Fig. 34.38 Poor oral hygiene in the patient shown in Fig. 34.37.

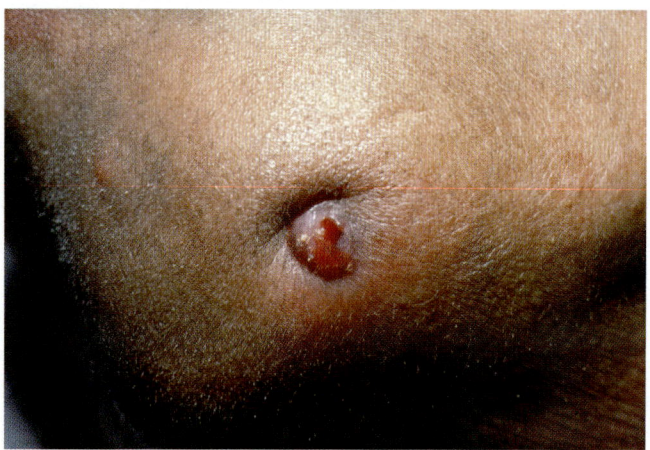

Fig. 34.39 Cutaneous dental sinus.

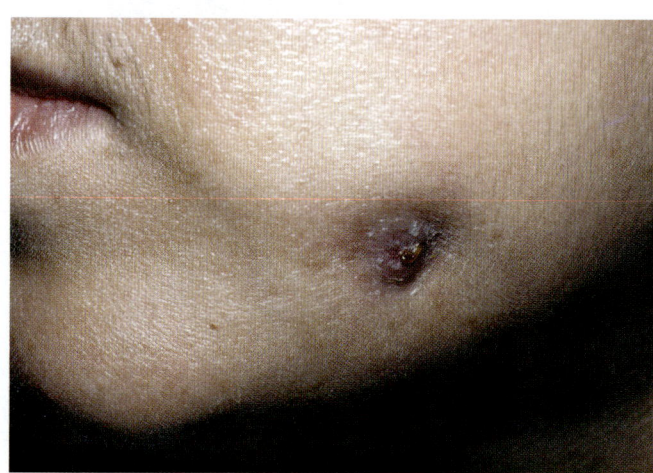

Fig. 34.40 Cutaneous dental sinus. *Courtesy Steven Binnick, MD.*

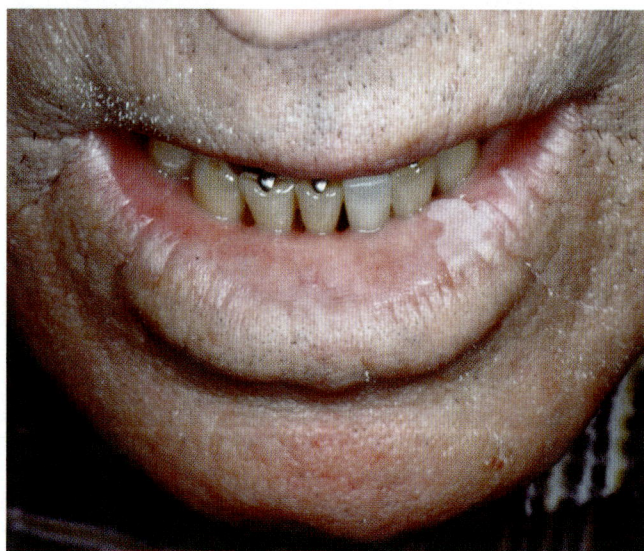

Fig. 34.41 Leukoplakia.

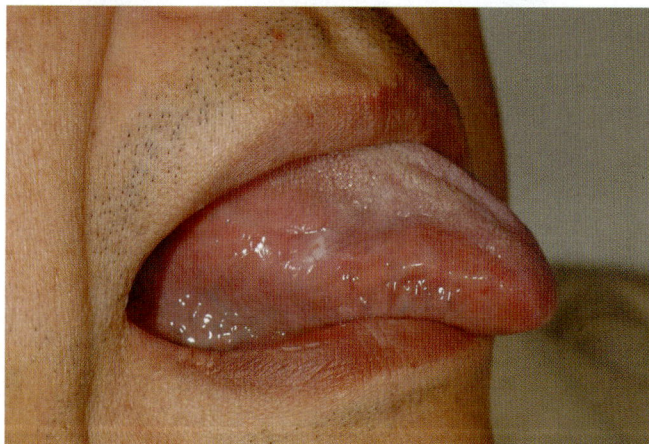

Fig. 34.42 Leukoplakia. *Courtesy Kaohsiung Chang Gang Memorial Hospital, Taiwan.*

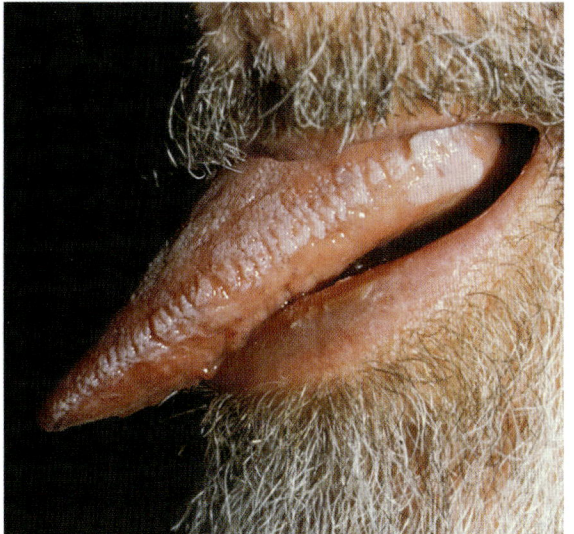

Fig. 34.43 Oral hairy leukoplakia.

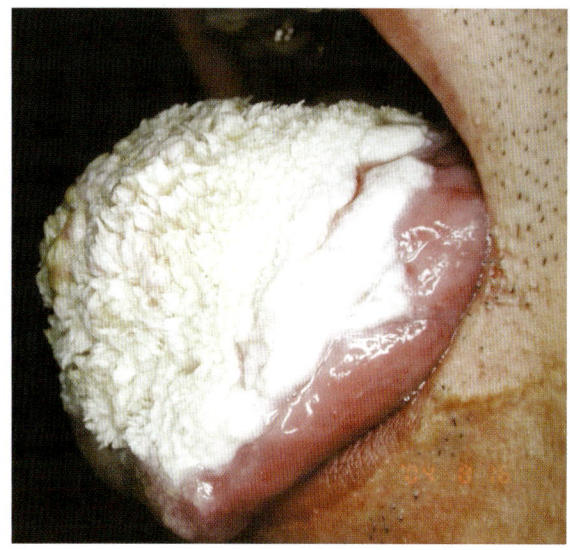

Fig. 34.44 Oral florid papillomatosis. *Courtesy National Cheng Kung University, Taiwan.*

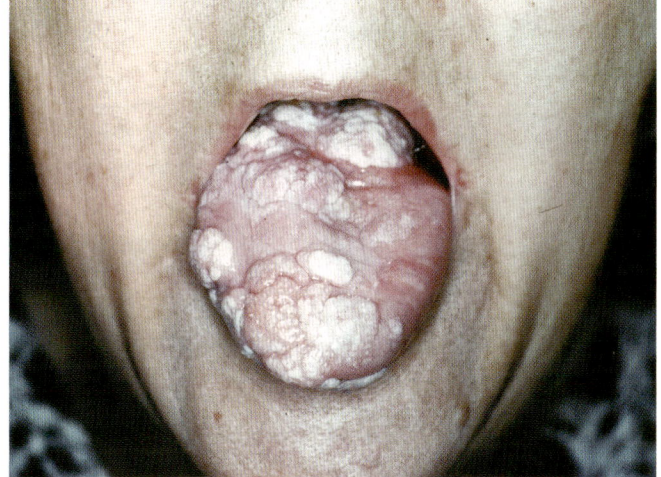

Fig. 34.45 Oral florid papillomatosis. *Courtesy Steven Binnick, MD.*

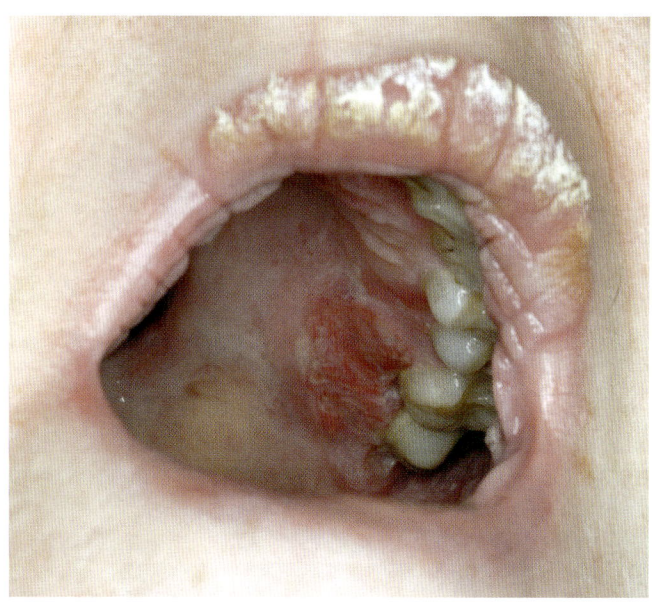

Fig. 34.46 Proliferative verrucous leukoplakia.

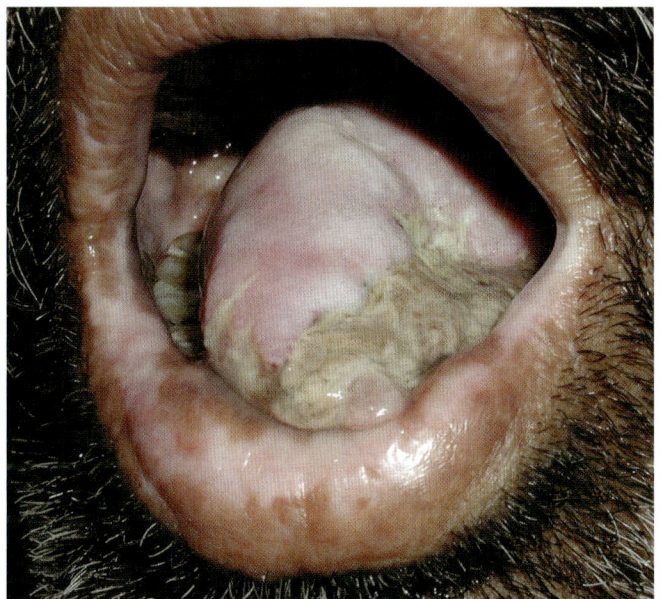

Fig. 34.47 Squamous cell carcinoma secondary to chewing betel nut. *Courtesy Shyam Verma, MBBS, DVD.*

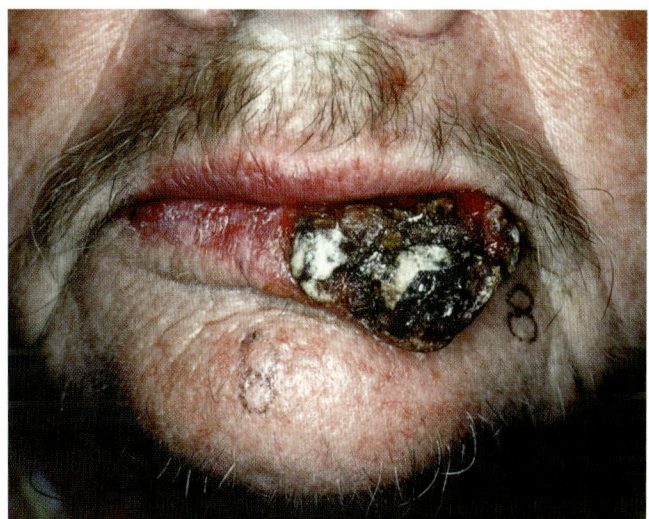

Fig. 34.48 Squamous cell carcinoma.

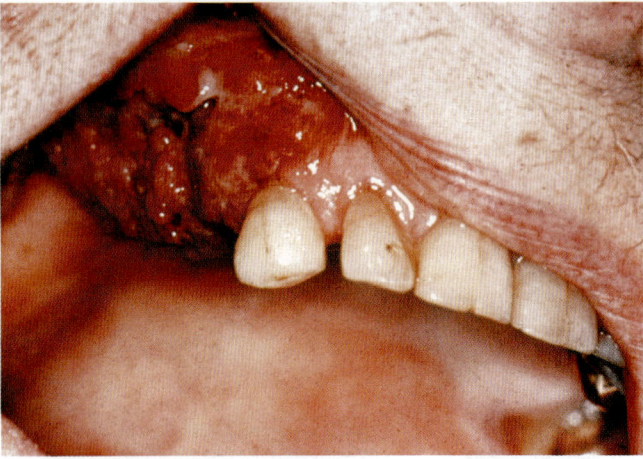

Fig. 34.49 Squamous cell carcinoma.

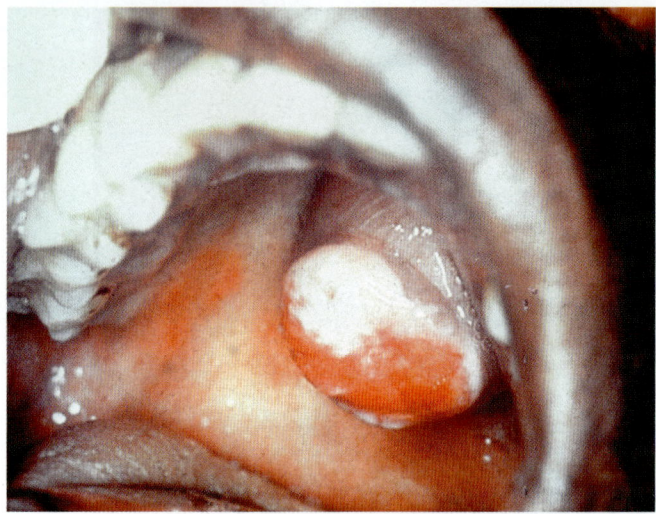

Fig. 34.50 Squamous cell carcinoma.

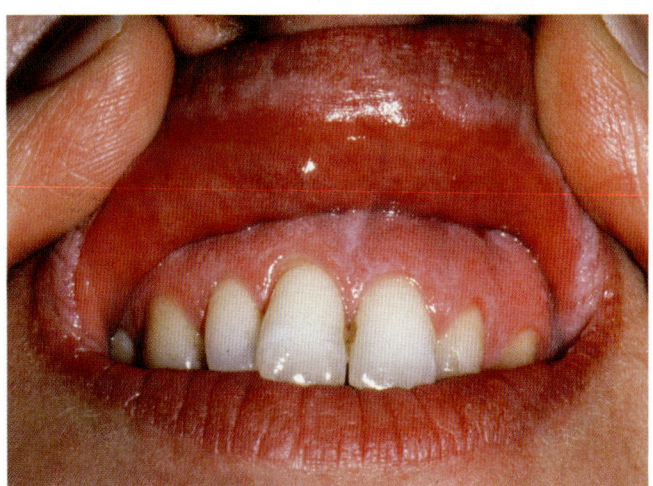

Fig. 34.51 Acquired dyskeratotic leukoplakia.

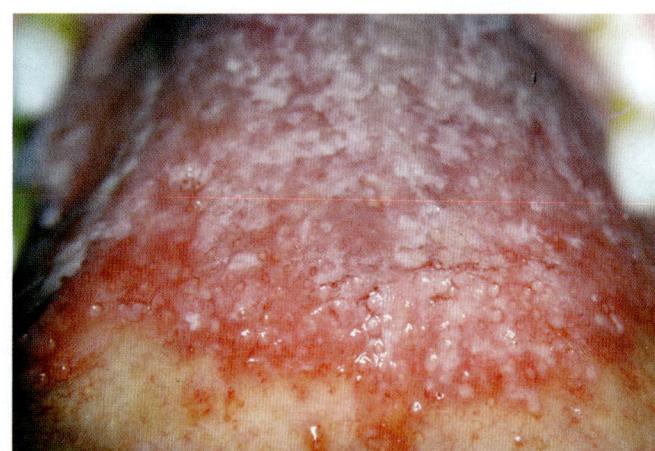

Fig. 34.52 Acquired dyskeratotic leukoplakia, gingiva.

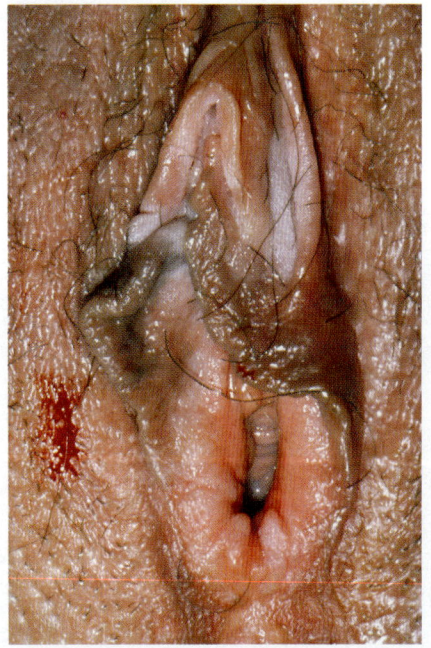

Fig. 34.53 Acquired dyskeratotic leukoplakia, genital involvement.

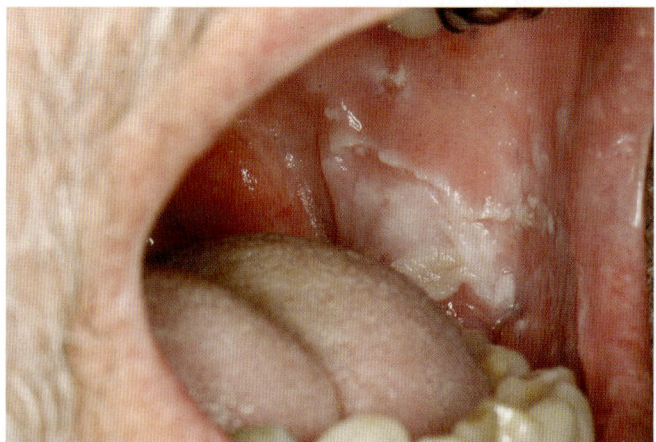

Fig. 34.54 Morsicatio buccarum.

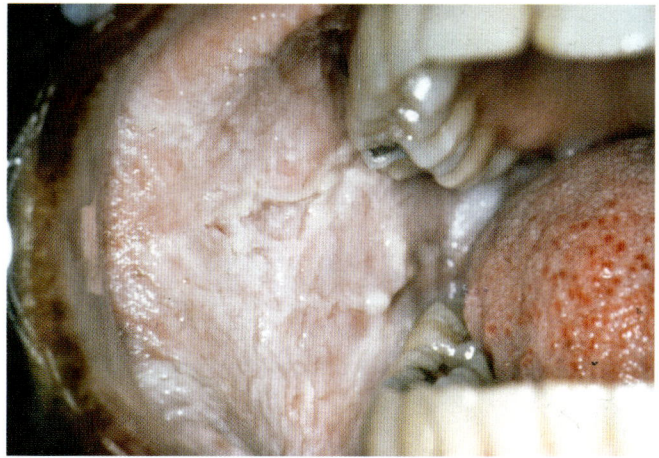

Fig. 34.55 White sponge nevus.

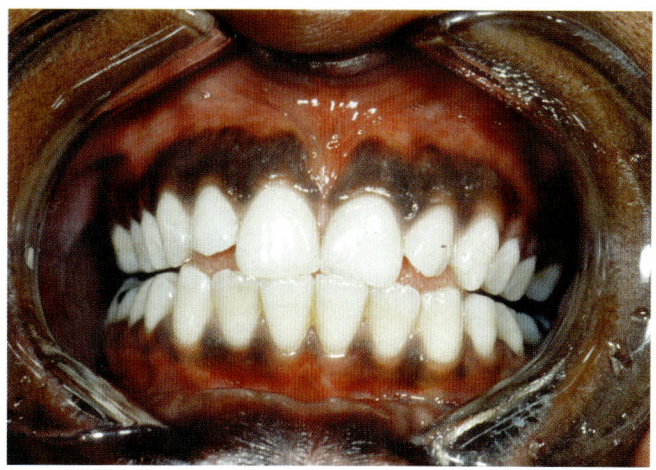

Fig. 34.56 Physiologic pigmentation.

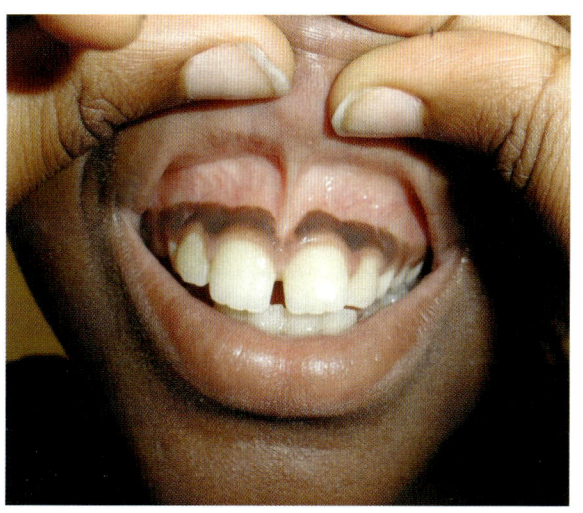

Fig. 34.57 Physiologic oral pigmentation. *Courtesy Scott Norton, MD.*

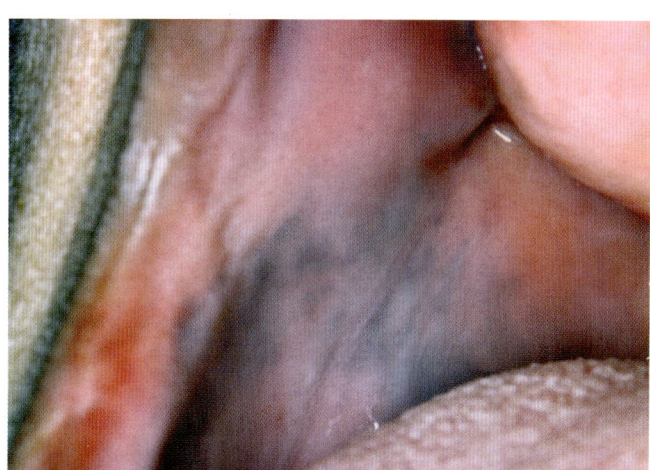

Fig. 34.58 Physiologic oral pigmentation.

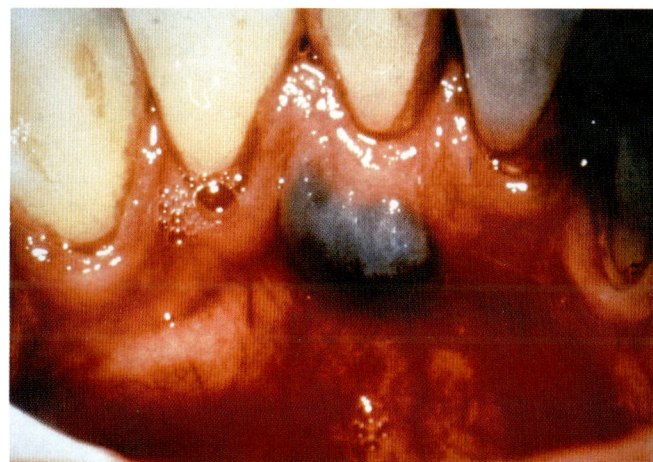

Fig. 34.59 Oral nevus.

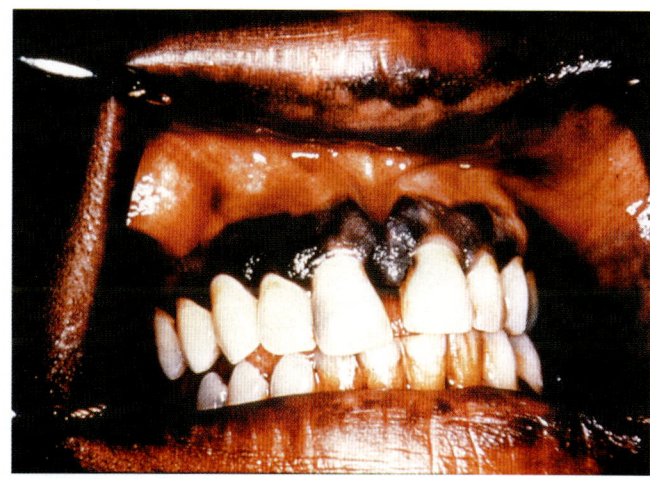

Fig. 34.60 Melanoma.

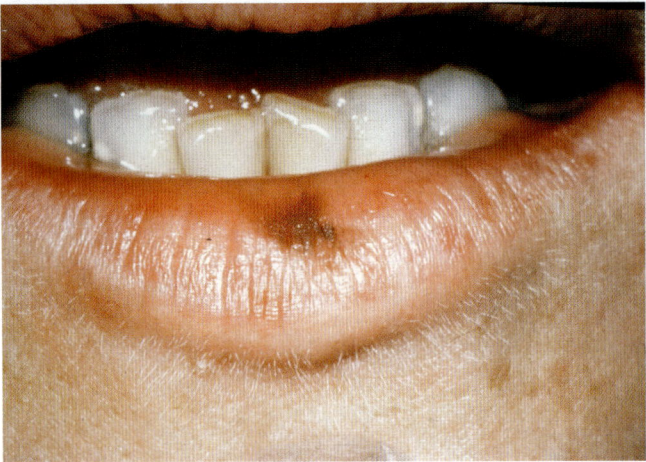

Fig. 34.61 Oral melanotic macule.

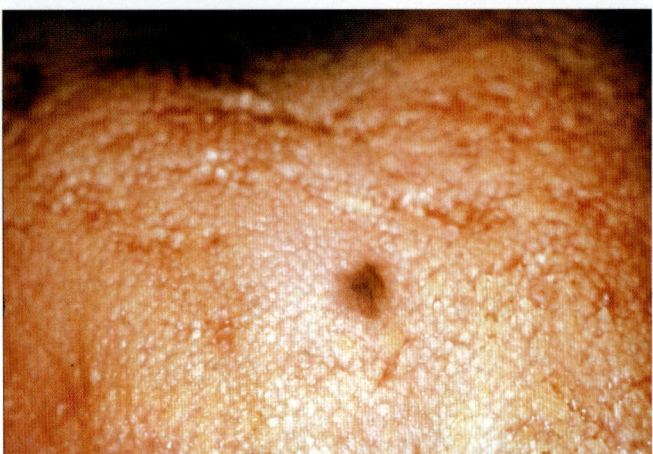

Fig. 34.62 Oral melanotic macule.

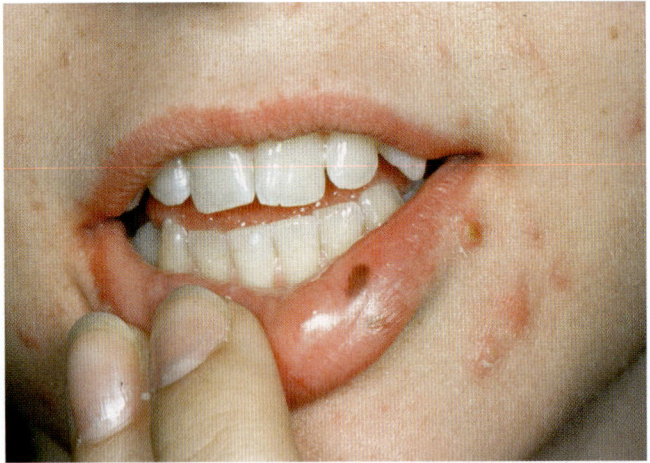

Fig. 34.63 Oral melanotic macule.

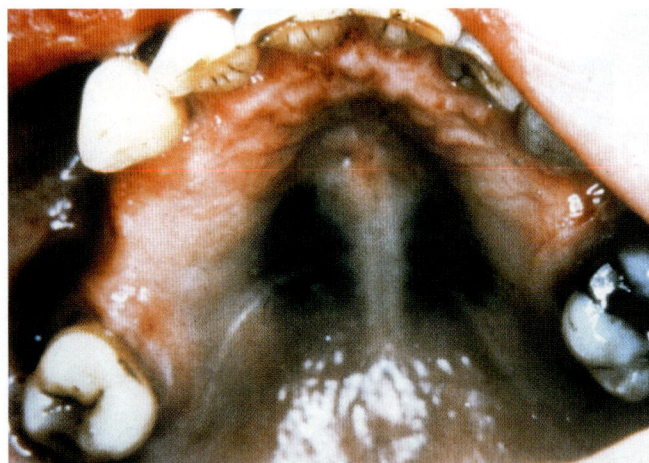

Fig. 34.64 Chloroquine hyperpigmentation.

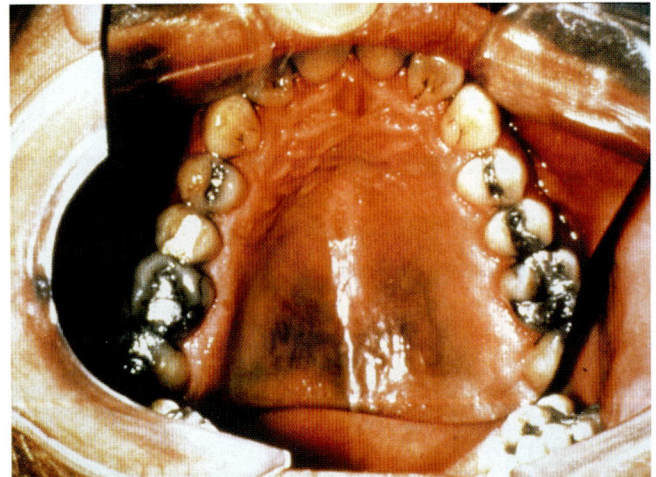

Fig. 34.65 Chlorpromazine hyperpigmentation.

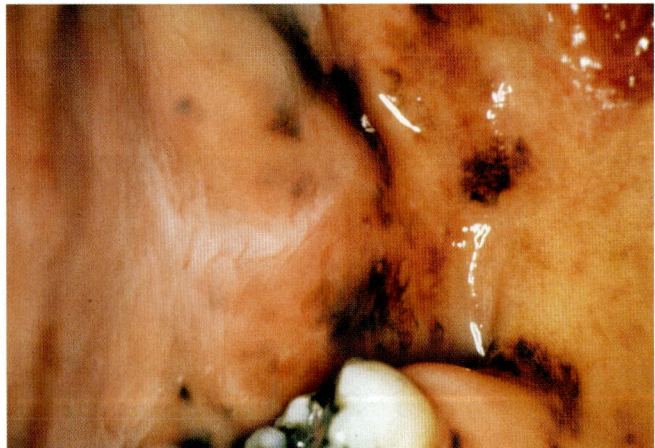

Fig. 34.66 Minocycline hyperpigmentation.

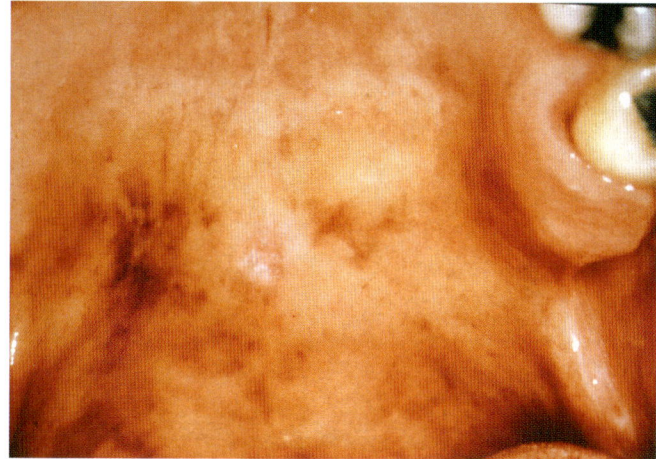

Fig. 34.67 Oat cell carcinoma–associated pigmentation.

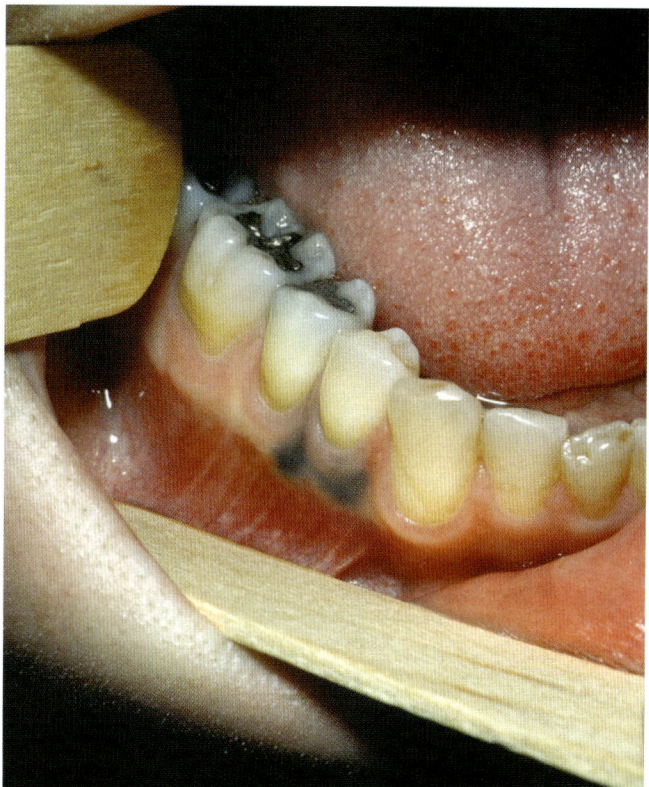

Fig. 34.68 Amalgam tattoo.

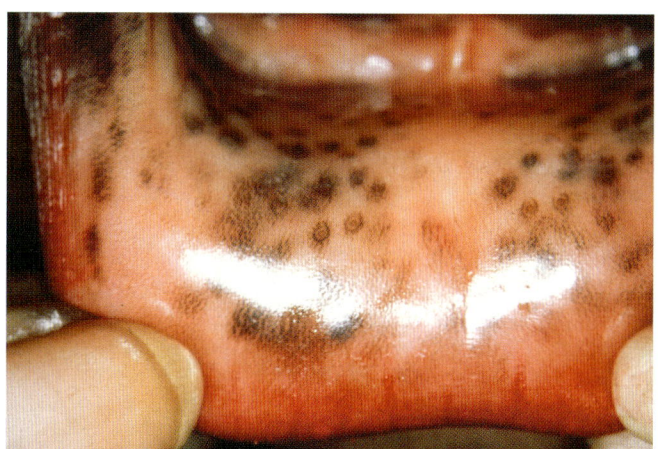

Fig. 34.69 Multiple oral melanoacanthomas.

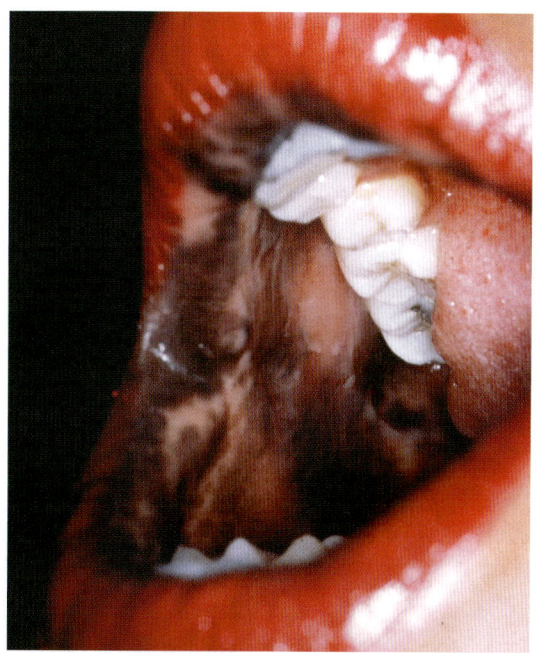

Fig. 34.70 Progressive involvement with multiple melanoacanthomas.

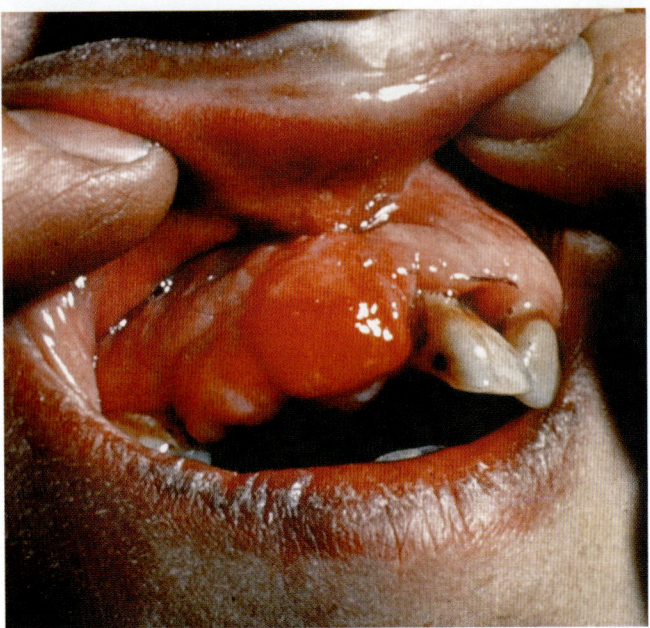

Fig. 34.71 Epulis.

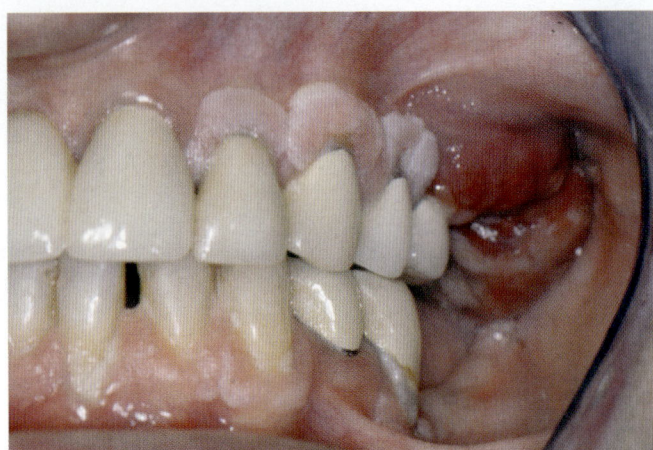

Fig. 34.72 Pyogenic granuloma.

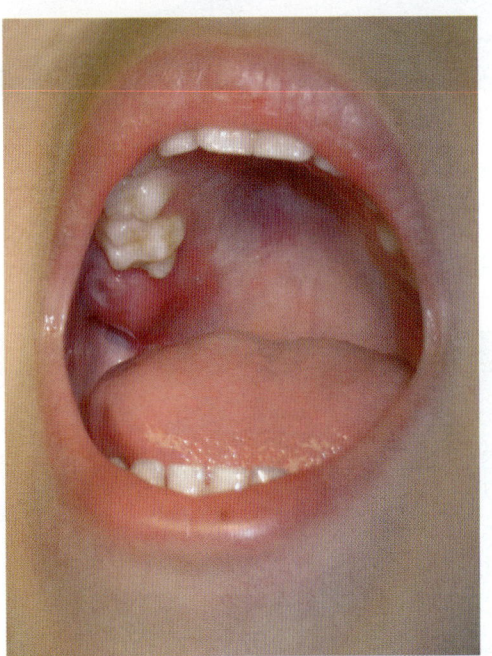

Fig. 34.73 Pyogenic granuloma.

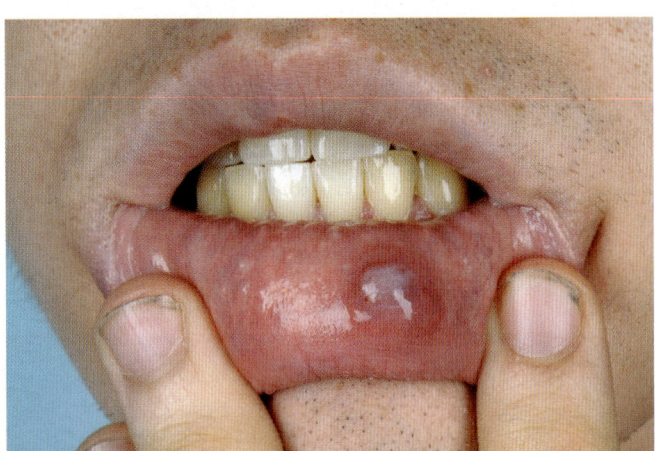

Fig. 34.74 Mucocele.

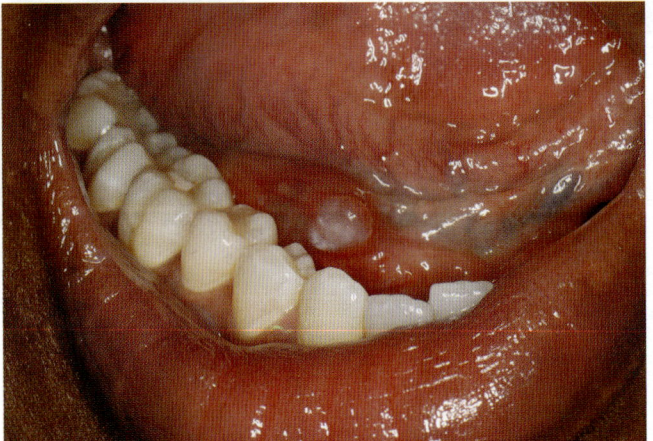

Fig. 34.75 Mucocele.

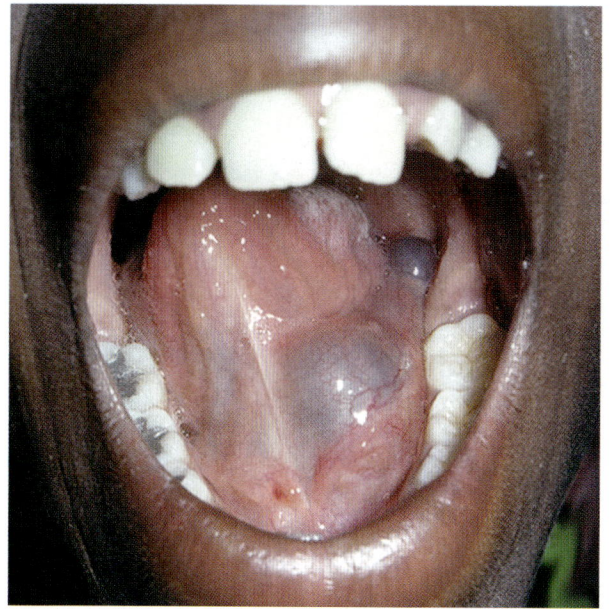

Fig. 34.76 Ranula.

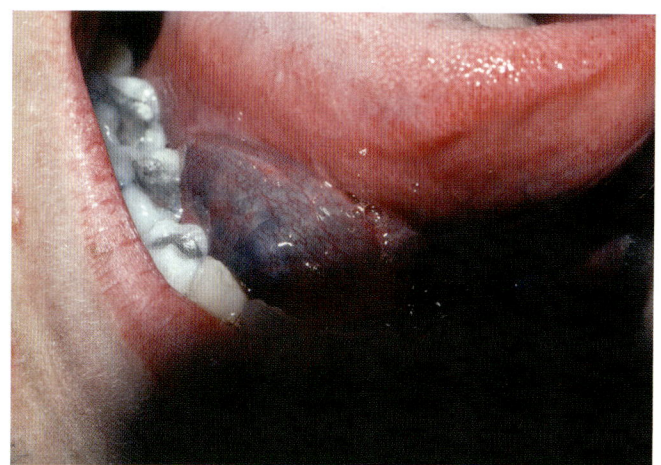

Fig. 34.77 Ranula. *Courtesy Steven Binnick, MD.*

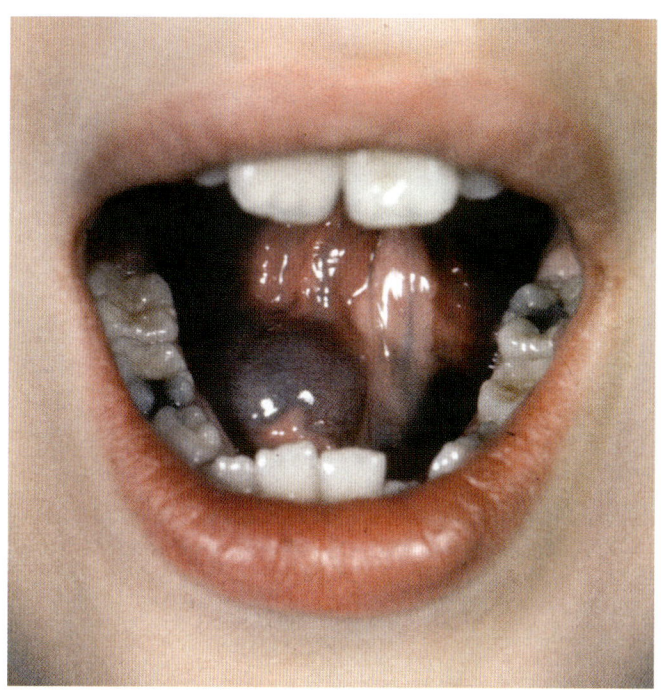

Fig. 34.78 Ranula. *Courtesy Steven Binnick, MD.*

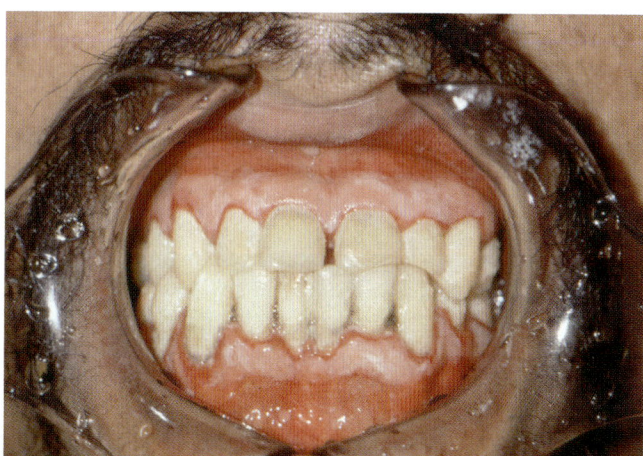

Fig. 34.79 Acute necrotizing ulcerative gingivostomatitis. *Courtesy Department of Oral Medicine, University of Pennsylvania School of Dentistry.*

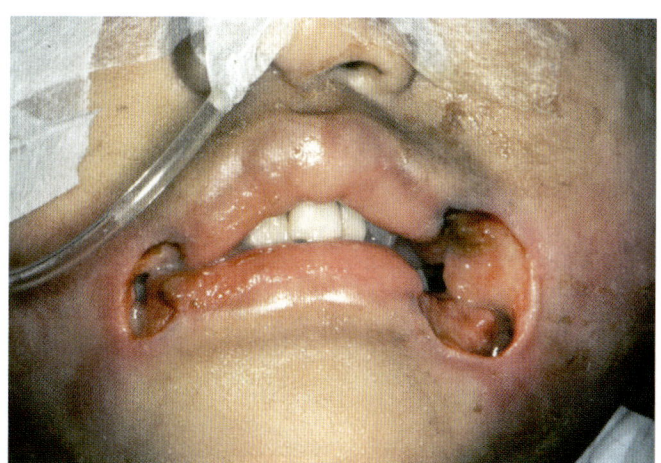

Fig. 34.80 Noma.

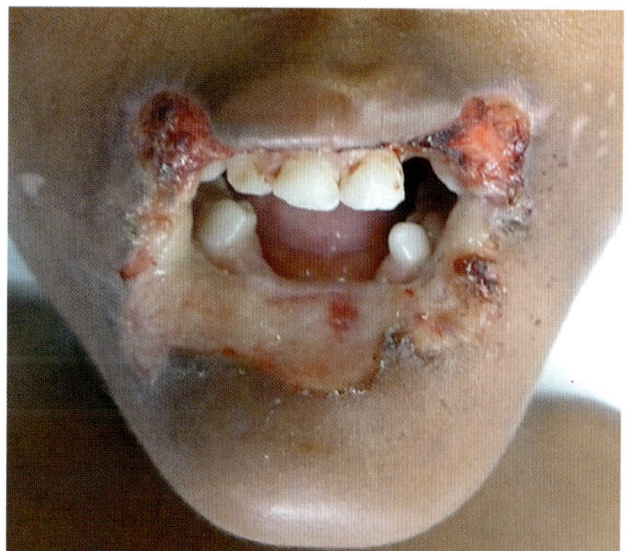

Fig. 34.81 Noma.

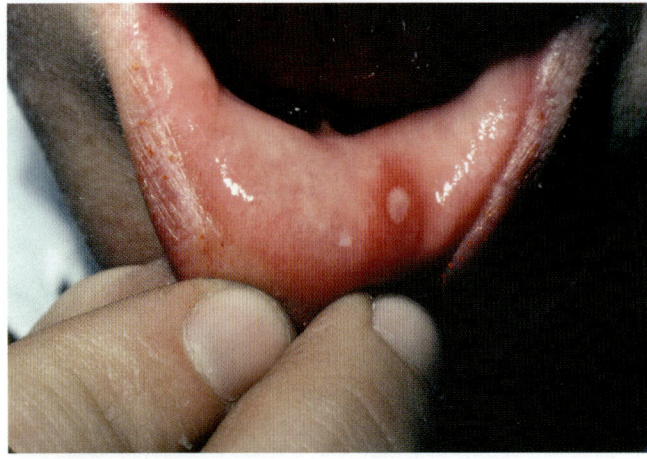

Fig. 34.82 Aphthous stomatitis. *Courtesy Steven Binnick, MD.*

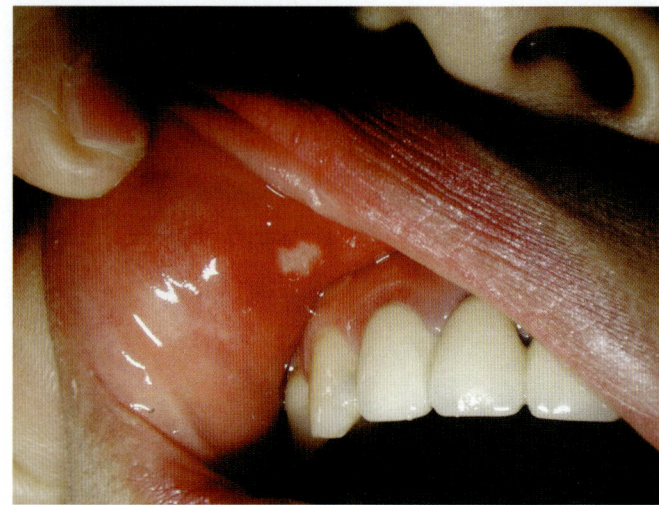

Fig. 34.83 Aphthous stomatitis. *Courtesy National Cheng Kung University, Taiwan.*

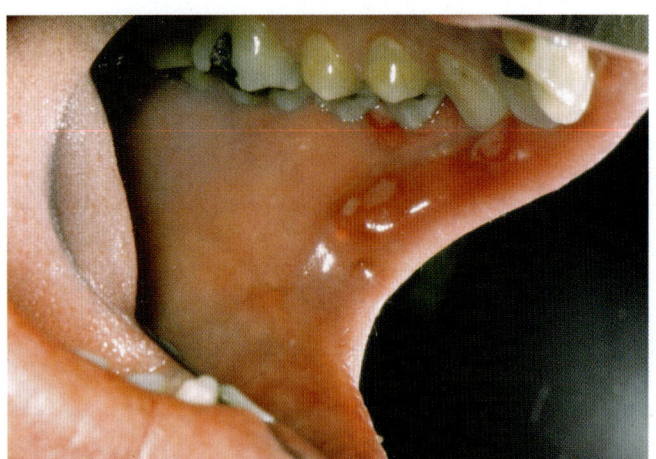

Fig. 34.84 Aphthous stomatitis. *Courtesy Steven Binnick, MD.*

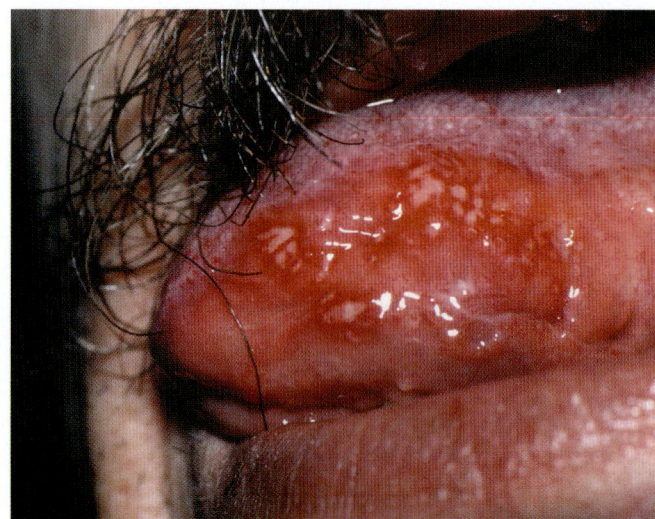

Fig. 34.85 Aphthous stomatitis. *Courtesy Steven Binnick, MD.*

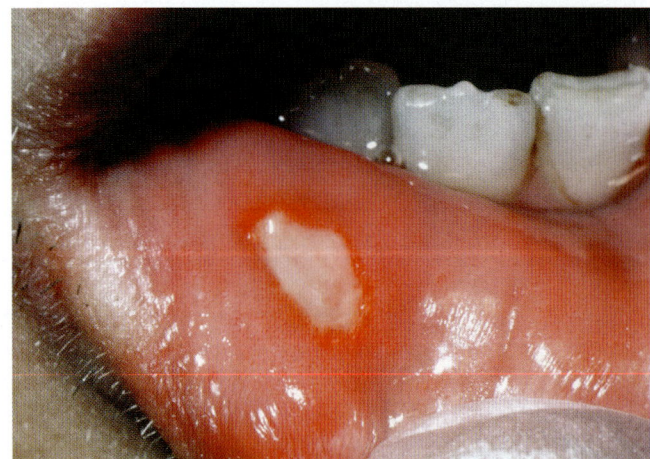

Fig. 34.86 Major aphthous stomatitis.

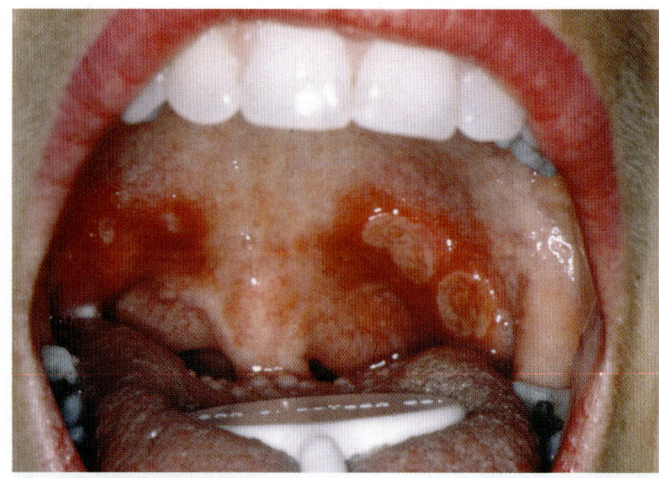

Fig. 34.87 Major aphthous stomatitis.

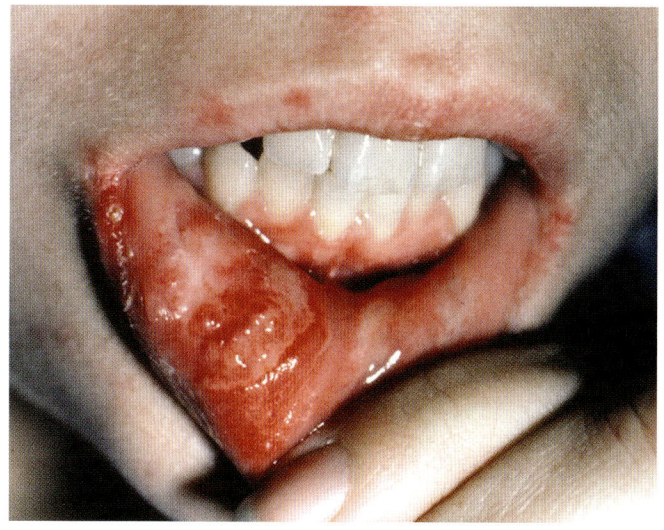

Fig. 34.88 Behçet disease. *Courtesy Ken Greer, MD.*

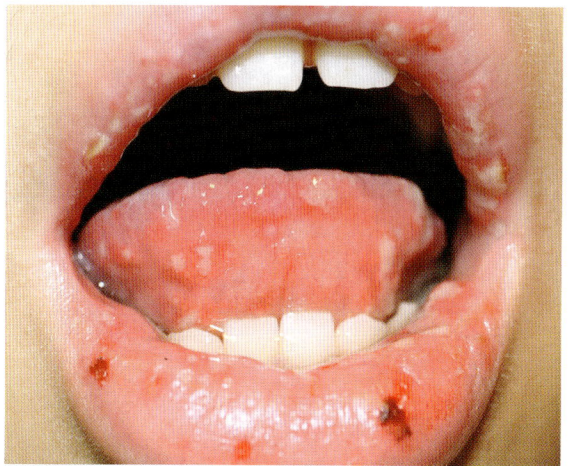

Fig. 34.89 Behçet disease. *Courtesy Yung-Tsu Cho, MD.*

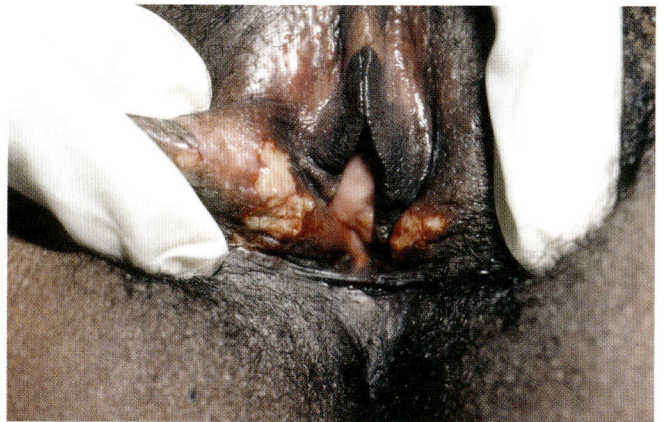

Fig. 34.90 Behçet disease. *Courtesy Ken Greer, MD.*

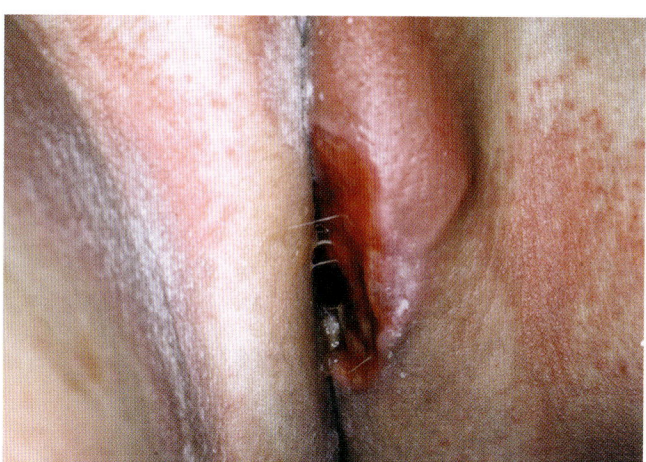

Fig. 34.91 Behçet disease.

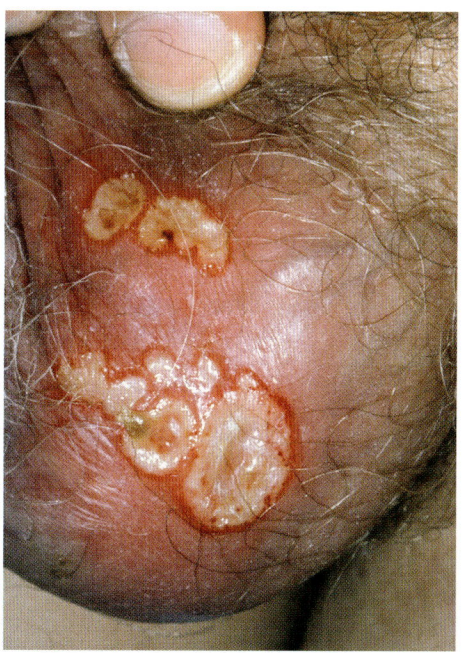

Fig. 34.92 Behçet disease.

Cutaneous Vascular Diseases 35

This section of the atlas will focus on vascular disorders of the skin, including such entities as Raynaud disease, erythromelalgia, livedo racemosa, livedoid vasculopathy, cryoglobulinemia, purpura fulminans, superficial thrombophlebitis, purpura, and vasculitis. As with other disorders of skin, the color, morphology, and distribution of skin lesions are critical to establishment of an accurate diagnosis. Immune complex–mediated disease often affects dependent areas of skin, whereas embolic and vasoconstrictive phenomena affect acral sites. Diseases affecting the post–capillary venule or capillaries seldom result in cutaneous necrosis and tend to produce lesions with a round-to-oval configuration, whereas diseases affecting arterioles commonly result in angular stellate infarcts and retiform purpura. Postcapillary venule disease results in petechiae, or palpable or macular areas of purpura, whereas chronic capillaritis presents with hemosiderin staining and thumbprint, annular, eczematous, or lichenoid-containing petechiae. Forms of vasculitis associated with a stellate or retiform morphology include antineutrophil cytoplasmic antibody–associated vasculitis, rheumatoid vasculitis, and septic vasculitis. Ischemic disease is often associated with pain, and severe or prolonged ischemia results in necrosis. Vasodilatation may relate to temperature regulation, abnormal shunting of blood, or small-fiber neuropathy, as in the case of erythromelalgia. The morphology and distribution of the lesions suggest the correct site and appropriate depth for a biopsy.

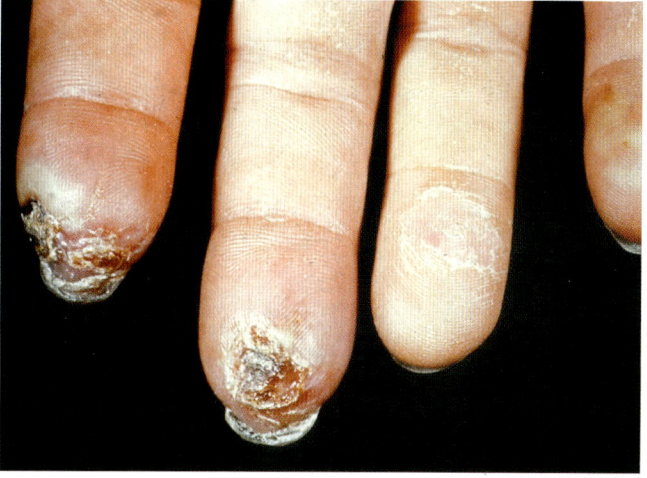

Fig. 35.2 Raynaud phenomenon with digital ulcers.

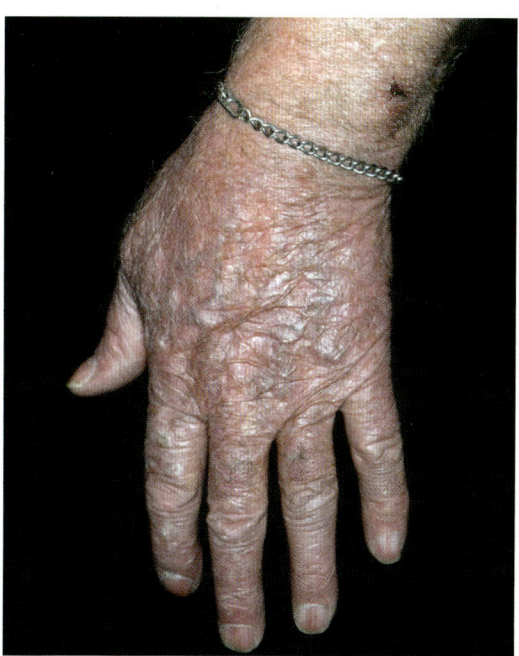

Fig. 35.3 Erythromelalgia.

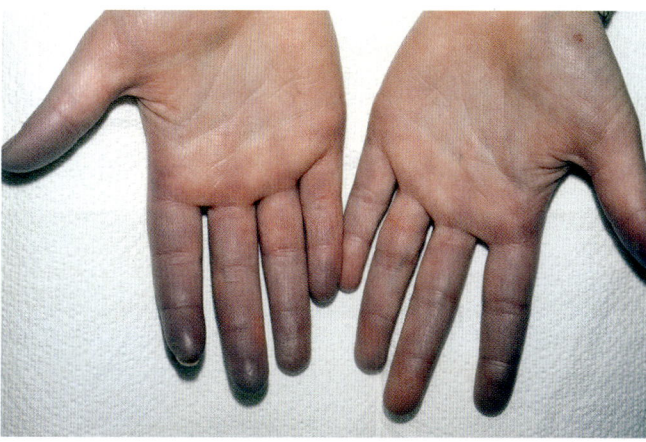

Fig. 35.1 Raynaud phenomenon secondary to mixed connective tissue disease.

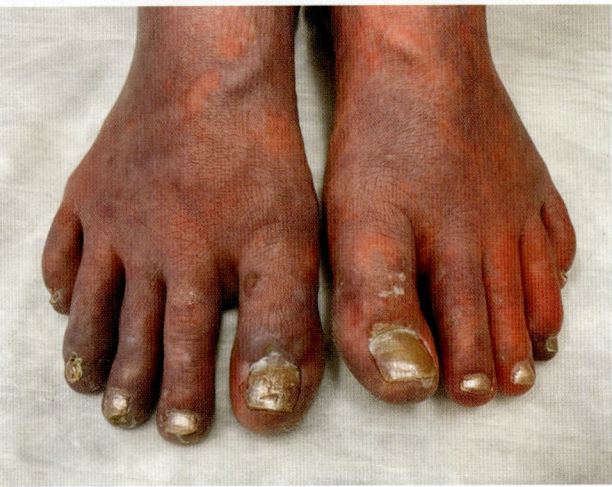

Fig. 35.4 Erythromelalgia.

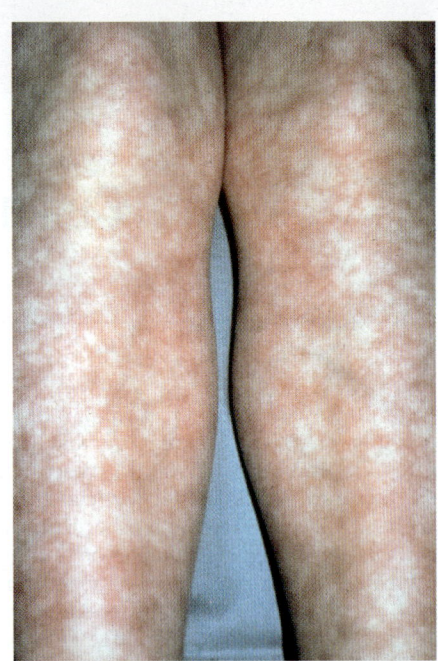

Fig. 35.5 Livedo reticularis.

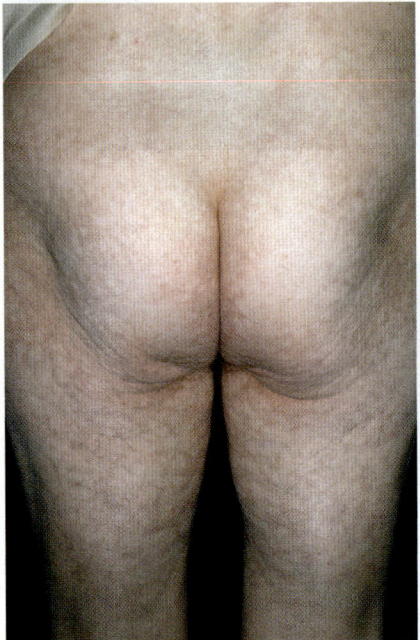

Fig. 35.6 Livedo reticularis caused by amantadine.

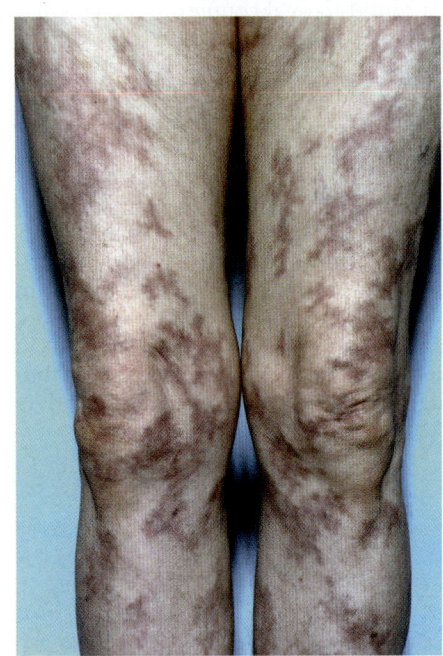

Fig. 35.7 Livedo racemosa.

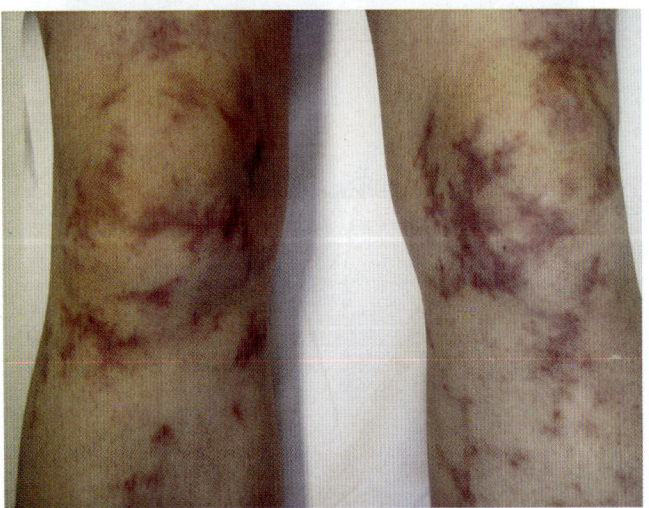

Fig. 35.8 Livedo racemosa. *Courtesy Rui Tavares Bello, MD.*

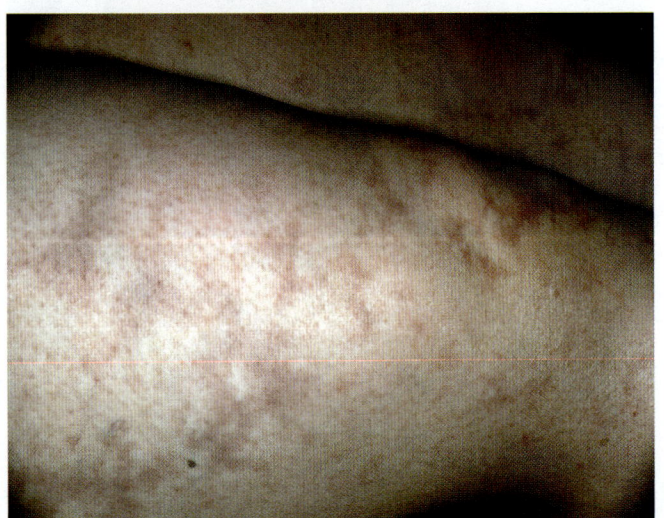

Fig. 35.9 Sneddon syndrome.

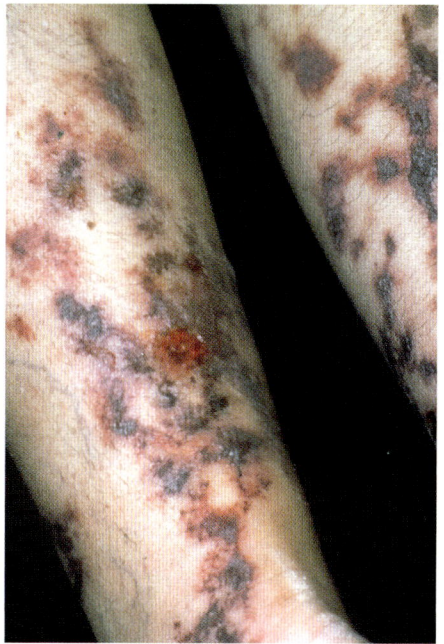

Fig. 35.10 Necrotizing livedo.

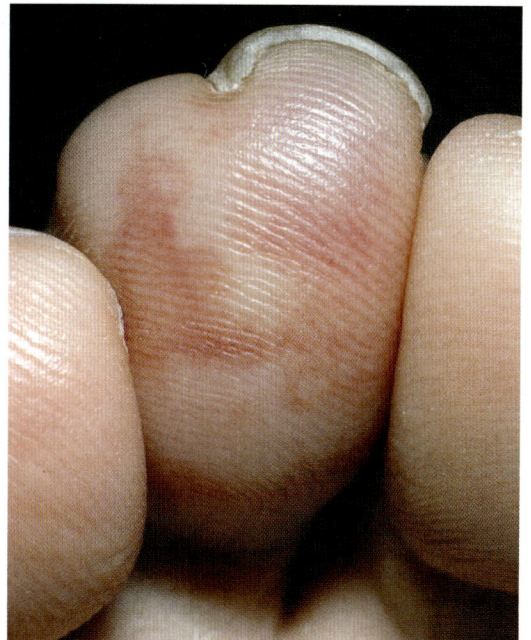

Fig. 35.11 Purple toe secondary to cholesterol emboli.

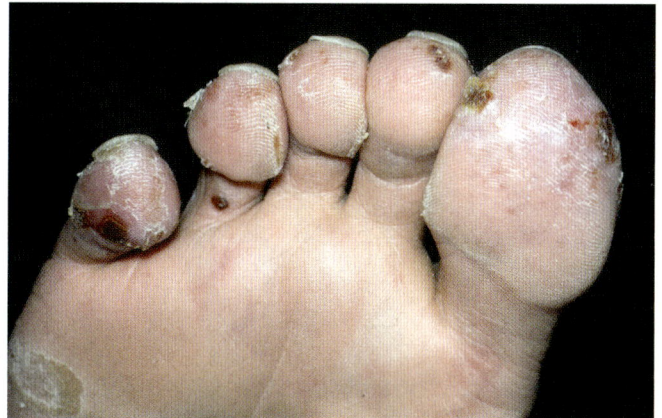

Fig. 35.12 Cholesterol emboli. *Courtesy Curt Samlaska, MD.*

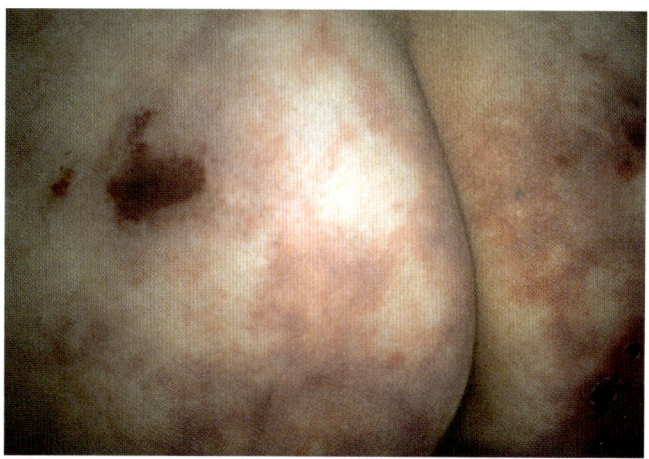

Fig. 35.13 Cholesterol emboli.

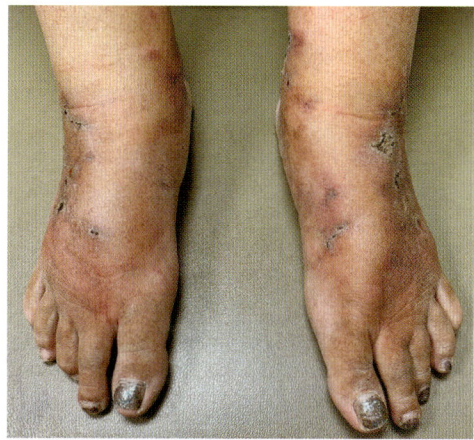

Fig. 35.14 Livedoid vasculopathy.

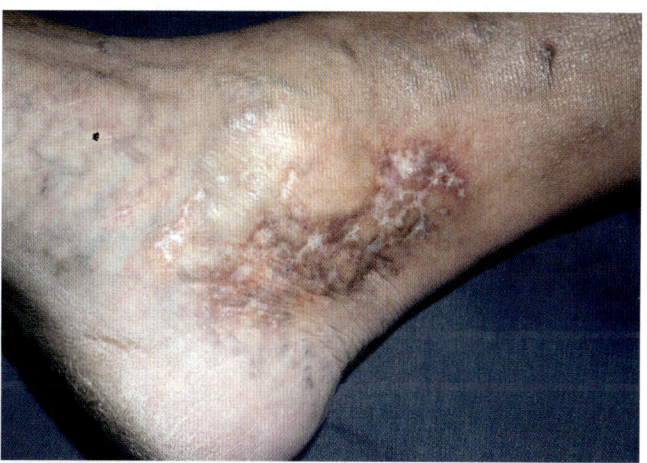

Fig. 35.15 Atrophy blanche.

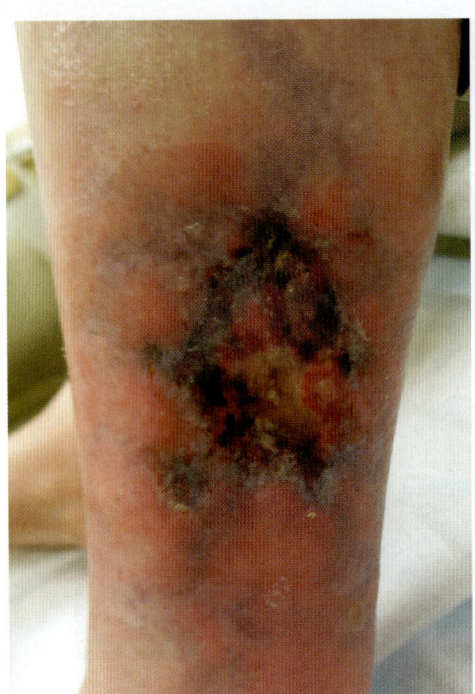

Fig. 35.16 Calciphylaxis.

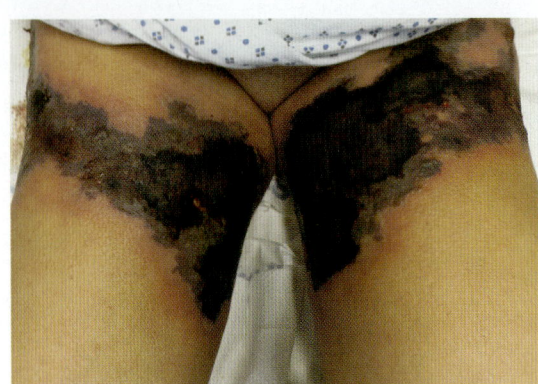

Fig. 35.17 Calciphylaxis.

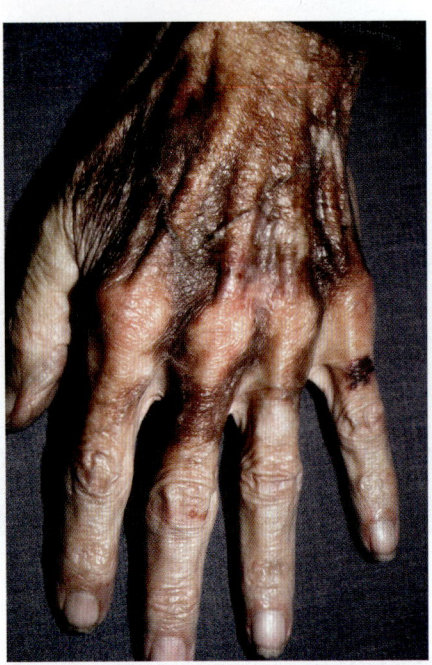

Fig. 35.18 Purpura in old age.

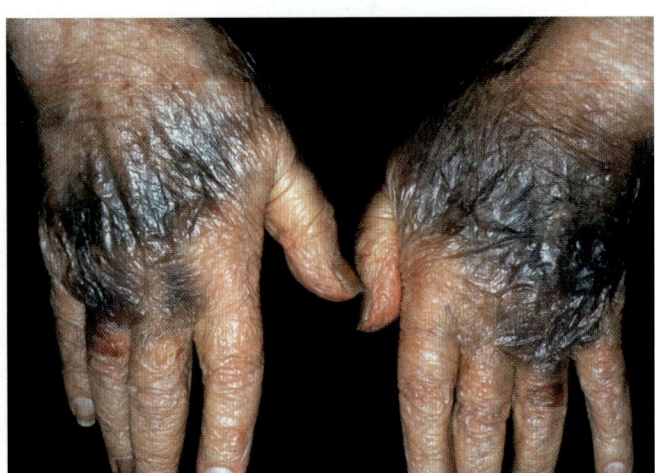

Fig. 35.19 Purpura in old age.

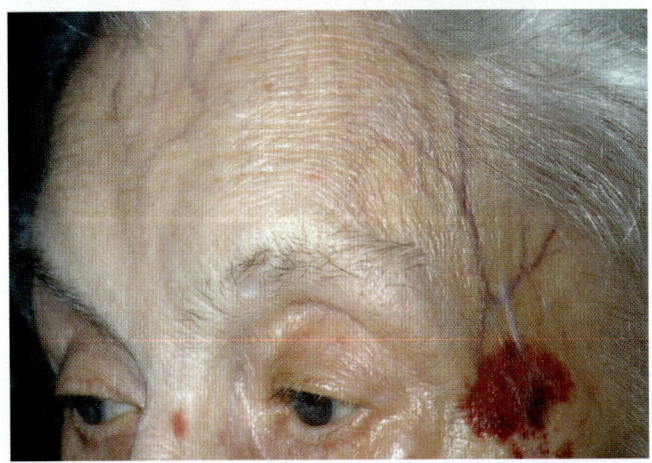

Fig. 35.20 Purpura in old age.

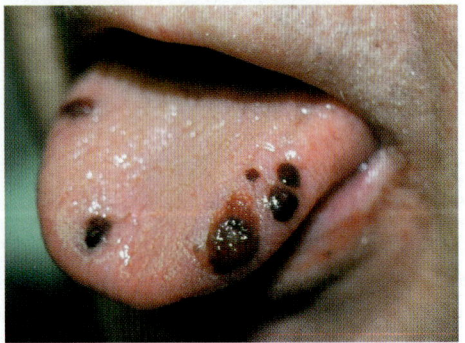

Fig. 35.21 Immune thrombocytopenic purpura.

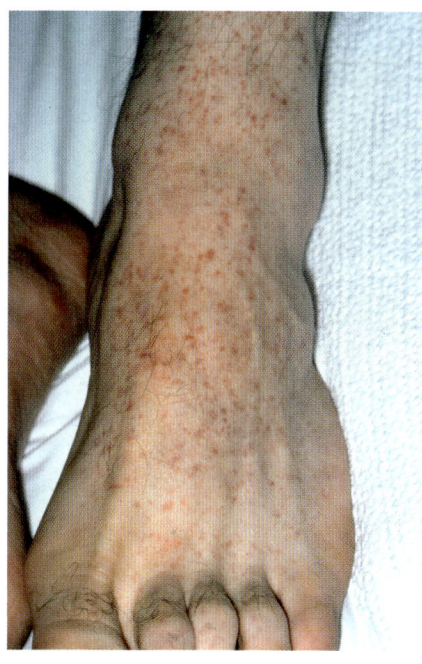

Fig. 35.22 Immune thrombocytopenic purpura.

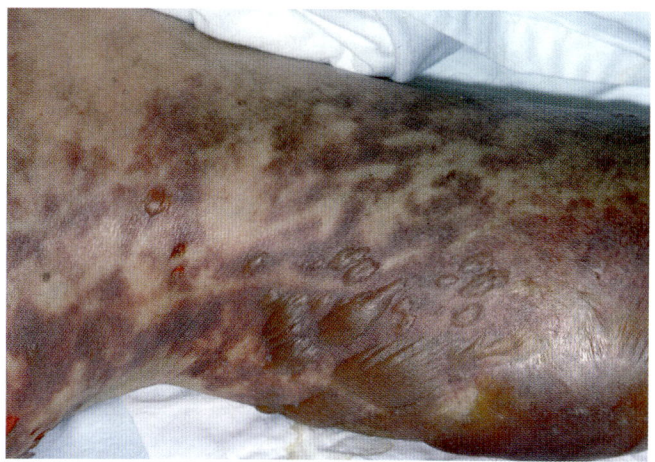

Fig. 35.23 Thrombotic thrombocytopenic purpura.

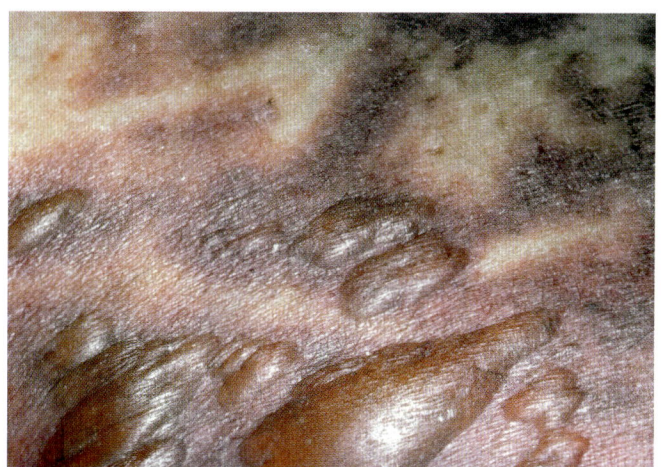

Fig. 35.24 Thrombotic thrombocytopenic purpura.

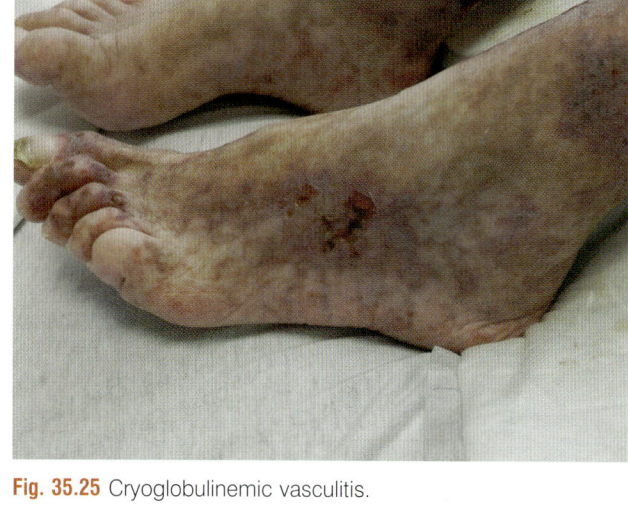

Fig. 35.25 Cryoglobulinemic vasculitis.

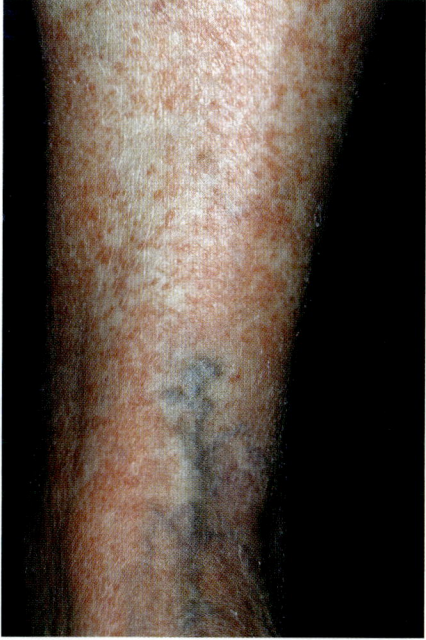

Fig. 35.26 Waldenström hypergammaglobulinemic purpura.

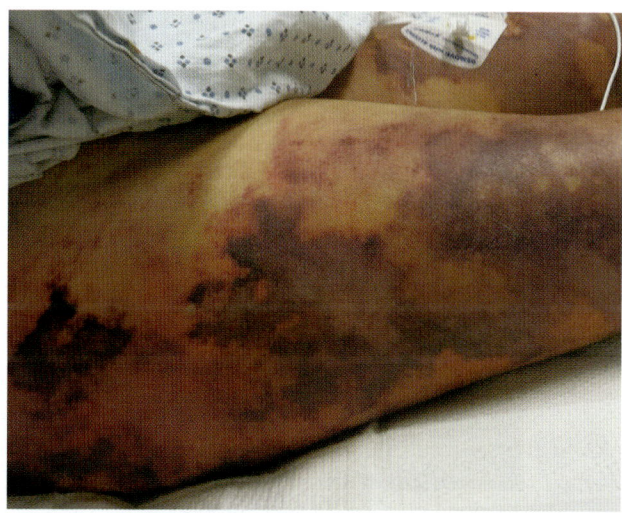

Fig. 35.27 Purpura fulminans secondary to *Escherichia coli* sepsis.

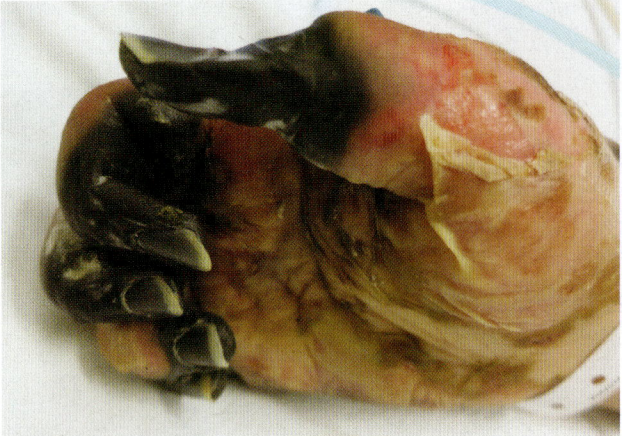

Fig. 35.28 Vasopressor-induced ischemia.

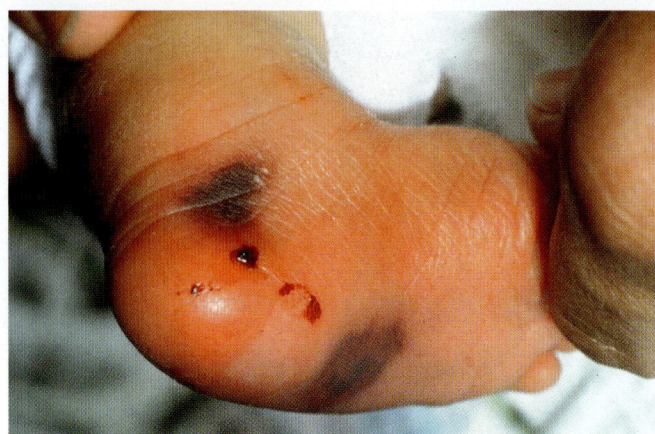

Fig. 35.29 Homozygous protein C deficiency.

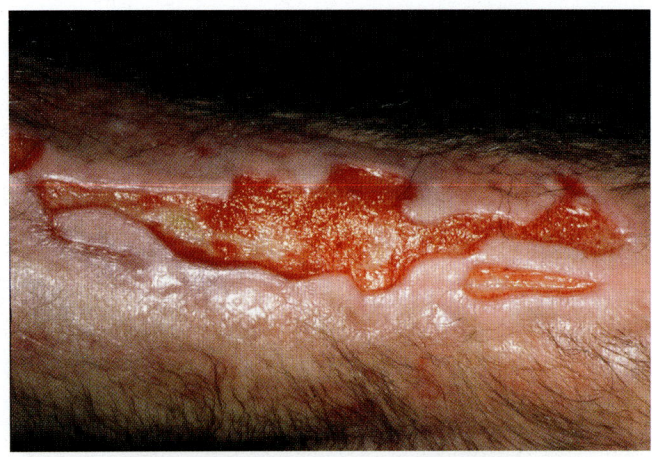

Fig. 35.30 Protein S deficiency.

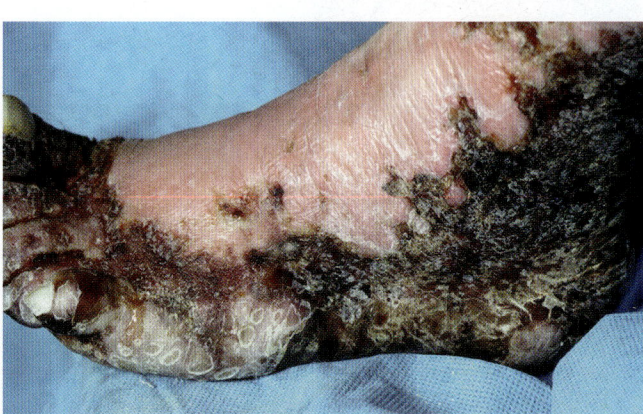

Fig. 35.31 Catastrophic antiphospholipid antibody syndrome.

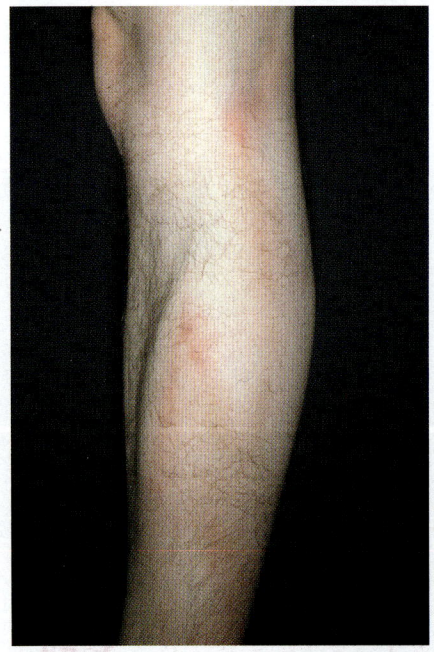

Fig. 35.32 Superficial thrombophlebitis.

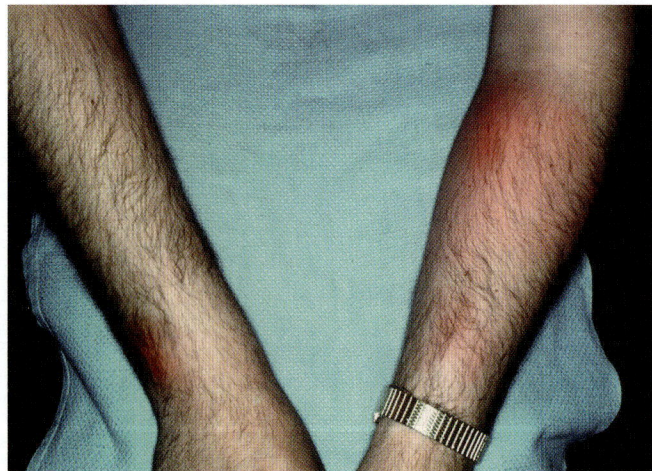

Fig. 35.33 Migrating superficial thrombophlebitis.

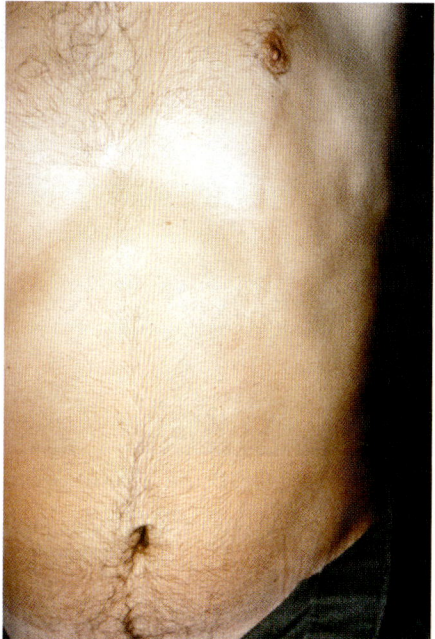

Fig. 35.34 Mondor disease.

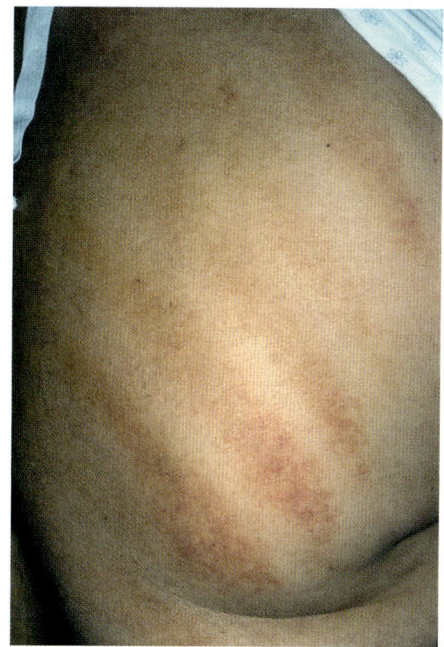

Fig. 35.35 Purpura from coin rubbing. *Courtesy Steven Binnick, MD.*

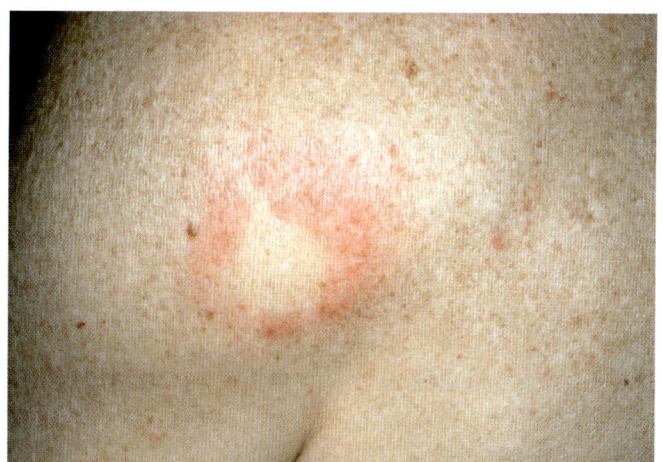

Fig. 35.36 Racquetball-induced purpura.

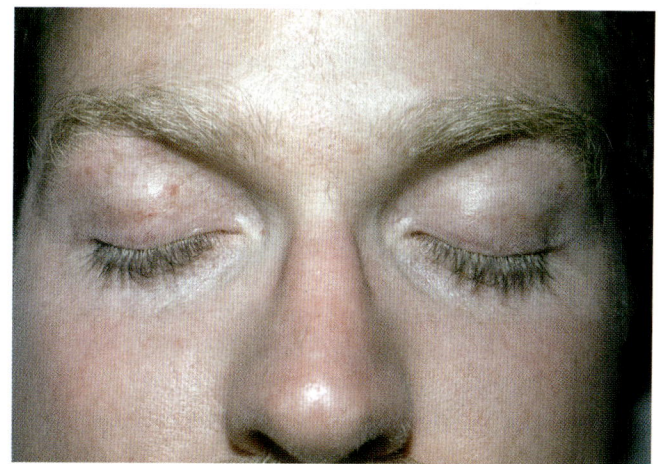

Fig. 35.37 Purpura after vomiting. *Courtesy Steven Binnick, MD.*

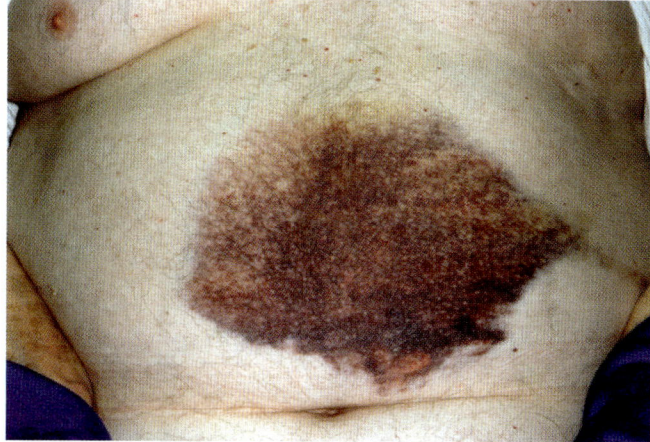

Fig. 35.38 Cough-induced purpura.

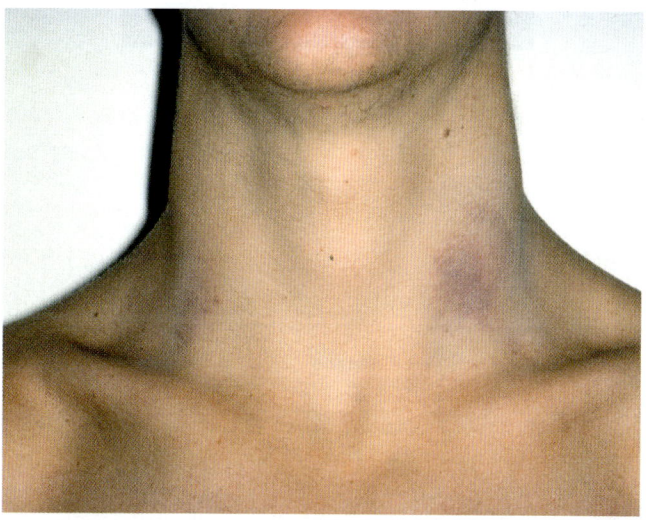

Fig. 35.39 Passion purpura.

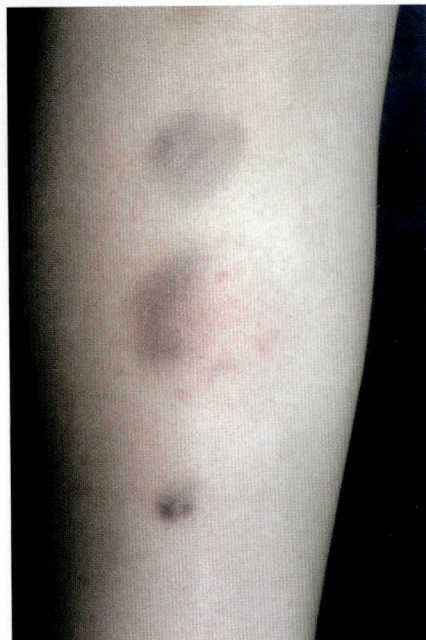

Fig. 35.40 Psychogenic purpura. *Courtesy Steven Binnick, MD.*

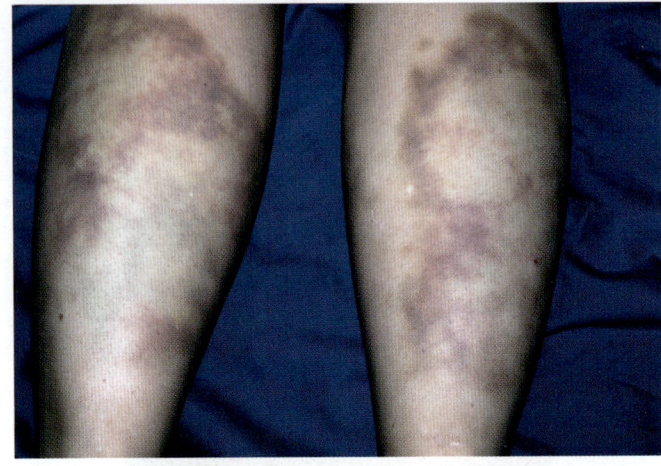

Fig. 35.41 Psychogenic purpura. *Courtesy Steven Binnick, MD.*

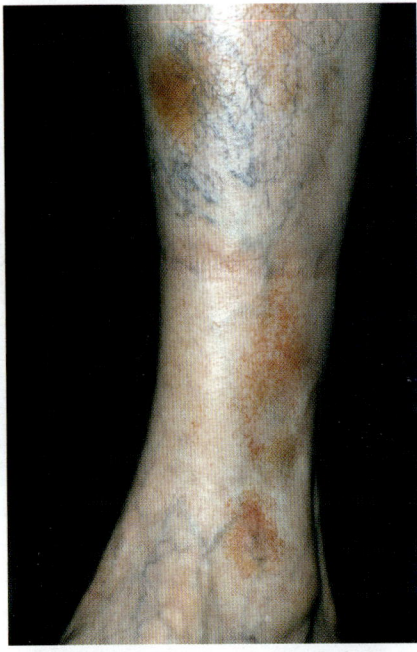

Fig. 35.42 Schamberg disease.

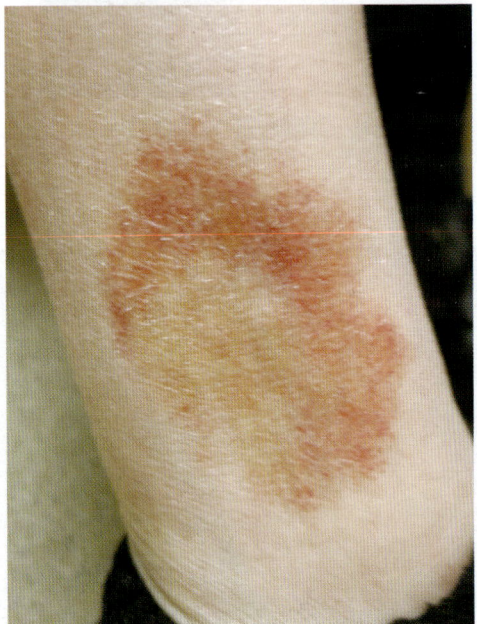

Fig. 35.43 Purpura annularis telangiectodes.

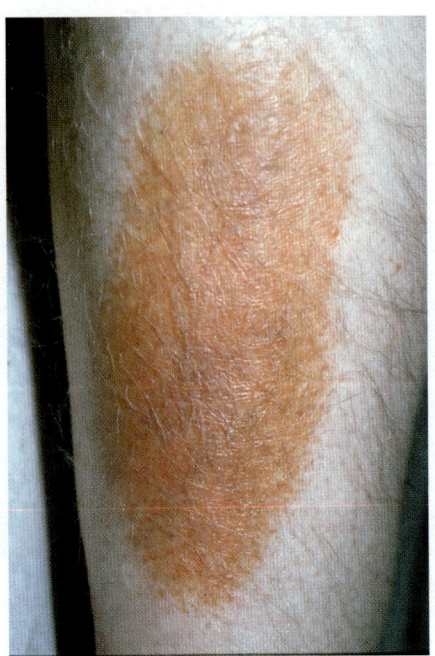

Fig. 35.44 Lichen aureus.

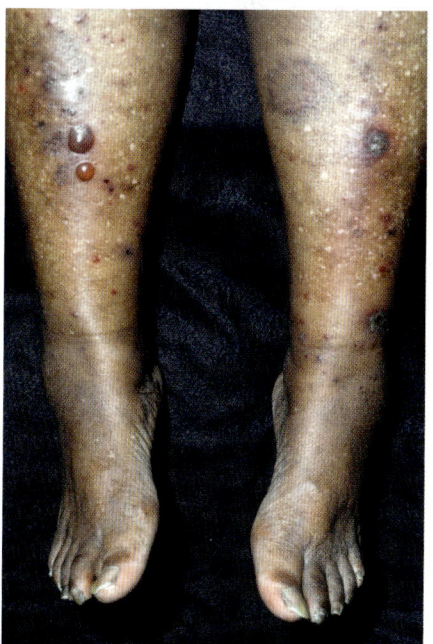

Fig. 35.45 Leukocytoclastic vasculitis.

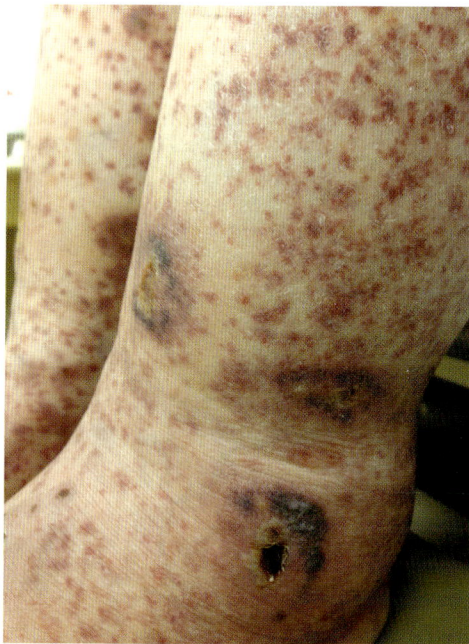

Fig. 35.47 Leukocytoclastic vasculitis (cutaneous small vessel vasculitis).

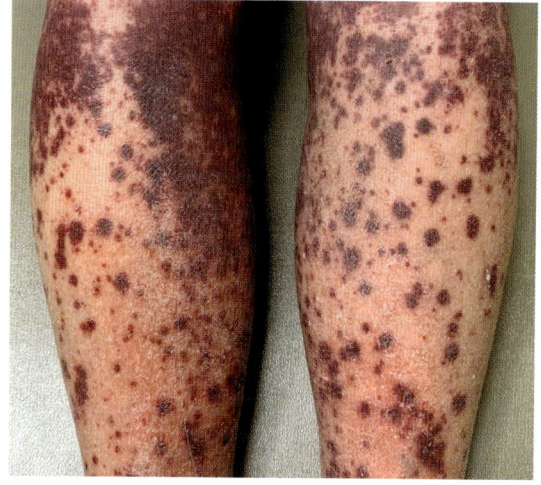

Fig. 35.46 Leukocytoclastic vasculitis (cutaneous small vessel vasculitis).

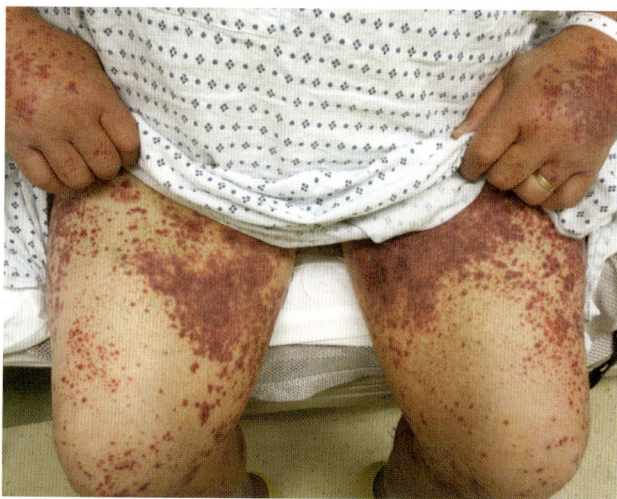

Fig. 35.48 Leukocytoclastic vasculitis (cutaneous small vessel vasculitis).

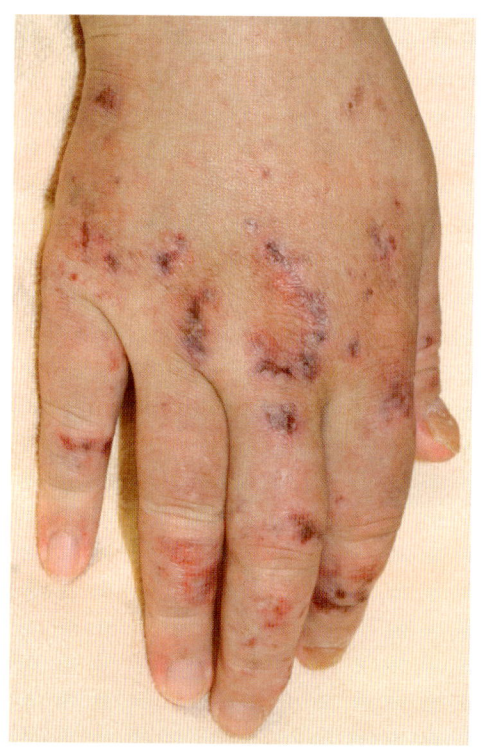

Fig. 35.49 Vasculitis in lupus erythematosus. *Courtesy Yung-Tsu Cho, MD.*

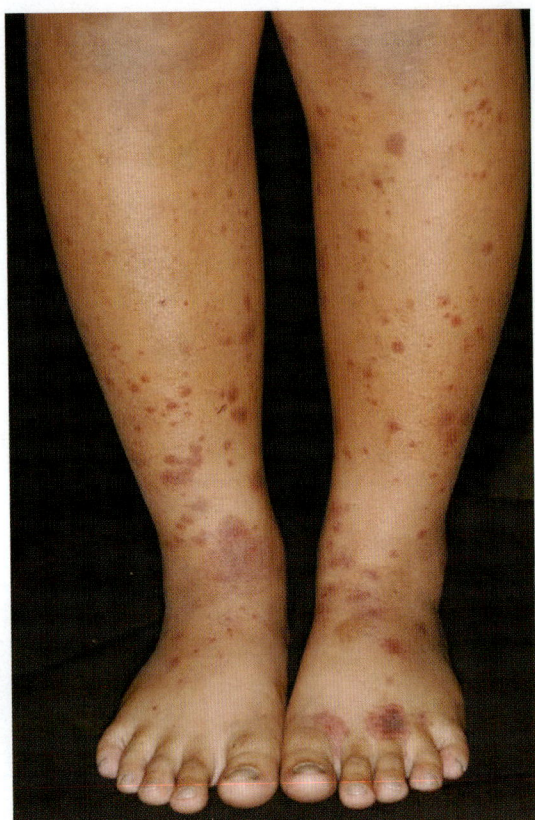

Fig. 35.50 Henoch-Schönlein purpura (IgA vasculitis). *Courtesy Kaohsiung Chang Gang Memorial Hospital, Taiwan.*

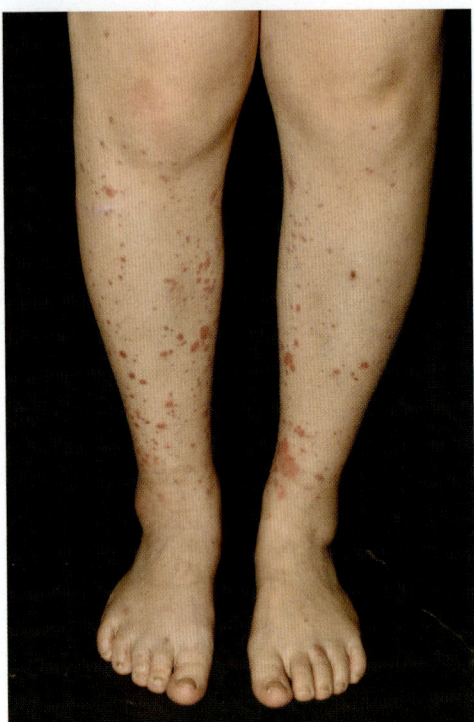

Fig. 35.51 Henoch-Schönlein purpura. (IgA vasculitis). *Courtesy National Taiwan University Hospital.*

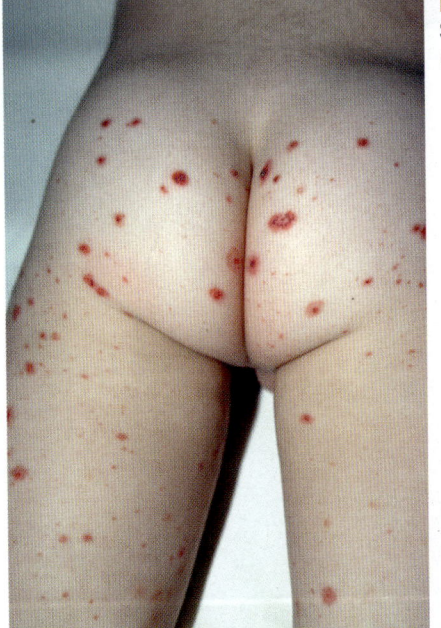

Fig. 35.52 Henoch-Schönlein purpura (IgA vasculitis).

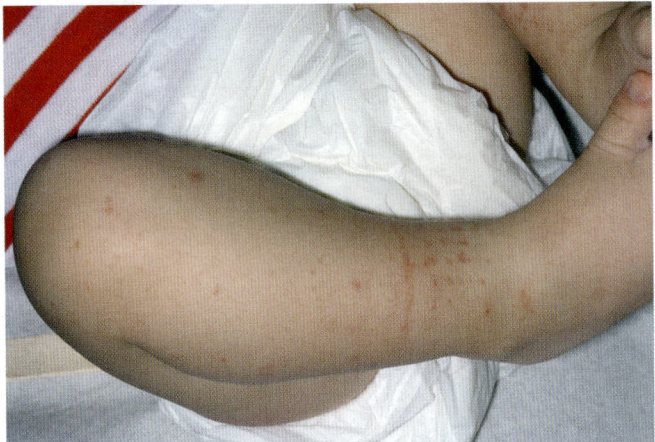

Fig. 35.53 Henoch-Schönlein purpura. Note lesions at site of pressure.

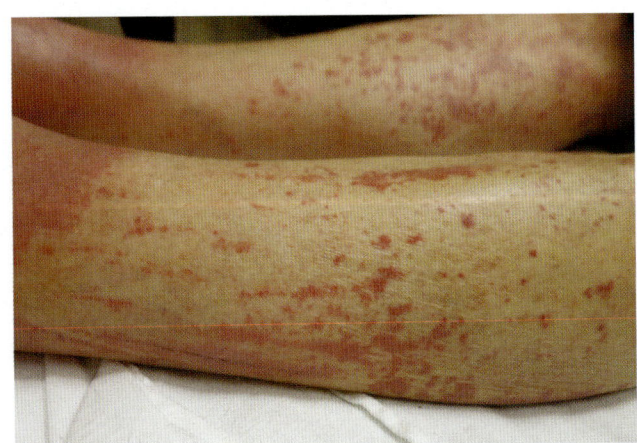

Fig. 35.54 IgA vasculitis in an adult patient.

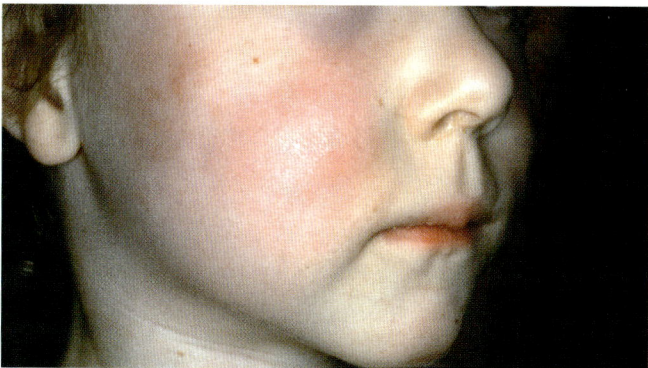

Fig. 35.55 Acute hemorrhagic edema of infancy.

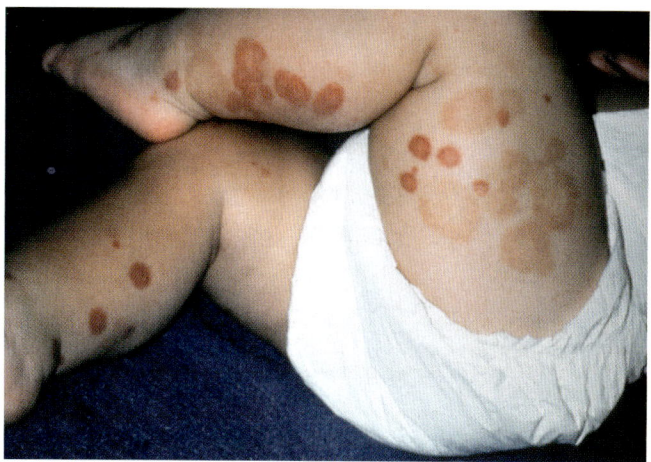

Fig. 35.56 Acute hemorrhagic edema of infancy.

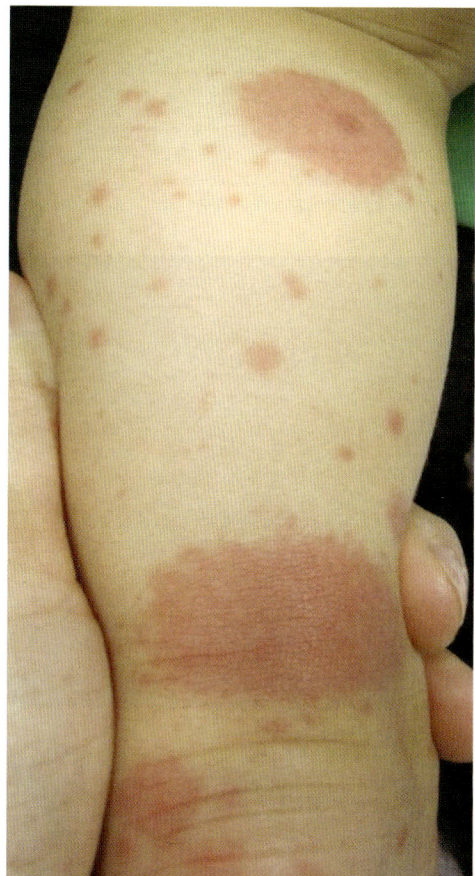

Fig. 35.57 Acute hemorrhagic edema of infancy.

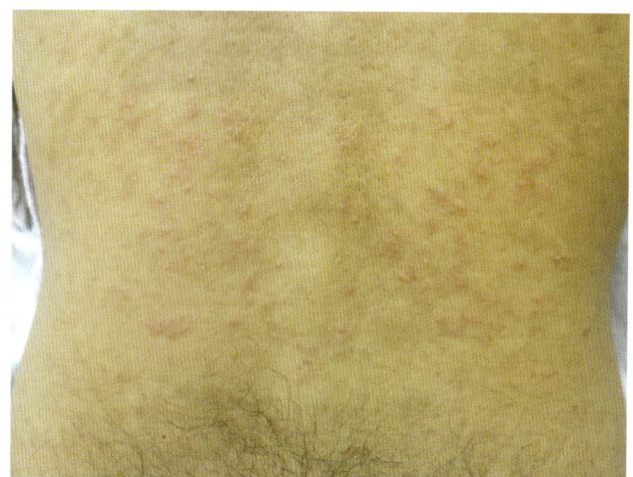

Fig. 35.58 Urticarial vasculitis.

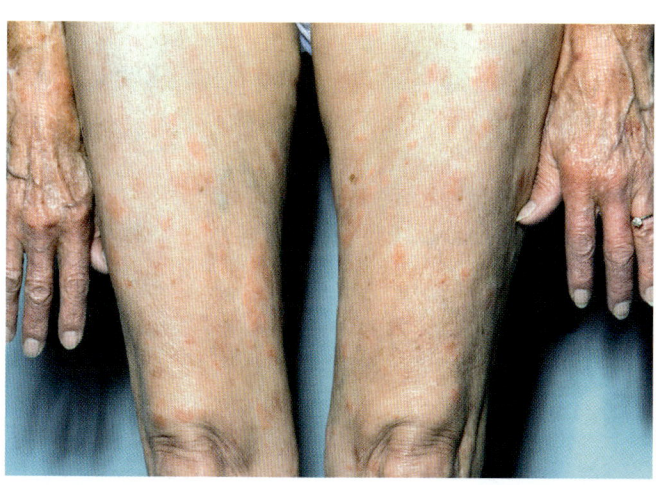

Fig. 35.59 Urticarial vasculitis.

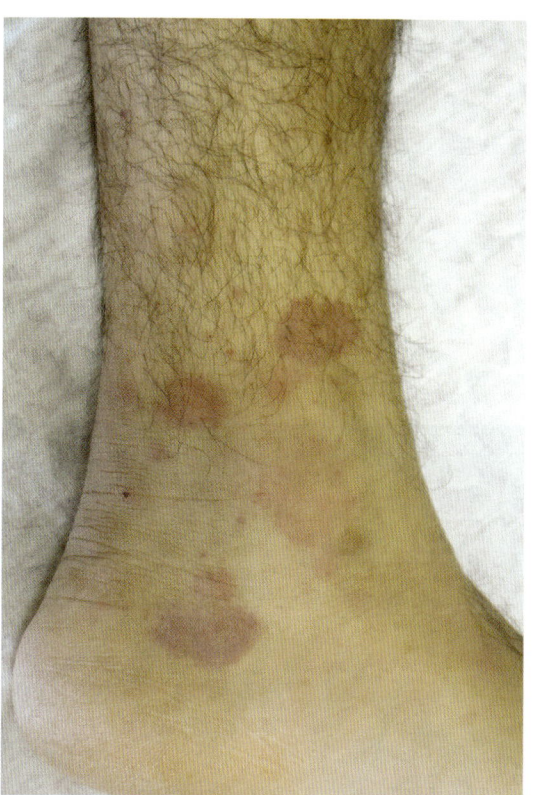

Fig. 35.60 Urticarial vasculitis.

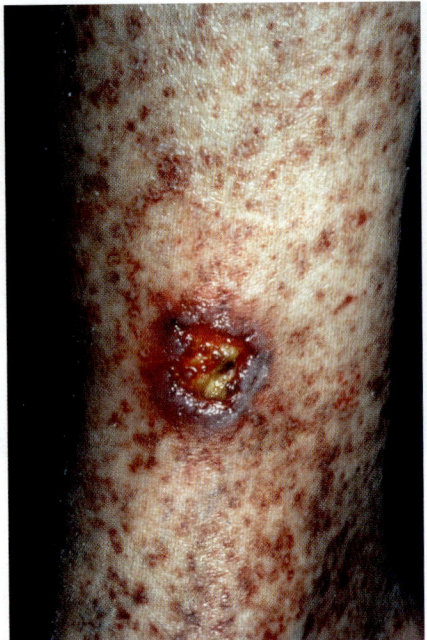

Fig. 35.61 Cryoglobulinemic vasculitis.

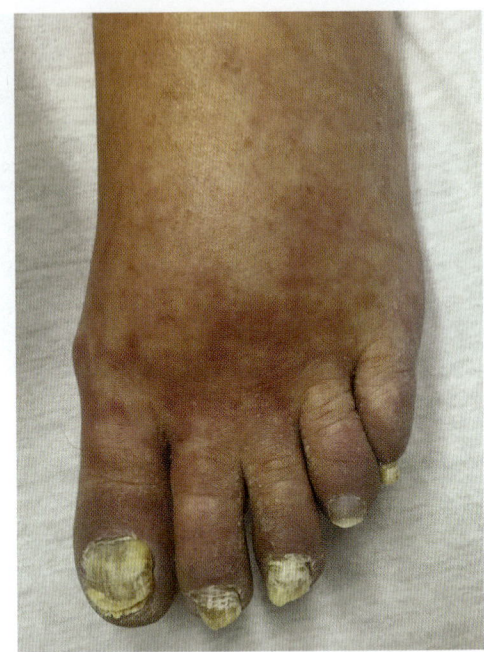

Fig. 35.62 Cryoglobulinemic vasculopathy secondary to multiple myeloma.

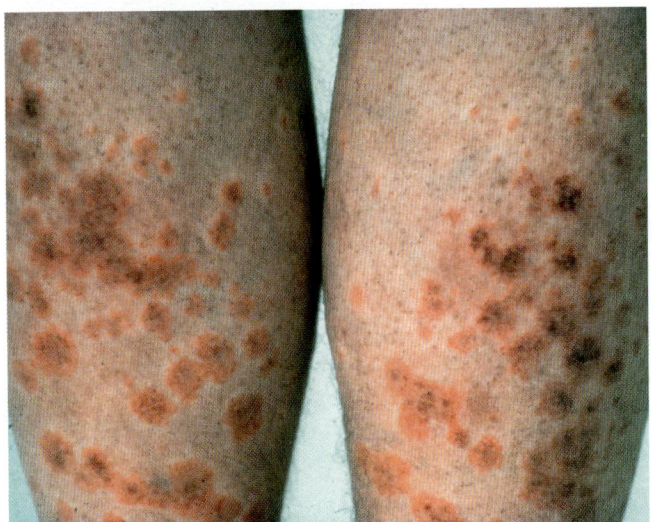

Fig. 35.63 Erythema elevatum diutinum.

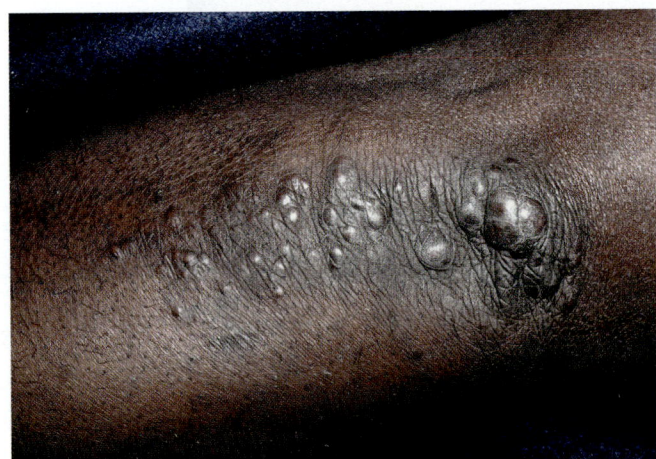

Fig. 35.64 Erythema elevatum diutinum.

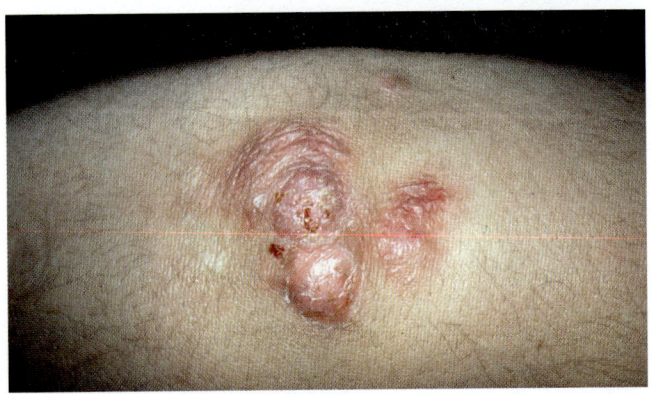

Fig. 35.65 Erythema elevatum diutinum.

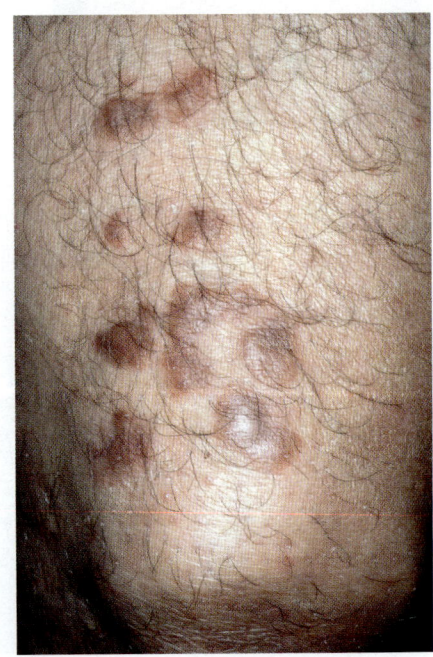

Fig. 35.66 Erythema elevatum diutinum.

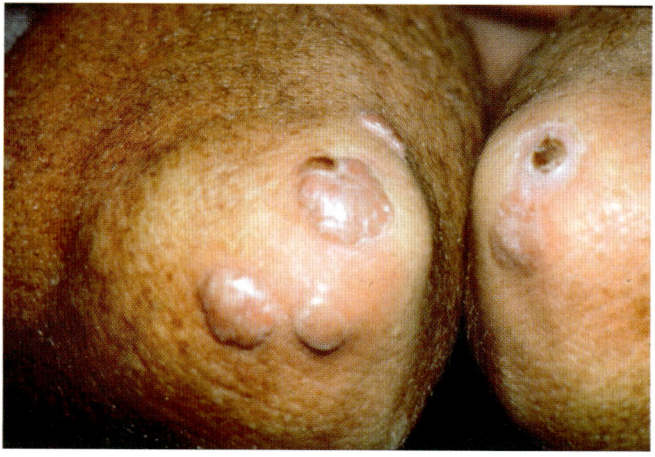

Fig. 35.67 Erythema elevatum diutinum.

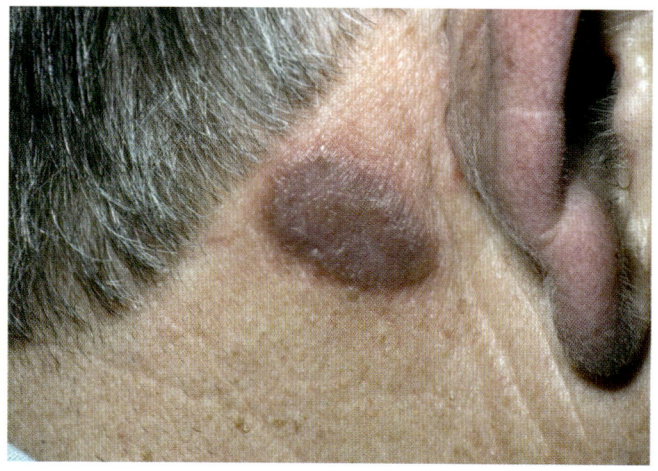

Fig. 35.68 Granuloma faciale. *Courtesy Steven Binnick, MD.*

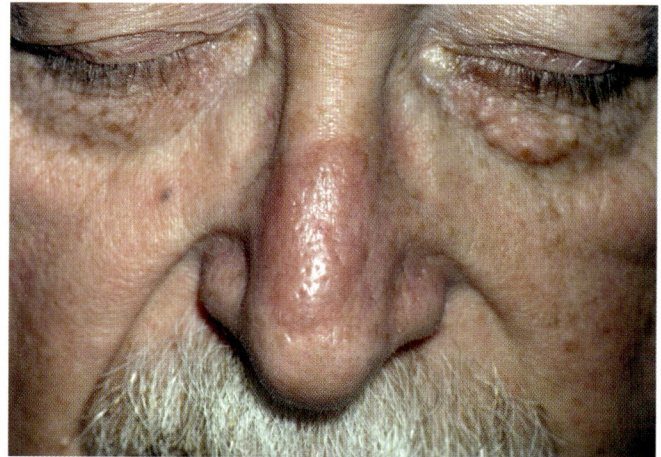

Fig. 35.69 Granuloma faciale. *Courtesy Steven Binnick, MD.*

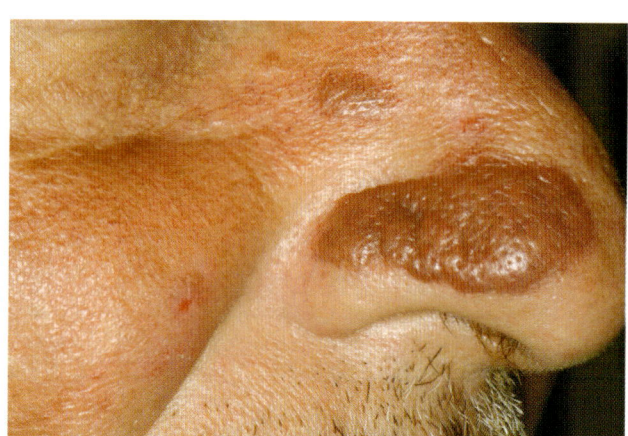

Fig. 35.70 Granuloma faciale.

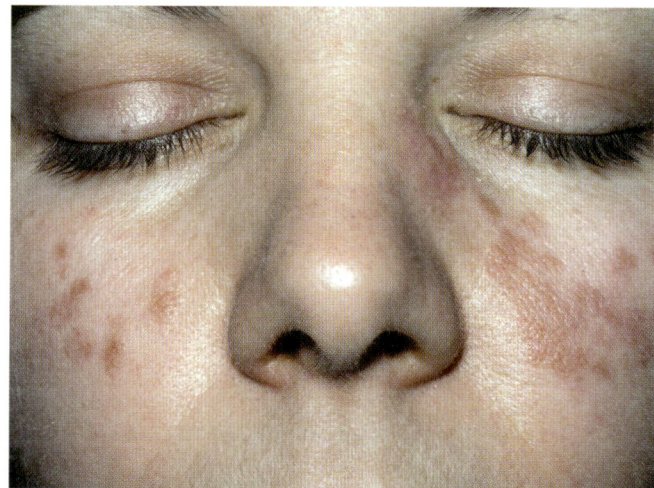

Fig. 35.71 Granuloma faciale.

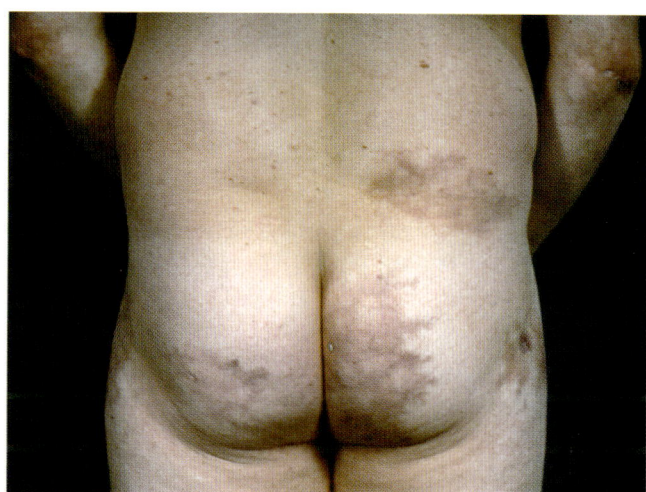

Fig. 35.72 Polyarteritis nodosa.

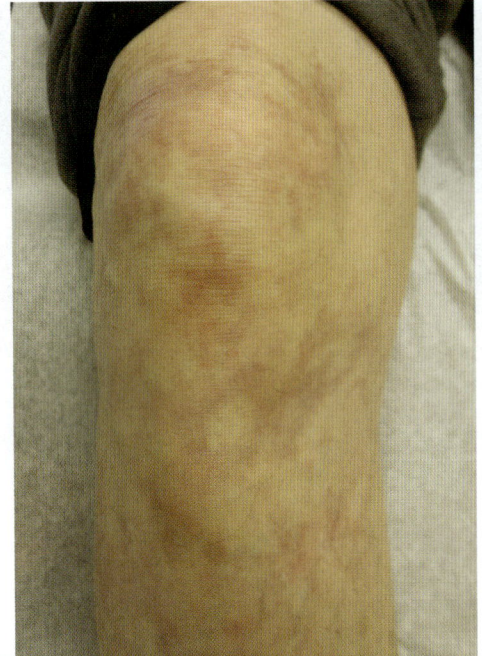

Fig. 35.73 Polyarteritis nodosa.

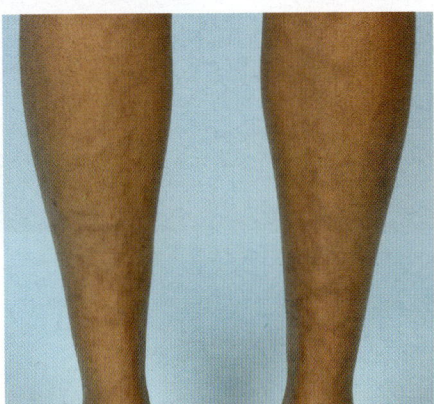

Fig. 35.75 Polyarteritis nodosa.

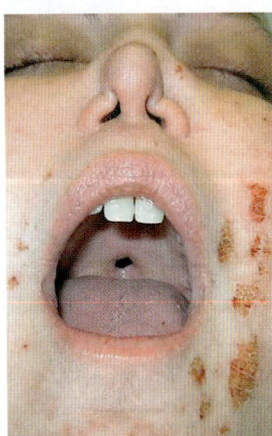

Fig. 35.78 Granulomatosis with polyangiitis. *Courtesy Campbell Stewart, MD.*

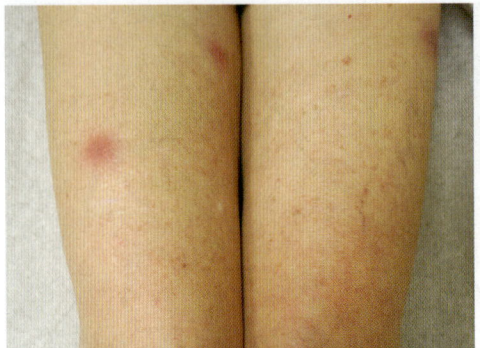

Fig. 35.74 Polyarteritis nodosa.

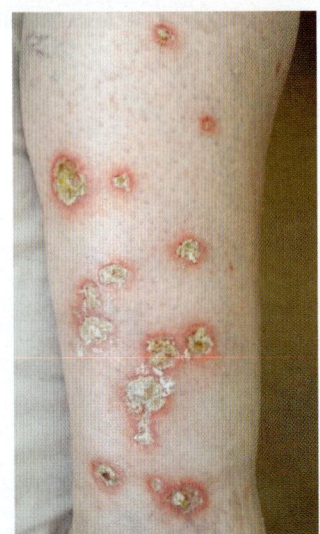

Fig. 35.76 Drug-induced antineutrophil cytoplasmic antibody-positive vasculitis.

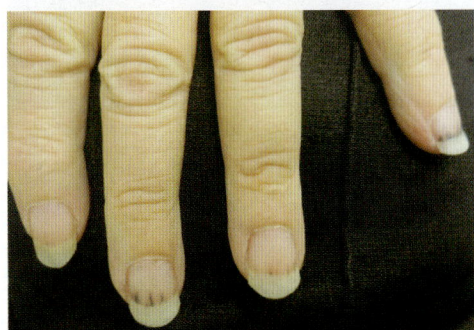

Fig. 35.77 Splinter hemorrhages in granulomatosis with polyangiitis.

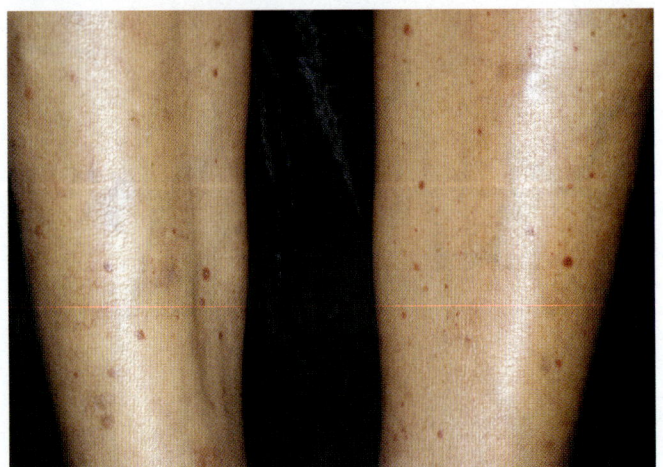

Fig. 35.79 Granulomatosis with polyangiitis.

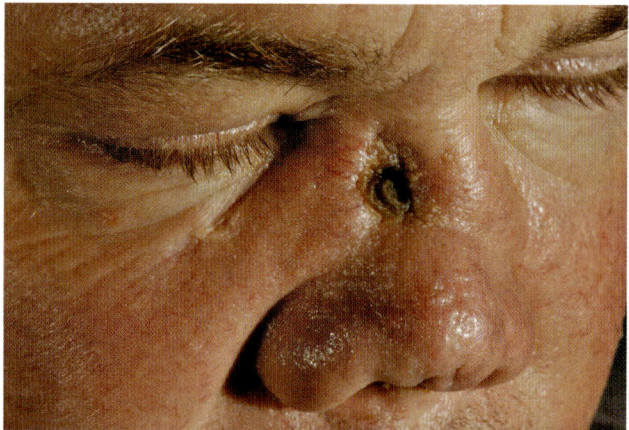

Fig. 35.80 Granulomatosis with polyangiitis. *Courtesy Curt Samlaska, MD.*

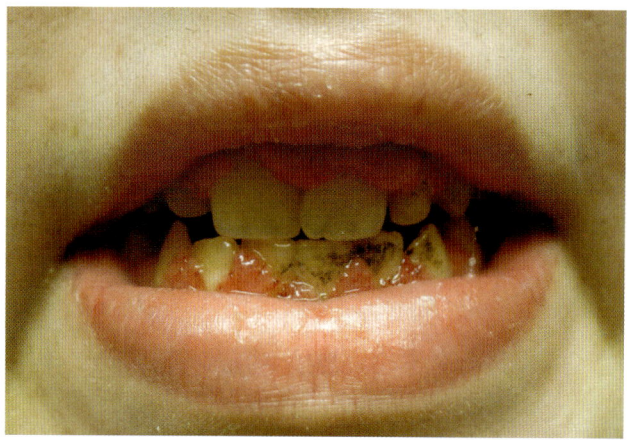

Fig. 35.81 Strawberry gingiva in granulomatosis with polyangiitis.

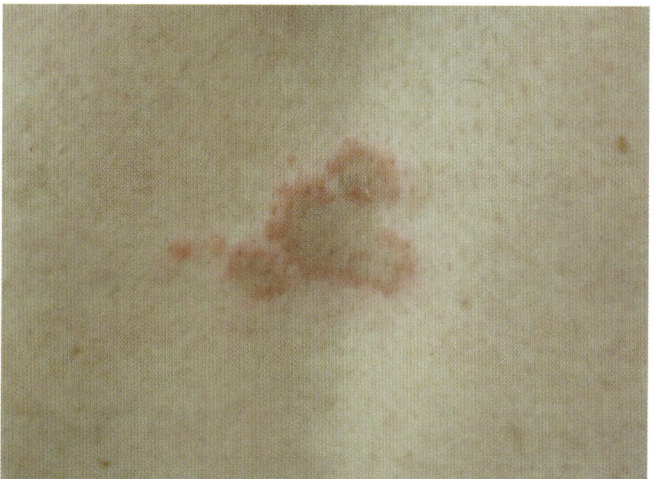

Fig. 35.82 Urticarial plaques in a patient with eosinophilic granulomatosis with polyangiitis.

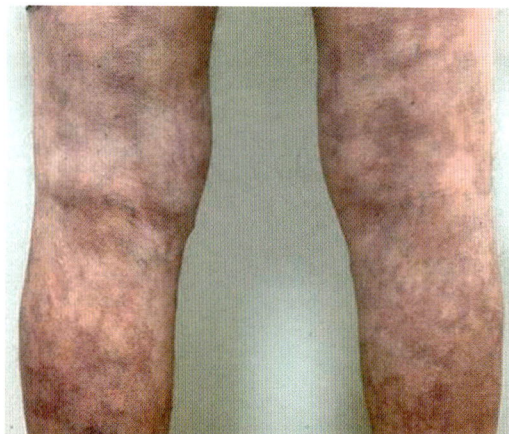

Fig. 35.83 Eosinophilic granulomatosis with polyangiitis.

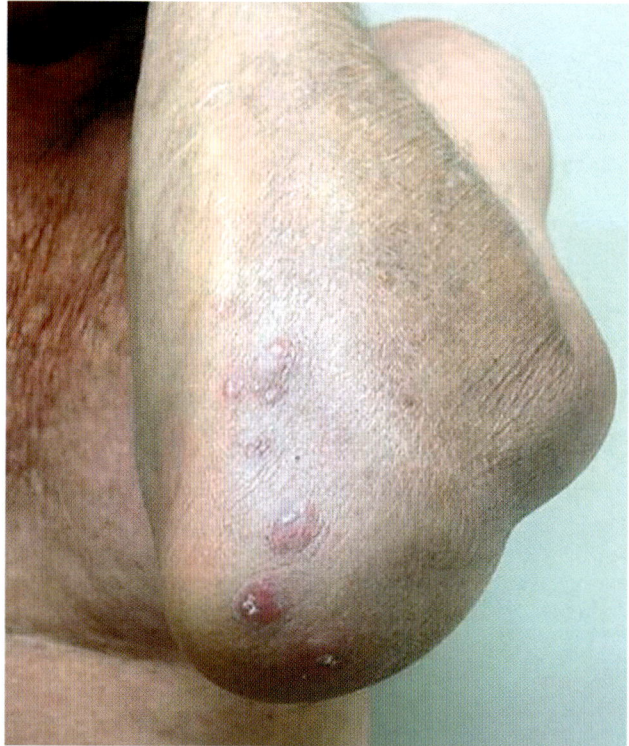

Fig. 35.84 Churg-Strauss nodules in eosinophilic granulomatosis with polyangiitis.

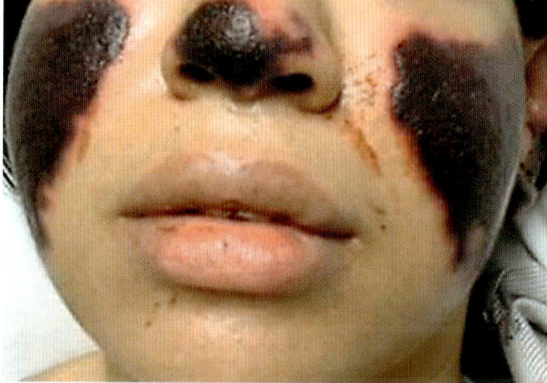

Fig. 35.85 Levamisole-induced vasculopathy. *Courtesy Antoine Sreih, MD.*

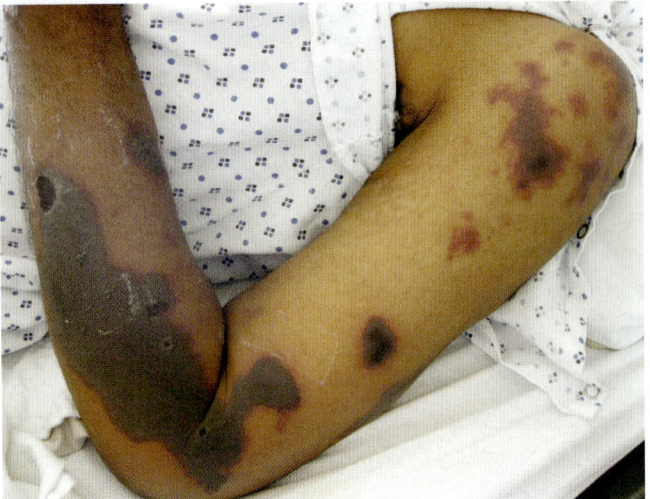

Fig. 35.86 Levamisole-induced vasculopathy. *Courtesy Misha Rosenbach, MD.*

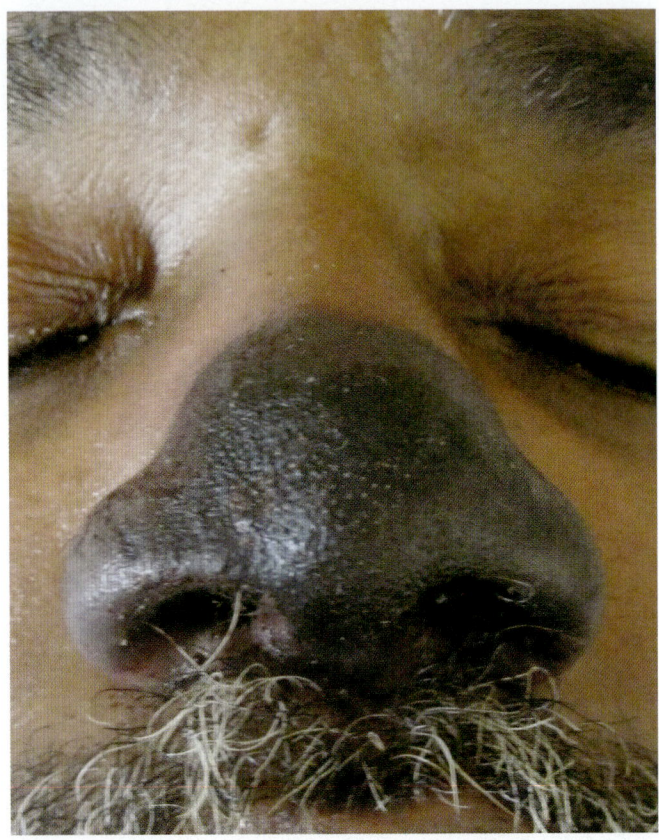

Fig. 35.87 Levamisole-induced vasculopathy. *Courtesy Misha Rosenbach, MD.*

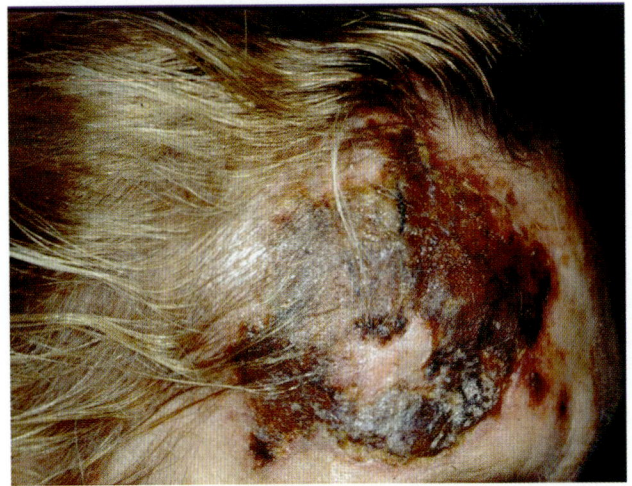

Fig. 35.88 Temporal arteritis.

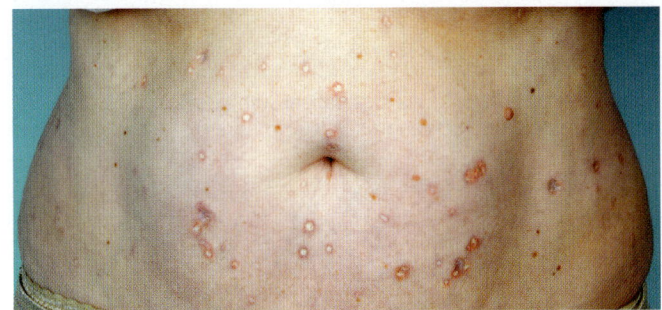

Fig. 35.89 Degos disease.

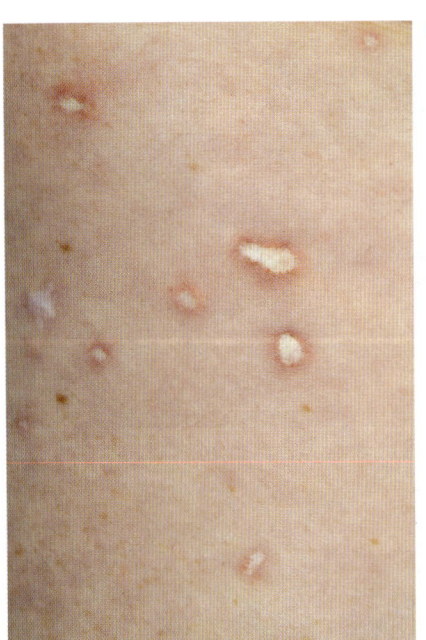

Fig. 35.90 Degos disease.

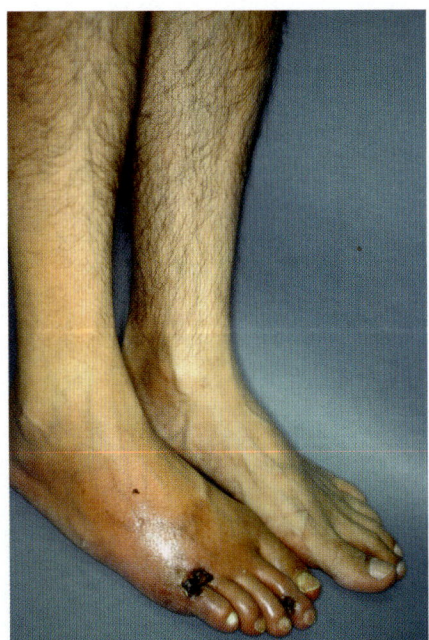

Fig. 35.91 Buerger disease.

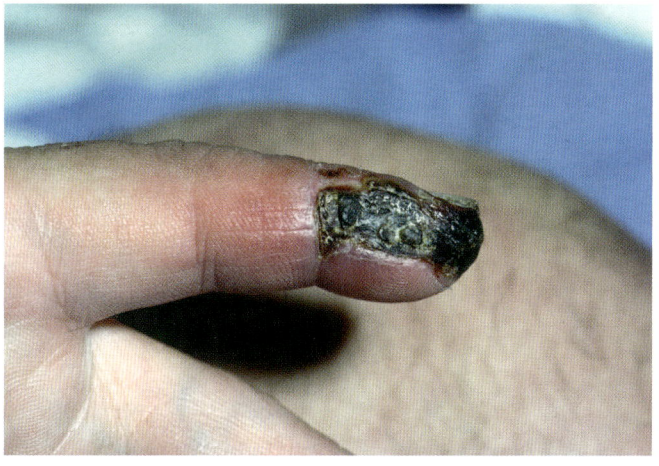

Fig. 35.92 Buerger disease.

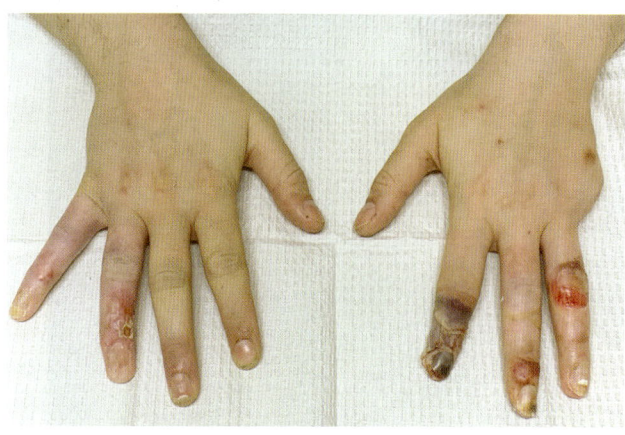

Fig. 35.93 Cannabis arteritis.

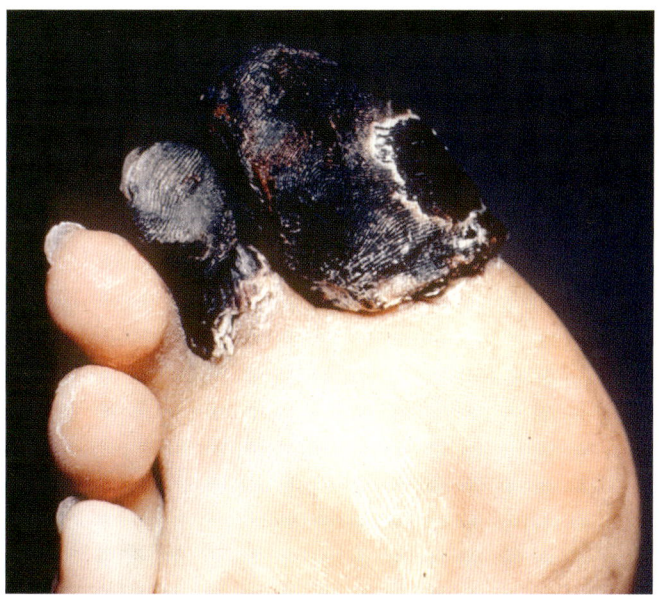

Fig. 35.94 Arteriosclerosis obliterans.

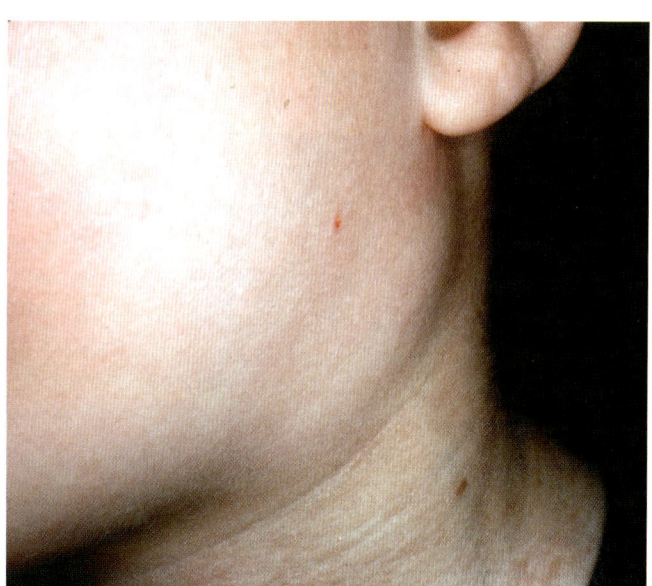

Fig. 35.95 Kawasaki disease.

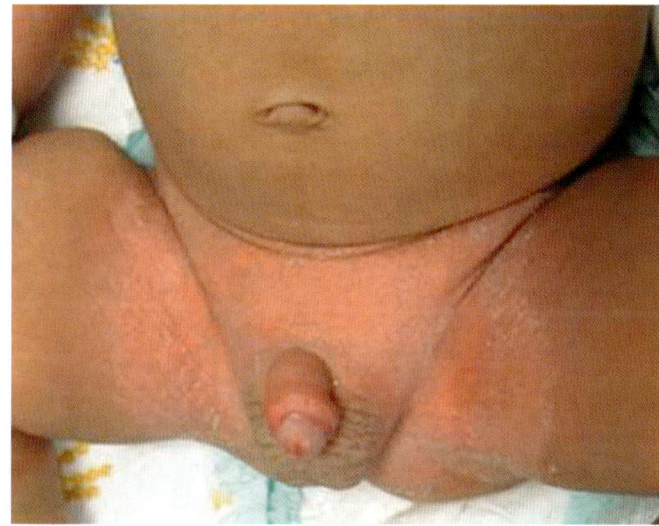

Fig. 35.96 Kawasaki disease.

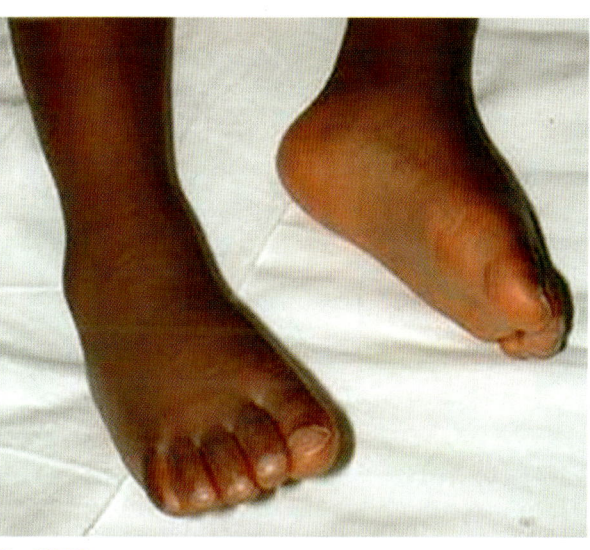

Fig. 35.97 Kawasaki disease.

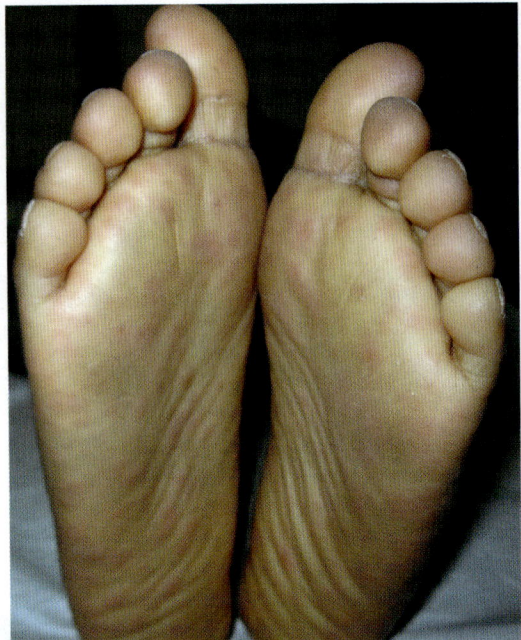
Fig. 35.98 Kawasaki disease.

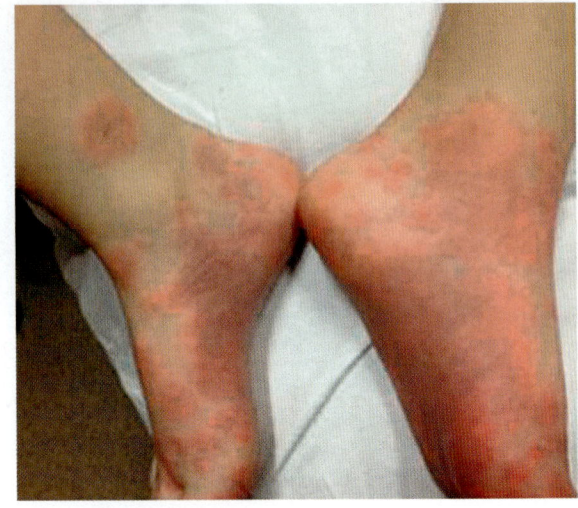
Fig. 35.99 Kawasaki disease.

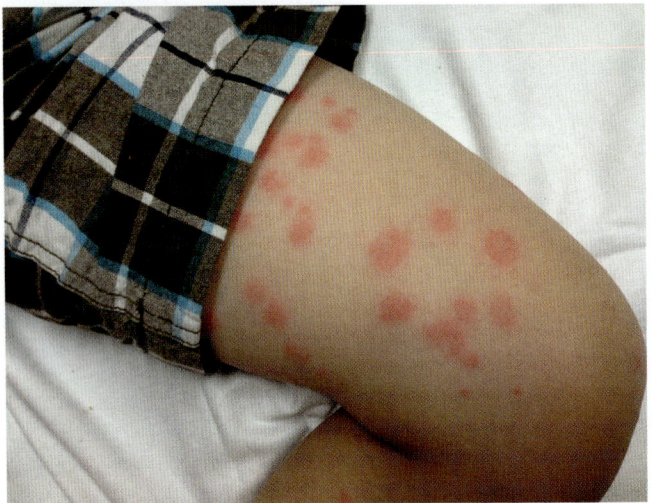
Fig. 35.100 Kawasaki disease.

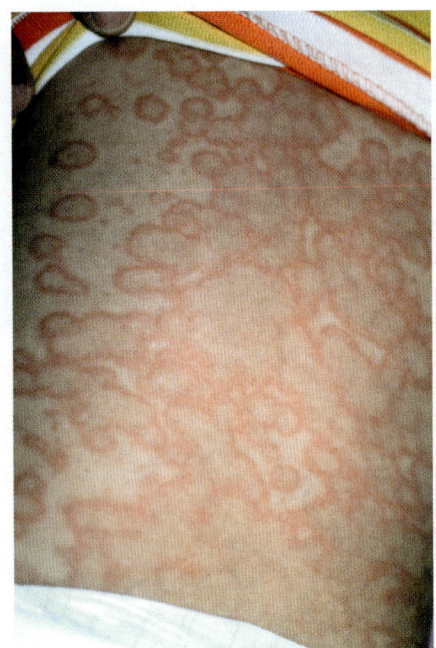
Fig. 35.101 Kawasaki disease.

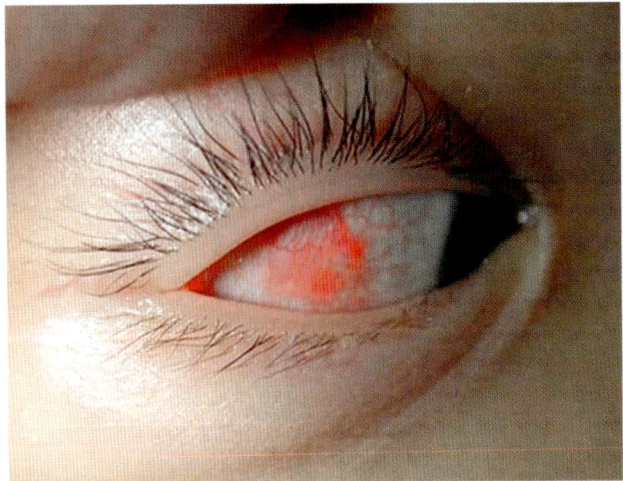
Fig. 35.102 Kawasaki disease.

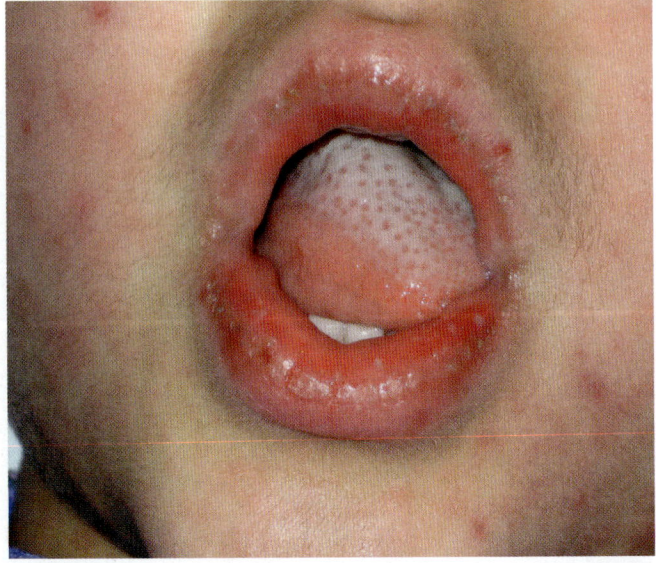
Fig. 35.103 Kawasaki disease.

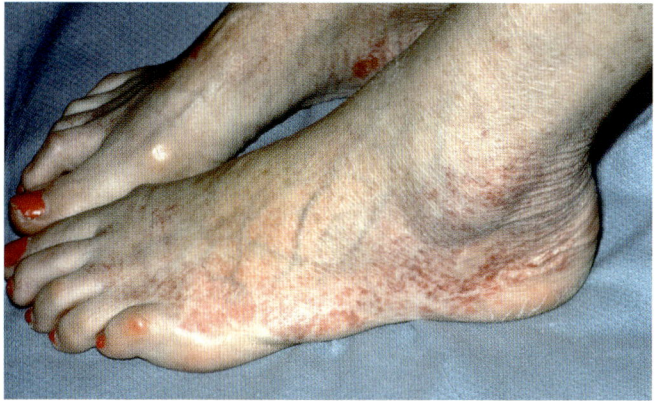

Fig. 35.104 Generalized essential telangiectasia.

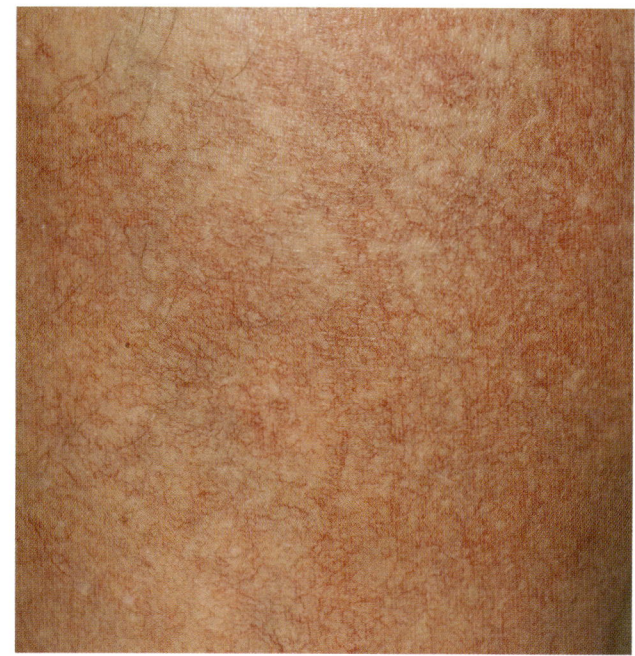

Fig. 35.105 Cutaneous collagenous vasculopathy.

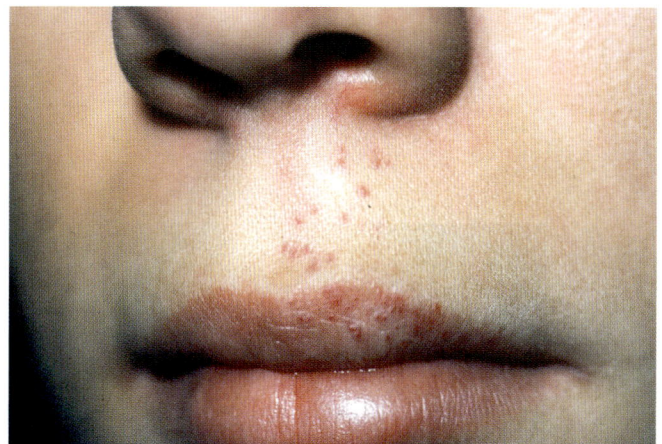

Fig. 35.106 Unilateral nevoid telangiectasia.

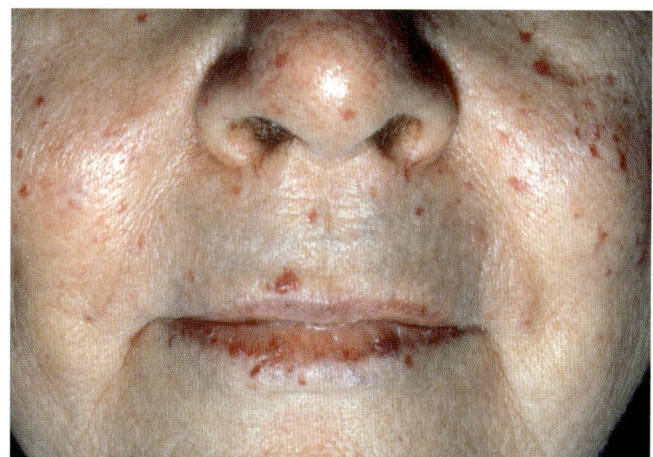

Fig. 35.107 Osler-Weber-Rendu disease.

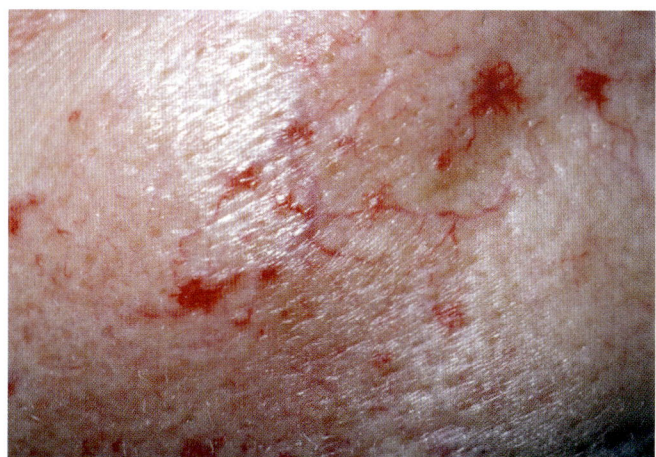

Fig. 35.108 Osler-Weber-Rendu disease.

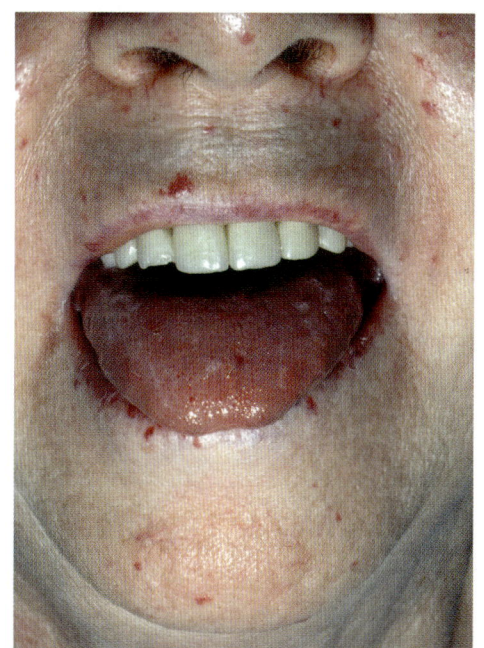

Fig. 35.109 Osler-Weber-Rendu disease.

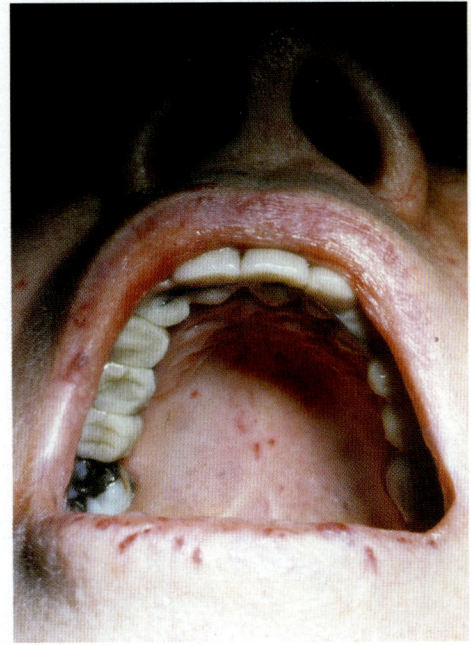

Fig. 35.110 Osler-Weber-Rendu disease.

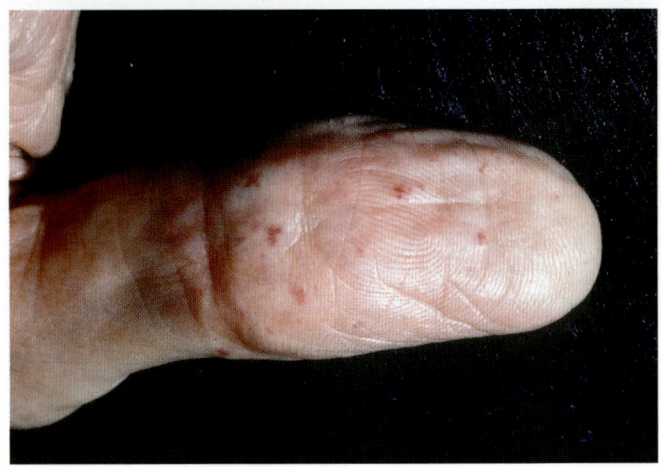

Fig. 35.111 Osler-Weber-Rendu disease.

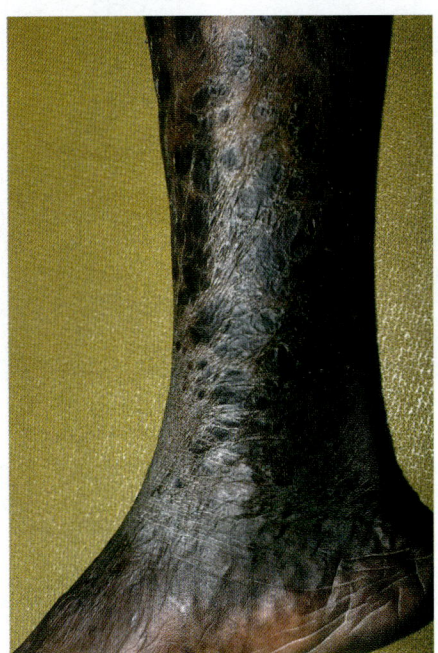

Fig. 35.112 Stasis dermatitis.

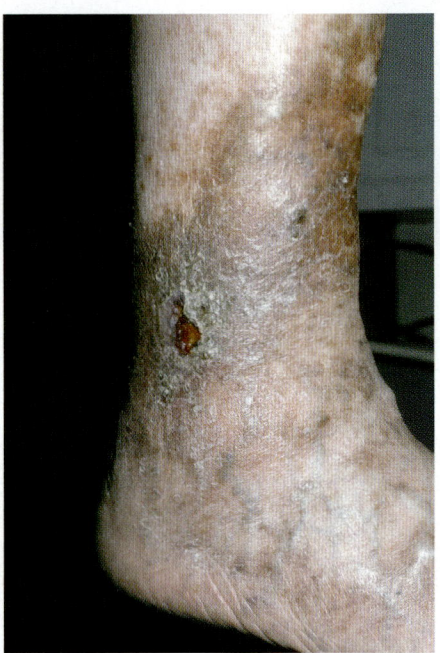

Fig. 35.113 Stasis dermatitis with early ulceration.

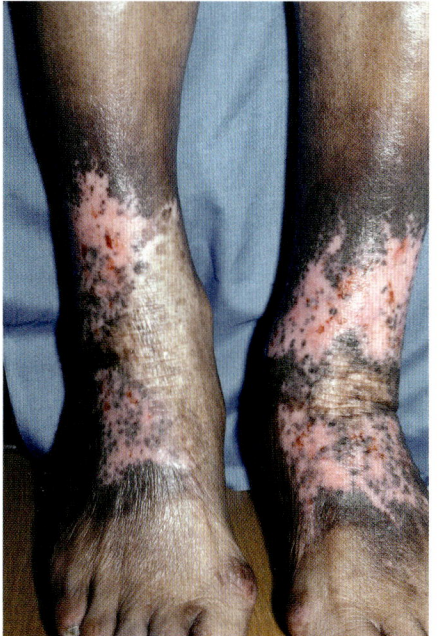

Fig. 35.114 Stasis dermatitis.

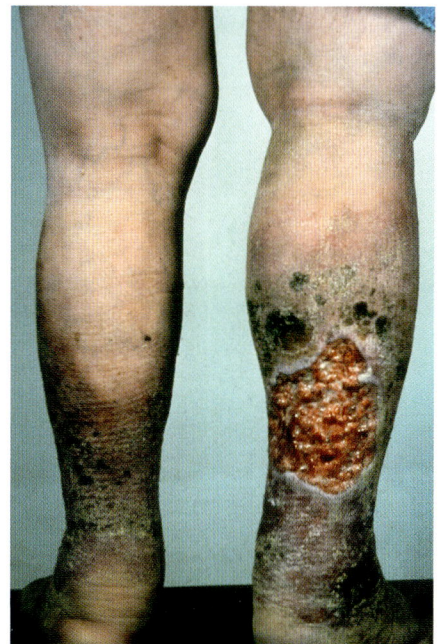

Fig. 35.115 Stasis dermatitis with ulceration.

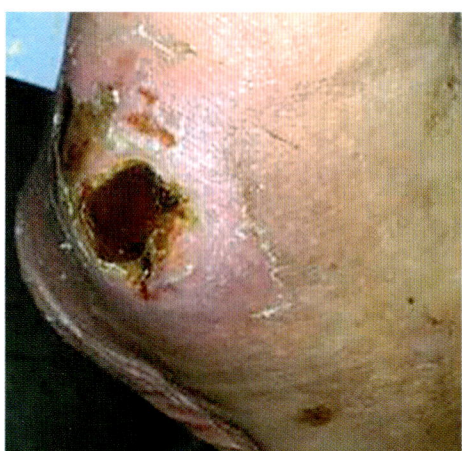

Fig. 35.116 Arterial ulceration.

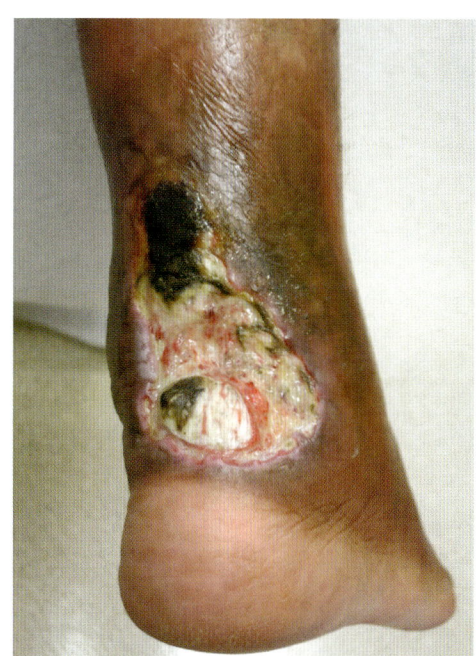

Fig. 35.117 Martorell hypertensive-ischemic ulcer.

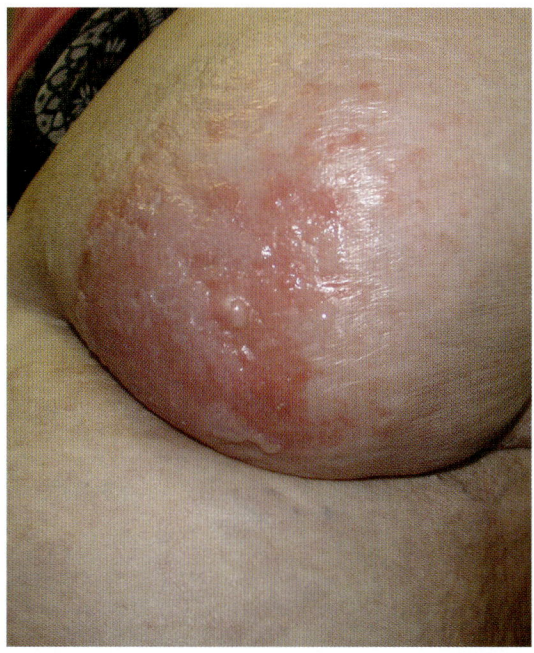

Fig. 35.118 Obesity-related lymphedema.

Disturbances of Pigmentation 36

Pigmentary disorders of the skin may present with depigmentation, hypopigmentation, or hyperpigmentation. The color, morphology, and distribution of the lesions help to suggest the correct diagnosis. Vitiligo may be segmental (blaschkoid), acral (lips and tips), or truncal in distribution. Each presentation has implications for treatment. The lesions of vitiligo must be distinguished from those of pityriasis alba, hypopigmented mycosis fungoides, leprosy, and the confetti-like depigmentation and ash-leaf macules of tuberous sclerosis. Hyperpigmented lesions cover a similar spectrum of disorders from lichenoid dermatoses to melasma and the café-au-lait macules of neurofibromatosis. This section of the atlas will focus on disorders of pigmentation not found in other chapters of the book, including vitiligo, piebaldism, pigmentary demarcation lines, melasma, and Galli-Galli disease. A Wood's lamp is of value in these disorders, as accentuation of the pigment suggests epidermal pigment alternation, whereas a decrease in the appearance of the pigmentary anomaly suggests dermal pigment deposition. Topical treatments can address many forms of epidermal dyspigmentation, whereas laser treatment is often more appropriate for the treatment of dermal pigment. When the clinical examination fails to provide a specific diagnosis, addition of a directed history or biopsy may be required. Fontana staining indicates the presence of melanin, and immunostains such as Mart-1 and Sox-10 confirm the pattern and distribution of melanocytes within the lesion.

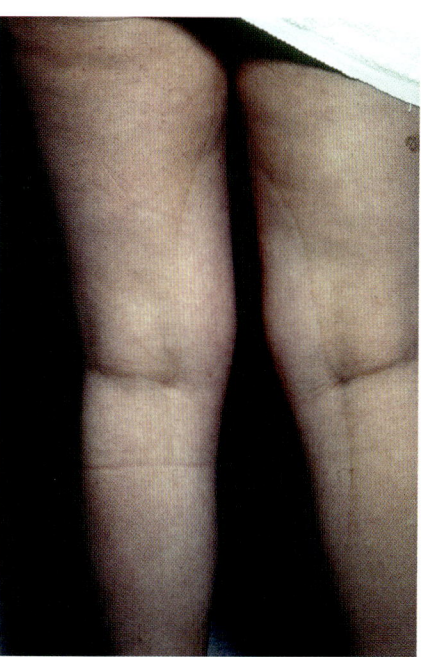

Fig. 36.2 Type B pigmentary demarcation lines

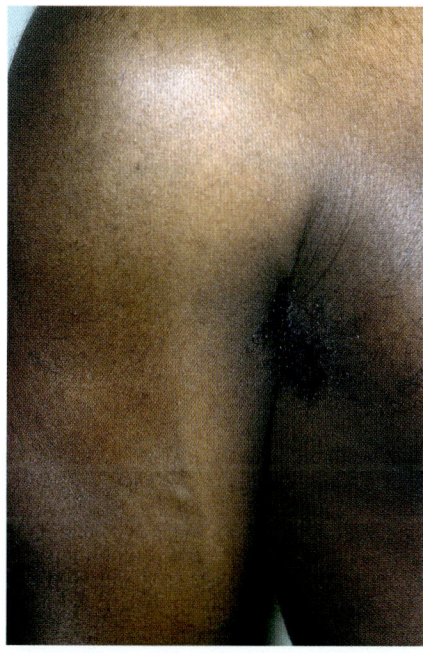

Fig. 36.1 Type A pigmentary demarcation.

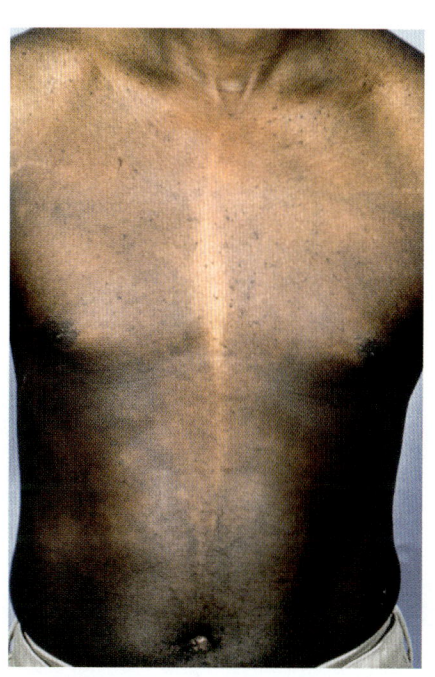

Fig. 36.3 Type C pigmentary demarcation.

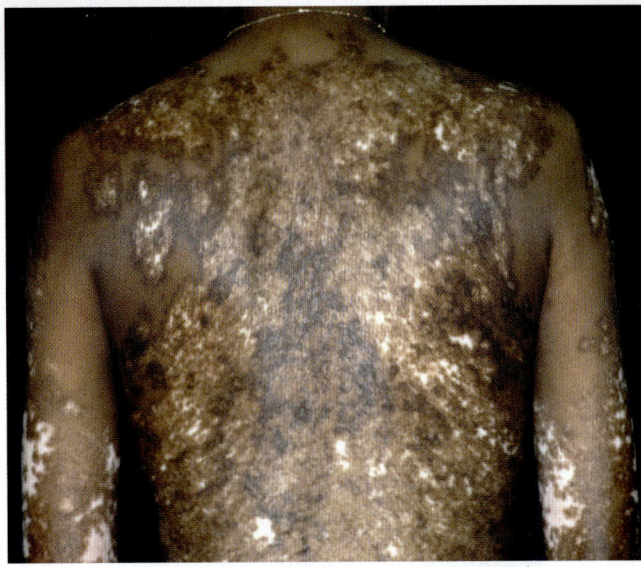

Fig. 36.4 Postinflammatory dyspigmentation secondary to lupus erythematosus.

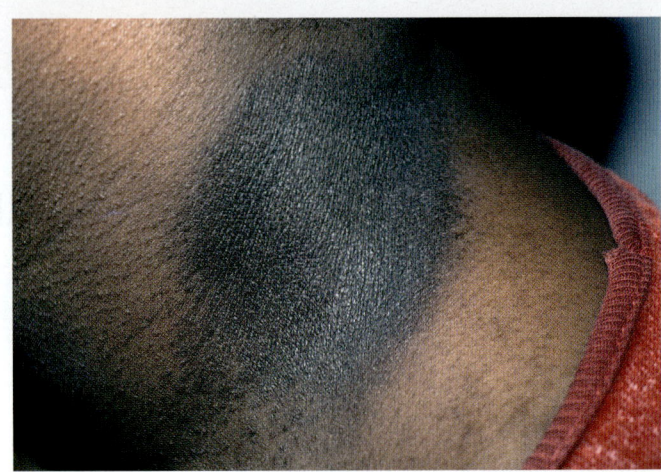

Fig. 36.5 Postinflammatory hyperpigmentation. *Courtesy Steven Binnick, MD.*

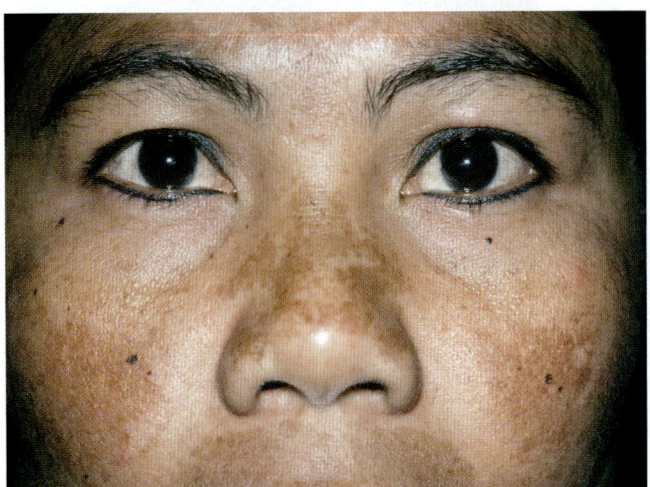

Fig. 36.6 Melasma.

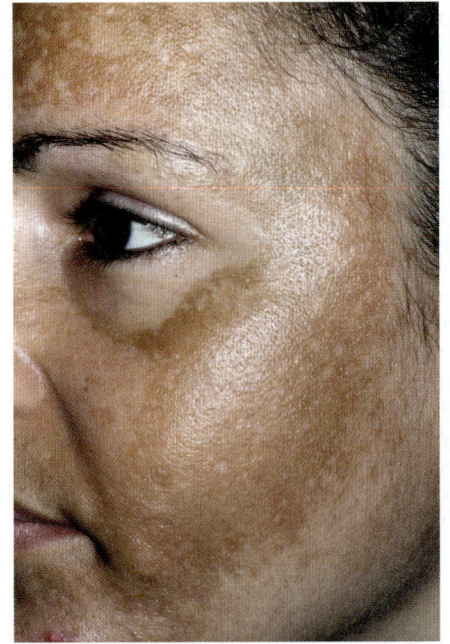

Fig. 36.7 Melasma.

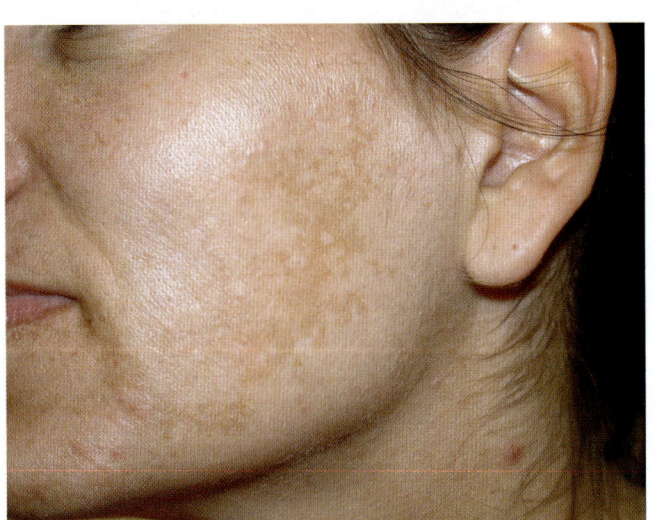

Fig. 36.8 Melasma.

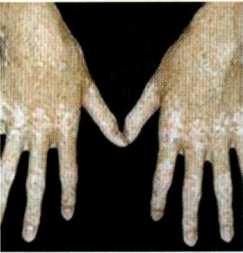

Fig. 36.9 Dyschromatosis symmetrica hereditaria. *Courtesy Department of Dermatology, Keio University, School of Medicine, Tokyo, Japan.*

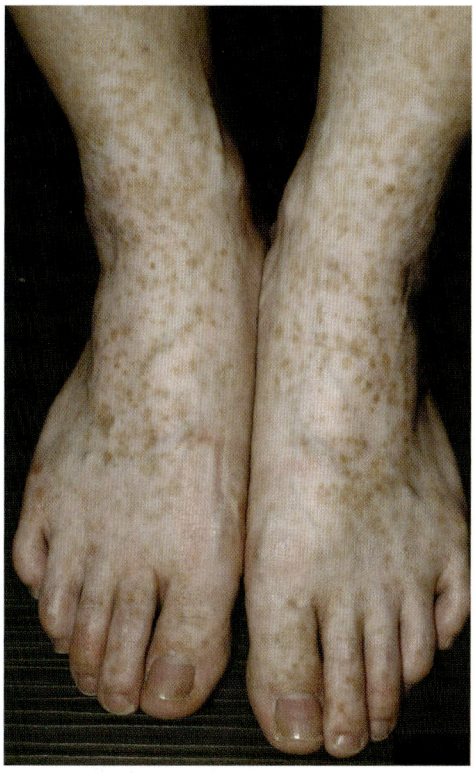

Fig. 36.10 Dyschromatosis symmetrica hereditaria. *Courtesy National Cheng Kung University, Taiwan.*

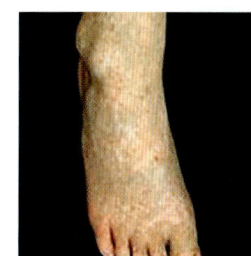

Fig. 36.11 Dyschromatosis symmetrica hereditaria. *Courtesy Department of Dermatology, Keio University, School of Medicine, Tokyo, Japan.*

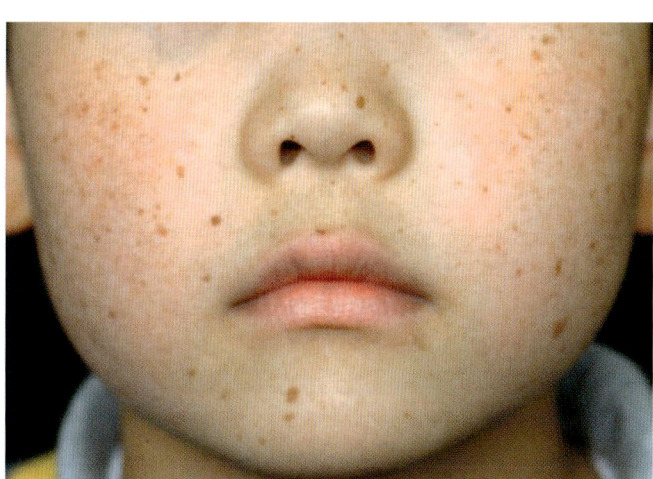

Fig. 36.12 Dyschromatosis symmetrica hereditaria. *Courtesy Department of Dermatology, Keio University, School of Medicine, Tokyo, Japan.*

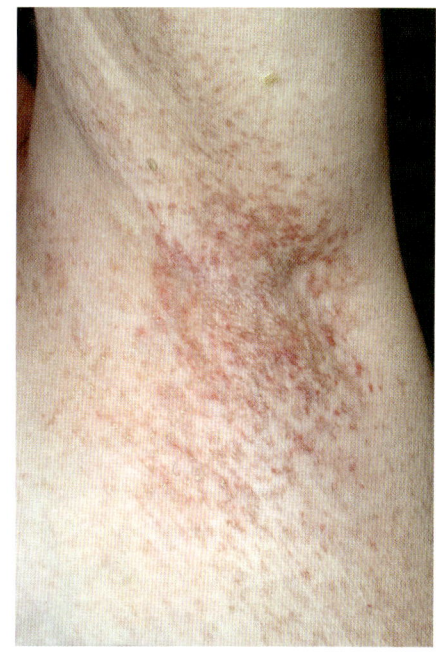

Fig. 36.13 Galli-Galli disease.

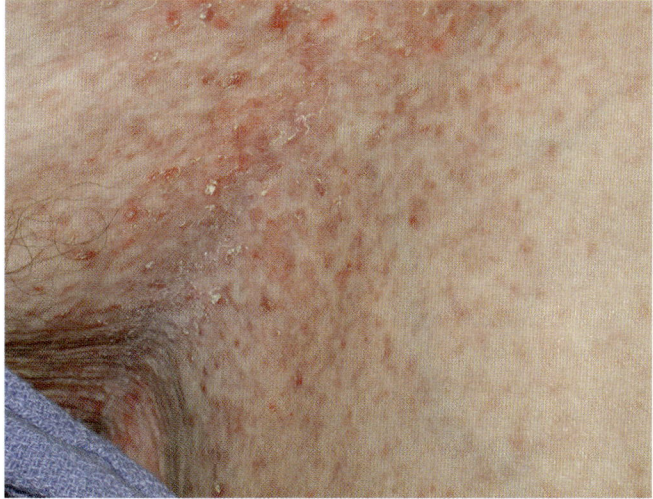

Fig. 36.14 Galli-Galli disease.

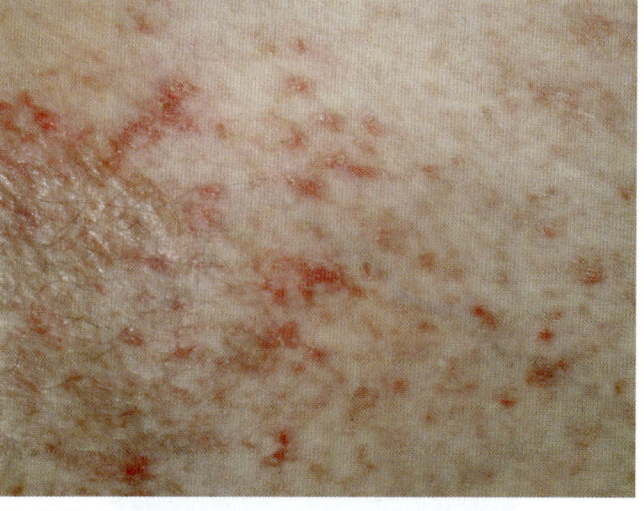

Fig. 36.15 Galli-Galli disease.

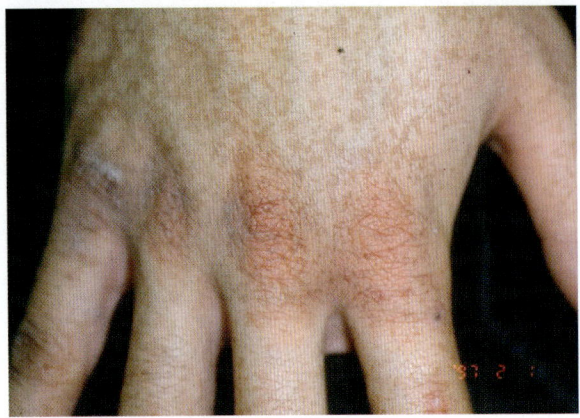

Fig. 36.16 Reticulate acropigmentation of Kitamura. *Courtesy Department of Dermatology, Keio University, School of Medicine, Tokyo, Japan.*

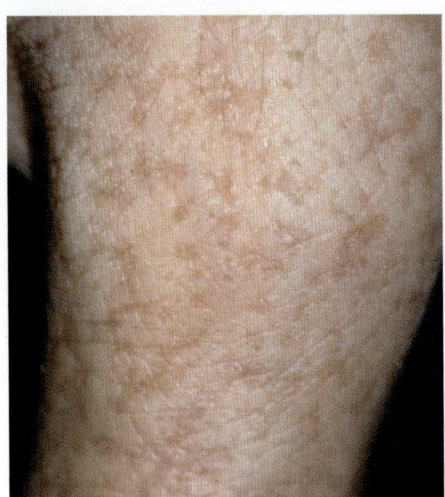

Fig. 36.17 Reticulate acropigmentation of Kitamura. *Courtesy Department of Dermatology, Keio University, School of Medicine, Tokyo, Japan.*

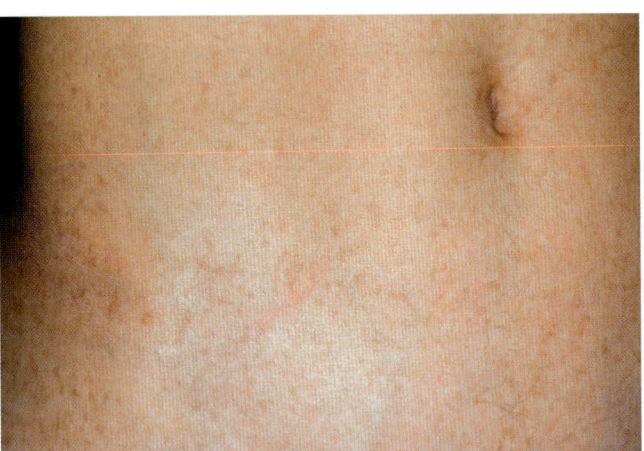

Fig. 36.18 Dermatopathia pigmentosa reticularis.

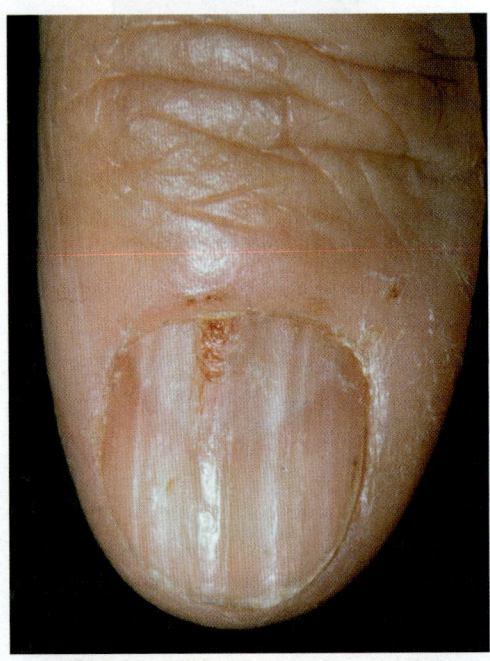

Fig. 36.19 Dermatopathia pigmentosa reticularis.

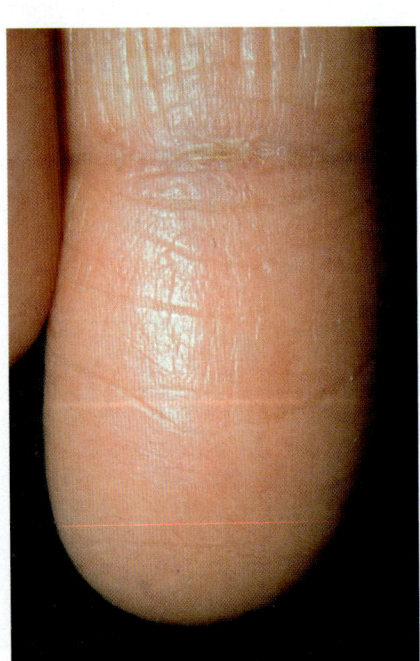

Fig. 36.20 Dermatopathia pigmentosa reticularis.

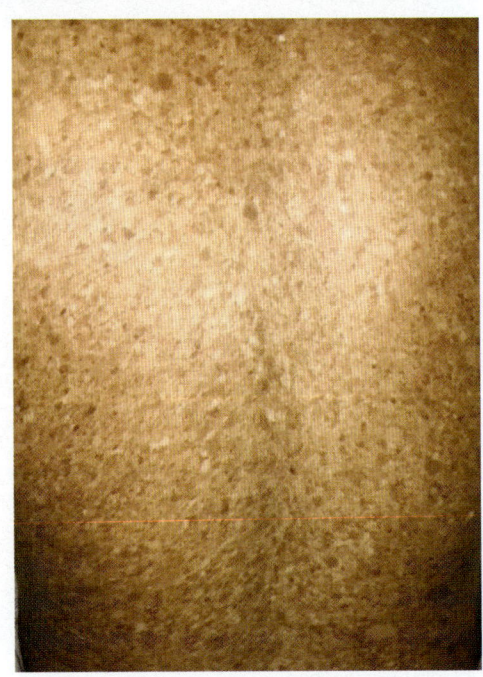

Fig. 36.21 Back of a patient with dyschromatosis universalis hereditaria.

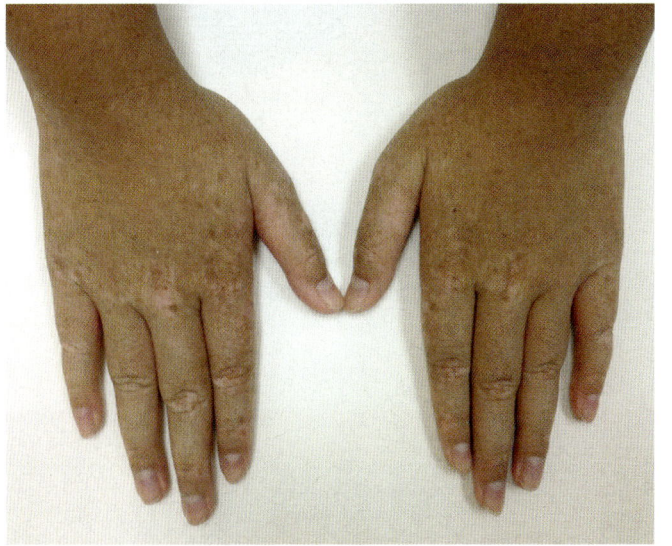

Fig. 36.22 Dyschromatosis universalis hereditaria. *Courtesy Vasanop Vachiramon, MD.*

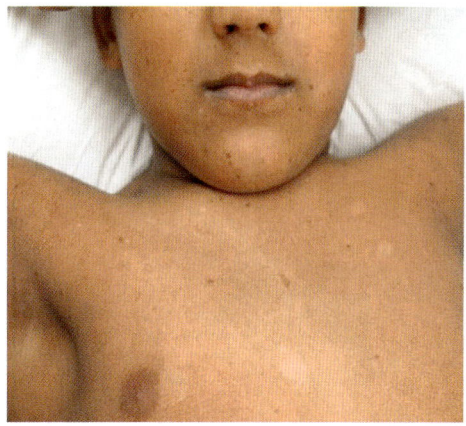

Fig. 36.23 Familial progressive hypopigmentation and hyperpigmentation (*KITLG* mutation). *Courtesy Lara Wine-Lee, MD, PhD.*

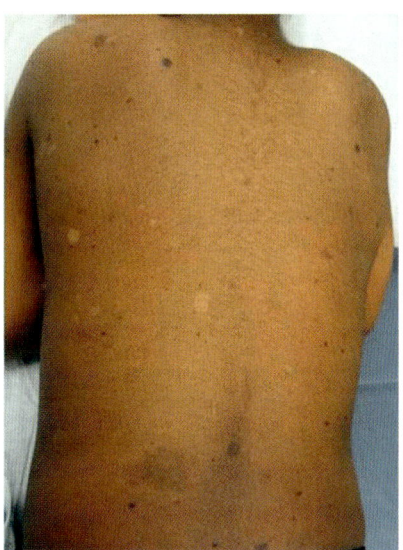

Fig. 36.24 Familial progressive hypopigmentation and hyperpigmentation (*KITLG* mutation). *Courtesy Lara Wine-Lee, MD, PhD.*

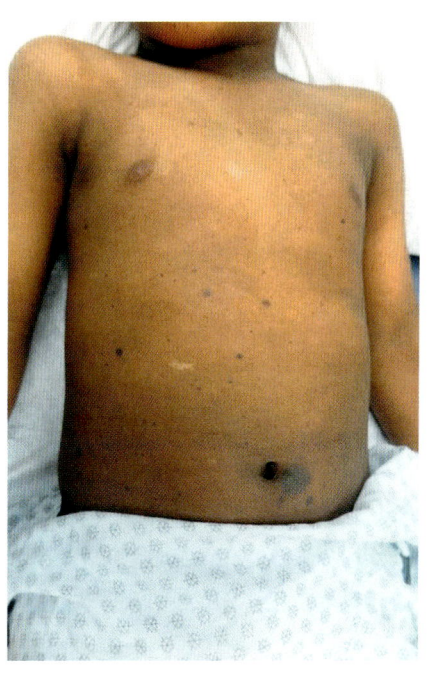

Fig. 36.25 Familial progressive hypopigmentation and hyperpigmentation (*KITLG* mutation). *Courtesy Lara Wine-Lee, MD, PhD.*

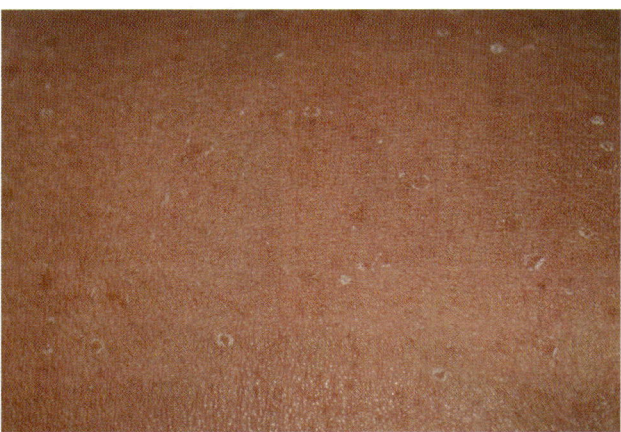

Fig. 36.26 Transient neonatal pustular melanosis.

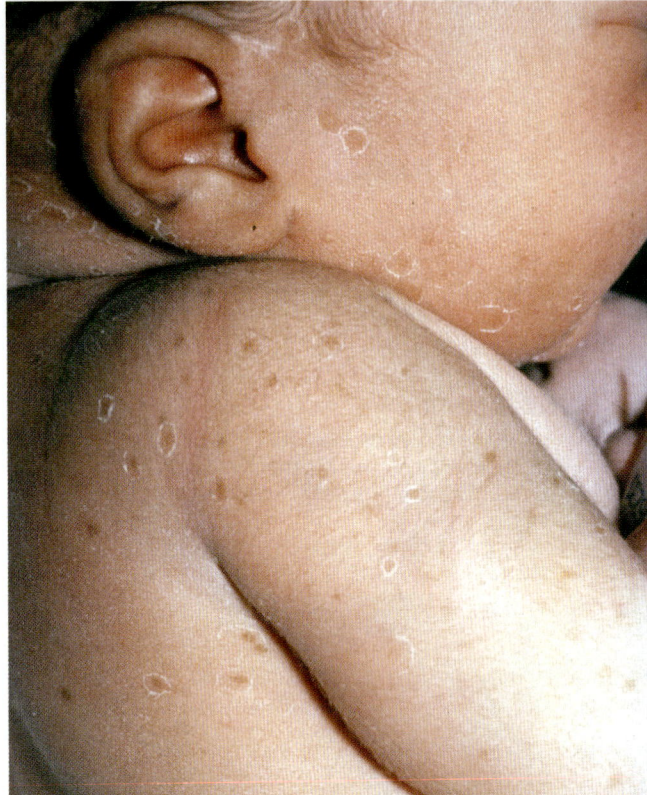

Fig. 36.27 Transient neonatal pustular melanosis.

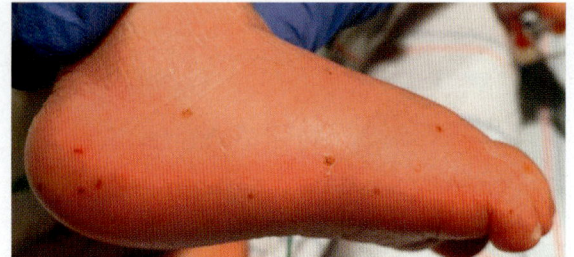

Fig. 36.28 Transient neonatal pustular melanosis.

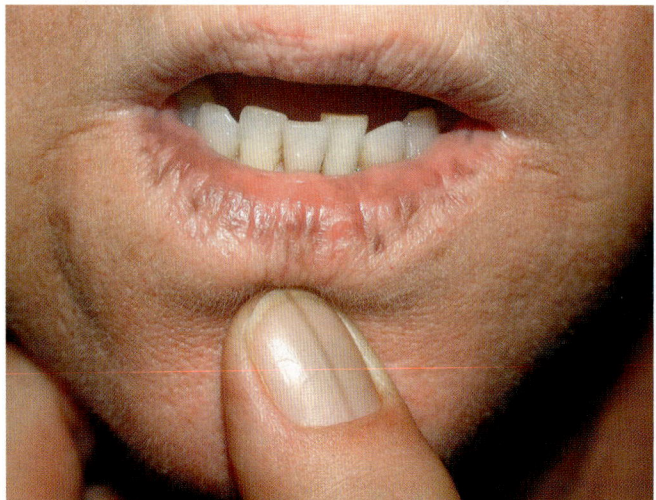

Fig. 36.30 Laugier-Hunziker syndrome.

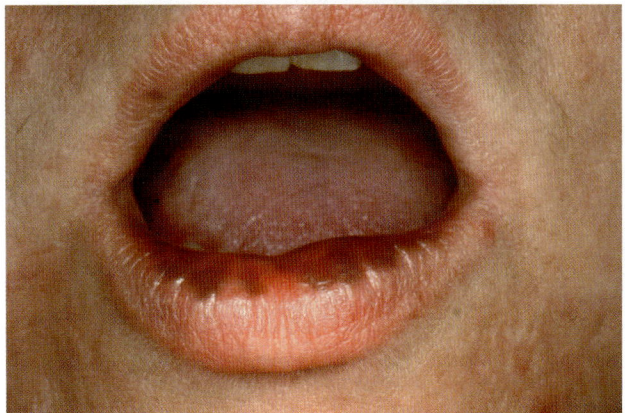

Fig. 36.29 Peutz-Jeghers syndrome. *Courtesy The University of Utah and Oregon Health Sciences University Leonard Swinyer MD image collection.*

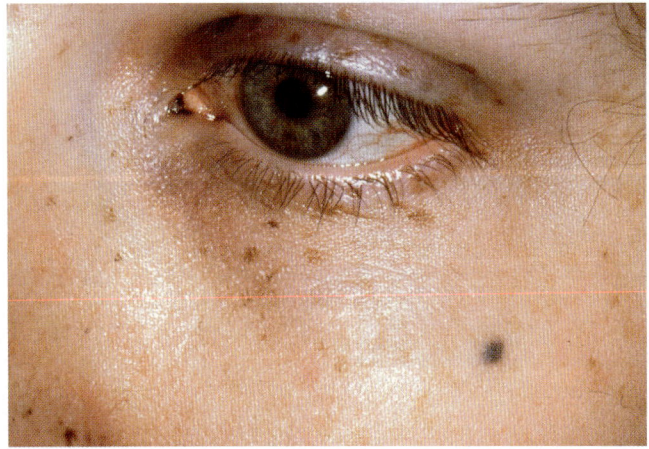

Fig. 36.31 Carney syndrome.

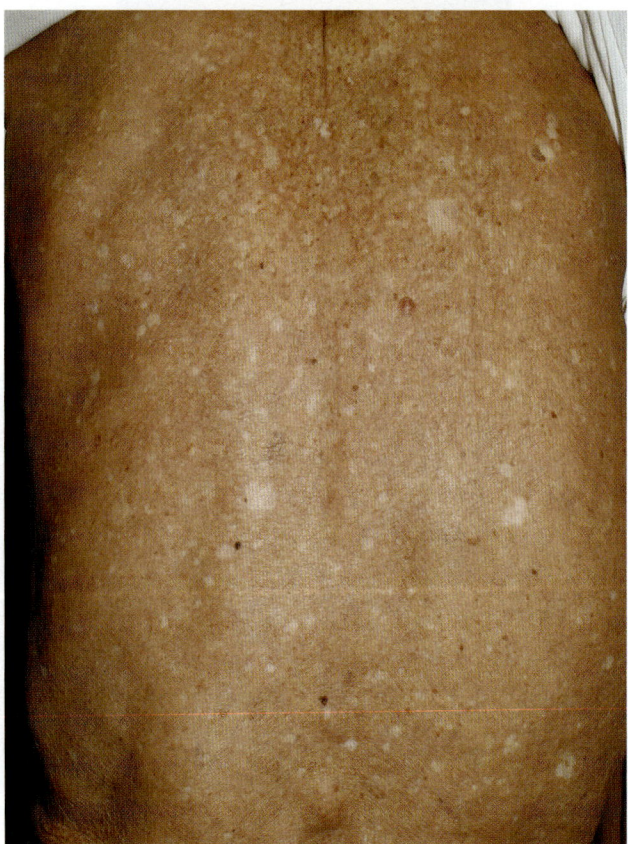

Fig. 36.32 Arsenic-induced leukomelanosis. *Courtesy National Cheng Kung University, Taiwan.*

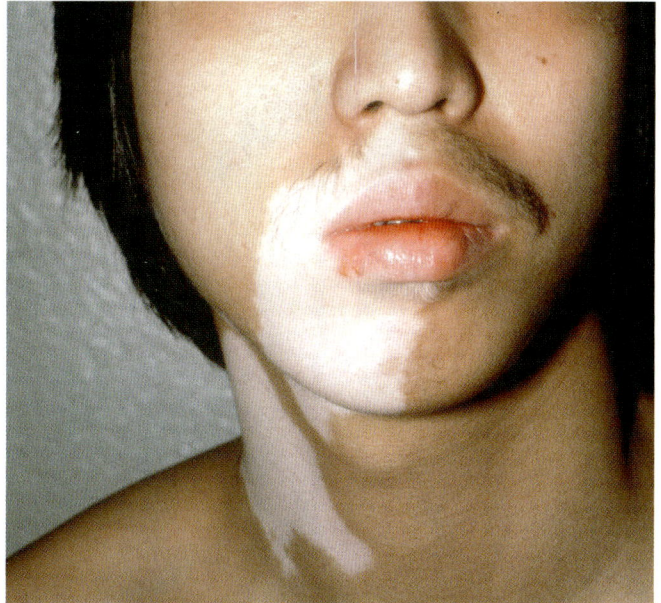

Fig. 36.33 Segmental vitiligo.

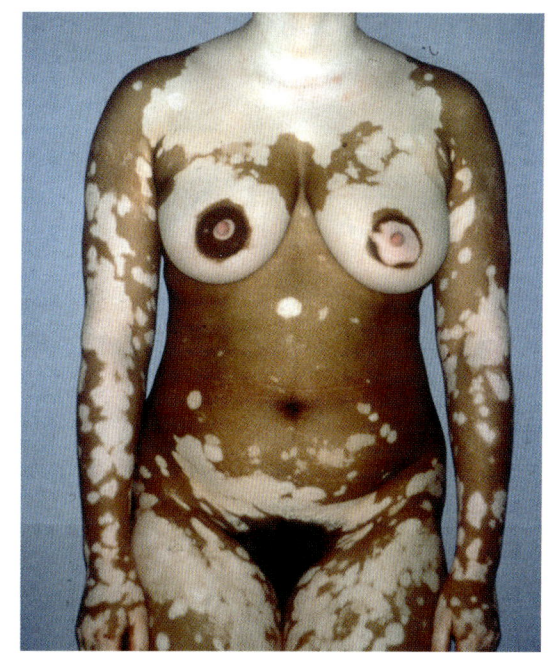

Fig. 36.34 Vitiligo.

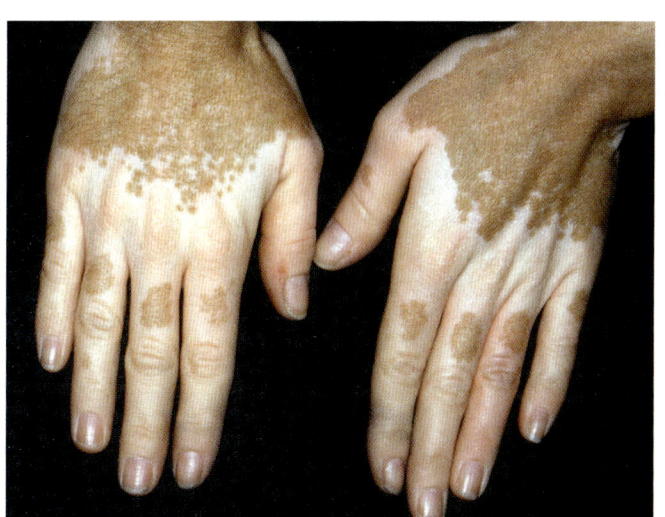

Fig. 36.35 Vitiligo.

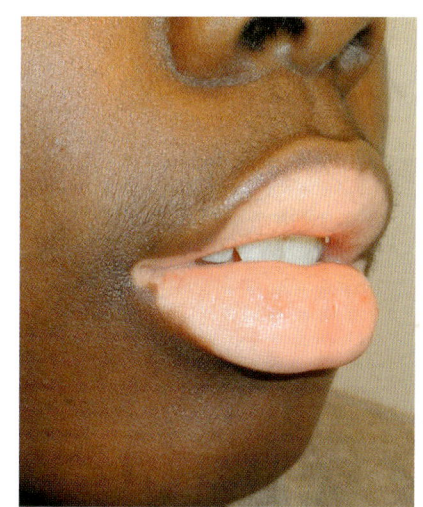

Fig. 36.36 Vitiligo.

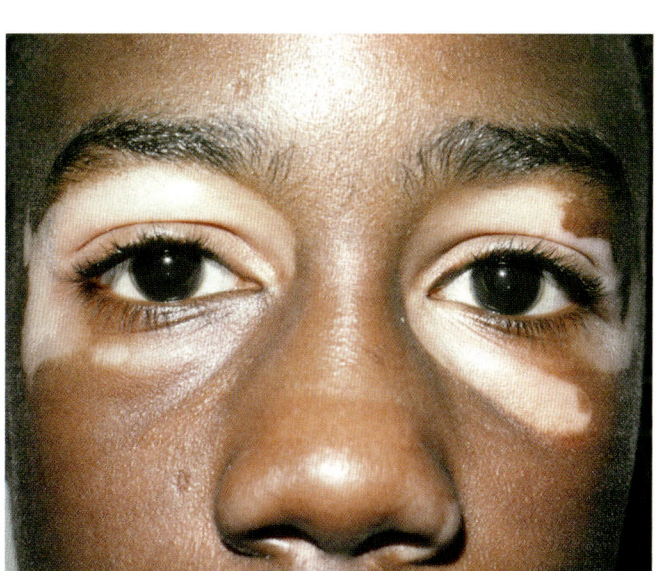

Fig. 36.37 Vitiligo. *Courtesy Steven Binnick, MD.*

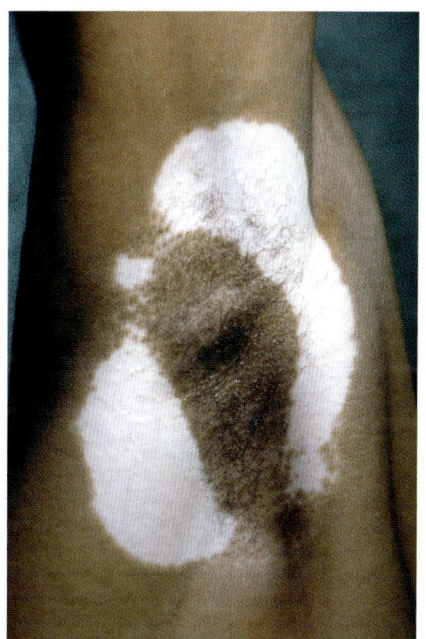

Fig. 36.38 Vitiligo.

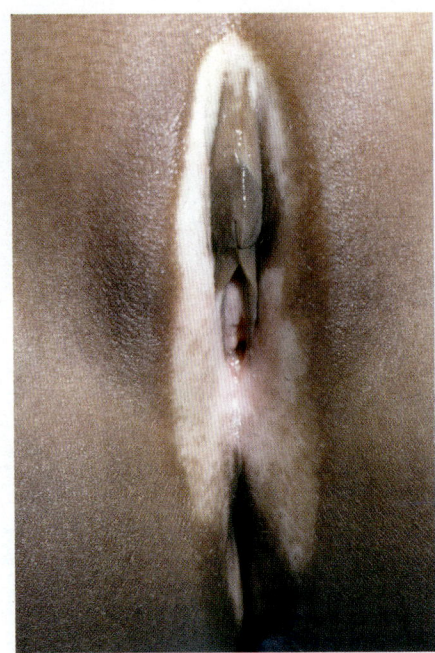

Fig. 36.39 Vitiligo.

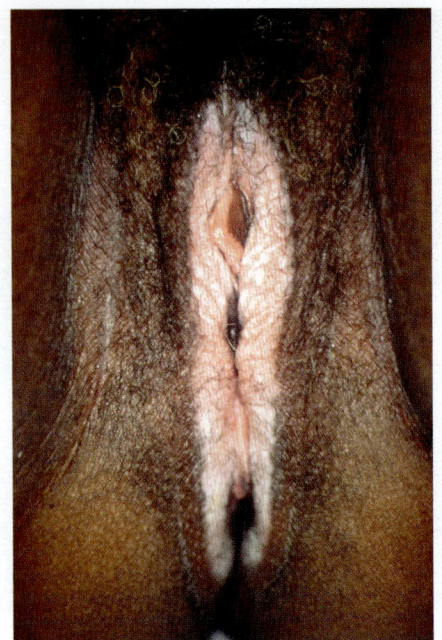

Fig. 36.40 Vitiligo. *Courtesy Steven Binnick, MD.*

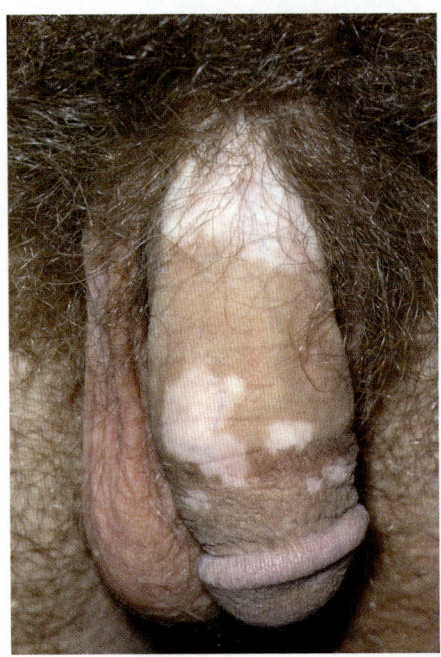

Fig. 36.41 Vitiligo.

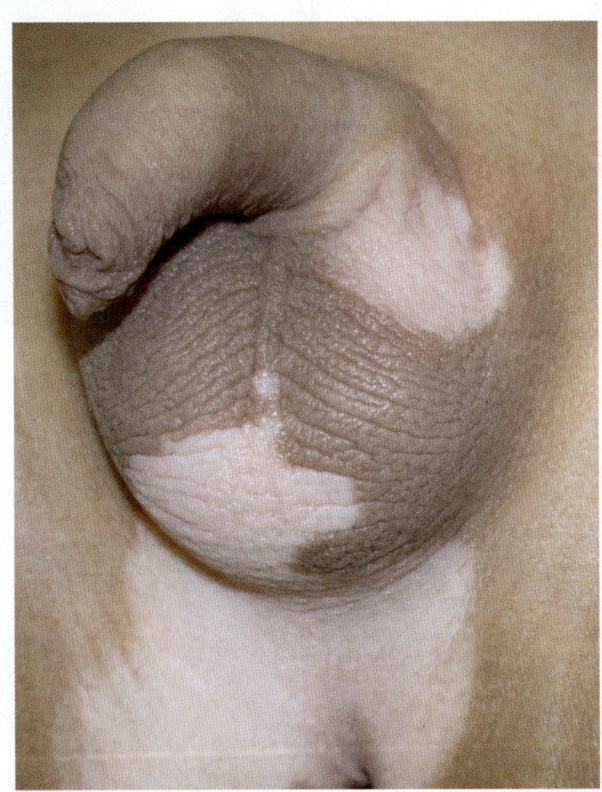

Fig. 36.42 Vitiligo.

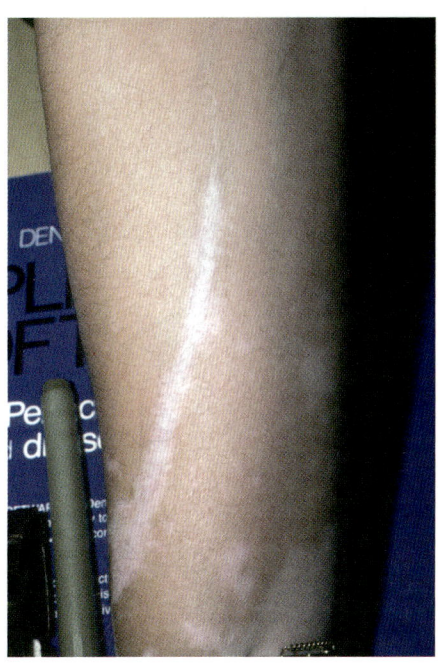

Fig. 36.43 Vitiligo with koebnerization.

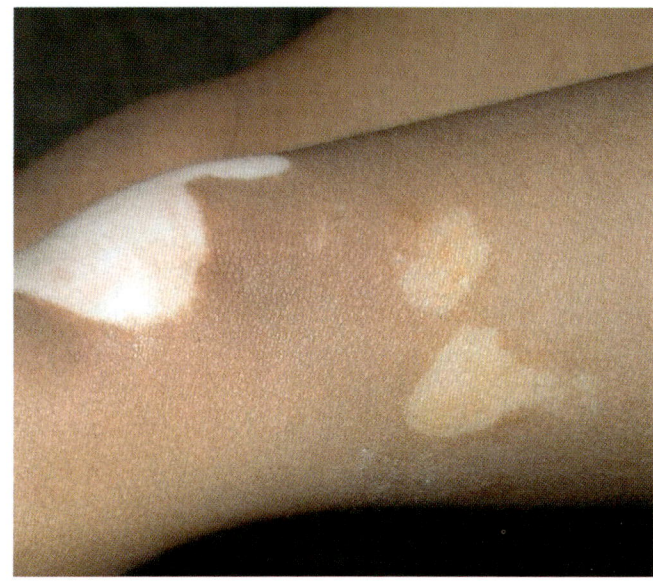

Fig. 36.44 Trichrome vitiligo. *Courtesy Scott Norton, MD.*

Fig. 36.45 Vitiligo, guttate pattern.

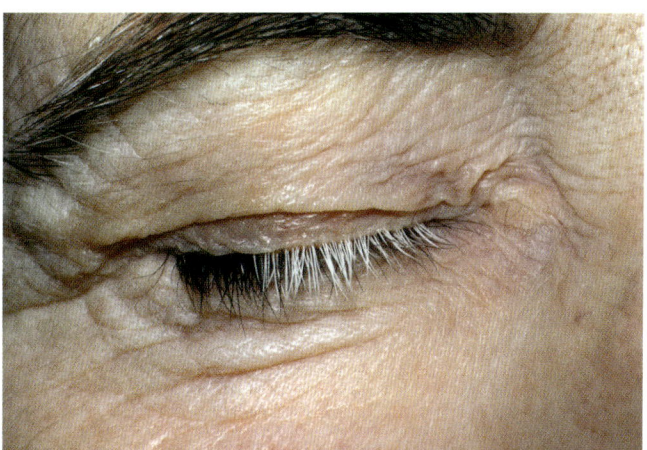

Fig. 36.46 Poliosis in vitiligo.

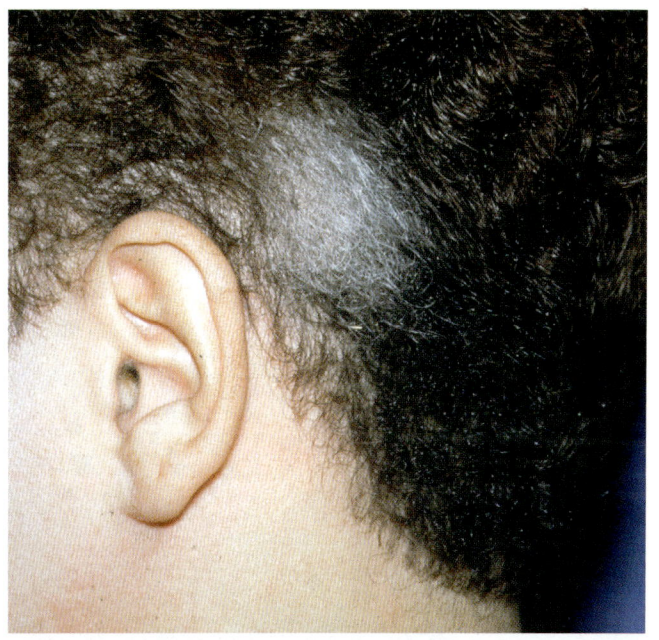

Fig. 36.47 Poliosis.

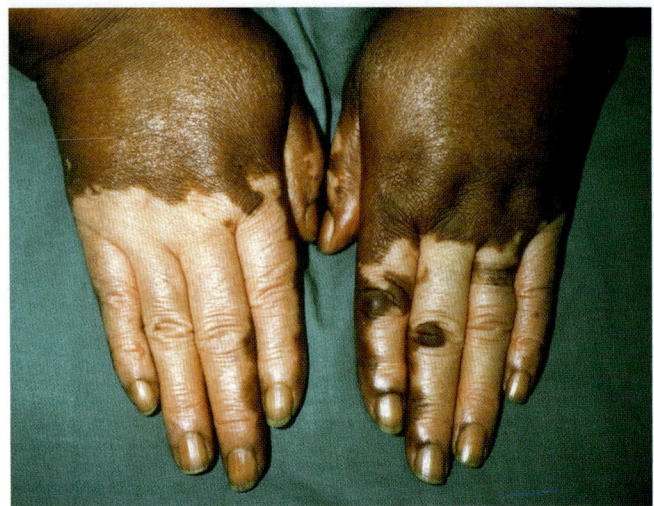

Fig. 36.48 Phenolic depigmentation.

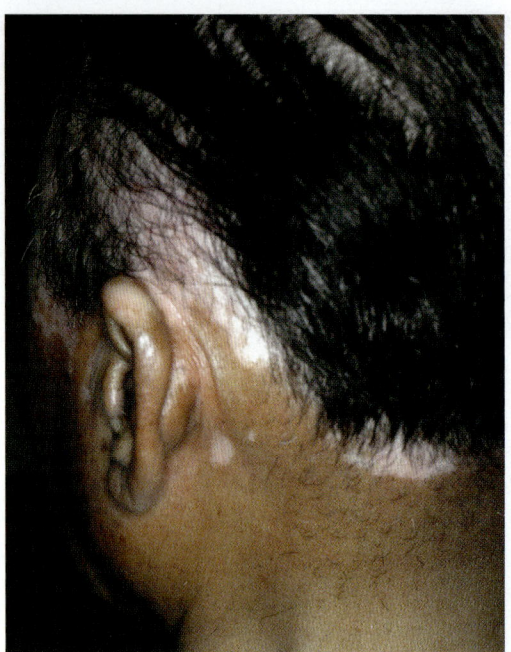

Fig. 36.49 Depigmentation secondary to paraphenylenediamine exposure.

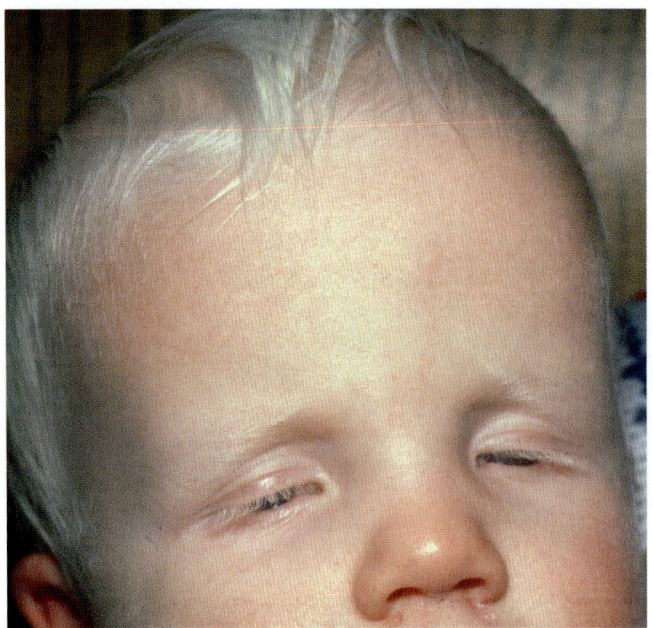

Fig. 36.50 Albinism.

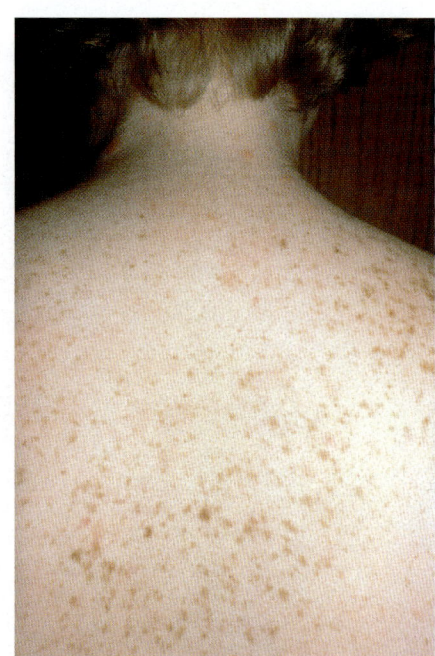

Fig. 36.51 Hermansky-Pudlak syndrome.

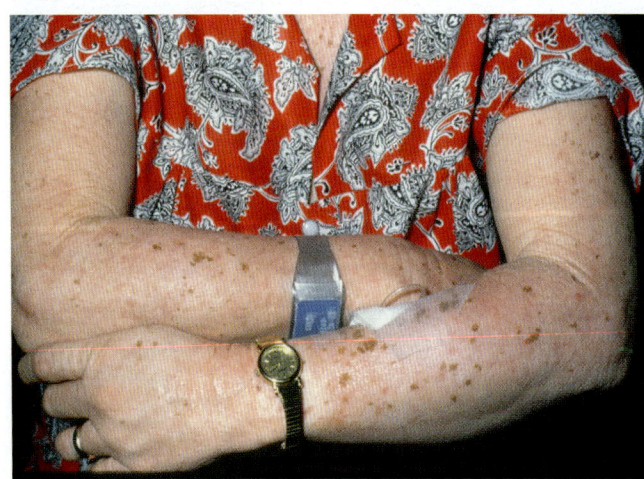

Fig. 36.52 Hermansky-Pudlak syndrome.

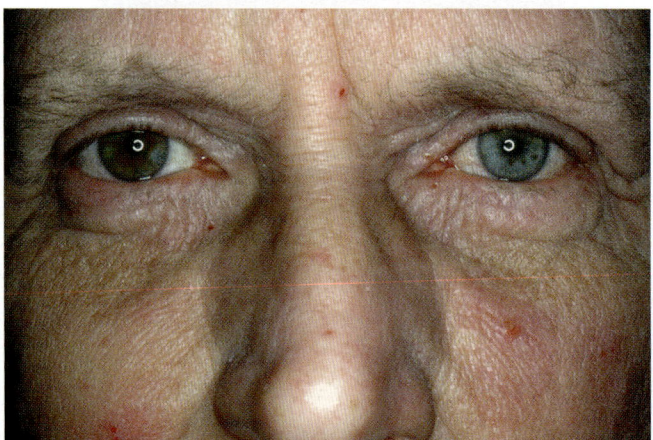

Fig. 36.53 Heterochromia.

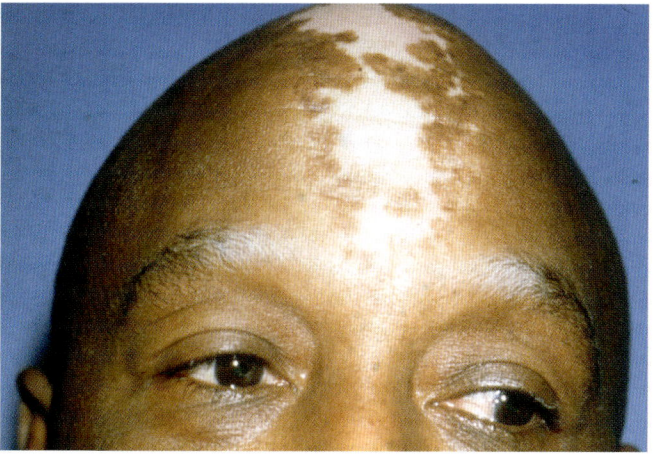

Fig. 36.54 Piebaldism.

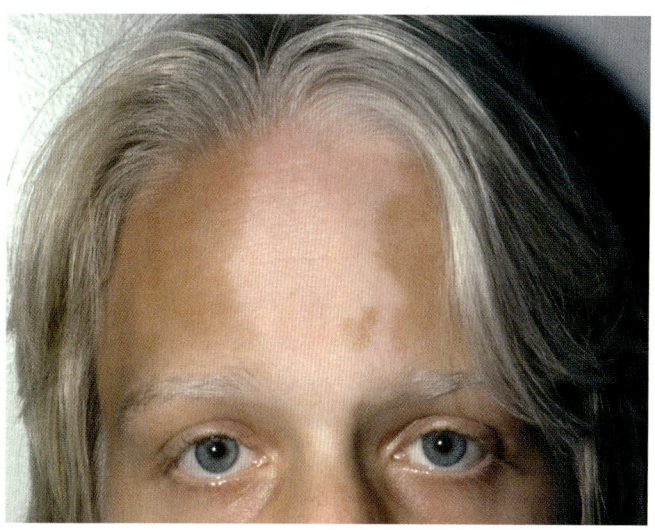

Fig. 36.55 Piebaldism.

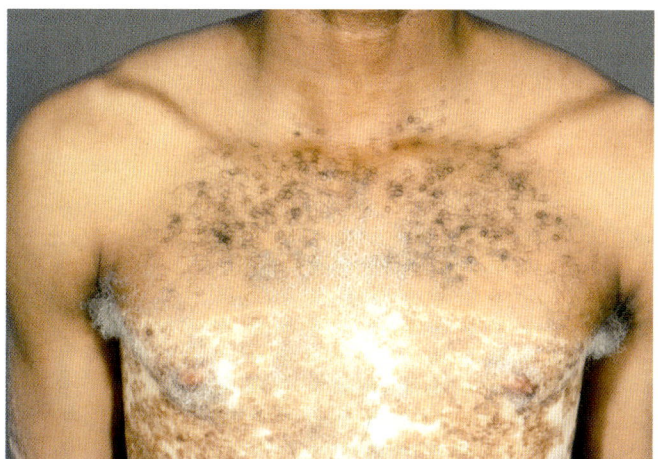

Fig. 36.56 Piebaldism.

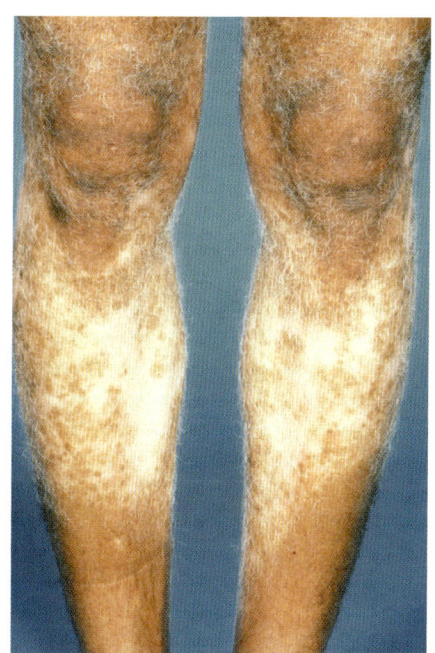

Fig. 36.57 Piebaldism.

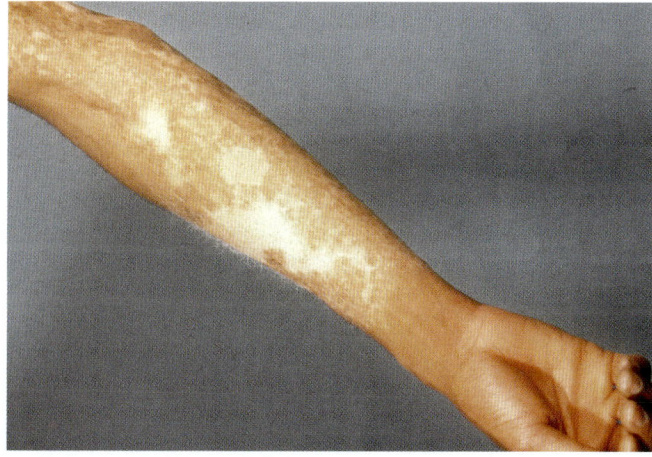

Fig. 36.58 Piebaldism.

INDEX

Page numbers followed by "*f*" indicate figures.

A

"ABCDs" of melanoma, 463
Acanthoma, 438*f*
Acanthosis
   in breast skin, 3*f*
   neoplasms with, 437
Acanthosis nigricans, 347*f*–348*f*
   with malignancy, 348*f*
Acid burn, 65*f*
Acne, 169–183
   with 21-hydroxylase deficiency, 174*f*
   childhood, 170*f*
   cosmetica, 176*f*
   cyst with scarring, 173*f*
   excoriée, 176*f*
   fulminans, 174*f*–175*f*
   hirsutism and, 527*f*
      with Cushing disease, 174*f*
   with hyperpigmentation, 173*f*
   keloidalis, 178*f*
   keloids resulting from, 175*f*
   mechanica, 176*f*
   mild to moderate, 171*f*–172*f*
   moderate to severe, 172*f*
   neonatal, 169*f*
   pomade, 176*f*
   preadolescent, 171*f*
   scarring, 175*f*
   severe, 172*f*–173*f*
   severe infantile, 170*f*
   severe truncal, 173*f*
      with hyperpigmentation, 173*f*
   steroid, 177*f*
Acquired dyskeratotic leukoplakia, 552*f*
Acquired partial lipodystrophy, 336*f*–337*f*
Acral lentiginous melanoma, 541
Acral persistent papular mucinosis, 121*f*
Acrodermatitis chronica atrophicans, 202*f*
Acrodermatitis continua, 137*f*
Acrodermatitis enteropathica, 326*f*–327*f*
Acrokeratoelastoidosis, 148*f*
Acrokeratosis verruciformis of Hopf, 395*f*
Acromegaly, 339*f*–340*f*
Acropachy, thyroid, 346*f*
Acrospiroma, 453*f*
Actinic cheilitis, 543*f*
Actinic dermatitis, chronic, 35*f*
Actinic granuloma, 485*f*
Actinic prurigo, 34*f*
Actinomycosis, 195*f*
Acute generalized exanthematous pustulosis, 76*f*–77*f*
Acute hemorrhagic edema, of infancy, 571*f*
Acute myelogenous leukemia, 17*f*
Acute necrotizing ulcerative gingivostomatitis, 557*f*
Acute paronychia, 187*f*
Acute shoe dermatitis, 68*f*
Acute systemic lupus erythematosus, 106*f*–107*f*
Acute urticaria, 18*f*
AD. *see* Atopic dermatitis (AD).
Adenomas, sebaceous, of Muir Torre syndrome, 450*f*
Adrenogenital syndrome, 342*f*–343*f*
Adult linear IgA disease, 320*f*
Aerosolized contact dermatitis, 67*f*
Ainhum, 421*f*
Alagille disease, lichen simplex chronicus in, 42*f*
Alagille syndrome, palmar striae in, 373*f*
Albinism, 592*f*
Alkaptonuria, 376*f*–377*f*
Allergic contact cheilitis, to topical steroids, 543*f*
Allergic shiners, 53
Alopecia
   androgenetic
      in man, 519*f*
      in woman, 519*f*
   central centrifugal cicatricial, 521*f*–522*f*
   congenital triangular, 520*f*
   frontal fibrosing, 521*f*
   in sarcoidosis, 492*f*
   scarring, secondary to discoid lupus erythematosus, 521*f*
   secondary syphilis, 258*f*
   in systemic lupus erythematosus, 107*f*
   traction, 522*f*–523*f*
Alopecia areata, 26*f*, 517*f*
   of beard, 517*f*
   in Down syndrome patient, 518*f*
   nails of patient with, 519*f*
   ophiasis type of, 518*f*
   recurrent, 518*f*
Alopecia mucinosa, 520*f*
   associated with mycosis fungoides, 507*f*
Alopecia neoplastica, from metastatic breast cancer, 432f, 523*f*
Alopecia universalis, 518*f*
Amalgam tattoo, 555*f*
Amantadine, livedo reticularis caused by, 562*f*
Amblyomma americanum, 303*f*
Amiodarone hyperpigmentation, 79*f*
Amyloidosis, 361, 361*f*–363*f*
   dyschromic, 365*f*
   lichen, 363*f*–364*f*
   macroglossia in, 362*f*
   macular, 363*f*
   nodular, 364*f*–365*f*
Anaplastic large cell lymphoma with acquired ichthyosis, 511*f*
Androgenetic alopecia
   in man, 519*f*
   widened central part, 519*f*
Anemia, smooth tongue in, 328*f*
Anergic leishmaniasis, 293*f*–294*f*
Anetoderma, 358*f*
Angioedema, 99*f*
Angioimmunoblastic T-cell lymphoma, 516*f*
Angiokeratoma
   circumscriptum, 411*f*
   of Fordyce, 411*f*–412*f*
   of Mibelli, 411*f*
Angiokeratoma corporis diffusum. *see* Fabry disease.
Angiolymphoid hyperplasia, with eosinophilia, 412*f*
Angiomas
   cherry, 415*f*
   circumscriptum, 411*f*
   serpiginosum, 413*f*
   spider, 410*f*
   tufted, 416*f*
Angiomatosis, diffuse dermal, 417*f*
Angiosarcoma, 418*f*–419*f*
Angular artery and vein, 13*f*
Angular cheilitis, 203, 544*f*
   in iron deficiency, 328*f*
Ankyloblepharon-ectodermal dysplasia-clefting, 398*f*
Annular atrophic panniculitis, 337*f*
Annular elastolytic granuloma, 484*f*–485*f*
Annular genital sarcoid, 488*f*
Annular lichen planus, 160*f*
Annular psoriasis, 133*f*
Annular sarcoidosis, 488*f*
Anonychia, 532*f*
Anthrax, with severe edema, 193*f*
Antibiotic allergy, leg ulcer with contact dermatitis due to, 72*f*
Antiphospholipid antibodies, in systemic lupus erythematosus, 109*f*
Apert syndrome, 403*f*
Aphthous stomatitis, 558*f*
Aplasia cutis congenita, 399*f*
Apocrine glands, in axillary skin, 3*f*
Aquagenic wrinkling, 150*f*
Arsenic-induced leukomelanosis, 588*f*
Arterial ulceration, 581*f*
Arteriosclerosis obliterans, 577*f*
Arteriovenous fistula, 409*f*
Arteriovenous malformation syndrome, RASA1-associated, capillary malformation due to, 408*f*
Arteritis, temporal, 576*f*
Ascher syndrome, blepharochalasis in, 357*f*
Aspergillosis, 227*f*
Aspergillus infection, 203, 226*f*–227*f*
Asymmetric periflexural exanthem, of childhood, 279*f*
Ataxia telangiectasia, 60*f*, 386*f*
Atopic dermatitis (AD), 53–64, 53*f*–56*f*
   chronic, 54*f*–55*f*
      with hyperpigmentation, 55*f*
   with Dennie-Morgan lines, 56*f*
   erythroderma from, 56f, 151*f*
   with excoriations, 54*f*
   hyperlinear palms in patient with, 57*f*
   lichenification, 55*f*
   papular, 56*f*
   with secondary infection, 54*f*–55*f*

595

Atrichia, with papular lesions, 523f
Atrophic lichen planus, 160f
Atrophic tongue, in vitamin B deficiencies, 323f
Atrophoderma, 24f
　of Pasini and Pierini, 113f
Atrophy blanche, 563f
Atypical fibroxanthoma, 425f
Atypical mycobacterial infections, 229
Auricular nerve, 14f
Auriculotemporal nerve, 10f
Autoinoculation vaccinia, 20f
Autosomal-recessive congenital ichthyosis due to transglutaminase gene mutation
　with collodion membrane, 390f
　lamellar phenotype, 390f
Axillary freckling neurofibromatosis, 15f
Axillary granular parakeratosis, 348f
Axillary skin, 3f

B

Bacillary angiomatosis, 199f
Bacterial infections, 185–202
Bandage, contact allergy to adhesive in, 70f
Bart syndrome, 387f
Basal cell cancer, chronic radiodermatitis with, 35f
Basal cell carcinoma, 443f–444f
　aggressive, 444f
　large, 444f
　morpheaform, 444f
　pigmented, 444f
　in radiation site, 445f
　skin tag-like, basal cell nevus syndrome with, 445f
　superficial, 443f
　tumor, 18f
　ulcer, 22f–23f
Basal cell nevus syndrome, 445f
Bazex syndrome, 434f
B-cell lymphoma, 513f
　leg type, 514f
Beau lines, 533f
Becker nevus, 467f
Bedbug bites, 300f
Bee sting, 302f
Behçet disease, 559f
Bejel, 251–261, 260f
Benign follicular mucinosis, 122f–123f
Benzocaine, allergy to, 71f
Biliary cirrhosis
　palmar striae xanthoma in, 373f
　plane xanthoma in, 373f
　primary, tuberoeruptive xanthomas and, 372f
Birt-Hogg-Dubé syndrome, 458f
Bites, 291–307
　of bedbug, 300f
　of brown recluse spider, 307f
　of *Cheyletiella* mite, 306f
　of chigger, 306f
　of flea, 302f–303f
　of insect, 299f
　of Russell pit viper, 307f
　of snake, 307f
　of spider, 307f
　of tick, 303f
　of Triatome, 294f
Black dermatographism, 69f

Black dot poison ivy dermatitis, 67f
Black hairy tongue, 549f
Black heel, 37f
Blastomycosis, North American, 220f–221f
Bleomycin-associated flagellate hyperpigmentation, 81f
Blepharochalasis, in Ascher syndrome, 357f
Blistering and atrophy, in complex regional pain syndrome, 51f
Blistering dactylitis, 192f
Blisters, factitial, 49f
Blistik, contact cheilitis to, 72f
Bloom syndrome, 403f
Blue rubber bleb syndrome, 408f
Borderline tuberculoid leprosy, 248f
Botryomycosis, 188f
Boutonneuse fever, 201f
Bowen disease, 447f–448f
　of nail bed, 540f
Bowenoid papulosis, 284f
BRAF inhibitor-induced hand-foot reaction, 83f
Breast
　nevus on, 469f
　Paget disease of, 448f–449f
Breast cancer
　ductal, 431f
　inflammatory, 432f
　male, metastases, 432f
Breast skin, 3f
Brocq, pseudopelade of, 522f
Brooke-Spiegler syndrome, 456f
Brown pigments, in cutaneous eruption, 1
Brown recluse spider bite, 307f
Bruising, factitial, 49f
Brunsting-Perry pemphigoid, 318f
Buccinators muscle, parotid duct piercing of, 11f
Buerger disease, 576f–577f
Buffalo hump, 341f
Bulb, hair, 5f–6f
Bulimia, vomiting with, enamel erosion secondary to, 47f
Bullous diabetic dermatosis, 376f
Bullous impetigo, 189f
Bullous mastocytosis, 426f
Bullous pemphigoid, 19f, 315f
　erosion, 22f
　vesicles and bullae, 19f
Bullous systemic lupus erythematosus, 107f–108f
Bullous tinea, 208f
Bullous tinea pedis, 208f
Burn scar, 28f
Burns
　acid, 65f
　cement, 65f
　dig, from acid solution, 66f
　pesticide, 66f
　senna, 66f
Buruli ulcer, 235f
Buschke-Lowenstein tumor, 284f
Buschke-Ollendorff syndrome, 422f

C

Calabar swelling, 298f
Calcinosis cutis, 361, 369f
Calciphylaxis, 368f, 564f
Candidal infections, 203

Candidal sepsis, 214f
Candidiasis, 210f–213f
　chronic, common variable immunodeficiency with, 61f
　chronic mucocutaneous, 213f–214f
　thrush in, 210f
　congenital, 203, 212f
　oral, 210f
Cannabis arteritis, 577f
Capillary, in papillary dermis, 5f
Capillary malformation (port-wine stain), 407f
　with Sturge-Weber syndrome, 407f
Carbon stain, in gunshot wound, 39f
Carcinoid syndrome, 436f
Carcinoma
　adnexal, microcystic, 455f
　basal cell, 443f–444f
　　aggressive, 444f
　　large, 444f
　　morpheaform, 444f
　　pigmented, 444f
　　in radiation site, 445f
　　skin tag-like, basal cell nevus syndrome with, 445f
　　superficial, 443f
　　tumor, 18f
　　ulcer, 22f–23f
　Merkel cell, 449f
　sebaceous, 450f
　squamous cell, 446f
　　Bowen disease with, 447f
　　verrucous, 447f
Carcinoma erysipeloides, 432f
Carney syndrome, 465f, 588f
Carotenemia, 330f
Cartilage, in early spine formation, 1f
Cat scratch disease, 199f
Catastrophic antiphospholipid antibody syndrome, 566f
Cavernous venous malformation, 408f
CD30+ anaplastic T-cell lymphoma, 511f
Cellulitis, 180f, 191f
Cement burns, 65f
Central centrifugal cicatricial alopecia, 521f–522f
Cephalic histiocytosis, benign, 494f, 497f
Cerebrotendinous xanthomas, 373f
Ceruminous glands, in ear canal, 2f
Chagas disease, Romana sign in, 294f
Chancroid, 197f
Cheilitis
　actinic, 543f
　allergic contact, to topical steroids, 543f
　angular, 203, 544f
　granulomatous, 547f
　plasma cell, 544f
　secondary to lip licking, 543f
Cheilitis glandularis, 544f
Chemotherapy
　toxic erythema of, 82f
　transverse nail bands secondary to, 537f
Chemotherapy-induced transverse nail hyperpigmentation, 80f
Cherry angiomas, and costal fringe telangiectases, 415f
Cheyletiella mite bites, 306f
Chigger bites, 306f
Chikungunya fever, 281f
Chilblain systemic lupus erythematosus, 107f

Childhood, asymmetric periflexural exanthem in, 279f
Childhood acne, 170f
Childhood linear IgA disease, 321f
Childhood pityriasis rubra pilaris, 144f
Chloracne, 177f
Chloroquine hyperpigmentation, 81f, 554f
Chlorpromazine hyperpigmentation, 79f, 554f
Cholesterol emboli, 563f
Cholinergic urticaria, 97f–98f
Chondrodermatitis nodularis chronica helices, 423f
Chromomycosis, 223f
Chronic actinic dermatitis, 35f
Chronic blistering dermatoses, 309–322
Chronic graft-versus-host disease, angiomatosis, 64f
Chronic hand dermatitis, from cement, 21f
Chronic mucocutaneous candidiasis, 213f–214f
Chronic solar damage, 32f
Chrysiasis, 79f
Cicatricial pemphigoid, 317f–318f
Cigarette burn, factitial, 48f
Circumferential ulceration, lipodermatosclerosis with, 342f
Circumscribed juvenile pityriasis rubra pilaris, 145f
Cirrhosis, primary biliary, hyperpigmentation in, 42f
Claw hand, 247f
Clonidine patch allergy, 71f
Closed comedones, 171f
Clostridial ulcer, 194f
Clothing contact dermatitis, 68f
CLOVE syndrome, 408f, 438f
Clubbing, 531f
Coccidioidomycosis, 203, 218f–219f
Cockayne syndrome, 402f
Cockayne-xeroderma pigmentosum syndrome, 402f
Coin rubbing, purpura from, 567f
Cold panniculitis, 335f–336f
Cold urticaria, 97f
Collagenous and elastotic marginal plaques, of hands, 148f
Colloid milium, 32f
Comedones
    closed, 171f
    open, 170f–171f
Complex regional pain syndrome, 50f–51f
Compositae dermatitis, 68f
Compulsive finger biting, 46f
Condyloma lata, 257f
Condylomata acuminata, 283f
Confluent and reticulated papillomatosis, 140f
Congenital anomalies, genodermatoses and, 379–404
Congenital candidiasis, 203, 212f
Congenital hemidysplasia, with ichthyosiform erythroderma and limb defects syndrome, 392f
Congenital hypothyroidism, 343f
Congenital ichthyosiform erythroderma, 21f
Congenital ichthyosis, collodion membrane in, 389f
Congenital onychodysplasia, of index finger, 532f
Congenital syphilis, 259f
    with Hutchinson teeth, 259f

with mulberry molar, 259f
with scars from rhagades, 260f
Congenital triangular alopecia, 520f
Conjunctiva, lipodermoid of, Schimmelpenning syndrome with, 438f
Conjunctival erythema, reactive arthritis with, 135f
Connective tissue disease, 101–118
Connective tissue nevus, 421f–422f
Conradi-Hunermann syndrome, 380f
Contact allergy
    to steroids, 72f
Contact cheilitis, to Blistex, 72f
Contact dermatitis, 65–85
    to eye drops, 72f
    leg ulcer with, 72f
    toilet seat cleaner, 70f
Contact urticaria, to surgical gloves, 72f
Coral granuloma, 296f
Costal fringe telangiectases, cherry angiomas and, 415f
Cotton granuloma, 38f
Cough-induced purpura, 567f
Cowden syndrome, 457f
Coxsackie A6 hand-foot-and-mouth disease, 277f
Cradle cap, 126f
Crohn disease, cutaneous, 545f–546f
Crusted scabies, in HIV-infected patient, 306f
Cryoglobulinemic vasculitis, 565f, 572f
Cryopyrin-associated periodic fever syndrome
    with atypical pernio-like lesion, 96f
    with Muckle-Wells syndrome, 96f
Cryptococcal infection, 220f
    in an HIV-infected patient, 220f
Cuboidal periderm, in early fetal life, 1f
Culprit swim goggles, 70f
Curth-Macklin with keratin 1 mutation, ichthyosis hystrix of, 147f
Cushing disease, 340f
    hypertrichosis in, 341f
    skin thinning and ecchymoses in, 341f
Cutaneous collagenous vasculopathy, 579f
Cutaneous Crohn disease, 545f–546f
Cutaneous dental sinus, 550f
Cutaneous diphtheria, 193f
Cutaneous larva migrans, 291, 297f
Cutaneous mucin deposition, 119
Cutaneous *Mycobacterium avium-intracellulare* infection, 237f
Cutaneous *Mycobacterium kansasii* infection, 237f
Cutaneous vascular diseases, 561–581
Cutis laxa, 357f
Cutis marmorata telangiectatica congenita, 406f
Cutis rhomboidalis nuchae, 31f
Cutis verticis gyrata, 399f
Cylindroma, 454f
Cysts
    acne, with scarring, 173f
    dermoid, 460f
    epidermal, 437–462
    epidermal inclusion, 459f
    eruptive vellus hair, 461f
    labial, 459f
    median raphae, 462f
    pilar, 460f
    pilonidal, 183f, 460f
    scrotal, 459f
    thyroglossal duct, 462f

Cytomegaloviral infection, in newborn, 272f
Cytomegaloviral ulcer, in HIV-infected patient, 272f

D

Darier disease, 16f, 394f–395f
    longitudinal erythronychia, 536f
    of nail, 531f
Decubitus ulcer, 37f
Deep lymphatic malformation, 410f
Degos disease, 576f
Delayed pressure urticaria, 98f
Delusions of parasitosis, 47f
Demodex mites, in facial skin, 2f
Dengue, 280f
Dennie-Morgan lines, atopic dermatitis with, 56f
Dental impression material allergy, stomatitis due to, 70f
Depigmentation, secondary to paraphenylenediamine exposure, 592f
Dermal and subcutaneous tumors, 405–435
Dermal dendrocyte hamartoma, 424f
Dermal duct tumor, 453f
Dermal fibrous tissue, abnormalities of, 351–359
Dermatitis
    actinic, chronic, 35f
    acute shoe, 68f
    atopic, 53–64, 53f–56f
        chronic, 54f–55f
        with Dennie-Morgan lines, 56f
        erythroderma from, 56f
        with excoriations, 54f
        hyperlinear palms in, 57f
        with hyperpigmentation, chronic, 55f
        lichenification, 55f
        papular, 56f
        with secondary infection, 54f–55f
    chronic hand, from cement, 21f
    clothing contact, 68f
    contact, 65–85
        to eye drops, 72f
        leg ulcer with, 72f
    earbud, 70f
    eyelid, 71f
    factitial, 48f
    finger, from primrose allergy, 58f
    fire coral, 295f
    hand, 71f
        with secondary infection, 58f
    herpetiformis, 309, 319f–320f
    irritant, from kerosene, 66f
    irritant diaper, 59f
    jellyfish, 295f
    Katayama fever-associated, 296f
    nickel, 69f
    oral lichenoid, 70f
    Paederus, 302f
    phytophotodermatitis, 33f
    poison ivy, 65, 67f
    Portuguese man of war, 295f
    radiodermatitis, chronic, 35f
    rubber, 70f
    sea wasp, 295f
    seaweed, 296f
    stasis, 580f–581f

Dermatitis (Continued)
   tea tree oil, 67f
   vulvar, 71f
Dermatofibroma, 405, 423f–424f
   multiple, 424f
   sarcoma protuberans, 424f–425f
Dermatographism, 87, 98f–99f
   white, 56f
Dermatology, field of, 517
Dermatomyositis (DM), 111f
   anti-MDA-5, 112f
   Gottron's papules, 110f
   heliotrope, 109f
   lateral thigh, 112f
   mechanic's hands, 111f
   Samitz sign, 110f
   shawl sign, 111f
   ulcerated inverse Gottron's papules, 112f
Dermatopathia pigmentosa reticularis, 586f
Dermatophyte infections, 203
Dermatophytoma, 209f
Dermatoses, resulting from physical factors, 27–39, 33f
Dermatosis papulosa nigra, 440f
Dermoscopy, 463
Desmosome, 6f
Diabetic dermopathy, 376f
Diabetic gangrene, 376f
Diffuse hyperkeratosis, of the soles, 147f
Diffuse large B-cell lymphoma, 513f
Diffuse leprosy of Lucio, 246f
Digital sarcoidosis, 490f
Digital ulcers, Raynaud phenomenon with, 561f
Digitate parapsoriasis, 139f
Dilated follicular orifices, 119
Discoid lupus erythematosus, 23f, 101f–103f
   generalized, 103f
   of scalp, 520f
   scarring alopecia secondary to, 521f
Disseminated herpes simplex infection, 267f
Disseminated Lyme disease, 202f
Disseminated sporotrichosis, 223f
Disseminated vaccinia, 274f
Disseminated varicella, 270f
DM. see Dermatomyositis (DM).
DOCK8 immunodeficiency, warts in, 61f–62f
Dominant dystrophic epidermolysis bullosa, 387f
Doxorubicin hyperpigmentation, 79f–80f
Doxycycline, photoonycholysis secondary to, 33f
Drip burn, from acid solution, 66f
Drug eruptions, 16f, 65–85, 73f
   in leukemic patient, 73f
Drug-induced antineutrophil cytoplasmic antibody-positive vasculitis, 574f
Dryness, secondary to compulsive hand washing, 46f
Ductal breast cancer, 432f
Dupuytren contracture, 420f
Dyschromatosis symmetrica hereditaria, 584f–585f
Dyschromatosis universalis hereditaria, 587f
   patient, back of, 586f
Dyschromic amyloidosis, 365f
Dyshidrosis, 19f
Dyskeratomas, warty, 439f
Dyskeratosis congenita, 396f–397f
Dyspigmentation, in systemic sclerosis, 115f
Dystrophic calcinosis cutis, 367f

E

Ear
   anatomy of, 10f
   juvenile spring eruption of, 34f
   polymorphous light eruption, 34f
   skin of, 2f
Ear canal, skin of, 2f
Ear eczema, 58f
Early follicular hyperkeratosis, pityriasis rubra pilaris with, 142f
Early scleromyxedema, 119f
Earphone dermatitis, 70f
Earrings, nickel dermatitis with, 69f
Eccrine acrospiroma, 453f
Eccrine carcinoma, 455f
Eccrine glands, in volar skin, 5f
Eccrine porocarcinoma, 454f
Eccrine poroma, 452f–453f
Eccrine spiradenoma, 453f
Ecthyma, 190f
Ecthyma gangrenosum, 195f–196f
Ectrodactyly ectodermal dysplasia-clefting, 398f
Eczema, 53–64
   ear, 58f
   eyelid, 58f
   herpeticum, 57f, 267f
   nipple, in atopic child, 58f
   nummular, 59f
   xerotic, 59f
Edema
   acute hemorrhagic, of infancy, 570f–571f
   rounded scars and, from skin popping, 23f
   in severe rosacea, 181f
EDS. see Ehlers-Danlos syndrome (EDS).
Ehlers-Danlos syndrome (EDS), 354f–357f
Elastic tissue, abnormalities of, 351–359
Elastosis, solar, of the forehead, 32f
Elastosis perforans serpiginosa, 352f, 354f
Elastotic striae, 359f
Electrical burn, from biting electrical cord, 28f
Emphysema, subcutaneous, 37f
Enamel erosion secondary to vomiting with bulimia, 47f
Encephalocele, 429f
Endocrine diseases, 339–349
Endometriosis, cutaneous, 431f
Enterovirus hand, foot, and mouth disease, 277f
Eosinophil, 7f
Eosinophilia, phenytoin-induced drug reaction with, 73f–74f
Eosinophilic annular erythema, 92f
Eosinophilic fasciitis, 116f
Eosinophilic folliculitis, in HIV-infected patient, 289f
Eosinophilic granulomatosis with polyangiitis, 575f
Eosinophilic pustular folliculitis of Ofuji, 136f, 137f
Epidemic typhus, 200f
Epidermal growth factor inhibitor-induced acneiform reaction, 83f
Epidermal growth factor inhibitor-induced paronychia, 83f
Epidermodysplasia verruciformis, in HIV-infected patient, 285f

Epidermolysis bullosa
   dominant dystrophic, 387f
   junctional, 386f
   recessive dystrophic, 387f
Epidermolysis bullosa acquisita, 318f–319f
Epidermolysis bullosa simplex
   generalized, 386f
   localized, 386f
Epidermolytic ichthyosis, 390f–391f
Epithelioid sarcoma, 425f
Epulis, 556f
Erb point, 13f
Erosio interdigitalis blastomycetica, 213f
Erosions, factitial, 49f
Erosive lichen planus, 159f
Erosive pustular dermatitis, of scalp, 522f
Eruptive histiocytomas, generalized, 494f
Eruptive xanthomas, 16f, 369f–370f
Erysipelas, 190f–191f
Erysipeloid, 193f
Erythema, 87–99
Erythema ab igne, 25f, 29f
Erythema annulare centrifugum, 91f
Erythema dyschromicum perstans, 162f–163f
Erythema elevatum diutinum, 573f
Erythema gyratum repens, 91f
Erythema induratum, 229, 233f, 331, 333f
Erythema infectiosum, 279f–280f
Erythema marginatum, 192f–193f
Erythema migrans, 201f–202f
Erythema multiforme, 88f–89f
   recurrent oral, 90f–91f
Erythema nodosum, 18f, 331f–333f
Erythema nodosum leprosum, 239
Erythema nodosum-like sarcoidosis, 491f
Erythema toxicum neonatorum, 88f
Erythematotelangiectatic rosacea, 180f
Erythrasma, 193f–194f
Erythroderma, 125–138
   from atopic dermatitis, 56f, 151f
Erythrodermic bullous pemphigoid, 316f
Erythrodermic psoriasis, 134f
Erythrodermic sarcoidosis, 492f
Erythrokeratoderma variabilis, 393f
Erythromelalgia, 561f–562f
Erythroplasia of Queyrat, 448f
Erythropoietic protoporphyria, 366f–367f
Excoriation, 41
   atopic dermatitis with, 54f
   Hodgkin disease, secondary to pruritus of, 41f
   prurigo nodularis with, 46f
   psychogenic, 47f
Exercise-induced urticaria, 97f
Exogenous nail staining, 538f
Exogenous ochronosis, 377f
Extensive warts, 282f–283f
External carotid artery, 13f
External jugular vein, 13f–14f
Extremities, skin tension lines in, 9f
Eyelid, anatomy of, 4f
Eyelid dermatitis, 71f
Eyelid eczema, 58f
Eyelid lichen planus, 161f

F

Fabry disease, 375f
Face, arterial and venous supply of, 13f
Facial artery and vein, 13f–14f

Facial dermatitis, granulomatous, 182f–183f
Facial expression, muscles of, 11f
Facial nerve, anatomy of, 11f
Facial skin, 2f
  innervation of, 12f
  major anatomic landmarks in, 10f
Facial swelling reaction, hyaluronic acid filler, 39f
Factitial blisters, 49f
Factitial bruising, 49f
Factitial dermatitis, 48f
Factitial erosions, 49f
Factitial lacerations, 49f
Factitial ulcers, 48f–49f
Fasciitis, 191f–192f
  in chronic graft-versus-host disease, 64f
Fat, subcutaneous, lobules of, 5f
Favre-Racouchot syndrome, 31f
Fibroepithelioma of pinkus, 443f
Fibrokeratoma, acquired digital, 422f
Fibroma
  sclerotic, 458f
  secondary to chronic tongue biting, 47f
Fibrous papule, of nose, 422f
Filariasis, 297f–298f
Finger biting, compulsive, 46f
Finger dermatitis, from primrose allergy, 58f
Fire ant stings, 302f
Fire coral cuts, 36f
Fire coral dermatitis, 295f
Fissured tongue, 548f
Fixed cutaneous sporotrichosis, 222f
Fixed drug reaction, 75f–76f
Flag sign, 524f
Flea bites, 302f–303f
Flegel disease, 440f
Fluoroscopy-induced radiodermatitis, 36f
Flushing, 87f
Focal acral hyperkeratosis, 148f–149f
Focal cutaneous mucinosis, 124f
Focal palmoplantar keratoderma, 146f
Fogo selvagem, 21f, 313f
Follicular accentuation, 1
Follicular iododerma, 84f
Follicular mucinosis, 119
  associated with mycosis fungoides, 123f
Folliculitis, 1
  Pityrosporum, 218f
  staphylococcal, 20f
Folliculitis decalvans, 522f
Foot, immersion, tropical, 30f
Fordyce spots, 547f
Forehead, medial, 12f
Forschheimer spots, in rubella, 278f
Fox-Fordyce disease, 529f
  with xanthomatous change, 529f
Frontal fibrosing alopecia, 161f, 521f
Frostbite, 30f
Fungal infections, 203
Fungi, diseases resulting from, 203–227
Fusarium infection, 203, 226f

G

GA. *see* Granuloma annulare (GA).
Galli-Galli disease, 585f
Gamma delta T-cell lymphoma, 512f
Gastric adenocarcinoma, 349f
Generalized discoid lupus erythematosus, 103f
Generalized essential telangiectasia, 579f
Generalized *Mycobacterium avium-intracellulare* infection, 237f
Genital lymphedema, 180f
Genital sarcoidosis, 488f
Genodermatoses, 379–404
Geographic tongue, 548f
Gianotti-Crosti syndrome, 263, 273f–274f
Giant cell tumor, of tendon sheath, 421f
Giant molluscum contagiosum, 275f–276f
Glandular rosacea, 181f
  with rhinophyma, 181f
Glioma, nasal, 428f
Globi, 239
Glomangioma, 416f–417f
Glucagonoma, 434f
Glucocorticoid excess, striae in, 341f
Gnathostomiasis, 297f
Gold, oral lichenoid dermatitis due to, 70f
Goltz syndrome, 399f–400f
Gonococcal infection, 198f
Gonococcemia, 198f
Gout, 377f–378f
Graft-*versus*-host disease
  acute, 62f–63f
  chronic, 63f–64f
  fasciitis in, 64f
  grade 2, acute, 62f
  grade 4, acute, 62f
  lichenoid, 63f
  sclerodermoid type, chronic, 63f–64f
Graham-Little-Piccardi syndrome, 162f
Gram-negative folliculitis, 177f–178f
Gram-negative toe web infection, 196f
Granular cell tumor, 405, 428f
  multiple, 428f
Granulation tissue, on isotretinoin, 176f
Granulocyte colony stimulating factor reaction, 84f
Granuloma, pyogenic, 18f, 412f–413f, 556f
Granuloma annulare (GA), 24f, 479, 479f–483f
  deep, 483f
  disseminated, 482f–483f
  facial, 484f
  perforating, 483f
  subcutaneous, 484f
Granuloma faciale, 573f
Granuloma inguinale, 197f–198f
Granulomatosis with polyangiitis, 574f–575f
  splinter hemorrhages, 574f
  strawberry gingiva, 575f
Granulomatous cheilitis, 547f
Granulomatous facial dermatitis, 182f–183f
Granulomatous lesion, in ataxia telangiectasia, 61f
Granulomatous slack skin, 509f
Graves ophthalmopathy, 346f
Greater auricular nerve enlargement, in leprosy, 241f
Green nail, 538f
  from *Pseudomonas* infection, 26f
Guttate psoriasis, 132f

H

Haemophilus influenzae cellulitis, 197f
Hailey-Hailey disease, 20f, 387f–388f
Hair
  anatomy of, 5f–6f
  diseases of, 517
  progressive kinking of, 526f
Hair collar sign, aplasia cutis congenita with, 399f
Hair follicles, in scalp skin, 3f
Hair granuloma, in barber, 38f
Hairy leukoplakia, 271f
Half-and-half nails, 533f
Hamartoma
  basiloid follicular, 459f
  smooth muscle, 431f
Hand, neuropathic ulcer of, 51f
Hand dermatitis
  with secondary infection, 58f
Hand washing, compulsive, dryness secondary to, 46f
Hand-foot-and-mouth disease, 276f–277f
Hansen disease, 239–250
Hard corn, 36f
Harlequin ichthyosis, 390f
Headlight sign, 53
Heel, black, 37f
Heel stick calcinosis, 368f
Hemangioma
  infantile, 413f–414f
    involuting, 414f–415f
    with ulceration, 414f
  spindle cell, 417f
  targetoid hemosiderotic, 415f
Hemangiomatosis, diffuse neonatal, 415f
Henoch-Schönlein purpura, 570f
Hepatic cholestasis, xanthomas of the palmar crease in, 42f
Hermansky-Pudlak syndrome, 592f
Herpangina, 276f
Herpes genitalis, 266f
Herpes gladiatorum, 265f
Herpes simplex infection, 25f
  disseminated, 267f
  intrauterine, 267f
  primary, 263f–264f
  recurrent, 264f–265f
  ulcerative, 268f
Herpes zoster, 269f–271f
Herpetic geometric glossitis, 267f
Herpetic sycosis, 265f
Herpetic whitlow, 265f
Heterochromia, 592f
Hidradenitis suppurativa, 169, 178f
Hidradenoma, nodular, 453f
Hidrocystoma, 452f
Hidrotic ectodermal dysplasia, 398f
Hirsutism, acne and, 527f
Histiocytoid leprosy, 246f
Histiocytoid Sweet syndrome, 94f
Histiocytosis
  cephalic, 494f, 497f
  Langerhans cell. *see* Langerhans cell histiocytosis (LCH).
  malignant, 514f
  progressive nodular, 495f
Histoplasmosis, 203, 219f
HIV-infected patient
  acquired ichthyosis in, 289f
  chronic herpes simplex in, 286f
  condylomata acuminatum in, 287f
  crusted scabies in, 288f, 306f
  cryptococcal infection in, 220f
  cytomegaloviral ulcer in, 272f
  eosinophilic folliculitis in, 289f
  epidermodysplasia verruciformis in, 285f, 287f

HIV-infected patient *(Continued)*
  generalized *Mycobacterium avium-intracellulare* infection in, 237f
  hair straightening in, 288f
  herpes simplex and seborrheic dermatitis in, 286f
  herpes zoster in, 271f, 287f
  Kaposi sarcoma in, 272f, 288f
  long eyelashes in, 289f
  molluscum contagiosum in, 287f
  oral hairy leukoplakia in, 288f
  proximal white onychomycosis in, 286f
  reactive arthritis in, 289f
  secondary syphilis in, 255f
  sulfa allergy in, 75f
  thrush in, 286f
  ulcerative herpes simplex in, 268f, 287f
Hodgkin disease, excoriations secondary to pruritus of, 41f
Homozygous familial hypercholesterolemia, xanthomas in, 17f
Homozygous protein C deficiency, 566f
Horn, cutaneous, 441f
Hot oil burn, 28f
Hot tub folliculitis, 196f-197f
Hot water bottle injury, 27f
Hot water burn, 27f
HTLV-1 dermatosis, 285f
Hunter syndrome, 377f
Hutchinson teeth, congenital syphilis with, 259f
Hydroa vacciniforme, 34f
Hydroa vacciniforme-like natural killer T-cell lymphoma, 512f-513f
Hydrofluoric acid burn, 65f
Hypercholesterolemia
  homozygous familial, xanthomas in, 17f
  with intertriginous xanthomas, 371f-372f
Hypereosinophilic syndrome, 516f
Hyperkeratosis
  diffuse, 147f
  focal acral, 148f-149f
  neoplasms with, 437
  spiny, 146f
  in volar skin, 4f
Hyperkeratotic diseases, 139-151
Hyperlinear palms, in atopic dermatitis, 57f
Hyperpigmentation
  in Addison disease, 341f-342f
  chronic atopic dermatitis with, 55f
  familial progressive, 587f
  of hand and cheek after phytophotodermatitis, 33f
  in primary biliary cirrhosis, 42f
  seborrheic dermatitis with, 126f
Hyperplasia, sebaceous, 450f
Hypersensitivity, piroxicam, 19f
Hypertrichosis
  in Cushing disease, 341f
  localized, 527f
  from minoxidil, 527f
Hypertrichosis cubiti, 527f
Hypertrophic lichen planus, 156f-157f
Hypertrophic lupus erythematosus, 17f
Hypertrophic osteoarthropathy, from lung cancer, 435f
Hypohidrotic X-linked ectodermal dysplasia, 397f-398f
Hypopigmentation
  after intralesional steroid injection, 85f
  familial progressive, 587f
  overlying sarcoidosis, 490f
  seborrheic dermatitis with, 127f
Hypopigmented mycosis fungoides, 502f-503f
Hypothyroidism, 344f

I

Ichthyosiform erythroderma, congenital, 21f
Ichthyosiform sarcoidosis, 491f-492f
Ichthyosis
  acquired
    in leprosy, 247f
    in myeloma patient, 435f
  autosomal-recessive congenital
    with collodion membrane, 390f
    lamellar phenotype, 390f
  epidermolytic, 390f-391f
  vulgaris, 388f-389f
    with hyperlinear palms, 389f
  X-linked, 21f, 389f
Ichthyosis hystrix, of Curth-Macklin with keratin 1 mutation, 147f
Id reaction, 59f, 204f
Idiopathic eruptive macular hyperpigmentation, with papillomatosis, 163f
IgA-mediated disease, 309
IgA vasculitis in adult patient, 570f
Immersion foot, tropical, 30f
Immune thrombocytopenic purpura, 564f-565f
Immunobullous dermatoses, 309
Impetiginized atopic dermatitis, 56f
Impetigo, 20f, 188f
Incontinentia pigmenti
  early inflammatory phase, 379f
  with pigmentary lesions, 380f
  with verrucous lesions, 379f-380f
Indeterminate leprosy, 239f
Infantile acne, 170f
Infantile bullous pemphigoid, 316f
Infantile digital fibromas, 421f
Infantile hemangioma, 413f-414f
  involuting, 414f-415f
  with ulceration, 414f
Infantile psoriasis, 131f-132f
Infected human bite, 199f
Infections
  Aspergillus, 226f-227f
  atypical mycobacterial, 229
  bacterial, 185-202
  candidal, 203
  cryptococcal, 220f
    in HIV-infected patient, 220f
  dermatophyte, 203
  fungal, 203
  Fusarium, 226f
  gonococcal, 198f
  Gram-negative toe web, 196f
  mold, 203
  perianal streptococcal, 192f
  Rhizopus, 226f
  Vibrio vulnificus, 199f
Inferior labial artery, 13f-14f
Inflammatory bowel disease (IBD), mucosal diseases in, 543
Inflammatory breast cancer, 432f
Infraorbital crease, 10f
Infraorbital foramen, and related structures, 12f

Infundibulofolliculitis, disseminate and recurrent, 528f
Infundibulum, follicular, tumor of, 459f
Ink spot lentigo, 464f
Inoculation tuberculosis, primary, 229f
Insect bite reaction, 299f
Insulin lipohypertrophy, 338f
Interdigital tinea, 207f
Internal jugular vein, 13f
Intertriginous xanthomas, hypercholesterolemia with, 371f-372f
Intertrigo, 194f
Intraepidermal neutrophilic IgA dermatosis, 314f
Intrauterine herpes simplex infection, 267f
Intravenous extravasation, with necrosis, 79f
Invasive *Candida parapsilosis*, 214f
Inverse lichen planus, 156f
Inverse psoriasis, 131f
Iron deficiency, angular cheilitis in, 328f
Irritant dermatitis, from kerosene, 66f
Irritant diaper dermatitis, 59f
Isomorphic (Koebner) phenomenon, 41
Isoniazid-induced pellagra-like reactions, 326f
Isotretinoin, granulation tissue on, 176f
Isotretinoin skin fragility, 22f
Itch, winter, 43f

J

Janeway spot, in staphylococcal endocarditis, 185f
Jaundice, 42f
Jellyfish dermatitis, 295f
Jessner lymphocytic infiltrate, of skin, 502f
Job's syndrome, 60f
Junctional epidermolysis bullosa, 386f
Juvenile spring eruption, of ears, 34f
Juvenile xanthogranulomas (JXG), 479, 493f
  large, 494f
  multiple, 494f
  plaque, 494f

K

Kaposi sarcoma, 26f
  in HIV-infected patient, 272f, 417f-418f
  secondary syphilis and, 255f
Kaposiform hemangioendothelioma, 416f
Kasabach-Merritt syndrome, 416f
Katayama fever-associated dermatitis, 296f
Kawasaki disease, 577f-578f
Keloids, 18f, 23f, 419f
  ulcerated, 419f
Keratinocytes, pale, 5f
Keratitis ichthyosis deafness syndrome, 392f
Keratoacanthoma, 442f
Keratoderma climactericum, 147f
Keratoderma of Vohwinkel, mutilating, 147f-148f
Keratolysis exfoliativa, 145f
Keratoses
  actinic, 441f
  arsenical, 440f
  lichenoid, benign, 440f
  seborrheic, 439f
  stucco, 440f
Keratosis follicularis spinulosa decalvans, 404f, 523f

Keratosis pilaris, 57f, 404f
Keratosis pilaris rubra faciei, 57f
Keratosis punctata, of palmar creases, 145f–146f
Kerion, 204f
Klippel-Trenaunay syndrome, 409f
Knuckle pads, 420f
Koebner phenomenon, 130f, 153, 155f
Koilonychia, 531f
  with trachyonychia, 531f
Koplik spots, 278f
Kwashiorkor, 328f–330f

L

Labiomental crease, 10f
Lacerations, factitial, 49f
Lamotrigine, toxic epidermal necrolysis to, 74f–75f
Langerhans cell, with Birbeck granules, 6f
Langerhans cell histiocytosis (LCH), 479, 497f–498f
  in adult, 499f
  congenital, 496f–497f
  nail involvement with, 497f
Larva migrans, cutaneous, 25f
Lateral nasal artery and vein, 13f
Laugier-Hunziker syndrome, 588f
LCH. see Langerhans cell histiocytosis (LCH).
Leiomyomas, 430f–431f
  multiple, 430f–431f
Leiomyosarcoma, 431f
Leishmaniasis
  anergic, 293f–294f
  mucocutaneous, 293f
  New World, 291f–293f
  Old World, 291f
  post-kala-azar dermal, 294f
Lentigines
  in LEOPARD syndrome, 465f
  solar, 464f
Lentiginosis
  generalized, 465f
  inherited patterned, 465f–466f
Lentigo maligna, 472f
Lentigo maligna melanoma, 472f
Lentigo simplex, 464f
LEOPARD syndrome, 381f
  lentigines in, 465f
Lepromatous leprosy, 244f–246f
  borderline, 243f–244f
Leprosy
  acquired ichthyosis in, 247f
  erythema nodosum leprosum, lepromatous leprosy with, 249f
  histiocytoid, 246f
  indeterminant, 239f
  lepromatous, 244f–246f
    borderline, 243f–244f
  of Lucio, 246f
  nerve enlargement in, 241f
    greater auricular, 241f
  neuropathic ulcer in, 247f
  secondary changes due to neurologic disease in, 247f
  tuberculoid, 239, 240f
    borderline, 241f–243f
    early, 239f
    type 1 reactional, 248f
    type 2 reactional, 249f

Leukemia, acute myelogenous, 17f
Leukemia cutis, 515f, 516f
Leukemic patient
  Aspergillus in, 226f–227f
  Fusarium infection in, 226f
Leukocytoclastic vasculitis, 569f
Leukonychia, 536f
  transverse, 536f
Leukoplakia, 550f
  acquired dyskeratotic, 552f
  cheilitis glandularis with, 544f
  oral hairy, 17f
Levamisole-induced vasculopathy, 575f–576f
Levator palpebrae superioris, 12f
Lichen amyloidosis, 363f–364f
Lichen aureus, 568f
Lichen nitidus, 153, 163f–165f
Lichen planopilaris, 161f, 521f
Lichen planus actinicus, 153, 162f
Lichen planus (LP), 24f, 153–168, 153f–157f, 159f–161f
  actinicus, 153, 162f
  after radiation therapy, 161f
  annular, 160f
  atrophic, 160f
  desquamative gingivitis, 158f
  eyelid, 161f
  hyperpigmentation, 156f
  hypertrophic, 156f–157f
  oral, 158f
Lichen planus lupus erythematosus overlap, 104f
Lichen planus pigmentosus, 153, 162f
Lichen sclerosus, 153, 166f–168f
Lichen scrofulosorum, 233f
Lichen simplex chronicus, 24f, 44f–45f
  in Alagille disease, 42f
  with dyspigmentation and early nodule formation, 45f
  in pruritus ani, 43f
  of scrotum, 43f
  of vulva, 43f
Lichen striatus, 153, 165f–166f
Lichenification, 41, 53
  of atopic dermatitis, 55f
Lichenoid drug reaction, 81f
Lichen planus–like chronic graft-versus-host disease, 63f
Lid margin, 4f
Linear epidermal nevus, 25f
Linear psoriasis, 132f
Lingual papillitis, 548f
Lip lichen planus, 159f
Lip licking, chronic, 46f
Lipoatrophy, after steroid injection, 85f
Lipodermatosclerosis, 331, 333f–334f
  circumferential ulceration, 334f
Lipodystrophy, acquired partial, 336f–337f
Lipofuscin, 437
Lipohypertrophy, insulin, 338f
Lipoid proteinosis, 374f–375f
Lipoma, 429f–430f
  multiple, 429f
Lisch nodule, 383f
Livedo racemosa, 562f
Livedo reticularis, 562f
Livedoid vasculopathy, 563f
Lobomycosis, 225f
Lobules, of subcutaneous fat, 5f
Loiasis, 298f

Longitudinal erythronychia in Darier disease, 536f
Loose anagen hair syndrome, 519f
Lower face acne, in adult woman, 174f
LP. see Lichen planus (LP).
Lucio phenomenon, 239, 250f
LUMBAR syndrome, linear perianal hemangioma associated with, 415f
Lung cancer
  hypertrophic osteoarthropathy from, 435f
  metastases, 432f–433f
Lupus erythematosus
  discoid, 23f, 101f–103f
    generalized, 103f
  hypertrophic, 17f, 103f
  neonatal, 105f–106f
    with scarring, 106f
  oral, 108f–109f
  postinflammatory hyperpigmentation secondary to, 584f
  subacute, in complement deficiency disorder, 62f
  systemic, 25f
  tumid, 104f–105f
Lupus patient, disseminated *Mycobacterium marinum* infection in, 235f
Lupus pernio, 488f–489f
Lupus profundus, 104f
  with resultant atrophy, 104f
Lupus vulgaris, 230f–232f
Lyme disease, 202f
Lymphangiectasia, acquired, 410f
Lymphangitis, 191f
Lymphangitis, sclerosing, 37f
Lymphedema, obesity-related, 581f
Lymphocytic Sweet syndrome, 94f
Lymphogranuloma venereum, 202f
Lymphoid hyperplasia, cutaneous, 501–516
  bandlike T-cell pattern, 501f
  nodular B-cell pattern, 501f
Lymphoma
  B-cell lymphoma. see B-cell lymphoma.
  gamma delta, 512f
  secondary cutaneous, 513f
  T-cell lymphoma. see T-cell lymphoma.
Lymphomatoid papulosis, 509f–510f

M

Macroglossia, in amyloidosis, 362f
Macrophage/monocyte disorders, 479–499
Maculae ceruleae, 301f
Macular amyloidosis, 363f
Macule, labial melanotic, 464f
Maffucci syndrome, 409f
Majocchi granuloma, 206f
Major aphthous stomatitis, 558f
Mal de Meleda, 149f
Malignant lymphomas, 501–516
Mammary duct, 3f
Mammary glands, secretory portion of, 3f
Marasmus, 328f
Marfan syndrome, 351, 357f
Marginal mandibular nerve, 13f
Marginal plaque, collagenous and elastic, of hands, 148f
Martorell hypertensive-ischemic ulcer, 581f
Mast cell, 8f
Mastectomy and breast reconstruction, cellulitis after, 191f

Mastocytoma
  Darier sign, 426f
  solitary, 425f
Mastocytosis, 426f–427f
  generalized adult, 427f
Median nail dystrophy, 535f
Median rhomboid glossitis, 549f
Mee lines, 533f
Melanoacanthoma, 467f
Melanocytosis, dermal, 476f
Melanoma, 471f, 541f, 553f
  acral, 473f
  acral lentiginous, 473f
  amelanotic, 474f
    metastatic, 475f
  color variegation, 26f
  large, 474f–475f
  lentigo maligna, 472f
  metastatic, 475f
  nodular, 474f
  oral, 474f
  satellite metastases from, 475f
  with satellitosis, 472f
  superficial spreading, 472f–473f
  tumor, 18f
Melanonychia, longitudinal, secondary to junctional nevus, 467f
Melanonychia striata
  benign, 537f
  caused by melanoma in situ, 537f
Melanosis
  diffuse, in metastatic melanoma, 475f
  penile, 465f
  vulvar, 464f
Melasma, 584f
Melkersson-Rosenthal syndrome, 547f
Melolabial crease, 10f
Meningococcemia, 198f
Menkes kinky hair syndrome, 524f
Mental foramen, and related structures, 13f
Mercury granuloma, from thermometer, 38f
Mercury toxicity, 84f
Merkel cell, 8f
Merkel cell carcinoma, 449f
Mesenchyme, in early spine formation, 1f
Metabolism, errors in, 361–378
Metastases
  ileum, metastatic adenocarcinoma of, 434f
  lung cancer, 433f
  metastatic breast cancer, 433f
  metastatic cholangiocarcinoma, 433f
  metastatic renal cell carcinoma, 433f
  prostate cancer, 433f
  uterine cancer, 434f
Metastatic breast cancer, alopecia neoplastica from, 523f
Metastatic tuberculosis, 233f
Methotrexate-induced oral ulcers, 82f
Methotrexate-induced vascular hyperpigmentation, 81f
Methotrexate, sunburn recall reaction induced by, 82f
Microcystic lymphatic malformation, 409f
Miescher granuloma, 485f
Milia, 461f
Milia en plaque, 461f
Miliaria crystallina, 28f
Miliaria pustulosa, secondary to childbirth, 29f
Miliaria rubra, 28f–29f

Milker nodule, 275f
Minocycline hyperpigmentation, 79f–80f, 554f
Minocycline pigmentation, 176f
Minocycline-induced photosensitivity, 77f
Mixed connective tissue disease, 116f
  Raynaud phenomenon secondary to, 561f
Modiolus, elevators, and depressors, 12f
Mold infections, 203
Moll glands, in eyelid, 4f
Molluscoid pseudotumor, 356f
Molluscum contagiosum, 275f–276f
Molluscum dermatitis, 276f
Mondor disease, 567f
Monilethrix, 525f
Mononucleosis, 271f
Morgellans disease, 21f
Morphea, 112f
  generalized, 112f
  with lichen sclerosis overlap, 112f
  linear, 113f–114f
Morsicatio buccarum, 552f
Mucinoses, 119–124
  benign follicular, 122f–123f
  focal cutaneous, 124f
  follicular, associated with mycosis fungoides, 123f
  reticular erythematous, 122f
Mucinous papules, 121f
Mucocele, 556f
Mucocutaneous leishmaniasis, 293f
Mucormycosis, 225f, 226f
Mucous membranes, diseases of, 543–559
Muehrcke lines, 533f
Muir Torre syndrome, sebaceous adenomas of, 450f
Mulberry molar, congenital syphilis with, 259f
Multicentric reticulohistiocytosis, 495f–496f
Multiple carboxylase deficiency, 326f
Multiple endocrine neoplasia type 1 angiofibromas, 347f
Multiple mucosal neuroma syndrome, 428f
Mycetoma, 224f–225f
Mycobacterial diseases, 229–237
Mycobacterium abscessus infection, 236f
Mycobacterium avium-intracellulare infection
  cutaneous, 237f
  generalized, 237f
Mycobacterium chelonae infection, 236f
Mycobacterium fortuitum infection, 235f–236f
Mycobacterium haemophilum cellulitis, 235f
Mycobacterium kansasii infection, cutaneous, 237f
Mycobacterium marinum infection, 233f–234f
  disseminated, in lupus patient, 235f
  in sporotrichoid pattern, 234f–235f
Mycoplasma infection, Stevens-Johnson syndrome secondary to, 74f
Mycosis fungoides, 24f
  alopecia mucinosa associated with, 507f
  follicular, 507f
  palmar plantar, 506f
  patch stage, 502f–504f
    with poikiloderma, 504f
  plaque stage, 504f–505f
  tumor stage, 505f–506f
Myelogenous leukemia cutis, acute, 515f
Myelomonocytic leukemia, 515f
  cutis, acute, 514f
Myiasis, 301f
Myrmecia, 285f

Myxedema, 119, 343f–344f
  preradial, 346f
  pretibial, 344f–345f
Myxoid cyst, 124f

N

Nail, Darier disease of, 531f
Nail dystrophy
  median, 535f
  nail patella syndrome with, 534f
  with washboard nail, 535f
Nail groove, from mucous cyst, 26f
Nail lichen planus, 529f–530f
Nail patella syndrome, 534f
  with nail dystrophy, 534f
Nail pemphigus vulgaris, 311f
Nail pits, in psoriatic nail, 530f
Nail polish, eyelid dermatitis secondary to, 71f
Nail psoriasis, 131f
  in patient with psoriatic arthritis, 530f
Nail units, examination of, 517
Nasal ala, 10f
Nasal glioma, 428f
Nasal tip, 10f
Nasoalar crease, 10f
Nasofacial sulcus, 10f
Natural killer T-cell lymphoma, 512f
Neck, posterior triangle of, anatomy of, 13f
Necrobiosis lipoidica, 375f–376f
Necrobiotic xanthogranuloma, 485f–486f
  with upper and lower eyelid involvement, 486f
Necrolysis, toxic epidermal, 21f
Necrolytic acral erythema, 272f–273f
Necrosis
  intravenous extravasation with, 79f
  subcutaneous fat, of newborn, 334f–335f
Necrotizing livedo, 563f
Neonatal cephalic pustulosis, 169, 169f
Neonatal lupus erythematosus, 105f–106f
  with scarring, 106f
Neoplasms
  epidermal, 437–462
  melanocytic, 463–477
Nephrogenic systemic fibrosis, 116f
Nerve enlargement, in leprosy, 241f
Netherton syndrome, 391f–392f
  trichorrhexis invaginata in, 392f, 525f
Neurilemmoma, 428f
Neurocutaneous diseases, 41–51
Neurofibroma, solitary, 427f
Neurofibromatosis, 18f, 383f
  with axillary freckling, 15f, 384f
  with café-au-lait macule, 384f
  with malignant peripheral nerve sheath tumor, 385f
  nevus anemicus, 406f
  with plexiform neurofibroma, 384f
  segmental, 385f
Neuroma, 428f
Neuropathic ulcer
  of the hand, 51f
  in leprosy, 247f
Neutrophilic dermatosis, of dorsal hand, 94f
Nevi/nevus, 468f
  acral, junctional, 467f
  anemicus, 406f
  Becker, 466f–467f
  blue, 477f

on breast, 469f
congenital, 469f-470f
dysplastic, 471f
epidermal, 437-462, 437f-438f
in genital area, 469f
halo, 469f
intradermal, 468f
junctional, 467f
lipomatosis superficialis, 430f
melanocytic, 463-477
ocular, 468f
oral blue, 468f
simplex, 406f-407f
spindle cell, 471f
spitz, 470f-471f
Nevus comedonicus, 438f
Nevus depigmentosus, 16f
Nevus of Ota, 15f, 476f-477f
Nevus sebaceous, 449f-450f
desmoplastic trichilemmoma, 450f
syringocystadenoma papilliferum in, 455f
Nevus spilus, 463f
New World leishmaniasis, 291f-293f
Nickel dermatitis, 69f
Nicotine stomatitis, 547f
Nilotinib, diffuse keratosis pilaris caused by, 82f
Nipple eczema, in atopic child, 58f
Nipple skin, 3f
Nocardia, 195f
Nodular amyloidosis, 364f-365f
Nodular sarcoidosis, 487f
Nodular scabies, 304f
Nodules, weathering, 32f
Noma, 557f
Nonbullous congenital ichthyosiform erythroderma, 390f
Noninfectious immunodeficiency disorders, 53-64
Nonkeratinizing epithelium, 5f
Noonan syndrome, 381f
Normal digit, 115f
North American blastomycosis, 220f-221f
Nose
fibrous papule of, 422f
lateral ridge of, 10f
Notalgia paresthetica, 50f
Nummular eczema, 59f
Nutritional diseases, 323-330
acrodermatitis enteropathica as, 326f-327f
anemia as, 328f
carotenemia as, 330f
iron deficiency as, 328f
kwashiorkor as, 328f-330f
marasmus as, 328f
multiple carboxylase deficiency as, 326f
pellagra as, 325f-326f
phrynoderma as, 323f
scurvy as, 324f-325f
vitamin B deficiencies as
atrophic tongue in, 323f
perléche in, 324f

O

Oat cell carcinoma-associated pigmentation, 555f
Obesity-related lymphedema, 581f
Occipital artery, 13f
Occipital vein, 13f
Oil burn, hot, 28f

Old World leishmaniasis, 291f
Older skin, skin tension lines in, 8f
Olmsted syndrome, 148f
Onchocerciasis, 298f-299f
Onchocercoma, 299f
Onychogryphosis, 532f
Onycholysis, 535f
Onychomadesis
after hand-foot-mouth disease, 533f
after toxic epidermal necrolysis, 533f
Onychomatricoma, 540f
Onychomycosis, 209f
Onychopapilloma, 540f
Onychophagia, 534f
Onychoschizia, 534f
Open comedones, 170f-171f
Oral candidiasis, 210f
Oral Crohn disease, 546f
Oral erythema, reactive arthritis with, 134f
Oral florid papillomatosis, 551f
Oral hairy leukoplakia, 17f, 551f
Oral lichen planus, 158f
Oral lichenoid dermatitis, 70f
Oral lupus erythematosus, 108f-109f
Oral lymphatic malformation, 409f
Oral melanosis, 555f
Oral melanotic macule, 554f
Oral nevus, 553f
Oral pemphigus vulgaris, 310f
Oral wart, 284f
Orf, 274f
Orificial tuberculosis, 232f
Osler-Weber-Rendu disease, 579f-580f
Osseous sarcoidosis, 490f
Osteogenesis imperfecta, 359f
Osteoma cutis, 175f, 369f

P

Pachydermodactyly, 420f
Pachydermoperiostosis, 436f
Pachydermoperiostosis, secondary to cancer, 435f
Pachyonychia congenita, 26f, 396f
follicular keratotic papules in, 396f
plantar keratoderma in, 396f
Pacinian corpuscle, in volar skin, 5f
Paederus dermatitis, 302f
Paget disease
of breast, 448f-449f
extramammary, 449f
Pain, 15
Palisaded neutrophilic granulomatous dermatitis, 108f
Palm, herpetic infection of, 266f
Palmar crease, xanthomas of, in hepatic cholestasis, 42f
Palmar hyperhidrosis, 528f
Palmar pits, in basal cell nevus syndrome, 445f
Palmar plantar mycosis fungoides, 506f
Palmar striae xanthoma, in biliary cirrhosis, 373f
Palmoplantar pustulosis, 138f
Pancreatic panniculitis, 336f
Panhypopituitarism, 342f
Panniculitis
annular atrophic, 337f
cold, 335f-336f
pancreatic, 336f

Pansclerotic morphea, 114f
Papillary dermis, 5f
Papillitis, 543
Papillomas, oral, in Cowden syndrome, 457f
Papillomatosis
confluent and reticulated, 140f
neoplasms with, 437
Papillon-Lefevre syndrome, 149f-150f
Papular atopic dermatitis, 56f
Papular mucinosis, 119
acral persistent, 121f
self-healing, 121f
Papular sarcoidosis, 486f-487f
Papuloerythroderma of Ofuji
with deck chair sign, 44f
Papulonecrotic tuberculid, 233f
Papulosquamous diseases, 139-151
Paracoccidiomycosis, 221f-222f
Paraneoplastic pemphigus, 20f, 314f, 435f
Parapheylenediamine allergy, hair dye, 71f
Paraphenylenediamine exposure, depigmentation secondary to, 592f
Parapsoriasis
digitate, 139f
small plaque, 139f
Parasitic infestations, 291-307
Parasitosis, delusions of, 47f
Paronychia, chronic, 213f
Parotid duct, anatomy of, 11f
Parotid gland, anatomy of, 10f
Parry-Romberg syndrome, 114f
Parvovirus B19 gloves and socks syndrome, 280f
Passion purpura, 567f
Pearly penile papules, 422f
Pediculosis, 300f
Pediculosis capitis, 300f
Pediculosis corporis, 300f
Pediculosis pubis, 301f
Pellagra, 325f-326f
Pembrolizumab-associated lichenoid reaction, 81f
Pembrolizumab-associated vitiligo, 83f
Pemphigoid, bullous
erosion, 22f
vesicles and bullae, 19f
Pemphigoid gestationis, 316f-317f
Pemphigus erythematosus, 313f
Pemphigus foliaceus, 309, 312f-313f
Pemphigus vegetans, 309, 311f-312f
Pemphigus vulgaris, 309, 309f-311f
Penicillamine elastopathy, 354f
Perforating collagenosis, reactive, 529f
Perforating disorder, of renal failure, 529f
Perianal condylomata acuminate, 284f
Perianal fissure, 22f
Perianal streptococcal infection, 192f
Perianal tinea, 207f
Perichondrium, in skin of ear, 2f
Perioral dermatitis, 182f
Periungual warts, 282f
Perléche, 210f
in vitamin B deficiencies, 324f
Pernio, 29f-30f
Pesticide burn, 66f
Petrolatum, extraction of larva after treating with, 301f
Peutz-Jeghers syndrome, 466f, 588f
PHACE syndrome, 415f
Phacomatosis pigmentovascularis, 405f

Phaeohyphomycosis, 224f
Phenolic depigmentation, 592f
Phenytoin plus radiation-induced reaction, 75f
Philtral crest, 10f
Photo onycholysis, secondary to doxycycline, 33f
Photosensitivity, to quinine, 78f
Phrynoderma, 323f
Physiologic oral pigmentation, 553f
Phytophotodermatitis, 33f
Piebaldism, 593f
Piezogenic papules, 37f
Pigmentary mosaicism, 380f
Pigmentation, disturbances of, 583–593
PIK3CA-related segmental overgrowth syndrome, 405f–406f
Pili annulati, 525f
Pili multigemini, 526f
Pili torti, 524f
Pilomatricoma, 455f–456f
Pilonidal cyst, 183f
Pincer nail, 536f
Pink disease, 84f
Pinta, 251–261, 261f
Piroxicam hypersensitivity, 19f
Piroxicam photosensitivity, 77f
Pitted keratolysis, 194f
Pityriasis alba, 57f
Pityriasis lichenoides chronica, 511f
Pityriasis lichenoides et varioliformis acuta, 510f
Pityriasis rosea, 139–151, 141f
  herald patch, 141f
Pityriasis rubra pilaris (PRP), 139–151, 142f–144f
  childhood, 144f
  circumscribed juvenile, 145f
  with early follicular hyperkeratosis, 142f
Pityrosporum folliculitis, 218f
Plane xanthoma, 372f
  in biliary cirrhosis, 373f
Plantar fibromatosis, 420f
Plantar pustulosis, 20f
Plantar warts, 282f
Plaque psoriasis, 125f
Plaque sarcoidosis, 487f–488f
Plasma cell cheilitis, 544f
Plasmacytoma, 514f
Platelet count, low, drug eruption in leukemic patient with, 73f
Poikiloderma, patch stage, mycosis fungoides with, 504f
Poikiloderma of Civatte, 31f
Poison ivy dermatitis, 65, 67f
Poliosis, 523f, 591f
Polyarteritis nodosa, 573f–574f
Polychondritis, relapsing, 118f
Polymorphous light eruption, 33f–34f
Pomade acne, 176f
Pompholyx, 58f–59f
Pore of Winer, 458f
Porokeratosis, 393f
  disseminated superficial actinic, 393f
Porokeratotic eccrine and osteal duct nevus, 394f
Porphyria cutanea tarda, 365f–366f
  hypertrichosis in, 366f
  milia and scarring, 365f
  sclerodemoid lesions in, 366f
Porphyrins, 361
Portuguese man of war dermatitis, 295f
Positive patch test, 66f

Postcapillary venule, in papillary dermis, 5f
Posterior auricular artery, 13f
Posterior auricular vein, 13f
Postinflammatory dyspigmentation, secondary to lupus erythematosus, 584f
Postinflammatory hypopigmentation, secondary to lip licking, 544f
Post-kala-azar dermal leishmaniasis, 294f
Post-steroid injection atrophy, 337f
Prader-Willi syndrome, skin picking in, 48f
Preadolescent acne, 171f
Pregnancy, pruritic urticarial papules and plaques of, 317f
Premelanosome, 7f
Prepuce, 4f
Preradial myxedema, 346f
Preservatives, vulvar dermatitis secondary to, 71f
Pretibial myxedema, 119, 344f–345f
Primary cutaneous aggressive epidermotropic CD8+ T-cell lymphoma, 512f
Primary herpes simplex infection, 263f–264f
Primary HIV infection, 286f
Primary inoculation tuberculosis, 229f
Primary syphilis, 251f–253f
  chancre on patient's left palate, 253f
  with secondary lesions on palms, 253f
  on upper lip, 253f
Primrose allergy, finger dermatitis from, 58f
Progeria, 401f
Progressive nodular histiocytosis, 495f
Progressive symmetric erythrokeratoderma, 393f
Proliferative verrucous leukoplakia, 551f
Prostate cancer, metastases, 433f
Protein C deficiency, homozygous, 566f
Protein S deficiency, 566f
Proteus syndrome, 385f
  with connective tissue nevus, 385f
  with epidermal nevus, 385f
Proximal trichorrhexis nodosa, 524f
PRP. *see* Pityriasis rubra pilaris (PRP).
Prurigo nodularis, 42f, 46f
Prurigo pigmentosa, 43f–44f
Pruritus, 41–51
  chronic, 22f
Pruritus ani, lichen simplex chronicus in, 43f
Pseudocyst, auricular, 462f
Pseudofolliculitis barbae, 526f
Pseudohypoparathyroidism, 346f–347f
Pseudopelade, of Brocq, 522f
Pseudo-porphyria cutanea tarda, 366f
Pseudoscars, stellate, 32f
Pseudoxanthoma elasticum (PXE), 351, 352f–353f
Pseudoxanthoma elasticum-like papillary dermal elastolysis, 354f
Psoriasis, 17f, 125–138, 127f–130f
  annular, 133f
  erythrodermic, 134f
  guttate, 132f
  in HIV-infected patient, after zoster, 133f
  infantile, 131f–132f
  inverse, 131f
  linear, 132f
  nail, 131f
    oil spot and subungual hyperkeratosis in, 131f
  nail pitting in, 130f
  pustular, 133f
Psoriatic arthritis, 134f

nail psoriasis in patient with, 530f
Psoriatic erythroderma, 151f
Psoriatic nail, 530f
  nail pits in, 530f
  oil spot in, 530f
Psychogenic excoriations, 47f
Psychogenic purpura, 568f
Pterygium inversum unguis, 535f
Pterygium unguis, 535f
Punctate keratoderma, 146f
Punctate palmoplantar keratoderma, **146f**
Purple toe, secondary to cholesterol emboli, 563f
Purpura
  after vomiting, 567f
  from coin rubbing, 567f
  cough-induced, 567f
  Henoch-Schönlein, 570f
  immune thrombocytopenic, 564f–565f
  in old age, 564f
  passion, 567f
  psychogenic, 568f
  racquetball-induced, 567f
  thrombotic thrombocytopenic, 565f
  Waldenström hypergammaglobulinemic, 565f
Purpura annularis telangiectodes, 568f
Purpura fulminans, 565f
  Escherichia coli, 565f
Purpuric glove-sock syndrome, 280f
Pustular dermatitis, 125–138
Pustular psoriasis, 133f
PXE. *see* Pseudoxanthoma elasticum (PXE).
Pyoderma faciale, 182f
Pyoderma gangrenosum, 22f, 95f
  breast surgery, 95f
  early, 95f
  vegetative, 95f
Pyogenic granuloma, 18f, 412f–413f, 556f
  with satellite lesions, 413f
Pyostomatitis vegetans, 546f

Q

Quinidine photo-induced livedo reticularis, 78f
Quinine, photosensitivity to, 78f

R

Racquet nails, 534f
Racquetball-induced purpura, 567f
Radiodermatitis, chronic, 35f
Ranula, 557f
RASA1-associated capillary malformation, due to arteriovenous malformation syndrome, 408f
Raynaud phenomenon, 561f
Reactive arthritis, 135f–136f
  with conjunctival erythema, 135f
  with oral erythema, 134f
  with urethral inflammation, 135f
Reactive perforating collagenosis, 352f
Recalcitrant palmoplantar eruptions, 125–138
Recessive dystrophic epidermolysis bullosa, 387f
Recurrent herpes simplex buttock, 266f
Recurrent herpes simplex infection, 264f–265f
Recurrent palmoplantar pustulosis, 138f

Red collagen bundles, in skin of young children, 2f
Red lunula, 538f
Red pigment, in cutaneous eruption, 1
Red tattoo reaction, 38f
Reeve sign, 24f
Relapsing polychondritis, 118f
Renal failure
    acquired perforating disease in, 41f-42f
    perforating disorder of, 529f
Reticular dermis, 5f
Reticular erythematous mucinosis, 122f
Reticulate acropigmentation of Kitamura, 586f
Reticulohistiocytoma, 495f
Reticulohistiocytosis
    congenital self-healing, 496f
    multicentric, 495f-496f
Retronychia, 536f
Rheumatoid nodules, 117f
Rheumatoid vasculitis, 117f
Rhinoscleroma, 199f
Rhizopus infection, 226f
Rickettsial pox, 201f
Rocky Mountain spotted fever, 201f
Romana sign, in Chagas disease, 294f
Rosacea, 169, 181f
    edema, in severe, 181f
    with erythema, 180f
    papules and pustules, 180f
    by topical steroids, 182f
Rosai-Dorfman disease, 516f
Rothmund-Thomson syndrome, 403f
Rubber dermatitis, 70f
Rubella, 278f
Rubeola (measles), 278f
Russell spider bite, 307f

S

Sarcoid
    annular genital, 488f
    in tattoo, 493f
Sarcoidosis, 16f, 479, 491f
    alopecia in, 492f
    annular, 488f
    digital, 490f
    erythema nodosum-like, 491f
    erythrodermic, 492f
    exocrine gland swelling, 489f
    genital, 488f
    hypopigmentation overlying, 490f
    ichthyosiform, 491f-492f
    nodular, 487f
    osseous, 490f
    papular, 486f-487f
    plaque, 487f-488f
    scar, 493f
    ulcerative, 490f-491f
Scabies, 303f-305f
Scalp
    discoid lupus of, 520f
    erosive pustular dermatitis of, 522f
    layers of, 14f
    skin of, 3f
Scalp pemphigus vulgaris, 310f
Scar
    burn, 28f
    posttraumatic, 23f
Scar sarcoidosis, 493f
Scarlet fever, 190f
Scarring
    after scrofuloderma, 233f
Scarring alopecia, secondary to discoid lupus erythematosus, 521f
Schamberg disease, 568f
Schimmelpenning syndrome, with lipodermoid of conjunctiva, 438f
Schnitzler syndrome, 96f
Sclerodactyly
    in limited scleroderma, 114f
    in systemic sclerosis, 115f
Scleredema, 122f
    calcinosis of knee in patient with, 114f
    limited, 24f
    in sclerodactyly, 114f
Sclerodermoid graft-versus-host disease, 63f-64f
Scleromyxedema, 119f-121f
    early, 119f
Sclerosing lymphangitis, 37f
Sclerotic digit, 115f
Scombroid poisoning, 87f
Scrofuloderma, 232f-233f
    linear scarring after, 233f
Scrotal calcinosis, 368f
Scrotum, lichen simplex chronicus of, 43f
Scrub typhus, 200f
Scurvy, 324f-325f
Sea urchin injury, 296f
Sea wasp dermatitis, 295f
Seabather eruption, 295f
Seaweed dermatitis, 296f
Sebaceous glands, in facial skin, 2f
Seborrheic dermatitis, 125-138, 125f-126f
    in HIV-positive patient, 126f
    with hyperpigmentation, 126f
    with hypopigmentation, 127f
Secondary syphilis, 253f-256f
    alopecia, 258f
    in HIV-infected patient, 255f
    Kaposi sarcoma and, 255f
    mucous patch, 256f
    of tongue, 256f
Segmental neurofibromatosis, 385f
Self-healing papular mucinosis, 121f
Senna burn, 66f
Sepsis, candidal, 214f-215f
Serum sickness-like reaction, 81f
Severe acne, 172f-173f
Severe infantile acne, 170f
Severe truncal acne, 173f
    with hyperpigmentation, 173f
Sézary syndrome, 508f-509f
Silica granuloma, 39f
Silicone granuloma, 38f
Sitosterolemia, 373f
Sjogren syndrome, 117f
    annular erythema of, 117f
Sjögren-Larsson syndrome, 392f
Skin
    axillary, 3f
    breast, 3f
    ear, 2f
    ear canal, 2f
    facial, 2f
        innervation of, 12f
        major anatomic landmarks in, 10f
    nipple, 3f
    older skin, skin tension lines in, 8f
    structure and function of, 1-14
    volar, 4f-5f
    in young children, 2f
Skin appendages, disease of, 517-541
Skin biopsies, for connective tissue disease, 101
Skin disease
    cutaneous signs and diagnosis of, 15-26
    diagnosis of, based on skin structure and function, 1
Skin fragility, isotretinoin, 22f
Skin lesion
    in systemic lupus erythematosus, 109f
    viral diseases and, 263
Skin picking, in Prader-Willi syndrome, 48f
Skin tag, 423f
Skin-popping, 38f
SLE. see Systemic lupus erythematosus (SLE).
Small hairs, in skin of young children, 2f
Small plaque parapsoriasis, 139f
Smallpox scarring, 274f
Smooth muscle, in breast skin, 3f
Smooth muscle hamartoma, 431f
Snake bite, 307f
Sneddon syndrome, 562f
Soft corn, 36f
Solar damage, chronic, 32f
Solar elastosis, of the forehead, 32f
Solar lentigo, 464f
Solar urticaria, 34f, 98f
Solid facial edema, 175f
Solitary congenital myofibroma, 421f
Sphagnum moss, sporotrichosis from, 222
Spider angioma, 410f
Spider bite, 307f
Spindle cell hemangioma, 417f
Spindle cell nevi, 471f
Splinter hemorrhage, 539f
Sporotrichoid pattern, *Mycobacterium marinum* infection in, 234f-235f
Sporotrichoid spread, nocardia with, 195f
Sporotrichosis, 222f
    disseminated, 223f
    fixed cutaneous, 222f
Spotted lunula, 539f
Squamous cell carcinoma, 17f, 446f, 540f, 551f-552f
    Bowen disease with, 447f
    dorsal forearm, 446f
    lupus vulgaris, 231f
Staphylococcal abscess, 187f
Staphylococcal emboli, 185f
Staphylococcal folliculitis, 20f, 186f
Staphylococcal scalded skin syndrome, 189f-190f
Staphylococci, 55f
Stasis dermatitis, 580f-581f
Steatocystoma multiplex, 460f-461f
Stellate pseudoscars, 32f
Steroid acne, 177f
Steroids, contact allergy to, 72f
Stevens-Johnson syndrome, 74f, 90f
    dilantin-induced, 74f
    secondary to *Mycoplasma infection*, 74f
Still disease, 118f
Stings, 291-307
Stomatitis, 70f
Stratum corneum, in eyelid, 4f
Stratum lucidum, in volar skin, 4f
Strawberry tongue, 190f
Streptococcal intertrigo, 192f
Streptococci, 55f

Striae distensae, 358f–359f
Sturge-Weber syndrome, capillary malformation (port-wine stain) with, 407f
Subacute cutaneous lupus erythematosus, 105f
Subacute lupus erythematosus, in complement deficiency disorder, 62f
Subcorneal pustular dermatosis, 136f
Subcutaneous emphysema, 37f
Subcutaneous fat
  diseases of, 331–338
    necrosis, of newborn, 334f–335f
Subepidermal calcified nodule, 368f
Subungual exostosis, 423f
Subungual hematoma, 539f
Subungual wart, 282f
Sulfa, erythema multiforme secondary to, 88f
Sulfa allergy, in HIV-infected patient, 75f
Sunburn, 30f
Superficial lymphatic malformation, 409f
Superficial muscular aponeurotic system, 11f
Superficial temporal artery, 10f
  and vein, 13f
Superficial thrombophlebitis, 566f
Superior labial artery, 13f–14f
Supraorbital artery and vein, 13f
Supratrochlear artery and vein, 13f
Surgical gloves, contact urticaria to, 72f
Sweet syndrome, 92f–94f
  in acute leukemia, 93f, 94f
  with acute myelogenous leukemia, 92f–93f
  histocytoid, 94f
  in leukemia, 93f
  lymphocytic, 94f
  in patient with systemic lupus erythematosus, 93f
Swimmer itch, 296f
Sycosis barbae, 186f
Syphilis, 251–261
  congenital, 259f
    with Hutchinson teeth, 259f
    with mulberry molar, 259f
    with scars from rhagades, 260f
  primary, 251f–253f
    chancre on patient's left palate, 253f
    with secondary lesions on palms, 253f
    on upper lip, 253f
  secondary, 253f–256f
    alopecia, 258f
    in HIV-infected patient, 255f
    Kaposi sarcoma and, 255f
    of lip with mucous patch of tongue, 256f
    mucous patch, 256f
  tertiary, 258f
Syringocystadenoma papilliferum, 455f
Syringomas, 451f–452f
  chondroid, 454f
  eruptive, 451f
Systemic lupus erythematosus (SLE), 25f, 107f
  acute, 106f–107f
  alopecia in, 107f
  bullous, 107f–108f
  chilblain, 107f
  with dyspigmentation, 107f
Systemic sclerosis
  dyspigmentation in, 115f
  mat telangiectasias in, 115f
  reduced oral aperture, 115f
Systemic symptoms, phenytoin-induced drug reaction with, 73f–74f

T

Tache noire, 201f
Tangier disease, 374f
Targetoid hemosiderotic hemangioma, 415f
TB. *see* Tuberculosis (TB).
T-cell lymphoma
  angioimmunoblastic, 516f
  CD30+ anaplastic, 511f
  cutaneous, 501–516
  hydroa vacciniforme-like natural killer, 512f–513f
  natural killer, 512f
  subcutaneous panniculitis-like, 512f
Tea tree oil dermatitis, 67f
Telangiectasia
  generalized essential, 410f
  in systemic sclerosis, 115f
  unilateral nevoid, 411f
Telangiectasia macularis eruptiva perstans (TMEP), 427f
Temporal arteritis, 576f
Tendinous xanthomas, 371f
Teratoma, 432f
Terry nail, 534f
Tertiary syphilis, 258f
Thermal burn, from child abuse, 27f
Thrombophlebitis, superficial, 566f
Thrombotic thrombocytopenic purpura, 565f
Thrush, 203
  in chronic mucocutaneous candidiasis, 210f
Thyroglossal duct cyst, 462f
Thyroid acropachy, 346f
Tick bite, 303f
Tinea, 203
  one hand involvement with, 209f
Tinea amiantacea, 528f
Tinea barbae, 204f
Tinea capitis, 203, 203f–204f
Tinea corporis, 25f, 203, 205f, 207f
Tinea cruris, 206f
Tinea faciei, 203, 205f
Tinea imbricata, 206f
Tinea manuum and onychomycosis, 205f
Tinea nigra, 215f
Tinea pedis, 207f–208f
  bullous, 208f
Tinea versicolor, 215f–217f
Tongue biting, chronic, fibroma secondary to, 47f
Tongue, herpes simplex infection of, 266f
Tonofibrils, 7f
Topical antibiotic, allergy to, 72f
Topical steroid atrophy, 85f
Topical steroid-induced atrophy, 84f
Topical steroids, allergic contact cheilitis to, 543f
Torus mandibularis, 548f
Torus palatinus, 547f
Toxic epidermal necrolysis, 75f, 90f
  to Lamictal, 74f–75f
Toxic erythema, of chemotherapy, 82f
Toxicodendron dermatitis, 65
Toxin-mediated conditions, 185
Toxoplasmosis, 294f

Trachyonychia, 532f
  with koilonychia, 531f
Traction alopecia, 522f–523f
Transient acantholytic dermatosis, 322f
Transient neonatal pustular melanosis, 587f–588f
Transverse facial artery and vein, 13f
Transverse leukonychia, 536f
Transverse nail bands, secondary to chemotherapy, 537f
Triatome bite, 294f
Trichilemmoma, 457f
Trichodysplasia spinulosa, 285f
Trichoepithelioma, 456f–457f
Trichofolliculoma, 456f
Trichomycosis axillaris, 528f
Trichorhinophalangeal syndrome, 404f
Trichorrhexis invaginata, in Netherton syndrome, 392f, 525f
Trichostasis spinulosa, 527f
Trichothiodystrophy, 402f
Trichotillosis, 50f, 519f–520f
Trichrome vitiligo, 591f
Trigeminal trophic syndrome, 51f
Tropical immersion foot, 30f
Trunk, skin tension lines in, 9f
TS. *see* Tuberous sclerosis (TS).
Tuberculoid leprosy, 239, 240f
  borderline, 241f–243f
  early, 239f
Tuberculosis (TB), 229
  metastatic, 233f
  primary inoculation, 229f
  verrucosa cutis, 229f–230f
Tuberoeruptive xanthomas, biliary cirrhosis and, 372f
Tuberous sclerosis (TS)
  with angiofibromas, 381f
  with ash leaf macule, 382f
  with dental enamel pit, 383f
  with fibrous forehead plaque, 382f
  with paintbrush-type white streaks, 382f
  with periungual fibromas, 382f
  with shagreen plaque, 382f
Tuberous xanthomas, 370f–371f
Tufted angioma, 416f
Tufted folliculitis, 522f
Tularemia, ulceroglandular, 200f
Tumid lupus erythematosus, 104f–105f
Tumor necrosis factor inhibitor-related psoriasiform reaction, 83f
Tumoral calcinosis cutis, 369f
Tumors
  dermal and subcutaneous, 405–435
  dermal duct, 453f
  of follicular infundibulum, 459f
  giant cell, of tendon sheath, 421f
  granular cell, 405, 427f
    multiple, 427f
Tungiasis, 303f
Turner syndrome lymphedema, 381f
Tylosis, with lung cancer, 147f
Type A pigmentary demarcation, 583f
Type B pigmentary demarcation, 583f
Type B syndrome, 348f–349f
Type C pigmentary demarcation, 583f
Type I hyperlipidemic eruptive xanthoma, 370f

U

Ulceration
  dermatomyositis with, 112f
  in systemic sclerosis, 115f
Ulcerations and bacterial superinfection secondary to skin popping, 38f
Ulcerative herpes simplex, 268f
  in HIV-infected patient, 287f
Ulcerative sarcoidosis, 490f–491f
Ulceronecrotic Mucha-Habermann disease, 510f
Ulcers
  Buruli, 235f
  factitial, 48f–49f
  neuropathic, in leprosy, 247f
Ulerythema ophrogenes, 404f
Uncombable hair syndrome, 525f
Unilateral nevoid telangiectasia, 579f
Urethral inflammation, reactive arthritis with, 135f
Urticaria, 19f, 77f, 87–99, 96f–97f
  cholinergic, 97f–98f
  cold, 97f
  delayed pressure, 98f
  exercise-induced, 97f
  solar, 34f, 98f
Urticaria multiforme, 90f
Urticaria pigmentosa, 426f, 427f
Urticarial bullous pemphigoid, 315f–316f
Urticarial vasculitis, 571f
Uterine cancer, metastases, 433f

V

Vaccinia vaccination, 274f
Varicella, 268f–269f
Vascular tumors, 405
Vasculitis
  cryoglobulinemic, 565f, 571f
  drug-induced antineutrophil cytoplasmic antibody-positive, 574f
  leukocytoclastic, 569f
  lupus erythematosus, 569f
  urticarial, 571f
Vasculopathy
  cryoglobulinemic, 572f
  cutaneous collagenous, 579f
  levamisole-induced, 575f–576f
  livedoid, 563f
Vasopressor-induced ischemia, 566f
Vegetating pyoderma, 188f
Venolymphatic malformation, 410f
Venous lakes, 410f
Venous malformation, 408f
Vermillion border, 10f
Verruca vulgaris, 17f
Verruciform xanthoma, 374f
Verruga peruana, 200f
Vesicular bullous pemphigoid, 316f
Vibrio vulnificus infection, 199f
Viral diseases, 263–289
Vitamin B deficiencies
  atrophic glossitis in, 323f
  perléche in, 324f
Vitamin K injection site reaction, 78f
Vitiligo, 15f, 589f–591f
  granulomas in, common variable immunodeficiency with, 61f
  with koebnerization, 591f
  poliosis in, 591f
  segmental, 589f
  trichrome, 591f
Volar skin, 4f–5f
Vomiting, purpura after, 567f
Voriconazole phototoxicity, 77f
Voriconazole-induced lentigines, 15f
Vulva, lichen simplex chronicus of, 43f
Vulvar dermatitis, 71f
Vulvovaginal-gingival syndrome, 158f

W

Waldenström hypergammaglobulinemic purpura, 565f
Warfarin-induced necrosis, 78f
Warts, 281f
  in DOCK8 immunodeficiency, 61f–62f
WAS. *see* Wiskott-Aldrich syndrome (WAS).
Washboard nails
  nail dystrophy with, 535f
  secondary to habitual trauma to the matrix, 46f
Wasp sting, 302f
Weathering nodules, 32f
Wells syndrome, 92f
Werner syndrome, 400f
White dermatographism, 56f
White piedra, 215
White sponge nevus, 553f
Winter itch, 43f
Wiskott-Aldrich syndrome (WAS), 60f
Wooly hair, 526f

X

Xanthelasma, 372f
Xanthoma disseminatum, 494f
Xanthomas
  eruptive, 16f
  in homozygous familial hypercholesterolemia, 17f
  palmar, hepatic cholestasis, 42f
Xeroderma pigmentosum, 401f–402f
Xerotic eczema, 59f
X-linked ichthyosis, 21f, 389f

Y

Yaws, 251–261, 260f
Yeasts, diseases resulting from, 203–227
Yellow nail syndrome, 539f
Yellow pigments, in cutaneous eruption, 1

Z

Zeiss glands, in eyelid, 4f
Zidovudine pigmentation, 538f
Zoon balanitis, 448f
Zosteriform lentiginous nevus, 463
Zygomycosis, 203
Zyplast granuloma, 39f